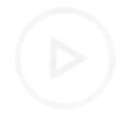

IMPORTANT:

HERE IS YOUR REGISTRATION CODE TO ACCESS
YOUR PREMIUM McGRAW-HILL ONLINE RESOURCES.

For key premium online resources you need THIS CODE to gain access. Once the code is entered, you will be able to use the Web resources for the length of your course.

If your course is using **WebCT** or **Blackboard**, you'll be able to use this code to access the McGraw-Hill content within your instructor's online course.

Access is provided if you have purchased a new book. If the registration code is missing from this book, the registration screen on our Website, and within your WebCT or Blackboard course, will tell you how to obtain your new code.

Registering for McGraw-Hill Online Resources

TO gain access to your McGraw-Hill web resources simply follow the steps below:

1. USE YOUR WEB BROWSER TO GO TO: **www.mhhe.com/payne8e**

2. CLICK ON **FIRST TIME USER**.

3. ENTER THE REGISTRATION CODE* PRINTED ON THE TEAR-OFF BOOKMARK ON THE RIGHT.

4. AFTER YOU HAVE ENTERED YOUR REGISTRATION CODE, CLICK **REGISTER**.

5. FOLLOW THE INSTRUCTIONS TO SET-UP YOUR PERSONAL UserID AND PASSWORD.

6. WRITE YOUR UserID AND PASSWORD DOWN FOR FUTURE REFERENCE. KEEP IT IN A SAFE PLACE.

TO GAIN ACCESS to the McGraw-Hill content in your instructor's **WebCT** or **Blackboard** course simply log in to the course with the UserID and Password provided by your instructor. Enter the registration code exactly as it appears in the box to the right when prompted by the system. You will only need to use the code the first time you click on McGraw-Hill content.

Thank you, and welcome to your McGraw-Hill online Resources!

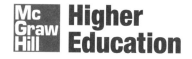

* YOUR REGISTRATION CODE CAN BE USED ONLY ONCE TO ESTABLISH ACCESS. IT IS NOT TRANSFERABLE.

0-07-297398-6 T/A PAYNE/HAHN/MAUER: UNDERSTANDING YOUR HEALTH, 8/E

ONLINE RESOURCES

REGISTRATION CODE

CM2D-2QCS-S00U-QALK-6J3W

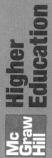

McGraw Hill — Learning to Go: HEALTH

Welcome to Learning to Go: Health!

Learning to Go: Health is an Internet-based learning reinforcement system that delivers fun, interactive lessons to help you retain and practice what you learn in your Personal Health course.

Each lesson includes 3 action steps that will help you boost your retention of one core skill – reinforced through quizzes, exercises, tips, and web links. Each lesson takes 10 to 15 minutes.

YOU choose when you want your lessons to arrive, and they are pushed to your browser at that time each day or week. Each bite-sized lesson puts the skills to work for you – and helps you build the habits of success.

STUDY TODAY'S PRINCIPLE IN-DEPTH ▶

Learning to Go: Health is provided in addition to the premium content resources located on your text's Online Learning Center.

To register:

- Go to the Online Learning Center that accompanies this book (the URL is listed on the back cover or inside cover of the text).

- Select the Register Link.

- Follow the registration instructions, which indicate where you'll need to enter your password/registration code.

- Once you're registered, you'll receive instructions for how to download and install Learning to Go: Health to your PC.

- Access is provided if you have purchased a new book. This code may be used only once. If you have purchased a used book, select the Register Link and then click on the link for used book owners.

P/N 292078-5

Your Learning To Go: Health password/registration code is:

u3bsa-b3yrf-3c4jg

understanding your health

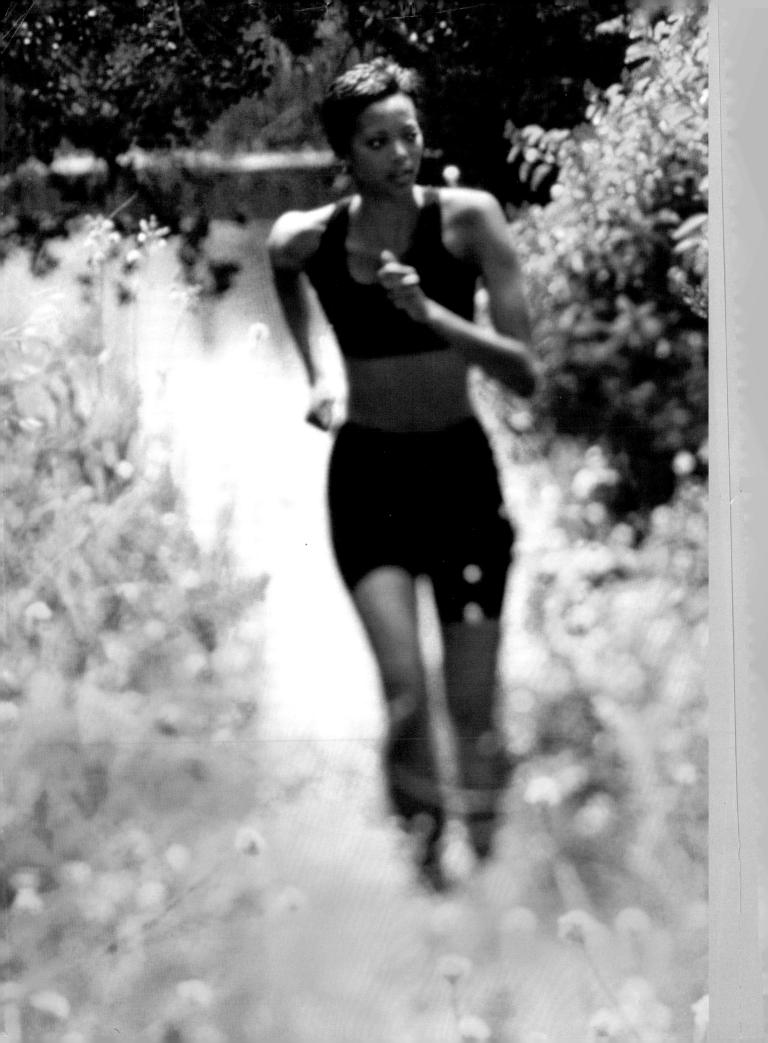

Understanding your health

Eighth Edition

Wayne A. Payne, Ed.D.

Dale B. Hahn, Ph.D.

Ellen B. Mauer, Ph.D.

All of Ball State University,
Muncie, Indiana

Boston   Burr Ridge, IL   Dubuque, IA   Madison, WI   New York   San Francisco   St. Louis
Bangkok   Bogotá   Caracas   Kuala Lumpur   Lisbon   London   Madrid   Mexico City
Milan   Montreal   New Delhi   Santiago   Seoul   Singapore   Sydney   Taipei   Toronto

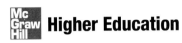

Higher Education

A Division of the McGraw-Hill Companies

UNDERSTANDING YOUR HEALTH
Published by McGraw-Hill, a business unit of The McGraw-Hill Companies, Inc., 1221 Avenue
of the Americas, New York, NY, 10020. Copyright © 2005, 2002, 2000, 1998, 1995,
1992, 1989, 1986, by The McGraw-Hill Companies, Inc. All rights reserved. No part of
this publication may be reproduced or distributed in any form or by any means, or stored in a
database or retrieval system, without the prior written consent of The McGraw-Hill Companies,
Inc., including, but not limited to, in any network or other electronic storage or
transmission, or broadcast for distance learning.
Some ancillaries, including electronic and print components, may not be available to customers
outside the United States.

This book is printed on acid-free paper.

1 2 3 4 5 6 7 8 9 0 WCK/WCK 0 9 8 7 6 5 4

ISBN 0-07-284437-X

Vice president and editor-in-chief: *Emily Barrosse*
Publisher: *William Glass*
Sponsoring editor: *Nicholas Barrett*
Director of development: *Kate Engelberg*
Developmental editor: *Ann Kirby-Payne*
Executive marketing manager: *Pamela S. Cooper*
Media producer: *Lance Gerhart*
Project manager: *Jill Moline-Eccher*
Senior production supervisor: *Carol A. Bielski*
Senior designer: *Kim Menning*
Associate media project manager: *Meghan Durko*
Manager, photo research: *Brian Pecko*
Art editor: *Emma C. Ghiselli*
Photo researcher: *Alexandra Ambrose*
Art director: *Jeanne Schreiber*
Cover design: *Yvo Riezebos*
Cover image: © *Anne-Marie Weber/Getty Images/Taxi*
Interior design: *Jeanne Calabrese*
Typeface: *10.5/12 Minion*
Compositor: *The GTS Companies, Inc.*
Printer: *Quebecor World Versailles Inc.*

The credits section for this book begins on page C-1 and is considered an extension
of the copyright page.

Library of Congress Cataloging-in-Publication Data

Payne, Wayne A.
 Understanding your health/Wayne A. Payne, Dale B. Hahn, Ellen B. Mauer.—8th ed
  p. cm.
 Includes index.
 ISBN 0-07-284437-X (softcover: alk. paper)
 1. Health. 2. College students—Health and hygiene. I. Hahn, Dale B. II. Mauer, Ellen B.
III. Title.
RA777.3.P39 2005
613'.0434—dc22
                                                                              2004045696

www.mhhe.com

To all of our students, with the hope that the decisions they make will be healthy ones.

contents in brief

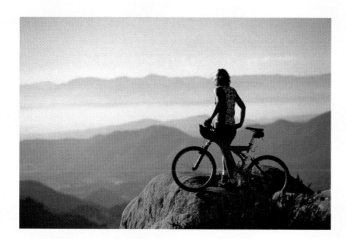

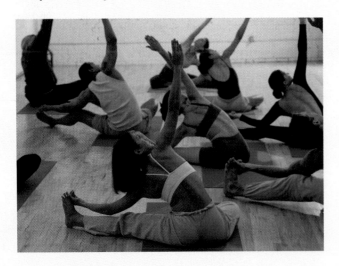

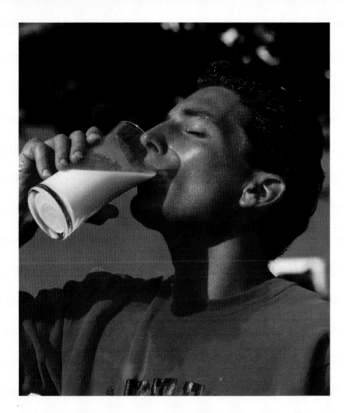

part two: the body 97

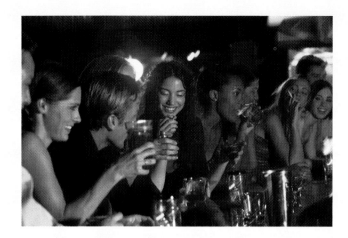

part three: preventing drug abuse and dependence 223

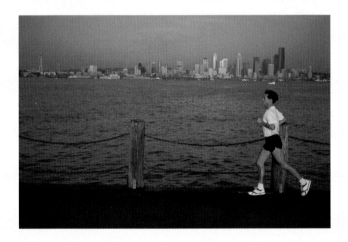

part four:
preventing diseases 331

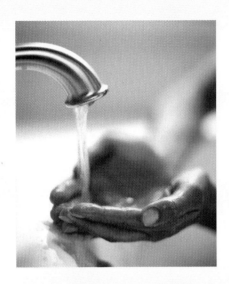

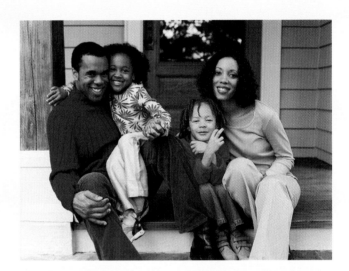

part five: sexuality and reproduction 471

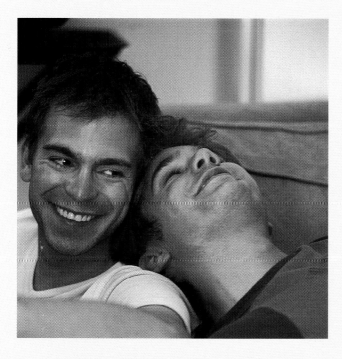

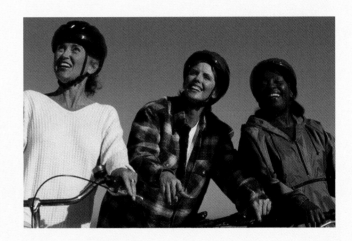

part six: Consumer and safety issues 579

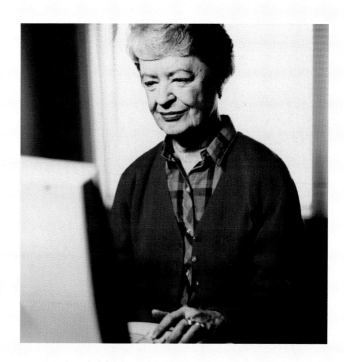

preface

As a health educator, you already know that personal health is one of the most exciting courses a college student will take. Today's media-oriented college students are aware of the critical health issues of the new millennium. They hear about environmental issues, substance abuse, sexually transmitted diseases, fitness, and nutrition virtually every day. The value of the personal health course is its potential to expand students' knowledge of these and other health topics. Students will then be able to examine their attitudes toward health issues and modify their behavior to improve their health and perhaps even prevent or delay the onset of certain health conditions.

Understanding Your Health accomplishes this task with a carefully composed, well-documented text that addresses the health issues most important to both instructors and students. As health educators, we understand the teaching issues you face daily in the classroom and have written this text with your concerns in mind.

We are pleased that this eighth edition of *Understanding Your Health* has been infused with an exciting new perspective through the major contributions of a third author. Ellen B. Mauer, Ph.D., serves as the Associate Director of the Ball State University Counseling Center. In this capacity she is responsible for coordinating the campus outreach activities of this comprehensive mental health center. Each academic year she connects with thousands of Ball State students through classroom presentations on her specialty areas of emotional health, stress management, eating disorders, and positive body image. As a licensed psychologist, Dr. Mauer regularly counsels students and also maintains a private clinical practice. For this eighth edition, Dr. Mauer wrote significant revisions for Chapters 2 (Achieving Psychological Health), 3 (Managing Stress), 5 (Understanding Nutrition and Your Diet), and 6 (Maintaining a Healthy Weight). We are proud to have this dynamic new author join our team.

Hallmarks of the Text

Several unique themes and features set *Understanding Your Health* apart from other personal health texts. These successful features continue to define *Understanding Your Health* in its eighth edition.

A Text for All Students

This book is written for college students in a wide variety of settings, from community colleges to large four-year universities. The content is carefully constructed to be meaningful to students of all ages. We have paid special attention to the increasing numbers of nontraditional-age students (those over age 25) who have decided to pursue a college education. *Understanding Your Health* continues to encourage students of all ages and backgrounds to achieve their goals.

Two Central Themes

Throughout the text, two central themes—the multiple dimensions of health and the developmental tasks—offer students a foundation for understanding their own health and achieving positive behavior change. The multiple dimensions of health are introduced in Chapter 1 and revisited in each part opener, where they are discussed in the context of the chapters that follow. The developmental tasks are also introduced in Chapter 1, where they are applied to young, middle, and older adulthood. These important milestones are then revisited in the part-ending Mastering Tasks sections, which help students evaluate their own progress in completing them. A helpful illustration (Figure 1-1 on page 6) depicts the role of health in the completion of developmental tasks.

Flexible Organization

The eighth edition of *Understanding Your Health* has twenty chapters. The first stands alone as an introductory chapter that explains the focus of the book. The arrangement of the remaining chapters follows the recommendations of both the users of previous editions of the book and reviewers for this edition. Of course, professors can choose to cover the chapters in any sequence that suits the needs of their courses.

Wellness and Disease Prevention

Throughout this new edition, students are continually urged to be proactive in shaping their future health. Even the chapter titles invite students to take control of their own health behavior.

Integrated Presentation of Aging

Topics of interest to midlife and older adults are integrated into appropriate chapters according to subject. This organization allows both traditional-age and nontraditional-age students to learn about the physical and emotional changes that take place as we age. Similarly, issues related to death and dying —from considering organ donation to preparing a living will—have been incorporated into relevant chapters.

Separate Coverage of Cancer and Chronic Conditions

Rapid developments in cancer prevention, diagnosis, and treatment warrant a single comprehensive chapter on cancer, in which we present the latest research and information. In addition, *Understanding Your Health* features a separate chapter in which more than twenty of the most common chronic conditions are discussed.

Technology: The Key to Teaching and Learning

Just a quick glance through the pages of *Understanding Your Health* shows that technology is woven throughout every chapter, both in the content and in the chapter pedagogy. Similarly, the package of supplements that accompanies the text emphasizes technology while acknowledging that printed materials also have merit. Together, the text and its supplements offer the ideal approach to teaching and learning—one that integrates the best tools that technology has to offer, challenging both instructors and students to reach higher.

Updated Coverage: New and Expanded Topics

As experienced health educators and authors, we know how important it is to provide students with the most current information available. The eighth edition of *Understanding Your Health* has been thoroughly updated with the latest information, statistics, and findings. Throughout each chapter, we have incorporated new examples and discussions, from information on newly available prescription drugs and medications (Chapters 2, 3, 11, and 12), to the latest information on dieting and supplements (Chapters 5, 6, and 19), to recent findings on air quality and health (Chapter 20).

Another exciting change in this edition of *Understanding Your Health* is the addition of a new Chapter 20, The Environment and Your Health. Prepared by David

LeBlanc, Ph.D., Professor of Biology at Ball State University, this chapter presents pertinent information on a variety of environmental factors—ranging from naturally occurring hazards like radon and ultraviolet radiation to human-made problems like water and air pollution—that can adversely affect personal health. Even more importantly, the chapter includes practical advice for protecting oneself from harmful environmental factors and proactive measures for working toward environmental change.

In addition to these topics, we have once again included chapter-ending "As We Go To Press" boxes in relevant chapters. These unique boxes allow us to comment on breaking news right up to press time, ensuring that the most current issues in health are addressed. For example, we discuss changes to fast food menus in response to consumer and government concerns over obesity in Chapter 5, and the controversy over gay marriages in Chapter 15. Following is a sampling of topics that are either completely new to this edition or are covered in greater depth than in the previous edition:

Chapter 1: Shaping Your Health

- Chapter introduction revised to more clearly emphasize the costs of failing health
- Prochaska's six stages of change
- Keys to living longer
- Episodic health care

Chapter 2: Achieving Psychological Health

- Psychological issues related to the Internet
- Taking positive steps toward psychological health
- Nonverbal communication
- Self-esteem, self-concept, emotional intelligence, and personality
- Laughter and enhancing psychological health
- Managing conflict
- Learned helplessness and learned optimism
- Treatments and drug therapies for specific disorders
- Mood disorders, including depression, bipolar disorder, postpartum depression, and seasonal affective disorder
- Anxiety disorders, including generalized anxiety disorder, panic disorder, posttraumatic stress disorder, obsessive-compulsive disorder, and phobias
- Schizophrenia

Chapter 3: Managing Stress

- Stress management techniques
- Technology and stress

- Three stages of stress
- Costs and benefits of stress
- Yerkes-Dodson law
- Student stress
- Perfectionism
- Type A and Type B personalities
- Stress in the aftermath of 9/11
- Melatonin

Chapter 4: Becoming Physically Fit

- New definitions for exercise, physical activity, and physical fitness
- Health-related physical fitness
- Performance-related physical fitness
- High-intensity aerobic activity
- Benefits of physical activity/aerobic fitness in reducing some health risks
- Muscular fitness and muscular endurance
- Isotonic resistance exercise
- Developing a cardiorespiratory fitness program
- Calculating your target heart rate
- Stretching and flexibility
- Childhood obesity

Chapter 5: Understanding Nutrition and Your Diet

- Food facts vs. food fiction
- Artificial sweeteners
- Religious food restrictions
- The importance of fats in satisfying appetite
- Trans fats
- Benefits of fiber
- New figures on current USDA food guidelines vs. the average American diet
- Healthy eating pyramid
- Fast food restaurant choices
- Probiotic products
- Food allergies and food intolerance
- Reading food labels
- Food safety
- Vegetarianism
- Antioxidants

Chapter 6: Maintaining a Healthy Weight

- Food and emotions
- The weight loss industry
- Obesity and underweight
- Body dysmorphic disorder
- Lifestyle change for weight management

- The meaning of thinness in American culture
- Supplements and appetite suppressants, including Phenylpropanolamine (PPA), and dietary supplements, including Ephedrine, Aristolochia Fangchi, Meridia, Orlistat
- Gastric band surgery
- Eating disorders

Chapter 7: Making Decisions About Drug Use

- Gamma-hydroxybutyrate (GHB), aka liquid ecstasy or Georgia Home Boy
- Ephedra
- Crystal meth
- Ritalin abuse
- Date rape depressants
- Long- and short-term effects of marijuana
- Medical marijuana
- Oxycontin

Chapter 8: Taking Control of Alcohol Use

- Moderate drinking
- Process of distillation added to section on the nature of alcoholic beverages
- New Star box on low-carbohydrate beer
- Effects of alcohol by number of drinks
- Hangovers

Chapter 9: Rejecting Tobacco Use

- Tobacco settlement results
- Chippers and part-time smokers
- Genetic influences on nicotine addiction
- Toxic and carcinogenic components of cigarette smoke
- Passive smoke
- Parental influences on smoking
- New tobacco/nicotine products: "safe" cigarettes and nontobacco sources of nicotine (nico water, patches, etc.)
- Smoking cessation programs and aids

Chapter 10: Enhancing Your Cardiovascular Health

- New statistics on hypertension, smoking, diabetes, and overweight/obesity as risk factors for heart disease
- New information on link between estrogen replacement therapy and heart attacks and strokes
- C-reactive protein
- Cholesterol screening and treatments for high cholesterol

- New information on defibrillators and CPR
- Echocardiography
- Diagnostic techniques such as positron emission tomography (PET), electron beam computed tomography (EBCT), and magnetic resonance imaging (MRI)
- Hypertension and pre-hypertension

Chapter 11: Living with Cancer

- Survivability
- Staging cancer and naming conventions for cancers
- Risk factors and treatments
- Breast self examination (BSE) and mammography
- Hormone replacement therapy and cancer
- Genetic links to cancer
- Tamoxifen
- Thinprep pap test
- Uterine cancer among African American women
- Prostate cancer and overtreatment
- Alternative screening tests for colorectal cancer
- Progress in the "War On Cancer"

Chapter 12: Managing Chronic Conditions

- Klinefelter's Syndrome
- Turner's Syndrome updated with more information on treatment
- Cystic fibrosis
- Scoliosis
- Diabetes
- Reactive and functional hypoglycemia
- Autoimmune/hypersensitivity disorders (fibromyalgia, asthma, Crohn's, lupus, multiple sclerosis)
- Degenerative diseases (Parkinson's, Alzheimer's)
- Drug therapies for chronic conditions

Chapter 13: Preventing Infectious Diseases

- SARS
- Stem cell research and treatments
- Adult immunizations
- Pneumococcal infections and vaccine
- Influenza and flu shots
- Hepatitis B infections and immunizations
- New AIDS medications, information on AIDS vaccines
- Monkeypox
- T cells and B cells
- West Nile virus and Lyme disease
- Herpes vaccines in clinical trials

Chapter 14: Exploring the Origins of Sexuality

- Responsible sexual behavior by 2010
- Effects of aging on the male reproductive system
- Female genital mutilation
- Endometriosis discussion thoroughly updated and revised
- Alternatives to hormone replacement therapy
- Link between cancer and hormone replacement therapy

Chapter 15: Understanding Sexual Behavior and Relationships

- Gay and lesbian partnerships and same-sex marriage
- Roots/causes of sexual orientation
- 2003 U.S. Supreme Court Texas sodomy law ruling
- Advertising pitched at lesbians and gay men
- The challenges bisexuals face
- Cohabitation arrangements vs. marriage

Chapter 16: Managing Your Fertility

- Nonoxynol-9 concerns
- New 5-year IUD
- Lunelle taken off the market
- Contraceptive ring
- Contraceptive patch
- Emergency contraception
- Updates on abortion laws

Chapter 17: Becoming a Parent

- Human cloning
- Becoming a parent through a stepfamily
- FDA concerns about ultrasound
- Intracytoplasmic sperm injection

Chapter 18: Becoming an Informed Health Care Consumer

- Communicating with physicians
- Acupuncture
- Reflexology, with references to recent studies in Israel, Britain, and Denmark
- Homeopathy
- Herbal supplements and recent FDA efforts to tighten control over their sale and use
- Nursing shortage
- Self-care and when to see a physician
- Medicare and prescription drug plans for Medicare recipients
- Medicaid/Medicare fraud

- Prescription drug issues
- Over-the-counter drugs
- Advance medical directives and living wills
- Organ donation
- Prepaying a funeral

Chapter 19: Protecting Your Safety

- Domestic/child abuse
- Gun violence
- Guns on campus
- Identity theft
- Watch dogs
- Recreational safety
- Firearm safety
- Motor vehicle safety

Chapter 20: The Environment and Your Health

Topics in this new chapter include:

- Indoor air quality
- Drinking water
- Noise
- Radio frequency radiation
- Air pollution
- Water pollution
- Land pollution
- Loss of green space
- Radiation
- Human population explosion
- Global climate change
- Stratospheric ozone depletion
- Loss of natural habitats and species extinction
- Ecoterrorism
- The high-tech revolution and e-waste

Student-Friendly Chapter Pedagogy

Each chapter of *Understanding Your Health* is rich with pedagogical features that offer a variety of ways to address new and emerging health issues and to pique student interest in particular topics.

Chapter Objectives (NEW)

Each chapter begins with a set of clear objectives that help students distill the most important concepts in the pages that follow.

Taking Charge of Your Health (NEW)

Located at the end of each chapter, these bulleted lists invite students to put the knowledge and information they've gleaned from the chapter to work in their everyday lives. Cross-referencing the text with Internet links and real-world situations allows students to see how what they've learned can be applied in their own lives.

Online Learning Center Resources

Online Learning Center boxes, found on the opening page of each chapter, direct students toward the useful resources available on the Online Learning Center that accompanies this text. These resources include chapter key terms and definitions, student interactive question-and-answer sites, and self-scoring chapter quizzes.

Talking It Over

This feature focuses on communication and health issues. It encourages students to begin each chapter by thinking about how they would discuss a specific health topic with their friends, their doctor, or their family. It also prompts them to think about controversial health issues from different viewpoints. Topics vary from how to communicate your sexual needs to your partner to the pros and cons of legalization of marijuana. CommunicationLinks suggest websites that students can explore to learn more about each topic.

Eye on the Media

Face it—a student's world revolves around media of all types, especially the web. Students get most of their health information not from instructors and textbooks, but from television, self-help books, popular news magazines, the web, and the radio. To meet students on this familiar ground, we've included Eye on the Media boxes, which take a critical look at these media sources of health information.

Discovering Your Spirituality

Spirituality has become an important focus in health courses. Discovering Your Spirituality boxes highlight the spiritual dimension of health and its effect on overall wellness. The boxes cover topics such as body image, living well with cancer or a chronic infectious disease, making decisions about sex, and having an enjoyable social life without abusing alcohol or other drugs.

Considering Complementary Care

This feature highlights nontraditional approaches to health care. Topics include the use of herbal supplements, biofeedback, meditation, and dietary aids. Students are encouraged to critique these approaches, weighing their possible advantages and disadvantages. Although methods that are known to be dangerous are clearly identified as such, students are invited to consider new approaches that are becoming more accepted because they show promising results. An underlying theme is patient responsibility coupled with a physician's advice.

Talking Points (NEW)

Interspersed throughout each chapter, Talking Points offer students opportunities to explore how they might start a dialogue about specific health-related issues and situations.

Changing for the Better

These unique question-and-answer boxes show students how to put health concepts into practice. Each box begins with a real-life question, followed by helpful tips and practical advice for initiating behavior change and staying motivated to follow a healthy lifestyle.

Health on the Web Behavior Change Activities

Today's computer-savvy students can find reliable health information at their fingertips when they search the world wide web. New activities direct students to important health websites related to the material in each chapter. For each activity, students explore a website and then complete a quiz or self-assessment offered at the site. These activities help students think critically about valuable health information.

HealthQuest Activities

Many chapters contain an activities box to complement the HealthQuest CD-ROM that accompanies the text. These activities allow students to assess their health behavior in each of nine different areas. HealthQuest's exciting graphics and interactive approach will encourage students to learn about topics such as condom use, cancer prevention, and healthy eating behavior as they complete the activities.

Learning from Our Diversity

These boxes expose students to alternative viewpoints and highlight what we can learn from the differences that make us unique. Topics include the Mediterranean Food Pyramid, the male contraceptive pill, and special issues related to infectious disease among older adults.

Focus On . . . Articles

The Focus On . . . articles examine current issues that students are hearing about in today's news, such as genetically modified food, drinking and violence, extreme sports, and job-related illness. These often controversial health-related topics are a perfect starting point for class or group discussions. Because these essays are placed at the end of each chapter, they can be covered or not at the instructor's option.

InfoLinks

InfoLinks boxes placed at the end of many of the Changing for the Better boxes and Focus On . . . articles give students a starting point for exploring health information on the Internet. Log onto the MADD website to learn how to host a party responsibly. Get tips on the most healthful menu choices at ethnic restaurants. Check out helpful advice for preparing for exams and coping with test anxiety. InfoLinks will get students plugged in to the possibilities for learning about health online.

Star Boxes

In each chapter, special material in Star boxes encourages students to delve into a particular topic or closely examine an important health issue.

Personal Assessments

Each chapter contains at least one Personal Assessment inventory. These self-assessment exercises serve three important functions: to capture students' attention, to serve as a basis for introspection and behavior change, and to provide suggestions for carrying the applications further.

Definition Boxes

Key terms are set in boldface type and defined in corresponding boxes. Pronunciation guides are provided where appropriate. Other important terms in the text are set in italics for emphasis. Both approaches facilitate student vocabulary comprehension.

Chapter Summaries

Each chapter concludes with a bulleted summary of key concepts and their significance or application. The student can then return to any topic in the chapter for clarification or study.

Review Questions

A set of questions appears at the end of each chapter to aid the student in review and analysis of chapter content.

Comprehensive Health Assessment

The Comprehensive Health Assessment at the beginning of the book allows students to take a close look at their current state of health, typical health behavior, and risk factors. Using this assessment, students can pinpoint trouble spots in their own health behavior and find out what they can do to reduce their risk of disease or other health conditions. At the end of the semester, they can take a look at their previous answers to see how their behavior changed as they learned more about health and wellness issues.

Health Reference Guide

The updated Health Reference Guide at the back of the book lists many commonly used health resources. Internet addresses, phone numbers, and mailing addresses of various organizations and government agencies are provided as available. The guide is perforated and laminated, making it durable enough for students to keep for later use.

Vegetarian Food Pyramid

Many students now follow or are considering a vegetarian diet. To help them understand how such a diet meets nutrient needs, we have printed a vegetarian food pyramid along with the USDA Food Guide Pyramid in Chapter 5.

Comprehensive Glossary

At the end of the text, all terms defined in boxes, as well as pertinent italicized terms, are merged into a comprehensive glossary.

"Exam Prep" Guide

A perforated exam preparation section is included in the back of the book. The multiple-choice and true/false questions test students' retention of the material they have read. The critical thinking questions allow them to integrate the concepts introduced in the text with the information presented in class lectures and discussions.

Appendixes

Understanding Your Health includes four appendixes that are valuable resources for the student:

- **First Aid.** This updated appendix outlines important general first-aid measures, such as what to do when someone is choking, bleeding, or in shock. It includes a special section on recognition and first-aid treatment of epileptic seizures.

- **Body Systems.** The systems of the human body have been clearly and accurately rendered in this appendix to make difficult anatomical concepts easier for students to understand.
- **Canadian Health.** Written by Canadian health educator Don Morrow, this section provides a comprehensive overview of the health promotion movement in Canada. It presents the historical background of the movement, including an explanation of important documents such as *A New Perspective on the Health of Canadians,* the *Ottawa Charter for Health Promotion,* and the theoretical model of *A Framework for Health Promotion.* It also discusses the *Action Statement for Health Promotion in Canada,* current provincial perspectives, recent initiatives, and future directions.
- **Canada's Food Guide to Healthy Eating.** This well-known and respected guide offers an interesting comparison with the USDA Food Guide Pyramid.

Supplements

An extensive supplements package is available to qualified adopters to enhance the teaching-learning process. We have made a concerted effort to produce supplements of extraordinary utility and quality. This package has been carefully planned and developed to help instructors derive the greatest benefit from the text. We encourage instructors to examine them carefully. Many of the products can be packaged with the text at a discounted price. Beyond the following brief descriptions, additional information about these supplements is available from your McGraw-Hill sales representative.

Integrated Instructor's Resource CD

Organized by chapter, the Instructor's Resource CD includes resources to help you teach your course. The CD will work in both Windows and Macintosh environments and includes the following elements:

- **Course Integrator Guide.** This guide includes all the useful features of an instructor's manual, such as learning objectives, suggested lecture outlines, suggested activities, media resources, and web links. It also integrates the text with all the related resources McGraw-Hill offers, such as the Online Learning Center, the HealthQuest CD-ROM, and the Health and Human Performance Discipline Page. The guide also includes references to relevant print and broadcast media.
- **Test Bank.** This file includes more than 1000 questions, including multiple-choice, true/false, and short essay. It has been rewritten to enhance clarity, and it now includes critical thinking questions and more applications questions.

- **Computerized Test Bank.** McGraw-Hill's Computerized Testing is the most flexible and easy-to-use electronic testing program available in higher education. The program allows instructors to create tests from book-specific test banks and to add their own questions. It accommodates a wide range of question types, and multiple versions of the test can be created. The program is available for Windows, Macintosh, and Linux environments.
- **PowerPoint.** A complete set of PowerPoint lecture slides for the course is included on the Instructor's Resource CD, as well as on the instructor's portion of the Online Learning Center. This presentation, ready to use in class, was prepared by a professional in the field of health and fitness. It corresponds to the content in each chapter of *Understanding Your Health*, making it easier for you to teach and ensuring that your students can follow your lectures point by point. You can modify the presentation as much as you like to meet the needs of your course.

Online Learning Center

The Online Learning Center to accompany this text offers a number of additional resources for both students and instructors. Many study tools are open to all students. Premium content such as assessments and PowerWeb require student registration using the pass code that comes free with new books. Visit this website to find useful materials such as the following:

For the instructor:

- Downloadable PowerPoint presentations
- Course Integrator Guide

For the student:

- Self-scoring chapter quizzes and online study guides
- Flash cards and crossword puzzles for learning key terms and their definitions
- Learning objectives
- Interactive activities
- Web links for study and exploration of topics in the text
- Online labs
- Wellness worksheets
- PowerWeb
- Newsfeeds
- Internet guide

HealthQuest CD-ROM, by Bob Gold and Nancy Atkinson

The HealthQuest CD-ROM helps students explore their wellness behavior using state-of-the-art interactive technology. Students can assess their current health status, determine their risks, and explore options for positive lifestyle change. Tailored feedback gives students a meaningful and individualized learning experience without using valuable classroom time. Modules include the Wellboard (a health self-assessment); Stress Management and Mental Health; Fitness; Nutrition and Weight Control; Communicable Diseases; Cardiovascular Health; Cancer; Tobacco, Alcohol, and Other Drugs. An online Instructor's Manual presents ideas for incorporating HealthQuest into your course.

Fitness and Nutrition Log

This logbook helps students track their diet and exercise programs. It serves as a diary to help students monitor their behaviors. It can be packaged with any McGraw-Hill textbook for a small additional fee.

PowerWeb

www.dushkin.com/online

The PowerWeb website is a reservoir of course-specific articles and current events. Students can visit PowerWeb to take a self-scoring quiz, complete an interactive exercise, click through an interactive glossary, or check the daily news. An expert in each discipline analyzes the day's news to show students how it relates to their field of study.

PowerWeb is part of the Online Learning Center. Students are also granted full access to Dushkin/McGraw-Hill's Student Site, where they can read study tips, conduct web research, learn about different career paths, and follow links on the web.

Wellness Worksheets

This collection of activities and assessments helps students become more involved in their own wellness and better prepared to implement behavior change programs. It includes 120 assessments under the topics of General Wellness and Behavior Change; Stress Management; Psychological and Spiritual Wellness; Intimate Relationships and Communication; Sexuality; Addictive Behaviors and Drug Dependence; Nutrition; Physical Activity and Exercise; Weight Management; Chronic Diseases: Cardiovascular Disease and Cancer; Infectious Diseases: Aging, Dying and Death; Consumer Health; Personal Safety; and Environmental Health. They are available online in the premium content or may be packaged with the text at minimal cost.

NutritionCalc Plus

http://nutritioncalc.mhhe.com

NutritionCalc Plus (ISBN 0-07-292084-X) is a dietary analysis program with an easy-to-use interface that allows users to track their nutrient and food group intakes, energy expenditures, and weight control goals. It generates a variety of reports and graphs for analysis, including comparisons with the Food Guide Pyramid and the latest Dietary Reference Intakes (DRIs). The database includes thousands of ethnic foods, supplements, fast foods, and convenience foods, and users can add their own foods to the food list. NutritionCalc Plus is available on CD-ROM or in an online version.

Video Library

The McGraw-Hill Video Library contains many quality videotapes, including selected videos from the *Films for Humanities* series and all the videos from the award-winning *Healthy Living: Road to Wellness* series. Digitized video clips are also available (see Healthy Living Video Clips CD-ROM). The library also features *Students on Health,* a unique video filmed on college campuses across the country that includes eight brief segments, 8 to 10 minutes long, featuring students involved in discussion and role play on health issues. Finally, an additional video—*McGraw-Hill Health Video*—is available. This video features brief clips on a wide range of topics of interest in personal health courses. Contact your McGraw-Hill sales representative to discuss eligibility to receive videos.

PageOut: The Course Website Development Center

www.pageout.net

PageOut, free to instructors who use a McGraw-Hill textbook, is an online program you can use to create your own course website. PageOut offers the following features:

- A course home page
- An instructor home page
- A syllabus (interactive and customizable, including quizzing, instructor notes, and links to the text's Online Learning Center)
- Web links
- Discussions (multiple discussion areas per class)
- An online gradebook
- Links to student web pages

Contact your McGraw-Hill sales representative to obtain a password.

Course Management Systems

www.mhhe.com/solutions

Now instructors can combine their McGraw-Hill Online Learning Center with today's most popular course management systems. Our Instructor Advantage program offers customers access to a complete online teaching website called the Knowledge Gateway, prepaid, toll-free phone support, and unlimited e-mail support directly from WebCT and Blackboard. Instructors who use 500 or more copies of a McGraw-Hill textbook can enroll in our Instructor Advantage Plus program, which provides on-campus, hands-on training from a certified platform specialist. Consult your McGraw-Hill sales representative to learn what other course management systems are easily used with McGraw-Hill online materials.

Classroom Performance System

Classroom Performance System (CPS) brings interactivity into the classroom/ lecture hall. It is a wireless response system that gives instructors and students immediate feedback from the entire class. The wireless response pads are essentially remotes that are easy to use and that engage students. CPS is available for both IBM and Mac computers.

Primis Online

www.mhhe.com/primis/online

Primis Online is a database-driven publishing system that allows instructors to create content-rich textbooks, lab manuals, or readers for their courses directly from the Primis website. The customized text can be delivered in print or electronic (eBook) form. A Primis eBook is a digital version of the customized text (sold directly to students as a file downloadable to their computer or accessed online by a password). *Understanding Your Health,* eighth edition, is included in the database.

You Can Make a Difference: Be Environmentally Responsible, Second Edition, by Judith Getis

This handy text is organized around the three parts of the biosphere: land, water, and air. Each section contains descriptions of the environmental problems associated with that part of the biosphere. Immediately following the problems, or challenges, are suggested ways in which individuals and communities can help solve or alleviate them.

Annual Editions

Annual Editions is an ever-enlarging series of more than seventy volumes, each designed to provide convenient, low-cost access to a wide range of current, carefully selected articles from some of the most important magazines, newspapers, and journals published today. The articles, drawn from more than 400 periodical sources, are written by prominent scholars, researchers, and commentators. All *Annual Editions* have common organizational features, such as annotated tables of contents, topic guides, unit overviews, and indexes. In addition, a list of annotated websites is included. An Instructor's Resource Guide with testing suggestions for each volume is available to qualified instructors.

Taking Sides

www.dushkin.com/takingsides

McGraw-Hill/Dushkin's *Taking Sides* series currently consists of twenty-two volumes, with an instructor's guide with testing material available for each volume. The *Taking Sides* approach brings together the arguments of leading social and behavioral scientists, educators, and contemporary commentators, forming eighteen to twenty debates, or issues, that present the pros and cons of current controversies in an area of study. An Issue Introduction that precedes the two opposing viewpoints gives students the proper context and historical background for each debate. After reading the debate, students are given other viewpoints to consider in the Issue Postscript, which also offers recommendations for further reading. *Taking Sides* fosters critical thinking in students and encourages them to develop a concern for serious social dialogue.

Acknowledgments

The publisher's reviewers made excellent comments and suggestions that were very useful to us in writing and revising this book. Their contributions are present in every chapter. We would like to express our sincere appreciation for both their critical and comparative readings.

For the Eighth Edition:

Srijana Bajracharya,
Ithaca College

Steve G. Gabany
Indiana State University

Rosann L. Poole
Tallahassee Community College

Kerry J. Redican
Virginia Polytechnic Institute and State University

Andrew L. Shim
Southwestern College

Lucille Talbot
William Paterson University

For the Seventh Edition:

Charles R. Baffi
Virginia Tech

M. Basti
Cuesta College

Susan T. Burge
Cuyahoga Community College

Karen Camarata
Eastern Kentucky University

Kim Clark
California State University, San Bernardino

David P. Diaz
Cuesta College

Mark Doherty
University of Louisiana-Monroe

Bridget Driscoll
California State University, Fullerton

Boyd Foster
Eastern Washington University

Sara Geist
Ohio University

Stephen Green
Mississippi State University

Kathryn Hilgenkamp
Coastal Carolina University

Kimberley Hyatt
Weber State University

Laurie Merges
Kent State University

Ron Murray
University of Virginia

Bill E. Pride
Arizona State University

DawnElla Rust
Stephen F. Austin State University

M. Ann Smith
Chadron State College

Charles Tucker
Valdosta State University

Karen Vail-Smith
East Carolina University

Kathy Webster
California State University, Fullerton

Holly Willey
Mississippi State University

For the Sixth Edition:

Srijana Bajracharya
University of Maine-Presque Isle

Gary Chandler
Gardner-Webb University

Patricia Cost
Weber State University

John Downey
Long Beach City College

Emogene Fox
University of Central Arkansas

Jolynn Gardner
Anoka Ramsey Community College

Ann Wertz Garvin
University of Wisconsin-Whitewater

Patricia Gordon
Arkansas Tech University

Rene Gratz
University of Wisconsin-Milwaukee

Loretta Herrin
Benedict College

Norm Hoffman
Bakersfield College

Carol Johnson
University of Richmond

Susan MacLaury
Kean University

Lori Marti
Mankato State University

Randy McGuire
Eastern Kentucky University

Phyllis Murray
Eastern Kentucky University

Carol Parker
University of Central Oklahoma

Alan Peterson
Gordon College

Kerry Redican
Gordon College

McKay Rollins
Brigham Young University

For the Fifth Edition:

Lori Dewald
Shippensburg University

Chester A. Halterman
Northern Virginia Community College

Richard Hurley
Brigham Young University

John Janowiak
Appalachian State University

Jacquelynn K. Lott
Antelope Valley College

Rosalie D. Marinelli
University of Nevada

For the Fourth Edition:

Rosemary C. Clark
City College of San Francisco

Marianne Frauenknecht
Western Michigan University

Nancy Geha
Eastern Kentucky University

Jeffrey Hallam
Ohio State University

Dawn Larsen
Mankato State University

Loretta M. Liptak
Youngstown State University

Bruce M. Ragon
Indiana University

For the Third Edition:

Charles A. Bish
Slippery Rock University

G. Robert Bowers
Tallahassee Community College

Donald L. Calitri
Eastern Kentucky University

Shae L. Donham
Northeastern Oklahoma State University

P. Tish K. Doyle
University of Calgary

Judy C. Drolet
Southern Illinois University-Carbondale

Dalen Duitsman
Iowa State University

Mary A. Glascoff
East Carolina University

Sonja S. Glassmeyer
California Polytechnic State University-San Luis Obispo

Health Education Faculty
Cerritos College

Norm Hoffman
Bakersfield College

C. Jessie Jones
University of New Orleans

Jean M. Kirsch
Mankato State University

Duane Knudson
Baylor University

Doris McLittle-Marino
University of Akron

Juli Lawrence Miller
Ohio University

Victor Schramske
Normandale Community College

Janet M. Sermon
Florida A&M University

Myra Sternlieb
DeAnza College

Mark G. Wilson
University of Georgia

Focus Group Participants:

Danny Ballard
Texas A&M University

Robert C. Barnes
East Carolina University

Jacki Benedik
University of Southwestern Louisiana

Kathie C. Garbe
Youngstown State University

Virginia Peters
University of Central Oklahoma

Les Ramsdel
Eastern Kentucky University

James Robinson III
University of Northern Colorado

Linda Schiller-Moening
North Hennepin Community College

For the Second Edition:

Dan Adame
Emory University

Judith Boone Alexander
Evergreen Valley College

Judy B. Baker
East Carolina University

Robert C. Barnes
East Carolina University

Loren Bensley
Central Michigan University

Ernst Bleichart
Vanier College

Shirley F. B. Carter
Springfield College

Vivien C. Carver
Youngstown State University

Cynthia Chubb
University of Oregon

Janine Cox
University of Kansas

Dick Dalton
Lincoln University

Sharron K. Deny
East Los Angeles College

Emogene Fox
University of Central Arkansas

George Gerrodette
San Diego Mesa College

Ray Johnson
Central Michigan University

James W. Lochner
Weber State College

Linda S. Myers
Slippery Rock University

Virginia Peters
University of Central Oklahoma

James Robinson III
University of Northern Colorado

Merwin S. Roeder
Kearney State College

James H. Rothenberger
University of Minnesota

Ronald E. Sevier
El Camino Community College

Reza Shahrokh
Montclair State College

Albert Simon
University of Southwestern Louisiana

Dennis W. Smith
University of North Carolina-Greensboro

Loretta R. Taylor
Southwestern College

For the First Edition:

Stephen E. Bohnenblust
Mankato State University

Neil Richard Boyd, Jr.
University of Southern Mississippi

William B. Cissell
East Tennessee State University

Victor A. Corroll
University of Manitoba

Donna Kasari Ellison
University of Oregon Umpqua Community College

Neil E. Gallagher
Towson State University

Susan C. Girratano
California State University-Northridge

Raymond Goldberg
State University of New York College at Cortland

Marsha Hoagland
Modesto Junior College

Carol Ann Holcomb
Kansas State University

Sharon S. Jones
Orange Coast College

Daniel Klein
Northern Illinois University

Susan Cross Lipnickey
Miami University of Ohio

Gerald W. Matheson
University of Wisconsin-La Crosse

Hollis N. Matson
San Francisco State University

David E. Mills
University of Waterloo

Peggy Pederson
Montana State University

Valerie Pinhas
Nassau Community College

Jacy Showers
Formerly of Ohio State University

Parris Watts
University of Missouri-Columbia

Wayne E. Wylie
Texas A&M University

Special Acknowledgments

Authors do not exist in isolation. To publish successful textbooks, an entire team of professionals must work together for a significant time. During the past three decades, we have worked with many talented people to publish seventeen successful textbooks.

For this edition of *Understanding Your Health*, we used the professional expertise and writing talents of a team of four contributing authors. Leonard Kaminsky, Ph.D., Professor and Coordinator of Ball State University's Adult Fitness and Cardiac Rehabilitation Programs, took on the task of revising and updating Chapter 4 (Becoming Physically Fit) and Chapter 10 (Enhancing Your Cardiovascular Health). Chapter 7 (Making Decisions About Drug Use) and Chapter 8 (Taking Control of Alcohol Use) were revised by Alison Cockerill, M.S., Health Educator in the Ball State Student Health Center. Robert Pinger, Ph.D., Professor and Chairperson of the Department of Physiology and Health Science at Ball State, revised Chapter 19 (Protecting Your Safety). And our new Chapter 20, The Environment and Your Health, was written by David LeBlanc, Ph.D.,

Professor of Biology at Ball State University. We thank these contributors for their professional dedication to this book and their personal commitment to the health of college students with whom they work on a daily basis.

There are many others whom we would like to thank for their contributions to this book. Ann Kirby-Payne did an exceptional job as our developmental editor. She took over the project at a rather challenging point but "rallied the troops" and always maintained her excitement and positive outlook. Ann found engaging ways to incorporate the revisions and perspectives of our new author, Ellen B. Mauer, and the four contributing authors. We believe that this eighth edition is a major reflection of Ann's insight, vision, and determination.

We remain grateful to Vicki Malinee, who saw us through nine book projects. This latest edition of *Understanding Your Health* also bears the imprint of Nick Barrett, Executive Editor, Health and Human Performance. Although Nick joined this project in its final stages, his infectious enthusiasm for *Understanding Your Health* and his positive vision for the future of our personal health texts make us especially proud to be McGraw-Hill authors. We look forward to working with Nick on upcoming projects.

Special recognition goes to Pam Cooper, Executive Marketing Manager, who is as energetic a person as we have seen in college publishing. We are confident that her experience, expertise, and talent will allow this book to reach many of our teaching colleagues.

We are also grateful to those who worked behind the scenes at McGraw-Hill on the production of this book. Lynda Huenefeld made a major contribution to the development of both the book and its supplements package. Project Manager Jill Moline-Eccher juggled this book and its brief version simultaneously with remarkable grace and good humor, all the while keeping watch over every detail and deadline. Senior Designer Kim Menning created an exciting, dynamic new look for the eighth edition. And Photo Research Coordinator Alexandra Ambrose culled a fine selection of colorful, thought-provoking images.

Finally, we would like to thank our families for their continued support and love. More than anyone else, they know the energy and dedication it takes to write and revise textbooks. To them we continue to offer our sincere admiration and loving appreciation.

Wayne A. Payne
Dale B. Hahn
Ellen B. Mauer

a visual guide to understanding your health

Whether you're trying to get in shape, looking for sound health advice, trying to interpret the health information you see in the media, or just working toward a good grade, *Understanding Your Health* is designed to help you succeed. Here's a brief guide to some of the useful and eye-opening features you'll find inside.

Chapter Objectives
Each chapter opens with a set of clear learning goals; check them out before you begin reading the chapter, and use them for review once you've completed it.

Online Learning Center Resources
A wealth of study aids and other resources to help you prepare for exams and improve your grade are available at **www.mhhe.com/payne8e**

Talking It Over
How would you approach a doctor, family member, friend, or partner about a specific health problem? Where do you stand on today's controversial health issues? Are you honest with yourself about your own health? Use these boxes to role play and sharpen your communication skills.

Eye on the Media
Curious about all those ads you see for various drugs? Wondering about the reliability of the health information you find on the Internet? This feature investigates the way that written, broadcast, and electronic media shape our perceptions about health, health care, and wellness.

Health on the Web Behavior Change Activities
Surfing the web can be good for your health! These activities guide you to interactive self-assessments on the web. How much stress are you under? What form of contraception is best for you? Log on and find out!

HealthQuest Activities
You received a free HealthQuest CD-ROM with your new copy of *Understanding Your Health.* This feature provides activities to help you explore HealthQuest and assess your health behavior in areas like cancer prevention, fitness, and nutrition.

chapter twenty
the environment and your health

Chapter Objectives

After reading this chapter, you should be able to:

■ Identify several environmental factors that can impact your personal health in either positive or adverse ways.

■ explain how your personal health is influenced by different environmental factors on several scales, including personal environment, the community and regional environment, and the global environment.

■ describe specific actions that you can take to minimize health risks associated with your personal environment—your home, your automobile, your workplace.

■ describe the distinction between a "point source" versus a "nonpoint source" of community/regional air or water pollution.

■ detail several specific actions that you can take to minimize environmental health risks at the community and regional level.

■ describe several global environmental health issues, and offer several actions that you might take to foster positive change.

Online Learning Center Resources

www.mhhe.com/payne8e

Log on to our Online Learning Center (OLC) for access to these additional resources:

- Chapter key terms and definitions
- Learning objectives
- Student interactive question-and-answer sites
- Self-scoring chapter quiz
- Online assessments
- Key term flash cards

Talking It Over

Talking—and Acting—Like an Environmentalist

One of your classmates claims to be an avid environmentalist who loves hiking, camping, and other outdoor activities. He is involved with several organizations that lobby the government for environmental reform. So, when you see him drive a large, gas-guzzling SUV up to the recycling center, where he deposits neatly sorted paper, bottles, and cans for recycling, does this image strike you as contradictory? Do you think he recycles to ease a guilty conscience about driving an SUV? Would it matter more if you were standing in the middle of New York City (far from any dirt roads), or in Salt Lake City (surrounded by vast wildlands)? If his love of the great outdoors requires a larger vehicle (to haul camping gear, kayak, etc.), might he have made a more environmentally sound choice?

CommunicationLinks:
www.thedetroitproject.com
http://www.ecocenter.org/auto.shtml

Eye on the Media

Does Eco-Terrorism Really Work to Protect Our Environment?

On August 23, 2003, several automobile dealerships were attacked by arsonists who left graffiti claiming that they destroyed or damaged gas-guzzling SUVs to protect the environment. The unknown perpetrators claimed to be acting in accordance with the Earth Liberation Front, or ELF. According to their Internet website, ELF is an international underground organization that uses "direct action" (called eco-terrorism by others) in the form of economic sabotage to stop the destruction of the natural environment. Since 1997, the ELF in North America ha~ ~d over $100 million in damages to entities who profit from the destruction of life and the planet. ELF-linked arson fires have destroyed many buildings associated with urban sprawl and economic developments in previously natural habitats.

Many people are angered by the degradation of our shared natural environment, but is direct action/eco-terrorism ever justified in a democratic society? For some, the degradation or destruction of a lo~ ~land, a

Health on the Web

Behavior Change Activities

Learn about Lead Poisoning

Lead poisoning has been a predominant topic in environmental health news in recent years. Lead is a very harmful substance, especially to young children as it is easily absorbed into their bodies. However, lead can be harmful to anyone who comes in contact with large quantities of it. Go to **http://www.wmeac. ~/learn/toxics.~** ~West Michigan Environmental Council and scroll down to the section on Lead. Click on the "self-test" link to learn whether you or your child should be tested for lead poisoning.

Automobiles and Air Pollution

Did you know that if you "top off" your gas tank on a hot day, you are actually creating smog, ~h you then brea~ ~ur lungs? Did ~ know that a full bus is six times more energy efficient than each person on the bus driving his or her own car? Learn more fascinating air pollution facts with this air pollution quiz from Car Talk at Cars.com. Go to **http://cartalk. cars.com/About/Pollution-Quiz/**, take the quiz, ~nd then learn how ~h fight air pollution!

HealthQuest Activities

What would you do if the person you were with collapsed and stopped breathing? Would you know how to perform CPR? CPR is an important skill to have—it could save someone's life. Go to the *CPR Exploration* in the Cardiovascular module. Complete the tutorial, and then complete the exploration. It could mean the difference between life and ~~th. (The materials fo~~ ~ in this tutorial

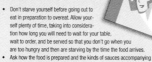

Changing for the Better

Learn to put health concepts into practice by following these useful tips. This feature provides practical advice for making positive changes and staying motivated to follow a healthy lifestyle.

Talking Points

Throughout each chapter, you'll find these tips for starting a dialogue about sensitive health topics.

Discovering Your Spirituality

A healthy body and a healthy mind go hand in hand. This feature will help you tap into your spiritual side to improve your self-esteem, foster good relationships with others, and jump-start your physical health.

Considering Complementary Care

Interested in nontraditional approaches to health care? What really works? What's really safe? This feature invites you to take a critical look at alternative approaches to health care and make up your own mind.

Learning from Our Diversity

These unique boxes invite you to explore the rich diversity of your own campus, and to gain perspective on the way such characteristics as age, racial/ethnic background, physical abilities, and sexual orientation can shape individuals' lives and well-being.

Personal Assessment

Do you eat too much fat? What's the best method of birth control for you if you are sexually active? Are you a perfectionist? Each chapter in *Understanding Your Health* includes an assessment to help you learn the answers to these and many other questions.

personal assessment

how stressed are you?

A widely used life stress scale called the Social Readjustment Rating Scale by Holmes and Rahe has been used to determine the degree of stress that you are experiencing due to life events over the past year. It also projects your chances of developing an illness- or stress-related health condition. Stress can lead to some serious health problems, and the more stress you have in your life, the more vulnerable you are to being susceptible to illness. Let's see how you score.

Life-Stress Scale

Check off the events which have happened to you **within the last year**. Then add up your total number of stress units for each life stress event. The number on the right-hand side represents the amount, duration, and severity of change required to cope with each item. See the point scale at the bottom of the inventory to determine your health risk associated with your stress level.

Life Event	Value	Score
Death of a partner	100	___
Divorce	73	___
Relationship separation	65	___
Jail term	63	___
Death of a family member	63	___
Personal injury/illness	53	___
Marriage	50	___
Fired from job	47	___
Reconciliation with partner	45	___
Retirement	45	___
Illness—family member	44	___
Pregnancy	40	___
Sexual difficulties	39	___
Addition of a family member	39	___
Change in financial situation	38	___
Death of a close friend	37	___
Change in job	36	___
...ent arguments...	35	
...ov...	31	

	Value	Score
Begin or end school	26	___
Partner begins/stops working	26	___
Change in living conditions	25	___
Change in personal habits	24	___
Trouble with supervisor	23	___
Change in work hours	20	___
Change in residence	20	___
Change in schools	20	___
Change in recreation	19	___
Change in church activities	19	___
Change in social activities	18	___
Mortgage/loan less than $10,000	17	___
Change in sleeping habits	16	___
Change in family visits	15	___
Change in eating habits	15	___
Vacation	13	___
Christmas	12	___
Minor violations of the law	11	___
TOTAL SCORE		___

What Is Your Health Risk?

Notice that positive events such as outstanding personal achievements, vacations, Christmas, can be as stressful as negative ones. Think of events in your life that are not listed on this inventory. For example, where would you put running in a marathon or going on a diet?

⇒ If your score was 150 points or less . . .
You are on reasonably safe and healthy ground. You have about a one-in-three chance of a health change in the next 2 years.

⇒ If your score was between 150–300 points . . .
You have about a 50/50 chance of developing an illness related to stress in the next 2 years.

...core was 30...

Focus On...

Every day you hear the buzz about hot health topics ranging from extreme sports to emerging diseases. Read these articles and decide where you stand on these controversial issues.

focus on

gay and lesbian unions: how close is our society to same-sex marriages?

What is the definition of a marriage? Must the marriage partners be only a man and a woman? Would allowing same-sex marriages weaken our society? Or would it make for a stronger society that is capable of recognizing commitments that legally bond men with men and women with women? These questions are being debated now on a scale that could not have been predicted even 5 years ago.

Same-sex marriages would grant gay couples an array of legal and economic benefits, including joint parental custody, insurance and health benefits, joint tax returns, alimony and child support, inheritance of property, hospital visitation rights, family leave, and a spouse's Social Security and retirement benefits.

Same-sex unions have been debated for many years. Some U.S. clergy were presiding over gay "marriages" in the 1980s, and hundreds of companies, businesses, associations and universities now offer benefits to same-sex partners of employees. Gay publications debated the subject in the 1950s. In his book *Same-Sex Unions in Premodern Europe*, late John Boswell, a V... ..., sugge...

..., sugge... over 800 civil unions, with three-quarters of the couples coming from out-of-state.[2] This trend has continued since the law has been in effect. By the summer of 2003, 85% of Vermont's civil unions were granted to out-of-state couples.[3]

The law permits same-sex couples to obtain civil union licenses from the town clerk, similar to the way opposite-sex couples obtain marriage licenses. A judge, justice of the peace, or clergy member certifies the civil unions. Divorces between civil union partners are called "dissolutions" and are handled in family court, similar to opposite-sex divorces.[4]

Vermont's law confers on same-sex couples all the benefits that the state presently allows heterosexual married couples. However, Vermont's law does not affect federal programs, such as Social Security. Additionally, civil unions that take place in Vermont are not generally recognized by other states. In fact thirty-seven states and the federal government have passed laws that deny the recognition of gay and lesbian marriages. These laws are called Defense of Marriage Acts (DOMAs) and ... ... as the union ... ...[5]

to happen, Canada would be following the path set by Germany (in 2001),[7] Holland (in 2001), and Belgium (in January 2003).[8]

In the United States, a State Supreme Court ruling in Massachusetts was expected in late summer 2003 in a case (*Goodridge v Department of Public Health*) in which seven gay and lesbian couples sued to have Massachusetts expand the definition of marriage to include same-sex couples. Another same-sex marriage suit was pending in New Jersey. While efforts to promote same-sex marriages in Hawaii and Alaska were unsuccessful, the California legislature was in the process of broadening the definition of domestic partnerships to include committed gay and lesbian couples. Such legislation, if passed, would grant to same-sex couples about one-third of the "rights, privileges, and obligations that the state automatically grants to married couples."[8]

Opponents of same-sex marriage were concerned that a June 2003 U.S. Supreme Court ruling (*Lawrence and Garner v Texas*) which struck down a Texas sodomy law banning private consensual sex between same-... ...would open the door, ...sbian mar...

Social and Occupational Health

	Not true/ rarely	Somewhat true/ sometimes	Mostly true/ usually	Very true/ always
1. I feel loved and supported by my family.	1	2	3	4
2. I establish friendships with ease and enjoyment.	1	2	3	4
3. I establish friendships with people of both genders and all ages.	1	2	3	4
4. I sustain relationships by communicating with and caring about my family and friends.	1	2	3	4
5. I feel comfortable and confident when meeting people for the first time.	1	2	3	4
6. I practice social skills to facilitate the process of forming new relationships.	1	2	3	4
7. I seek opportunities to meet and interact with new people.	1	2	3	4
8. I talk with, rather than at, people.	1	2	3	4
9. I am open to developing or sustaining intimate relationships.	1	2	3	4
10. I appreciate the importance of parenting the next generation and am committed to supporting it in ways that reflect my own resources.	1	2	3	4
11. I recognize the strengths and weaknesses of my parents' childrearing skills and feel comfortable modifying them if I choose to become a parent.	1	2	3	4
12. I attempt to be tolerant of others whether or not I approve of their behavior or beliefs.	1	2	3	4
13. I understand and appreciate the contribution that cultural diversity makes to the quality of living.	1	2	3	4
14. I understand and appreciate the difference between being educated and being trained.	1	2	3	4
15. My work gives me a sense of self-sufficiency and an opportunity to contribute.	1	2	3	4
16. I have equal respect for the roles of leader and subordinate within the workplace.	1	2	3	4
17. I have chosen an occupation that suits my interests and temperament.	1	2	3	4
18. I have chosen an occupation that does not compromise my physical or psychological health.	1	2	3	4
19. I get along well with my coworkers most of the time.	1	2	3	4
20. When I have a disagreement with a coworker, I try to resolve it directly and constructively.	1	2	3	4

Points _____

Spiritual and Psychological Health

	Not true/ rarely	Somewhat true/ sometimes	Mostly true/ usually	Very true/ always
1. I have a deeply held belief system or personal theology.	1	2	3	4
2. I recognize the contribution that membership in a community of faith can make to a person's overall quality of life.	1	2	3	4

3. I seek experiences with nature and reflect on nature's contribution to my quality of life.	1	2	3	4
4. My spirituality is a resource that helps me remain calm and strong during times of stress.	1	2	3	4
5. I have found appropriate ways to express my spirituality.	1	2	3	4
6. I respect the diversity of spiritual expression and am tolerant of those whose beliefs differ from my own.	1	2	3	4
7. I take adequate time to reflect on my own life and my relationships with others and the institutions of society.	1	2	3	4
8. I routinely undertake new experiences.	1	2	3	4
9. I receive adequate support from others.	1	2	3	4
10. I look for opportunities to support others, even occasionally at the expense of my own goals and aspirations.	1	2	3	4
11. I recognize that emotional and psychological health are as important as physical health.	1	2	3	4
12. I express my feelings and opinions comfortably, yet am capable of keeping them to myself when appropriate.	1	2	3	4
13. I see myself as a person of worth and feel comfortable with my own strengths and limitations.	1	2	3	4
14. I establish realistic goals and work to achieve them.	1	2	3	4
15. I understand the differences between the normal range of emotions and the signs of clinical depression.	1	2	3	4
16. I know how to recognize signs of suicidal thoughts and am willing to intervene.	1	2	3	4
17. I regularly assess my own behavior patterns and beliefs and would seek professional assistance for any emotional dysfunction.	1	2	3	4
18. I accept the reality of aging and view it as an opportunity for positive change.	1	2	3	4
19. I accept the reality of death and view it as a normal and inevitable part of life.	1	2	3	4
20. I have made decisions about my own death to ensure that I die with dignity when the time comes.	1	2	3	4

Points _____

Stress Management

	Not true/ rarely	Somewhat true/ sometimes	Mostly true/ usually	Very true/ always
1. I accept the reality of change while maintaining the necessary stability in my daily activities.	1	2	3	4
2. I seek change when it is necessary or desirable to do so.	1	2	3	4
3. I know what stress-management services are offered on campus, through my employer, or in my community.	1	2	3	4
4. When necessary, I use the stress-management services to which I have access.	1	2	3	4
5. I employ stress-reduction practices in anticipation of stressful events, such as job interviews and final examinations.	1	2	3	4
6. I reevaluate the way in which I handled stressful events so that I can better cope with similar events in the future.	1	2	3	4
7. I turn to relatives and friends during periods of disruption in my life.	1	2	3	4
8. I avoid using alcohol or other drugs during periods of stress.	1	2	3	4
9. I refrain from behaving aggressively or abusively during periods of stress.	1	2	3	4

		Not true/ rarely	Somewhat true/ sometimes	Mostly true/ usually	Very true/ always
10.	I sleep enough to maintain a high level of health and cope successfully with daily challenges.	1	2	3	4
11.	I avoid sleeping excessively as a response to stressful change.	1	2	3	4
12.	My diet is conducive to good health and stress management.	1	2	3	4
13.	I participate in physical activity to relieve stress.	1	2	3	4
14.	I practice stress-management skills, such as diaphragmatic breathing and yoga.	1	2	3	4
15.	I manage my time effectively.	1	2	3	4

Points _____

Fitness

		Not true/ rarely	Somewhat true/ sometimes	Mostly true/ usually	Very true/ always
1.	I participate in recreational and fitness activities both to minimize stress and to improve or maintain my level of physical fitness.	1	2	3	4
2.	I select some recreational activities that are strenuous rather than sedentary in nature.	1	2	3	4
3.	I include various types of aerobic conditioning activities among the wider array of recreational and fitness activities in which I engage.	1	2	3	4
4.	I engage in aerobic activities with appropriate frequency, intensity, and duration to provide a training effect for my heart and lungs.	1	2	3	4
5.	I routinely include strength-training activities among the wider array of fitness activities in which I engage.	1	2	3	4
6.	I routinely vary the types of strength-training activities in which I participate in order to minimize injury and strengthen all of the important muscle groups.	1	2	3	4
7.	I do exercises specifically designed to maintain joint range of motion.	1	2	3	4
8.	I believe that recreational and fitness activities can help me improve my physical health and my emotional and social well-being.	1	2	3	4
9.	I include a variety of fitness activities in my overall plan for physical fitness.	1	2	3	4
10.	I take appropriate steps to avoid injuries when participating in recreational and fitness activities.	1	2	3	4
11.	I seek appropriate treatment for all injuries that result from fitness activities.	1	2	3	4
12.	I believe that older adults should undertake appropriately chosen fitness activities.	1	2	3	4
13.	My body composition is consistent with a high level of health.	1	2	3	4
14.	I warm up before beginning vigorous activity, and I cool down afterward.	1	2	3	4
15.	I select properly designed and well-maintained equipment and clothing for each activity.	1	2	3	4
16.	I avoid using performance-enhancing substances that are known to be dangerous and those whose influence on the body is not fully understood.	1	2	3	4
17.	I sleep seven to eight hours daily.	1	2	3	4
18.	I refrain from using over-the-counter sleep-inducing aids.	1	2	3	4
19.	I follow sound dietary practices as an important adjunct to a health-enhancing physical activity program.	1	2	3	4
20.	My current level of fitness allows me to participate fully and effortlessly in my daily activities.	1	2	3	4

Points _____

Nutrition and Weight Management

	Not true/ rarely	Somewhat true/ sometimes	Mostly true/ usually	Very true/ always
1. I balance my caloric intake with my calorie expenditure.	1	2	3	4
2. I obtain the recommended number of servings from each of the food groups.	1	2	3	4
3. I select a wide variety of foods chosen from each of the food groups.	1	2	3	4
4. I understand the amount of a particular food that constitutes a single serving.	1	2	3	4
5. I often try new foods, particularly when I know them to be healthful.	1	2	3	4
6. I select breads, cereals, fresh fruits, and vegetables in preference to pastries, candies, sodas and fruits canned in heavy syrup.	1	2	3	4
7. I limit the amount of sugar that I add to foods during preparation and at the table.	1	2	3	4
8. I consume an appropriate percentage of my total daily calories from carbohydrates.	1	2	3	4
9. I select primarily nonmeat sources of protein, such as peas, beans, and peanut butter, while limiting my consumption of red meat and high-fat dairy products.	1	2	3	4
10. I consume an appropriate percentage of my total daily calories from protein.	1	2	3	4
11. I select foods prepared with unsaturated vegetable oils while reducing consumption of red meat, high-fat dairy products, and foods prepared with lard (animal fat) or butter.	1	2	3	4
12. I carefully limit the amount of fast food that I consume during a typical week.	1	2	3	4
13. I consume an appropriate percentage of my total daily calories from fat.	1	2	3	4
14. I select nutritious foods when I snack.	1	2	3	4
15. I limit my use of salt during food preparation and at the table.	1	2	3	4
16. I consume adequate amounts of fiber.	1	2	3	4
17. I routinely consider the nutrient density of individual food items when choosing foods.	1	2	3	4
18. I maintain my weight without reliance on over-the-counter or prescription diet pills.	1	2	3	4
19. I maintain my weight without reliance on fad diets or liquid weight loss beverages.	1	2	3	4
20. I exercise regularly to help maintain my weight.	1	2	3	4

Points _____

Alcohol, Tobacco, and Other Drug Use

	Not true/ rarely	Somewhat true/ sometimes	Mostly true/ usually	Very true/ always
1. I abstain or drink in moderation when offered alcoholic beverages.	1	2	3	4
2. I abstain from using illegal psychoactive (mind-altering) drugs.	1	2	3	4
3. I do not consume alcoholic beverages or psychoactive drugs rapidly or in large quantities.	1	2	3	4
4. I do not use alcohol or psychoactive drugs in a way that causes me to behave inappropriately.	1	2	3	4
5. My use of alcohol or other drugs does not compromise my academic performance.	1	2	3	4

		Not true/ rarely	Somewhat true/ sometimes	Mostly true/ usually	Very true/ always
6.	I refrain from drinking alcoholic beverages or using psychoactive drugs when engaging in recreational activities that require strength, speed, or coordination.	1	2	3	4
7.	I refrain from drinking alcoholic beverages while participating in occupational activities, regardless of the nature of those activities.	1	2	3	4
8.	My use of alcohol or other drugs does not generate financial concerns for myself or for others.	1	2	3	4
9.	I refrain from drinking alcohol or using psychoactive drugs when driving a motor vehicle or operating heavy equipment.	1	2	3	4
10.	I do not drink alcohol or use psychoactive drugs when I am alone.	1	2	3	4
11.	I avoid riding with people who have been drinking alcohol or using psychoactive drugs.	1	2	3	4
12.	My use of alcohol or other drugs does not cause family dysfunction.	1	2	3	4
13.	I do not use marijuana.	1	2	3	4
14.	I do not use hallucinogens.	1	2	3	4
15.	I do not use heroin or other illegal intravenous drugs.	1	2	3	4
16.	I do not experience blackouts when I drink alcohol.	1	2	3	4
17.	I do not become abusive or violent when I drink alcohol or use psychoactive drugs.	1	2	3	4
18.	I use potentially addictive prescription medication in complete compliance with my physician's directions.	1	2	3	4
19.	I do not smoke cigarettes.	1	2	3	4
20.	I do not use tobacco products in any other form.	1	2	3	4
21.	I minimize my exposure to secondhand smoke.	1	2	3	4
22.	I am concerned about the effect that alcohol, tobacco, and other drug use is known to have on developing fetuses.	1	2	3	4
23.	I am concerned about the effect that alcohol, tobacco, and other drug use is known to have on the health of other people.	1	2	3	4
24.	I seek natural, health-enhancing highs rather than relying on alcohol, tobacco, and illegal drugs.	1	2	3	4
25.	I take prescription medication only as instructed, and I use over-the-counter medication in accordance with directions.	1	2	3	4

Points _____

Disease Prevention

		Not true/ rarely	Somewhat true/ sometimes	Mostly true/ usually	Very true/ always
1.	My diet includes foods rich in phytochemicals.	1	2	3	4
2.	My diet includes foods rich in folic acid.	1	2	3	4
3.	My diet includes foods that are good sources of dietary fiber.	1	2	3	4
4.	My diet is low in dietary cholesterol.	1	2	3	4
5.	I follow food preparation practices that minimize the risk of food-borne illness.	1	2	3	4
6.	I engage in regular physical activity and am able to control my weight effectively.	1	2	3	4
7.	I do not use tobacco products.	1	2	3	4
8.	I abstain from alcohol or drink only in moderation.	1	2	3	4
9.	I do not use intravenously administered illegal drugs.	1	2	3	4
10.	I use safer sex practices intended to minimize my risk of exposure to sexually transmitted diseases, including HIV and HPV.	1	2	3	4

	Not true/ rarely	Somewhat true/ sometimes	Mostly true/ usually	Very true/ always
11. I take steps to limit my risk of exposure to the bacterium that causes Lyme disease and to the virus that causes hantavirus pulmonary syndrome.	1	2	3	4
12. I control my blood pressure with weight management and physical fitness activities.	1	2	3	4
13. I minimize my exposure to allergens, including those that trigger asthma attacks.	1	2	3	4
14. I wash my hands frequently and thoroughly.	1	2	3	4
15. I use preventive medical care services appropriately.	1	2	3	4
16. I use appropriate cancer self-screening practices, such as breast self-examination and testicular self-examination.	1	2	3	4
17. I know which chronic illnesses and diseases are part of my family history.	1	2	3	4
18. I know which inherited conditions are part of my family history and will seek preconceptional counseling regarding these conditions.	1	2	3	4
19. I am fully immunized against infectious diseases.	1	2	3	4
20. I take prescribed medications, particularly antibiotics, exactly as instructed by my physician.	1	2	3	4

Points _____

Sexual Health

	Not true/ rarely	Somewhat true/ sometimes	Mostly true/ usually	Very true/ always
1. I know how sexually transmitted diseases are spread.	1	2	3	4
2. I can recognize the symptoms of sexually transmitted diseases.	1	2	3	4
3. I know how sexually transmitted disease transmission can be prevented.	1	2	3	4
4. I know how safer sex practices reduce the risk of contracting sexually transmitted diseases.	1	2	3	4
5. I follow safer sex practices.	1	2	3	4
6. I recognize the symptoms of premenstrual syndrome and understand how it is prevented and treated.	1	2	3	4
7. I recognize the symptoms of endometriosis and understand the relationship of its symptoms to hormonal cycles.	1	2	3	4
8. I understand the physiological basis of menopause and recognize that it is a normal part of the aging process in women.	1	2	3	4
9. I understand and accept the range of human sexual orientations.	1	2	3	4
10. I encourage the development of flexible sex roles (androgyny) in children.	1	2	3	4
11. I take a mature approach to dating and mate selection.	1	2	3	4
12. I recognize that marriage and other types of long-term relationships can be satisfying.	1	2	3	4
13. I recognize that a celibate lifestyle is appropriate and satisfying for some people.	1	2	3	4
14. I affirm the sexuality of older adults and am comfortable with its expression.	1	2	3	4
15. I am familiar with the advantages and disadvantages of a wide range of birth control methods.	1	2	3	4
16. I understand how each birth control method works and how effective it is.	1	2	3	4
17. I use my birth control method consistently and appropriately.	1	2	3	4
18. I am familiar with the wide range of procedures now available to treat infertility.	1	2	3	4

	Not true/ rarely	Somewhat true/ sometimes	Mostly true/ usually	Very true/ always
19. I accept that others may disagree with my feelings about pregnancy termination.	1	2	3	4
20. I am familiar with alternatives available to infertile couples, including adoption.	1	2	3	4

Points _____

Safety Practices and Violence Prevention

	Not true/ rarely	Somewhat true/ sometimes	Mostly true/ usually	Very true/ always
1. I attempt to identify sources of risk or danger in each new setting or activity.	1	2	3	4
2. I learn proper procedures and precautions before undertaking new recreational or occupational activities.	1	2	3	4
3. I select appropriate clothing and equipment for all activities and maintain equipment in good working order.	1	2	3	4
4. I curtail my participation in activities when I am not feeling well or am distracted by other demands.	1	2	3	4
5. I repair dangerous conditions or report them to those responsible for maintenance.	1	2	3	4
6. I use common sense and observe the laws governing non-motorized vehicles when I ride a bicycle.	1	2	3	4
7. I operate all motor vehicles as safely as possible, including using seat belts and other safety equipment.	1	2	3	4
8. I refrain from driving an automobile or boat when I have been drinking alcohol or taking drugs or medications.	1	2	3	4
9. I try to anticipate the risk of falling and maintain my environment to minimize this risk.	1	2	3	4
10. I maintain my environment to minimize the risk of fire, and I have a well-rehearsed plan to exit my residence in case of fire.	1	2	3	4
11. I am a competent swimmer and could save myself or rescue someone who was drowning.	1	2	3	4
12. I refrain from sexually aggressive behavior toward my partner or others.	1	2	3	4
13. I would report an incident of sexual harassment or date rape whether or not I was the victim.	1	2	3	4
14. I would seek help from others if I were the victim or perpetrator of domestic violence.	1	2	3	4
15. I practice gun safety and encourage other gun owners to do so.	1	2	3	4
16. I drive at all times in a way that will minimize my risk of being carjacked.	1	2	3	4
17. I have taken steps to protect my home from intruders.	1	2	3	4
18. I use campus security services as much as possible when they are available.	1	2	3	4
19. I know what to do if I am being stalked.	1	2	3	4
20. I have a well-rehearsed plan to protect myself from the aggressive behavior of other people in my place of residence.	1	2	3	4

Points _____

Health Care Consumerism

	Not true/ rarely	Somewhat true/ sometimes	Mostly true/ usually	Very true/ always
1. I know how to obtain valid health information.	1	2	3	4
2. I accept health information that has been deemed valid by the established scientific community.	1	2	3	4

3. I am skeptical of claims that guarantee the effectiveness of a particular health care service or product.	1	2	3	4
4. I am skeptical of practitioners or clinics who advertise or offer services at rates substantially lower than those charged by reputable providers.	1	2	3	4
5. I am not swayed by advertisements that present unhealthy behavior in an attractive manner.	1	2	3	4
6. I can afford proper medical care, including hospitalization.	1	2	3	4
7. I can afford adequate health insurance.	1	2	3	4
8. I understand the role of government health care plans in providing health care to people who qualify for coverage.	1	2	3	4
9. I know how to select health care providers who are highly qualified and appropriate for my current health care needs.	1	2	3	4
10. I seek a second or third opinion when surgery or other costly therapies are recommended.	1	2	3	4
11. I have told my physician which hospital I would prefer to use should the need arise.	1	2	3	4
12. I understand my rights and responsibilities as a patient when admitted to a hospital.	1	2	3	4
13. I practice adequate self-care to reduce my health care expenditures and my reliance on health care providers.	1	2	3	4
14. I am open-minded about alternative health care practices and support current efforts to determine their appropriate role in effective health care.	1	2	3	4
15. I have a well-established relationship with a pharmacist and have transmitted all necessary information regarding medication use.	1	2	3	4
16. I carefully follow labels and directions when using health care products, such as over-the-counter medications.	1	2	3	4
17. I finish all prescription medications as directed, rather than stopping use when symptoms subside.	1	2	3	4
18. I report to the appropriate agencies any providers of health care services, information, or products that use deceptive advertising or fraudulent methods of operation.	1	2	3	4
19. I pursue my rights as fully as possible in matters of misrepresentation or consumer dissatisfaction.	1	2	3	4
20. I follow current health care issues in the news and voice my opinion to my elected representatives.	1	2	3	4

Points _____

Environmental Health

	Not true/ rarely	Somewhat true/ sometimes	Mostly true/ usually	Very true/ always
1. I avoid use of and exposure to pesticides as much as possible.	1	2	3	4
2. I avoid use of and exposure to herbicides as much as possible.	1	2	3	4
3. I am willing to spend the extra money and time required to obtain organically grown produce.	1	2	3	4
4. I reduce environmental pollutants by minimizing my use of the automobile.	1	2	3	4
5. I avoid the use of products that contribute to indoor air pollution.	1	2	3	4
6. I limit my exposure to ultraviolet radiation by avoiding excessive sun exposure.	1	2	3	4
7. I limit my exposure to radon gas by using a radon gas detector.	1	2	3	4

	1	2	3	4
8. I limit my exposure to radiation by promptly eliminating radon gas within my home.	1	2	3	4
9. I limit my exposure to radiation by agreeing to undergo medical radiation procedures only when absolutely necessary for the diagnosis and treatment of an illness or disease.	1	2	3	4
10. I avoid the use of potentially unsafe water, particularly when traveling in a foreign country or when a municipal water supply or bottled water is unavailable.	1	2	3	4
11. I avoid noise pollution by limiting my exposure to loud noise or by using ear protection.	1	2	3	4
12. I avoid air pollution by carefully selecting the environments in which I live, work, and recreate.	1	2	3	4
13. I do not knowingly use or improperly dispose of personal care products that can harm the environment.	1	2	3	4
14. I reuse as many products as possible so that they can avoid the recycling bins for as long as possible.	1	2	3	4
15. I participate fully in my community's recycling efforts.	1	2	3	4
16. I encourage the increased use of recycled materials in the design and manufacturing of new products.	1	2	3	4
17. I dispose of residential toxic substances safely and properly.	1	2	3	4
18. I follow environmental issues in the news and voice my opinion to my elected representatives.	1	2	3	4
19. I am aware of and involved in environmental issues in my local area.	1	2	3	4
20. I perceive myself as a steward of the environment for the generations to come, rather than as a person with a right to use (and misuse) the environment to meet my immediate needs.	1	2	3	4

Points _____

YOUR TOTAL POINTS _____

Interpretation

770–880 points

Congratulations! Your health behavior is very supportive of high-level health. Continue to practice your positive health habits, and look for areas in which you can become even stronger. Encourage others to follow your example, and support their efforts in any way you can.

550–769 points

Good job! Your health behavior is relatively supportive of high-level health. You scored well in several areas; however, you can improve in some ways. Identify your weak areas and chart a plan for behavior change, as explained at the end of Chapter 1. Then pay close attention as you learn more about health in the weeks ahead.

330–549 points

Caution! Your relatively low score indicates that your behavior may be compromising your health. Review your responses to this assessment carefully, noting the areas in which you scored poorly. Then chart a detailed plan for behavior change, as outlined at the end of Chapter1. Be sure to set realistic goals that you can work toward steadily as you complete this course.

Below 330 points

Red flag! Your low score suggests that your health behavior is destructive. Immediate changes in your behavior are needed to put you back on track. Review your responses to this assessment carefully. Then begin to make changes in the most critical areas, such as harmful alcohol or other drug use patterns. Seek help promptly for any difficulties that you are not prepared to deal with alone, such as domestic violence or suicidal thoughts. The information you read in this textbook and learn in this course could have a significant effect on your future health. Remember, it's not too late to improve your health!

To Carry This Further . . .

Most of us can improve our health behavior in a number of ways. We hope this assessment will help you identify areas in which you can make positive changes and serve as a motivator as you implement your plan for behavior change (see Chapter 1). If you scored well, give yourself a pat on the back. If your score was not as high as you would have liked, take heart. This textbook and your instructor can help you get started on the road to wellness. Good luck!

understanding your health

chapter one

shaping your health

Chapter Objectives

Upon completing this chapter, you should be able to:

▌ understand how your health affects your lifestyle.

▌ recognize how the delivery of health care influences definitions of health.

▌ detail some of the health concerns outlined by the Institute of Medicine and Healthy People 2010.

▌ suggest additional reasons why health behavior change is difficult, beyond those outlined in your textbook.

▌ speculate on strategies for encouraging health behavior change.

▌ list Prochaska's six stages of change.

▌ describe and compare the range of traditional and nontraditional students on your campus.

▌ describe the developmental tasks of adulthood, and assess your current level of progress in mastering them.

▌ monitor your own activities, and list the dimensions of health from which resources were drawn.

▌ compare wellness and health promotion, noting both the differences and the similarities between the two concepts.

▌ describe your textbook's new definition of health, and compare it with definitions of episodic health care and health promotion.

Online Learning Center Resources

www.mhhe.com/payne8e

Log on to our Online Learning Center (OLC) for access to these additional resources:

- Chapter key terms and definitions
- Learning objectives
- Student interactive question-and-answer sites

- Self-scoring chapter quiz
- Online assessments
- Key term flash cards

Talking It Over

Getting in Shape Together: That's What Friends Are For

Shaping up can be a lonely business—unless you use the buddy system. But convincing a friend to get out and walk, run, or play volleyball can be tricky. Even a good friend might think you're saying he's flabby or lazy.

Try this approach: Say that *you* need to get in shape and want your friend's help and support. Make it clear to your friend that you don't want to become a marathon runner, just improve your cardiovascular fitness.

Tell your friend that it won't be punishment—it might even be fun! Check out the websites below for ideas on getting started.

CommunicationLinks
www.healthfinder.gov
www.healthworld.com

Eye on the Media

Where Does Our Health Information Come From?

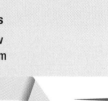

Today our health information comes from a variety of media—some more reliable than others. Media in the Spotlight will appear in each chapter of this text, highlighting the important issue of which ones are good (in other words, valid and reliable) sources for learning about health.

Radio and Television

When you think of radio, the first thing that may come to mind is your favorite music. But two areas of radio are especially important for news and information: talk radio and public radio networks, such as National Public Radio (NPR) and Public

Radio International (PRI). Talk radio raises the question of validity of information. For example, if you're listening to a talk show about HIV exposure, the perceptions and opinions of the host (which may be strong or even extreme) are an important part of the show. When this point of view is combined with the opinions of callers, whose "facts" may come from unauthoritative sources, what you're hearing is probably not solid information. It's certainly not a good basis for making your health decisions.

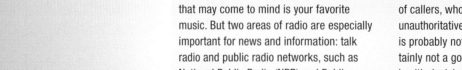

NPR and PRI, on the other hand, take a scholarly approach to news, featuring experts who do not always agree on an issue. In general, the news reports on NPR and PRI are long enough to present an in-depth, balanced treatment of health-related topics.

Television too, is often an important source of health information. Coverage ranges from brief health-related segments on national or local news programs to entire cable programs devoted to health topics, such as those seen on the Learning and Discovery channels. While these programs can be timely and accurate, television also provides an array of "Infomericals" promoting health products that should be evaluated more critically.

Newspapers and Magazines

Let's assume that most people read only one or two newspapers a day—their local paper and perhaps a national newspaper such as *The New York Times* or *USA Today.* If so, the health information they are receiving is typically from wire services like the Associated Press; it is condensed and simplified but accurate within these limitations. When health-related information in newspapers is accompanied by illustrations and identification of the original source (such as a professional journal), it is more helpful to the reader.

Unlike newspapers, magazines are so diverse in terms of ownership, intended audience, and standards of validity that it is difficult to determine the reliability of their health-related content. In general, the national news magazines, such as *Time* and *Newsweek,* are very careful about the accuracy of their reporting, often including primary (original) sources. Their content is considered "state of the art." In contrast, the checkout-lane tabloids, such as *The Globe* and *The National Enquirer,* are known for printing stories with "health" content that few readers take seriously. Between these two extremes is a wide array of general content magazines, such as *The Saturday Evening Post,* and health-oriented magazines, such as *Prevention,* that vary greatly in validity and reliability.

Professional Journals

Your college library probably offers a broad selection of professional journals. Through these publications, the members of an academic discipline share the latest developments and issues in their field with their colleagues and other readers. Because the study of health is so multifaceted, drawing on different disciplines for information, health-related journals are plentiful. The vast majority of articles that appear in publications such as *The New England Journal of Medicine* and *The Journal of the American Dietetic Association* are peer-reviewed. This means that professionals in the particular field review and judge the content of a submitted article to determine whether or not it should be published. Then, if a study being reported was not carefully controlled, or if its underlying theory seems to be flawed, the article is returned to the author(s) for refinement. This process greatly reduces the risk of publishing invalid information. Currently, journals are beginning to appear in fields such as complementary (alternative) health care. When reading such publications, you need to consider whether they are backed by a peer-review process.

Government Documents

Each year various departments of the federal government, particularly the Department of Health and Human Services (DHHS), release the results of research being done under the oversight of its many divisions and agencies. These documents, such as the annual *Surgeon General's Report on Smoking and Health,* become the source of much of the health-related news reported by other media sources, including textbooks and professional journals. These publications generally can be purchased through the U.S. Government Printing Office. They are also available through urban public libraries and large university libraries. With few exceptions, the information in these publications is reviewed by the most respected authorities in each field.

Books

Books continue to be a vast source of information on health-related topics. Today's health books, in addition to academic health textbooks such as *Understanding Your Health,* fall into three categories: reference books, medical encyclopedias, and single-topic trade (retail) books.

Included in the category of reference books are important professional publications such as *The Merck Manual* and the *Physicians' Desk Reference.* These books, intended for professionals in various health fields, contain the most current information on specific aspects of health. Although these books can be purchased by the general public, their content is technical and complex, and their language is often difficult for nonprofessional readers to follow.

More valuable to the typical American household are the various medical (health) encyclopedias, such as *The Johns Hopkins Home Medical Handbook* and *The Mayo Clinic Family Health Book.* Such books usually include a wide array of medical conditions and offer valuable information about health promotion and disease prevention. Their clear writing styles and highly valid information make these books excellent home references.

Single-topic health-related trade books, such as those about diets and health problems, are readily available from retail outlets like bookstores and the Internet. Like magazines, these books are difficult to assess because of their quantity and the varying backgrounds of the authors. Some are very sound in terms of content and philosophy. Others may be misleading and may contain advice that could be dangerous to your health. Included in this group are self-help books, the best-selling health books of all.

The Internet

Today, at least 60% of all U.S. households can access the Internet directly, with 72% of those headed by college graduates having direct Internet access. Internet access is also available through libraries, educational institutions, and the workplace. With just a few clicks, you can reach many health-related websites that offer a wide range of health information. Chat rooms provide a forum for individuals to share their personal health

Eye on the Media *continued*
experiences. Because the Internet is such an important source of health information for both professionals and the general public,

this textbook highlights helpful websites in all chapters. To learn about criteria for assessing the validity and reliability of Internet information, see Chapter 18.

Sources: Percentage on Internet-connected Households Soars to 60% in 2000; In-Stat Reveals Results in Buying and Internet Usage Trends. *In-Stat MDR Press Release.* March 28, 2000. http://www.in-stat.com

"Take care of your health, because you'll miss it when it's gone," younger people hear often from their elders. This simple and heartfelt advice is given in the belief that young people take their health for granted and assume that they will always maintain the state of health and wellness they now enjoy. Observation and experience should, however, remind all of us that youth is relatively brief, and health is always changing—often in a downward direction. In fact, as health deteriorates, our ability to participate in meaningful life activities can be compromised or even lost. Consider, for example, how failing health might affect the following activities:

- Your ability to pursue an education or career
- Your opportunity to socialize with friends and family
- The chance to travel—for business, relaxation, or adventure
- The opportunity to meet and connect with a spouse or partner
- The ability to conceive children or the opportunity to raise a family
- Participation in hobbies or physical activities, from skydiving to stamp collecting
- Your enjoyment of a wide range of foods
- The opportunity to enjoy a high-level of physical activity

It is quality-of-life issues such as these that your parents and grandparents are thinking about when they advise you to take care of your health. As you will learn in this chapter, health is intertwined with activities such as these—indeed, your authors will present a new definition of health specifically related to accomplishing these important life tasks. But fiirst, a few familiar perceptions of health, each of which is concerned primarily with illness and death, will be reviewed, and strategies for changing health behaviors will be discussed.

Definitions of Health

By the time they reach college age, most Americans are familiar with the many ways in which health care is provided. Here are some easily recognizable examples, all of which serve to reinforce our traditional definition of health. As you will learn, these definitions are centered in the cure or management of illness and the extension of life. Note the concerns over **morbidity** and **mortality** present in the descriptions that follow.

Episodic Health Care

The vast majority of Americans use the services of professional health care providers during periods (episodes) of illness and injury, that is, when we are "unhealthy." We consult providers, seeking a diagnosis that will explain why we are not feeling well. Once a problem is identified, we expect to receive effective treatment from the practitioners that will lead to our recovery (the absence of illness) and a return to health. If we are willing to be compliant with the care strategies prescribed by our practitioner, we should soon be able to define ourselves as "healthy" once again.

The familiarity of episodic health care is evident in the 823.5 million times that Americans visited physicians during 2000. Although some of these visits were for preventive health care (see discussion below), the vast majority were in conjunction with illness. When viewed by racial groups, Whites averaged 3.2 visits, Asians 2.9, Blacks 2.1 and Native Americans 0.8 visits during that year.[1]

 TALKING POINTS Would you be hesitant to talk to your doctor about health advice you found on the Internet? How would you approach the subject?

Preventive or Prospective Medicine

Simple logic suggests that it makes more sense to prevent illness than to deal with it through episodic health

> **Key Terms**
>
> **morbidity** pertaining to illness and disease.
>
> **mortality** pertaining to death.

Factors That Affect Well-Being

Which factors do today's adults associate with the ability to feel good about their lives? Check the list below for the answers given to this question. Note that virtually none makes direct reference to being free of illness and disease or to living long into the future. Rather, they are more aligned with a personally defined sense of being adequately independent, self-sufficient, responsible, respected by others, and nurturing.

- A sense of *personal satisfaction* (82%) was identified as the most important feeling that should be experienced during adulthood.
- A sense of *being in control* of one's life (80%) was the second most identified index of adult well-being.
- A sense that one was a partner in a *good marriage* (78%) appeared as the third most important component of living well as an adult.
- A sense that one was *competent at one's job* (69%) placed employment in fourth position—important but clearly below the factors listed above. Also, note that *making a lot of money* was selected by only 25 percent as being of primary importance in defining adult life satisfaction.
- A sense that one's *children were (or would be) successful* was cited by 63 percent of the adults sampled as an important factor in feeling a sense of well-being.

Having studied these responses, you also may appreciate more fully the meaning we assign to having a sense of well-being and the role health plays in making it possible.

(medical) care. This philosophy characterizes **preventive or prospective medicine**. Unfortunately, however, many physicians say they have little time to practice preventive medicine because of the large number of episodically sick people who fill their offices every day.

When physicians do practice preventive or prospective medicine, they first attempt to determine their patient's level of risk for developing particular conditions. They make this assessment by identifying **risk factors** (and **high-risk health behaviors**) with a variety of observational techniques and screening tests, some of which may be invasive (taking tissues from the body such as a biopsy or blood draw). Additionally, an important tool in assessing risk is an accurate family health history, something that over one-third of all adults cannot adequately provide to their health care providers.[2] However, when you are certain that any of the conditions shown in Figure 1-1 have occurred in your family, this information should be shared with your health care provider.

Once they have identified levels of risk in patients, health practitioners try to lower those risk levels through patient education, lifestyle modification, and, when necessary, medical intervention. Continued compliance on the part of the patients will result in a lower level of risk that will continue over the years. Note that preventive medicine is guided by practitioners, and patients are expected to be compliant with the direction they are given.

Although preventive medical care appears to be a much more sensible approach than episodic care in reducing morbidity and mortality, third-party payers (insurance plans) traditionally have not provided coverage for these services. Managed health care plans that earn a profit by preventing sickness, such as health maintenance organizations, or HMOs (see Chapter 18), should be much more receptive to the concept and practice of preventive medicine.

Health Promotion

Throughout the United States, YMCA/YWCA-sponsored wellness programs, commercial fitness clubs, and corporate fitness centers offer risk-reduction programs under the direction of qualified instructors, many of whom are university graduates in disciplines such as exercise science, wellness management, and **health promotion**. Using approaches similar to those employed in preventive medicine, these nonphysician health professionals attempt to guide their clients toward activities and behaviors that will lower their risk of chronic illness. Unlike preventive medicine, with its sometimes invasive assessment procedures and medication-based therapies, health promotion programs are not legally defined as medical practices and thus do not require the involvement of physicians.

Key Terms

preventive or prospective medicine physician-centered medical care in which areas of risk for chronic illnesses are identified so that they might be lowered.

risk factor a biomedical index such as serum cholesterol level, or a behavioral pattern such as smoking, associated with a chronic illness.

high-risk health behavior a behavioral pattern, such as smoking, associated with a high risk of developing a chronic illness.

health promotion movement in which knowledge, practices, and values are transmitted to people for use in lengthening their lives, reducing the incidence of illness, and feeling better.

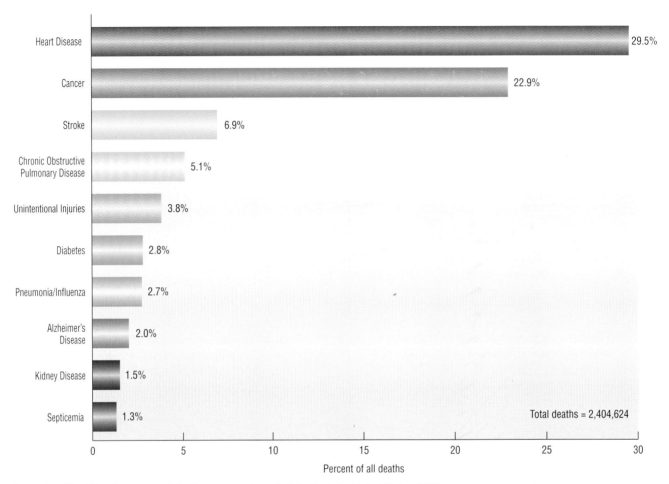

Figure 1-1 The 10 leading causes of death as a percentage of all deaths in the United States, 2000.

Source: *Deaths and death rates by leading causes of death and ages: 2000.* U.S. National Center for Health Statistics. Vital Statistics of the United States, Annual: National Vital Statistics Report (NVSR). 2002.

In addition, the fitness focus, social interaction, and healthy lifestyle orientation these programs provide tend to mask the emphasis on preventing chronic illness that would be the selling point of such efforts if they were undertaken as preventive medicine. In fact, it is likely that people receiving health promotion in these settings do not recognize it as such. Rather, they are only submitting to assessments and listening to health-related information as incidental parts of personal goals, such as losing weight, preparing for their first marathon, or simply meeting friends for lunch-hour basketball.

Community Health Promotion

In addition to the practices just described, a group-oriented form of health promotion is offered in many communities. This approach to improving health through risk reduction is directed at empowering community groups, such as church congregations or a neighborhood

association, so they can develop, operate, and financially sustain their own programs with little direct involvement of health promotion specialists.[3,4]

The key to successful community-based health promotion is **empowerment**.[5,6] In the context of health, empowerment refers to a process in which individuals or groups of people gain increasing control over their health. To take control over health matters, individuals and groups must learn to "liberate" themselves from a variety of barriers that tend to restrict health enhancement. In this sense, people learn to take charge of their lives, regardless of any current forces that discourage positive health changes. Empowered people and groups do not

---

Key Terms

empowerment the nurturing of an individual's or group's ability to be responsible for their own health and well-being.

At age 34, I find that I'm getting lazy about good health habits. How can I start to refocus my thoughts and actions on good health?

Prescriptions for good health usually place considerable importance on *risk reduction.* Health care professionals stress the importance of identifying behavioral patterns and biomedical indexes that suggest the potential for illness or death. Each of us has the opportunity to receive information, counseling, behavior change strategies, and medical therapies designed to lower our risk. The extent to which we act on this opportunity is our degree of *compliance.*

Some risk factors cannot be reduced. For example, gender, race, age, and genetic predisposition make developing certain conditions more likely. Being aware of these risk factors is important.

To refocus on good health, concentrate on these actions, which can reduce risk factors:

- *Refrain from using tobacco in any form.* This rule is so critically important that the surgeon general of the United States has identified smoking as the single most important reversible factor contributing to illness and early death.

- *If you drink alcohol, do so in moderation.* This is particularly important for people who must drive or operate machinery, women who are pregnant or planning to become pregnant, and people taking certain medications.

- *Engage in regular exercise designed to train the cardiorespiratory system as well as maintain muscle strength.* You can use a wide array of exercises as the basis of a fitness program, and you can develop specific programs around recommendations about frequency, duration, and intensity of activity.

- *Eat a balanced diet that includes a wide array of choices from each of the food groups.* Pay attention to the recommended amounts of carbohydrate, protein, and fat, as well as the specific food items that supply these three nutrients.

- *Develop effective coping techniques for use in moderating the effects of stress.* Effective coping can reduce the duration of physiological challenge the body faces during periods of unexpected change. Remember, however, that some forms of coping can themselves be sources of additional stress.

- *Maintain normal body weight.* Persons who are excessively overweight or underweight may experience abnormal structural or

functional changes, predispose themselves to chronic illnesses, and unnecessarily shorten their lives. Lifelong weight management is preferable to intermittent periods of weight gain and loss.

- *Receive regular preventive health care from competent professionals.* This care should include routine screening and risk-reducing lifestyle management, early diagnosis, and effective treatment if needed.

- *Maintain an optimistic outlook.* Anger, cynicism, and a pessimistic outlook on life can erode the holistic basis on which high-level health is built. Several chronic conditions, including cardiovascular diseases and cancers, occur more frequently in persons who lack a positive outlook on their own lives and life in general.

- *Establish a personally meaningful belief system.* Over the course of long life the presence of such a system and the supportive faith community usually associated with it may prove to be the most beneficial health resource we will possess.

InfoLinks

www.cdc.gov/nccdphp/index.htm

blame individuals or environmental realities for health conditions but focus on producing constructive change through dialogue and collaboration.

Empowerment programs have produced positive health consequences for individuals and groups that traditionally have been underserved by the health care system, such as minority populations. Once such people are given needed information, inroads into the political process, and skills for accessing funding sources, they become better able to plan, implement, and operate programs tailored to their unique health needs. In many communities, empowered people have organized grassroots campaigns to prevent neighborhood violence, improve childhood nutrition, promote healthy lifestyles, or prevent drug use among youth. When successful, these programs stand as excellent examples of the reality that people can make a difference when they become empowered.

Healthy People 2000 and Healthy People 2010

To identify all of the health-related concerns identified by members of the health community would be a monumental undertaking far beyond the scope of this book. However, in 2003, the Institutes of Medicine released a list of priority health concerns that they believe need particular attention. Among these priority concerns are:[7]

- treatment of asthma
- coordination of care for the 60 million persons with chronic health conditions
- reduction in the development of diabetes
- development of evidence-based cancer screening
- enhanced rates of immunization, particularly for flu and pneumonia

- improved detection of depression, which is now inadequately diagnosed and treated
- aggressively promoted prevention of cardiovascular disease, presently the leading killer of American adults
- concerted efforts to reduce the rate of nosocomial infections (infections that occur as a result of medical care) that kill an estimated 100,000 Americans annually
- reduction of tobacco dependence through cessation and prevention of smoking
- widened availability of prenatal care

While improvements in these areas are greatly needed, the Institutes of Medicine have no specific programs in place at this time to address them. In comparison, a well-established and ongoing program, Healthy People 2000, has established specific goals and objectives to improve the health of Americans in many of these areas. A brief descripton of this ongoing program follows.

In 1991 a U.S. government document titled *Healthy People 2000: National Health Promotion and Disease Prevention Objectives*[8] outlined a strategic plan for promoting the health of the American public. The plan included 300 health objectives in twenty-two priority areas. Forty-seven of the 300 objectives were defined as "sentinel" ones, that is, particularly significant goals that could be used to measure the progress of the 1990s health promotion objectives.

Progress toward achieving the objectives was assessed near the middle of the decade and reported in a document titled *Healthy People 2000: Midcourse Review and 1995 Revisions*.[9] Although progress was reported in some areas, little or no progress was reported in many. Subsequently, a new plan, called *Healthy People 2010: Understanding and Improving Health*,[10] was formulated, refined, and is now being implemented.[11]

Healthy People 2010: Understanding and Improving Health is a health promotion program intended to be implemented at all levels, ranging from individual involvement through multinational cooperative efforts, including *Health for All in the 21st Century*,[12] a World Health Organization health promotion initiative. Although the goals of *Healthy People 2000: National Health Promotion and Disease Prevention Objectives* and *Healthy People 2010: Understanding and Improving Health* are similar, the latter focuses on the projected needs of the United States during the first decade of the new century. Newly emerging demographics, such as the increasing number of older adults, and technologies, including new vaccines and HIV antiviral drugs, are better addressed in *Healthy People 2010: Understanding and Improving Health*.

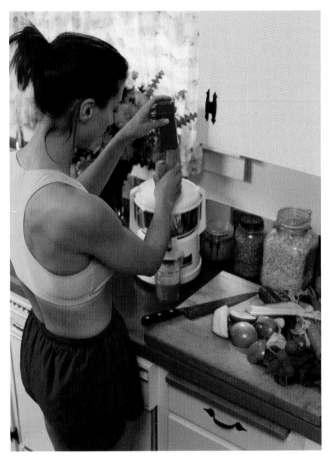

Many students have been able to change a specific health-related behavior, such as replacing poor eating habits with nutritious food choices.

Central to the design of *Healthy People 2010: Understanding and Improving Health* are two paramount goals: (1) increasing quality and years of life, and (2) eliminating health disparities in areas such as gender, race, and ethnicity, as well as income and education level. These goals in turn provide twenty-eight more focused objectives. Progress in accomplishing these objectives is anticipated through the manipulation of the behavioral, biological, and environmental determinants of health as they relate to ten of the leading health indicators: (1) physical activity, (2) weight management, (3) tobacco use, (4) substance abuse, (5) responsible sexual behavior, (6) mental health, (7) injury and violence, (8) environmental quality, (9) immunization, and (10) access to health care.

The success of *Healthy People 2010: Understanding and Improving Health* will not be known until nearer the end of the decade. However, if its goals are ultimately reached, Americans can anticipate an improved quantity and quality of life.

Changing Health-Related Behavior

Although some health concerns can be successfully addressed through local, state, national, or international efforts, such as those just outlined, most are ultimately based on the willingness and ability of persons to change aspects of their own behavior.

Why Behavior Change Is Often Difficult

Several factors can strongly influence a person's desire to change high health-risk behaviors, including those listed below.

1. A person must know that a particular behavioral pattern is clearly associated with (or even causes) a particular health problem. For example: Cigarette smoking is the primary cause of lung cancer.
2. A person must believe (accept) that their behavioral pattern will make (or has made) them susceptible to this particular health problem. For example: My cigarette smoking will significantly increase my risk of developing lung cancer.
3. A person must recognize that risk-reduction intervention strategies exist and that should they adopt these in a compliant manner they too will reduce their risk for a particular health condition. For example: Smoking cessation programs exist, and following such a program could help me quit smoking.
4. A person must believe that benefits of newly adopted health-enhancing behaviors will be more reinforcing than the behaviors being given up. For example: The improved health, lowered risk, and freedom from dependence resulting from no longer smoking are better than the temporary pleasures provided by smoking.
5. A person must feel that significant others in their lives truly want them to alter their high-risk health behaviors and will support their efforts. For example: My friends who are cigarette smokers will make a concerted effort to not smoke in my presence and will help me avoid being around people who smoke.

When one or more of the conditions listed above is not in place, the likelihood that persons will be successful in reducing health-risk behaviors will be greatly diminished.

Stages of Change

The process of behavioral change unfolds over time and progresses through defined stages.[13,14] James Prochaska, John Norcross, and Carol DiClemente outlined six predictable stages of change. They studied thousands of individuals who were changing long-standing problems such as alcohol abuse, smoking, and gambling. While these people used different strategies to change their behavior, they all proceeded through six consistent stages of change in the process referred to as **Prochaska's Stages of Change** .[15]

Precontemplation Stage

The first stage of change is called *precontemplation,* during which a person might think about making a change, but ultimately finds it too difficult and avoids making it. For example, during this phase a smoker might tell friends, "Eventually I will quit," but has no real intention of stopping within the next 6 months.

Contemplation Stage

For many, however, progress toward change begins as they move into a *contemplation* stage, during which they might develop the desire to change but have little understanding of how to go about it. Typically, they see themselves taking action within the next 6 months.

Preparation Stage

Following the contemplation stage, a *preparation* begins, during which change begins to appear to be not only desirable but possible as well. A smoker might begin making plans to quit during this stage, setting a quit date for the very near future (a few days to a month), and perhaps enrolling in a smoking cessation program.

Action Stage

Plans for change are implemented during the *action* stage, during which changes are made and sustained for a period of about 6 months.

Maintenance Stage

The fifth stage is the *maintenance* stage, during which new habits are consolidated and practiced for an additional 6 months.

Termination Stage

The sixth and final stage is called *termination,* which refers to the point at which new habits are well established and so efforts to change are complete.

Key Terms

Prochaska's Stages of Change the six predictable stages—precontemplation, contemplation, preparation, action, maintenance, and termination—people go through in establishing new habits and patterns of behavior.

Table 1.1 Leading Causes of Death in the United States by Age Group, 2000

1–4 Years	Number of Deaths
Unintentional injuries	1,780
Birth defects	471
Cancer	393
5–14 Years	
Unintentional injuries	2,878
Cancer	1,017
Homicide	364
15–24 Years	
Unintentional injuries	13,616
Homicide	4,796
Suicide	3,877
25–44 Years	
Unintentional injuries	24,817
Cancer	20,200
Heart disease	15,267
45–64 Years	
Cancer	136,363
Heart disease	97,334
Unintentional injuries	18,252
65 Years and Older	
Heart disease	595,440
Cancer	392,082
Stroke	146,725

Source: Deaths and death rates by leading causes of death and ages: 2000. U.S. National Center for Health Statistics. Vital Statistics of the United States, Annual: National Vital Statistics Report (NVSR). 2002.

Today's Health Concerns

To this point in the chapter your textbook has identified some health concerns and addressed the desirability of health-related behavior change. Later in the chapter, your textbook will look at those illnesses that are the major causes of death that afflict the American public. Beyond those mentioned, it is evident that, in spite of astonishing progress on many fronts, we continue to face a number of serious health challenges. Heart disease, cancer, accidents, drug use, and mental illness all are important concerns for each of us, even if we are not directly affected by them. Also becoming increasingly troublesome are the complex problems of environmental pollution, violence, health care costs, and the international scope of the HIV/AIDS epidemic, as well as other sexually transmitted diseases. Figure 1-1 on page 6 lists the ten leading causes of death in the United States expressed as a percentage of all deaths. Table 1.1 depicts the leading causes of death at various age levels. World hunger, over-population, and the threat of domestic and international terrorism are other health-related issues that will affect us, as well as the generations that follow.

The health concerns just mentioned are by no means unmanageable. Fortunately, we as individuals can reduce the likelihood of encountering many of these conditions by making choices in the way we live our lives. On a personal level, we can decide to pursue a plan of healthful living to minimize the incidence of illness and disease and to extend life.

Health: More Than the Absence of Illness?

What exactly is health? Is it simply the absence of disease and illness, as Western medicine has held for centuries—or does health embrace other elements we ought to consider now that the twenty-first century has begun?

Rather routinely national news magazines (and other media) feature articles describing advances in modern medicine.[16,17] These articles describe vividly in words and images the impressive progress being made in fields such as cancer treatment, gene manipulation, computer-aided surgery, and complementary medical care. Because of articles like this that relate health to medical care, most of us continue to hold to our traditional perception of health as (1) the virtual absence of disease and illness (low levels of morbidity) and (2) the ability to live a long life (reduced risk of mortality). However, in striving to be fully "health educated" in the new century, perhaps we need to consider a broader definition that more accurately reflects the demands associated with becoming functional and satisfied persons as we transition through each adult stage of life—*young adulthood, middle adulthood,* and, finally, *older adulthood.* With this in mind, look forward to another definition of health—one that recognizes the importance of the more familiar definitions of health, but is focused on the demands of our own growth and development. However, before looking at this newer perception of health and its relationship to life stages (as labeled above), let's meet the readers of this book, today's college students, each of whom will fall into one of the adult life stages.

Today's College Students

Readers of this textbook are college students, but they are also young adults, middle age adults, or even older adults. In some cases their decision to be a student has placed them in settings far different from those being experienced by other people their age. For many students, college classes are sandwiched in between other obligations—for example, a full-time job, parenting, community involvement, even the care of older parents. Some might be the first members of their families to pursue higher education. Many students come from eco-

Ages of Undergraduate College Students (Full- and Part-time), Projected for 2001

Age	Number	Percentage of Total
14–17	170,000	1.1
18–19	3,543,000	23.1
20–21	3,101,000	20.2
22–24	2,457,000	16.1
25–29	1,863,000	12.2
30–34	1,223,000	8.0
35+	2,943,000	18.8
		99.5

Source: *Total fall enrollment in degree-granting institutions, by attendance status, sex, and age: 1970 to 2011.* U.S. Census Bureau. *Statistical Abstract of the United States: 2002* (122nd Edition)

nomic, racial, or ethnic backgrounds quite different from that of the majority of their classmates. Thus, today there is no one type of college student, but nevertheless, all of them are progressing through life in predictable yet unique ways.

Traditional-Age Undergraduate College Students

Statistics indicate that more than 13.4 million students were enrolled in degree-granting U.S. colleges and universities in 2003.[18] Nearly 60% of these students are women. Minority students make up approximately 28% of American college students and foreign students total 10.1%.[18] Approximately 60% of students attend college on a full-time basis.[19]

Because two-thirds (66%) of all undergraduates are traditional-age students,[19] this book is directed first at these students. However, because of significant growth in the proportion of older students, we will also address a variety of life experiences and developmental tasks appropriate to these students. Unquestionably, the nontraditional-age students in our classes help our traditional-age students understand the wide and varied role that health plays throughout the life cycle.

TALKING POINTS You are in charge of a campus event for students of various ages from several cultural groups. How would you go about finding out what would make the event attractive to students with backgrounds different from your own?

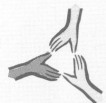

Learning from Our Diversity

Back to the Future: Nontraditional-Age Students Enrich the College Experience

To anyone who's visited an American college campus in the last ten years, it's abundantly clear that the once typical college student—white, middle class, between the ages of eighteen and twenty-four—is no longer in a majority on campus. In most institutions of higher learning, today's student body is a rich tapestry of color, culture, language, ability, and age. Wheelchair-accessible campuses roll out the welcome mat for students with disabilities; the air is filled with the music of a dozen or more languages spoken by students from virtually every part of the world; students in their 60s chat animatedly with classmates young enough to be their grandchildren.

Of all the trends that are changing the face of college enrollment in the United States, perhaps the most significant is the increasing diversity in the age of students now on campus. Older students today are both a common and welcome sight in colleges and universities across the country. Many women cut short their undergraduate education—or defer graduate school—to marry and raise children. Divorcees, widows, and women whose children are grown often return to college, or enroll for the first time, to prepare for professional careers. And increasingly, both men and women are finding it desirable, if not essential, to

further their education as a means of either keeping their current job or qualifying for a higher position.

Just as children are enriched by the knowledge and experience of their grandparents and other older relatives, so too is today's college classroom a richer place when many of the seats are filled by students of nontraditional age. Without being didactic or preachy, older students can provide valuable guidance and direction to younger classmates who may be uncertain of their career path, or who may be wrestling with decisions about marriage and parenthood. In doing so, nontraditional-age students can gain helpful insights about young people's feelings, attitudes, challenges, and aspirations.

Among the many important benefits of today's increasingly diverse college campus, surely one of the most significant is the enhanced opportunity for intergenerational communication and understanding made possible by the growing numbers of students of nontraditional age.

In your classes, how would you characterize the interactions between traditional-age students and those of nontraditional age? In what ways are they enriching each other's college experience?

Nontraditional-Age Undergraduate College Students

In 1999, nearly 33% of American undergraduate college students were classified as **nontraditional-age students.**[18] Included in this vast overlapping group are part-time students, military veterans, students returning to college, single parents, older adults, and evening students. These students enter the classroom with a wide assortment of life experiences and observations. Most of these students are twenty-five to forty years old. Read the Learning from Our Diversity box for a closer look at nontraditional-age students.

Many nontraditional-age students are trying to juggle an extremely demanding schedule. The responsibilities of managing a job, a schedule of classes, and perhaps a family present formidable challenges. Performing these tasks on a limited budget compounds the difficulty. For nontraditional-age students, concerns over paying next month's rent, caring for aging parents, or finding affordable child care are as common as the challenges that confront students of traditional age.

For these reasons, we want to make this textbook meaningful for both traditional-age and nontraditional-age students. Much of the information we present applies to both categories of students. We ask nontraditional-age students to do two things as you

read this book: (1) reflect on your own young adult years, and (2) examine your current lifestyle to see how the decisions you made as a younger adult are affecting the quality of your life now. As a nontraditional-age student, you may have young adult children whose lives you can observe in light of the information you will find in this book.

Minority Students

Although enrollment patterns at colleges and universities vary, the overall number of minority students is increasing. In 1999, slightly over 26% of all college students were minority students, with African Americans, Hispanic Americans, Asian Americans, and Native Americans representing the largest groups of minority

---

> **Key Terms**
>
> **nontraditional-age students** administrative term used by colleges and universities for students who, for whatever reason, are pursuing undergraduate work at an age other than that associated with the traditional college years (18–24).

In addition to the two episodic and preventive forms of medical care described here, a variety of other forms of health care, both curative and preventive, are moving more progressively into the medical care mainstream. Among these are chiropractic, reflexology, homeopathy, naturopathy, and herbalism (see Chapter 18), to mention but a few. Although the established medical community has long scoffed at these practices as being unscientific and ineffective, they are increasingly attractive to a growing segment of the population. Initially referred to collectively as *alternative* forms of health care, and more recently as *complementary* forms of care, today they are increasingly referred to as *integrative* forms of health care. This last term suggests a fusion (or integration) of various forms of care into traditional treatment/prevention approaches.

The increasing acceptance of integrative forms of health care is also seen in two relatively recent developments. The first is the formation in the mid-1990s of an Office of Complementary and Alternative Medicine within the National Institutes of Health. Created and funded by Congress, this office has been charged with the objective and systematic study of the effectiveness of selected forms of nontraditional care. To date, reports from this office, some supportive and others critical, have been released on acupuncture, chiropractic, therapeutic massage, St. John's Wort, garlic, and glucosamine/chondroitin sulfate. Subsequent assessments will be released as they are completed.

A second expression of the growing popularity of integrative forms of health care is the increasing tendency of health insurance companies and HMOs (Health Maintenance Organizations; see Chapter 18) to provide reimbursement of services from providers of nontraditional care. Today approximately 65% of all HMOs and several major insurance companies, including Blue Cross and Blue Shield of Massachusetts, Kaiser Permanente of Colorado, and Prudential HealthCare, provide coverage for selective forms of integrative care.

As impressive as the "rush to coverage" described above might appear, consumers of medical care services should remember that at this time relatively little carefully controlled research is available on the *efficacy* (effectiveness) of most forms of integrative care. Therefore, until such research is completed and disseminated, we must assume that the increased availability of insurance coverage for integrative care is, in fact, being driven by market forces, which are themselves based on a desire for alternatives to traditional medical care that seems too expensive and impersonal to be the sole basis of our health care system.

---

students.[20] These students bring a rich variety of cultural influences and traditions to today's college environment.

Students with Disabilities

People with reported disabilities are another rapidly growing student population, currently comprising 9.3% of all undergraduates.[21] Improved diagnostic, medical, and rehabilitation procedures coupled with improved educational accommodations have opened up opportunities for these students at an increasing rate. In addition to students who have visible disabilities, such as blindness, deafness, or a physical disability requiring use of a wheelchair, a greater number of students with "hidden" disabilities are appearing on campuses. Examples are students with learning disabilities (including attention deficit disorders), those with managed psychiatric and emotional problems, and those recovering from alcohol and substance abuse. Interestingly, many students with reported "hidden disabilities" often do not consider themselves to be disabled.[21]

 TALKING POINTS When controversial subjects are discussed in class, do you think that your opinions (or how you present them) are affected by the fact that students of different cultural backgrounds are involved in the discussion?

Developmental Tasks of Young Adulthood

Because most of today's undergraduate college students range between the ages of eighteen and perhaps forty, we will address several areas of growth and development (defined as *developmental tasks*) that characterize the lives of people in this age group (Figure 1-2). When people sense that they are making progress in some or all of these areas, they are likely to report a sense of life satisfaction or, as we describe it, a sense of well-being.

Forming an Initial Adult Identity

For most of childhood and adolescence, most young people are seen by adults in their neighborhood or community as someone's son or daughter. With the onset of young adulthood, that stage has almost passed; both young people and society are beginning to look at each other in new ways.

As emerging adults, most young people want to present a unique identity to society. Internally they are constructing perceptions of themselves as the adults they wish to be; externally they are formulating the behavioral patterns that will project this identity to others.

Completion of this first developmental task is necessary for young adults to establish a foundation on which

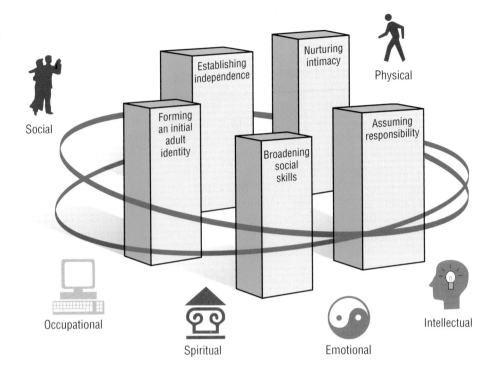

Figure 1-2 Mastery of the developmental tasks through a balanced involvement of the six dimensions of health will lead to your enjoying a more productive and satisfying life.

to mature identity during later stages of adulthood. As a result of their experiences in achieving an initial adult identity, they will become capable of answering the central question of young adulthood: "Who am I?" Most likely, many nontraditional-age students are also asking themselves this question as they progress through college and anticipate the changes that will result from completing a high level of formal education.

Establishing Independence

In contemporary society the primary responsibility for socialization during childhood and adolescence is assigned to the family. For nearly two decades the family is the primary contributor to a young person's knowledge, values, and behaviors. By young adulthood, however, students of traditional college age should be demonstrating the desire to move away from the dependent relationship that has existed between themselves and their families.

 TALKING POINTS What does being an adult mean to you at this point? How would you explain this to your best friend?

Travel, peer relationships, marriage, military service, and, of course, college have been traditional avenues for disengagement from the family, although most undergraduates return home during summers.[22] Generally the ability and willingness to follow one or more of these paths will help a young adult establish independence. Success in these endeavors will depend on the willingness to use a variety of resources we will explore later.

Assuming Responsibility

The third developmental task in which traditional-age college students are expected to progress is the assumption of increasing levels of responsibility. Young adults have a variety of opportunities to assume responsibility. College-age young adults may accept responsibility voluntarily, such as when they join a campus organization or establish a new friendship. Other responsibilities are placed on them when professors assign term papers, when dating partners exert pressure on them to conform to their expectations, or when employers require consistently productive work. In other situations they may accept responsibility for doing a particular task not for themselves but for the benefit of others. As important and demanding as these areas of responsibility are, a more fundamental responsibility awaits young adults: the responsibility of maintaining and improving their health and the health of others.

Broadening Social Skills

The fourth developmental task of the young adult years is broadening the range of appropriate and dependable social skills. Adulthood ordinarily involves "membership" in a variety of groups that range in size from a marital pair to a national political party or international corporation. These memberships will require the ability to function in many different social settings and with a wide variety of people.

The college experience traditionally has prepared students very effectively in this regard, but interactions in friendships, work relationships, or parenting may require that they make an effort to grow and develop beyond levels they achieved by belonging to a peer group. Young adults will need to refine a variety of social skills, including communication, listening, and conflict management.

Nurturing Intimacy

The task of nurturing intimacy usually begins in young adulthood and continues through midlife. During this

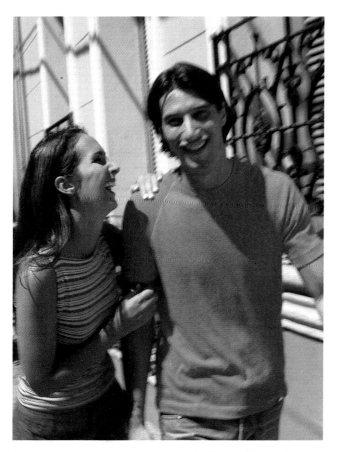

Intimacy can occur in many forms, including traditional dating relationships.

time it is developmentally important to establish one or more intimate relationships. Most people in this age group are viewing intimacy in its broadest sense as a deeply close, sharing relationship. Intimacy may unfold in the context of dating relationships, close friendships, and certainly mentoring relationships.

Involvement in intimate relationships varies, with some people having many relationships and others having only one or two. The number does not matter. From a developmental standpoint, what matters is that we have others with whom to share our most deeply held thoughts and feelings as we attempt to validate our own unique approach to living.

Related Developmental Tasks of Young Adulthood

In addition to the five developmental tasks of young adulthood just described, two additional areas of growth and development seem applicable to 18- to 24-year-olds. These include obtaining *entry-level employment* and the *developing of parenting skills.*

For at least the last sixty years, students in increasing numbers have pursued a college education in large part to gain entry into many occupations and professions. Students of today certainly anticipate that a college degree will open doors for their first substantial employment or entry-level employment.

In many respects employment needs go beyond those associated purely with money. Employment provides the opportunity to assume new responsibilities in which the skills learned in college can be applied and expanded. Employment also involves taking on new roles (such as colleague, mentor, *mentee,* or partner) that may play an important part in the way we define ourselves for the remainder of our lives. In addition, employment provides a new, more independent arena in which friendships (intimacy) can be pursued. By no means least important, entry-level employment provides the financial foundation on which we can establish independence.

For many people, young adulthood marks the entry to parenthood, one of the most important responsibilities anyone can choose to assume. The multitude of decisions associated with this lifetime commitment will, naturally, shape the remainder of one's life. Examples of these decisions are whether to parent or not, and, if so, when to begin, how many children to have, what interval between children, and what role parenting will play in the context of overall adulthood. The ability to make sound decisions and to develop the skills and insights necessary to parent effectively may be the most challenging aspect of growth and development that confronts young adults.

Developmental Tasks of Middle Adulthood

If you are a traditional-age student, have you wondered what it would be like to be twenty or thirty years older than you are now? What would you be doing, feeling, and thinking if you were the age of your parents? What are your parents thinking about and trying to accomplish as they move through their midlife years?

One thought that probably recurs all too often is the reality of their own eventual death. Their awareness that they will not live forever is a subtle but profoundly influential force that can cause them to be restless, to renew their religious faith, and to be more highly motivated to master the developmental tasks of middle adulthood. This motivation and the awareness of the reality of death combine to produce the dynamic concept of being at "the prime of life"—a time when there seems to be a great deal to accomplish and less time in which to accomplish it.

Achieving Generativity

In a very real sense, people in middle adulthood are asked to do something they have not been expected to do previously. As a part of their development as unique people, they are expected to "pay back" society for the support it has given them. Most people in middle adulthood begin to realize that the collective society, through its institutions (families, schools, churches), has been generous in its support of their own growth and development and that it is time to replenish these resources.[23] Younger and

older people may have needs that middle-aged people can best meet. By meeting the needs of others, people in middle adulthood can fulfill their own needs to grow and develop. *Generativity* reflects this process of contributing to the collective good.

The process of repaying society for its support is structured around familiar types of activities.[24] Developmentally speaking, people in middle adulthood are able to select the activities that best use their abilities to contribute to the good of society.

The most traditional way in which people in middle adulthood repay society is through parenting. Children, with their potential for becoming valuable members of the next generation, need the support of people who recognize the contribution they can make. By supporting children, either directly through quality parenting or through institutions that function on behalf of children, middle-aged people repay society for the support they have themselves received. As they extend themselves outward on behalf of the next generation, they ensure their own growth and development. In a similar fashion, their support of aging parents and institutions that serve older adults provides another means to express generativity.

For people who possess artistic talent, generativity may be accomplished through the pleasure brought to others. Artists, craftspeople, and musicians have unique opportunities to speak directly to others through their talents. Volunteer work serves as another avenue for generativity. Most people in middle adulthood also express generativity through their jobs by providing quality products or services and thus contribute to the well-being of those who desire or need these goods and services.

Reassessing the Plans of Middle Adulthood

People in middle adulthood must also begin coming to terms with the finality of their own deaths. In conjunction with doing this, they often feel compelled to take time to think about their goals for adulthood they formulated twenty-five or more years previously. Their dreams are thus revisited. This reassessment constitutes a second developmental task of people in middle adulthood.

By carefully reviewing the aspirations they had as young adults, middle-aged people can more clearly study their short- and long-term goals. Specifically, strengths and limitations that were unrecognizable when they were young adults are now more clearly seen. The inexperience of youth is replaced by the insights gained through experience. A commitment to quality often replaces the desire for quantity during the second half of the life cycle. Time is valued more highly because it is now seen in a more realistic perspective. The dream for the future is more sharply focused, and the successes and failures of the past are more fully understood as this developmental task of reassessing earlier plans of young adulthood is accomplished.

Developmental Tasks of Older Adulthood

In this section, we focus on the developmental tasks confronted by older adults. Accepting the physical changes of aging, maintaining a high level of physical function, and establishing a sense of integrity are tasks of the older adulthood period.

Accepting the Changes of Aging

The general decline associated with the latter part of the life cycle is particularly serious between the seventh and eighth decades. Physically, emotionally, socially, intellectually, and occupationally, older adults must accept at least some decline. For example, a person may no longer be able to drive a car, which could in turn limit participation in social activities. Even a spiritual loss may be encountered at those times when life seems less humane. Clearly, a developmental task to be accomplished by the older adult is to accept the nature and extent of these changes.

Maintaining High Levels of Function

Because each segment of the life cycle should be approached with the fullest level of involvement possible, the second developmental task of the older adult is to maintain as much functionality in each segment as possible, particularly, those that support independence.

For areas of decline in which some measure of reversal is possible, older adults are afforded an opportunity to seek *rehabilitation*. Whether through a self-designed and individually implemented program or with the aid of a skilled professional, older adults can bring back some function to a previously high level.

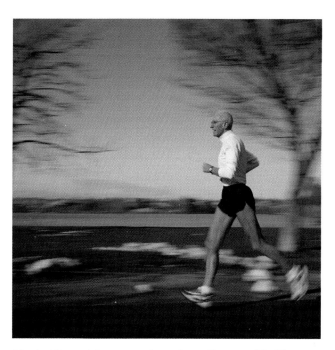

Physical fitness is important throughout all stages of the life span, including older adulthood.

The second approach, often used in combination with rehabilitation, is *remediation*, whereby an alternative to the area of loss is introduced. Examples of remediation include the use of hearing aids, audiocassettes, and caregivers or home health aids. By using alternative resources, function can often be returned.

For a growing number of older adults, rehabilitation and remediation are rarely necessary because of the high level of health that they enjoy. For most, only minor modifications are necessary to enjoy full independence.

Establishing a Sense of Integrity

The third major developmental task that awaits the older adult is to establish a sense of integrity, or a sense of wholeness, concerning the journey that may be nearly complete.[25] The elderly must look back over their lives to see the value in what they were able to accomplish. They must address the simple but critical questions, "Would I do it over again?" "Am I satisfied with what I managed to accomplish?" "Can I accept the fact that others will have experiences to which I can never return?"

If the elderly can answer these questions positively, then they will feel a sense of wholeness, personal value, and worth. Having established this sense of integrity, they will believe that their lives have had meaning and that they have helped society.

Since they have already experienced so much, many older adults have no fear of death, even though they may

Why Men Die Young

The extra longevity of women in our society is well established. In fact, the difference in life expectancy for infants born today is projected to be 80 years for females and only 75 for males. This 5-year difference has commonly been attributed to genetic factors. However, new evidence demonstrates that this discrepancy may be affected more by male behavior rather than genetic traits.

Men outrank women in all of the top fifteen causes of death except for Alzheimer's disease. Men's death rates are twice as high for suicide, homicide, and cirrhosis of the liver. In every age group, American males have poorer health and higher risk of mortality than do females. Common increased risks include:

- More men smoke than women
- Men are twice as likely to be heavy drinkers, or to engage in other risky behaviors such as abusing drugs and driving without a seatbelt.
- More men work in dangerous settings than women, and men account for 90% of on-the-job fatalities.
- More men drive SUVs that are rollover prone and suffer fatalities in motorcycle accidents.

Perhaps some of these increased risks are associated with deep-seated cultural beliefs, which reward them for taking risks and facing danger head-on. This "macho" attitude seems to extend to the care that men take of their own physical and mental health. Women are twice as likely to visit their doctor on an annual basis and explore preventative medical treatments than are men. Men are more likely to ignore symptoms and less likely to schedule checkups or seek follow-up treatment. Psychologically, men tend to internalize their feelings or stressors, or even self-medicate to deal with stress, while women tend to seek psychological help. Almost all stress-related diseases are more common in men.

In the final analysis, men and women alike must be responsible for their own health and well-being. By making sound choices regarding diet, exercise, medical care, and high-risk behaviors, both genders can attempt to maximize the full potential of their life expectancy.

---

fear the process of dying. Their ability to come to terms with death thus reinforces their sense of integrity.

Like all of the other developmental tasks, this critical area of growth and development is a personal experience. Older adults must assume this last developmental task with the same sense of purpose they used for earlier tasks. When older adults can feel this sense of integrity, their reasons for having lived will be more fully understood.

The Multiple Dimensions of Health

In an earlier section of the chapter your authors promised a new definition of health that would be less focused on morbidity (illness) and mortality (death) than most others. Before we do this, however, let us introduce a multidimensional concept of health (or **holistic health**)—a requirement for any definition of health that moves beyond the cure/prevention of illness and the postponement of death.

Although our modern health care community too frequently acts as if the structure and function of the physical body is the sole basis of health, common experience supports the validity of a *holistic* nature to health. In this section we will examine six component parts, or dimensions, of health, all interacting in a synergistic manner allowing us to engage in the wide array of activities of daily living.

Physical Dimension

Most of us have a number of physiological and structural characteristics we can call on to aid us in accomplishing the wide array of activities that characterize a typical day, and, on occasion, a not-so-typical day. Among these physical characteristics are our body weight, visual ability, strength, coordination, level of endurance, level of susceptibility to disease, and powers of recuperation. In certain situations the physical dimension of health may be the most important. This almost certainly is why traditional medicine for centuries has equated health with the design and operation of the body.

Emotional Dimension

We also possess certain emotional characteristics that can help us through the demands of daily living. The emotional dimension of health encompasses our ability to cope with stress, remain flexible, and compromise to resolve conflict.

For young adults, growth and development often give rise to emotional vulnerability, which may lead to feelings of rejection and failure that can reduce productivity and satisfaction. To some extent we are all affected by feeling states, such as anger, happiness, fear, empathy, guilt, love, and hate. People who consistently try to improve their

> **Key Terms**
>
> **holistic health** a view of health in terms of its physical, emotional, social, intellectual, and occupational makeup.

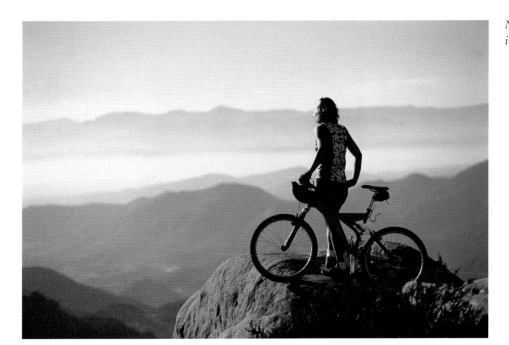

emotional health appear to enjoy life to a much greater extent than do those who let feelings of vulnerability overwhelm them or block their creativity.

Social Dimension

A third dimension of health encompasses social skills and insights. Initially, family interactions, school experiences, and peer group interactions foster social skill development, but future social interactions will demand additional skill development and refinement of already existing skills and insights. In adulthood, including young adulthood, the composition of the social world changes, principally because of our exposure to a wider array of people and the expanded roles associated with employment, parenting, and community involvement.

The social abilities of many nontraditional-age students may already be firmly established. Entering college may encourage them to develop new social skills that help them socialize with their traditional-age student colleagues. After being on campus for a while, nontraditional-age students are often able to interact comfortably with traditional-age students in such diverse places as the library, the student center, and the bookstore. This interaction enhances the social dimension of health for both types of students.

Intellectual Dimension

The ability to process and act on information, clarify values and beliefs, and exercise decision-making capacity ranks among the most important aspects of total health. For many college-educated persons, this dimension of health may prove to be the most important and satisfying of the six. In fact, for all of us, at least on certain occasions, this will hold true. Our ability to analyze, synthesize, hypothesize, and then act upon new information enhances the quality of our lives in multiple ways.

Spiritual Dimension

The fifth dimension of health is the spiritual dimension. Although certainly it includes religious beliefs and practices, many young adults would expand it to encompass more diverse belief systems, including relationships with other living things, the nature of human behavior, and the need and willingness to serve others. All are important components of spiritual health.

Through nurturing the spiritual dimension of our health, we may develop an expanded perception of the universe and better define our relationship to all that it contains, including other people. To achieve growth in the spiritual dimension of health, many people undertake a serious study of doctrine associated with established religious groups and will assume membership in a community of faith, believed by some. For others, however, spiritual growth is believed to occur, in the absence of a theist-based belief system, as they open themselves to new experiences that involve nature, art, body movement, or stewarding of the environment.

Interestingly, the role of the spiritual dimension of health was recently given an increased measure of credence

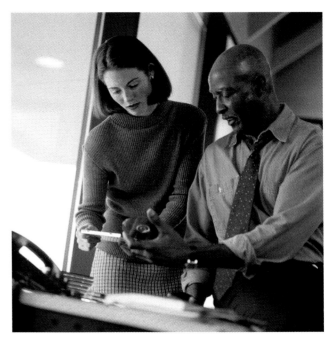

Discovering Your Spirituality

How Does Your Faith Affect Your Life?

Faith can include religious practice, but it can also be quite distinct from it. Faith is the most fundamental stage in the human quest for the meaning of life. It's a developing focus of the total person that gives purpose and meaning to life.

By the time people reach college age, their faith may have already placed them in uncomfortable situations. Taking seriously their responsibility for their own commitments, lifestyles, beliefs, and attitudes, they've had to make some difficult personal decisions. This demands objectivity and a certain amount of independence. It requires finding a balance between personal aspirations and a developing sense of service to others. Finally, the symbols and doctrines of faith must be translated into personalized spiritual concepts that become part of everyday living.

- Have you had any experiences that show you're growing in your faith?
- Do you consider yourself more spiritual or less spiritual than your friends or family members?
- What school-related experiences have affected the spiritual dimension of your health most powerfully?

The occupational dimension of health is especially important to nontraditional-age students, who often have to balance school with work, parenting, and other responsibilities.

when studies published in the scientific literature, including a statistical review of forty-two earlier studies, demonstrated a consistently longer life for persons who regularly participated in religious practices, particularly for women.[26,27] This was true even when factors such as smoking, alcohol use, and income were statistically eliminated. Contradictory to these findings, however, was a report suggesting that the ability of prescriptive prayer (prayers of intercession) to enhance healing and extend life could not be supported by current research due to design flaws in the studies made to date.[28]

Occupational Dimension

A significant contribution made by the currently popular wellness movement is that it defines for many people the importance of the workplace to their sense of well-being. In today's world, employment and productive efforts play an increasingly important role in how we perceive ourselves and how we see the "goodness" of the world in which we live. In addition, the workplace serves as both a testing ground for and a source of life-enhancing skills. In our place of employment we gain not only the financial resources to meet our demands for both necessities and luxuries, but also an array of useful skills like conflict resolution, experiences in shared responsibility, and intellectual growth that can be used to facilitate a wide range of

non-employment-related interactions. In turn, the workplace is enhanced by the healthfulness of the individuals who contribute to its endeavors.

Wellness

Expanded perceptions of health are the basis for **wellness**. Recall that episodic health care, preventive medicine, and community health promotion are directly aligned with concerns over morbidity and mortality, while health promotion at the individual level is focused on aspects of appearance, weight management, body composition, and physical performance capabilities. Wellness differs from these kinds of health care because it has virtually no interest in morbidity and mortality.

Practitioners describe wellness as a process of extending information, counseling, assessment, and lifestyle modification strategies, leading to a desirable change in

> ### Key Terms
>
> **wellness** the promotion and achievement of optimal health, including physical, emotional, social, spiritual, intellectual, and occupational well-being.

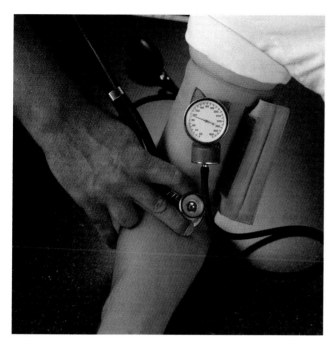

Although not primarily interested in illness or premature death, wellness practitioners consider it essential to inform their clients about the role of elevated blood pressure in the development of cardiovascular disease.

the recipients' overall lifestyle, or the adoption of a wellness lifestyle. Once adopted, the wellness lifestyle produces a sense of well-being (also called wellness) that in turn enables recipients to unlock their full potential.

This explanation of how wellness differs from episodic health care, preventive medicine, and health promotion does, on first hearing, seem progressive and clearly devoid of interest in morbidity and mortality concerns. But in practice, wellness programs are not all that different from other kinds of health care. Your authors have consistently noted that wellness programs, as carried out on college campuses, in local hospital well centers, and in corporate settings, routinely transmit familiar health-related information and engage in the same risk-reduction activities that characterize preventive medicine and health promotion. It is in the final aspect of wellness, the "unlocking of full potential," that wellness differs from other concepts of health. More than the absence of chronic illness, it involves achieving optimal health across all six of the dimensions of health discussed in the previous section.

A New Definition of Health

At the beginning of the chapter we asked you to consider a new way to view health—a view that would be far less centered in morbidity and mortality concerns than tradi-

tional concepts of health and even of wellness. The definition that we propose takes into account the differences between *what health is for* (its role) and *what health is* (its composition).

The Role of Health

The role of health in our lives is very similar to the role of a car. Much as a car (or other vehicle) takes us to the place we need or want to be at, health enables us to accomplish the activities that transition us into and through developmental tasks associated with each stage of adulthood (see pages 13 through 17). Recall that the process of moving through each stage of adulthood does not occur simply because of the passage of time, but rather because we actively participate, on a day-to-day basis, in demands of life appropriate to our life stage.

The Composition of Health

Now that you know what the role of health is, its composition can be seen as being more than simply having a body free of illness and apparently destined for a long life. Rather, the composition of health is that of a collection of resources, from each dimension of health (see pages 18 through 20), determined to be necessary for the successful accomplishment of activities that you need or want to do. Some of these needed resources will already be within you (intrinsic), while others will need to come from outside (extrinsic). However, regardless of their origin, once they are accessed and applied to activities, small forward growth steps will occur. Obviously, to recognize what resources are needed, you must be a student of society's expectations for persons of your age, as well as your own highly personalized developmental aspirations.

Our Definition of Health

By combining the role of health with the composition of health, we offer a new definition of health that we believe is unique to this textbook.

> Health is a reflection of your ability to use the **intrinsic** and **extrinsic** resources related to each dimension of health to participate fully in the activities that contribute to your growth and development, with the goal of feeling a sense of well-being as you evaluate your progress through life.

In light of this definition, do not be surprised when your textbook asks whether you are resourceful (healthy) enough for the goals you wish to reach, or whether you are healthy enough to sustain a particular behavioral pattern that you have adopted, or whether you are experiencing the sense of well-being to which you aspire.

- Complete the Comprehensive Health Assessment on page xxxvii. Develop a plan to modify your behavior in the areas in which you need improvement.
- Take part in a new spiritual activity, such as meditating, creating art or music, or appreciating nature.
- To promote the social dimension of your health, try to meet one new person each week during the semester.

- Choose one developmental task you would like to focus on, such as assuming responsibility, and plan the steps you can follow to progress in this area.
- Volunteer to be an assistant in a community service program, such as a literacy project or a preschool program.

Summary

- When used to define health, morbidity and mortality relate to the prevalence of particular diseases and illnesses and to death resulting from those diseases and illnesses.
- When we seek the services of health care practitioners because of symptoms of illness or disease, we are said to be seeking episodic health care.
- Preventive medical care attempts to minimize the incidence of illness and disease by identifying early indicators of risk to bring them under control.
- Individual health promotion involves risk-reduction activities similar to those used in preventive medical care, except that the techniques cannot be invasive, and are directed by professionals who are not physicians.
- Community health promotion involves the empowerment of individuals so that they can organize and participate in their own health promotion activities.
- Healthy People 2010 is a federally funded program to improve the nation's health, increase life expectancy, and expand access to comprehensive health care.
- A decision to change a health behavior is often difficult to make because of multiplicity factors underlying the behavior, making the behavior one that results in immediate gratification.
- Health behavior change requires movement through a multistaged process, including precontemplation, contemplation, preparation, action, maintenance, and termination.
- A wide array of health problems (for example, cancer, cardiovascular disease, HIV/AIDS) persist despite today's highly sophisticated health care technology.
- Today's college campus is a dynamic blend of students of both traditional and nontraditional ages and of diverse backgrounds, cultures, and attributes.
- Complementary and integrative medicine involves the integration of alternative forms of care, such as acupuncture and therapeutic massage, into traditional medical practices. Today several forms of

complementary care are under careful study by the Office of Complementary and Alternative Medicine of the National Institutes of Health.
- Young adulthood is characterized by five key developmental tasks: forming an initial adult identity, establishing independence, assuming responsibility, broadening social skills, and nurturing intimacy.
- Each phase of the life cycle involves a set of personal developmental tasks that are common to all, yet may be undertaken differently by each individual.
- Multidimensional definitions of health, including holistic health, have existed for decades—although the primary emphasis has always been on the physical dimension.
- Current multidimensionals definitions of health may include many or all of the following dimensions: physical, emotional, social, intellectual, spiritual, and occupational.
- Wellness contends a disinterest in morbidity and mortality, rather emphasizing living a wellness lifestyle that leads to a sense of well-being.
- The role of health, as seen by your textbook, is to enable individuals to participate in the activities that collectively constitute growth and development.
- The composition of health, as seen by your textbook, is the intrinsic and extrinsic resources on which individuals can draw to participate fully in their own growth and development.

Review Questions

1. What are morbidity and mortality, and how are they involved in the more traditional definitions of health?
2. When and from whom do people seek episodic health care?
3. In preventive medical care, who determines a person's level of risk and decides what risk-reduction techniques should be implemented?
4. In terms of professional personnel and the type of risk reduction techniques used, how does health promotion at the individual level differ from preventive medical care?
5. What does the term empowerment mean and how would it appear as a component of a community-based health promotion program?
6. What are the two primary goals of *Healthy People 2010*, the federally funded program to improve the health of the American population?
7. What factors could underlie the inability or unwillingness of persons to change their health behavior?
8. What are the six stages that persons pass through as they consider and then attempt to change their health behavior?
9. What are several of the more pressing health problems that confront the American people?
10. In what ways is the current American college student population more diverse than any that came before?
11. What is implied by the terms *alternative, complementary,* and *integrative* when applied to health care practices?
12. What are the five developmental tasks of young adulthood and how can the accomplishing of one influence the accomplishing of any of the remaining four?
13. What is implied by the statement, "growth and development are predictable yet unique"?
14. How does the term *multidimensional* apply to the concept of holistic health?
15. What are the most frequently included dimensions within a holistically centered definition of health?
16. What is the underlying reason that proponents of wellness give for being uninterested in morbidity and mortality?
17. In the view of wellness practitioners, what will eventually be experienced by persons who adopt a wellness lifestyle.
18. How does your textbook's definition of health differ from traditional definitions?
19. How does your textbook define the role of health?
20. How is composition of health defined by your textbook? What would be examples of resources from each of the five dimensions of health?
21. Why is it necessary to understand developmental expectations before we can answer the question, "Are you healthy enough to . . . ?"

References

1. Centers for Disease Control and Prevention. *National Ambulatory Medical Care Survey: 2000.* July 2002.
2. Roper Center for Public Opinion Research (for Pfizer Women's Health), University of Connecticut. *Adults know their family history. USA Today.* May 30, 2000. p.5D.
3. Cottrell RR, Girvan JT, McKenzie JF. *Principles and foundations of health promotion and education.* Benjamin Cummings, 2002.
4. Kreuter MW, Lezin NA, Kreuter MW, Green LW. *Community health promotion ideas that work: a field-book for practitioners.* Jones and Bartlett Publishers, 2003.
5. McKenzie JF, Smeltzer JL. *Planning. implementing and evaluating health promotion programs,* 3rd ed. Allyn and Bacon, 2001.
6. Bensley RJ, Brookins-Fisher J (Editors). *Community health education methods: a practitioner's guide.* Jones and Bartlett Publishers, 2003.
7. *Priority areas for national action: transforming healthcare quality (2003).* The National Academies Press, 2003.
8. *Healthy people 2000: national health promotion and disease prevention objectives* (full report with commentary). U.S. Department of Health and Human Services. Public Health Service, 1991.
9. *Health people 2000: midcourse review and 1995 revisions.* Department of Health and Human Services. Public Health Service, 1995.
10. *Health people 2010: understanding and improving health.* Department of Health and Human Services. Public Health Service, 2000.
11. *Health people 2010: understanding and improving health.* 2nd ed. Department of Health and Human Services. Public Health Services, 2000.
12. Health for all in the 21st century. World Health Organization, 1979. **www.who/int/archives/hfa/policy.htm**

13. Prochaska JO, Velicer WF: The transtheoretical model of health behavior change. *Am J of Health Promotion* 12:38–48, 1994.

14. Norcross JC, Prochaska JO. Using the stages of change. *Harv Ment Health Lett* 18(11):507, 2002.

15. Prochaska JO, Norcross JC, DiClemente CC. *Changing for good.* William Morrow and Company, 1994.

16. *Drugs of the future. Time* (special issue). 157:02, January 15, 2001.

17. *The science of alternative medicine. Newsweek,* December 02, 2002.

18. U.S. Census Bureau. *Statistical Abstract of the United States: 2002* (122nd Edition).

19. U.S. Department of Education. National Center for Education Statistics. Integrated Postsecondary Education Data System, "Fall Enrollment, 1999" Survey. 2001.

20. U.S. Department of Education. National Center for Education Statistics, Integrated Postsecondary Data System (IPEDS). *Fall enrollment in institutions of higher education: projections of education statistics to 2009,* July 1999. **http://nces.ed.gov/[ibs2000/digest99/**

21. U.S. National Center for Education Statistics. *Profile of undergraduates in U.S. postsecondary education institutions, 1999–2000.* July 2000.

22. *Most college students living with the folks. USA Today.* August 27, 2002. p.5D. Source: *Collegeclub.com* online survey of 3,188 self-selected respondents. June 7, 2002.

23. McAdams DP, St Aubin, ED (Editors). *Generativity and adult development: How and why we care for the next generation.* American Psychology Association, 1998.

24. Peterson BE, Stewart AJ. *Antecedents and contexts of generativity motivation at midlife. Psychol Aging* (1):21–33. 1996.

25. Erikson EH. *Childhood and society.* (reissue edition). W.W. Norton, 1993.

26. Strawbridge WJ, Cohen RD, Shema SJ: Comparative strength of association between religious attendance and survival. *Int J Psychiatry Med* 30(4):299–308, 2000.

27. Oman D, et al: Religious attendance and cause of death over 31 years. *Int J Psychiatry Med* 32(1):69–89, 2002.

28. Sloan RP, et al: Should physicians prescribe religious activities? *N Engl J Med.* 342(25):1913–16, 2000.

As We Go to Press

At the heart of preventive medical care is the need on the part of physicians to identify areas of risk that foretell chronic illnesses for their patients. The taking of detailed family medical histories, combined with the results of an array of screening procedures assessing biomedical indices, augment physicians' observational skills in identifying areas of concern and the high-risk behaviors associated with each. From the information gleaned, physicians should counsel their patients toward risk reduction. But how frequently does this important patient education occur?

In a recent assessment of patient education efforts made by physicians practicing in Derby, Connecticut, and reported in *Preventive Medicine,* the results were not encouraging. For example, about one-half of the physicians failed to discuss with their patients two important areas of behavior related to the potential for chronic illness: dietary practices and exercise. Even more discouraging, only three-fourths of physicians reported talking to their patients about the importance of discontinuing cigarette smoking—the single most powerful high-risk health behavior relating to the development of cancer and cardiovascular disease. Researchers concluded that competing priorities for physicians' time, the lack of physician self-efficacy, and financial restraints might be the underlying factors reducing the likelihood of physicians' engaging in important patient education.

In spite of the less than ideal level of patient education reported above, it is encouraging to note that when physicians did counsel (educate) their patients regarding exercise and dietary practices, patients were encouragingly compliant. In contrast, however, patient education regarding the importance of stopping cigarette smoking was largely ignored. Thus, the authors concluded that patient education was a moderately motivating factor in changing patients' high-risk health behaviors.

chronic daily headaches

Initial public attention to chronic daily headaches (CDH), or (CDHA), occurred in 2003 when a series of newspaper articles were published describing the condition. Unique to CDH is the population in which it is seen, elementary-age girls and boys (in about equal numbers) but my late adolescences, predominately young women. Current estimates are that 5 to 10% of the population in this age range are afflicted with this condition. Beyond young adulthood, some women continue to experience the condition. The condition has been recognized for decades, but until recently little focused attention has been directed to it.

Central to the diagnosis of chronic daily headache is a persistent pattern of incapacitating migraine-like headaches and gripping spasms in the muscles of the neck on at least half the days of each month. Like more traditional migraine headaches, these headaches quickly result in increased sensitivity to light, episodes of nausea, and profound fatigue. So debilitating are these headaches that many students will miss dozens, if not a hundred or more, of days of school during a typical school year. Sustained college course work proves almost impossible to accomplish in the absence of effective management.

Since the majority of persons with CDH, beyond elementary school age, are young women, the underlying cause of the headaches is thought to be hormonal. Additionally, in many but not all cases of CDH, and in both genders, symptoms of depression are frequently present, as well as a family history of migraine headaches. High levels of stress are also commonly seen in persons who experience chronic daily headaches.

The management of CDH is most often approached from two perspectives: the use of migraine-controlling pharmaceuticals known as "triptans" (Maxalt, Imitrex, Zomig, and Amerge) and antidepressants, since depression appears to be an underlying cause. In conjunction with the above medications, Botox injections have been used to relieve neck muscles spasms and acupuncture has been employed.

Having read Chapter 1 of your textbook, you can clearly see that the treatment of CDH involves primarily episodic medical care, featuring treatment of the headaches once they begin, along with some attempt to prevent them or at least respond to their occurrence with effective quickness. To date, preventive medical care of CDH is limited to a recognition of a family history and the treatment of depression, along with some assistance in learning stress-management techniques.

the mind

The first part in this textbook covers two topics that are closely linked to how we handle change in our lives. Chapter 2 discusses psychological health, and Chapter 3 deals with stress management. As explained below, your personal growth closely relates to each of the six dimensions of your health.

1. Physical Dimension

The physical dimension of health is concerned with the structure and function of all body systems. Many of the experiences that will shape your feelings about yourself are made possible by good physical health. In addition, effective coping skills often require us to draw on the physical dimension of health.

2. Psychological Dimension

Our responses to stress are primarily emotional. Feelings of uneasiness arising from the demands of college, relationships, parenting, or work are the hallmarks of stress. Fortunately, you can cope with change by using the resources of your psychological dimension of health. Your sense of humor, capacity for empathy, and attitude towards adversity will help you cope with demanding changes in your life.

3. Social Dimension

Growth and development are influenced by the people with whom you interact. When things go well with roommates, coworkers, or your spouse or children, you begin to feel capable as a social person. Occasional failures in social relationships can produce stress but can also remind you that emotional growth and coping skills take time to develop.

4. Intellectual Dimension

As you grow older, you will call on your intellectual resources with increasing frequency. These resources will help you enjoy life more fully and understand your emotional and spiritual growth. During difficult times, your mind may be your most dependable coping source. A book, concert, or art exhibit may be a refuge from the stress of the classroom, family, or office.

5. Spiritual Dimension

Many of today's students are searching for a deeper understanding of the meaning of life. Some students feel pressured to accept the spiritual beliefs of the majority. The uncertainties of exploring what to believe and how to express those beliefs can create stress. Your spirituality can be a valuable resource during periods of stress. Meditation, introspection, and prayer can free people from some of the stress of living in a fast-paced, sometimes uncaring world. To believe deeply in something and to act on that belief by serving others leads to personal growth.

6. Occupational Dimension

The vocation you choose will have a lasting effect on shaping the person you will become. Many people choose an occupation that allows them to serve others. However, work can be a primary source of life stress. Some of this stress is unwelcome and can be harmful. But occupational stress can also challenge you to perform at your peak, generating a sense of pride and accomplishment.

chapter two

achieving psychological health

Chapter Objectives

Upon completing this chapter, you will be able to:

▌ define the terms *self-esteem* and *self-concept*, and describe how they apply to you.

▌ describe the characteristics of psychologically healthy people.

▌ define the terms *emotional intelligence* and *learned optimism*, and explain how they relate to psychological health.

▌ explain Maslow's hierarchy of needs and how it can apply to your daily activities.

▌ describe strategies to enhance communication skills.

▌ describe mood disorders, including the difference between having "the blues" and clinical depression.

▌ describe anxiety disorders.

▌ explain the treatment modalities for psychological disorders.

▌ explain the differences between a psychiatrist, psychologist, social worker, and counselor.

▌ list four types of psychotherapy and their accompanying techniques.

Online Learning Center Resources

www.mhhe.com/payne8e

Log on to our Online Learning Center (OLC) for access to these additional resources:

- Chapter key terms and definitions
- Learning objectives
- Student interactive question-and-answer sites
- Self-scoring chapter quiz
- Online assessments
- Key term flash cards

Talking It Over

Becoming More Assertive

While visiting your home, which has a "smoke-free" policy, your friend lights up a cigarette. How would you handle this situation? If you're an assertive person, you would firmly but courteously ask your friend to smoke outside. If you tend to be passive, you might remain silent but feel angry. If you're an aggressive person, you might yell.

Regardless of the communication style you grew up with, you can learn to become more assertive, asking for what you need or want while respecting other people. When you become an assertive person, your psychological health and self-esteem will soar.

CommunicationLinks

www.lifeclinic.com/focus/stress/communicating.asp
www.wellsource.com

Eye on the Media

Self-Help via the Internet—Guidance to Wellness or Path to Destruction?

Some people feel more comfortable accessing psychological information and asking questions regarding their mental health via the Internet. According to a recent poll conducted by Harris Interactive, about 98 million American adults use the Internet to find health-related information.[1] There are also self-help and support groups, counseling, and assessments available through the Web.

However, much of the information available on the Web is not accurate and may cause harm if the reader accepts the information without question. The Internet can potentially be a dangerous tool as people can diagnose themselves through taking online surveys, which may lack validity or reliability. In fact, a study conducted by the UCLA Internet project[2] reported that half of the information they accessed on the Internet was reliable and accurate. A person reading about bulimia may self-diagnose and decide that he or she does not meet the criteria

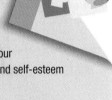

when in fact s/he may be developing this disorder. You may purchase a herbal medicine that claims to alleviate depression when there is no research to support this, and it may actually cause harm. There are also websites that instruct people on how to commit suicide or become better anorexics, again causing greater distress rather than offering assistance to improving psychological health.

The number of resources on the Internet is growing by leaps and bounds, doubling in size about every year. In addition, anyone can publish on the Internet and since there are over 800 million Internet sites, the accuracy of what is out on the Net is difficult if not impossible to regulate. Unfortunately, many people believe that if it is on the Internet, it must be true which is not necessarily the case.

How can you be reasonably sure that the information you are reading is correct? Here are some important questions to consider:

- What are the author's qualifications and credentials? Is the resource from an expert or scholar in the field or from an individual's own opinion and experience?

- Is there any evidence of quality control? This would be more likely if the information is part of an official organizational website, such as an affiliation with a college or university or recognized professional organization like the American Psychological Association.

- What is the reliability of the information presented? Does it seem consistent with other things you have read? Is it error free? Are the sources listed?

- What is the motivation of the author? Does the author stand to gain financially from the way the information is presented? Is there evidence of bias—was some information omitted, or was the material presented in a one-sided way?

- How current is the information? What was the last date the information was revised? Are there up-to-date links listed?

There are of course many positive reasons for accessing the Internet for information, support, and help. For example, Ball State University has started a new program in which students can ask health-related questions using their computers. They can receive medical advice without leaving their residence hall room! The students can see the nurse but the nurse cannot see them. The nurse can also present pictures, video clips, or documents to the student via Web browser to help discuss and diagnose the student's condition.[3]

There have been some efforts from American Accreditation HealthCare Commission towards organizing an advisory committee from a variety of groups such as the Internet Healthcare Coalition, Hi-Ethics, and the American Medical Association to begin developing standards for accrediting health websites. Until this group or some other agency is formed to regulate the credibility or the information on the Internet, it is advisable to be a wise consumer of Internet information.

1. International Food Information Council Foundation. *Navigating for Health: Finding Accurate Information on the Internet.* Nov/Dec. 2000.
2. The UCLA Internet Report Surveying the Digital Future. *Internet Access and Use: 2000, 2001, and 2002.*
3. *The Chronicle of Higher Education,* April 11, 2003. Ball State Tests System for Answering Students' Health Questions Online.

Have you recently been frustrated, angry, fearful, content, excited, or happy? Have you occasionally felt anticipation or anxiety about doing something new? These feelings are all part of the psychological dimension of health. The terms *emotional wellness* or *psychological health* have been used interchangeably to describe how people function in the affective and cognitive realms of their lives. This includes how people express their emotions, cope with stress, adversity, and success, and adapt to changes in themselves and their environment. Psychological health also addresses cognitive functioning—the way people think and behave in conjunction with their emotions. There is some debate about whether thoughts influence feelings or feelings cause us to think and behave a certain way. However, the most accepted view is that the way we think can directly change how we feel about an event or situation. Thus you can change your feelings about something by changing your attitude and perspective about a situation. This has implications for how we can increase our self-esteem, and confidence level, and enhance our interactions with others. You will learn more about psychological health as you study this chapter.

Psychological Health

How do you feel about yourself? When you apply resources from the multiple dimensions of health (see Chapter 1) in ways that allow you to direct your growth, assess deeply held values, deal effectively with change, and have satisfying relationships with others, you are psychologically healthy.

Research in the area of health psychology has shown that there is a mind-body connection in which biological, psychological, and social factors interact to influence health

Key Terms

psychological health a broadly based concept pertaining to cognitive functioning in conjunction with the way people express their emotions, cope with stress, adversity, and success and adapt to changes in themselves and their environment.

or illness. This is referred to as the **biopsychological** model.[1] We know that your psychological state has a significant effect on physical health; stress, depression, and anxiety have been associated with how your immune system responds and can impair physical health. Studies have shown that terminally ill cancer patients who had better psychological health lived longer lives and reported having higher quality of lives.[2]

Psychological health has also been associated with developing and maintaining a positive **self-concept,** positive **self-esteem,** and a higher level of **emotional intelligence.** Each of these concepts will be explained further. However, as you will see, psychological health is much more than just the absence of mental illness.

Changing for the Better

Fostering Your Emotional Growth

As a 32-year-old college student, I feel as though I'm being pulled in too many different directions. Sometimes I think I'm losing my sense of self or wonder if I ever had one. What can I do to help myself grow emotionally?

Emotional growth requires both knowing about yourself and learning from new experiences. The activities listed below can be used in support of these requirements:

Keep a daily journal. Writing down your thoughts and making note of experiences are effective tools in fostering greater self-understanding. Once written, the information that these accounts contain can be reprocessed for an even greater awareness of self.

Join a support group. Sharing experiences and feelings in the presence of people who can "stand in your shoes" creates an environment that will support your efforts to grow as a more interesting and self-directed person. Additionally, being an active participant in a support group also functions as a "new experience" through which new insights into your sense of self-worth can be gained.

Take an assertiveness course. Learning how to greet others, give and receive compliments, use "I" statements, express spontaneity, and state your feelings of disagreement are important tools in developing self-confidence. Very likely, an assertiveness course is or will be offered on your campus.

Seek counseling. Nowhere is counseling generally more available and affordable than on a college campus. Clearly, much can be learned about your sense of self and the psychological factors that have shaped it. Contact the campus health center or the psychological services center for referral to an experienced psychologist or counselor.

InfoLinks

www.mhsource.com/healthieryou.html

Characteristics of Psychologically Healthy People

Some of the characteristics most people associate with being psychologically healthy are listed on page 31. Psychologically healthy people:

- Accept themselves and others
- Like themselves
- Appropriately express the full range of human emotions, both positive and negative
- Give and receive care, love, and support
- Accept life's disappointments
- Accept their mistakes
- Express empathy and concern for others
- Take care of themselves
- Trust others as well as themselves
- Establish goals, both short and long term
- Can function both independently and interdependently
- Lead a health-enhancing lifestyle that includes regular exercise, good nutrition, and adequate sleep

The Changing for the Better box above suggests some activities that may enhance your current level of emotional health.

Self-Esteem

What is self-esteem? How do you know when someone is lacking in self-esteem? Most people answer this question by saying that they define positive self-esteem as:

Key Terms

biopsychological model a model that addresses how biological, psychological, and social factors interact and affect psychological health.

self-concept an individual's internal picture of him or herself; the way one sees oneself.

self-esteem an individual's sense of pride, self-respect, value, and worth.

emotional intelligence the ability to understand others and act wisely in human relations and measure how well you know your emotions, manage your emotions, motivate yourself, recognize emotions in others, and handle relationships.

- Having pride in yourself
- Treating yourself with respect
- Considering yourself valuable, important, worthy
- Feeling good about yourself
- Having self-confidence, being self-assured
- Accepting yourself

People with lower levels of self-esteem tend to allow others to mistreat them, don't take care of themselves, have difficulty being by themselves, and have little self-confidence. In addition, people with low self-esteem tend to take things personally and are sometimes seen as overly sensitive; they tend to be perfectionists who are highly critical of themselves and others. These individuals often have a pessimistic outlook on life and see themselves as undeserving of good fortune. We will explore the concepts of optimism and pessimism as they relate to psychological health in a later section of this chapter.

Self-Concept

Where do we get our self-esteem? Most people would say from their parents, teachers, peers, siblings, religious institutions, and the media. While these factors certainly can positively or negatively affect our self-esteem, they are all *external* factors. Self-esteem relates to our *internal* self-perception. People with low self-esteem tend to have a poor self-concept, meaning that their internal picture of themselves is very negative. Because of this poor self-concept, people with low self-esteem tend to allow others to mistreat or abuse them and fail to be assertive. Many psychological problems have their underpinnings in low self-esteem, including eating disorders, substance abuse problems, and depression.

Many people who suffer from low self-esteem do tend to focus on outside factors. If self-esteem truly came from outside ourselves, then we would need to change our environment and the people around us. Thus, many people believe that if they had more money, a nicer car, a better re-lationship, etc., they would feel better about themselves. This can become a vicious cycle, leaving the person always seeking more and perpetually unsatisfied with his or her self. This can also lead to perfectionism and not accepting oneself.

It is generally accepted that self-esteem comes from within ourselves and is ultimately within each individual's control. In addition, self-esteem is not an all-or-none commodity, as most people have varying degrees of self-esteem, depending upon their stage of development, events in their lives, and their environment.[3]

Emotional Intelligence

A third aspect of psychological health is the degree of emotional intelligence you possess. Emotional intelligence refers to "the ability to understand others and act wisely in human relations."[4] Furthermore, emotional intelligence can be broken down into five main domains:

- **Knowing your emotions.** This is considered the cornerstone of emotional intelligence and relates to how much self-awareness and insight you have. How quickly you are able to recognize and label your feelings as you feel them determines the level of your emotional intelligence.
- **Managing your emotions.** How well can you express your feelings appropriately and cope with your emotions? People who have trouble coping with anxiety, distress, and failures tend to have lower levels of emotional intelligence.
- **Motivating yourself.** People who can motivate themselves tend to be more highly productive and independent than those who rely on external sources for motivation. The more you can self-motivate and engage in goal-directed activities, the higher your emotional intelligence.
- **Recognizing emotions in others.** Another aspect of emotional intelligence is the degree of empathy you have or how sensitive you are to the feelings of others and how you come across to other people.
- **Handling relationships.** This refers to your level of social skills. The more interpersonally effective you are and able to negotiate conflict and build a social support network, the more emotional intelligence you possess.

Of course people have differing levels of emotional intelligence and may have higher levels in one domain than in another. People with overall high levels of emotional intelligence tend to take on leadership roles, are confident, assertive, express their feelings directly and appropriately, feel good about themselves, are outgoing, and adapt well to stress.[4]

The Importance of Forgiveness

In an excellent video titled *Late Frost,* an elderly gentleman muses the important lessons of life that are finally recognized by those who have lived to reach old age. A particularly poignant moment occurs when the man thanks God for having given him the ability to forget. On closer examination, however, we can see that forgetfulness is not a strange attribute for us to want or to be thankful for. This is because frequently our ability to forget harmful events reflects the fact that we have first been able to forgive those who have hurt us so deeply.

Experts in the field of mind-body connectedness suggest we can eventually forgive, but only when we truly want to do so. In other words, we must be willing to work in order to forgive and thus forget our pain. Accordingly, we must master a process involving these difficult but necessary steps:

The ability to embrace our anger. Anger is a human attribute that is both natural and important in its ability to lead us toward positive change. Its initial strongly felt presence must be recognized and accepted as such. Anger can be a positive emotion, validating our self-esteem and self-worth. It is important to manage and express our anger in appropriate, constructive ways rather than in a destructive, abusive manner.

The ability to look beyond our own pain. In spite of the fury that rages inside us, the person whose actions have caused us such unbearable pain is a person of value as well. We must at some point look for the redeeming qualities this person possesses.

The ability to refrain from speaking derogatorily. In spite of the hurt others have caused us, to continue speaking in demeaning ways about others negates our ability to see them as having redeeming value as people.

The ability to see a future free from anger. Much as athletes visualize their own "perfect" performance, when deeply injured we must stay focused on what life will be like when we have finally moved beyond our anger and hurt.

The ability to begin wishing well to those who have hurt us. Earlier we were told to see our offenders as people of value. Now we must internalize this attitude to the extent that we can begin to truly wish these people well.

The ability to persevere. Even though the offense against us may have taken only seconds, it may require months or even years for us to replace our pain and anger with a sense of forgiveness. We cannot rush the process, nor can we give up on it.

When we can forgive those who have hurt us, particularly those who have been close and dear, the debilitating effects of stress stemming from anger eventually will subside. Forgiving will then lead to greater peace, less stress, and the ability to feel hopeful about the future.

Personality

What is meant when someone says, "She has a good personality"? Is it possible to have no personality? **Personality** is generally defined as a specific set of consistent patterns of behavior and traits that helps to identify and characterize an individual. Personality is comprised of thoughts, feelings, behaviors, motivation, instinct, and temperament.[5] Isn't it likely that you associate someone's "good" personality with the existence of psychological health?

There is some debate about how personality is formed and where we acquire our personality traits. A general consensus is that two factors, **nature** and **nurture,** influence the shaping of personality. Nature refers to the innate factors we are born with that genetically determine our personality traits. Nurture is the effect that the environment, people, and external factors have on our personality.[6] While it is agreed that both nature and nurture influence personality development, there is some debate about how much each one plays a role in its formation. We all know people who are introverted or quiet or shy "by nature" or "naturally outgoing." We seem to be born with a predisposition toward certain personality traits that often resemble our parents. "She is serious like her father" or "He is funny like his mother" are remarks people may make alluding to this genetic link. Environmental factors such as social relationships, family harmony, financial resources, job and academic concerns, particular situations, and even the weather can influence your personality.

Often assumptions are made about an individual's personality based largely on someone's appearance. Studies have shown that physically attractive people are seen as warm, friendly, and intelligent, and unattractive people are viewed as cold, humorless, and not as bright.[7] First impressions also play a major role in how we perceive other people's personalities. Research shows that we tend

> ### Key Terms
>
> **personality** a specific set of consistent patterns of behavior and traits that helps to identify and characterize an individual; personality is comprised of thoughts, feelings, behaviors, motivation, instinct, and temperament.
>
> **nature** the innate factors that genetically determine personality traits.
>
> **nurture** the effect that the environment, people, and external factors have on personality.

I keep getting into unhealthy romantic relationships and have come to expect that the person I am dating will eventually find something wrong with me and leave me. What can I do to feel better about myself and change my attitude toward my chances of having a successful relationship?

As the saying goes, it is hard to allow others to love you when you don't love yourself. So the first step is to start accepting and liking yourself and develop a more positive self-concept. The activities listed below can help you to start the process of enhancing your self-esteem:

Write down three things you like about yourself every day. Ask yourself what you did well today—not what you did wrong.

Share this list with a friend. It is generally more accepted to share your flaws and problems rather than your successes or positive qualities. We often hear people say, "That was a stupid thing for me to say" or "I'm having a bad hair day" rather than "I was proud of how I was able to answer a question in class today."

Accept compliments. Frequently we deflect or laugh away compliments rather than accept them. One of the ways to test yourself to see if you took in a compliment is to see if you remember what that person said about you an hour later. Another way is to focus on how you are feeling—do you feel more positive, confident, happier with yourself?

Give compliments. Sometimes people with low self-esteem criticize others in order to feel better about themselves. To get out of this pattern, look for positives in other people and share your feedback, without belittling yourself. Instead of saying, "You do that so much better than I do" just say "You are really good at that."

Watch your body posture. Making eye contact with others, keeping your head up, shoulders back, and not folding your arms in front of you, but keeping an open body posture helps to build self-esteem and confidence and projects this image to others.

Take a risk, do something different. People with lower levels of self-esteem tend to tell themselves, "I can't do that" and so don't even try. Don't be afraid of making a mistake or looking foolish. Take a risk and do something new and different—you might surprise yourself and be more successful than you anticipated.

Disarm the critic. Don't listen to the critical voice in your head that tells you that you are stupid, lazy, or not good enough. Sometimes this critical voice is the voice of our parents, teachers, or someone else in our lives who told us these negative messages. Replace the negative statements with positive ones and tell the critic to ease up a bit.

Reward yourself and be good to yourself. We frequently do nice things for other people or wait for others to reward us. Do something fun or nice for yourself every day.

Signs and symbols of self-worth. Keep your list of positive qualities where you will see it—in your room or in your car. Have things around you that remind you that people care about you and that you are a worthwhile person, such as notes from friends, pictures of enjoyable times with others, or an item that is special to you in some way.

Set realistic goals and expectations for yourself. Changing patterns takes time and practice. You didn't develop your self-concept overnight, and it will take some time to change the way you talk to yourself and see yourself. Notice how much progress you have made rather than how much more you have to go.

InfoLinks

www.self-esteem-nase.org

to make a decision about someone's personality within 4 minutes of meeting them. Once an impression is formed, it is difficult to change, regardless of how the person behaves or of new information that you receive that might contradict what you initially perceived.[6] Thus, people can make errors in judgment because they have not taken the context into consideration or taken enough time to get to know someone over the course of several months and in a variety of settings.

The Normal Range of Emotions

You probably know people who seem to be cheerful all the time. These people appear to be confident, happy, and full of good feelings twenty-four seven. Although some people like this may exist, they are truly the exceptions. For most people, emotions are more like a roller coaster ride. At times, they feel good about themselves and others; other times, nothing seems to be going right. Once you know them better, these same people may show that they feel happy, sad, pleased, uncertain, confident, excited, and afraid all in the same day or week. To outsiders, they might even appear to be moody. To the mental health professional, however, these same people would probably seem to be normal, since the feeling states that they are demonstrating all fall within a normal range of emotions.

Everyone, not only college students, experiences a range of emotions. This is normal and healthy. Experiencing a range of emotions is an important part of experiencing life. You should not expect to remain calm and rational every minute of the day. You also should not expect to adjust effectively to every situation with which you are confronted. Life has its ups and downs, and the concept of the *normal range of emotions* reflects this. If one concept is important for you to understand about being psychologically healthy, it is this one.

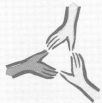
Happiness and a Sense of Humor

Perhaps the most prized emotion to be experienced is a feeling of happiness about life—a feeling that is more likely to occur when day-to-day events are entered into with an underlying sense of humor.

Maintaining a sense of humor is now known to be a critically important component of the emotional dimension of health.[8] People who possess this resource understand that life is not meant to be one long, boring exercise. Part of the reason for living is to have fun. Life taken too seriously can be the most miserable life imaginable.

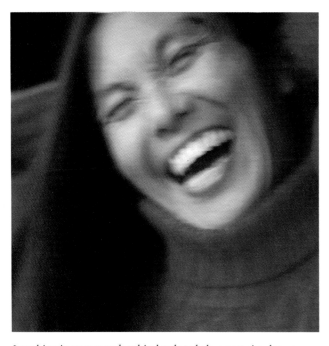

Laughing increases endorphin levels to help ease pain, decrease stress, and release tension from your body.

Recognizing the humor in daily situations and occasionally being able to laugh at yourself will make you feel better not only about others but also, more importantly, about yourself. Others will enjoy being associated with you, and your ability to perform physically and to recover from injuries and illnesses will also be enhanced.[9] In addition, laughter reduces stress,[10] boosts the immune system,[11] alleviates pain,[12] stabilizes mood,[13] decreases anxiety,[14] enhances communication,[15] and inspires creativity.[16] The research suggests that we need to laugh 30 minutes total in a 24-hour period in order to attain these benefits. This is an easy task for children who on average laugh 250 times a day but more challenging for adults who tend to only laugh 15 times a day.[17] Employers have been putting the benefits of laughter to good use to increase productivity in factories. Factories in India have created "laughing clubs" in which people laugh together for 20 minutes a day, resulting in less absenteeism and better performance among the workers.[18]

 TALKING POINTS How would you describe your personality? How do you think your friends or family would describe you? Do you think they would be the same or different?

Developing Communication Skills

Shyness and loneliness, two of the more common conditions suggesting a less-than-optimal level of psychological health, will be described later in the chapter. Both of these conditions can be a consequence of feeling uncomfortable with others. When people find it difficult to initiate or even participate in conversations with others, it is likely, in part, that they have not developed some of the communication skills with which others feel comfortable.

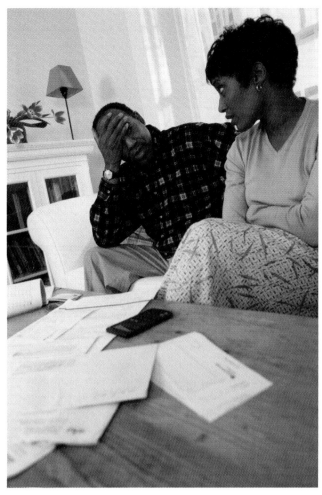

Nonverbal communication can be a powerful tool in sending messages to others through body language and posture as well as facial expressions.

In this section of your textbook, we will investigate how speaking and listening can foster improved social relationships. We will also look at the use of unspoken communication as an aid to social interaction. Remember that how people see themselves (their self-concept) influences how they feel about themselves (their self-esteem).

Verbal Communication

Communication between people can be viewed in terms of a particular person's role as sender or receiver of the spoken language. You can enhance your effectiveness as a sender of verbal information by implementing several important steps:[3]

- Take the time to think before speaking. Effective communication requires that you know what you want to say.

- Focus your words on your most important thoughts and ideas. Your main message may get lost in too many details or too long a story.

- Speak clearly and concisely. This will aid the listener, particularly when ideas are complex or new.

- Talk with, rather than at, the listener. Speaking with other people encourages listeners to share freely and comfortably with those speaking.

- Start on a positive note. Even when the message is negative, a more positive atmosphere is established when a conversation begins in this manner.

- Seek feedback from listeners. Provide frequent intervals between ideas to allow listeners to respond.

- Use other forms of communication to transmit important ideas when face-to-face conversation is not effective. Written communication or the use of a carefully selected third person is often highly effective.

Verbal communication requires that you function as skillfully as a listener, or receiver, as you do as a sender of spoken ideas. Certainly, there are skills for structuring the exchange of information. The following are a variety of listening approaches:

- Listen with attention. In many situations it will be important to hear and understand everything that is being said.

- Ask for clarification and summarize what you think you heard the speaker saying to ensure you have received the message accurately.

- On some occasions, it may be necessary to guide the speaker to ensure that excessive or confusing information is not being transferred. This is accomplished by asking carefully worded questions intended to stay on the topic and not get too far off on a tangent.

Nonverbal Communication

Information can be communicated verbally and nonverbally. Nonverbal communication is what is communicated by your facial expressions, body posture, tone of voice, movements, and even the way you breathe, such as when you sigh or yawn. Nonverbal communication is a very powerful and sometimes more important aspect of the message than what is verbally communicated. In fact, people use information from facial cues more than any other source.[19] Facial cues, particularly from the eyes, are attended to more than any other type of nonverbal communication, even when information from other sources, such as hand and body movements, may provide a more accurate picture of what the person is feeling. The following suggestions can enhance your non-verbal communication skills:

- *Facial expressions.* Facial expressions have been cited as one of the most important sources of nonverbal communication in terms of a person's emotional state.[19] When people speak with their eyebrows raised, they tend to be seen as more animated, excited, and happier. Flushing of one's face can indicate embarrassment, and crinkling one's nose can mean that you don't like something. Every part of your face can communicate some type of emotional reaction.

- *Eye contact.* Maintaining eye contact is an important component of positive nonverbal communication, while looking away or shifting your eyes can be read as seeming dishonest. But don't stare—5 to 7 seconds seems to be the maximum amount of time to look at someone's eyes before they begin to feel scrutinized.

- *Personal space.* There are cultural differences in how much personal space or distance is comfortable and accepted when sitting or standing next to another person. For example, Americans' personal space—about 3 to 4 feet for a casual conversation—tends to be much greater than that of Arabs or Italians, but less than Japanese or Britons. Gender and age and degree of familiarity are other factors that can determine the amount of personal space you are comfortable having between you and another person.

- *Body posture.* Assertiveness is equated with people who carry themselves with their heads up, shoulders back, and maintain eye contact. Folding your arms, crossing your legs, and turning your body away from the speaker can indicate defensiveness and rejection.

As with verbal communication, when nonverbal components are recognized and controlled, communication is undertaken more effectively.

Managing Conflict

Communication can be especially challenging when there is a conflict or disagreement. Emotions such as anger, hurt, and fear might alter your ability to communicate as effectively as you would like. Some techniques for managing angry or upset people or conflictual situations are:

- *Listen and acknowledge the other person's point of view, even if it differs from your own.* To ensure that you have heard the person accurately and to let that person know you are listening to them, repeat back or summarize what you heard and ask if you misunderstood something that was said.

- *Use assertive communication.* Using "I" statements rather than "You" helps to avoid putting people on the defensive and is especially helpful when negotiating conflict or disagreements. Rather than saying, "You are inconsiderate," you can say, "I feel upset when you're late and don't call to let me know."

- *Focus not just on what you say but how you say it.* Pay attention to your tone of voice and speak in a conversational tone. People tend to talk louder because they think they will be better heard that way. This can result in a shouting match in which neither person hears the other.

- *Acknowledge the others person's feelings.* Use statements like, "I can understand why this is so frustrating for you."

- *Watch your body posture.* Don't fold your arms in a closed, defensive posture, maintain eye contact, be aware of your facial expression so that you are not conveying hostility nonverbally. Make sure your nonverbal communication matches your verbal communication.

- *Accept valid criticism.* If you made a mistake, admit to it, apologize for whatever you think you did to contribute to the misunderstanding or conflict. This will open the door for the other person to take responsibility for his/her part in the conflict as well.

- *Focus on the problem at hand.* If you try to resolve every disagreement you have ever had with this person, you will become overwhelmed and won't accomplish much. Stay on track by talking about the present situation.

- *Take a team approach by engaging in mutual problem solving.* Avoid the winner versus loser paradigm, and look for areas of compromise. Find a middle ground you can both agree to and live with.

- *Agree to disagree.* There is probably more than one right answer and you can agree that you will not persuade the other to change his or her point of view.

- *Agree to discuss this at a later time.* If the conversation becomes too volatile and heated, take some time to calm down and think about the situation. Some time and distance from the problem can be beneficial.

Maslow's Hierarchy of Needs

Abraham Maslow has been among the significant contributors to the understanding of personality and emotional growth. Central to Maslow's contribution to twentieth-century American psychological thought is

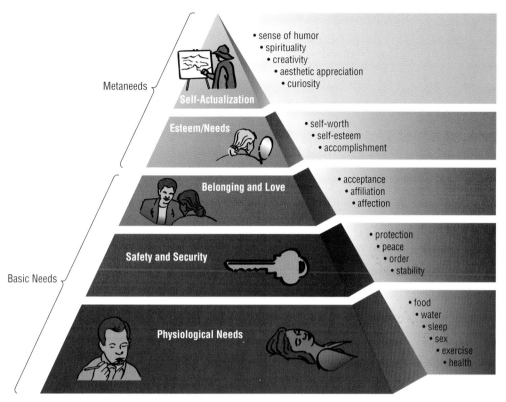

Figure 2-1 Maslow's hierarchy of needs.

his view of psychological health in terms of the individual's attempt to meet inner needs, what he called *the hierarchy of needs.*[20] Maslow's hierarchy of needs is outlined in Figure 2-1. Maslow's theory is a positive, optimistic theory of human behavior. He believed that people are motivated to grow and fulfill their potential, referring to this phenomenon as **self-actualization.** He described self-actualization as "the need to become more and more what one is, to become everything that one is capable of becoming."[21] Maslow differentiated between two different categories of needs: **basic needs** and **metaneeds.** Basic needs—physiological needs, belonging and love, and esteem needs—are the deficiency needs and are essential and urgent. Metaneeds come into play once the basic needs are met and include spirituality, creativity, curiosity, beauty, philosophy, and justice. Maslow's hierarchy of needs is arranged with the basic needs on the bottom, as they are the most fundamental and powerful needs. Lower level needs must be met before the next level of needs can be satisfied. Maslow believed that the fulfillment of metaneeds is needed to become a completely developed human being. Left unfulfilled, people can become cynical, apathetic, and lonely.[24]

Maslow arrived at this model by examining what he considered to be exceptionally healthy people, people he defined as having developed to their fullest potentials. Self-actualized people that Maslow identified included Albert Einstein, Albert Schweitzer, Eleanor Roosevelt, and Abraham Lincoln. He perceived these people to share similar personality characteristics, such as being self-assured principled, innovative, compassionate, altruistic, goal-oriented, and internally motivated.[22] There are

---

Key Terms

self-actualization the highest level of psychological health at which one reaches his or her highest potential and values truth, beauty, goodness, faith, love, humor, and ingenuity.

basic needs deficiency needs that are viewed as essential and fundamental, including physiological needs, belonging and love, and esteem needs.

metaneeds secondary concerns, such as spirituality, creativity, curiosity, beauty, philosophy, and justice, that can be addressed only after the basic needs are met.

some similarities between having reached self-actualization and having high self-esteem. The Health on the Web on page 43 will help you to foster your psychological health and, in doing so, help you on your journey towards self-actualization.

Creative Expression

Another characteristic of people who have developed their psychological health is creativity. Allowing yourself to express your thoughts, feelings, and individuality in a creative manner entails having self-confidence, self-esteem, and flexibility. Confidence and self-esteem are essential so that you don't feel embarrassed by your creativity and feel free to share your creative side with others. Children can easily do this when they draw a picture or make up a dance and say, "Look at me; look at what I made." However, as we age, some of us become inhibited and don't allow ourselves to be creative or to share this part of ourselves. Like muscles, if you don't exercise your creative side, it can begin to atrophy.

What are some resources that you might need to develop in order to foster your creativity?

- *Nonconformity.* Creative individuals aren't terribly concerned about what other people think of them. They are willing to risk looking foolish or proposing ideas that are divergent from others or traditional ways of thinking.

- *Independence.* Highly creative people tend to work well alone and sometimes prefer this to working in a group. As children, they often were encouraged to solve problems on their own rather than having someone else to do so for them.

- *Motivation.* Creative people are motivated by intrinsic rather than external rewards, meaning they like to be creative for their own pleasure, not to please others or because it is expected of them. They don't fear failure and success is not the main goal. They enjoy creativity for creativity's sake alone and not to reap rewards or praise from others.

- *Curiosity.* Creative people have a wide range of interests and a broad base of knowledge. They are open to new experiences and question things that other people ignore or take for granted.

- *Persistence.* This is seen as one of the most important traits of a creative person. As Thomas Edison said, "Genius is one-tenth inspiration and nine-tenths perspiration." Persistence requires not giving up when your first efforts are not successful and continually to think of new ways of doing something, problem solving, or thinking "outside of the box."[40]

Some people reviewing the preceding list may recognize many of these characteristics as being already well developed in their own personalities. Others may not have demonstrated some of the traits listed, and they may appear far beyond their reach. Nevertheless, most people can increase their creativity by giving themselves permission to be creative. Some people state, "I'm not a creative person" and yet they haven't explored that part of their personality, perhaps since childhood. There are many avenues of creativity and the first step is to experiment, to be open and spontaneous. In this way, you can gain greater psychological health from accessing your inner strengths and resources.

Spiritual Health

Having a sense of purpose, direction, and awareness are some of the dimensions of spiritual health. This aspect of psychological health also refers to how well we integrate our beliefs and values with our behavior. People with spiritual health seek meaning and purpose in their lives and have a deep appreciation for a sense of unity and community. Spiritual health also includes one's morals, ethics, intrinsic values, and beliefs. It also refers to an awareness and appreciation of the vastness of the universe, and recognition of a dimension beyond the natural and rational, involving, perhaps, a belief in a force greater than oneself.[23] Spirituality has been found to increase psychological health, as people that incorporate it into their lives reported better psychological coping, increased well-being, increased satisfaction with life, lower anxiety and depressive symptoms, less hostility and anger, and greater happiness in general.[24] Similarly, spirituality has also been related to better physical health. Studies have shown that no matter how spirituality was defined or measured, it has a positive effect on reducing coronary heart disease, high blood pressure, stroke, cancer, and increasing life expectancy.[25]

As a resource in the spiritual dimension of health, the existence of spirituality provides a basis on which your belief system can mature and your expanding awareness of life's meaning can be fostered. In addition, the existence of spirituality gives meaning to your career and assists you in better understanding the consequences of your vocational efforts. Further, spirituality in something (or someone) can influence many of the experiences that you will seek throughout life and can temper the emotional relationships that you have with these experiences. In virtually all cultures, spirituality provides individuals and groups with rituals and practices that foster the development of a sense of community. In turn, the community provides the authority and

Solitude: Time to Reflect, Regroup, Renew

Have you taken a moment today to be quiet and just be with yourself? Time alone can help you step away from a busy, fragmented world and draw inward for renewal. It provides an opportunity to reflect and to have new and deeper observations. Having strengthened awareness of yourself in both mind and body allows you to experience the fullness of the moment, even to feel in sync with the universe.

Solitude can also help you establish your identity, clarify what's important to you, and strengthen your independence. Because most of our time is spent living with, caring for, or responding to others, it is only when we are alone that we have the opportunity to fully emerge and become ourselves.

Any time you take for this meditation will be restorative. You may start with just five minutes every morning. You will need a place where you feel comfortable to be alone with your own thoughts, whether it be at the kitchen table, in bed, in the bath, at a coffee shop, in the library, or in the garden. Go for a walk, listen to music, weed the garden, write a letter to a friend, paint, read a poem, or just be still and concentrate on your breathing. All of these are solitary actions that, in the end, reconnect you to a life force and to others. Pretty soon you may feel that your time of solitude is more energizing than sleep! When you are faced with a difficult project, a household disaster, or something more serious, such as sickness or death, these reflective moments will give you mental and spiritual renewal.

It's not selfish to carve out whatever time you need alone to refresh yourself. By claiming solitude regularly, you're reconnecting to your inner self. This nourished spirit is what you can share with others, whether family, friends, coworkers, or strangers. Through your appreciation of a deep, rich, inner reality, you will feel rapture in the mystery and gift of just *being* here.

guidance that nurtures the emotional stability, confidence, and sense of competence needed for living life fully.[26]

TALKING POINTS How well do your actions reflect your beliefs and values? How can you better integrate your values, beliefs, and behavior? How much time and energy do you devote to what is most important to you?

Taking an Optimistic Approach to Life

Is your happiness within your control? Are people born naturally happy or sad? One important key to psychological health is the way that you think about and interpret events in your life. For example, if you say "hello" to someone and you don't get a response, do you begin to wonder if that person is angry with you? Or do you surmise that he or she didn't hear you or perhaps was distracted? Research shows that having a positive interpretation of life's events, particularly how you cope with adversity, can make a significant difference in terms of your health, academic and work performance, as well as how long you will live.[27] Do you see the glass half empty, as pessimists do, or half full, like optimists? Does it matter? Again studies overwhelmingly contend that your perspective makes a tremendous difference in your psychological health. Compared to pessimists, optimists tend to:

- Contract fewer infectious diseases
- Have better health habits
- Possess stronger immune systems
- Be more successful in their careers
- Perform better in sports, music, and academics

We do know that people can learn to be helpless and ultimately become depressed and even suicidal. Pavlov demonstrated the concept of **learned helplessness** in his classic study in which he administered an electric shock to dogs that were harnessed and couldn't escape the shock. When he moved the dogs to another room and delivered the shocks, the dogs lay down and whimpered and didn't try to avoid the shocks. This time the dogs were not harnessed and could have easily escaped the shocks by moving to another side of the room. This reaction has been referred to as learned helplessness, as the dogs learned that there was nothing they could do to affect their situation, and they lost hope and felt trapped and powerless.[28] We have seen this same phenomenon with humans. College students volunteered for an experiment in which they were subjected to an earsplitting noise and their efforts to stop the noise were unsuccessful. Later, when they were placed in another situation where they could have easily pulled a control lever to turn off the noise, they made no effort to do so and just suffered with the noise until the experimenter stopped it.[29] Battered women have demonstrated this same sense of powerlessness and helplessness in their ability to escape the abuse they are subjected to by their partners.

> **Key Terms**
>
> **learned helplessness** a theory of motivation explaining how individuals can learn to feel powerless, trapped, and defeated.

So if people can learn to be helpless and pessimistic, can they also learn to feel more optimistic, powerful, and in control? Martin Seligman conducted studies to prove that this is possible, and called this concept **learned optimism.** He identified three key factors that contribute to having an optimistic or pessimistic perspective. Learned optimism refers to your explanatory style—in other words, if you describe the glass as being half full or half empty. These crucial dimensions are **permanence, pervasiveness,** and **personalization.**

The first dimension is *permanence.* When something bad happens, pessimists tend to give up easily because they believe the causes of bad events are *permanent.* They say things like "Things never work out for me," "That won't ever work," or "He's always in a bad mood." They use permanent language—words like *never, always* and *forever*—which implies that this negative situation is not temporary, but will continue on indefinitely. Optimists tend to use temporary language—such words as *sometimes, frequently,* and *often*—and they blame bad events on transient conditions. Examples of optimistic language are "It didn't work out this time," "Doing it that way didn't work," or "He's in a bad mood today." Optimists see failure as a small, transitory setback and are able to pick themselves up, brush themselves off, and persevere towards their goals.

The second factor that affects our outlook is *pervasiveness.* This refers to whether you perceive negative events as universal and generalize them to everything in your life, or if you can compartmentalize and keep them defined to the specific situation. Pessimists tend to make universal explanations for their problems and when something goes wrong in one part of their lives, they give up on everything. While a pessimist would say that they are not good at math, an optimist would say that they didn't perform well in that particular class with that type of math: "I'm good at algebra but not as good with geometry."

The last aspect of an optimistic or pessimistic explanatory style is determined by whether you blame bad things on yourself or on other people or circumstances.

Pessimism and low self-esteem tend to come from personalizing events—blaming oneself and having an internal explanatory style for negative events. An optimist might say, "The professor wrote a very poor exam and that is the reason I received a lower score," while the pessimist would say, "I am stupid" or "I didn't study enough." This is different from not taking responsibility for one's actions and blaming other people for your problems or mistakes: the idea is to have a balanced perspective and outlook on life. Pessimists tend to give credit to other people or circumstances when good things happen and blame themselves when bad events occur. For example, a pessimist would say, "That was just dumb luck," rather than taking credit for a success. However, if pessimists fail, they read-ily blame themselves, saying, "I messed up." On the other hand, optimists tend to give themselves credit for their accomplishments, saying, "I worked hard and did a good job," and don't belittle themselves when things go wrong.

Seligman conducted many studies to test out how an optimistic explanatory style might be useful in daily living. For example, he worked with a swimming team from the University of California, Berkeley, to see how optimism or pessimism might affect their performance. He has their coaches tell the athletes that their times were slower than they actually were. The swimmers were then asked to swim the event again as fast as they could. The performance of the pessimists deteriorated in their 100-yard event by 2 seconds, the difference between winning the event and finishing dead last. The optimists got faster by 2 to 5 seconds, again enough to be the difference between losing and winning the race.[27] So how you interpret events, your attribution style, can make a tremendous difference in the eventual success or failure in your endeavors.

How can you learn to be more optimistic? Albert Ellis developed a cognitive framework for positive thinking called the ABC method. When you encounter adversity, the "A" part of the formula, you try to make sense out of it and explain what has happened. For example, if you receive a notice from the bank that you have overdrawn your checking account, you start to think, "How did this happen?" These thoughts are associated with your beliefs, the "B" in ABC. Your beliefs affect your feelings, and so you can control your emotions by changing your beliefs and thoughts.[30] So if you think, "I'm irresponsible for letting this happen. I can't manage my money," then you will feel badly about yourself. But if you said, "The bank

Key Terms

learned optimism an attribution style comprised of permanence, pervasiveness, and personalization; how people explain both positive and negative events in their lives, accounting for success and failure.

permanence the first dimension of an individual's attribution style, related to whether certain events are perceived as temporary or long-lasting.

pervasiveness the second dimension of an individual's attribution style, related to whether they perceive events as specific or general.

personalization the final dimension of attribution style, related to whether an individual takes things personally or is more balanced in accepting responsibility for positive and negative events.

probably made a mistake" or "I might have added something incorrectly," you will most likely feel much better about yourself and the situation.

The "C" aspect is the consequence of the event, how you end up feeling about the situation. When someone feels depressed, he or she feels hopeless, trapped, and powerless. By adopting a more positive way of reframing or thinking about events, you create options, hope, and a strategy for solving problems rather than remaining stuck, like the whimpering dogs lying down and putting up with being shocked. In the previously described scenario with the overdraft, you can generate ideas such as "I need to check with the bank, go over my bank statement, be more careful in recording and calculating my balances, and request overdraft protection to prevent this from becoming a problem again."

Everyone encounters adversity sometime in his or her life. You can become discouraged by these events, blame yourself for these problems, and feel hopeless, worthless, and cynical about the world. Or you can be persistent and become stronger by overcoming these obstacles by having positive beliefs, and seeing these problems as short-lived, specific, and not as a flaw in your character. When you embrace an optimistic perspective, you will feel more hopeful, stronger, and confident. You will be able to accept new challenges and take risks in your life.

TALKING POINTS Think about something bad that has happened in your life recently. What were your beliefs about this event? How did you feel? Using the concepts of permanence, pervasiveness, and personalization, how can you change your beliefs about this situation? How do you feel differently about the event?

Taking a Proactive Approach to Life

In addition to the approaches already discussed, the plan that follows is intended to give you other strategies for enhancing your psychological health. The following is a four-step process that continues throughout life: constructing perceptions of yourself, accepting these perceptions, undertaking new experiences, and reframing your perceptions based on new information.

Constructing Mental Pictures

Actively taking charge of your psychological health begins with constructing a mental picture of what you're like. Use the most recent and accurate information you have about yourself—what is important to you, your values, and your abilities.

To construct this mental picture, set aside a period of uninterrupted quiet time for reflection. Before proceeding to the second step, you also need to construct mental pictures about yourself in relation to *other people and material objects;* including your residence and college or work environment, to clarify these relationships.

For example, after graduating from college with a degree in fine arts, Allison moved to a large city to become a jewelry designer. Two years later, her small business was thriving and she was living in a spacious loft apartment with room for her studio. Still, Allison felt that something was missing. She constructed a mental picture in which she saw herself as a resourceful, creative, independent person who was comfortable in her new surroundings. However, Allison realized that she wanted a partner to share her success and her life.

Accepting Mental Pictures

The second step of the plan involves an *acceptance* of these perceptions. This implies a willingness to honor the truthfulness of the perceptions you have formed about yourself and other people. For example, Allison acknowledges her professional success and her artistic ability, and she also accepts that she has been unable to establish a satisfying long-term romantic relationship.

Emotional development is rarely a passive process. You must be willing to be *introspective* (inwardly reflective) about yourself and the world around you.

Undertaking New Experiences

The next step of the plan is to test your newly formed perceptions. This *testing* is accomplished by *undertaking a new experience* or by reexperiencing something in a different way.

New experiences do not necessarily require high levels of risk, foreign travel, or money (see Learning from Our Diversity, above). They may be no more "new" than deciding to move from the dorm into an apartment, to change from one shift at work to another, or to pursue new friendships. The experience itself is not the goal; rather, it's a means of collecting information about yourself, others, and the objects that form your material world.

For instance, Allison volunteered to teach art therapy classes to chronically ill patients at a local hospital. This work was enjoyable and fulfilling for her, and she formed friendships with a few of the other hospital volunteers. Allison also met and began dating Mark, a staff physical therapist.

Reframing Mental Pictures

When you have completed the first three steps in the plan, the new information about yourself, others, and objects becomes the most current source of information. Regardless of the type of new experience you have undertaken and its outcome, you are now in a position to modify the initial perceptions constructed during the first step. Then you will have new insights, knowledge, and perspectives.

Allison reframed her mental pictures in light of the changes that had taken place in her life. Her volunteer work gave her a renewed appreciation for art. Also, she now saw herself as part of a circle of friends and as a partner in a long-term relationship with Mark. With her proactive approach to life, Allison had created challenges for herself that allowed her to change and grow.

Psychological Disorders

In the course of one year, an estimated 22% of Americans, about one in five, suffer from a diagnosable mental disorder.[31] This translates to 44.3 million people being diagnosed with a mental disorder each year, with many people suffering from more than one mental disorder at a given time.[32] In addition, four of the ten leading causes of disability in the United States and other developed countries are mental disorders.[33] However, two-thirds of these people will not receive treatment due to the stigma and cost associated with mental health treatment.[34] Overall, minorities share the same prevalence rate of mental disorders as Caucasians; however, there are great disparities in the rate of mental health care for minorities as compared to the nonminority population.

How common are these disorders? Quite common, as the figures just mentioned suggest. In addition, the lives of millions of other people who work, live, and have relationships with people with mental illness also suffer the impact of these disorders. While there are over 300 different types of mental illness that can be diagnosed, we will cover three major categories of mental disorders: mood disorders, including depression and bipolar disorder; anxiety disorders, including panic disorder, obsessive-compulsive disorder, and post-traumatic stress disorder; and schizophrenia.[35] Over 450 million people worldwide are affected by mental disorders at any given time, and these numbers are expected to increase in the future.[36]

In the sections that follow, we will investigate selected disorders, identify professionals who are trained to treat these conditions, and take a look at the techniques they employ to help those who are afflicted.

Mood Disorders

Mood disorders, such as depression, seasonal affective disorder, and bipolar disorder, refer to psychological problems in which the primary symptom is a disturbance in mood.[35] You might see someone as moody, unable to predict if the person will be in a good or bad mood from one day to the next.

Depression

According to the World Health Organization (WHO), more than 340 million people worldwide, 18 million in the United States alone, are estimated to suffer from **clinical depression.**[36] WHO further contends that this will only worsen in the future, predicting that depression will become the second leading cause of disability worldwide by the year 2020, after heart disease, unless strides are made in prevention and treatment. We have already begun to see this trend, as the number of college students with depression has doubled over the last 13 years.[37] About one in ten Americans suffer some form of depression, with women experiencing depression twice as often as men.[38] While depression can develop at any age, the average age of onset is the mid-twenties.

How can you tell the difference between having the blues and clinical depression? The symptoms of depression are:

Key Terms

clinical depression a psychological disorder in which individuals experience a lack of motivation, decreased energy level, fatigue, social withdrawal, sleep disturbance, disturbance in appetite, diminished sex drive, feelings of worthlessness, and despair.

- Depressed mood most of the day, nearly every day
- Frequent crying
- Withdrawing, isolating oneself from others
- Lack of interest in activities that are typically enjoyable
- Increase or decrease in appetite resulting in significant weight loss or weight gain
- Insomnia, disturbed or restless sleep, or sleeping more than usual
- Feeling tired most of the time, regardless of how much sleep you have had
- Low self-esteem, feelings of hopelessness and worthlessness
- Difficulty concentrating, remembering things, and focusing on a task, and indecisiveness
- Frequent thoughts of suicide

Most people have experienced some of these symptoms at one point or another in their lives; however, clinically depressed individuals experience most of these symptoms every day and have felt this way for at least two weeks. Most people can find ways of pulling themselves out of feeling down, but for those suffering from clinical depression, the normal methods used to cope with the blues don't work. Clinical depression can range from mild to severe depression and can result in significant impairment in functioning, for example, not being able to get out of bed to attend classes or go to work, lacking the energy or motivation to take care of your basic needs for food, hygiene, and rest. Some people tend to become irritable, negative, and uncommunicative, which can cause greater stress and conflict in their relationships. Depression has been described as constantly having a black cloud over your head, not being able to get out from underneath it no matter what you do.

There are several causes or triggers for depression. Research suggests that if you have a family history of depression or any type of mood disorder, you are more prone to developing a depressive disorder. In fact, rates of depression for a child with a depressed parent are two to four times greater than for children without this type of heredity.[39] While there is no single gene that causes depression, your genetic makeup can make you more vulnerable to depression. Neurotransmitters and hormone levels play a major role in the way your brain regulates your mood and emotions. Two neurotransmitters, serotonin and norepinephrine, are often found to be deficient in people with depression.

However, biological processes are not the only explanation for depression. You may have a family history of depression and never develop depressive symptoms, although this puts you in a higher risk category for this disorder. Other life events, stressors, and losses can activate this predisposition, causing depression. In addition, you may have no genetic predisposition and still become clinically depressed. Depression can be caused by many factors such as:

- loss of a significant relationship
- death of a family member or friend
- physical or sexual abuse or assault
- serious illness or health problems
- experiencing numerous setbacks and problems simultaneously

Having a support system, effective coping strategies, and a positive attributional style can make the difference between succumbing to depression or being protected during stressful and adverse times in our lives.

There are many ways to treat depression, but the most efficacious treatment approach is a combination of counseling and medication. Counseling can help people develop effective and healthy coping skills, learn stress management strategies, focus on developing an optimistic explanatory style, and improve relationships and social skills. Medication, such as antidepressants, have been found to be very helpful in the treatment of depression, as they act to increase the serotonin or norepinephrine levels to a normal and functional range. Some of the newer antidepressants are Prozac, Paxil, Zoloft, Serzone, Remeron, Effexor, and Lexapro. It takes 4 to 6 weeks for an

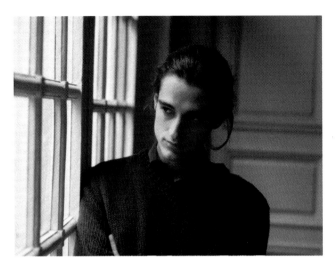

People who suffer from depression tend to feel hopeless and unmotivated, and withdraw from others, which then increases their feelings of being trapped and stuck.

antidepressant to be fully effective, and there may be side effects such as dry mouth, decreased sexual drive, drowsiness, constipation, or diarrhea. Most of these side effects will disappear after 2 weeks of taking the medication. Interestingly, while the percentage of people taking antidepressants has increased from 37% to 75% of people with depression, those receiving psychotherapy has declined from 71% to 60%.[40] The use of antidepressants for youths 2 to 19 years of age has increased three to fivefold over the past 7 years.[41] Most people take an antidepressant for 6 months to a year and then are able to taper off the medication without a reoccurrence of symptoms. If you have had three separate episodes of depression, recovering from each episode and then relapsing, this can be a sign that your depression has a biological basis and an indication that you may need to continue taking an antidepressant medication long term.

Herbal supplements, such as St. John's Wort, have also been touted as a treatment for depression, although there is some debate as to how effective they truly are. Most clinicians agree that St. John's Wort can be somewhat effective in alleviating mild depression, but not for more moderate or severe types of depression. As is the case with all herbal supplements, St. John's Wort is not subject to FDA approval nor has it been put through the clinical trials prescription medication has undergone to establish its therapeutic dose and efficacy. However, the National Institute of Mental Health, the National Center for Complementary and Alternative Medicine, and the Office of Dietary Supplements are currently conducting a $4 million collaborative 4-year study to investigate the safety and effectiveness of St. John's Wort, and so more definitive information will be available in the near future.

Exercise and activity level also play a significant role in alleviating and insulating people from depression. Again it seems that the endorphin levels and effects on brain chemistry and hormonal levels are part of the explanation for why this is a powerful antidote for depression.[42]

Electroconvulsive therapy (ECT) is another form of treatment for depression, with 100,000 Americans receiving this treatment each year. While ECT has fallen out of favor in the past 25 years (due in part to depictions of it in films such as *One Flew over the Cuckoo's Nest*), it has recently enjoyed a resurgence in popularity. The procedure involves delivering a 90-volt burst of electricity, equal to the electricity in a 40-watt light bulb, for about a minute to the brain causing a grand mal seizure. The patient is under anesthesia and receives muscle relaxants prior to administering the shock, and the heart rate and oxygen level are constantly monitored during the treatment. Most patients receive three ECT treatments each week, for a total of six to twelve sessions. Proponents of ECT claim that it is an effective treatment for depression when no other antidepressant or treatment regime has worked. Critics of ECT say that it causes brain damage, and memory loss, and that the decrease in depressive symptoms are only temporary.[43] Although ECT has been used for the past 60 years, no one knows exactly how it works or why it alleviates depression.

TALKING POINTS Have you ever felt depressed? If so, what did you do to cope with these feelings? What did you do that worked and/or didn't help you to feel better?

Seasonal Affective Disorder

In addition to the types of depression just described, some people may be especially vulnerable to depression on a seasonal basis. **Seasonal Affective Disorder (SAD)** is a form of depression that develops in relation to the changes in the seasons. While most people with SAD begin to feel increasing depressed in October and report their depression lifts in March or April, about one in six SAD sufferers experience Summer SAD, beginning in May or June and ending in the fall months. Twice as many women as men are affected with SAD.[47]

Key Terms

seasonal affective disorder (SAD) a form of depression that develops in relation to the changes in the seasons.

SAD seem to be related to environmental factors such as the amount of light, temperature, and situational stressors. Weight gain, fatigue, increased sleep, diminished sex drive, and mood swings are some of the symptoms of Winter SAD, while agitation, loss of appetite, insomnia, and increased suicidal thoughts are characteristic of Summer SAD. Seasonal depression in the winter seems linked to increases in the production of melatonin, a chemical that helps set the brain's daily rhythm, set off by the decrease in light. Antidepressants, counseling, and light therapy have been used to treat SAD. Light therapy for Winter SAD involves sitting in front of a white fluorescent bulb, housed in a plastic diffusing screen, for 20 to 90 minutes each day so that the light is falling on your eyes.[44] For Summer SAD, which tends to occur in hotter locales, individuals are instructed to travel to cooler climates, to swim in cool water, and to stay in darkened, air-conditioned rooms.

Postpartum Depression

Another unique form of depression is **postpartum depression,** a more severe kind of depression from the commonly experienced "baby blues" that many women feel following childbirth. Postpartum depression occurs in one out of eight mothers who give birth and can last from a few days to over a year, but most commonly lasts for 2 weeks. Postpartum depression is characterized by fatigue, frequent crying, emotional withdrawal, anxiety, and other symptoms associated with depression. This should be differentiated from postpartum psychosis, which is marked by hallucinations and delusions. Sometimes people with postpartum depression have been associated with psychotic behavior, as was the situation with the much publicized case of Andrea Yates who in 2002 drowned her five children, ages 6 months to 7 years. Reportedly, Yates suffered from postpartum depression after the birth of her fourth child, and with the birth of her fifth child along with the death of her own father, became increasingly depressed and psychotic.

Suicide

Suicide is the third leading cause of death for young adults 15 to 24 years old and the eleventh leading cause of all deaths in the United States. Men commit suicide four times more often than women do, and 72% of all suicides are committed by white men. Suicide occurs most often among Americans age 65 and older.[48] However, women are three times more likely than men to attempt suicide. Men tend to employ more lethal methods such as using firearms, hanging, or jumping from high places, while women tend to use methods of suicide such as overdosing with pills or cutting their wrists, which are slower methods and allow more time for medical attention. Twice as many Caucasians complete suicide as African Americans, with Asian Americans being one of the lowest risk groups in terms of ethnicity. The suicide rate for the Hispanic population is lower than for Caucasians but higher than for African Americans.

Key Terms

postpartum depression a form of depression that affects women in the weeks and months following childbirth.

Why do people attempt or commit suicide? The majority of suicidal people have depressive disorders and feel helpless and powerless over their lives. They say things like "I just wanted the pain to stop" and don't see any other options available to them. There are some risk factors associated with suicidal behavior such as having:

- little to no support system
- made previous suicide attempts
- a family history of mental illness, including substance abuse
- a family history of suicide
- problems with drugs or alcohol
- possession of a firearm
- been exposed to the suicidal behavior of others, including through the media

It is estimated that there are 300,000 suicide attempts made each year in the United States, or one every 2 minutes. Some people say that suicidal gestures or threats are a "cry for attention" or a "cry for help" and think it is better to ignore the person. But left ignored, the person may go ahead and take the next step to attempt suicide because no one seems to care. It is always best to take any threats or talk about suicide seriously and act accordingly. What should you do if a friend or family member talks to you about thoughts of suicide? See the Star Box for the Do's and Don'ts of Suicide Intervention.

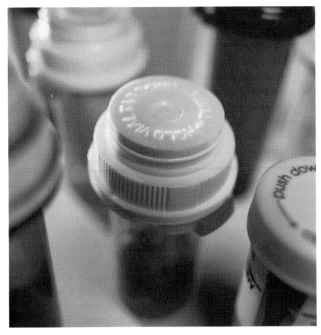

Women tend to overdose on pills as a method of suicide while men tend to use more lethal means such as firearms, hanging, or jumping from high places.

Bipolar Disorder

Another important mood disorder is **bipolar disorder,** a condition that was previously known as manic depression. The term *bipolar* refers to the extreme mood swings individuals with this disorder experience, from feeling euphoric, energetic, and reckless to feeling depressed, powerless, and listless. An estimated 2.3 million Americans suffer from bipolar disorder, with men and women equally likely to develop this condition. It is the least common of the mood disorders. The average age of onset for the first manic episode typically occurs in the early twenties. This change in mood or "mood swing" can last for hours, days, weeks, or months. Bipolar disorder is found across all ages, races, ethnic groups, and social classes. When one parent has bipolar disorder, the risk to each child is estimated to be 15 to 30%, when both parents have bipolar disorder, the risk increases to 50 to 75%.[35]

We have already described depression a great deal in the previous section. Bipolar disorder involves both having depressive periods and manic episodes. **Mania** is characterized by the following:

- Excessive energy, needing little sleep, being highly excitable
- Racing thoughts, feeling as though your mind is going 50 mph
- Rapid speech, changing from topic to topic quickly in conversation
- Easily irritated and distracted
- Impulsive and reckless in behavior: for example, going on spending sprees, increased involvement in sexual activity and drug and alcohol use
- Trying to do too much, feeling as though you can accomplish a great deal

Many people with bipolar disorder will tell you that they enjoy the "highs" but dread the lows. However, manic behavior can become very destructive because when people are in a manic phase, they can create enormous credit card debt, abuse drugs and alcohol, drive recklessly, and often feel invincible. They stay up all night and feel very little need for rest or food and eventually their bodies can't

---

Key Terms

bipolar disorder a mood disorder characterized by alternating episodes of depression and mania.

mania an extremely excitable state characterized by excessive energy, racing thoughts, impulsive and/or reckless behavior, irritability, and being prone to distraction.

The Do's and Don'ts of Suicide Intervention

Don't . . .

1. Avoid talking about suicide or dancing around the topic. Talking about suicide doesn't upset people more. In fact, often people who are thinking about killing themselves say it is a relief to talk about it and it helps them to let go of this idea, not pursue it further.

2. Be judgmental or argumentative. Now is not the time to debate the morality of suicide—you will lose the debate and possibly the person.

3. Assume that the person is not serious. Saying "You're not serious" or "You don't mean that" may inadvertently encourage the person to show you how serious she or he truly is.

4. Argue that things aren't that bad or people have it worse and they should be happy about their life. This can make people feel worse about themselves and guilty about their feelings of unhappiness.

5. Don't promise not to tell anyone. If you keep this promise and something happens to this person, how will you feel?

Do . . .

1. Remain calm and talk about the person's feelings of sadness and helplessness.

2. Offer support and assistance. Tell them they are not alone.

3. Encourage problem solving and taking positive steps.

4. Emphasize the temporary nature of the problem. Suicide is a permanent solution to a temporary problem.

5. Seek help and don't try to handle this problem on your own. This might involve the person's family, religious advisor, friends, and teachers, or calling a mental health agency for consultation.

6. Make a no-suicide contract. Ask the person to promise not to hurt or kill him/herself.

7. If possible, stay with the person until you can get further assistance.

---

function and they collapse. Mood stabilizers such as Lithium, Lithobid, and anticonvulsant medications, such as Depakote, Neurontin, Topomax, and Lamictal, have been used to treat bipolar disorder along with psychotherapy.

Anxiety Disorders

Bill, a very talented and bright twenty-six year old, has a very promising career as an executive in a large accounting firm. However he is in jeopardy of losing his job because of his absenteeism and tardiness. It can take him hours to get to work even though he lives 15 minutes away, and sometimes he doesn't go to work even though he is in the car and ready to go. Bill has a routine in the morning that involves checking the windows, doors, iron, stove, and garage door five times to ensure that things are secure and safe. Sometimes he drives away and then returns to the house to check again. He feels a need to turn the handles on doors five times, and if he loses track, he starts all over again.

Susan has been having such severe panic attacks in the car while driving to work that she has needed to pull over. Her heart races, her breathing is labored, and she sometimes feels as though she is having a heart attack and might die. She is frightened of being in the car alone and having an attack and not being able to get help or having a car accident. She is beginning to be afraid to leave her house and feels safer at home. She has declined invitations to go out with her friends and on vacations and only goes out when absolutely necessary. She feels as though she is losing control of her life.

John worries constantly about what other people think of him. When he passes a group of people who are laughing, he assumes that they are laughing at him. He has trouble having conversations with people because he believes whatever he says will sound "stupid" and people will not like him. He also plays conversations over and over in his head when he is trying to go to sleep, thinking about what he should have said and worrying about how people are judging him.

Bill, Susan, and John are all suffering from *anxiety disorders.* While everyone tends to feel nervous or worry about something at some point in their lives, people with anxiety disorders feel anxious most, if not all, of the time. They also feel powerless to alleviate their anxiety, and tend to worry about becoming anxious, so their anxiety causes them even greater anxiety. Anxiety is related to fear and is part of daily life. Some anxiety can even be helpful and motivating at times. Anxiety is a physiological, adaptive response to danger or potential threat and can enhance performance and keep us out of harm's way. In Chapter 3, Managing Stress, we will discuss the flight or fight response and how the stress response is related to anxiety. Anxiety disorders are differentiated from daily stress as being:

1. intense, often debilitating, in which people sometimes think they are going to die

2. long lasting, persisting after the danger or stressful event has passed

3. dysfunctional, causing significant interference in daily functioning

Anxiety disorders include generalized anxiety disorder, obsessive-compulsive disorder (such as Bill's problem), post-traumatic stress disorder, panic disorder (which describes Susan's symptoms), and phobias such as the social phobia John suffered from in the example above.[46] Approximately 19 million Americans have an anxiety disorder, and women are twice as likely as men to suffer from panic disorder, post-traumatic stress disorder, generalized anxiety disorder, agoraphobia, and specific phobias. There are no gender differences with obsessive-compulsive disorder or social phobia.[47]

Generalized Anxiety Disorder (GAD)

Generalized Anxiety Disorder (GAD) involves experiencing anxiety for at least 6 months in which the intensity and frequency of the worry is excessive and out of proportion to the situation. GAD can be distinguished from specific phobias in which people feel worried about a par-

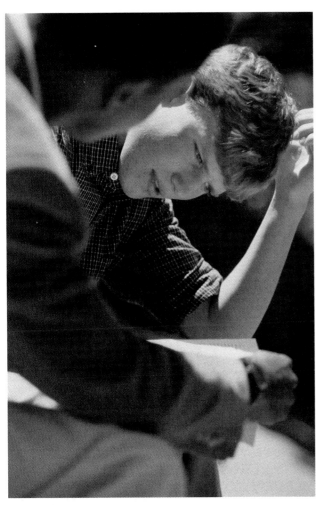

Anxiety is one of the three most frequent problems students report experiencing during college.

ticular situation or stimulus. An individual with GAD appears to worry all the time about everything, thinks the worst, and overreacts to situations. Restlessness, fatigue, irritability, difficulty concentrating, muscle tension, and trouble sleeping are some of the symptoms associated with GAD. Physical symptoms include excessive sweating, nausea, diarrhea, being easily startled, shortness of breath, racing heart, and feeling shaky.[35] Because people with GAD are tense and anxious much of the time, they experience impairment in their relationships, work performance, and general functioning. Most people with GAD say that they are afraid of losing control, of failing, of rejection or abandonment, and death or disease. In addition, they feel unable to cope with their fears and thus out of control in managing their anxiety.

Panic Disorder

Shortness of breath, pounding heart, dizziness, trembling, sweating, nausea, tingling in hands and feet, hot and cold flashes, chest pain, and a feeling of choking are the symptoms of **Panic Disorder,** exemplified by Susan's situation. Many panic disorder sufferers feel as though they are going to die, are losing control or going crazy which of course makes them feel more anxious and panicked. Frequently, these individuals go to the emergency room thinking they are having a heart attack. This can seemingly occur out of the blue or because of some trigger, and can last for a few minutes or for hours. Because people become fearful of having a panic attack and don't know when the next attack might occur, they may develop **agoraphobia.** Agoraphobia is a fear of being in situations in which you can't escape or get help if you suddenly had a panic attack, and avoiding being in these situations or places.[46]

Panic disorder is often treated with antidepressant medications such as imipramine and tranquilizers such as

---

Key Terms

generalized anxiety disorder (GAD) an anxiety disorder that involves experiencing intense and nonspecific anxiety for at least 6 months, in which the intensity and frequency of worry is excessive and out of proportion to the situation.

panic disorder an anxiety disorder characterized by panic attacks, in which individuals experience severe physical symptoms; these episodes can seemingly occur "out of the blue" or because of some trigger, and can last for a few minutes or for hours.

agoraphobia a fear of being in situations from which there is no escape or where help would be unavailable should an emergency arise; often associated with panic disorder.

Xanax. Counseling can help individuals learn to recognize when a panic attack may be starting and to minimize and ward if off before it becomes a full blown attack, using relaxation and stress management exercises, as well as positive self statements such as "I'm not going to die. I can get through this."

Obsessive-Compulsive Disorder (OCD)

Obsessive-compulsive disorder, or OCD (such as Bill's), affects 3 million Americans and symptoms often begin during childhood or adolescence.[48] OCD involves more than just being neat and orderly: symptoms include having recurring thoughts and behaviors that seem irrational and out of control, and which can be extremely time consuming. Obsessions are intrusive thoughts, images, or impulses causing a great deal of distress. Most people recognize that their obsessions are ungrounded and senseless but can't seem to push them out of their minds. Obsessions may occur by themselves without being attached to compulsive behavior, but compulsions are associated with 25% of those with obsessive thoughts.[46] Compulsions refer to repetitive behaviors aimed at reducing anxiety or stress that is associated with the obsessive thoughts, such as checking that the iron is off, praying for your parent's good health, or washing your hands. Some compulsions seem relevant to a particular fear (such as handwashing out of a fear of germs), but others might seem unrelated—for example, having to do something an odd number of times in order that your parents will not come to any harm. The most common compulsions are washing, checking, and counting.[35]

Even though the goal of compulsive behavior is to alleviate distress brought about by obsessions, it is in itself a source of shame and anxiety. Individuals with OCD, like Bill in the earlier example, realize that their behavior is excessive and unreasonable but are unable to resist engaging in this behavior. This can cause great distress in their relationships, problems completing their work, and getting to places on time. In addition, once they have performed the compulsive behavior, their anxiety is only temporarily alleviated and then the obsessive thoughts return and the cycle continues.

Treatment for OCD includes antidepressant medication such as Prozac and also counseling. Counseling might involve response prevention strategies such as exposing the individual to the situations that trigger the obsessive thoughts and then preventing the person from engaging in the compulsive behaviors to break this vicious cycle. For example, the individual might be exposed to a dirty environment and then allowed to wash his or her hands only once.

Phobias

John is suffering from one of the most common anxiety disorders, **social phobia,** previously called social anxiety disorder.[46] Social phobia refers to feelings of extreme dread and embarrassment in situations in which public speaking or social interaction is involved because the person worries she/he will be seen as stupid, clumsy, or lacking in some way. The most common social phobia is fear of public speaking. Commonly called stage fright, it is the most common of all phobias; many successful actors and performers suffer from this disorder, including actor Donny Osmond, gold medallist swimmer Susie O'Neill, and actresses Kim Basinger and Barbara Streisand.

Social phobia differs from another disorder called **Specific Phobia** in which the person has a strong fear and avoids one particular situation or object such as snakes, high places, or airplanes. Specific phobias affect 10 percent of the population and often begin as childhood fears that were never outgrown.[46] Sometimes a phobic reaction develops as a result of a traumatic event such as an accident, a particularly difficult visit to the doctor or dentist, or from an illness. Specific phobias tend to be easily treated with counseling in which the individual learns relaxation techniques and then is gradually exposed, first in imagery, then in real life situations, to the feared situation.

Post-Traumatic Stress Disorder (PTSD)

The essential feature of **post-traumatic stress disorder** is the development of symptoms following exposure to an extreme stressor involving threat of death or serious

Key Terms

obsessive-compulsive disorder an anxiety disorder characterized by obsessions—intrusive thoughts, images, or impulses causing a great deal of distress—and compulsions—repetitive behaviors aimed at reducing anxiety or stress that is associated with the obsessive thoughts.

social phobia a phobia characterized by feelings of extreme dread and embarrassment in situations in which public speaking or social interaction is involved.

specific phobia an excessive and unreasonable fear about a particular situation or object that causes anxiety and distress and interferes with a person's functioning.

post-traumatic stress disorder an anxiety disorder that sometimes develops following exposure to an extreme stressor involving threat of death or serious injury; symptoms include recurrent and distressing thoughts or nightmares about the event, emotional numbness, feelings of detachment, sleep disturbance, hypervigilance and irritability.

injury. This threat may be directly experienced or from witnessing an event that is life threatening and dangerous.[35] This disorder was first identified during World War I when soldiers were observed to be suffering from anxiety, flashbacks, and nightmares. They were also easily startled, had angry outbursts, experienced difficulty concentrating, and were hypervigilant. Post-traumatic stress can be the result of not only combat, but any trauma that produces intense fear, horror, terror, and feelings of helplessness, such as sexual assault; natural disasters like an earthquake or tornado; a car accident; life-threatening illness; or a mugging. The symptoms associated with PTSD are:

- Recurrent and distressing thoughts about the event
- Nightmares about the event
- Flashbacks—feeling as though one is reliving the event
- Emotional numbness, feeling detached from oneself and one's feelings
- Avoidance of anything that reminds one of the event
- Detachment from others
- Difficulty expressing one's feelings
- Sleep disturbance
- Irritability, angry outbursts
- Being easily startled
- Difficulty concentrating
- Hypervigilence—extreme awareness of one's environment

People with PTSD tend to be highly anxious and depressed, have problems with their relationships with others, have difficulty trusting other people, and may restrict their activities because of their fearfulness. It is also not uncommon to experience panic attacks when exposed to something that triggers a memory of the trauma. Again counseling to express and resolve the feelings, losses, and negative thoughts associated with the trauma as well as antidepressant medications or tranquilizers are beneficial in treating PTSD.

Schizophrenia

Schizophrenia is one of the most severe mental disorders as it is characterized by profound distortions in one's thought processes, emotions, perceptions, and behavior. People with schizophrenia experience hallucinations (seeing things that are not there, hearing voices), delusions (believing that you are Jesus, the CIA is after you, or that radio waves are controlling your mind), and disorganized thinking (wearing multiple coats, scarves, and gloves on a warm day, shouting and swearing at passersby, maintaining a rigid posture and not moving for hours). There are several types of schizophrenia: paranoid, disorganized,

catatonic, and undifferentiated. This disabling illness affects 1 percent of the U.S. population, and symptoms typically surface in people in their late teens and early twenties. Men and women are equally likely to develop schizophrenia, and it seems to run in families. The movie *A Beautiful Mind* gives a glimpse into the life of one schizophrenic, John Nash, and his recovery.

Schizophrenia is often confused with multiple personality disorder, which is an entirely separate and distinct mental illness. While people with multiple personality disorder display two or more distinct identities or personalities that take control of the person's life, people with schizophrenia do not have multiple, separate, enduring personalities.

While there is no cure for schizophrenia, there are antipsychotic medications, such as Seroquel, Risperidone, Zyprexa, Ability, and Geodon, that can effectively treat this illness and enable people to live functional, satisfying lives. Psychotherapy can be helpful in developing problem-solving approaches, in addition to identifying stressors, triggers, and early detection of a psychotic episode. Unfortunately, some people with schizophrenia are unable to recognize that they are delusional or irrational and so do not get treatment or take their medications on a regular basis.

Health Providers Involved in the Treatment of Psychological Disorders

As in other areas of health care, a variety of practitioners, each of whom has unique training and uses specific therapies, treat and manage the mental health conditions just described.

Psychiatrists

A **psychiatrist** is a health care provider with a medical degree and has specialized in the field of psychiatry. Since psychiatrists are medical doctors, they may prescribe

---

Key Terms

schizophrenia one of the most severe mental disorders, characterized by profound distortions in one's thought processes, emotions, perceptions, and behavior; symptoms may include hallucinations, delusions, disorganized thinking, and/or maintaining a rigid posture and not moving for hours.

psychiatrist a medical doctor with specialized training in the diagnosis and treatment of psychological disorders through the use of biological and medical interventions.

drugs and perform medical procedures such as electroshock therapy. Psychiatrists tend to treat psychological disorders through medical management and take a biological approach to addressing psychological disorders. They tend to give less focus to talking about one's problems, and treat more severely and chronically ill patients.

Psychologists

A **psychologist** is a mental health care provider whose educational background includes a doctoral level degree in the field of counseling or clinical psychology. Psychologists practice general psychology and their clients range from those with severe pathology to those with more temporary problems of living. There is a variety of subspecialties such as children and adolescents, neurological disorders and assessments, psychological evaluations and assessments, forensic psychology, industrial psychology, health psychology, career counseling, and marriage counseling. Until recently, one difference between psychiatrists and psychologists was that psychologists did not have prescription privileges and so couldn't use drug therapies in their treatment interventions. However, the lines are beginning to blur, as there has been a push in many states for legislation that would allow psychologists to prescribe psychiatric medicines; such legislation exists in New Mexico already. In general, psychologists treat psychological disorders using behavior therapy, problem-solving approaches and talk therapy that focuses on changing the client's attitudes, behavior, affect, and cognitions. A psychologist must be licensed in the state in which s/he practices, and this typically requires passing a national certification examination and having a specific number of hours practicing psychology under the supervision of a licensed psychologist.

Counselors

Counselors typically have a master's degree in counseling or clinical psychology. People with master's degrees usually work in group counseling practices, clinics, and schools and may specialize in areas such as substance abuse, divorce recovery, vocational rehabilitation, school counseling, marriage and family therapy, sexual assault, domestic violence, and employee assistance programs. In some states people with master's degrees must be supervised by a licensed doctoral level psychologist. However, there is a relatively new trend in licensure laws allowing masters level counselors to become licensed as professional mental health counselors. This has been passed in forty states to date. These licensing laws establish a standard of care and regulate the practice of counseling so that master's counselors can practice without being supervised by a psychologist.

Social Workers

Social workers have a master's degree in social work, and must be licensed to use the title social worker. While psychologists, mental health counselors, and psychiatrists

Key Terms

psychologist a doctoral level practitioner with specialized training in the diagnosis and treatment of psychological disorders through the use of psychotherapy.

social worker a professional with a master's degree in social work; social workers provide both mental health and social services to the community and are the largest group of professional to provide psychological services.

A New Problem . . . Internet Addiction

The Internet has changed the way we work, socialize, and educate ourselves. While the Internet has provided connections that otherwise could not be made very easily with people all around the world, it has also created unique psychological problems for some individuals. There is some question about the psychological implications the Internet may be having on our society as we are moving from a world in which we used to know our neighbors and interact with people face to face to developing serious and deep relationships with people from a distance. Marriages have broken up, affairs have taken place, and teenagers have been kidnapped by people they met over the Internet. In fact, one teenager was encouraged to overdose on drugs by his Internet friends and died while communicating over the Net to this group.

There is a feeling of anonymity that is created by talking on the Web. You can be who you want to be, reveal as much or as little as you want, and not be judged by your appearance. Of course, this also means people can be deceitful and dishonest about who they are and what they want from you. In addition, there is a blending of home and work and increased solitude. Studies show that greater use of the Internet is associated with less communication among family members, decreased socializing with local friends, and increased depression and loneliness.[50] One study showed that using the Internet more than 5 hours a week resulted in less time with friends, family, and social activities.[51]

In fact, there is such concern about the potential adverse effects of spending too much time on the Internet that there are mental health professionals that propose adding "Internet addiction" as a diagnosable mental disorder. How can you tell if you are addicted? Here are some warning signs:

1. Preoccupation with the Internet—planning and thinking about the next time you can get online.
2. Increased use of the Internet over time.
3. Repeatedly making unsuccessful attempts to curtail your use of the Internet.
4. Feeling irritable, restless, and moody when you attempt to cut down your use of the Internet or are prevented from getting online when you would like.
5. Unaware of how much time you are spending on the Internet, staying online longer than you originally intended.
6. Lying to family members and friends about your use of the Internet.
7. Jeopardizing your job or risking losing a relationship because of the time you are spending on the Web.
8. Using the Internet as a way of escaping from problems and coping with depression.
9. Declining invitations to spend time with family and friends because you would rather be online.

Of course, answering "yes" to one of these questions does not indicate a concern. However, if you can answer "yes" to more than half of these questions, then you may want to examine your use of the Internet. Here are some ways you can avoid being an Internet addict:

- Decide how much time you want to spend on the Internet before you get online and set an alarm for that time. Stick to that time allotment.
- Take frequent breaks. Spend at least 5 minutes out of every hour or 15 to 20 minutes of every 3 hours on unwired activity. Take a walk, stretch your body, eat a snack, or listen to music.
- Visit the Net with a purpose and a strategy. Surfing the Web aimlessly can lead to being online for longer than you anticipated.
- Interact with people in a nonwired world. Make a commitment to socially interact at least once a day with someone who is not online.
- Don't let the Internet be the center of your existence or the most important, enjoyable part of your day. Remind yourself of your life goals, values, and interests. What are other ways to achieve these goals besides via the Web?[52]

tend to focus on the individual's problems, social workers look at the bigger picture and take into consideration the environment, community, and system the individual is living in. Social workers provide both mental health and social services to the community and are the largest group of professionals to provide psychological services.

Social workers typically consult and counsel clients and arrange for services that can help them. Often, they refer clients to specialists in services such as debt counseling, childcare or eldercare, public assistance, or alcohol or drug rehabilitation. Social workers then follow through with the client to assure that services are help-

ful and that clients make proper use of the services offered. Social workers may review eligibility requirements, visit clients on a regular basis, and provide support during crises.[49]

Approaches in Treating Psychological Disorders

There are over 200 approaches to treating psychological disorders and new variations and models are continuing to develop. Most approaches have their foundations based upon a few basic therapeutic models, which we will look at in the section that follows. These therapies can be utilized with individuals, families, or couples.

Dynamic Therapy

Dynamic therapy is based upon the belief that effective treatment must focus on the psychological forces underlying the individual's problems. They view these forces as beginning in early childhood and having great significance on later behavior and personality development. Because this type of therapy focuses on the person's childhood years to uncover the source of the current problem, it usually is a long-term, intensive, and expensive form of therapy that many insurance companies refuse to cover.

Humanistic Therapy

Humanistic treatment approaches are based on the belief that people, left to their own devices, will naturally grow in positive and constructive ways. The job of the therapist is to help clients unearth their natural potential and gain greater self-awareness and self-acceptance. **Humanistic therapy** has its roots in Carl Rogers's "client-centered therapy" and in Abraham Maslow's hierarchy of needs. In client-centered therapy, the client, not the therapist, is responsible for behavior change. The task of the therapist is to facilitate in a nondirective manner the process of helping individuals resolve their problems.[7] Rogers further believed that when people accept themselves, they will also accept other people.

Behavior Therapy

Behavior therapy focuses not on one's thoughts or feelings but on behavior modification. Thus the goal of treatment is not to uncover the reasons underlying the problems an individual is having but to eliminate the symptoms and change behavior. Insight, awareness, and past history are unimportant in behavior therapy. The idea is that behavior has been learned and so can be unlearned and different, more adaptive behavior can be taught. This can be especially effective for the treatment of anxiety such as phobias, panic disorder, and anxiety.

Cognitive-Behavioral Therapy

Cognitive-behavioral therapy focuses on changing an individual's thoughts or cognitive patterns in order to change his or her behavior and emotional state. Pioneered by psychologists Aaron Beck and Albert Ellis in the 1960s, cognitive therapy assumes that maladaptive behaviors and disturbed mood or emotions are the result of inappropriate or irrational thinking patterns. As with behavior therapy, cognitive-behavioral therapy does not explore why someone is thinking or behaving in a particular way, nor does it look at the client's past history. Instead, cogni-

tive therapists attempt to make the client aware of distorted thought patterns and change them through strategies such as cognitive restructuring, cognitive reframing, challenging irrational beliefs, and thought stopping. This type of treatment has been especially effective in treating obsessive-compulsive disorder, eating disorders, anxiety disorders, and mood disorders. The learned optimism paradigm discussed earlier in this chapter was also based on cognitive-behavioral concepts.

Solution-Focused Therapy

Solution-focused therapy is a goal-oriented therapeutic approach that helps clients change by looking for solutions rather than dwelling on problems. Similar to cognitive-behavioral therapy, attention is directed towards the present and the future, rather than on the past. Solution-focused therapists have confidence in the client and focus on the strength and resources within the individual. Clients are encouraged to envision a future in which their problems are no longer a dominant force in their lives, and in partnership with the therapist, treatment interventions are formulated in an effort to reach that goal.

Couples and Family Therapy

Couples counseling and family therapy includes premarital counseling, marital therapy, conflict mediation, and divorce counseling. Communication skills, assertiveness

---

Key Terms

dynamic therapy an intensive therapy based upon the belief that effective treatment must focus on the psychological forces underlying the individual's problems.

humanistic therapy a treatment approach based on the belief that people, left to their own devices, will naturally grow in positive and constructive ways.

behavior therapy a behavior modification therapy based upon the learning principles of reinforcement therapy, stimulus-response, and conditioning responses to change behavior.

cognitive-behavioral therapy an action-oriented form of therapy that assumes that maladaptive, or faulty, thinking patterns cause maladaptive behavior and negative emotions; treatment focuses on changing an individual's thoughts or cognitive patterns in order to change his or her behavior and emotional state.

solution-focused therapy a goal-oriented approach that helps clients change by looking for solutions rather than dwelling on problems.

skills, sexual disorders, intimacy and commitment, anger management, step-parenting, and blended families are some of the psychological issues that are typically addressed by these therapies.

Group Therapy

Group therapy usually is comprised of five to eight people who meet regularly with a therapist to focus on the psychological problems with which they are struggling. Often the group members share common problems such as eating disorders, childhood sexual abuse, substance abuse, or divorce recovery, and so they can support each other and understand each other's experiences. The group members can help and learn from each other and don't feel so alone in their problems. Group therapy is very beneficial in breaking your sense of isolation and challenging the belief that you are the only one having this type of problem. The idea behind group therapy is that you can learn new ways of behaving and practice these skills and behaviors in a safe, supportive atmosphere. In fact, the research strongly suggests that group therapy can be superior to individual therapy or at least is a necessary next step after individual therapy for particular psychological problems, such as sexual abuse, eating disorders, substance abuse, and interpersonal relationship problems.

 TALKING POINTS How do you think change occurs in people or yourself? What form of treatment described fits best with your perceptions of problems and behavior change?

Psychological Health: A Final Thought

As you can see, psychological health involves how your emotions, thoughts, and behavior interplay with each other and with the world around you. There is an important mind–body connection in terms of your psychological health having a significant impact on your physical health and vice versa. Psychological health is not just the absence of mental illness, and there is a range or continuum of psychological health. Possessing a positive self-concept, developing high self-esteem, and cultivating an optimistic attitude towards life can promote psychological health and enhance relationships with others. While heredity plays a role in the development of personality and psychological health, environmental factors and stressors seem to have an equally important role. As people age and come across developmental milestones, they encounter new challenges, obstacles, and resources in continuing to maintain their psychological health.

Taking Charge of Your Health

Assess how effective and healthy your style of communication is by considering the following questions:

- Do you know the difference between passive, aggressive, and assertive behavior?
- Do you use assertive language such as "I" statements rather than "you" statements?
- Do you have assertive body language such as making eye contact and keeping an open body posture without crossing your arms in front of you?
- Are you aware of your nonverbal communication?
- Are you aware of the volume and tone of your voice and the message you might be conveying?

- Do you acknowledge the other person's feelings and point of view before stating your own?
- Do you feel comfortable saying "no" to requests?
- Do you feel comfortable asking for someone's help, disagreeing with someone, or giving your opinion about something?

Having a positive and effective communication style is an important aspect of psychological health and can have a significant impact on your relationships, success at work, and your self-worth. Learn to be more optimistic in your attitude and communication by considering the characteristics of an optimist on page 40.

Summary

- There is a mind–body connection in which biological, psychological, and social factors interact to influence health or illness. This is referred to as the biopsychological model.

- Psychological health has also been associated with developing and maintaining a positive self-concept, positive self-esteem, and emotional intelligence.

- Psychologically healthy people display a wide range of emotions.
- There is a continuum for self-esteem, and people can enhance their self-esteem through the use of several effective techniques.
- Personality is generally defined as a specific set of consistent patterns of behavior and traits that helps to identify and characterize an individual. Personality is comprised of thoughts, feelings, behaviors, motivation, instincts and temperament.
- People with overall high levels of emotional intelligence tend to take on leadership roles, are confident and assertive, express their feelings directly and appropriately, feel good about themselves, are outgoing, and adapt well to stress.
- Two factors, nature and nurture, influence the shaping of personality. Nature refers to the innate factors we are born with that genetically determine our personality traits while nurture is the effect that the environment, people, and external factors have on our personality.
- Maintaining a sense of humor is a key to psychological health and well-being.
- Nonverbal communication is what is communicated by your facial expression, body posture, tone of voice, and movements.
- Maslow's theory is a positive, optimistic theory of human behavior. He believed that people are motivated to grow and fulfill their potential, referring to this phenomenon as self-actualization.

- People with spiritual health seek meaning and purpose in their lives and have a deep appreciation for a sense of unity and community.
- Having a positive interpretation of life's events, particularly how you cope with adversity, can make a significant difference in terms of your health and academic and work performance, as well as how long you will live.
- Clinical depression can range from mild to severe and can result in significant impairment in functioning.
- The majority of suicidal people have depressive disorders and feel helpless and powerless over their lives. It is always best to take any threats or talk about suicide seriously and act accordingly.
- Anxiety disorders include generalized anxiety disorder, obsessive-compulsive disorder, post-traumatic stress disorder, panic disorder, and phobias.
- The most common phobia is fear of public speaking.
- Schizophrenia is one of the most severe mental disorders, as it is characterized by profound distortions in one's thought processes, emotions, perceptions, and behavior.
- A number of different health care professionals are trained to treat mental disorders, including psychiatrists, psychologists, social workers, and counselors.
- Treatments for psychological illnesses include dynamic, humanistic, behavioral, cognitive-behavioral, and solution-focused therapies, as well as drug therapies.

Review Questions

1. What is the name of the model that talks about a mind–body connection in which biological, psychological, and social factors interact to influence health or illness?
2. What are three factors that have been associated with psychological health?
3. What are the characteristics commonly demonstrated by psychologically healthy people?
4. What is the definition of self-esteem and how can self-esteem be enhanced?
5. What is the definition of personality and what is it comprised of?
6. What characterizes people with overall high levels of emotional intelligence?
7. What are the main two factors thought to influence the shaping of personality?
8. What relationship is there between humor and psychological health?
9. What is nonverbal communication?
10. Describe Maslow's theory of the hierarchy of needs.
11. What traits are associated with people with spiritual health?
12. How can having a positive interpretation of life's events make a significant difference in people's health?
13. How is clinical depression different from having the "blues"?
14. How should you respond to someone threatening or talking about committing suicide?
15. List five different types of anxiety disorders.
16. What is the most common phobia?
17. What disorder is considered one of the most severe mental disorders?
18. How does a psychiatrist differ from a psychologist?
19. Who are the largest group of professionals to provide psychological services?
20. What does dynamic therapy focus on in treating psychological problems?
21. Humanistic treatment approaches are based on what belief?

22. What therapy is based upon the learning principles of reinforcement therapy, stimulus-response, and conditioning responses to change behavior?
23. What therapy is an action-oriented form of therapy that assumes that maladaptive, or faulty,

thinking patterns cause maladaptive behavior and negative emotions?
24. What does solution-focused therapy focus on in the treatment of psychological disorders?

References

1. Papalia D and Olds S. *Psychology* (2nd edition). New York: McGraw-Hill, 1988.
2. Seligman M. *Learned Optimism.* New York: Simon & Schuster Inc., 1990.
3. McKay M and Fanning P. *Self-Esteem* (3rd edition). Oakland, CA: New Harbinger Publications, 1992.
4. Goleman D. *Emotional Intelligence.* New York: Bantam Books, 1997.
5. Wade C and Tavris C. *Psychology.* New York: Harper & Row Publishers, 1987.
6. Spear P, Penrod S, and Baker T. *Psychology: Perspectives on Behavior.* New York: John Wiley & Sons, 1988.
7. Kagan J and Segal J. *Psychology: An Introduction,* 6th edn. Orlando, Florida: Harcourt Brace Jovanovich Inc., 1988.
8. Thorson JA, et al. Psychological health and sense of humor. *Journal of Clinical Psychology* 53(6), 605–619, 1997.
9. Yoshino S, Fujimori J, Kohda M. Effects of mirthful laughter on neuroendocrine and immune systems in patients with rheumatoid arthritis. *Journal Rheumatol* 23(4), 793–794, 1996.
10. Castro B, Eshleman J, Shearer R. Using humor to reduce stress and improve relationships. *Seminar Nurse Management* 7(2), 90–92, 1999.
11. Berk LS, et al. Immune System Changes During Humor Associated Laughter. *Clinical Research* 39, 124a, 1991.
12. Cogan R, et al. Effects of Laughter and Relaxation on Discomfort Thresholds. *Journal of Behavioral Medicine,* 139–144, 1987.
13. Martin RA and Lefcourt HM. Sense of Humor as a Moderator Between Stressors and Moods. *Journal of Personality and Social Psychology* 45, 1313–1324, 1983.
14. Nezu A, Nezu C, and Blissett S. Sense of humor as a moderator of the relationship between stressful events and psychological distress. *Journal of Personality and Social Psychology* 54, 520–525, 1988.
15. Miller J. Jokes and joking: A serious laughing matter, in Durant J and Miller J, Eds. *Laughing Matters: A Serious Look at Humor.* Essex England: Longman Scientific and Technical, 1988.
16. Lefcourt HM and Martin RA. *Humor and Life Stress: Antidote to Adversity.* New York: Spring-Verlag, 1986.
17. Kuhn C. *Humor Techniques for Health Care Professionals,* Presentation at Ball Memorial Hospital, April 22, 1998.
18. Nair M. A Documentary, *The Laughing Clubs of India,* 2001.
19. Collier G. *Emotional Expression.* Hillsdale, NJ: Lawrence Erlbaum Associates, 1985.
20. Maslow A H. *The Farthest Reaches of Human Nature.* Peter Smith, 1983.
21. Maslow A H. *Motivation and Personality,* 2nd edn. New York: Van Nostrand, 1970.
22. Lindzey G, Thompson R, and Spring B. *Psychology,* 3rd edn. New York: Worth Publishers, Inc. 1988.
23. May R. Values, myths, and symbols. *American Journal of Psychiatry,* 132, 703–706, 1975.
24. Hemenway J E, et al. *Assessing Spiritual Needs: a Guide for caregivers.* Augsburg Press, 1993.
25. Ayele H, Mulligan T, Gheorghiu S, and Reyes-Ortiz C. Religious activity improves life satisfaction for some physicians and older patients. *Journal of the American Geriatrics Society* 43, 453–455, 1999.
26. Levin JS. Religion and health: Is there an association, is it valid and is it causal? *Social Science Medicine* 38(11), 1475–1482, 1994.
27. Seligman M. *Learned Optimism.* New York: Pocket Books, 1990.
28. Pavlov I P. *Conditioned Reflexes.* New York: Oxford University Press, 1927.
29. Hiroto D. Locus of control and learned helplessness. *Journal of Experiential Psychology* 102, 187–93, 1974.
30. Ellis A. *Reason and Emotion in Psychotherapy.* New York: Lyle Stuart, 1962.
31. Regier DA. Narrow WE, Rae DS, et al. The de facto mental and addictive disorders service system. Epidemiologic Catchment Area prospective 1-year prevalence rates of disorders and services. *Archives of General Psychiatry* 50(2): 85–94, 1993.
32. Narrow WE. *One-year prevalence of mental disorders, excluding substance use disorders, in the U.S.: NIMH ECA prospective data.* Population estimates based on U.S. Census estimated residential population age 18 and over on July 1, 1998, unpublished.
33. Murray CJL, Lopez AD, eds. *Summary: The global burden of disease: a comprehensive assessment of*

mortality and disability from diseases, injuries, and risk factors in 1990 and projected to 2020. Cambridge, MA: Published by the Harvard School of Public Health on behalf of the World Health Organization and the World Bank, Harvard University, 2003.

34. Lehrer J. Transcript from On Line News Hour. *Living with Mental Illness,* December 13, 1999.

35. American Psychiatric Association. *Diagnostic and Statistical Manual on Mental Disorders, fourth edition (DSM-IV-TR).* Washington, DC: American Psychiatric Press, 2000.

36. World Health Organization. *Mental Health,* 2003.

37. Dramatic Increases Seen in College Students' Mental Health Problems over Last 13 Years. *Journal of Professional Psychology: Research and Practice,* February 2003.

38. National Institute of Mental Health, 2003.

39. Peterson K. Resilience, talking can help kids beat depression, in *USA Today,* June 4, 2002.

40. Tanner L. With less stigma, more drugs, treatment for depression soars, in *USA Today,* January 9, 2002.

41. Presentation of the *American Psychological Association* in New Orleans, 2001.

42. Exercise Better than Drugs for Depression. *British Journal of Sports Medicine* 35, 114–117, April 2001.

43. Study puts spotlight on electroshock therapy, in *USA Today,* March 13, 2001.

44. Rosenthal NE. *Winter Blues.* New York: The Guilford Press, 1998.

45. Understanding Depression: A Special Health Report from *Harvard Medical School,* 2003.

46. Bourne E. *The Anxiety and Phobia Workbook.* Oakland CA: New Harbinger Publications Inc., 1995.

47. Robins L, Regier D, eds., *Psychiatric disorders in America: the Epidemiologic Catchment Area Study.* New York: *The Free Press,* 1991.

48. Narrow W, Raie D, and Regier D. NIMH epidemiology note: prevalence of anxiety disorder. *One year prevalence best estimates calculated from ECA and NCS data.* Population estimates based on U.S. Census estimated residential population age 18 to 54 on July 1, 1998.

49. Occupational Outlook Handout, U.S. Department of Labor Bureau of Labor Statistics, 2002–2003.

50. Kraut R, Patterson M, Lundmark V, Kiesler S, Mukopadyay T, and Scherlis W. Internet Paradox: A social technology that reduces social involvement and psychological well-being? *American Psychologist* 53(9), 1998.

51. Streitfeld D. Study finds heavy Internet users are isolated. *Washington Post,* February 16, 2000.

52. Goldstein D and Flory J. Best of the Net: *Online Guide Book Series.* New York: McGraw-Hill, Irwin Professional Publishing Inc. 1996.

As We Go to Press

When teenagers seem irritable, sullen or complain of unhappiness, it is often dismissed as a "passing phase" or a normal stage of development, such as the "rebellious teenage years." However, this may be a sign of something much more serious and potentially lethal. Having trouble sleeping, eating more or less than usual, moodiness, being critical of oneself and losing interest in things you normally like to do may be a sign of clinical depression. With suicide being the third leading cause of death for ten to twenty-year-olds, this is certainly a group that is at risk for depression. It is no wonder that the use of anti-depressants has dramatically increased for this age group, along with the FDA's nod of approval for use of Prozac to treat depression for children and adolescents. There is some debate if kids are more depressed today (as 8% of adolescents and 2% of children are clinically depressed), or if there is just a greater recognition of this problem. With the increased divorce rate, violence and rising social and academic pressures facing adolescents, it is no wonder that we are seeing more teenagers succumb to what was once thought of as an "adult disease."

The NIMH recently launched a major 12-city initiative called the "Treatment for Adolescents with Depression Study" to further investigate the reasons behind teenage depression and effective treatment interventions. While there is evidence supporting that short-term behavioral therapy can be helpful in treating depression, along with anti-depressants, this seems to work for only 60% of the cases. In addition, half of those who improve relapsed within a year of stopping treatment. The NIMH research study is hoping to find which treatment is best for particular individuals with specific types of symptoms, as all people do not exhibit depressive symptoms in the same way. There is also a continuum in terms of severity of the symptoms and so they are examining what type of treatment might work best for different levels of depression. Hopefully we will soon find a way to detect who might be at risk and how to intervene before we lose more victims to this illness.

Source: "Young and Depressed," *Newsweek,* October 7, 2002. "FDA Approves Prozac for Children," *USA Today,* January 3, 2003.

lending a hand: becoming a volunteer

Service is the rent each of us pays for living—the very purpose of life and not something you do in your spare time or after you have reached your personal goals.

—Marian Wright Edelman

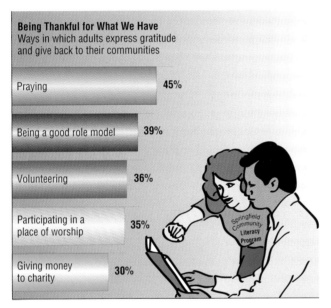

Being Thankful for What We Have
Ways in which adults express gratitude and give back to their communities

Praying	45%
Being a good role model	39%
Volunteering	36%
Participating in a place of worship	35%
Giving money to charity	30%

Many of us have been fortunate enough not to experience poverty, serious illness, or lack of education. Do you think it's important to express gratitude by giving something back to your community?

Finding homes for abandoned animals . . . dishing out hot food in a shelter for the homeless . . . rehabbing a house for a low-income family . . . teaching adults to read . . . comforting infants with AIDS . . .

What do all of these activities have in common? Simply put, each of them is about helping and serving others, without pay, without glory, often without recognition—at least not in the tangible ways we associate with top performance in school or at work. In fact, for most volunteers, it's the intangible rewards of

service that keep them motivated and keep them coming back.

Ever since the United States was founded, Americans have freely expended their time, talents, and energy in support of others in an ever-widening array of endeavors. From well-established, federally funded organizations like the Peace Corps,[1] VISTA (Volunteers in Service to America),[2] and AmeriCorps[3] to hometown scout troops, tree-planting projects, and creating and staffing shelters for battered women, tens of millions of

Americans put their idealism into action by using their skills in service to others. For college students and new graduates, hundreds—if not thousands—of programs at the local, state, national, and international levels provide a host of volunteer opportunities.

Amigos de las Americas[4] (a program for teens to live and volunteer in Latin America), International Executive Service Corps[5] (a program for retired U.S. executives to help businesses in more than one hundred twenty foreign nations), and World Teach[6] (a program for college graduates to teach English in a foreign country) are just a few examples of agencies that are using the skills of Americans to improve conditions in other parts of the world. And in today's tech-savvy times, it's no surprise that a community of cyber-volunteers is springing up on the Internet, spearheaded by efforts like The Virtual Volunteering Project[7] in which experienced volunteers provide expertise to groups and agencies via the Internet.

Helping Others and Improving Yourself

While service benefits those in need, volunteering is also good for the volunteer. It provides companionship, friendship, and fellowship in working toward a common goal. It allows us to use skills and talents we normally don't use in our daily jobs. In this way, volunteering encourages us to branch out, learn new things, and become more well rounded. By volunteering, we can help someone achieve more power over his or her life. When working for a cause of deep personal concern, volunteers can become involved with information gathering and decision making that allows them to feel less helpless when confronting that issue.

Motivations for volunteering vary almost as widely as do the volunteers themselves. Some who have benefited from the help of others in the past, such as receiving the support and comfort of a hospice program in caring for a terminally ill loved one, may want to give something back by providing the same service for others in need. Some simply want to make their neighborhood, hometown, or the world a better place; they feel a strong sense of community and hurt when others hurt.[8]

More important than why or how people serve is that they *do* serve. Hungry people are fed and trees are saved one by one—and it makes a difference. It also makes a difference in the lives of the volunteers. Providing service is good for the human psyche. It brings people from different backgrounds together, makes them feel useful, and raises the aspirations of all involved.

Helping others also may help your career. You can make business contacts when you meet other volunteers, and you may develop and enhance skills you'll find useful in your job. What's more, becoming a volunteer can identify you to your employer as someone with a balanced life who contributes creative solutions and displays strong leadership skills. Volunteer work can even boost your academic career by improving your performance through the structure, planning, and discipline you learn while volunteering. Gaining in popularity and participation is the concept of service learning, in which college students make a commitment to volunteer as part of their higher education experience. Find out what programs are available to you by visiting the websites of the Learn & Serve America National Service-Learning Clearinghouse[9] and the International Partnership for Service Learning.[10]

Diversity Among Volunteers

Like the people they help, volunteers themselves are a highly diverse group. Among recipients of the American Institute of Public Service's Jacqueline Kennedy Onassis Awards for outstanding local community service is Isaac Pope, who overcame a segregated boyhood in Tennessee to earn a medical degree. After being diagnosed with cancer 10 years ago, he sold his medical practice to open a clinic for severely disabled children.

What John Beal of Seattle did was try to restore environmentally crippled streams in the Duwamish River watershed in South Seattle. In 23 years of tireless work, he's brought teeming life back to Hamm Creek.

Another Onassis Award recipient is Lenny Larson who has helped people with AIDS to cope with the deadly disease, providing support through the Northwest AIDS Foundation, the Chicken Soup Brigade, and the Seattle AIDS Support Group, three organizations he co-founded.

Elizabeth Thomas, another award recipient, provided care and comfort to children in need as a dedicated pediatric nurse practitioner at the Odessa Brown Children's Clinic in Seattle.

Peter Truong of Burien, a war refugee who fled his native Vietnam in 1975, volunteers his time to assist Asian immigrants in dealing with an unfamiliar culture and country—when he's not working as a community service officer for the King County Sheriff's Office.

Just as important are the unsung volunteers who receive no official recognition for their efforts: the college dropout who volunteers at the Center for Democracy and Technology, a group that fights for the preservation of free speech on the Internet; the college students who spend their summers at housing projects in Hartford, Connecticut, to counsel, tutor, and play with the children who live there; and people of all ages, who work with the Missouri Humane Society to find loving homes for abused, neglected, and unwanted animals. Thankfully, the list goes on and on with the names of mothers,

fathers, sisters, brothers, sons, daughters, neighbors, and friends whose gift of time and caring truly benefits us all.

Ways to Volunteer

No matter what your interests, abilities, or time commitments, there's much you can do to serve your community or your country. Here are just a few of the many opportunities you might want to pursue:

AIDS
Animal welfare
Arts/cultural enrichment
Business assistance
Citizenship
Civic affairs
Consumer services/legal rights
Day care/Head Start
Disaster response/emergency
    preparedness
Drug abuse/alcoholism
Education
Employment
Health issues
Law enforcement/crime prevention
Literacy
Mental health
Nutrition
Parenting
Physical environment
Psychosocial support services
Recreation and sports
Teen pregnancy prevention
Transportation and safety
Women's crisis centers

You can make a difference alone, with a few friends, or as part of an organization. The Student Environmental Action Coalition has chapters at more than two thousand high schools and colleges. VISTA, the Peace Corps, AmeriCorps, United Way, Salvation Army, and Red Cross are jut a few of the national organizations in need of volunteers. To volunteer, you can contact one of these organizations or your local place of worship, hospital, nursing home, city recreation department, or scout council directly, or call the Nationwide Hotline on Volunteer Opportunities at 800-424-8867 or the Points of Light Foundation at 800-879-5400.

For Discussion . . .

Do you currently volunteer? Why or why not? If you decided to become a volunteer, what areas of service would most interest you? Can you think of a volunteer who has touched your life? How do you feel about compulsory volunteer service?

References

1. Peace Corps: *Today's Peace Corps is still the toughest job you'll ever love.* **www.peacecorps.gov/home.html,** August 2000.
2. Catalog of Federal Domestic Assistance. *Volunteers in Service to America.* August 2000.
3. Corporation for National Service: AmeriCorps. **www.americorps.org,** August 2000.
4. Amigos de las Americas. **info@amigoslink.org,** August 2000.
5. International Executive Service Corps. **www.iesc.org,** August 2000.
6. World Teach. **worldteach@hiid. harvard.edu,** August 2000.
7. The Virtual Volunteering Project. **www.serviceleader.org,** August 2000.
8. Morris T. Volunteerism & the community: a win-win situation, *Work & Learning Network News* 1998; 1(1):1–2.
9. Learn & Serve America National Service-Learning Clearinghouse. **www.nicsl.coled.umn.edu/home. htm,** August 2000.
10. International Partnership for Service Learning. **www.ipsl.org,** August 2000.

InfoLinks

www.heartsandminds.org/home.htm
www.cns.gov/learn/about/
service_learning.html

personal assessment

how does my self-concept compare with my idealized self?

Below is a list of fifteen personal attributes, each portrayed on a 9-point continuum. Mark with an X where you think you rank on each attribute. Try to be candid and accurate; these marks will collectively describe a portion of your sense of self-concept. When you are finished with the task, go back and circle where you *wish* you could be on each dimension. These marks describe your idealized self. Finally, in the spaces on the right, indicate the difference between your self-concept and your idealized self for each attribute.

Decisive				Indecisive				
9	8	7	6	5	4	3	2	1

Anxious | | | | Relaxed
9 8 7 6 5 4 3 2 1

Easily influenced | | | | Independent thinker
9 8 7 6 5 4 3 2 1

Very intelligent | | | | Less intelligent
9 8 7 6 5 4 3 2 1

In good physical shape | | | | In poor physical shape
9 8 7 6 5 4 3 2 1

Undependable | | | | Dependable
9 8 7 6 5 4 3 2 1

Deceitful | | | | Honest
9 8 7 6 5 4 3 2 1

A leader | | | | A follower
9 8 7 6 5 4 3 2 1

Unambitious | | | | Ambitious
9 8 7 6 5 4 3 2 1

Self-confident | | | | Insecure
9 8 7 6 5 4 3 2 1

Conservative | | | | Adventurous
9 8 7 6 5 4 3 2 1

Extroverted | | | | Introverted
9 8 7 6 5 4 3 2 1

Physically attractive | | | | Physically unattractive
9 8 7 6 5 4 3 2 1

Lazy | | | | Hardworking
9 8 7 6 5 4 3 2 1

Funny | | | | Little sense of humor
9 8 7 6 5 4 3 2 1

To Carry This Further . . .

1. Overall, how would you describe the difference between your self-concept and your self-ideal (large, moderate, small, large on a few dimensions)?

2. How do these differences for any of your attributes affect your sense of self-esteem?

3. How do you think someone who knows you well would rate you? Would they rate you in a similar way to how you see yourself? If not, why not?

4. Identify several attributes that you realistically believe can be changed to narrow the gap between your self-concept and your self-ideal and, thus, foster a well-developed sense of self-esteem.

chapter three

managing stress

Chapter Objectives

Upon completing this chapter, you will be able to:

■ define stress, the stress response, and chronic stress.

■ describe the flight or fight response.

■ list at least ten physical responses to stress.

■ discuss the general adaptation syndrome including three stages of stress: the alarm, resistance, and exhaustion stages.

■ discuss at least five different types of student stress explored in this chapter.

■ describe the differences between Type A and Type B personalities.

■ describe the physical aspects of stress management.

■ describe the social aspects of stress management.

■ describe the environmental aspects of stress management.

■ describe the psychological aspects of stress management.

■ describe relaxation and deep breathing, progressive muscle relaxation, guided imagery and visualization, meditation and hypnosis, biofeedback, stress inoculation, and cognitive self-talk as tools for stress management.

Online Learning Center Resources

www.mhhe.com/payne8e

Log on to our Online Learning Center (OLC) for access to these additional resources:

- Chapter key terms and definitions
- Learning objectives
- Student interactive question-and-answer sites

- Self-scoring chapter quiz
- Online assessments
- Key term flash cards

Talking It Over

Communication and Stress

You just found out that your sister has been diagnosed with cancer, and you're feeling very stressed. You need to talk to someone, but who? First, figure out what you want. Is it emotional support, advice, affection, or help with errands? The answer will lead you to the best person. Second, explain what you're going through as clearly as you can. Tell the person what you need—whether it's a sympathetic ear or someone to drive you to the hospital.

Third, talk to your sister as normally as possible. She needs you to talk—and listen—to her now more than ever.

CommunicationLinks

www.wellsource.com
www.webmd.com
www.cancer.org

Eye on the Media

New Technology, New Stresses

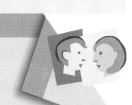

The Internet has connected an estimated 13 million computers in 195 countries on every continent, even Antarctica. The way we work, shop, access information, take classes, and socialize with others has all changed thanks to the Internet. While the Internet has connected the world in ways once unimaginable, along with the convenience and easy access to information have come new risks, and subsequently, new stress. Vulnerability to hackers, identity thieves, and viruses—not to mention endless piles of junk e-mail—can make the Internet a scary place. Your private journal or letter to someone might be read by someone you didn't intend to read it, your credit card information might fall into the wrong hands, or information about your medical records might be disbursed to people you didn't authorize to have this information.[1]

Information can be corrupted when it is available on an insecure network. This means that unauthorized changes are made to information, whether by human error or intentional tampering. If you pay your bills online, or use the Internet for activities such as electronic funds transfers and financial accounting, this could cause you considerable stress should the information become corrupted. It is important to ascertain what is a hoax and what is legitimate on the Internet, as there is a great deal of information conveyed that is incorrect. Financial stress can also result from purchasing something on the Web from an unscrupulous company and not receiving the goods you thought you were purchasing.

The number of reported security incidents has grown dramatically over the past few years. While human error accounts for some of the problems on the Web, financial gain is often the reason people receive hundreds of scam e-mails. There are also people who intentionally tamper with the Internet to cause problems. A hacker may seek entertainment, intellectual challenge, a sense of power, political attention, or financial gain. This may be someone who is curious about what he or she can do on the Internet, has created a new software tool, or seeks personal gain or a feeling of power. It could also be a disgruntled former employee or a consultant who gained network information while working with a company.[2]

Losing hours of work on your computer due to a virus or worm tends to create a sense of powerlessness and hopelessness for the victims of this kind of attack. When word spreads that there is a new virus circulating, people become increasingly anxious and on the alert. People can become angry with friends, co-workers, and family members for spreading a virus to their computer when they were unaware of doing so.

Some tips for protecting yourself against viruses, worms, and hackers are:

- Install antivirus software and make sure you update it regularly as new viruses appear frequently.
- Install security patches for your software. Microsoft offers patches for the Windows operating system at *windowsupdate. Microsoft.com* or *Microsoft.com/security*.
- Be very cautious about opening e-mail attachments, particularly from senders you don't recognize. The same caution should be taken with downloading from the Internet.
- Consider installing a firewall program to further protect your computer.
- Use a hard-to-guess password and change it frequently.
- Make sure you back up important documents.[3]

While new advances are being made every day to increase the security and integrity of the Internet, it still has the potential to cause stress in your life. While new technology offers many advantages, it also creates new types of stress in our lives. It is important to be aware of the potential risks and to protect yourself from the stress associated with Internet use as much as you can.

Sources: 1. Levy S. *Hackers: Heroes of the Computer Revolution.* Garden City, NY: Anchor Press/Doubleday, 1984. 2. Stoll C. *The Cuckoo's Egg: Tracking a Spy Through the Maze of Computer Espionage.* New York: Doubleday, 1989. 3. Denning PJ (ed). *Computers Under Attack: Intruders, Worms, and Viruses.* New York: ACM Press, Addison-Wesley, 1990.

What Is Stress?

How do you know when you are stressed? You might experience headaches, stomach aches, or back and neck aches, or you might feel irritable, tired, anxious, and depressed. Some people eat more, while others find eating difficult when they are stressed. **Stress** refers to physiological and emotional responses to a significant or unexpected change or disruption in one's life. It can be brought on by real or imagined factors or events.

Stress was first described in the 1930s by Hans Selye. During his second year of medical school, Selye observed that, although his patients suffered from a variety of illnesses, they all showed common symptoms, such as fatigue, appetite disturbance, sleep problems, mood swings, gastrointestinal problems, and diminished concentration and recall. He began developing his now-famous theory of the influence of stress on people's ability to cope with and adapt to the pressures of injury and disease. He discovered that patients with a variety of ailments manifested many similar symptoms, which he ultimately attributed to their bodies' efforts to respond to the stresses of being ill. He called this collection of symptoms—this separate stress disease—stress syndrome, or the **general adaptation syndrome (GAS).** He also described this as "the syndrome of being ill."[1] We'll discuss Selye's discovery further later in the chapter.

Selye defines stress as "the nonspecific response of the body to any demand whether it is caused by or results in pleasant or unpleasant conditions." Stress can be both

---

Key Terms

stress the physiological and psychological state of disruption caused by the presence of an unanticipated, disruptive, or stimulating event.

general adaptation syndrome (GAS) sequenced physiological responses to the presence of a stressor, involving the alarm, resistance, and exhaustion stages of the stress response.

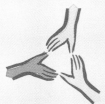

Learning from Our Diversity

Communicating with Students Who Have a Disability

For many college students, interacting with classmates who have a disability is uncomfortable and stressful. The students with the disability feel this discomfort, and it is a source of stress for them. They are also dealing with the demands of college in the context of their unique disability.

What approach could be taken to minimize the discomfort for all parties involved? The following list contains some suggestions:

- Remember that everyone is a *person first.* In addition, that person may have a disability. Think in terms of a student with a learning disability, not a learning-disabled student.
- Always make *eye contact* with the person. This simple courtesy is very important in assuring the individual with a disability that he or she is a part of your college experience.
- *Talk with* the person with the disability rather than with the accompanying attendant or assistant.

- Keep in mind that the person in the attendant/assistant role may know only certain aspects of the individual with a disability.
- Don't *"fake it"* or *"smile it off."* If you can't understand the person with a disability, simply say: "I'm sorry. Give that to me one more time."
- If verbal communication is very difficult or simply ineffective, *do what it takes* to interact with the person with a disability. For example, sit down at the computer and write a note.
- If you think that the person with a disability needs assistance, just ask: *"May I assist you?"* The worst that can happen is that the person might say no. If the person says yes, he or she might even tell you how you can help.
- *Don't generalize* from a single negative and stressful experience about interacting with someone with a disability. Expect no more or no less from that person than you would from your able-bodied classmates.

positive or negative: again it is our response to stress—how we manage stress—that makes a difference in terms of how it affects us. Stress resulting from unpleasant events or conditions is called **distress** (from the latin *dis,* meaning bad, as in displeasure). Stress resulting from pleasant events or conditions is called **eustress** (from the Latin *eu,* meaning good, as in euphoria). Both eustress and distress elicit the same physiological responses in the body, as noted in Selye's general adaptation syndrome model.

While stress may not always be negative, our responses to it can be negative, problematic, or unhealthy. Both positive and negative stressful situations place extra demands on the body—your body is reacting to an unexpected change or a highly emotional experience, regardless of whether this change is good or bad. If the duration of your stress is relatively short, the overall effect is minimal and your body will rest, renew itself, and everything returns to normal. But as you will learn in this chapter, long-lasting stress, experiencing multiple stressors simultaneously, and not managing your stress effectively, can take a toll on your body.

Stress is actually normal and healthy at a certain level. With functional, healthy levels of stress, your overall physiological equilibrium is maintained at a balanced level. You will learn in this chapter that you really don't want to eliminate all of your stress because stress is adaptive, functional, and can be beneficial. You need to understand

how you uniquely deal with stress and what works and doesn't work well for you in coping with day-to-day pressures and problems.

How We Respond to Stress

When we are stressed, we react in specific ways. The **stress response** is the result of learned and conditioned habits adopted early in life as a way of coping with problems, conflict, and disruptive events. But many of our responses to stress are innate, basic human survival mechanisms left over from our primordial roots. In prehistoric times, the best response to perceived danger, such as

> ### Key Terms
>
> **distress** stress that diminishes the quality of life; commonly associated with disease, illness, and maladaptation.
>
> **eustress** stress that enhances the quality of life.
>
> **stress response** the physiological and psychological responses to positive or negative events that are disruptive, unexpected, or stimulating.

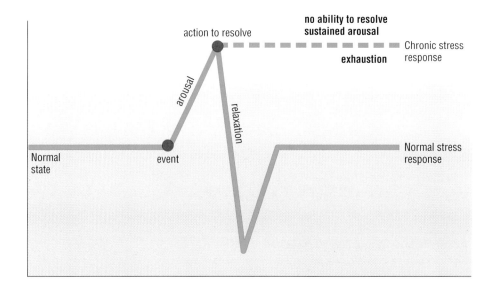

Figure 3-1 Resolving Stress There is a tremendous difference in how long your body remains at a high level of physiological arousal depending upon how quickly and effectively you act to resolve the stress.

Source: Selye H. "The Stress of Life."

Fight or Flight Response

seeing a saber-tooth tiger coming your way, might be to either fight the animal or to run away. Stress in modern times remains the same except that we are responding to 21st century threats and dangers rather than to saber-tooth tigers. Again it is not the events that determine how stressed we will feel but our response to these stressors. We will discuss the way that this innate stress response affects our modern lives in the section that follows.

Fight or Flight Response

Our response to stress involves many physiological changes that are collectively called the **fight or flight response.** In situations in which you must react immediately to danger, it is advisable to either fight off the danger or flee. For example, you are walking back from class at night, thinking about all the studying you need to do and you begin to cross the street. Suddenly, out of nowhere, you see a car with its headlights coming right at you. Since your best response is probably not to fight the car, you run as fast as you can to the other side of the road. In that split second, when you see the car careening quickly towards you, your muscles tense, your heart beats faster, your adrenaline is pumping faster and being released at higher levels into your blood stream, your breathing becomes more shallow and rapid, and your pupils dilate to see the car better.

This is the fight or flight response. Receiving alert signals from the brain, the sympathetic nerves signal most of the organs of the body, and the adrenal glands are activated. Within the brain itself, neural pathways, involved in increased attention and focus, are activated. In this way, performance and learning can be heightened. Again, all of these changes are very adaptive and helpful

to your survival in getting out of harm's way. In the above example, when you get to the other side of the road and realize that you are okay, your body begins to relax and return to its normal state. You take a large, deep breath, expressing a big sigh of relief. Your muscles may feel even weaker than usual, your breathing may become deeper and heavier than is typical, and you may feel shaky as your body goes from extreme arousal to relaxing very quickly. Figure 3-1 depicts these changes from your normal state to an arousal state to a very relaxed state then back to normal.

Accompanying this fight or flight reaction is a slower response. During stressful events, the pituitary secretes a peptide called adrenocorticotrophin, or ACTH, into the blood. ACTH travels through the blood to the adrenal, where it signals the production of a hormone called cortisol.[2] Cortisol aids the body in recovering stressful experiences by freeing up energy stores. The logic behind the slower stress response is that the quick fight or flight response uses up a lot of the body's available energy. The slower response helps to replenish the available energy. The body usually has some small amount of cortisol circulating in the blood at all times. When the stress response lasts too long or is initiated too frequently, the cortisol level is increased. After enough of

> **Key Terms**
>
> **fight or flight response** the physiological response to a stressor that prepares the body for confrontation or avoidance.

these small increases, the body soon resets its control mechanism to maintain a higher constant amount of cortisol in the body.

Chronic Stress

Now let's consider a different situation. You have a test in a week that you are very concerned about. It seems to be preoccupying your every waking thought and you have trouble sleeping as well. You are worried that you won't perform well on the test and you really need to do better than you did on your last test. Your parents have been putting a great deal of pressure on you to do better in school in general. Because our bodies respond similarly to perceived or anticipated threat, you can have the same response to something that hasn't yet occurred. In other words, your heart races, breathing becomes labored, muscles are tense, body sweats, and blood flow is constricted to the extremities and digestive organs and increases to the major muscles and brain. Your body is becoming ready to fight or flee the danger. However, you cannot take any action and make a fight or flight response, because nothing has really happened. You haven't taken the test yet, and even once you do, you don't know your grade. So your body remains at this high level of arousal.

Remaining in a continued state of physiological arousal for an extended period of time is called **chronic stress.** This high level of arousal is similar to putting your foot on the accelerator of your car while it is in park and not letting up on the gas pedal. Since the fight or flight response is meant to be a very quick, short acting response, your body begins to wear down if kept at this physiological state of arousal for too long; eventually, you will begin to experience the physical and psychological symptoms of chronic stress. This is also the reason that people cope better with anxiety by taking some action, doing something about whatever they are worried about rather than stewing about their problems. Thus the fight or flight response can be triggered inappropriately in response to phobias, irrational beliefs, an overactive imagination, or hallucinations or delusions.

The Three Stages of Stress

Once under the influence of a stressor, people's bodies respond in remarkably similar, predictable ways. For example, when asked to give a speech for a class, your heart rate may increase, your throat becomes dry, palms sweat, and you may feel lightheaded, dizzy, and nauseous. If an individual lost her or his job or discovered that her or his partner wanted to terminate their relationship, s/he might experience similar sensations. It is clear that different stressors are able to evoke these common physical reactions.

Selye described the typical physical response to a stressor in his general adaptation syndrome model[3] discussed earlier in the chapter. Selye stated that the human body moves through three stages when confronted by stressors as follows.

Alarm Stage

Once exposed to any event that is perceived as threatening or dangerous, the body immediately prepares for difficulty, entering what Selye called the **alarm stage.** These involuntary changes, described in Figure 3-2, are controlled by the hormonal and nervous system, and trigger the fight or flight response. For example, you realize that the final exam you thought was today was actually scheduled for yesterday. You may begin to experience: fear, panic, anxiety, anger, depression, and restlessness.[4]

Resistance Stage

The second stage of a response to a stressor is the **resistance stage,** during which the body attempts to reestablish its equilibrium or internal balance. The body is geared for survival, and because staying in the alarm stage for a prolonged amount of time is not conducive for the body's optimal functioning; it will resist or attempt to resolve the problem and reduce the intensity of the response to a more manageable level. Specific organ systems, such as the cardiovascular and digestive systems, become the focus of the body's response.[5] During this phase, you might take steps to calm yourself down and relieve the stress on your body: You might deny the situation, withdraw and isolate yourself from others, and shut down your emotions. Thus, in the example above, you may not tell anyone about missing the exam, may tell yourself that you don't care about that class anyway, and go back to bed.

> ### Key Terms
>
> **chronic stress** refers to remaining at a high level of physiological arousal for an extended period of time; it can also occur when an individual is not able to immediately react to a real or perceived threat.
>
> **alarm stage** the first stage of the stress response involving physiological, involuntary changes that are controlled by the hormonal and nervous system; the fight or flight response is activated in this stage.
>
> **resistance stage** the second stage of a response to a stressor, during which the body attempts to reestablish its equilibrium or internal balance.

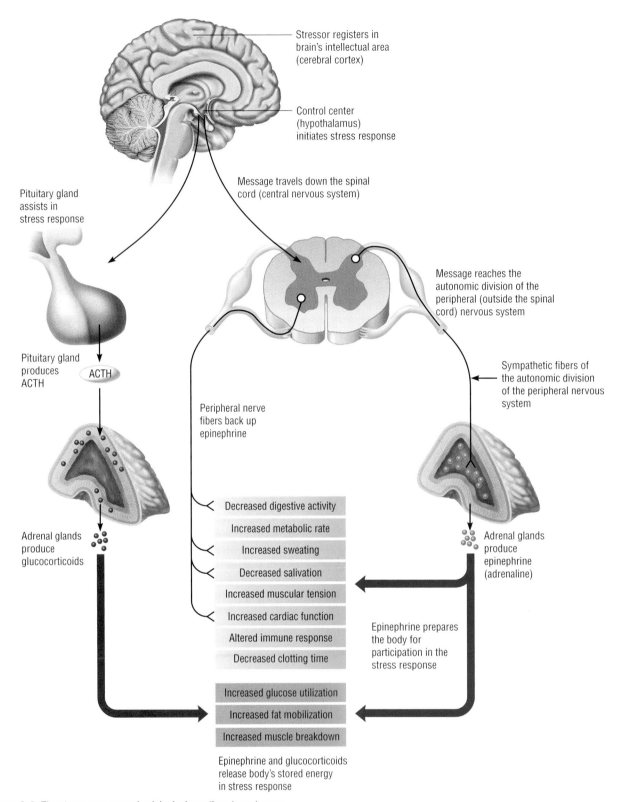

Stressor registers in brain's intellectual area (cerebral cortex)

Control center (hypothalamus) initiates stress response

Message travels down the spinal cord (central nervous system)

Pituitary gland assists in stress response

Message reaches the autonomic division of the peripheral (outside the spinal cord) nervous system

Pituitary gland produces ACTH

ACTH

Sympathetic fibers of the autonomic division of the peripheral nervous system

Peripheral nerve fibers back up epinephrine

Adrenal glands produce glucocorticoids

Decreased digestive activity

Increased metabolic rate

Increased sweating

Decreased salivation

Increased muscular tension

Increased cardiac function

Altered immune response

Decreased clotting time

Adrenal glands produce epinephrine (adrenaline)

Epinephrine prepares the body for participation in the stress response

Increased glucose utilization

Increased fat mobilization

Increased muscle breakdown

Epinephrine and glucocorticoids release body's stored energy in stress response

Figure 3-2 The stress response: physiological reactions to a stressor.

Stress and Psychoneuroimmunology

Can Stress Affect Our Immune System?

The newly emerging field of psychoneuroimmunology addresses the apparent interplay of the mind, the nervous system (the hypothalamus and autonomic nervous system), and the immune system (see Chapter 13).[1]

On the basis of clinical observation and laboratory studies, it is recognized that feelings associated with stress (depression and anxiety) and the disruption of social support systems relate to the weakening of the immune response and the development of some illnesses. For example, a study involving self-assessment of stress levels and the occurrence of colds demonstrated that as levels of chronic stress increase, colds become more common.[2] In another study, immunizations were less effective in producing an immune response in students stressed by upcoming examinations than in those not scheduled to take examinations.

As such studies are replicated and new studies are designed, it is increasingly apparent that the changes initially reported in the immune system of animals during periods of stress can be applied to humans. Our growing understanding of the interfacing of thoughts (negatively affected during periods of distress), the nervous system, and the functional status of the immune system enhances our insight into illnesses and their relationship to stress. As this understanding continues to mature, we will develop more effective coping strategies that enhance the connection between our feelings and their impact on nervous system and endocrine system function and the maintenance of immune system capabilities.

Sources:
1. Masek K et al. Past, present and future of psychoneuroimmunology. *Toxicology* 2000; 142(3): 179–188.
2. Cohen S et al. Types of stressors that increase susceptibility to the common cold in healthy adults. *Health Psychol* 1998; 17(3): 214–223.

Exhaustion Stage

Your ability to move from the alarm stage to a less damaging resistance stage will determine the impact that the stressor has on your physical and psychological health. As you gain more control and balance is reestablished, you can begin to recover from the stress.

The length of time, energy, and effort demanded in accomplishing this will decide how exhausted your body becomes as a result of the stressor. Of course, the longer the body is under stress and out of balance, the more negative impact this will have on your body. Long-term exposure to a stressor or coping with multiple stressors at the same time often results in overloading your system. Specific organs and body systems that were called upon during the resistance stage may not be able to resist a stressor indefinitely. When all the psychological and physical resources we rely on to deal with stress are used up, an **exhaustion stage** results, and the stress-producing hormones such as adrenaline rise again. This is when chronic and serious illnesses can begin to develop. In the above example, the individual may develop clinical depression.

Sources of Stress

There are other causes of stress besides experiencing positive or negative events in your life.[6] What events or situations trigger stress for you? For some it is financial worries, for others it might be relationship conflict, and for others it is work-related stress. Even positive events, such as getting married, starting a new job, or moving to a new place, can be **stressors.** Going on vacation can be stressful as you get things done ahead of time to prepare for being away, pack your belongings, spend money on the trip, and completely change your routine. Any type of change in your life has the potential to trigger a stressful response.

Because stress involves a physiological response, it has a direct link to your physical and psychological health. The work of Thomas Holmes and Richard Rahe have found direct connections between changes in people's lives and physical illness. They developed a widely used inventory, called the Social Readjustment Rating Scale, to assess the degree of stress people experience in connection with particular life events. While one of these events alone might be tolerable, a combination of too many life changes within a short period of time is more likely to lead to illness.[7] To assess your level of stress and potential vulnerability to illness, complete the personal assessment inventory at the end of this chapter.

> ### Key Terms
>
> **exhaustion stage** the point at which the physical and psychological resources used to deal with stress have been consumed.
>
> **stressors** factors or events, real or imagined, that elicit a state of stress.

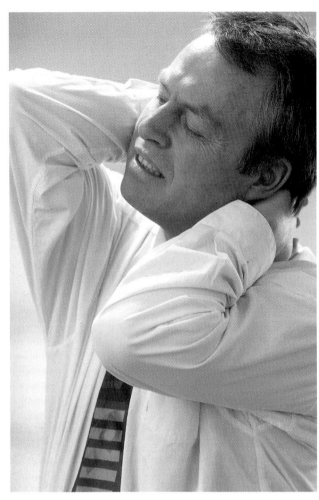

Tension and pain in the neck, shoulders, and back are common reactions when people experience stress.

The Costs and Benefits of Stress

Stress can be costly, taking a toll on our physical and mental health as well as our finances.

The Physical Toll of Stress

Constant arousal and increased levels of adrenaline in your system will eventually wear down your body's immunological system. As this occurs, you will be less able to cope with stress, and so it takes less and less to cause a stress reaction. When you are chronically stressed, it takes very little to frustrate you and you feel easily irritated and stressed at the littlest thing. Your body is both psychologically as well as physically less able to cope with stress. This can cause your immune system to become compromised, and you may become ill more easily. It may also take longer for you to recover from illness.

The following medical problems have been associated with stress[8] (to examine stress indicators for your personal stress, complete the rating scale at the end of this chapter):

- Cardiovascular problems (heart attacks, strokes, hypertension)
- Gastrointestinal problems (ulcers, irritable bowel syndrome, diarrhea, constipation, diverticulitis)
- Headaches and migraines
- Muscle spasms and cramps
- Sleep disorders
- Anxiety
- Jaw problems (temporomandibular joint [TMJ] syndrome)
- Allergies
- Cancer
- Back pain
- Asthma
- Kidney disease
- Sexual dysfunction
- Infertility
- Alcoholism and drug abuse

Other Costs of Stress

Stress can be very costly, not just in physical and psychological wellness but financially as well. While you can't put a price tag on your quality of life, we do know that stress-related accidents, disease, early death, and absenteeism have had a devastating impact. Stress-related symptoms and illnesses are costing industry a conservatively estimated $150 billion a year in absenteeism, company medical expenses, and lost productivity.[9] For example, researchers at the American Institute of Stress estimate that 75 to 90% of all visits to health-care providers result from stress-related disorders.[10] The American Heart Association says that more than 50 million workdays a year, totaling $8 billion, are lost annually to heart-related diseases.[11] The National Council on Compensation Insurance says that stress-related claims account for almost one-fifth of all occupational disease.[12] Researchers estimate that 60 to 80% of all industrial accidents are related to stress.[13]

Benefits of Stress

While too much stress can have a negative impact and cause some serious health problems, a moderate level of stress is positive and beneficial. Stress can be very motivating and energizing. Without some stress, many of us may not get much accomplished in our day or even get

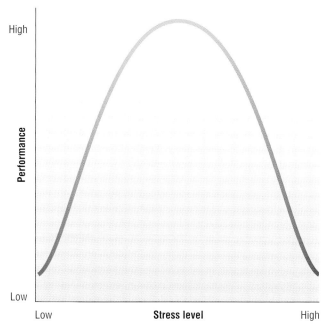

Figure 3-3 The Yerkes-Dodson Law. Too little or too much stress is not helpful, but a moderate level of stress encourages peak performance.

Source: Hebb DO. Drive and the CNS (conceptual nervous system). *Psychological Review* 62(4), 243–254, 1955.

out of bed! Look at the diagram in Figure 3-3 on this page. What do you notice? Too little and too much stress is not helpful. When you are not stressed at all, you can be apathetic and lethargic. When you are too stressed, you are paralyzed with fear, like deer in the headlights. This is referred to as the **Yerkes-Dodson Law** that shows a bell-shaped curve, demonstrating that there is an optimal level of stress for peak performance (see Figure 3-3). This holds true for any type of performance from academic or work activities to music or athletics.[14] Recognizing your appropriate level of stress for your ideal performance level is important in reaching your potential.

Student Stress

Going to college has been likened to "crossing into a new culture," and there are unique challenges and stressors that students face[6]. Similar to going to live in another country, students must learn new customs and traditions, new ways of doing things, a new language, and must leave comfortable and familiar surroundings. This can cause a high level of stress for students, many of whom have left their support system behind to live in a place where they know few people. In the sections that follow, we will cover some of the specific stressors college students face and offer ways to manage these situations.

Coping with Homesickness

Homesickness is one of the most common problems facing college students—which is understandable given that you are separated from your friends and family and learning to live in an entirely new environment. When undergoing a great deal of change in your life, it is helpful to have the comfort and security of your home base remaining stable and consistent. Moving from home to college can disrupt this sense of safety. While this can be an exciting and challenging time in your life, you may be missing your friends and family at home with whom you normally share these events. You may have also lost your sense of belonging while you struggle with finding a way to fit in with and navigate your new surroundings.

Often homesickness doesn't hit until a few weeks or maybe a month after you have moved, as the first few weeks are filled with meeting new people, social activities, and unpacking. After the dust settles, some people begin to feel lonely and alone. See Changing for the Better on page 73 for advice on how to deal with homesickness.

Relationship Problems

Along with homesickness, another very common stressor for students is relationship problems. Often students are separated by long distances from their best friends and romantic partners. While it can be difficult to maintain long distance relationships, it is not impossible. Studies show that the key to effective long distance relationships is communication. The quality of a long distance relationship is increased if you both are committed to each other, you can talk openly about your concerns, feelings, and fears, and you can agree on the rules of the relationship such as dating other people. In addition, there needs to be a strong level of trust between the couple, as this is often tested in long distance relationships. Both of you will change and it is important that you share these changes so that you can grow together, not apart. Communicate how often you will see each other, call or e-mail, and focus on spending quality time together.

It can be beneficial to have your friends visit you at college (rather than you going home) so that they can

Key Terms

Yerkes-Dodson Law a bell-shaped curve demonstrating that there is an optimal level of stress for peak performance; this law states that too little and too much stress is not helpful, while a moderate level of stress is positive and beneficial.

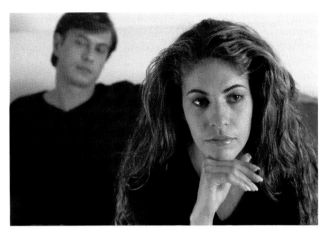

Stress caused by one aspect of your life can cause problems in other areas such as in your relationships.

interact with you in your new environment and meet your new friends. Often students feel as though they live in two worlds, home and school, and it can be stressful to negotiate going from one to the other. The more you can con-

nect these two worlds, the less stress you will experience. So it can be helpful to share what you are doing in your day—activities around campus, details of your classes, even who you ate lunch with—with your friends and family back home, and ask the same about them.

Balancing Work, Home, and School

It is estimated that about three-quarters of students work along with going to college and more students are working full-time to pay for the costs of tuition (see Figure 3-4). In addition it is estimated that between 5 to 10% of college students also have children. This, of course, adds more stress to a student's life in balancing time for school, children, work, and household responsibilities. This is partly as a result of a nationwide trend of more women in their mid-twenties or older who are starting or returning to college. In fact, a national study by the University of Michigan showed that the number of full-time female students over 25 years old grew by 500% over the past 30 years.[15]

While some campuses offer child care, many do not and this leaves students having to coordinate schedules

---

Discovering Your Spirituality

Journaling: Self-Help for Stress

Feeling anxious about your college experience? Trying to put past events in perspective? Want to record your experiences? Focused, regular writing—journaling—is growing in popularity as a way to approach these issues.

Writing in a journal each day slows down your pace. You sit and reflect. You connect with an experience by recalling details you may have forgotten, then write them down. For 15 to 30 minutes a day, you pause to make sense of your life.

Journaling generally gets easier the more you do it, so start by writing about nonthreatening topics. Try this: Each day, ask yourself a simple question, and then write the answer in your journal. As you gain experience, you may want to tackle more difficult issues.

Here are some journaling tips. Use an easy-to-carry spiral-bound notebook with a thick cover, so you can write anywhere. Or you may want to set aside a regular time and place so you won't be disturbed. Once you start writing, keep your pen moving continuously. Don't go back to correct spelling or punctuation. That will only slow you down and distract you from your thoughts, which are more important than perfect writing. Give yourself permission not to have to share your journal with others as this may inhibit your writing, making it less honest and open.

One powerful form of journaling is therapeutic or healing journaling, in which the individual writes about a traumatic event for 15 to 30 minutes a day, on three or four consecutive days. Studies by James W. Pennebaker, M.D., and colleagues noted lowered blood pressure and heart rates in healthy people who wrote about their innermost feelings for 20 minutes on three consecutive days.

Therapeutic writing can be very difficult and should be approached with caution. In particular, if you have been under medical treatment, check with your health-care professional before you begin a therapeutic journaling program. If you write about private events, you can shred or burn your pages. Be aware of not just writing about negative events or emotions. Don't allow this to be a journal about "how I messed up today."

Want to know more about journaling? *Personal Journaling Magazine (www.journalingmagazine.com)* is a good place to start. You'll find that journaling takes many forms, including memoirs, dream journals, chronicles of daily life, and "blogging" on the Internet.

In college, most of the things you write, such as papers and reports, are assigned and judged by an instructor. But when you write in a journal, it's for yourself—no judgments, no grades.

Tired of being stressed out all the time? Want to clear out the cobwebs in your head? Take out paper and pen and embark on one of the most exciting trips you'll ever take—the journey into yourself.

Balancing Work and School

More than half of the nation's 9.4 million college students under age 25 worked at paying jobs in recent years.

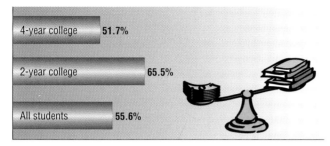

Figure 3-4 Percentages of college students who also work at paying jobs.

Source: Data from the U.S. Department of Labor.

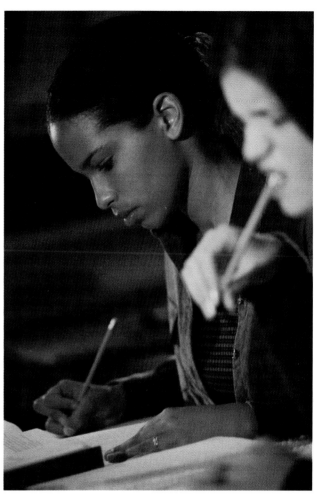

Test anxiety is related more to your confidence level than it is to how well you know the material.

and juggle responsibilities even more, causing potentially more stress. Also the cost of child care can be exorbitant for some and can certainly add to financial worries. Managing your time well and having a strong support system is essential for students with children, particularly single parents. Often there is little to no time available for relaxation, socializing, or exercising, and so employing these stress relief strategies can be challenging.

Test Anxiety

You have studied for the test you are about to take and are well prepared. You look at the first test question and suddenly your mind goes blank. The harder you try to think,

Changing for the Better

I just started college and my family and friends are 5 hours away from me. I tend to be on the shy side and don't know anyone at my college. I miss my friends and family and don't feel like I belong here. I am thinking about withdrawing from school and going home. What should I do?

The following are some strategies to combat these feelings:

- Get involved! Become active in noncurricular, social activities such as special interest clubs, student government, religious clubs, fraternities, and sororities. Clubs associated with your major are a great way to meet people, further your academic and career interests, and keep you from feeling homesick.

- Call, e-mail, or write your family and friends regularly and let them know you would like to hear from them.
- Be open to meeting new people. Introduce yourself to people in your classes, and exchange e-mail addresses and phone numbers. This is also an excellent way to get a study partner or study group together. Keep your door open when you are in your room, and spend time in public, common areas—not just hiding away in your room when you have spare time. Strike up a conversation while doing your laundry in the common laundry room area.
- Don't eat alone. Ask someone to join you to eat, or ask people at a table if you can eat with them.

- Don't go home on the weekends. Even though it may be tempting to visit your family and friends, the weekends are the best time to meet people and participate in the activities going on around campus.
- Be patient with yourself. Accept that loneliness and longing for home is normal and it will take some time for you to adjust to all of the changes you are experiencing. Don't decide to throw in the towel after the first few days! It may take a month before you begin to feel more comfortable in your new home. Give yourself some time to face this new challenge.

the more nervous and distressed you feel. You just can't think clearly and feel like you have some type of mental block—what is happening? One-fifth of students experience these feelings, referred to as **test anxiety.** Exams are one of the greatest sources of stress for college students. The physical sensations associated with test anxiety are similar to those of general anxiety, such as fidgeting, having the feeling of butterflies in your stomach, rapid heart rate, difficulty breathing, nausea, tension in your neck, back, jaw, and shoulders, headaches, sweaty palms, and feeling shaky. People suffering from test anxiety make more mistakes on their tests, don't read the test accurately, and tend to make simple mistakes, such as spelling errors or adding something incorrectly. Many don't pace themselves well, and have a hard time finishing exams. Test anxiety is a form of performance anxiety, as people anticipate that they will perform poorly on the test.[16]

 TALKING POINTS What are some problems with stress described in this chapter that you have experienced?

Speech Anxiety

As was mentioned in the previous chapter, speech anxiety, or fear of public speaking, is one of the most common anxiety disorders. Since students are frequently required to give oral presentations, expected to engage in class discussion, and graded on class participation points, this can present a problem for some.

In addition to the basic stress management techniques outlined in this chapter, it is also advised to do the following in coping with speech anxiety:

- Volunteer to go first. It is advisable to go first since anxiety is dealt with best by taking action. The pressure and expectations tend to mount with each person that takes a turn. Another advantage is that your performance is judged on its own merit without being compared to anyone else.

- Practice in front of a mirror and for your friends. Solicit feedback: do you need to slow down or speak louder? This will also help you to remember your talk so that you aren't reading it word for word which can seem less interesting to your audience.

- Engage in positive visualization. Taking deep, comfortable breaths, imagine yourself giving your speech with confidence and receiving positive feedback and compliments regarding your performance.

- Vary your presentation style and format. Use visuals such as slides, illustrations, or photographs, and engage your audience in discussion so that they are an active not a passive part of your presentation.

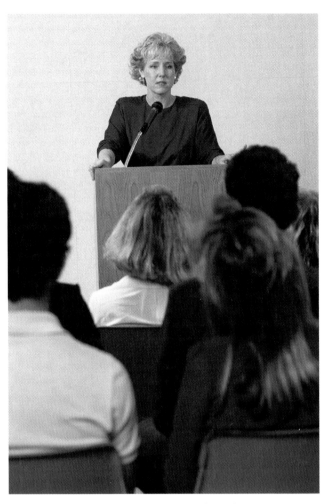

There are effective behavioral and psychological interventions to treat speech anxiety.

Math Anxiety

Another common stressor for college students is math anxiety. Math anxiety is an intense emotional feeling of anxiety that some people have about their ability to understand mathematics. People who suffer from math anxiety feel that they are incapable of performing well in activities and classes that involve math. The incidence of math anxiety among college students has risen significantly over the last decade. Many students have even chosen their college major on the basis of how little math is required for the degree. Math anxiety has become so

Key Terms

test anxiety a form of performance anxiety that generates extreme feelings of distress in exam situations.

Do You Suffer from Test Anxiety?

Test anxiety is a commonly experienced problem and can significantly impair your academic performance. Here are some questions you can ask yourself to help analyze if you might be suffering from test anxiety.

1. Are you aware of being really nervous on a test, maybe so nervous that you don't do your best and lose points, even though you know you've studied well and are prepared?
2. Does your stomach ever get tight or upset before or during a test? Hands cold and sweaty? Headaches? Do you have trouble sleeping the night before a test?
3. Do you ever find your mind racing or dull or cloudy so that you can't think clearly while taking a test?
4. During a test, do you ever forget material you studied and learned, only to remember it again after the test is over?
5. Do you overanalyze questions, see too many possibilities, choose the complex answer, and overlook the simpler, correct one?
6. Do you make many careless errors on a test?

7. Have you had some bad experiences with tests and made poor grades when you didn't expect them?
8. Do you spend a lot of time and energy studying and preparing for tests, yet fail to make grades that represent what you know?
9. Are tests and finals a particularly miserable time for you?

If you answered yes to more than half of these questions, you might want to consider getting some help in managing the anxiety associated with test taking. College counseling centers frequently offer stress management programs and can teach you techniques to manage your anxiety. Similar to managing other types of stress and anxiety, test anxiety can be coped with by using the following suggestions:

- Prepare well in advance. Don't cram at the last minute for the test. Rehearsal and repetition are the best ways of remembering information.
- Improve your odds by getting a good night's sleep before the test and eating a nutritious meal to give your brain needed energy.

- Have a positive attitude and watch your test talk. Don't talk about the test beforehand with friends as this tends to increase anxiety. Go into the test with a confident attitude, reminding yourself that you are well prepared and have taken many tests and performed satisfactorily in the past.
- Activity reduces anxiety. If you stumble on a question, don't linger over it; go onto the next question and return to that one later.
- Ask for clarification if you don't understand a question or something on the test.
- Don't pay attention to the people around you. Focus on the test and don't allow yourself to get distracted.
- Take deep breaths, allow your breathing to help you to relax, and bring more oxygen to the brain so you can think more clearly.
- Pace yourself and be aware of your time. Know when you need to be half-way through the test according to the time allotted for the exam.

Source: Newman E. *No More Test Anxiety.* Los Angeles, CA: Learning Skills Publications, 1996.

---

prevalent on college campuses that many schools have designed classes and special counseling programs to help math-anxious students.

Typically, people with math anxiety have the potential to perform well in math and it is more of a psychological, rather than intellectual, problem. However, since math anxiety interferes with a person's ability to learn math, it can create an intellectual problem. Often math anxiety is the result of a student's negative or embarrassing experience with math or a math teacher in previous years. Or perhaps the student was repeatedly told that he or she would not be able to perform well in math by a parent or teacher. Such an experience can leave a student believing him- or herself deficient in math ability. This belief can actually result in poor performance, which serves as confirming evidence to the student. This phenomenon is known as the self-fulfilling prophecy that is described more fully later in this chapter.

Students who fear math often avoid asking questions to save embarrassment, sit in the back of the classroom, fail to seek help from the professor, and usually put off studying math until the last moment. All of these negative behaviors are intended to reduce the student's anxiety but

actually result in more intense anxiety. However, you can take a number of positive steps to facilitate learning and performance in math classes. A student can use a number of the following strategies to overcome math anxiety:

1. Be sure to have developed a solid arithmetic foundation. As complex concepts build cumulatively on more simplistic ones, a remedial course or short course in arithmetic is often a significant first step in reducing the anxiety response to math.
2. If you have a choice, take an easier, slower math course as opposed to a faster-paced, more challenging one. It is better to stack the odds in your favor than to risk reinforcing your negative experiences with math.
3. Be aware of thoughts, feelings, and actions as they are related to math. Cultivate positive math talk rather than self-defeating, negative statements.
4. There is safety in numbers! Math anxiety is learned and reinforced over a long period of time and may take time to eliminate. You can reduce your anxiety with the help of a tutor, studying with a friend, or talking with your instructor.

5. Sit near the front of the class where you will experience fewer distractions and feel more a part of what is being discussed.

6. If you have questions or can't keep up with the instructor, ask for clarification and to repeat something you missed.[17]

7. Review the material. As with most things, skill in math comes from practice and repetition. Make sure you review the material covered in that class, and identify questions you need to ask the instructor as soon as possible after the class. Research shows that you will remember 50% of what you heard in class if you review it immediately after class, but only 20% is retained 24 hours later if you don't review it right away.[18]

Stress and Learning

How does stress affect learning? Research suggests that people that are highly anxious tend to perform better than others at simple learning tasks but less well than others at difficult tasks, particularly with reasoning activities and time-limited tests. An interesting study was conducted that showed college students with average scholastic ability earned significantly better grades when they had low levels of anxiety as compared to highly anxious average students.[19] When you are more stressed or anxious, you have a diminished ability to concentrate, to recall information, and to master problem-solving activities. You may find yourself reading the same page in your textbook over and over again and not knowing what you read.[16]

Using Time Effectively

An overwhelming number of students identify time management as the reason for their academic success or failure. Setting priorities and goals, balancing academic life with your social life, and finding time for sleeping, eating, exercising, and working along with studying is an essential aspect of managing your stress effectively.

Time Management

Managing your time effectively can help you cope with your stress by feeling more in control, having a sense of accomplishment, and having a sense of purpose in your life. Establishing good time management habits can take 2 to 3 weeks. By using specific systems, even the most disorganized persons can make their lives less chaotic and stressful.

Assess Your Habits

The first step is to analyze how you are spending your time. When is your more productive and least productive

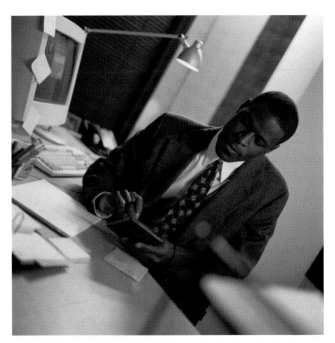

Managing your time well can greatly reduce your stress level.

time of day or night? Do you tend to underestimate how long something will take you to complete? Do you waste time or allow interruptions to take you off the task? Carrying a notebook with you for a week and writing down how you spend your time might provide you with some insight into the answers to these questions and how you spend your time. You might find that you've been devoting most of your time to less important tasks. Perhaps it is tempting to do your laundry rather than to start writing that term paper, but this is probably not the best use of your time.

Use a Planner

Keeping a daily planner to schedule your time is the next step in managing your time more effectively. First block off all of the activities that are consistent, regular, weekly activities such as attending classes, eating meals, sleeping, going to meetings, exercising, and working. Then look at the open, available time remaining. Schedule regular study time, relaxation time, and free time. Remember to schedule your study time during the more productive part of your waking hours. When you have a 1-hour block of time, what can you realistically get done in that time? This may be a good time to review your notes from class, pay bills, or get some reading done.

Set Goals and Prioritize

It is advisable to set goals for the week as well as for each day. If something unexpected interferes with your time schedule, modify your plans but don't throw out the entire schedule.

Making a to-do list can be helpful, but it is only the first step. Breaking the larger tasks into smaller, more manageable pieces and then prioritizing them is the key to effective time management. When you prioritize your tasks, it is beneficial to use the ABC method of task management. The A tasks are those items that are most urgent and must be done today. Then the B tasks are those things that are important but, if need be, could wait 24 hours. The C tasks are activities that can easily wait a few days to a week. Don't fall into the C trap which is when you do the less important tasks because they are quick and can be checked off your list with ease. This can lead to procrastinating the more important A activities, leaving them until you feel stressed and overwhelmed.[20] We will discuss more about procrastination in the next section.

Procrastination

Procrastination means postponing something that is necessary to do to reach your goal.[21] Putting things off is a common problem that plagues students and can cause stress. A survey of college students found that approximately 23% of students said they procrastinated about half of the time and 27% of students said they procrastinated most of the time.[22] Procrastination has been seen as a time management problem but it is really more than that, and so time management strategies tend to be ineffective in resolving this problem. Procrastination is also different from indecision, as people can make a decision but have trouble implementing their decisions.

Typically there is a psychological aspect to procrastination as we tend to delay doing things we don't want to do. Emotions such as anxiety, guilt, and dread often accompany thinking about the task. By putting the dreaded activity off, you can temporarily alleviate your anxiety and discomfort, and this is a reinforcing aspect of procrastination. In the short term, procrastination seems like a good solution and helps you to feel better. However, in the long run, procrastinating activities usually leads to bigger problems and more work. For example putting off paying your bills may feel good in the moment, but when your electricity is turned off and you have to pay late fees, and your roommates are upset with you because they thought you had paid the bill, your pleasurable feelings soon turn sour.

Procrastination occurs as frequently for men as for women, but more people in the mid to late twenties and sixty year olds procrastinate than any other age group.[23] Individuals who procrastinate are frequently referred to as "lazy" or "stupid" but actually there are no differences in levels of intelligence between procrastinators and non-procrastinators. However, students who procrastinate tend to perform less well and retain less than students

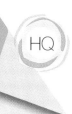
who do not. You might want to take the survey at the end of this chapter to assess your risk for procrastination.

Many people who procrastinate report feeling overwhelmed and highly anxious. They have difficulty tuning out external stimulation and concentrating on the task at hand. They also worry about how their performance will be judged by others and have perfectionistic standards for themselves. We will discuss perfectionism in the next section of this chapter.

Some techniques for combating procrastination involve time management, stress management, assertiveness training, and increasing self-esteem and self-acceptance. Specifically with regard to time management, procrastinators tend to both over- and underestimate how much time a task will take. When they underestimate the time, they feel justified in procrastinating because they erroneously believe they have plenty of time to complete the task. When they overestimate the time needed, they feel intimidated by the magnitude of the job, feel anxious, and so have trouble getting started. Most students explain that their anxiety stems from a fear of failure or being evaluated. Sometimes their anxiety manifests itself because they don't understand the material or what the instructor is wanting but are afraid to ask for clarification.

People also report procrastinating when they feel forced or pressured to do something they don't want to do. Rather than communicating assertively, they rebel by agreeing to do something but constantly put it off, which can be a passive-aggressive way of behaving. They fear the consequences of saying no or not fulfilling their obligations, but are also angry about what they perceive as unfair expectations and demands on them. This is where some assertiveness training may be helpful. Finally,

Key Terms

procrastination a tendency to put off completing tasks until some later time, sometimes resulting in increased stress.

increasing self-esteem can solve problems with procrastination as feeling better about yourself relieves you of worrying about what others think of you and having to prove yourself to them constantly. Some procrastinate because they think they need to do everything perfectly or not at all. With increased self-esteem, you are more accepting of mistakes and don't expect yourself to perform perfectly.

Perfectionism

Perfectionism leads to undue stress because perfection is an unattainable goal. By setting the standard at perfect, you will set yourself up to fail. Perfectionists tend to be their own worst critic; they are harder on themselves than anyone else is on them, and they are also critical of others. These individuals are described as neat and organized, seeming to "have it all together" and to be able to do more than most people and do it exceptionally well. Often people envy perfectionistic people because they seem very confident and competent; however, individuals who are perfectionistic never feel good enough and often feel out of control in their lives.[24] People who are perfectionists focus on what they haven't accomplished or haven't done right rather than on what they have completed or have done well. Making mistakes feels especially humiliating to persons who are perfectionistic, and they tend to feel a strong sense of shame and low self-esteem when someone catches them in error. They have difficulty with criticism or any negative feedback as much of their self-esteem is based upon being accurate, competent, and being the best. While striving to do your best is an admirable quality, expecting to be perfect in everything you do and never making a mistake places a great deal of stress and pressure on yourself.

People with perfectionistic behavior tend to be rigid in their thinking, saying "I must be perfect or else I am a failure," and tend to put in 100% of their effort into something or don't want to attempt it at all, which can lead to procrastination. In expecting perfection, there seems, to these individuals, to be a right and wrong way to do things. Thus, perfectionism can create a great deal of anxiety and distress.

The unreasonably high standards set by perfectionists can cause a great deal of anxiety, and perfectionism is often associated with obsessive-compulsive disorder as well as with eating disorders. Having perfectionistic tendencies can also create stress and conflict in relationships because people who interact with perfectionists feel as though nothing they do is good enough or will please that person.

In alleviating the stress of perfectionism, it is helpful to develop your self-esteem from who you are rather than what you do. This involves accepting yourself and others unconditionally, including the imperfections. Lowering your expectations of yourself and others and aiming for 80% rather than 100% is another strategy in battling perfectionism. Notice what you are doing well and have accomplished rather than what is still left to do. Time management strategies such as those

Key Terms

perfectionism a tendency to expect perfection in everything one does, with little tolerance for mistakes.

My girlfriend is a perfectionist and she is driving me crazy. Nothing I do seems good enough for her as much as I try to please her. Her unrealistic expectations are causing a great deal of stress in our relationship and our friends are beginning to stay away from us because they don't like to hear us argue. What can I do?

Sometimes people who are perfectionist tend to blame others for their own sense of failure or rejection. Here are some ways to respond better to your girlfriend:

1. Communicate how you feel when she is critical of you or shows her disapproval. Suggest more positive ways that she can give you feedback or share her disappointments.
2. Give specific examples of how she may be expecting too much and find a compromise between all or nothing.

3. Don't retaliate. It is tempting to point out her flaws when she is doing the same to you. Instead, reassure her that you think highly of her and point out her successes and accomplishments, as she is probably focusing on her failures.
4. Communicate your confidence in her abilities and ask her to have the same trust in you.
5. Model acceptance of imperfection in yourself and others. Show her that everybody is flawed, no one is perfect, and this makes us human.
6. Don't focus on her mistakes or tease her when she makes an error. Instead give positive reinforcement when she doesn't do something well.
7. Help her to relax and have fun even if all the work is not yet done.
8. Talk about how she is feeling rather than on the content of her message, such as

saying "You sound very stressed and overwhelmed."
9. Don't fall into the perfectionist trap yourself. It is easy to think, "If I just try harder, she will be happy with me." Perfectionism is an impossible goal to reach and so you are setting yourself up for failure and rejection.
10. Help her to see the forest rather than the trees. It is easy for perfectionists to get lost in the details and lose sight of the overall goal. It may help to alleviate her stress if you can help her to refocus on what is really important and what the overall goal is such as having fun at the party you are throwing and not having the house perfectly clean.

---

outlined on pages 76–77 can be useful in managing your expectations of yourself. Push yourself to take risks and allow yourself to make mistakes. It can be useful to make mistakes on purpose in order to get accustomed to this experience and realize that people still like and accept you and nothing bad will happen. Relaxation and stress management techniques such as the ones described at the end of this chapter can also help alleviate the stress that comes with perfectionism. You might want to take the survey at the end of this chapter to assess your level of perfectionism.

Type A and Type B Personalities

Cardiologists Meyer Friedman and Roy Rosenman identified two basic types of personalities when they interviewed individuals in order to ascertain people who may be susceptible to stress-related heart disease.[25] In the interview, they asked individuals the following questions:

1. Does your job carry heavy responsibility?
2. Is there any time when you feel particularly rushed or under pressure?
3. When you are under pressure, does it bother you?
4. Would you describe yourself as a hard-driving ambitious type of person in accomplishing the things you want or would you describe yourself as a relatively relaxed and easy-going person?

From the responses to these questions, Friedman and Rosenman were able to distinguish two types of personalities with respect to stress: type A and type B personalities. **Type A** individuals often feel pressured, are ambitious, impatient, competitive, walk and talk rapidly, and can be easily annoyed by delays. **Type B** individuals tend to be calm, relaxed, easy-going, and patient. They also found that many cases of heart disease couldn't be attributed to other cardiac risk factors such as smoking or dietary habits but could be linked to stress. Type A personalities tend to share qualities of workaholism and perfectionism such as having high expectations and feeling out of control, irritable and overwhelmed, stressed and pressured most of the time. There is a constant sense of needing to go faster and hurry through activities to get onto the next task. Thus type A people tend not to enjoy

---

Key Terms

type A personality a personalty type that tends to be competitive, ambitious, and impatient; often associated with heart attacks and other stress-related conditions.

type B personality a personality type that tends to be more relaxed and patient.

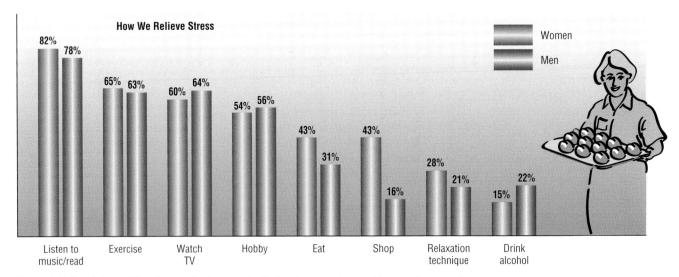

Figure 3-5 People have different ways of relaxing and relieving stress, such as cooking, reading a mystery novel, or swimming. How do you cope with stress?

what they are doing because they are thinking about the next activity rather than enjoying the present.[26] This can of course cause tension in their relationships as well. Type A people tend to drive themselves to exhaustion and stop only when they collapse or become ill.

While Friedman and Rosenman didn't describe type A personalitites as an illness but more as a personality type, they did find correlations with stress. As with perfectionism, type A people sometimes need to slow down, lower their expectations of themselves, delegate responsibilities to others, and prioritize their tasks. Type A individuals often complain that they have trouble relaxing and don't know how to relax. They also don't allow themselves to have fun until all of the work is done which rarely occurs. Scheduling social activities and time to relax is one important component in alleviating the stress that accompanies type A personalities. Exercising, meditation, massage, spiritual activities, and yoga are other ways to relax the mind and body and take a break from your busy day.

Managing Stress: Effective Coping Strategies

The research on how people cope with crisis and stress in their lives has shown that people tend to resolve problems within 2 weeks of experiencing a crisis. Because stress involves a disruption in your equilibrium, and the body does not function well in a chronic state of disequilibrium, it is human nature to seek a way to alleviate the stress your body is experiencing and return to a steady state. As discussed previously, our bodies cannot function for very long in the fight or flight response without serious damage, and so you will naturally strive to make changes to resolve the stress for survival. However, it is important to note that the way that you resolve your problems and alleviate your stress may be positive or negative.

There are a number of negative ways of dealing with stress that are quite common and often quite harmful. As indicated in Figure 3-5, some turn to alcohol and drugs to avoid their problems and numb their feelings, and cigarettes are also cited as a way of relieving stress. Many people use food to comfort themselves. Procrastinating distasteful tasks and avoiding stressful situations is another negative way of coping with stress. Some people use sleep as a way of escaping their problems, and certainly depression has been associated with not having the ability to effectively manage stress. In the next section, we will discuss ways of effectively managing stress.

What are some positive, effective methods to cope with stress? There are different strategies and methods for stress management involving the physical, social, environmental, and psychological aspects of your stress. We will review techniques and strategies within each of these dimensions, and you will need to practice and experiment to find the stress management techniques that are right for you.

The Physical Aspects of Stress Management

The physical aspects of stress management involve meeting your basic needs of nutrition, sleep, and exercise as was discussed in Chapter 2 under Maslow's Hierarchy of Needs.[27]

Nutrition

In Chapter 5 you will learn that nutrients provide the necessary fuel the body needs to function. When people are

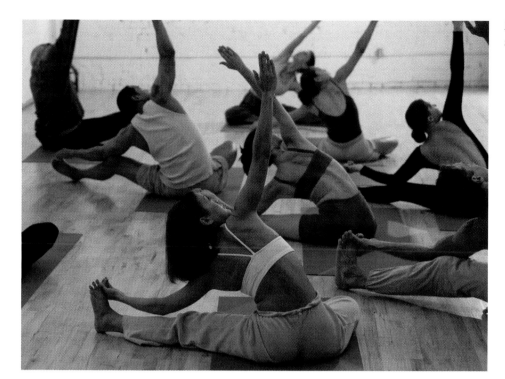

Exercising is one of the best ways to manage your stress.

stressed, they often skip meals or eat on the run. Since the fight or flight response requires more energy than is normally needed, it is even more essential that you eat a balanced, nutritious diet during stressful times. Without proper nutrition, the body will begin the breakdown of its own tissues in an effort to obtain the energy required to survive. The immune system can then become compromised and the body is more susceptible to disease. It is not a coincidence that many people who are under a great deal of stress for prolonged periods of time become ill and regaining their health takes longer than for those who are managing their stress well.

As was previously mentioned, people often use food to cope with stress and can overeat, typically eating high sugar and high fat foods such as chips, candy, and cookies, when under stress. Eating too much or too little is not an effective way to manage stress and can eventually lead to more serious health problems, such as obesity, eating disorders, diabetes, and hypertension.

Sleep

As with eating, too much sleep or too little is also an ineffective way of managing stress. Most adults require 7 to 8 hours of sleep a night.[28] Sometimes people get very little sleep during the week and they try to "catch up" over the weekend, sleeping 14 hours at a time or taking naps during the day. Sleep is not like a bank account in which you can make deposits and withdrawals, and so getting an average of 7 to 8 hours a night over a week's time is not the same thing as sleeping this amount each night.

It is also important that you experience uninterrupted sleep. Normal **circadian rhythms,** the biological process related to the 24-hour light/dark cycle, are necessary for normal sleep and optimal daytime functioning. Our sleep patterns relate to these biological cycles which also impact our patterns of hunger and eating, body temperature, and hormone release. It is important that these cycles be in harmony to have a sense of well-being during our waking hours.[29] Research also shows that sleeping too much can result in increased depression and decreased energy levels. Sleep deprivation has been found to cause losses in higher cognitive processing tasks, decline in the performance of simple tasks, memory loss, and, with prolonged sleep deprivation, temporary psychosis such as hallucinations and delirium.[25] So getting adequate rest is an essential aspect of stress management.

Exercise

Exercise is another physical aspect of stress management. Exercising aerobically at least three times a week for 20 to

30 minutes has been found to manage stress effectively for several reasons. First, exercising requires you to focus on your breathing and to breath deeply, the key to stress management. By tensing and releasing the muscles through exercise, you are allowing your body to relax and unwind. Secondly, exercise can alleviate stress through the release of endorphins, naturally occurring chemicals in the brain. Endorphins help to counter stress, subdue pain, and increase pleasure, which is the reason people talk about the runner's high. Hitting a racquet ball against the wall or playing basketball can be a great way to release the frustrations of the day and let go of tension and stress. Aerobic exercise includes walking briskly, running, bicycling, skating, and dancing. The benefits of exercise will be further discussed in Chapter 4.

The Social Aspects of Stress Management

It is also important in managing your stress effectively for you to make time to have fun and play. Like exercise, laughter increases the release of endorphins and requires you to breath deeply, and so having humor in your life is an essential part of stress management.[30] Research has shown that stress can be related to having inadequate social interactions.[31] Hugging and human contact have also been demonstrated as having a significant effect in reducing the harmful physical effects of stress.[32] Participating in social activities such as social organizations, sports, or just talking with friends can give you the break you need to rest your mind and focus on something other than work.

Actually you don't even have to have human contact to reduce stress—as just owning a pet can make the difference. Studies have shown that just petting an animal produces calming effects such as lowered blood pressure and decreased heart rate. Cardiac patients who own pets tend to live much longer than those who have no pets.[33]

The Environmental Aspects of Stress Management

To effectively manage your stress, you need to take into consideration environmental stressors such as the noise level, amount of light, and aesthetic quality of the space you inhabit. Stress has been linked to being exposed to prolonged, daily noise such as in a factory.[34] We know that depression can be related to the amount of light to which you are exposed, and this can also affect your circadian rhythms.[35] Natural light tends to elevate your mood while prolonged exposure to artificial lighting can increase your stress level. There is also research to suggest that different colors can raise or lower your stress and energy level. Some people associate the color red

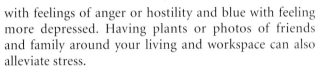

OnSITE/InSIGHT

Learning to Go: Health

Want to reduce your stress load? Click on Learning to Go: Health on the Online Learning Center at **www.mhhe.com/payne8e** and check out this lesson for some interesting suggestions:

Lesson 9: Learn how to manage your stress.

with feelings of anger or hostility and blue with feeling more depressed. Having plants or photos of friends and family around your living and workspace can also alleviate stress.

Smell can also play a significant role in managing stress. As the saying goes, "Stop and smell the roses." Studies have shown that aromatherapy, using different aromas or odors therapeutically, can lower stress levels. When you breathe in the oils, they send a direct message to your brain via your olfactory nerves, where they can then affect the endocrine and hormonal systems via the hypothalamus. Odors have an amazing effect on our emotional states because they hook into the emotional or primitive parts of our brains such as the limbic system. Aromatherapy has been used to relieve pain, enhance relaxation and stress relief, unknot tense muscles, soften dry skin, and enhance immunity. So it is wise to pay attention to your aromatic surroundings, as they may affect you much more than you may realize.

While social interaction has been shown to have positive results on lessening the effects of stress, it does make a difference as to the type of friends with whom you surround yourself. Spending time with negative, pessimistic people can increase your stress level rather than decrease it. It is obviously more advantageous to surround yourself with positive, optimistic friends to better manage your stress.[36] Feeling crowded in a room and not having enough personal space can also lead to an increase in stress.[37] Interestingly, it is not being in crowds itself but how familiar you are with the people, the activity that is taking place, and how much control you feel over your personal space that makes the difference. In other words, being in a crowded room filled with your friends during a party feels subjectively different than feeling trapped in a crowded restaurant filled with strangers.

Other important aspects of managing stress in your environment include having meaningful work and challenging and interesting classes. Having work that is stimulating but not beyond your abilities helps to keep your stress response at a moderate, optimal level for performance.

The Psychological Aspects of Stress Management

Lastly, you can effectively cope with stress by using a variety of cognitive and psychological strategies. There are several different techniques, but as you will see, many are focused on deep breathing, which is the key to managing stress.

Relaxation and Deep Breathing

The relaxation response, developed by Herbert Benson, M.D., is a powerful weapon in ensuring you do not remain in the stress response for too long. It is effective because it entails the opposite of the stress response. Rather than taking shallow breaths, you are required to breathe deeply, inhaling to a count of four and exhaling to a count of four while sitting in a comfortable position. As you breathe deeply, your muscles unwind and relax, again the opposite of the stress response. It is generally advised not to cross your legs or arms so that your muscles can relax easily. Blood flows to the extremities and your heart rate slows. In fact, experienced users of this technique can temporarily lower their breathing rate from a typical rate of fourteen to eighteen breaths per minute to as few as four breaths per minute. Body temperature decreases and blood pressure is lowered as well. The entire nervous system is slowed, in direct opposition to its role in the stress response. You are instructed to focus on your breathing and inner experience and become less aware of your external environment. To help to tune out the outside world, you are instructed to close your eyes and let go of the worries and concerns of the day.[38]

To try this technique, take a moment to focus on your breathing and breathe in for a count of four and out for four. After doing so a few times, tighten your body, clench your hands, teeth, and jaw, close your eyes tightly, and pull your shoulders up while you are still breathing deeply. Are you able to do so? It is virtually impossible to tense your body and breathe deeply, as they are mutually exclusive activities. Thus, the relaxation response is the foundation of most of the stress management techniques that will be described in this chapter. Deep breathing is the fundamental aspect of stress management.

Progressive Muscle Relaxation (PMR)

In 1929 Edmund Jacobson, M.D., published a book describing a simple procedure of deliberately tensing and releasing major muscle groups in sequence from head to toe to achieve total relaxation of the body. His technique, called Progressive Muscle Relaxation, still enjoys popularity today.[39] By learning to recognize the difference between contracted and relaxed muscles, Jacobson believed that people would be able to have more of a sense of control over their bodies and the stress response. Progressive

muscle relaxation enables you to intentionally put certain muscles into a controlled state of relaxation and reduce your overall stress level.

PMR is based on the use of positioning your body in a comfortable position, sitting or lying down, and concentrating on certain muscle groups. As you inhale, breathing in for a count of four, you contract your muscles starting with your forehead and counting to four as you exhale and relax your muscles. Continue to clench and relax the muscles, using your breathing to help you to tighten and release, working your way down your body all the way to your feet and toes. Concentrate on the sensations of relaxation and how different this feels from feeling tense and stressed. Fifteen minutes, twice a day, is the recommended schedule. In 1 to 2 weeks, you will have mastered the basics and will be aware of which muscles need more attention in order to relax. You will also be more sensitive to the buildup of tension in your body so that you will be able to decrease your stress level before it becomes overwhelming.[40]

Guided Imagery and Visualization

In the early 1900s, Emil Coué, a French pharmacist, first suggested using human suggestibility to overcome the stress syndrome, enhance recovery from illness, and facilitate the accomplishment of positive goals.[41] By forming an image of a peaceful, serene place or seeing yourself being successful in accomplishing a task, you can use guided imagery or visualization to manage your stress. Guided imagery involves having someone describe a beautiful, relaxing scene while focusing on taking deep, comfortable breaths. While in a comfortable position, in an environment free from interruptions and distractions, you breathe deeply, relaxing your muscles and imagining a pleasant scene. The imagery includes all of the senses, not just what you see, but pleasant smells, sounds, touch, and even taste. Guided imagery can be self-taught or you can listen to recordings of narrated scripts.

Visualization is similar to guided imagery with the scene being more specifically focused on something you are about to do, want to accomplish, or some performance or activity that may be causing you distress. Guided imagery and visualization techniques help you to consciously program change through positive mental images. For example, you might imagine yourself auditioning for a part in a play, seeing yourself go through your lines effortlessly and flawlessly, and feeling confident and proud of yourself. You are probably already skilled at visualization. Unfortunately we frequently engage in negative visualization and are unaware of doing so: we imagine ourselves making fools of ourselves or making mistakes.

Athletes are trained in using positive visualization to improve their performance and visualize their goals.[40] Positive visualization has also been used in managing pain, especially chronic pain management. This technique has also been effective in weight management, smoking cessation, insomnia, and for almost any type of behavior change. Some images commonly used to decrease stress are to visualize tightly twisted rope as uncoiling; hard, cold wax melting and softening, creaky hinges being oiled and becoming silent and gliding smoothly; or the feeling of sandpaper turning into silk. Again, guided imagery and visualization exercises have optimal benefit when practiced at least once a day, every day for 15 to 20 minutes.

Meditation and Hypnosis

Meditation allows the mind to transcend thought effortlessly when the person concentrates on a focal point. In Transcendental Meditation, a widely recognized approach to meditation, people repeat a mantra, or a personal word, while using deep breathing and relaxation techniques. In other meditation approaches, alternative focal points are used to establish the depth of concentration needed to free the mind from conscious thought. Physical objects, music relaxing environmental sounds or breathing can be used as focal points.

Hypnosis is an artificially induced state, resembling, but physiologically distinct from, sleep. It involves a heightened state of suggestibility that creates flexible and intensified attention and receptiveness, and an increased responsiveness to an idea or to a set of ideas. The focus is on the unconscious rather than on the conscious state of mind, using deep breathing and relaxation techniques. Hypnosis is perhaps the oldest and most misunderstood type of relaxation technique. It has been given a bad reputation by stage entertainers who use hypnosis to have unsuspecting audience members engage in embarrassing behavior.

Hypnosis is a natural state of mind that occurs spontaneously in nearly every person. It is a trancelike state, similar to those that you experience upon awakening, prior to falling asleep, or when you are engrossed in thought while performing other tasks—such as driving down a highway—on autopilot. It is possible to learn self-hypnosis from a trained professional or participate in hypnosis sessions with a qualified hypnotherapist.

Similar to the other techniques described, meditation and hypnosis are best when you are in a comfortable, quiet environment and are practiced at least once a day, every day, for 15 to 20 minutes.

Biofeedback

The word *biofeedback* was coined in 1969 to describe procedures to teach people to alter brain activity, blood pressure, muscle tension, heart rate, and other bodily functions that are not normally controlled voluntarily. Biofeedback is a training technique in which people are taught to improve their health and performance by using signals from their own bodies. It operates on the premise that individuals can alter their involuntary responses by being "fed back" information either visually or audibly about what was occurring in their bodies. In addition, studies have shown that we have more control over so-called involuntary bodily functions than we once thought possible.

One commonly used device, for example, picks up electrical signals from the muscles and translates the signals into a form that people can detect. This device triggers a flashing light or activates a beeper every time muscles become more tense. If one wants to relax tense muscles, one must try to slow down the flashing or beeping. People learn to associate sensations from the muscle with actual levels of tension and develop a new, healthy habit of keeping muscles only as tense as is necessary for as long as necessary. After treatment, individuals are then able to repeat this response at will without being attached to the sensors. Other biological functions that are commonly measured and used in a similar way to help people learn to control their physical functioning are skin temperature, heart rate, sweat gland activity, and brainwave activity. In this way, you can manage your stress by decreasing the physiological components of the stress response.

Stress Inoculation

Similar to being protected from influenza by injecting some of the flu strain into your system, stress inoculation involves exposing an individual to specific stressful situations, a little at a time, under controlled, safe conditions. Stress inoculation teaches individuals to relax using deep breathing and progressive muscle relaxation while exposing them to stressful situations rather than avoiding them.

The first step is to construct your personal list of stressful situations and arrange the list from the least to the most stressful items, and learn how to evoke each of these situations in your mind while at the same time focusing on your breathing and relaxing your muscles. The second step is to create an arsenal of stress-coping thoughts, such as "I'm going to be all right," "I've succeeded with this before," and "Getting started is the hardest part, then it will get easier for me," to counteract stress. The third step is to practice this *in vivo*, meaning in real life situations, while using the relaxation and cognitive techniques to minimize the stress response.[41] In addition to stress management, stress inoculation has also been helpful in anger management.

Cognitive Self-Talk

What we tell ourselves, our self-talk, has a tremendous impact upon how well we manage our stress. Stress can be generated from faulty conclusions, misinterpretations, and expecting the worst. Some people claim that if they expect the worst, they won't feel disappointed or hurt, but

Coping with the Stress in the Aftermath of 9/11

Certainly our country as a whole experienced a great deal of stress from the terrorist attacks of September 11, 2001. A poll of 560 adults conducted 3 to 5 days after Sept. 11 showed that 44% of adults reported one or more substantial symptoms of stress, such as having difficulty concentrating, having trouble falling or staying asleep, and feeling irritable or having angry outbursts. Children have also suffered increased stress from these events, reporting more nightmares and feeling more worried about their own safety since 9/11.

Researchers have found that people who used "active coping" strategies right after the attacks were experiencing fewer symptoms of stress than those who denied the events or avoided talking about them. Donating money or blood, attending memorials, and talking with people about their feelings after the attacks were some of the strategies that seemed to alleviate the stress people were feeling. Studies have also shown that there was an increase in the alcohol consumption, cigarette smoking, and marijuana use among Manhattan residents after the September 11 terrorist attacks, providing evidence that people were avoiding having thoughts or feelings about these events and not coping well with the stress they were experiencing.

Many people reported feeling a decreased sense of security and felt increasingly vulnerable and threatened. With the continual warnings of further terrorist attacks, people's stress levels could not return to a normal level and were constantly in a state of high stress, leading to chronic stress. Many people reported that they felt hopeless about the future and began to question the meaning and purpose of their lives.

Disaster reactions tend to follow a predictable sequence of phases for community groups. The initial "heroic" phase involves concerns for survival and altruistic efforts to help overcome reactions such as fear, anger, confusion, and numbness. A "honeymoon" phase occurs next, characterized by outpourings of community and professional support and assistance. As the aftermath of the crisis extends in time, many sources of initial support may be withdrawn as agencies complete their initial goals and normal routines are reestablished. This has been identified as a "disillusionment" phase. This may be characterized by a loss of a sense of shared experience in the community, and a sense of a more pervasive disappointment, anger, resentment, and abandonment. The final phase of disaster adaptation is to mourn what was lost, to reestablish relationships, and reconnect and reinvest one's energies into current life pursuits, relationships, and interests. This process can extend for years, depending on the magnitude of the losses sustained by individuals and communities. It is important to note that the honeymoon phase ends just at the point when persistent and severe post-traumatic stress reactions would be likely to emerge, about 1 to 3 months following the disaster.

Sometimes present loss or trauma can trigger past events. If you have been the victim of past abuse or trauma, the 9/11 terrorist attacks may have triggered these memories for you or made it more difficult to cope with the stress of these events.

What can you do to cope?

- Spend time with other people. Coping with stressful events is easier when people support each other.

- Talk about how you are feeling. Be willing to listen to others who need to talk about how they feel.
- Get back to your everyday routine. Familiar habits can be comforting.
- Take time to grieve if you need to. It is better to express your feelings rather than push them away or avoid them as feelings tend to emerge one way or another and it is better for you to have some say in how they are expressed.
- Ask for support and help from your family, friends, church, or other community resources. Join or develop support groups.
- Limit how much time you spend watching the news about the war or related events in order to avoid retraumatizing yourself.
- Find something positive you can do. Join efforts in your community to respond to this tragedy.
- Stay positive and watch your negative self-talk and expectations in terms of self-fulfilling prophecy.
- Get professional help if you continue to experience difficulties. College counseling centers offer excellent services in coping with grief and loss and trauma.

Sources: Vahvo D, Galea S, Resnick H, Ahern J, Boscarino J, Bucuvalas M, Gold J, Kilpatrick D. Increased Use of Cigarettes, Alcohol and Marijuana Around Manhattan, New York Residents After the September 11th Terrorist Attacks. *American Journal of Epidemiology* 155 (11), 988–996, 2002. Welzant V and Loewenstein R. Psychiatry and the Aftermath of 9/11, Vol. 28, No. 2; pp. 1, 4–6, 2002.

in reality, they still feel the pain from their disappointment. Also, it is important to be careful what you expect because you may inadvertently make it happen, a phenomenon referred to as **self-fulfilling prophecy.** [42] Self-fulfilling prophecy can work for you or against you. If you expect that work will be boring and uninteresting, you will tend to portray a negative, unmotivated attitude and will probably have a miserable time. However, if you

---

Key Terms

self-fulfilling prophecy the tendency to make something more likely to happen as a result of your own expectations and attitudes.

Melatonin: A Good Night's Sleep?

Melatonin is a natural hormone secreted by the pineal gland, a pea-size structure at the center of the brain. The production of melatonin goes hand in hand with the light-dark cycle. At night melatonin is produced to help our bodies regulate our sleep-wake cycles. As melatonin production rises, you begin to feel less alert. Body temperature starts to fall as well, and you begin to feel sleepier. Then melatonin levels drop quickly with the sunlight from the start of a new day. The amount of melatonin produced by our bodies seems to lessen as we get older. Scientists believe this may be why young people have less sleep problems than do older people.

Health food stores sell both synthetic and animal melatonin. Synthetic melatonin is made in factories where the manufacturing process is not controlled by the U.S. Food and Drug Administration (FDA). Melatonin is one of only two hormones not regulated by the FDA and sold over-the-counter without a prescription. (DHEA, or dehydroepiandrosterone, is the other.) Because melatonin does appear naturally in some foods, the U.S. Dietary Supplement and Health Education Act of 1994 allows it to be sold as a dietary supplement, and as such it does not need FDA approval.

Because melatonin has not undergone FDA approval or controlled laboratory studies, little is really known about its safety and efficacy. According to one report, "10 percent of the users said the hormone did nothing for them, and another 10 percent complained of side effects such as nightmares, headaches, morning grogginess, mild depression, and low sex drive." Information about reported side effects are not required to be listed on the product's packaging. Worsened fatigue and depression, constriction of the arteries to the heart, and possible effects on fertility have also been reported.

Without extensive research and testing, it is unclear as to how much to take, when to take it, and the overall effectiveness of melatonin. The doses listed on the bottles may not be accurate. In fact, one study found that a batch tested contained far more than the amount listed on the label. Furthermore, no one knows which dosage level might be the most effective.

As is true of all dietary supplements, you must be cautious and aware of the risks of taking melatonin, given that that are so many unanswered questions about its safety and effectiveness.

Sources: American Academy of Family Physicians. *Melatonin: Frequently Asked Questions,* 1999; *Newsweek,* November 6, 1995, pp. 60–63.

---

expect to enjoy yourself at work, you are more likely to go into work looking for challenge and making it more fun.

In looking more closely at how we make faulty conclusions and misinterpretations, there are many ways we can make cognitive distortions that lead to a more stressed filled life, such as:

1. Filtering—Selectively paying attention to the negative and disregarding the positive.
2. Polarized Thinking—Putting things into absolute, all-or-nothing categories with no middle ground. For example, you have to be right or else you are wrong.
3. Overgeneralization—From one isolated event, you make a general, universal rule. For example if you have failed once, you will always fail.
4. Mind Reading—Without people saying so, you believe you know what people are feeling and the reasons they behave the way they do. For example, if your friend seems tired, you think she doesn't really want to go out to the movies tonight as you had planned and so you cancel the plans thinking that is what she really wants.
5. Catastrophizing—Expecting disaster or the worst case scenario.
6. Personalization—Thinking that things people do or say is in reaction to you and comparing yourself with others. For example, you walk past a group of people laughing and assume that they are laughing at you.
7. Control Fallacies—Feeling either that you have total control and responsibility for events or no control whatsoever over what is happening. You feel responsible for other people's happiness or pain.
8. Fallacy of Fairness—Feeling resentful when situations don't seem fair or just. Believing that good things happen to good people and bad things happen to bad people.
9. Blaming—Consistently blaming yourself or others for things that may not be entirely your or their fault.
10. Shoulds—Telling yourself what you are supposed to do, what is expected of you, or what you feel obligated to do rather than what you want to do. This is often something we don't want to do but think we should do and feel somewhat pressured or forced to do.
11. Emotional Reasoning—Believing that what you feel must be true and what you feel is what you are. For example, if you feel bad, then you are bad.
12. Fallacy of Change—Expecting that other people will change to the way you believe they should be because you perceive your happiness is contingent upon their changing their behavior. For example, telling yourself, "I would be happy if my parents showed more approval towards me and my decisions."

13. Global Labeling—Applying stereotypes or labels to a whole group of people, behavior, or experiences, such as "I'm compulsive about my house."

14. Being Right—Continually proving that your opinions and actions are correct. Being wrong is unacceptable and means you are inferior and less worthy.[41]

In order to change these cognitive distortions, you need to generate some rebuttals to your negative self-statements. This entails finding middle ground between all-or-nothing thinking by asking yourself, "What is the evidence?" that this statement is true and identifying some exceptions to this statement. Look for balance in your statements by asking yourself what is the opposite of this negative self-statement? Rather than telling yourself what you "should" do, ask yourself what do you "want" to do. Be specific instead of generalizing and avoid labeling yourself and others. Instead of telling yourself "I'm lazy," you might say, "I wish I would have studied a few more hours for that test." Stick to the facts without blaming yourself or others. Question yourself as to how you know something is true and if you might be making an assumption or mind reading. Be mindful of your self-fulfilling prophecies. It may be wiser to acknowledge that you don't know or consider many different possible outcomes rather than to expect the worst.

Changing negative self-talk requires time, practice, and patience. We develop these patterns of thinking over years and they become almost automatic. It takes concentrated effort to be aware of and change this way of thinking. Remember that your rebuttals need to be strong, nonjudgmental, and specific. Practice developing more flexible and balanced thinking about people, behavior, and situations.

As you can see, there are many different aspects to consider in managing stress, such as the physical, social, environmental, and psychological component of stress. As you think about how you can more effectively manage your stress level, you will need to practice and experiment to find the stress management techniques that will be most beneficial for you.

 TALKING POINTS Think back to stressful times in your life. What were some positive ways you coped and what were some negative things you did to cope?

A Realistic Perspective on Stress and Life

The development of a realistic approach to today's fast-paced demanding lifestyle may best be achieved by fostering many of the following perspectives:[43]

Do not be surprised by trouble. Anticipate problems and see yourself as a problem solver. Although each specific problem is unique, it is, nevertheless, most likely similar to past experiences. Use these past experiences to quickly recognize workable approaches to resolving new problems.

Search for solutions. Act on a partial solution, even when a complete solution seems distant. By resolving some aspects of a problem, you can gain time for more focused consideration of the remaining difficulties. In addition, some progress is a confidence builder that can help you remain committed to finding a complete solution.

Take control of your own future. Set out to accomplish your goals. Do not view yourself as a victim. Also, recall from Chapter 2 that being proactive and optimistic is an excellent way to take charge of your life and recognize capabilities that you were previously unaware of.

Be cognizant of self-fulfilling prophecies. Do not extend or generalize difficulties from one area into another. Further, negativity about yourself, in the form of self-doubt and self-blame, is certain to erode your feelings of success.

Visualize success. Do not disregard the possibility of failure. Rather, focus on those things that are necessary and possible to ensure success. The very act of "imaging," in which a person sees himself or herself performing skillfully, has proven beneficial in a variety of performance-oriented activities.

Accept the unchangeable. Focus on taking control of what you can and letting go of the rest. The direction your life takes is only in part the result of your own doing. Cope as effectively as possible with those events over which you have no direct control; beyond a certain point, however, you must let go of those things over which you have little control.

Live each day well. Combine activity, contemplation, and a sense of cheerfulness when approaching the many things that must be done each day. Celebrate special occasions. Undertake new experiences. Learn from your mistakes. Recognize your accomplishments. Most importantly, however, remember that the fabric of our lives is far more heavily influenced by day-to-day events than it is by the occasional milestones of life.

Act on your capacity for growth. Undertake new experiences and then extract from them new information about your own interests and capacities. The multiple dimensions of health identified in Chapter 1 will, over the course of your lifetime, provide a wide array of resources that will allow growth to occur throughout your entire life.

Allow for renewal. Make time for yourself, and take advantage of opportunities to pursue new and fulfilling relationships. Foster growth in each of the multiple dimensions of health—physical, psychological, social, intellectual, spiritual, and occupational. Initial renewal in one dimension may serve as a springboard for renewal in others.

Accept mistakes. Both you and others will make mistakes. Recognize that these can cause anger, and learn to avoid feelings of hostility. Mistakes, carefully evaluated, can serve as the basis for even greater knowl-

edge and more likely success in those activities not yet undertaken.

Keep life simple. Keep the demands of life as orderly and manageable as you can. Just as adding too many appliances to an electrical circuit will quickly overload it and cause a power outage, excess demands and commitments added to our daily schedule can quickly burn out our psyches. Learning to prioritize and postpone activities is key to building a productive and enjoyable life.

Taking Charge of Your Health

- Analyze your past successes in resolving stressful situations, noting the resources that were helpful to you.
- Prioritize your daily goals in a list that you can accomplish, allowing time for recreational activities.
- Counteract a tendency to procrastinate by setting up imaginary (early) deadlines for assignments and rewarding yourself when you meet those dates.
- Add a new physical activity, such as an intramural team sport, to your daily schedule.

- Replace a negative coping technique that you currently use, such as smoking, with an effective alternative, such as deep breathing, relaxation exercises or yoga.
- List the positive aspects of your life, and make them the focus of your everyday thoughts.
- Explore the stress-reduction services that are available in your community, both on and off campus.

Summary

- Stress refers to physiological changes and responses your body makes in response to a situation. This can be a real or perceived threat.
- Both eustress and distress elicit the predictable stress response, also called the fight-or-flight response.
- The term *eustress* is assigned to the stress response when its presence is interpreted as being positive (such as stress experienced when riding a roller coaster).
- The term *distress* is assigned to the stress response when its presence is interpreted as being uncomfortable, threatening, or frightening.
- The fight or flight response is a physiological response to perceived, anticipated, or real threat; it causes the heart to race, breathing becomes labored, muscles are tense, the body sweats, and blood flow is constricted to the extremities and digestive organs and increases to the major muscles and brain.
- Chronic stress refers to remaining at a high level of physiological arousal too long and not being able to immediately react to the perceived or real threat.
- While too much stress can have a negative impact and cause some serious health problems, a moderate level of stress is positive and beneficial.

- Yerkes-Dodson Law refers to a bell-shaped curve demonstrating that there is an optimal level of stress for peak performance. This law states that too little and too much stress is not helpful, while a moderate level of stress is positive and beneficial.
- Constant arousal and increased levels of adrenaline in your system will eventually wear down your body's immunological system. You will be less able to cope with stress, and so it takes less and less to cause a stress reaction.
- General Adaptation Syndrome is a sequenced physiological response to the presence of a stressor, involving the alarm, resistance, and exhaustion stages of the stress response.
- Students can experience unique types of stress such as homesickness, relationship problems, test anxiety, speech anxiety, math anxiety, problems with learning, time management, procrastination, and perfectionism.
- When you are more stressed or anxious, you have a diminished ability to concentrate, recall information, and engage in problem solving activities.
- An overwhelming number of students identify time management as the reason for their academic success or failure. Setting priorities and goals, balancing academic

life with your social life, and finding time for sleeping, eating, exercising, and working along with studying is an essential aspect of managing your stress effectively.

- Procrastination means postponing something that is necessary to do to reach your goal. Typically, there is a psychological aspect to procrastination, as we tend to delay doing things we don't want to do.
- While striving to do your best is an admirable quality, expecting to be perfect in everything you do and never making a mistake places a great deal of stress and pressure on yourself.
- Type A individuals often feel pressured, are ambitious, impatient, competitive, walk and talk rapidly, and can be easily annoyed by delays. Type B individuals tend to be calm, relaxed, easy-going, and patient.
- Research has shown that stress can be related to having inadequate social interactions.
- To effectively manage your stress, you need to take into consideration environmental stressors such as the noise level, amount of light, and aesthetic quality of

the space you inhabit. It is also important to get adequate amounts of rest, nutrition, and exercise.
- The relaxation response is effective becuse it entails the opposite of the stress response. Rather than taking shallow breaths, you are required to breath deeply, inhaling to a count of four and exhaling to a count of four while sitting in a comfortable position.
- Effective psychological tools for stress management include progressive muscle relaxation, visualization, guided imagery, meditation, hypnosis, biofeedback, stress inoculation, and cognitive self-talk.
- Self-fulfilling prophecy is the tendency to make something more likely to happen as a result of your expectations and attitudes.
- Some of the ways people make cognitive distortions include filtering, polarized thinking, overgeneralization, mind reading, catastrophizing, personalization, control fallacies, fallacies of fairness, blaming, shoulds, emotional reasoning, fallacies of change, global labeling, and being right.

Review Questions

1. What is stress?
2. How does stress relate to your physical and psychological health?
3. What is the fight or flight response?
4. What are some long-term physiological effects of chronic stress?
5. Describe the Yerkes-Dodson Law.
6. Explain the three stages of the General Adaptation Syndrome.
7. List at least five unique types of stress characteristics students can experience.
8. What are some common effects of test anxiety?
9. What type of anxiety is one of the most common fears for people?
10. How does stress affect your ability to learn?

11. What do an overwhelming number of students identify as the reason for their academic success or failure?
12. Define procrastination, and explain how it relates to stress.
13. How can being perfectionistic cause stress?
14. Describe Type A and Type B personality traits.
15. How do social interactions affect your stress level?
16. List some environmental stressors, and explain, how higher levels of stress have been linked to environmental factors.
17. Describe the relaxation response and how it is effective for stress management.
18. Name seven cognitive and psychological stress management techniques, and explain how they work.

References

1. Selye H. *Stress Without Distress.* New American Library, 1975.
2. Scott LV, Dinan T6 Vasopressin and the regulation of hypothalamic-pituitary-adrenal functions: implications for the pathophysiology of depression. *Life Sci* 1998; 62(22): 1985–1998.
3. Selye, H. *The Stress of Life.* New York: McGraw-Hill Co. Inc. 1984.
4. Girdano DA, Everly GS, Dusek DE. *Controlling Stress and Tension.* Allyn & Bacon, 1996.
5. Raber M and Dyck G. *Managing Stress for Mental Fitness.* Menlo Park, CA: Crisp Publications, 1993.
6. Rowh M. *Coping with Stress in College.* New York: College Board Publications, 1989.
7. Holmes T and Rahe R. Social Readjustment Rating Scale. *Journal of Psychosomatic Research,* 11, 1967.
8. Kagan J and Segal J. *Psychology: An Introduction,* 6th edition. Orlando, Florida: Harcourt Brace Jovanovich Inc., 1988.

9. Padus, E. *Positive Living and Health: The Complete Guide to Brain/Body Healing and Mental Empowerment.* Emmaus, PA: Rodale Press, 1990.

10. Kiev A. Managing stress to achieve success. *Executive Health* 24(1): 1–4, 1987.

11. Lewen MK, Kennedy HL. The role of stress in heart disease. *Hospital Medicine,* 125–138, August 1986.

12. Byers SK. Organizational stress: Implications for health promotion managers. *American Journal of Health Promotion.* 21–26, Summer 1987.

13. O'Donnell MP, Ainsworth TH. *Health Promotion in the Workplace.* 185. New York: John Wiley & Sons, 1984,

14. Benson H and Allen R. How much stress is too much? *Harvard Business Review,* September/October, 1980.

15. Affordable Care for Kids Squeezes College Students. *The Detroit News,* November 23, 2001. Vandenbeele J.

16. Newman E. *No More Test Anxiety.* Los Angeles, CA: Learning Skills Publications, 1996.

17. Arem C. *Conquering Math Anxiety: A self-help workbook.* Pacific Grove: CA: Brooks/Cole Publishing Co., 1993.

18. Kahn N. *More Learning in Less Time.* Berkeley, CA. Ten Speed Press. 1992.

19. Lindzey G, Thompson R, and Spring B. *Psychology,* 3rd ed. New York: Worth Publishers, Inc. 1988.

20. Lakein A. *How to Get Control of Your Time and Your Life.* New York: New American Library, 1973.

21. Hill MB, Hill DA, Chabot AE, and Barrall JF. A Survey of College Faculty and Student Procrastination. *College Student Journal* 12, 256–262, 1978.

22. Roberts M. *Living Without Procrastination.* Oakland, CA: New Harbinger Publications, 1995.

23. Ferrari J, Johnson J, and McGown W. *Procrastination and Task Avoidance; Theory, Research and Treatment.* New York: Plenum. 1995.

24. Basco M. *Never Good Enough.* New York: Simon & Schuster, 1999.

25. Spear P, Penrod S, and Baker T. *Psychology: Perspectives on Behavior.* New York: John Wiley & Sons, 1988.

26. Robinson B. *Overdoing It. How to Slow Down and Take Care of Yourself.* Deerfield Beach, Florida: Health Communications Inc. 1992.

27. Maslow AH. *Motivation and Personality,* 2nd ed. New York: Van Nostrand, 1970.

28. Ferber R. *Solve Your Child's Sleep Problems.* New York: Simon & Schuster, 1985.

29. Saladin KS. *Anatomy & Physiology: the Unity of Form and Function.* McGraw-Hill, 2001.

30. Lefcourt HM and Martin RA. *Humor and Life Stress: Antidote to Adversity.* New York: Spring-Verlag, 1986.

31. Asterita MF. *The Physiology of Stress.* 4–5. New York: Human Sciences Press, 1985.

32. Hugging Warms the Heart and Also May Protect It. *USA Today,* March 10, 2003.

33. Allen K, Shykoff BE, Izzo JL, Jr. Pet Ownership but Not ACE Inhibitor Therapy Blunts Home Blood Pressure Responses to Mental Stress. *Hypertension 2001,* October, 38(4), 815–820.

34. Goliszek AG. *Breaking the Stress Habit.* Winston-Salem, NC: Carolina Press, 1987.

35. Rosenthal NE. *Winter Blues.* New York: The Guilford Press, 1998.

36. Seligman M. *Learned Optimism.* New York: Simon & Schuster Inc., 1990.

37. Wade C and Tavris C. *Psychology.* New York: Harper & Row Publishers, 1987.

38. Benson H. *The Relaxation Response.* New York: Avon, 1976.

39. Jacobson E. *Progressive Relaxation.* Chicago: University of Chicago Press, 1942.

40. Fanning P. *Visualization for Change.* Oakland, CA: New Harbinger Publications, Inc. 1988.

41. McKay M, Davis M, and Fanning P. *Thoughts and Feelings: the Art of Cognitive Stress Intervention.* Oakland, CA: New Harbinger Publications, 1981.

42. Jones RA. *Self-Fulfilling Prophecies.* Hillsdale, N.J.: John Wiley & Sons, 1977.

43. McGinnis L. *The Power of Optimism.* Harper & Row, 1990.

As We Go to Press

Can our stress levels be regulated by the government? Jeff Peckman, an activitist and author of the "Initiative for Safety Through Peace" or "Initiative 101" thought so. He was instrumental in putting a measure on the Denver ballot in the November 2003 election for a city ordinance to "ensure public safety by adopting and promoting stress reducing techniques or programs." His "anti-stress" legislation is the first of its kind in the nation, suggesting programs such as improving the nutritional quality of school meals, playing "peace promoting music" in elevators, waiting rooms and offices, offering meditation, yoga and relaxation programs for voters, and developing other stress friendly environments. He likened the city's obligation to reducing the public's stress level to hauling away trash in the city. Unfortunately, the measure only received 32% of the vote and didn't pass. Perhaps this ballot will pave the way for others to coordinate ways to reduce stress on a community level.

Source: "In Denver, stress is on the ballot" in USA Today, August 13, 2003. Telephone Conversation on February 18, 2004 with Jeff Peckman.

going it alone: managing the stress of single parenthood

No One to Help

"I've got too much to do and no one to help." Does this sound a lot like your life? Imagine having children depending solely on you. Then again maybe you don't have to imagine. Twenty-eight percent (20 million) of children under the age of 18 live in a single-parent family and 84% of these families are headed by women.[1] Single-parent families can be formed when parents separate or divorce, when a spouse dies, and when the parents chose not to get married and live separately. Increasingly, unmarried women over thirty are raising children without male partners. Other nontraditional families are headed by gay men, lesbians, or lesbian or gay couples.

From 1972 to the present time, the number of female-headed single-parent families more than tripled, reaching 9.8 million.[1] Not all single-parent families or single parents themselves are the same, but the following generalizations have been observed: (1) Single parents tend to be younger than married parents, and (2) single mothers tend to be younger than single fathers.[2] Since the vast majority of single parents are women and a large percentage of that group are young, it is not surprising that they are often in dire financial straits. Women still earn an average of $.78 to every dollar a man earns,[3] and women who become parents by the age of twenty have incomes 37% lower than those of women who become mothers after age twenty-seven.[4,5] The stress of single parenthood goes far beyond financial issues. Pressures of time, emotional strain, guilt, and social stigma weigh heavily on the parent going it alone.

The Financial Burden

Income tends to vary with family structure. In 2001, the median income for married households with children was $60,335; for single-mother households, $25,745; and for single-father households, $36,590. The federal poverty level for a family of four in 2003 is $18,400. Almost 12 million, or 16% of American children, lived in poverty in 2001. This is about the same number of children who lived in poverty in 1980. Seven percent of American children, 5 million, lived in extreme poverty. This was a 17% increase from 2000. Also consider that the poverty rate for young children remains far higher than that for any other age group. It continues to exceed the rate for older children, ages six through seventeen, and is more than double the rate for adults, ages eighteen through sixty-four, and the elderly, ages sixty-five and above. Making life more difficult, only one-third of single mothers are entitled to receive child support, and even those that do get child support, two-thirds of the payments are less than the court ordered.[4] Some states are redoubling their efforts to collect child support. In Illinois a person's driver's license can be revoked because of default on child support payments, and in Indiana wanted posters of the top offenders are posted at highway rest areas.

Many other government programs, such as welfare, AFDC (Aid to Families with Dependent Children), Medicaid, food stamps, education, training, and employment programs, are inadequate or counterproductive. On the other side of the equation, education can go a long way in fighting poverty. Socioeconomic contrasts of children of one- and two-parent families were not as dramatic when the parents had attended college or graduated from high school.[6]

Time to Learn

As the manufacturing jobs in this country are replaced by low and minimum wage service jobs, everyone, married and single alike, needs more and more education to earn an income that will support a family. Thus many single parents find themselves returning to school in order to improve their family's standard of living. At school, loans, scholarships, grants, subsidized day care, and on-campus housing may help ease the burden single parents feel—if these services exist at their university. In exchange, there are extra time demands unique to the school setting. Much of what is expected of college students is done outside of class on "their own time," but single parents are always on call for their kids, so they have little or no time of their own. Reading textbooks, studying for tests, and writing papers must be done while fixing dinner, helping with baths, and reading bedtime stories or put off to the few precious hours when everyone else is in bed. Group projects, papers, and study sessions require finding and paying for a sitter. In-class requirements may also create a conflict for single parents. What do you do when faced with a sick child on the day of the midterm exam if there is no chance for a makeup test?

Single parents often juggle their academic work with the pressures of employment. Seventy-nine percent of single parents with children ages six to seventeen work and 59% of those with children under six are employed.[6] Employers are sometimes less than sympathetic to the stress of balancing child care, household responsibilities, and educational requirements.

While having a good support system and social interaction is an effective way of managing stress, often single parents report feeling isolated and alone, especially those attending school. They describe feeling different from their classmates and don't have a sense of belonging or fitting in. In addition, they have little time for social activities.

Child Care and Parenting

If single parents can find child care, it is often costly and may not accommodate their work hours or class schedule. The expense of child care can consume 25% to 60% of the family income.[5] If the parent moves into his or her parents' house to cut costs and have grandparents readily available for child care, there may be child-rearing conflicts. If the parent and grandparent(s) set different rules, the children can become confused. Parental authority is weakened if the parent is viewed as a child again. A different blended household arises when a grandparent needs care and moves into the home of his or her child and grandchildren.

If the father is absent, the lack of a same-sex role model for male children may be of concern. The presence of a grandfather or uncle in the house eases this concern somewhat, but the involvement of playmates' or classmates' fathers in their children's lives may cause sadness or wistfulness. When a father is occa-sionally present, he may turn into a "Disneyland Dad," taking on the role of friend and entertainer, leaving Mom with the day-to-day responsibility.

Emotional Stress

With reduced finances, excessive demands on time, and reduced social supports, solo parents often experience emotional and parental isolation. Single parents experience responsibility overload from the tension, pressure, and confusion of their circumstances, task overload from social isolation, and emotional overload from having the sole responsibility of their children without anyone to step in to relieve them or problem solve with them.

Tips to Reduce Stress

Despite these overwhelming difficulties, many single parents have come up with creative ways to reduce their stress levels. A few suggestions are listed here:

- Investigate to see if you qualify for the child care connections program. The mission of this program is to promote quality, affordable child care.
- Join an organized group, such as Parents without Partners.
- Join or organize a group of neighborhood or workplace single parents.
- Trade child care time with other single parents.
- Arrange for a friend or relative to baby-sit sometime when you have nothing planned, and do something for yourself.
- Give yourself permission to ask family and friends for help.
- Set realistic goals and expectations for yourself. You don't need to do it all now or perfectly.

Perhaps most important is to remind yourself often that you are doing the best you can with the resources you have.

The Outlook

Although difficult, women and men across this country are making single parenthood work. New insights into both the strengths and causes of stress within single-parent families help give these families the support they need.

For Discussion . . .

Are you a single parent? If so, what is the most important thing that you wish people would understand about single parenting? Were you raised in a single-parent household? How did this affect you? If you do not fall into either of these two categories, what was your biggest misconception about single-parent families? What government policies on family issues need to be changed? How would you change them?

References

1. www.singleparentcentral.com/factstat2.htm
2. Ginglas M, Weinraub M. The more things change . . . single parenting revisited. *Fam Iss* 1995; 16(1):29–52.
3. Bureau of Labor Statistics. Women's earnings as a percent of men's, 1979–1997. *NEWS*, Washington, DC, 1998. (www.dol.gov/dol/wb/public/stats/main.htm)
4. Kissman K, Allen JA. *Single-parent families.* Sage, 1993.
5. Leslie MR, ed. *The single mother's companion.* Seal Press, 1994.
6. Mulroy EA. *The new uprooted.* Auburn House, 1995.

InfoLinks

www.parentsplace.com
www.parenthoodweb.com

personal assessment

how stressed are you?

A widely used life stress scale called the Social Readjustment Rating Scale by Holmes and Rahe has been used to determine the degree of stress that you are experiencing due to life events over the past year. It also projects your chances of developing an illness- or stress-related health condition. Stress can lead to some serious health problems, and the more stress you have in your life, the more vulnerable you are to being susceptible to illness. Let's see how you score.

Life-Stress Scale

Check off the events which have happened to you **within the last year.** Then add up your total number of stress units for each life stress event. The number on the right-hand side represents the amount, duration, and severity of change required to cope with each item. See the point scale at the bottom of the inventory to determine your health risk associated with your stress level.

Life Event	Value	Score
Death of a partner	100	____
Divorce	73	____
Relationship separation	65	____
Jail term	63	____
Death of a family member	63	____
Personal injury/illness	53	____
Marriage	50	____
Fired from job	47	____
Reconciliation with partner	45	____
Retirement	45	____
Illness—family member	44	____
Pregnancy	40	____
Sexual difficulties	39	____
Addition of a family member	39	____
Change in financial situation	38	____
Death of a close friend	37	____
Change in job	36	____
Frequent arguments with partner	35	____
Mortgage over $10,000	31	____
Foreclosure of mortgage/loan	30	____
Change in work responsibilities	29	____
Child leaving home	29	____
Trouble with in-laws	29	____
Outstanding personal achievement	28	____

Begin or end school	26	____
Partner begins/stops working	26	____
Change in living conditions	25	____
Change in personal habits	24	____
Trouble with supervisor	23	____
Change in work hours	20	____
Change in residence	20	____
Change in schools	20	____
Change in recreation	19	____
Change in church activities	19	____
Change in social activities	18	____
Mortgage/loan less than $10,000	17	____
Change in sleeping habits	16	____
Change in family visits	15	____
Change in eating habits	15	____
Vacation	13	____
Christmas	12	____
Minor violations of the law	11	____
TOTAL SCORE		____

What Is Your Health Risk?

Notice that positive events such as outstanding personal achievements, vacations, Christmas, can be as stressful as negative ones. Think of events in your life that are not listed on this inventory. For example, where would you put running in a marathon or going on a diet?

⇒ If your score was 150 points or less . . .
You are on reasonably safe and healthy ground. You have about a one-in-three chance of a health change in the next 2 years.

→ If your score was between 150 300 points . . .
You have about a 50/50 chance of developing an illness related to stress in the next 2 years.

⇒ If your score was 300 points or more . . .

You have a 90 percent chance of developing an illness due to stress that could seriously affect your health. You need to be very watchful in how you are managing your stress.

Based on Holmes and Rahe "Social Readjustment Scale".

personal assessment

am i a perfectionist?

Below are some ideas that are held by perfectionists. Which of these do you see in yourself? To help you decide, rate how strongly you agree with each of the statements below on a scale from 0 to 4.

0	1	2	3	4
I do not agree		I agree somewhat		I agree completely

_____ 1. I have an eye for details that others can miss.

_____ 2. I can get lost in details and forget the real purpose of the task.

_____ 3. I can get overwhelmed by too many details.

_____ 4. It stresses me when people do not want to do things the right way.

_____ 5. There is a right way and a wrong way to do most things.

_____ 6. I do not like my routine to be interrupted.

_____ 7. I expect a great deal from myself.

_____ 8. I expect no less of others than I expect of myself.

_____ 9. People should always do their best.

_____ 10. I am neat in my appearance.

_____ 11. Good grooming is important to me.

_____ 12. I do not like being seen before I have showered and dressed.

_____ 13. I do not like making mistakes.

_____ 14. Receiving criticism is horrible.

_____ 15. It is embarrassing to make mistakes in front of others.

_____ 16. Sharing my new ideas with others makes me anxious.

_____ 17. I worry that my ideas are not good enough.

_____ 18. I do not have a great deal of confidence in myself.

_____ 19. I'm uncomfortable when my environment is untidy or disorganized.

_____ 20. When things are disorganized it is hard for me to concentrate.

_____ 21. What others think about my home is important to me.

_____ 22. I have trouble making difficult decisions.

_____ 23. I worry that I may make the wrong decision.

_____ 24. Making a bad decision can be disastrous.

_____ 25. I often do not trust others to do the job right.

_____ 26. I check the work of others to make certain it was done correctly.

_____ 27. If I can control the process it will turn out fine.

_____ 28. I am a perfectionist.

_____ 29. I care more about doing a quality job than others do

_____ 30. It's important to make a good impression.

_____ **TOTAL SCORE**

Scoring

Add all thirty items together to get total score. If your score was less than 30, then you are probably not a perfectionist, although you may have a few of the traits. Scores from 31 to 60 suggest mild perfectionism. When you are stressed your score may be higher. Scores of 61 to 90 suggest moderate perfectionism. This probably means that perfectionism is causing you trouble in some specific areas, but is not out of control. Scores higher than 91 suggest a level of perfectionism that could cause you serious problems.

Adapted from: _Never Good Enough_ by Monica Ramirez Basco.

the body

Part Two comprises three chapters whose content is especially relevant to college students: fitness, nutrition, and weight management. This part will help you learn how to improve your health in these areas.

1. **Physical Dimension**

   Health experts believe that fitness, nutrition, and weight management are interrelated. How well our bodies work depends on what we eat and how we exercise. Healthy bodies allow us to participate in daily activities and recover more quickly from illness and injury.

2. **Psychological Dimension**

   When you start a fitness program or begin to pay attention to your diet, you learn about your level of motivation and commitment. You will be challenged, but the psychological rewards for your efforts, such as an improved self-concept and greater confidence, can be substantial.

3. **Social Dimension**

   The social dimension of health is closely related to fitness, nutrition, and weight management. Exercising with friends offers an opportunity for social interaction. Participation in most group fitness activities involves listening, sharing, and counseling. Food, like alcohol, can function as a "social lubricant" by bringing and holding people together. However, an excessive food intake and lack of exercise can hinder social relationships when a person is significantly above his or her desirable weight.

4. **Intellectual Dimension**

   Some evidence suggests that people feel mentally sharper after they exercise. Many students report that they can study more efficiently after a workout. People deprived of adequate exercise and proper nutrition may suffer intellectual impairment. Regular physical activity, a sound diet, and effective weight management will allow you to enjoy a wide range of new experiences that can lead to improved intellectual functioning.

5. **Spiritual Dimension**

   Throughout this text we emphasize that an important part of your spiritual growth is serving others. Staying physically fit, following a healthful diet, and managing your weight can enhance your ability to serve others. You can express your own spirituality and help others find meaning in their lives when you take proper care of your health.

6. **Occupational Dimension**

   Just as you can better serve others when you feel your best, you can also pursue a career and carry out daily occupational tasks when you take care of your body. Some job functions, such as traveling and heavy lifting, require that you be in good physical condition. In addition, being fit can help you deal more effectively with the stress that inevitably accompanies employment. Taking care of your body can increase your self-esteem and improve your confidence—a definite plus when you are trying to land a job or earn a promotion.

chapter four

becoming physically fit

Chapter Objectives

After reading this chapter, you should be able to:

- explain why cardiorespiratory fitness is more important to health than other types of fitness, including muscular strength, muscular endurance, and flexibility.
- describe the effects that regular aerobic exercise has on the heart, lungs, and circulatory system.
- assess your own level of fitness in the areas of body composition, cardiorespiratory capacity, muscular strength, and flexibility.
- define aerobic energy production and anaerobic energy production.
- list and discuss the health concerns of midlife adults and of elderly adults.
- discuss the requirements of a suitable cardiorespiratory fitness program, including the mode of activity, frequency, intensity, duration, and resistance.
- explain the role of the warm-up, conditioning, and cooldown in an exercise session.
- explain the role exercise should play in pregnancy.
- discuss the role of fluid replacement in exercise, including when one should consume fluids and the best types of fluids one should consume.
- discuss the contribution of sleep to overall wellness.
- explain five principles for the prevention and care of sports injuries.

Online Learning Center Resources

www.mhhe.com/payne

Log on to our Online Learning Center (OLC) for access to these additional resources:

- Chapter key terms and definitions
- Learning objectives
- Student interactive question-and-answer sites
- Self-scoring chapter quiz
- Online assessments
- Key term flash cards

Talking It Over

Fitness for Kids—A Great Start

Talking to kids about fitness isn't easy—especially if you're out of shape yourself. Here are some approaches to try:

- Be a good role model. Start getting in shape by walking. Tell your kids how much better you feel, and ask them to join you.
- When you buy gifts for your kids, choose items for active play, like a bike, rollerblades, a basketball, or a tennis racquet.
- Make time for play with your kids. Toss a football around in the backyard or throw a

Frisbee with them. Take your kids to the pool and get in the water with them. Show them—and tell them—that being active together is fun.

CommunicationLinks
www.intelihealth.com
www.mayohealth.org

Eye on the Media

Infomercials for Fitness Equipment

As you channel surf with your TV's remote control, it's difficult to avoid seeing an infomercial for some type of fitness equipment. These paid commercials generally last from 15 to 30 minutes and often have an easily recognizable, healthy, attractive person as the spokesperson. The fitness equipment often has a catchy name. You've probably heard of most of them: BowFlex, Nordic Trac, Thigh-Master, Soloflex, and every imaginable name for equipment to improve the abdominal muscles. One of these devices, called the Torso Track, is promoted by Suzanne Somers.

The equipment advertisers frequently promise that by using their fitness device you will develop a beautiful, slim, strong, and well-toned body like that of the person "modeling" the equipment. And here is the best part: "You can achieve the body you want in just a few minutes each day . . . with very little effort on your part."

Is this possible? Probably not, say the fitness experts. There aren't many shortcuts to achieving overall fitness. The most lasting levels of fitness come from carefully designed programs that use a variety of activities and fitness equipment and encourage gradual increases in exertion and weight loss, if indicated.

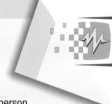

For many college students, the day begins early in the morning; continues with classes, assignments, study, a job, or recreational activities; and does not end until after midnight. This kind of pace demands that the student be physically fit. Even a highly motivated college student must have a conditioned, rested body to maintain such a schedule.

Of course, many college students do not look at physical fitness as a means to a more satisfying, exciting life. Instead, many students look for the cosmetic benefits of fitness. They want to look in the mirror and see the kind of body they see in the media: one with well-toned muscles, a trim waistline, and an absence of flabby tissue, especially on the arms, legs, abdomen, and hips. Thus, many students become motivated to start fitness programs because they hope that they can build a better body for themselves. Through their efforts to do so, students usually start to feel better, physically and mentally. They realize that physical fitness can improve every aspect of their lives, because they see it happening with each passing week.

Fortunately, you need not become a full-time athlete to enjoy the health benefits of fitness. Indeed, the Surgeon General has reported that significant health benefits can be achieved if you accumulate a moderate amount of physical activity on most, preferably all days of each week.[1]

Benefits of Fitness

Following a program of regular aerobic exercise improves the capacity of your cardiovascular and muscular systems. More specifically, regular aerobic exercise strengthens the muscles of your heart, enabling your heart to pump more blood with fewer strokes to meet the demands you place on it. As a result, your resting heart rate may become slower than in the past, indicating that you have become more physically fit. At the same time, your skeletal muscles develop improved metabolic machinery

to allow them to use more oxygen and thus produce more energy. This cardiorespiratory fitness enables you to deal with the routine and extraordinary demands of your daily life more easily.

Cardiorespiratory fitness is the foundation for whole-body fitness. This fitness increases your capacity to sustain a given level of energy for a prolonged period. Thus your body can work longer and at greater levels of intensity.

As you will see, cardiorespiratory fitness has important benefits for everyone, including children (page 120), pregnant women (page 113), and older adults (page 112).

In addition, improving your cardiorespiratory (aerobic) fitness has a variety of benefits that can improve nearly all parts of your life. Aerobic fitness can help you gain the following physical benefits:

- Control your weight
- Greater ability to perform a wide variety of activities throughout your life
- Ward off infections
- Improve the efficiency of your other body systems
- Reduce the concentration of triglycerides and increase the concentration of high-density lipoproteins ("good cholesterol") in your blood
- Reduce your risk of heart disease and certain types of cancer
- Increase the capillary network in your body
- Prevent hypertension and Type II diabetes
- Increase your longevity

Aerobic fitness also offers a variety of other benefits that, although not immediately obvious, are no less important. For example, the increased stamina that comes with cardiorespiratory fitness enables you to complete and better enjoy your daily activities. In addition, your improved fitness level may reduce the severity and

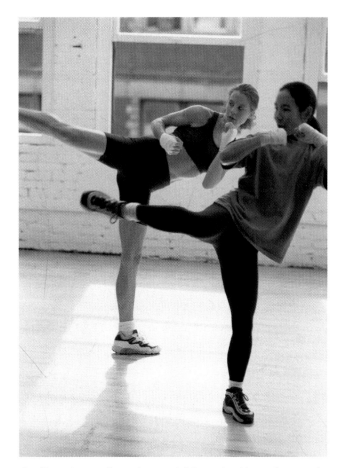

Cardiorespiratory fitness is essential for optimal heart, lung, and blood vessel function.

shorten the duration of common illnesses. Likewise, you will find your ability to cope with stressors to be increased with your fitness level. As a result, you may find your sense of well-being and confidence to be improved.

Older adults will find that improving their cardiorespiratory fitness enables them to enjoy their later years to a greater extent, giving them the energy and ability to participate in activities that they might have delayed for many years, such as traveling, or even activities they might never have considered, such as joining a square dance club or learning how to line dance.

When you become aerobically fit, you may be able to achieve a long-held goal, such as hiking part of the Appalachian Trail, climbing Mt. Rainier, or bicycling through Europe. Others might find that becoming physically fit reduces their dependence on substances such as alcohol, cigarettes, or other drugs and that they sleep more soundly.

Finally, while you are pursuing your physical fitness activities, you probably will meet other healthy, active

OnSITE/InSIGHT

Learning to Go: Health

Looking for a workout routine that's right for you? Click on Learning to Go: Health on the Online Learning Center at **www.mhhe.com/payne8e** to find these lessons, which offer valuable information and suggestions:

    Lesson 10: Discover the benefits of physical fitness.

    Lesson 11: Uncover the components of physical fitness.

    Lesson 12: Create a fitness program that works for you.

    Lesson 13: Choose the right athletic shoe.

    Lesson 14: Promote sound sleep for fitness.

people and find that you are expanding your circle of friends. The Learning from Our Diversity box on page 101 takes a look at the physical and social benefits for persons with disabilities who participate in the Special Olympics.

 TALKING POINTS If your screening tests indicate that you cannot start a vigorous fitness program, are you prepared to ask your doctor about alternative activities?

Components of Physical Fitness

People who **exercise** regularly often choose **physical activities** that fit their lifestyles and individual preferences (Figure 4-1). These activities have the potential for helping them achieve a state of physical fitness. **Physical fitness** is characterized by the ability to perform occupational and recreational activities without becoming unduly fatigued

---

Key Terms

exercise a subcategory of physical activity; it is planned, structured, repetitive, and purposive in the sense that an improvement or maintenance of physical fitness is an objective.[2]

physical activity any bodily movement produced by skeletal muscles that results in energy expenditure.[2]

physical fitness a set of attributes that people have or achieve that relates to the ability to perform physical activity.[2]

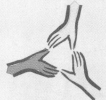

Learning from Our Diversity

A Different Kind of Fitness: Developmentally Disabled Athletes Are Always Winners in the Special Olympics

In America, as in many other countries around the world, physical fitness and athletic prowess carry a high degree of prestige, whereas lack of conditioning and poor sports performance often draw scorn and rejection. As anyone knows who's ever been picked last when sides were being chosen for a schoolyard game, few things are more damaging to youthful self-esteem than being the player nobody wants.

Some of these children blossom into accomplished athletes as they gain coordination or are inspired and guided by caring coaches. Others, lacking strong interest in sports, turn to less physical arenas in which they can excel—drama, debating, music, computers, science.

But what about people who want to be athletes at almost any cost, but who have no realistic hope of attaining the standards of athletic accomplishment set for those in top physical condition? The Joseph P. Kennedy Foundation created an arena in which these athletes could compete when it established the Special Olympics in 1968. Joseph Kennedy was the father of President John F. Kennedy, whose older sister Rosemary was virtually shut away from the world when her family discovered she was mentally retarded. Many people at that time shared the Kennedys' view that the kindest way to treat family members who were developmentally disabled was to "protect" them from stares and whispers by keeping them at home or placing them in institutions or residential facilities. Spearheaded by President Kennedy's sister Eunice Kennedy Shriver, the Special Olympics was intended to change the old attitudes toward developmentally disabled people by giving them an opportunity to compete at their own level and to celebrate their victories publicly.

Now, more than thirty years later, the Special Olympics holds both winter and summer games and boasts participation of more than 1 million developmentally disabled athletes in 140 countries around the world. The 2001 Special Olympics World Winter Games were held in Anchorage, Alaska.

The contests are open to athletes between the ages of eight and sixty-three, some of whom have proved wrong the specialists who claimed they would never walk, let alone compete internationally. "Mainstream" Olympic champions like figure-skating silver medalist Brian Orser and a host of well-known entertainers have attended opening-day ceremonies to cheer and inspire the special athletes.

But medals aren't what the Special Olympics is all about. No matter where a Special Olympian finishes in a contest, he or she is applauded and celebrated for the accomplishment of playing the game and seeing it through. The oath taken by each participant in the Special Olympics aptly states the credo of this remarkable group of athletes: "Let me win. But if I cannot win, let me be brave in the attempt."

In what ways other than physical conditioning do you think a developmentally disabled person might benefit from participating in the Special Olympics? What can the rest of us learn from these athletes' courage and perseverance?

and to have the capacity to handle unforeseen emergencies. In the following sections, we discuss cardiorespiratory endurance, muscular fitness, flexibility, and body composition.

These characteristics of physical fitness can be categorized as health-related physical fitness. Other characteristics, such as speed, power, agility, balance, and reaction time are associated with what would be called performance-related physical fitness. Although the latter type is most important for competitive athletes, it is the former type that has the most relevance to general population. Thus, it is health-related physical fitness that this chapter will focus on.

Cardiorespiratory Endurance

If you were limited to improving only one area of your physical fitness, which would you choose—muscular strength, muscular endurance, or flexibility? Which would a dancer choose? Which would a marathon runner select? Which would an expert recommend?

The experts, who are exercise physiologists, would say that another fitness dimension is of even greater importance than those just listed. These research scientists regard improvement of your heart, lung, and blood vessel function as the key focal point of a physical fitness program.

Cardiorespiratory endurance forms the foundation for whole-body fitness. Cardiorespiratory endurance increases your capacity to sustain a given level of energy production for a prolonged period. Development of cardiorespiratory endurance helps your body to work longer and at greater levels of intensity.

Occasionally your body cannot produce the energy it needs for long-term activity. Certain activities require performance at a level of intensity that outstrips your

Key Terms

cardiorespiratory endurance the ability of the heart, lungs, and blood vessels to transport oxygen required by muscle cells so that they can contract over a period of time. Cardiorespiratory endurance is produced by exercise that requires continuous, repetitive movements.

Figure 4-1 Running or working out in a gym is not for everyone. Which physical activities fit your preferences and lifestyle?

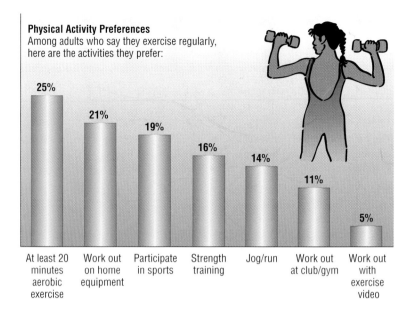

Physical Activity Preferences
Among adults who say they exercise regularly, here are the activities they prefer:

Activity	Percentage
At least 20 minutes aerobic exercise	25%
Work out on home equipment	21%
Participate in sports	19%
Strength training	16%
Jog/run	14%
Work out at club/gym	11%
Work out with exercise video	5%

cardiorespiratory system's ability to transport oxygen efficiently to contracting muscle fibers. When the oxygen demands of the muscles cannot be met, **oxygen debt** occurs. Any activity that continues beyond the point at which oxygen debt begins requires a form of energy production that does not depend on oxygen.

This oxygen-deprived form of energy production is called **anaerobic** (without oxygen) **energy production,** the type that fuels many intense, short-duration activities. For example, rope climbing, weight lifting for strength, and sprinting are short-duration activities that quickly cause muscle fatigue; they are generally considered anaerobic activities. The key factor is if the energy demand of the activity exceeds the aerobic energy production capability. Thus, even activities that typically are considered to be aerobic (walking or cycling) can require anaerobic energy if the intensity is high.

If you usually work or play at low intensity but for a long duration, you have developed an ability to maintain **aerobic** (with oxygen) **energy production.** As long as your body can meet its energy demands in this oxygen-rich mode, it will not convert to anaerobic energy production. Thus fatigue will not be an important factor in determining whether you can continue to participate. Marathon runners, serious joggers, distance swimmers, bicyclists, and aerobic dancers can perform because of their highly developed aerobic fitness. The cardiorespiratory systems of these aerobically fit people have developed a large capacity to take in, transport, and use oxygen.

Besides allowing you to participate in activities such as those mentioned, aerobic conditioning (cardiorespiratory endurance conditioning) may also provide certain structural and functional benefits that affect other dimensions of your life (see the Discovering Your Spirituality box on page 103). These recognized benefits have received considerable documented support. It is now well accepted that regular physical activity that produces aerobic fitness will reduce the risk of heart disease, Type 2 diabetes, osteoporosis, obesity, depression, and cancer of the breast and colon.[3] For many women, exercise reduces the number and severity of symptoms that come with premenstrual syndrome (PMS) (see Chapter 14 for information regarding PMS).

Key Terms

oxygen debt a physical state in which one's activity exceeds the body's ability to produce energy aerobically, causing the body to switch to anaerobic energy production. This produces an excess buildup of by-products, especially lactic acid, and a feeling of inability to "catch one's breath." Respiration and heart rate remain increased until the excess by-products are cleared and the body can return to aerobic energy production.

anaerobic energy production the body's alternative means of energy production, used when the available oxygen is insufficient for aerobic energy production. Anaerobic energy production is a much less efficient use of stored energy.

aerobic energy production the body's primary means of energy production, used when the respiratory and circulatory systems can process and transport sufficient oxygen to muscle cells to convert fuel to energy.

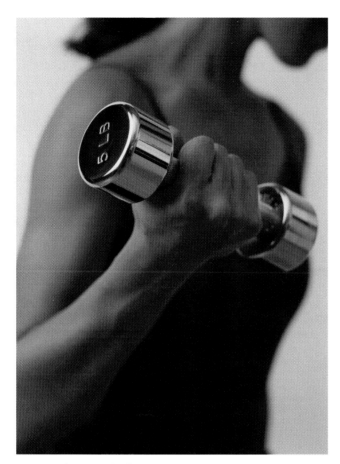

Exercises for muscular fitness are important for both functional and health reasons

Muscular Fitness

Muscular fitness is the term used to represent the capabilities of the skeletal muscles to perform contractions. The capacity of the muscles have two distinct yet integrated characteristics: muscular strength and muscular endurance. The strength of the muscle is related to its ability to perform at or near its maximum for a short period of time. Whereas the endurance of the muscle is related to its ability to perform at submaximal levels for a long period of time.

Muscular fitness is essential for your body to accomplish work. Your ability to maintain posture, walk, lift, push, and pull are familiar examples of the constant demands you make on your muscles to maintain or increase their level of contraction. The stronger you are, the greater your ability to contract muscles and maintain a level of contraction sufficient to complete tasks.

Muscular strength can best be improved by training activities that use the **overload principle.** By overloading, or gradually increasing the resistance (load, object, or

Harnessing the Spirit: The Saga of Lance Armstrong

In the summer of 1999, American cyclist Lance Armstrong made one of the most amazing sports comebacks in history. Armstrong won the Tour de France, the most grueling cycling event in the world. In October 1996, Armstrong had been diagnosed with advanced testicular cancer and was given less than a 50% chance of survival. At the time of the diagnosis, the cancer had already spread to Armstrong's abdomen, lungs, and brain.

After being diagnosed with cancer, but before starting aggressive therapy, Armstrong declared himself "a cancer survivor, not a cancer victim." He convinced himself, his family, and his medical support team that he could beat the long odds facing him. He even established the Lance Armstrong Foundation (**www.laf.org**) before he had surgery and chemotherapy. He battled through his therapy without giving up the hope that the cancer would be defeated.

Miraculously, Armstrong's cancer disappeared. He then stunned the cycling world by returning to active training and planning a comeback that included competing for the 1999 Tour de France title. As Armstrong's physical condition improved and his training regimen became more demanding, cycling enthusiasts believed that Armstrong might be able to compete in—but certainly not win— the world's most famous bike race.

Armstrong proved his doubters wrong by winning the 1999 Tour de France. Perhaps even more amazingly, he has won the Tour de France *again* in the years 2000, 2001, 2002, and 2003, and participated on the U.S. Olympic Cycling Team at the Sydney Olympics in 2000, winning a bronze medal in the Men's Individual Time Trial event. Armstrong chronicled his battle with testicular cancer in his best-selling book *It's Not About the Bike* (Putnam) and followed this with a cycling training book called *The Lance Armstrong Performance Program* (Rodale Press). Clearly, his powers of the mind and spirit worked to help him overcome his physical barriers. His success story has undoubtedly inspired others to take charge of their lives by doing their best to rise above mental and physical barrriers to pursue the dreams that sometimes seem impossible.

Key Terms

muscular strength the component of physical fitness that deals with the ability to contract skeletal muscles to a maximal level; the maximal force that a muscle can exert.

overload principle the principle whereby a person gradually increases the resistance load that must be moved or lifted; this principle also applies to other types of fitness training.

weight) your muscles must move, you can increase your muscular strength. The following three types of training exercises are based on the overload principle.

In **isometric** (meaning "same measure") **exercises,** the resistance is so great that your contracting muscles cannot move the resistant object at all. Thus your muscles contract against immovable objects, usually with increasingly greater efforts. Because of the difficulty of precisely evaluating the training effects, isometric exercises are not usually used as a primary means of developing muscular strength and can be dangerous for people with hypertension.

Isotonic resistance exercises, also called same-tension exercises, are currently the most popular type of strength-building exercises and include the use of traditional free weights (dumbbells and barbells), as well as many resistance exercise machines. People who perform progressive resistance exercises use various muscle groups to move (or lift) specific fixed resistances or weights. Although during a given repetitive exercise the weight remains the same, the muscular contraction effort required varies according to the joint angles in the range of motion.[4] The greatest effort is required at one angle (sticking point) in the range of motion of the movement.

Isokinetic (meaning "same motion") **exercises** use mechanical devices that provide resistances that consistently overload muscles throughout the entire range of motion. The resistance will move only at a preset speed regardless of the force applied to it. For the exercise to be effective, a user must apply maximal force. Isokinetic training requires elaborate, expensive equipment. Thus the use of isokinetic equipment may be limited to certain athletic teams, diagnostic centers, or rehabilitation clinics. The most common isokinetic machines are Cybex, Mini-Gym, Exergenie, KinCom, and Biodex.

Which type of strength-building exercise (machines or free weights) is most effective? Take your choice, since all will help develop muscular strength. Some people prefer machines because they are simple to use, do not require stacking the weights, and are already balanced and less likely to drop and cause injury.

Other people prefer free weights because they encourage the user to work harder to maintain balance during the lift. In addition, free weights can be used in a greater variety of exercises than can weight machines. Workouts with free weights are also associated with visual images and specialized sounds, which some lifters prefer.

Muscular endurance can be improved by performing repeated contractions of a less than maximal level. This aspect of muscular fitness is most related to common physical activities (postural muscles, leaf raking, pushing a lawn mower). Although it is not viewed to be as glamorous as the muscular strength component, it is an important part of muscular fitness.

Flexibility

The ability of your joints to move through their natural range of motion is a measure of your **flexibility.** This fitness trait, like so many other aspects of structure and function, differs from point to point within your body and among different people. Not every joint in your body is equally flexible (by design), and over the course of time, use or disuse will alter the flexibility of a given joint. Certainly gender, age, genetically determined body build, and current level of physical fitness will affect your flexibility.

One's inability to move easily during physical activity can be a constant reminder that aging and inactivity are the foes of flexibility. Failure to use joints regularly will quickly result in a loss of elasticity in the connective tissue and shortening of muscles associated with the joints. Benefits of flexibility include improved balance, posture, and athletic performance and reduced risk of low back pain.

As seen in young gymnasts, flexibility can be highly developed and maintained with a program of activity that includes regular stretching. Stretching also helps reduce the risk of injury. Athletic trainers generally prefer **static stretching** to **ballistic stretching** for people who wish to improve their range of motion, as ballistic stretching carries a higher risk of tears to soft tissue (see the Guidelines for Static Stretching on page 111.)

Key Terms

isometric exercises (eye so **met** rick) muscular strength-training exercises in which the resistance is so great that the object cannot be moved.

isotonic resistance exercises muscular strength-training exercises in which traditional barbells and dumbbells with fixed resistances are used.

isokinetic exercises (eye so kin **et** ick) muscular strength-training exercises in which machines are used to provide variable resistances throughout the full range of motion.

muscular endurance the aspect of muscular fitness that deals with the ability of a muscle or muscle group to repeatedly contract over a long period of time.

flexibility the ability of joints to function through an intended range of motion.

static stretching the slow lengthening of a muscle group to an extended stretch, followed by a holding of the extended position for 10–30 seconds.

ballistic stretching a "bouncing" form of stretching in which a muscle group is lengthened repetitively to produce multiple quick, forceful stretches.

Body Composition

Body composition is the analysis of what the body is made up of (muscle, bone, fat, water, minerals).[4] Of particular interest to fitness experts are percentages of body fat and fat-free weight. Health experts are especially concerned about the large number of people in American society who are overweight and obese. Cardiorespiratory fitness trainers increasingly are recognizing the importance of body composition and are including strength-training exercises to help reduce body fat. (See Chapter 6 for further information about body composition, health effects of obesity, and weight management.)

Aging Physically

With aging, physical decline occurs and the components of physical fitness become more difficult to maintain. From the fourth decade onward, a gradual decline in vigor and resistance eventually gives way to various types

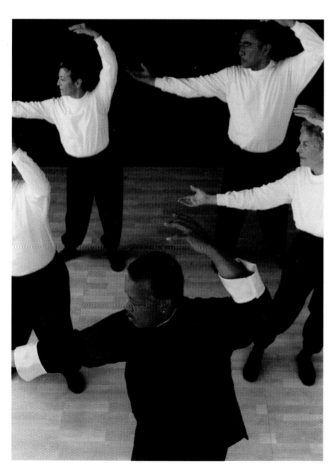

Exercising in a class can be fun and help you stick with your fitness program.

of illnesses. In the opinion of many authorities, people do not die of old age. Rather, old age worsens specific conditions responsible for death. However, physical decline can be slowed and the onset of illness delayed by staying physically active. The process of aging can be described on the basis of predictable occurrences,[5] as follows:

- Change is gradual. In aging, gradual changes occur in body structure or function before specific health problems are identified.

- Individual differences occur. When two people of the same age are compared for the type and extent of change that has occurred with age, important differences can be noted. Even within the same person, different systems decline at differing rates and to varying extents.

- Greatest change is noted in areas of complex function. In physiological processes involving two or more major body systems, the most profound effects of physiological aging can be noted.

- Homeostatic decline occurs with age. Becoming older is associated with a growing difficulty in maintaining homeostasis (the dynamic balance among body systems). In the face of stressors, the older adult's system takes longer to respond, does not respond with the same magnitude, and may take longer to return to baseline.

Like growth and development, aging is predictable yet unique for each person.

Health Concerns of Midlife Adults

The period between forty-five and sixty-four years of age brings with it a variety of subtle changes in the body's structure and function. When life is busy and the mind is active, these changes are generally not evident. Even when they become evident, they are not usually the source of profound concern. Nevertheless, your parents, older students in your class, and people with whom you will be working are experiencing these changes:[5]

- Decrease in bone mass and density
- Increase in vertebral compression
- Degenerative changes in joint cartilage
- Increase in adipose tissue—loss of lean body mass
- Decrease in capacity to engage in physical work
- Decrease in visual acuity
- Decrease in basal energy requirements
- Decrease in fertility
- Decrease in sexual function

For some midlife adults these health concerns can be quite threatening, especially for those who view aging with apprehension and fear. Some middle-aged people reject these physical changes and convince themselves they are sick. Indeed, hypochondriasis is much more common among midlife people than among young people.

Osteoporosis

Osteoporosis is a condition frequently seen in late middle-aged women. However, it is not fully understood why menopausal women are so susceptible to the increase in calcium loss that leads to fractures of the hip, wrist, and vertebral column. Approximately 80% of those with osteoporosis are women. Estimates from the National Osteoporosis Foundation are that half of women and one in eight men over age 50 will have an osteoporosis-related fracture in their lifetime.[6]

The endocrine system plays a large role in the development of osteoporosis. At the time of menopause, a woman's ovaries begin a rapid decrease in the production of estrogen, one of two main hormones associated with the menstrual cycle. This lower level of estrogen may decrease the conversion of the precursors of vitamin D into the active form of vitamin D, the form necessary for absorbing calcium from the digestive tract. As a result, calcium may be drawn from the bones for use elsewhere in the body.

Additional explanations of osteoporosis focus on two other possibilities—hyperparathyroidism (another endocrine dysfunction) and the below-average degree of muscle development seen in osteoporotic women. In this latter explanation the reduced muscle mass is associated with decreased activity, which in turn deprives the body of the mechanical stimulation needed to facilitate bone growth.

Premenopausal women have the opportunity to build and maintain a healthy skeleton through an appropriate intake of calcium. Current recommendations are for an intake of 1,200 mg of calcium per day. Three to four daily servings of low-fat dairy products should provide sufficient calcium. The diet also must contain adequate vitamin D because it aids in the absorption of calcium.

Many women do not consume an adequate amount of calcium. Calcium supplements, again in combination with vitamin D, can be used to achieve recommended calcium levels. It is now known that calcium carbonate, a highly advertised form of calcium, is no more easily absorbed by the body than are other forms of calcium salts. Consumers of calcium supplements should compare brands to determine which, if any, they should buy.

In premenopausal women, calcium deposition in bone is facilitated by exercise, particularly exercise that involves movement of the extremities. Today, women are encouraged to consume at least the recommended servings from the milk group and engage in regular physical activity that involves the weight-bearing muscles of the legs, such as aerobics, jogging, or walking.

Postmenopausal women who are not elderly can markedly slow the resorption of calcium from their bones through the use of estrogen replacement therapy. When combined with a daily intake of 1,500 mg of calcium, vitamin D, and regular exercise, estrogen therapy almost eliminates calcium loss. Of course, women will need to work closely with their physicians to monitor the use of estrogen because of continuing concern over the role of estrogen replacement therapy in the development of breast cancer and increased risk of coronary heart disease events and stroke.

Osteoarthritis

Arthritis is an umbrella term for more than one hundred forms of joint inflammation. The most common form is **osteoarthritis.** It is likely that as we age, all of us will develop osteoarthritis to some degree. Often called "wear and tear" arthritis, osteoarthritis occurs primarily in the weight-bearing joints of the knee, hip, and spine. In this form of arthritis, joint damage can occur to bone ends, cartilaginous cushions, and related structures as the years of constant friction and stress accumulate.

The object of current management of osteoarthritis (and other forms) is not to cure the disease but rather to reduce discomfort, limit joint destruction, and maximize joint mobility. Aspirin and nonsteroidal anti-inflammatory agents are the drugs most frequently used to treat osteoarthritis.

> ### Key Terms
>
> **osteoporosis** a decrease in bone mass which leads to increased incidence of fractures primarily in postmenopausal women.
>
> **osteoarthritis** arthritis that develops with age; largely caused by weight bearing and deterioration of the joints.

It is now believed that osteoarthritis develops most commonly in people with a genetic predisposition for excessive damage to the weight-bearing joints. Thus the condition seems to run in families. Further, studies comparing the occurrence of osteoarthritis in those who exercise and those who do not demonstrate that regular movement may decrease the likelihood of developing this form of arthritis.

Health Concerns of Older Adults

In older people, it is frequently difficult to distinguish between changes caused by aging and those caused by disease. For virtually every body system, biomedical indexes for the old and young can overlap. In the respiratory system, for example, the oxygen uptake capacity of a man of seventy years may be no different from that of a man fifty-five years old who has a history of heavy cigarette smoking. Is the level in the older man to be considered an indicator of a disease, or should it be considered a reflection of normal old age? In dealing with older adults, physicians frequently must make this kind of distinction.

In older people, as in midlife people, structural and physiological changes are routinely seen. In some cases, these are closely related to disease processes, but in most cases they reflect the gradual decline that is thought to be a result of the normal aging process. The most frequently seen changes include the following:

- Decrease in bone mass
- Changes in the structure of bone
- Decrease in muscle bulk and strength
- Decrease in oxygen uptake
- Loss of nonreproducing cells in the nervous system
- Decrease in hearing and vision abilities
- Decrease in all other sensory modalities, including the sense of body positioning
- Slower reaction time
- Gait and posture changes resulting from a weakening of the muscles of the trunk and legs

In addition to these changes, the most likely change seen in older adults is the increased sensitivity of the body's homeostatic mechanism. Because of this sensitivity, a minor infection or superficial injury can be traumatic enough to decrease the body's ability to maintain its internal balance. An illness that would be easily controlled in a younger person could even prove fatal to a seemingly healthy seventy-five-year-old person.

Continuing to follow a physical fitness plan throughout midlife and older adulthood is essential to minimizing age-related health problems. The plan should be modified as necessary to accommodate changes in physical functioning (see the following Star box for an example).

Older Adults and Tai Chi Chuan

Continuing to follow a program of physical fitness is vital throughout midlife and older age. However, which types of exercise are most appropriate for older adults?

Many older adults choose gentle aerobic activities that put less stress and strain on joints, such as walking or water aerobics. Another option is the Chinese discipline tai chi chuan. Practitioners say that the slow, gentle movements of tai chi provide a variety of health benefits, such as improving physical strength and balance. Now a recent study[1] supports these beliefs, reporting that geriatric practitioners of tai chi enjoy greater flexibility, lower body fat, and greater peak oxygen uptake (an indication of cardiorespiratory fitness). The study concludes that tai chi may be prescribed as a suitable conditioning exercise for older adults.

[1] Lan C. et al: Cardiorespiratory function, flexibility, and body composition among geriatric tai chi chuan practitioners. *Arch Phys Med Rehabil* 1996 June; 77(6): 612–616.

Developing a Cardiorespiratory Fitness Program

For people of all ages, cardiorespiratory conditioning can be achieved through many activities. As long as the activity you choose places sufficient demand on the heart and lungs, improved fitness is possible. In addition to the familiar activities of swimming, running, cycling, and aerobic dance, many people today are participating in brisk walking, rollerblading, cross-country skiing, swimnastics, skating, rowing, and even weight training (often combined with some form of aerobic activity). Regardless of age or physical limitations, you can select from a variety of enjoyable activities that will condition the cardiorespiratory system. Complete the Personal Assessment on pages 127–128 to determine your level of fitness.

Many people think that any kind of physical activity will produce cardiorespiratory fitness. Many people consider golf, bowling, hunting, fishing, and archery to be forms of exercise. If performed regularly and for sufficient periods of time, they may enhance your health. However, they do not meet the requirements to be called exercise, and would not necessarily improve physical fitness. The American College of Sports Medicine (ACSM), the nation's premier professional organization of exercise physiologists and sport physicians,[7] has well accepted guidelines for exercise training.

The ACSM's most recent recommendations for achieving cardiorespiratory fitness were approved in 1998 and include four major areas: (1) mode of activity, (2) frequency of training, (3) intensity of training, and (4) duration of training. ACSM has also made recommendations for muscular fitness and flexibility training. We summarize these recommendations. You may wish to compare your existing fitness program with these standards.

Mode of Activity

The ACSM recommends that the mode of activity be any continuous physical activity that uses large muscle groups and can be rhythmic and aerobic in nature. Among the activities that generally meet this requirement are continuous swimming, cycling, aerobics, basketball, cross-country skiing, rollerblading, step training (bench aerobics), hiking, walking, rowing, stair climbing, dancing, and running. Water exercise (water or aqua aerobics) has become a popular fitness mode, because it is especially effective for pregnant women and older, injured, or disabled people.[8]

Endurance games and activities, such as tennis, basketball, racquetball, and handball, are fine as long as you and your partner are skilled enough to keep the ball in play; walking after the ball will do very little for you. Softball and football are generally less than sufficient continuous activities—especially the way they are played by weekend athletes. An old coaching adage applies here: You get in shape to play the game, you do not play the game to get in shape. In other words, using recreational sports is not an effective method to develop physical fitness; however, it may be a useful (and enjoyable) way to maintain fitness.

Regardless of which continuous activity you select, it should also be enjoyable. Running, for example, is not for everyone—despite what some accomplished runners say!

Find an activity you enjoy. If you need others around you to have a good time, corral a group of friends to join you. Vary your activities to keep from becoming bored. You might cycle in the summer, run in the fall, swim in the winter, and play racquetball in the spring. To help you maintain your fitness program, see the suggestions in the Changing for the Better box on page 109. In addition, the Star box on page 109 provides information on exercising in an urban environment.

Frequency of Training

Frequency of training refers to the number of times per week a person should exercise. The ACSM recommends three to five times per week. For most people, participation in fitness activities more than five times each week does not significantly further improve their level of conditioning. Likewise, an average of only two workouts each week does not seem to produce a measurable improvement in cardiorespiratory conditioning. Thus, although you may have a lot of fun cycling twice each week, do not expect to see a significant improvement in your cardiorespiratory fitness level.

Intensity of Training

How much effort should you put into an activity? Should you run quickly, jog slowly, or swim at a comfortable pace? Must a person sweat profusely to become fit? These questions all refer to **intensity** of effort.

The ACSM recommends that healthy adults exercise at an intensity level of between 65% and 90% of their maximum heart rate (estimated by subtracting your age from 220 however, you should be aware that there could be a considerable difference between your estimated maximal heart rate and your actual maximal heart rate [measured during a maximal exercise test]) or between 50% and 85% of their heart rate range. This level of intensity is called the **target heart rate (THR)** (see the Changing for the Better box on page 110). This rate refers

---

Key Terms

frequency the number of exercise sessions per week; for aerobic fitness 3 to 5 days are recommended.

intensity the level of effort put into an activity; for aerobic fitness 50% to 85% of heart rate range is recommended.

target heart rate (THR) the number of times per minute the heart must contract to produce a cardiorespiratory training effect.

to the minimum number of times your heart needs to contract (beat) each minute to have a positive effect on your heart, muscles, and blood vessels. This improvement is called the training effect. Activity at an intensity below the THR will be insufficient to make a significant improvement in your fitness level. Although intensity below the THR will still help you expend calories and thus lose weight, it will probably do little to make you more aerobically fit. On the other hand, intensity that is significantly above your THR will probably cause you to become so fatigued that you will be forced to stop the activity before the training effect can be achieved.

Choosing a particular THR depends on your initial level of cardiorespiratory fitness. If you are already in relatively good physical shape, you might feel comfortable starting exercise at 70% of your heart rate range. A well-conditioned person needs to select a higher THR for his or her intensity level, whereas a person with a low cardiorespiratory fitness level will still be able to achieve a training effect at the lower THR of 50% of heart rate range.

Exercising in an Urban Environment

People who live in large cities face special challenges as they pursue fitness activities. Some of these challenges are just annoying, but some challenges can be life-threatening. News reports occasionally tell of someone who was seriously injured or killed (accidentally or intentionally) while trying to exercise in an urban environment. Visitors to cities can also be confronted with these difficulties, and visitors may be less experienced adjusting to these challenges than those who live year-round in the city.

Among the obstacles are pollution, heavy vehicular and pedestrian traffic, and the possibility of criminal activity. These problems may also exist in small towns, but more likely they exist to a lesser degree. Resist the temptation to use "the city" as an excuse not to exercise. Fortunately, you can tailor a fitness program to fit the urban environment in numerous ways. Consider these strategies as you plan your fitness activities in the city.

- If you are unfamiliar with the environment, exercise indoors. It can be dangerous to jog, rollerblade, or cycle in a place where

you could become lost. Exercise inside your home or apartment, a local health club or YMCA, or in your hotel. Many indoor exercise machines provide a good cardiorespiratory and strength-training workout. Some facilities also have swimming pools, indoor tracks, handball courts, and special fitness classes.

- If you plan to exercise outdoors, always do so with a partner. There is, indeed, safety in numbers. Exercising with a friend or two (or jogging with a large, leashed dog) can provide a measure of protection. If you become injured, friends can help summon medical assistance.

- Try to avoid heavily congested areas. Cycling or jogging in heavy traffic is dangerous not only for you but also for other pedestrians and motorists. This is especially true during rush hours (7–9 A.M., noon, and 4–6 P.M.). Try to locate a relatively quiet place that also seems secure. If you are a visitor to an area, make certain you know whether a particular area is safe for walking, cycling, or jogging. Don't

assume that every urban park is a safe haven for exercisers.

- Do not exercise outside at night. A city can take on an entirely different mood during the night. It is foolish to place yourself at risk by exercising outside when it is dark. Stick to the daylight hours.

- Be aware of pollution levels before you exercise. If there is a pollution warning, consider exercising indoors until the alert is over. If you are one who must exercise outside, you might wish to use a pollution mask; the mask will filter a significant amount of large particles. However, it may also serve to attract unnecessary attention.

- Consider carrying an alarm or protective spray device when exercising outdoors. This suggestion has both proponents and opponents. Carrying a protective spray device or alarm can be helpful, if you know how to use it in an emergency. Remember, some devices can be used against you, especially if an assailant surprises and overpowers you.

In the example in the Changing for the Better box, the younger person would need to participate in a continuous activity for an extended period while working at a THR of 158 beats per minute. The older person would need to function at a THR of 150 beats per minute to achieve a positive training effect.

Determining your heart rate is not a complicated procedure. Find a location on your body where an artery passes near the surface of the skin. Pulse rates are difficult to determine by touching veins, which are more superficial than arteries. Two easily accessible sites for determining heart rate are the carotid artery (one on each side of the windpipe at the front of your neck) and the radial artery (on the inside of your wrist, just above the base of the thumb).

You should practice placing the front surface of your index and middle fingertips at either of these locations and feeling for a pulse. Once you have found a regular pulse, look at the second hand of a watch. Count the number of beats you feel in a fifteen-second period. Multiply this number by four. This number is your heart rate. With a little practice, you can become very proficient at determining heart rate.

Duration of Training

The ACSM recommends that the **duration** of training be between twenty and sixty minutes of continuous aerobic activity. Generally speaking, the duration can be on the shorter end of this range for people whose activities use a high intensity of training (75% to 85% of heart rate range). Those who choose activities with a low range of intensity (50% to 60% of heart rate range) should maintain that activity for a longer time. Thus a fast jog and a moderate walk will require different amounts of time to accomplish the training effect. The fast jog might be maintained for twenty-five minutes, whereas the brisk walk should be kept up longer—perhaps for fifty minutes. The bottom line is to achieve what ACSM calls an adequate volume (total amount) of exercise. ACSM recommends that individuals should expend between 1000–2000 kilocalories per week in aerobic exercises to obtain a cardiorespiratory training effect. This total volume can be achieved in a variety of ways. For example, some may choose to exercise at a moderate intensity (50% to 60% of heart rate range) for a longer duration (40 minutes per session) and higher frequency (5 days per week). Whereas, others can get similar benefits by choosing higher intensity (75% to 80% of heart rate range) with a shorter duration (30 minutes per session) and lower frequency (4 days per week).

Resistance Training

Recognizing the important fact that overall body fitness includes muscular fitness, the ACSM now recommends resistance training in its current standards. The ACSM suggests participation in resistance training two or three times a week. This training should help develop and maintain a healthy body composition—one with an emphasis on lean body mass. The goal of resistance training is not to improve cardiorespiratory endurance but to improve overall muscle strength and muscular endurance. For some people (individuals with hypertension or type 2 diabetes), resistance training with heavy weights is not recommended because it can induce a sudden and dangerous increase in blood pressure.

> **Key Terms**
>
> **duration** the length of exercise time of each training session; for aerobic fitness 20–60 minutes per session are recommended.

The resistance training recommended by the ACSM includes one set of eight to twelve repetitions (ten to fifteen repetitions for individuals over age fifty) of eight to ten different exercises. Although any weight that produces an overload will result in improvement, the greatest muscular fitness gains will be achieved if the weight lifting results in fatigue of the muscle (i.e., more than twelve repetitions cannot be performed). These exercises should be geared to the body's major muscle groups (for example, legs, arms, shoulders, trunk, and back) and should not focus on just one or two body areas. Isotonic (progressive resistance) or isokinetic exercises are recommended (see p. 104). For the average person, resistance training activities should be done at a moderate-to-slow speed, use the full range of motion, and not impair normal breathing. With just one set recommended for each exercise, resistance training is not very time consuming.

Flexibility Training

To develop and maintain a healthy range of motion for the body's joints, the ACSM suggests that flexibility exercises be included in one's overall fitness program. Stretching can be done in conjunction with other (cardiorespiratory or muscular fitness) training or can be performed separately. It is important to note that if flexibility training is done separately, a general warm-up should be performed prior to stretching. For most individuals, static stretching is the best type. Flexibility improvements can be obtained by training as little as two days per week; however, stretching is an activity that can be safely performed daily. ACSM recommends that a flexibility program should include all the major muscle and/or tendon groups. The intensity of each stretch should be at a position where you feel mild discomfort in the muscle. Each stretch should be held for between ten to thirty seconds and should be repeated three to four times per training session. Stretching should be done according to safe and appropriate techniques. (See the Guidelines for Static Stretching below.)

Special Considerations

Warm-up, Conditioning, Cooldown

Each training session consists of three basic parts: the warm-up, the conditioning, and the cooldown.[4] The warm-up should last ten to fifteen minutes. During this period, you should begin slow, gradual, comfortable movements related to the upcoming activity, such as walking or slow jogging. If the upcoming activity requires specific types of movement, some range of motion exercises mimicking those movements are beneficial. All body

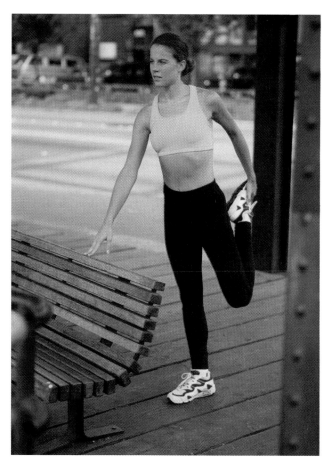

Flexibility exercises can be performed almost anywhere.

segments and muscle groups should be exercised as you gradually increase your heart rate. Near the end of the warm-up period, the major muscle groups should be stretched. This preparation helps protect you from muscle strains and joint sprains.

Guidelines for Static Stretching

Take the following precautions to reduce the possibility of injury during stretching:

- Warm up using a slow jog or fast walk before stretching.
- Stretch only to the point at which you feel tightness or resistance to your stretching. Stretching should not be painful.
- Be sure to continue normal breathing during a stretch. Do *not* hold your breath.
- Use caution when stretching muscles that surround painful joints. Pain is an indication that something is wrong—it should not be ignored.

The warm-up is a fine time to socialize. Furthermore, you can mentally prepare yourself for your activity or think about the beauty of the morning sky, the changing colors of the leaves, or the friends you will meet later in the day. Mental warm-ups can be as beneficial for you psychologically as physical warm-ups are physiologically.

The second part of the training session is the conditioning phase, the part of the session that involves improving muscular fitness, cardiorespiratory endurance, and flexibility. Workouts can be tailor-made, but they should follow the ACSM guidelines discussed previously in this chapter.

The third important part of each fitness session is the cooldown. Ideally, one should not abruptly stop exercise as this could cause circulatory problems (i.e., insufficient blood returning to the heart). The cooldown consists of a five- to ten-minute session of relaxing exercises, such as slow jogging, walking, and stretching. Note, this is the ideal time for flexibility training, since the muscles and joints are warmed from the conditioning phase. This activity allows your body to cool and return to a resting state. A cooldown period helps reduce muscle soreness.

Exercise for Older Adults

An exercise program designed for younger adults may be inappropriate for older people, particularly those over age fifty. Special attention must be paid to matching the program to the interests and abilities of the participants. Often, this is best achieved by having older individuals begin their exercise program under the supervision of a certified exercise professional. The goals of the program should include both social interaction and physical conditioning.

Older adults, especially those with a personal or family history of heart problems, should have a physical examination before starting a fitness program. This examination should include an evaluation of all the physiological systems of the body, especially the cardiovascular, respiratory, and musculoskeletal. Ideally, the evaluation should also include a maximal exercise test (a "stress" test). Participants should learn how to monitor their own cardiorespiratory status during exercise.

Well-designed fitness programs for older adults will include activities that begin slowly, are monitored frequently, and are geared to the enjoyment of the participants.[9] The professional staff coordinating the program should be familiar with the signs of distress (excessively elevated heart rate, nausea, breathing difficulty, pallor, and pain) and must be able to perform CPR. Warm-up and cooldown periods should be included. Activities to increase flexibility are beneficial in the beginning and ending segments of the program. Participants should wear comfortable clothing and appropriate shoes, and they should be mentally prepared to enjoy the activities.

A program designed for older adults will largely conform to the ACSM criteria specified previously in this chapter, including both cardiorespiratory and muscular fitness training. Certainly, specific modifications or restrictions to the exercise program may be required due to health concerns of the individual. For example, because of possible joint, muscular, or skeletal problems, certain activities may have to be done in a sitting position. Pain or discomfort should be reported immediately to the fitness instructor.

Fortunately, properly screened older adults will rarely have health emergencies during a well-monitored fitness program. Many fit older adults can also safely exercise alone.

Low Back Pain

A common occurrence among adults is the sudden onset of low back pain. Four out of five adults develop this condition at least once in their lifetime, which can be so uncomfortable that they miss work, lose sleep, and generally feel incapable of engaging in daily activities. Many of the adults who have this condition will experience these effects two to three times per year.

Although low back pain can reflect serious health problems, most low back pain is caused by mechanical (postural) problems. As unpleasant as low back pain is, the symptoms and functional limitations usually subside within a week or two. The services of a physician, physical therapist, or chiropractor are generally not required.

By engaging in regular exercise, such as swimming, walking, and bicycling, and by paying attention to your back during bending, lifting, and sitting, you can minimize the occurrence of this uncomfortable and incapacitating condition. Many commercial fitness centers and campus recreational programs are starting to offer specific exercises geared to muscular improvement in the lower back and abdominal areas.

Fitness Questions and Answers

Along with the six necessary elements to include in your fitness program, you should consider many additional issues when you start a fitness program.

Should I See My Doctor Before I Get Started?

First of all, we should state that it is highly desirable to have regular checkups with your family physician as part of your overall health plan. However, the question still applies to many. The Surgeon General suggested that most adults can safely increase their activity level to a moderate amount without the need for a comprehensive medical evaluation. Individuals with chronic diseases should consult with their physician prior to increasing their activity level.

If more vigorous forms of exercise are desired, then a medical exam is recommended for men over the age of forty and women over the age of fifty. It would also be recommended for individuals with more than one risk factor for coronary artery disease or if there were any other notable health problems. The American College of Sports Medicine would also recommend an exercise ("stress") test for these individuals.[10]

What Causes a "Runner's High"?

During or after exercise, a person occasionally experiences feelings of euphoria. Runners and joggers call these feelings the "runner's high." However, these positive feelings of relaxation, high self-esteem, and reduced stress are not limited to runners. Almost any fitness activity can leave participants with these intense positive feelings. Swimmers, aerobic exercisers, hikers, and cyclists all have reported exercise-induced highs.

Although these pleasurable feelings can be attributed in part to psychological causes, there is plenty of scientific evidence to suggest a physiological cause. During physical activity, the brain releases its own morphinelike (opiate-like) substances called *endorphins*. These chemicals are released by brain neurons and produce sensations that are pleasurable, and sometimes even numbing. Exercisers report that these episodes of euphoria are unpredictable. Sometimes they experience highs and sometimes they do not. However, endorphin highs are more likely to occur during or after a strenuous, challenging workout.

How Should "30-Somethings" Alter Their Exercise Programs?

People who are in their thirties need to make few if any significant adjustments in their fitness programs. Men and women can continue physical activities they have used since their twenties. If they feel mired in activities that now seem boring, "30-somethings" might try a new activity. However, any new activity (or increase in the intensity of a current activity) should be undertaken gradually.

Should Women Exercise During Pregnancy?

Pregnant women should continue to exercise.[11] During pregnancy a woman's entire body undergoes many physical changes. Muscles are stretched, joints are loosened, and tissues are subjected to stress. If a woman is in good physiological condition, she is more likely to handle these changes with few complications. The baby may also benefit. Studies have shown that women who exercise moderately during pregnancy tend to give birth to healthier babies.[12]

Some reports suggest that exercise during pregnancy can make delivery of the baby easier and faster. Exercise can also help control her weight gain and improve her balance during pregnancy, and make it easier to get back to normal weight after delivery.

The types of exercises a woman should perform during pregnancy depend on the individual and the stage of pregnancy.[11] Most pregnant women should perform general exercises that increase overall fitness and stamina, as well as exercises that strengthen specific muscle groups. Muscles of the pelvic floor, for example, should be exercised regularly, because these muscles will be supporting most of the extra weight of the baby.

A variety of exercises are appropriate, including walking, swimming, stretching, and strengthening exercises. Yoga and tai chi are also good forms of exercise for pregnant women. The muscles of the pelvic floor, abdomen, and back are especially subject to stress and strain during pregnancy and delivery, so certain exercises can also be performed to strengthen these muscles. Exercises can also be performed to speed up recovery after delivery. Such postpartum exercises can be started in some cases within twenty-four hours after delivery. Exercises can even be started before conception if a pregnancy is anticipated.

Some types of exercise can put the fetus at risk. A pregnant woman should avoid any activity in which she becomes overheated, because her elevated body temperature will warm up the fetal environment. Thus pregnant women should not use saunas or hot tubs, nor should they exercise in a hot, humid environment. During the last trimester of pregnancy, women should also avoid any strenuous or high-impact exercise that involves bouncing, jumping, or jarring motions. Obviously, pregnant women should first consult with their obstetricians to develop a safe, productive exercise routine.

How Beneficial Is Aerobic Dance Exercise?

One of the most popular fitness approaches is aerobic exercise, including aerobic dancing. Many organizations sponsor classes in this form of continuous dancing and movement. The rise in popularity of televised and videotaped aerobic exercise programs reflects the enthusiasm for this form of exercise. Because extravagant claims are often made about the value of these programs, the wise consumer should observe at least one session of the activity before enrolling. Discover for yourself whether the program meets the criteria outlined earlier in this chapter in terms of mode of activity, frequency, intensity, duration, resistance training, and flexibility training.

Street dancing, swing dancing, and Latino dancing are fast becoming some of the most popular aerobic exercises. Popularized by rap music, hip-hop music, and the growth of vigorous dancing in music videos, these forms of dancing provide an excellent way of having fun and maintaining cardiorespiratory fitness. Have you experienced the exhilaration that results from an hour or two of dancing?

What Are Low-Impact Aerobic Activities?

Because long-term participation in some aerobic activities (for example, jogging, running, aerobic dancing, and rope skipping) may lead to injury of the hip, knee, and ankle joints, many fitness experts promote low-impact aerobic activities. Low-impact aerobic dancing, water aerobics, bench aerobics, and brisk walking are examples of this kind of fitness activity. Participants still conform to the principal components of a cardiorespiratory fitness program. THR levels are the same as in high-impact aerobic activities.

The main difference between low-impact and high-impact aerobic activities is the use of the legs. Low-impact aerobics require having one foot on the ground at all times. Thus, weight transfer does not occur with the forcefulness seen in traditional, high-impact aerobic activities. In addition, low-impact activities may include exaggerated arm movements and the use of hand or wrist weights. All of these variations are designed to increase the heart rate to the THR without undue strain on the joints of the lower extremities. Low-impact aerobics are excellent for people of all ages, and they may be especially beneficial to older adults.

In-line skating (rollerblading) is one of the fastest-growing fitness activities. This low-impact activity has cardiorespiratory and muscular benefits similar to those of running without the pounding effect that running can produce. However, it should be recognized that it requires both skill and balance. Rollerblading requires important safety equipment: sturdy skates, knee and elbow pads, wrist supports, and a helmet. Obviously, the potential for falling makes this a higher-risk activity.

What Is the Most Effective Means of Fluid Replacement During Exercise?

Despite all the advertising hype associated with commercial fluid replacement products, for an average person involved in typical fitness activities, water is still the best fluid replacement. The availability and cost are unbeatable. However, when activity is prolonged and intense, commercial sport drinks may be preferred over water because they contain electrolytes (which replace lost sodium and potassium) and carbohydrates (which replace depleted energy stores). However, the carbohydrates in sports drinks are actually simple forms of sugar. Thus, sports drinks tend to be high in calories just like regular soft drinks. Regardless of the drink you choose, exercise physiologists recommend that you drink fluids before and at frequent intervals throughout the activity, particularly in warm, humid environments.

What Effect Does Alcohol Have on Sport Performance?

It probably comes as no surprise that alcohol use is generally detrimental to sport performance. Alcohol consumption, especially excessive intake the evening before an activity, consistently decreases the level of performance. Many research studies have documented the negative effects of alcohol on activities involving speed, strength, power, and endurance.[13]

Lowered performance appears to be related to a variety of factors, including impaired judgment, reduced coordination, depressed heart function, liver interference, and dehydration. Understandably, sports federations within the International Olympic Committee have banned the use of alcohol in conjunction with sports competition.

Only in the sports of precision shooting (pistol shooting, riflery, and archery) have studies shown that low-level alcohol use may improve performance, by reducing the shooter's anxiety and permitting steady hand movements. However, alcohol use has also been banned from these sports.[13]

Why Has Bodybuilding Become So Popular?

The popularity of bodybuilding has increased significantly in recent years for many reasons. Bodybuilders often start lifting weights to get into better shape—to improve muscle tone. They may just want to look healthier and feel stronger. When they realize that they can alter the shape of their bodies, they find that bodybuilding offers challenges that, through hard work, are attainable. Bodybuilders also report enjoying the physical sensations (the "pump") that result from a good workout. The results of their efforts are clearly visible and measurable. Some bodybuilders become involved in competitive events to test their advancements.

Perhaps we should dispel a few myths about bodybuilding. Are bodybuilders strong? The answer is emphatically—yes! Will muscle cells turn into fat cells if weight-lifting programs are discontinued? No, muscle cells are physiologically incapable of turning into fat cells. Will women develop bulky muscles through weight training? No, they can improve muscle size, strength, and tone, but unless they take steroids, their muscle mass cannot increase to the same degree as men's muscle mass. Is bodybuilding socially acceptable? Yes, for many people. Just observe all the health clubs and campus exercise rooms that cater to weightlifters and bodybuilders.

Where Can I Find Out About Proper Equipment?

College students are generally in an excellent setting to locate people who have the resources to provide helpful information about sports equipment. Contacting physical education, exercise science, or health education faculty members who have an interest in your chosen activity might be a good start. Most colleges also have a number of clubs that specialize in fitness interests—cycling, hiking, and jogging clubs, for example. Attend one of their upcoming meetings.

Sporting goods and specialty stores (for runners, tennis and racquetball players, and cyclists) are convenient places to obtain information. Employees of these stores should be knowledgeable about sports and equipment; however, keep in mind their primary job is selling a product. So *caveat emptor*. Try to gather as much information as you can so that you can make an informed decision. The Star box on pages 116–117 provides tips for choosing an athletic shoe, and the Star box on page 116 discusses various popular types of home fitness equipment.

How Worthwhile Are Commercial Health and Fitness Clubs?

The health and fitness club business is booming. Fitness clubs offer activities ranging from free weights to weight machines to step walking to general aerobics. Some clubs have saunas and whirlpools and lots of frills. Others have course offerings that include wellness, smoking cessation, stress management, time management, dance, and yoga. The atmosphere at most clubs is friendly, and people are encouraged to have a good time while working out.

If your purpose in joining a fitness club is to improve your cardiorespiratory fitness, measure the program offered by the club against the ACSM standards. If your primary purpose in joining is to meet people and have fun, request a trial membership for a month or so to see whether you like the environment.

Before signing a contract at a health club or spa, do some careful questioning. Find out when the business was established, ask about the qualifications of the employees, contact some members for their observations, and request a thorough tour of the facilities. You might even consult your local Better Business Bureau for additional information. Finally, make certain that you read and understand every word of the contract.

What Is Crosstraining?

Crosstraining is the use of more than one aerobic activity to achieve cardiorespiratory fitness. For example, runners may use swimming, cycling, or rowing periodically to

Aerobic Shoes

When selecting shoes for aerobic dancing, J. Lynn Reese, president of J. Lynn & Co. Endurance Sports, Washington, DC, advises the following:

- Check the width of the shoe at the widest part of your foot. The bottom of the shoe should be as wide as the bottom of your foot; the uppers shouldn't go over the sides.
- Look for leather or nylon uppers. Leather is durable and gives good support, but it can stretch. Nylon won't stretch and gives support, but it's not as durable. Canvas generally doesn't offer much support.
- Look for rubber rather than polyurethane or black carbon rubber soles. Treads should be fairly flat in the forefoot. If you dance on carpet, you can go with less tread; if you dance on gym floors, you may need more grab.

Basketball Shoes

What's most important when choosing a basketball shoe? John Burleson, of the Sports Authority, offers this advice:

- Cushioning. Cushioning is especially important in the forefoot area. Each shoe manufacturer has its own cushioning system. For example, Nike has "Air," and Reebok promotes its "Hexalite" material, composed of hexagonal air chambers.
- Side support. Side support, also called lateral and medial support, is important for making quick directional changes.
- Fit of heel cup. Try on the shoe, and then put your little finger in behind the heel. It should fit snugly.
- Traction. Keep in mind the surface on which you play most often. More traction is needed on asphalt than on hardwood.
- Socks. Socks should be breathable and pull moisture away from the foot.
- "Rope" laces. Rope laces are more convenient than the more traditional flat laces because pulling on the ends will tighten up the laces on the whole shoe at once.

Running Shoes

Need new running shoes? Here's advice from Jeff Galloway, former Olympic runner and founder and president of Phidippides International aerobic sports stores, headquartered in Atlanta.

- Take time to shop, and find a knowledgeable salesperson. Good advice is crucial.
- Check the wear pattern on your old shoes to see whether you have floppy or rigid feet. Floppy-footed runners wear out their soles on the outside and inside edges; rigid-footed runners wear out soles predominantly on the outside edges. Floppy-footed runners can sacrifice cushioning for support; rigid-footed runners can sacrifice support for cushioning.

- Know whether your feet are curved or straight and whether you have high arches or are flatfooted. The shoe should fit the shape of your foot.

Walking Shoes

Have you joined the millions of people who walk for fitness? If so, and if you are ready for a pair of athletic walking shoes, shoe manufacturer Nike has the following advice for you:

- Note where most of your weight falls on your foot when you walk. Are you landing mostly on the heel or on the forefoot? Where you land is where you will want cushioning.
- As with all other types of athletic shoes, take the time to find a knowledgeable salesperson who will provide good advice.
- Go for comfort. Stride in the different types of shoes at your typical walking pace and identify the shoes that are most comfortable.
- Choose shoes that are comfortable in the forefoot area, which will be carrying much of your weight.
- All-leather uppers are satisfactory for most walkers. If you are a serious walker, consider shoes with breathable uppers made of material such as mesh.

Crosstraining Shoes

Crosstraining shoes are a new hybrid, an all-purpose shoe for those who participate in a variety of fitness activities, such as basketball, weightlifting, or light trail hiking. If you tend to specialize in one type of activity (such as basketball), consider buying shoes designed specifically for that activity (for example, high-top basketball shoes for ankle support). To shop for an all-purpose crosstraining shoe, Nike recommends that you keep the following points in mind:

- Once again, comfort is paramount. Try to simulate the activity when you try on the shoe, such as rolling from side to side for court sports, fast movement for walking or running, or walking an incline for light hiking.
- If you tend toward one activity (such as running), look for crosstraining shoes that support that activity (for example, heel and forefoot cushioning for running).
- If you intend to use the shoes for activities with lots of lateral movement, such as court sports or aerobic classes, look for good lateral support.

Aerobic Shoes (*next page top*)

Flexibility: More at ball of foot than running shoes; less flexible than court shoes or running shoes; sole is firmer than running shoes. Uppers: Most are leather or leather-reinforced nylon. Heel: Little or no flare. Soles: Rubber if you dance on wood floors; polyurethane for other surfaces. Cushioning: More than court shoes; less than running

continued

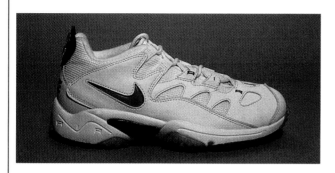

shoes. Tread: Should be fairly flat, especially on forefoot; may also have "dot" on the ball of the foot for pivoting.

Basketball Shoes (*below*)

Soles: Can be made from rubber for durability, EVA for lightweight cushioning, or polyurethane, which is both lightweight and durable. Flexibility: Should be most flexible in the forefoot, for making jump shots. Cushioning: Should absorb shock in the ball of the foot, for landing from jump shots. Heel: A snug-fitting heel cup is essential to keep the ankle in place; the shoe can be high-, mid-, or low-cut,

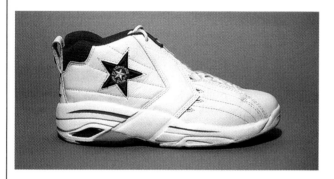

depending on the amount of ankle support desired. Tread: For playing outdoors, the sole should be harder and the tread deeper; a smoother tread works well for playing on a court. Uppers: Can be made of leather for durability or nylon or other synthetics for breathability.

Running Shoes (*below*)

Heel: Flare gives foot broader, more stable base. Soles: Usually carbon-based for longer wear. Cushioning: More than court shoes, especially at heel. Tread: "Waffle" or other deep-cut tread for grip on many surfaces.

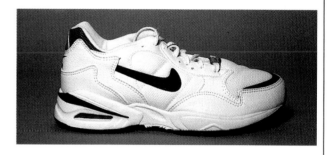

Walking Shoes

Cushioning: Can be forefoot and heel, or primarily forefoot or heel. Heel: May have some flare, similar to running shoes. Soles: Typically polyurethane for durability. Tread: Some tread for traction, but slightly flatter than running shoes.

Crosstraining Shoes

Cushioning: Can be forefoot and heel, or primarily forefoot or heel. Tread: Can be moderate to aggressive.

replace running in their training routines. Crosstraining allows certain muscle groups to rest and injuries to heal. In addition, crosstraining provides a refreshing change of pace for the participant. You will probably enjoy your fitness program more if you vary the activities.

What Are Steroids and Why Do Some Athletes Use Them?

Steroids are drugs that physicians can legally prescribe for a variety of health conditions, including certain forms of anemia, inadequate growth patterns, and chronic debilitating diseases. Steroids can also be prescribed to aid recovery from surgery or burns. **Anabolic steroids** are drugs that function like the male sex hormone testosterone. They can be taken orally or by injection (see the Considering Complementary Care box on page 119).

 TALKING POINTS If you suspected a young person you know was using steroids, what strategies would you use to encourage the person to change his or her behavior?

Anabolic steroids are used by athletes who hope to gain weight, muscular size and strength, power, endurance, and aggressiveness. Over the last few decades, many bodybuilders, weightlifters, track athletes, and football players

> **Key Terms**
>
> **anabolic steroids** (ann uh **bol** ick) drugs that function like testosterone to produce increases in weight, strength, endurance, and aggressiveness.

Home Cardiorespiratory Fitness Equipment

In the past ten years, there has been an explosion in the purchase and use of home fitness equipment. This equipment is especially helpful for those who do not have access to health/fitness clubs, who prefer to exercise alone and at home, and who must exercise at irregular hours. It is advisable to thoroughly test out the equipment prior to purchase. Unfortunately, many people purchase a machine and seldom use it. Most forms of equipment can provide a good cardiorespiratory workout. However, people looking for a complete workout may have to add some strength training, barbell work to their fitness program. A discussion of current popular devices follows.

Stationary Bicycles

Many models of stationary bikes are available, ranging in price from about $150 to $3,500 or more for a computerized exercise bike. Some upright bikes have a "dual action" component, whereby the user can "pump" extended handlebars for an upper-body workout. Other bikes allow the user to sit back while pedaling. These recumbent bikes take pressure off the lower back and permit the rider to exercise the hamstring muscles to a greater degree than upright bikes. Bike training stands that allow you to convert your regular bicycle into a stationary bike are also available.

Treadmills

Treadmills are relatively simple devices that consist of a moving belt stretched over two rollers. Two basic forms of treadmills are commonly used. The less expensive is the variety that is driven manually by the walking or running action of the user. Motorized treadmills are much more expensive and driven, of course, by an electric motor. The cost of a treadmill can range from several hundred dollars to nearly $15,000 for top-of-the-line models. Most electric models allow the user to change speeds and also the incline angle of the platform. Changing the incline angle can increase the intensity of the workout. First-time users are cautioned to start slowly and gradually become familiar with the motion of the motorized models. Getting on and off a moving belt can be a potentially dangerous task.

Stair Climbers

These devices allow the user to simulate climbing up a series of stair steps. This form of movement is much preferred to the actual, repetitive climbing of stairs that some people undertake in high-rise buildings. Stair climbers take much of the pressure off the knee joint. These machines vary in price from around $200 for the simplest lever model to $5,000 for a programmable model that varies the speed and amount of resistance. Some models come with an upper body component that allows the user to pump the arms while climbing.

Rowing Machines

Users of these machines exercise by simulating the movements involved in rowing a boat. Most brands have a sliding seat and movable handles that are similar to oars. Users push their feet against footplates while pulling back on the handles. The simplest models may cost around $300, and prices range up to more than $3,000 for health club models.

Elliptical Machines

Elliptical machines provide a movement pattern whereby the feet describe an ellipse, with the longer action aligned roughly parallel to the ground. This is the same pattern that we move when we walk or run. Recent studies have found that these types of machines actually can require more involvement of the gluteals (buttocks) and the thigh muscles than can be obtained from treadmill or stationary cycles. These machines are the fastest growing segment of all cardiovascular exercise equipment. Costs range from several hundred to several thousand dollars.

Which Machine Is Best for You?

The machine that is best for you is the one that you will enjoy using. All too often, these machines are given as birthday or holiday gifts and used consistently for only a short time. (Notice all the ads for used fitness equipment in the classified ads section of your local paper.) Remember that machines can be somewhat specific in their focus. You may wish to broaden your workout with additional exercises or strength-building activities.

In terms of which device produces the greatest level of energy expenditure, a recent *Journal of the American Medical Association* article indicated that treadmill users walking or running "somewhat hard" expended (burned) more calories per hour than users of five other common home exercise machines. In this study, exercisers using a dual-action stationary bike and a regular stationary bike expended the fewest calories per hour.[1]

[1] Zeni AL, et al. Energy expenditure with indoor exercise machines. *JAMA* 8 May 1996; 275(18).

---

have chosen to ignore the serious health risks posed by illegal steroid use. More recently, steroid use among high school and college campuses has reached epidemic levels. The mass media has begun to focus attention on the dangers of steroid use, but many young athletes choose to ignore these warnings.

The use of steroids is highly dangerous because of serious, life-threatening side effects and adverse reactions. These effects include heart problems, certain forms of cancer, liver complications, and even psychological disturbances. The side effects on female steroid users are as dangerous as those on men. Figure 4-2 shows the adverse effects of steroid use.

Steroid users have developed a terminology of their own. Anabolic steroids are called "roids" or "juice." "Roid rage" is an aggressive, psychotic response to chronic steroid use. "Stacking" is a term that describes the use of multiple steroids at the same time.

Popular Ergogenic Aids

Androstendione ("andro") and creatine have recently received much attention for their use as possible **ergogenic aids.** Ergogenic aids are supplements taken to improve athletic performance.[1] These products presently can be purchased legally in health food stores. Andro is a steroidlike precursor to the male hormone testosterone. When taken into the body, andro stimulates the body to produce more of its natural testosterone. Increased levels of testosterone help a person build lean muscle mass and recover more quickly from injuries.

Andro's primary use as an ergogenic aid is to build muscle tissue, improve overall body strength, and boost performance, especially in anaerobic sports. Andro is banned by the National Football League, the National Collegiate Athletic Association, and the International Olympic Committee. The health concerns that most physicians attribute to andro are similar to those of anabolic steroids.

Perhaps the most famous user of andro was Mark McGwire, baseball player for the St. Louis Cardinals. In the summer of 1998, McGwire rocked the baseball world by surpassing Roger Maris's home run record by hitting seventy home runs. It is interesting, though, that during the 1999 baseball season, McGwire opted to stop using andro but still managed to hit nearly seventy home runs. Further, at the time of this writing in the summer of 2000, McGwire leads the National League with 30 home runs at the midpoint of the season.

Creatine is an amino acid found in meat, poultry, and fish. In a person's body, creatine is produced naturally in the liver, pancreas, and kidneys. Typically, people consume 1 to 2 grams of creatine each day from their food intake.[1] As an ergogenic aid, creatine performs its work in the muscles, where it helps restore the compound adenosine triphosphate (ATP). ATP provides quick energy for muscle contractions. It also helps to reduce the lactic acid buildup that occurs during physical exertion. This buildup causes a burning sensation that limits the amount of intense activity one can perform.

Early studies suggest that creatine can help athletes in anaerobic sports, which require short, explosive bursts of energy. However, the increase in performance has been small, the long-term health impacts are unknown, studies have been restricted to highly trained subjects (not recreational athletes), and damage to the kidneys is possible with high dosages. Users are cautioned to consume ample amounts of water to prevent cramping and dehydration.

All in all, creatine is unlikely to prove as potentially dangerous as androstendione. If additional studies should indicate that creatine can consistently improve performance, this substance might be banned by many sports governing bodies. At the time of this writing, the safest, most prudent recommendation is for athletes to spend their time and energy improving their training programs rather than looking for a solution in a bottle.

[1] The creatine craze. *UC Berkeley Wellness Letter* 1998; 14(3):6.

Many organizations that control athletic competition (such as the National Collegiate Athletic Association [NCAA], The Athletics Congress, the National Football League, and the International Olympic Committee) have banned steroids and are testing athletes for illegal use. Fortunately, some athletes finally seem to be getting the message and are steering clear of steroids.

What Is the Female Athlete Triad?

In the early 1990s, the ACSM identified a three-part syndrome of disordered eating, **amenorrhea** (lack of menstruation), and osteoporosis as the female athlete triad.[14] The conditions of this syndrome appear independently in many women, but among female athletes they appear together. The female athlete triad is most likely to be found in athletes whose sport activities emphasize appearance (for example, diving, ice skating, or gymnastics).

Parents, coaches, athletic trainers, and teammates should be watchful for signs of the female athlete triad. This syndrome has associated medical risks, including inadequate fuel supply for activities, inadequate iron intake, reduced cognitive function, altered hormone levels, reduced mental health, early onset of menopause, increased likelihood of skeletal trauma, altered blood fat profiles, and increased vulnerability to heart disease.[14] Vitally important is an early referral to a physician who is knowledgeable about the female athlete triad. The physician will likely coordinate efforts with a psychologist, a nutritionist, or an athletic trainer to improve the health of the athlete and prevent recurrences.

Are Today's Children Physically Fit?

Major research studies published during the last ten years have indicated that U.S. children and teenagers lead very sedentary lives. Children ages six to seventeen score extremely poorly in the areas of strength, flexibility, and cardiorespiratory endurance. In many cases,

---

> **Key Terms**
>
> **ergogenic aids** supplements that are taken to improve athletic performance.
>
> **amenorrhea** cessation or lack of menstrual periods.

Figure 4-2 Effects of steroids on various parts of the body.

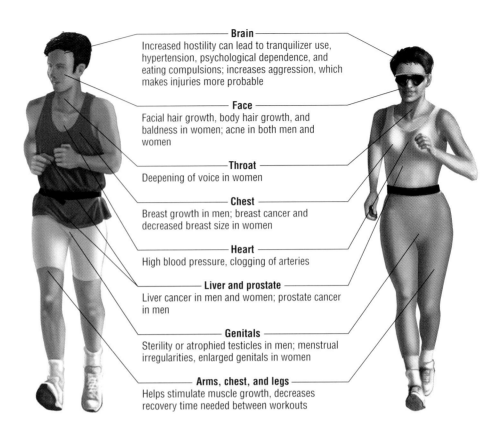

Brain
Increased hostility can lead to tranquilizer use, hypertension, psychological dependence, and eating compulsions; increases aggression, which makes injuries more probable

Face
Facial hair growth, body hair growth, and baldness in women; acne in both men and women

Throat
Deepening of voice in women

Chest
Breast growth in men; breast cancer and decreased breast size in women

Heart
High blood pressure, clogging of arteries

Liver and prostate
Liver cancer in men and women; prostate cancer in men

Genitals
Sterility or atrophied testicles in men; menstrual irregularities, enlarged genitals in women

Arms, chest, and legs
Helps stimulate muscle growth, decreases recovery time needed between workouts

parents are in better shape than their children. A major consequence of these sedentary habits in children is obesity. The 1999–2000 National Health and Nutrition Examination Survey (NHANES) indicates that 15% of children and adolescents ages 6–19 years are overweight. Indeed from NHANES II (1976–80) to NHANES III (1988–1994), the prevalence of overweight nearly doubled among children and adolescents and has continued to rise. The seriousness of these data is revealed by the fact that most obese children become obese adults.

This information presents a challenge to educators and parents to emphasize the need for strenuous play activity. Television watching and parental inactivity were implicated as major reasons in these studies. For students reading this text who are parents or grandparents of young children, what can you do to encourage more physical activity and less sedentary activity (see Talking It Over on page 98)?

How Does Sleep Contribute to Overall Fitness?

Sleep is an important adjunct to a well-planned exercise program (see the Changing for the Better box on page 121). Sleep is so vital to health that people who are unable to

sleep sufficiently (those with insomnia) or who are deprived of sleep experience deterioration in every dimension of their health. Fortunately, exercise is frequently associated with improvement in sleeping.

The value of sleep is apparent in a variety of positive changes in the body. Dreaming is thought to play an important role in supporting the emotional dimension of health. Problem-solving scenarios that occur during dreams seem to afford some carryover value in actual coping experiences. A variety of changes in physiological functioning, particularly a deceleration of the cardiovascular system, occur while you sleep. The feeling of being well rested is an expression of the mental and physiological rejuvenation you feel after a good night's sleep.

The amount of sleep needed varies among people. In fact, for any person, sleep needs vary according to activity level and overall state of health. As we age, the need for sleep appears to decrease from the six to eight hours young adults require. Elderly people routinely sleep less than they did when they were younger. This decrease may be offset by the short naps older people often take during the day. For all people, however, periods of relaxation, daydreaming, and even an occasional afternoon nap promote electrical activity patterns that help regenerate the mind and body.

Can we work at being better sleepers? The answer is yes. Many activities, when done at the appropriate time, will aid you in your quest for sound sleep.

Activities for the Day

Schedule. Maintain a consistent schedule of daily activities; a disrupted day makes sleeping difficult.

Physical activity. Regular vigorous activity promotes sleep; exercising too near bedtime, however, can make you too energized to sleep soundly.

Eating. A large meal taken late in the evening interferes with sleeping; avoid heavy late-night snacks as well.

Alcohol use. A single drink in the evening may be relaxing, but too many drinks during the day can make sleeping difficult.

Central nervous system (CNS) stimulants. Coffee, tea, soft drinks with caffeine, and some medications can disrupt normal sleeping patterns.

Worry. Problems and concerns should be put behind you by the time you retire for the night; practice leaving your concerns at the office or in the classroom.

Rituals. A ritualistic "winding down" over the course of the evening promotes sleep; watching television, listening to music, and reading during the evening are excellent ways to prepare the body for sleep.

Activities for the End of the Day

Bathing. For many people, a warm bath immediately before retiring promotes sleep.

Yoga. The quiet, relaxing exercises of yoga promote sleep by slowing the body's activity level.

Snack or nightcap. A light snack of foods high in l-tryptophan (for example, eggs, tuna, and turkey) and a glass of milk will help you fall asleep.

Muscular relaxation. Alternating contraction and relaxation of the large muscles of the extremities aids the body in falling asleep.

Imaging. Quieting images can distract the mind, thus allowing you to fall asleep more easily.

Fantasies. Escaping into fantasies slows the mind and encourages the onset of sleep.

Breathing. Slow, deep breaths set a restful rhythm the body can "ride" into sleep.

Thinking. By envisioning yourself as sleeping soundly, you may actually fall asleep quicker.

InfoLinks

www.sleepnet.com

What Exercise Danger Signs Should I Watch For?

The human body is an amazing piece of equipment. It functions well regardless of whether you are conscious of its processes. It also delivers clear signals when something goes wrong.

You should monitor any sign that seems abnormal during or after your exercise. "Listen to your body" is a good rule for self-awareness. The adjacent Changing for the Better box lists some common warning signs to monitor.

However, such occurrences are extremely unusual. Fear of developing these difficulties should not deter you from starting a fitness program. These risks are minimal—and the benefits far outweigh the risks. Sports injuries are discussed further in the following section.

Sports Injuries

At any time during your participation in fitness or sport activities, it is possible that you will become injured, even if you carefully warm up before your exercise and cool down after your exercise. If you are lucky, the injury will only be a minor one and after a short period of rest you will be able to resume your fitness interests. Sometimes, however, an injury can be significant and require you to seek medical care and undergo extensive rehabilitation.

It is beyond the scope of this textbook to provide a comprehensive discussion of the prevention, care, and treatment of sports injuries. (You can find this information in an athletic training textbook, a fitness textbook, or a popular sports medicine book.) We will try to provide you with some general principles related to the prevention and care of sports injuries and a table that lists many common fitness injuries.[15]

1. A *well-planned fitness program starts at a low level and progresses gradually and consistently.* This principle supports the concept of starting at a level of activity that can be handled comfortably. If the activity is a walking program, an unfit person should not begin with walks of five or six miles a day but should start with a shorter distance and gradually add addi-

tional distance in a consistent manner to avoid muscle, skeletal, or joint injuries.

2. *If you stop exercising for an extended time, do not restart the activity at the level at which you stopped.* Do not plan on returning to a high level of activity if you have been inactive for an extended time. Rather, reduce your activity significantly and gradually return to your earlier levels of activity.

3. *"Listen to your body."* Always be aware of the nature of your body as you are exercising. If you sense that something is wrong, stop the activity and assess the situation. For example, if you think you might be

Table 4.1 Common Injuries Associated with Physical Activity

Injury	Condition
Achilles tendinitis	A chronic tendinitis of the "heel cord" or muscle tendon, located on the back of the lower leg just above the heel. It may result from any activity that involves forcefully pushing off with the foot and ankle, such as in running and jumping. This inflammation involves swelling, warmth, tenderness to touch, and pain during walking and especially running.
Ankle sprains	Stretching or tearing of one or several ligaments that provide stability to the ankle joint. Ligaments on the outside or lateral side of the ankle are more commonly injured by rolling the sole of the foot downward and toward the inside. Pain is intense immediately after injury, followed by considerable swelling, tenderness, loss of joint motion, and some discoloration over a 24- to 48-hour period.
Groin pull	A muscle strain that occurs in the muscles located on the inside of the upper thigh just below the pubic area and that results from either an overstretch of the muscle or from a contraction of the muscle that meets excessive resistance. Pain will be produced by flexing the hip and leg across the body or by stretching the muscles in a groin-stretch position.
Hamstring pull	A strain of the muscles on the back of the upper thigh that most often occurs while sprinting. In most cases, severe pain is caused simply by walking or in any movement that involves knee flexion or stretch of the hamstring muscle. Some swelling, tenderness to touch, and possibly some discoloration extending down the back of the leg may occur in severe strains.
Patellofemoral knee pain	Nonspecific pain occurring around the knee, particularly the front part of the knee, or in the kneecap (patella). Pain can result from many causes, including improper movement of the kneecap in knee flexion and extension; tendinitis of the tendon just below the kneecap, which is caused by repetitive jumping; bursitis (swelling) either above or below the kneecap; and osteoarthritis (joint surface degeneration) between the kneecap and thigh bone. It may involve inflammation with swelling, tenderness, warmth, and pain associated with movement.
Quadriceps contusion "charley horse"	A deep bruise of the muscles in the front part of the thigh caused by a forceful impact or by some object that results in severe pain, swelling, discoloration, and difficulty flexing the knee or extending the hip. Without adequate rest and protection from additional trauma, small calcium deposits may develop in the muscle.
Shin splints	A catch-all term used to refer to any pain that occurs in the front part of the lower leg or shin, most often caused by excessive running on hard surfaces. Pain is usually caused by strain of the muscles that move the ankle and foot at their attachment points in the shin. It is usually worse during activity. In more severe cases it may be caused by stress fractures of the long bones in the lower leg, with the pain being worse after activity is stopped.
Shoulder impingement	Chronic irritation and inflammation of muscle tendons and a bursa underneath the tip of the shoulder, which results from repeated forceful overhead motions of the shoulder, such as in swimming, throwing, spiking a volleyball, or serving a tennis ball. Pain is felt when the arm is extended across the body above shoulder level.
Tennis elbow	Chronic irritation and inflammation of the lateral or outside surface of the arm just above the elbow at the attachment of the muscles that extend the wrist and fingers. It results from any activity that requires forceful extension of the wrist. Typically occurs in tennis players who are using faulty techniques hitting backhand ground strokes. Pain is felt above the elbow after forcefully extending the wrist against resistance or applying pressure over the muscle attachment above the elbow.

hurting your back or that a joint or muscle is becoming strained, stop and evaluate the situation. If you think something is wrong, by all means don't test your body by returning to the activity. (Have you ever seen a person with a suspected ankle injury "test" the ankle by hopping up and down on the injured leg? This makes no sense at all.) Pain indicates that something is wrong. If this is the case, seek a professional evaluation, perhaps from an athletic trainer or a physical therapist. A physician, especially one trained in sports medicine, can make an accurate diagnosis of the injury.

4. *Follow the rehabilitation instructions carefully.* Athletic trainers and physical therapists are trained to design effective rehabilitation programs. If you are injured, it is very important that you follow the advice of these professionals. This is especially true in cases where you start to feel better before the rehabilitation program is finished. Even though you feel better, your body may not be fully recovered. A return to activity too quickly may result in an even more serious injury than your original one. (This is especially true for adults over the age of forty.) The best advice is to resist the urge

to return to your activity until you are given full clearance from your trainer or therapist.

5. *Develop a prevention approach.* After you recover from an injury, try to discover ways to prevent that injury from happening again. Learn about proper stretching exercises, effective strength-training activities, appropriate equipment, and the proper mechanics for your selected sports/fitness activities. Use this collective knowledge to prevent the injury from recurring.

For example, if you have injured your hamstring muscles while running, you will need to learn how to effectively stretch these muscles in the future. You will also need to learn how to strengthen these muscles through resistance training. If your running shoes are old and worn, they may have to be replaced. Finally, if you are running too fast before warming up, you will want to start slowly and gradually increase your speed after the muscles are fully warmed up. Preventive actions like these will allow you to have a fitness program that is not regularly interrupted by a nagging injury.

For more information about specific sports injuries, look at Table 4.1 on page 122.

Taking Charge of Your Health

- Assess your level of fitness by completing the National Fitness Test on page 127.
- Start a daily stretching program based on the guidelines in this chapter.
- Implement or maintain a cardiorespiratory fitness program that uses the most recent American College of Sports Medicine recommendations.
- Examine your athletic shoes to determine their appropriateness for the fitness activities you do (see Choosing an Athletic Shoe on p. 116).

- Monitor your physical activities for potential danger signs indicating that you should consult an athletic trainer, physical therapist, or physician.
- For 2 weeks, keep track of the amount of sleep you are getting. Determine whether this is enough sleep, and make adjustments accordingly.

Summary

- Physical fitness allows one to avoid illness, perform routine activities, and respond to emergencies.
- The health benefits of exercise can be achieved through regular, moderate exercise.
- Fitness is composed of four components: cardiorespiratory endurance, muscular fitness, flexibility, and body composition.
- The American College of Sports Medicine's program for cardiorespiratory fitness has four components:

mode of activity, frequency of training, intensity of training, and duration of training. Additionally, ACSM now recommends that everyone also include resistance training and flexibility training.
- The target heart rate refers to the number of times per minute the heart must contract to produce a training effect.
- Training sessions should take place in three phases: warm-up, workout, and cooldown.

- Fitness experts are concerned about the lack of fitness in today's youth.
- Street dancing, swing dancing, step aerobics, and rollerblading are currently popular aerobic activities.
- College students who are interested in fitness should be as knowledgeable as possible about the important topics of steroid use, crosstraining, fluid replacement, body-building, and proper sleep.
- Following a few simple principles can help prevent many common sports injuries.

Review Questions

1. Identify the four components of fitness described in this chapter. How does each component relate to physical fitness?
2. What is the difference between anaerobic and aerobic energy production? What types of activities are associated with anaerobic energy production? With aerobic energy production?
3. List some of the benefits of aerobic fitness.
4. Describe the various methods used to promote muscular fitness.
5. What does the principle of overload mean in regard to fitness training programs?
6. Identify the ACSM's four components of an effective cardiorespiratory fitness program. Explain the important aspects of each component.
7. Under what circumstances should you see a physician before starting a physical fitness program?
8. Identify and describe the three parts of a training session.
9. Describe some of the negative consequences of anabolic steroid use.
10. How can people improve their sleeping habits?
11. Describe the three-part female athlete triad.
12. Discuss the five basic principles important in avoiding sports injuries.

References

1. U.S. Department of Health and Human Services. *Physical Activity and Health: A Report of the Surgeon General.* Atlanta, GA: U.S. Department of Health and Human Services, Centers for Disease Control and Prevention, National Center for Chronic Disease Prevention and Health Promotion, 1996.
2. Casperson C, et al. Public Health Reports 100: 126, 1985.
3. American Heart Association, Councils on Clinical Cardiology and Nutrition, Physical Activity and Metabolism. *Exercise and Physical Activity in the Prevention and Treatment of Atherosclerotic Cardiovascular Disease.* Circulation; 107:3109, 2003.
4. Brubaker PH, Kaminsky LA, Whaley HM. Coronary Artery Disease. *Human Kinetics,* 2002.
5. Ferrini AF, Ferrini RL. *Health in later years,* 2nd ed. Brown & Benchmark, 1992.
6. Rubin R. Brittle bones: promising strides against osteoporosis mean better, longer life for the elderly. *USA Today* 2000 March 28:1D.
7. American College of Sports Medicine. Position stand on the recommended quantity and quality of exercise for developing and maintaining cardiorespira-tory and muscular fitness and flexibility in healthy adults. *Med Sci Sports Exerc* 1998;30(6):975–991.
8. White MD. *Water exercise.* Human Kinetics, 1995.
9. An exercise prescription for older people. *Harvard Health Letter* 1998; 8(10):1–4.
10. American College of Sports Medicine. *Guidelines for Exercise Testing and Prescription,* 6th ed. Lippincott, Williams, and Wilkins, 2000.
11. Kaehler K, Tivers C. *Primetime pregnancy: the proven program for staying in shape before and after your baby is born.* Contemporary Books, 1997.
12. Williams RD. Healthy pregnancy, healthy baby. *FDA Consumer* 1999; 33(2):18–23.
13. Williams MH. Alcohol and sports performance. *Sports Sci Exch* 1992; 4(40): 1–4.
14. Stevens WC, Brey RA, Harris JE, Fowlkes-Godek S. The dangerous trio: a case study approach to the female athlete triad. *Athletic Therapy Today* 1997; 2(2):30–36.
15. Prentice WE. *Fitness for wellness and life,* 6th ed. McGraw-Hill College Division, 1998.

extreme sports: living on the edge

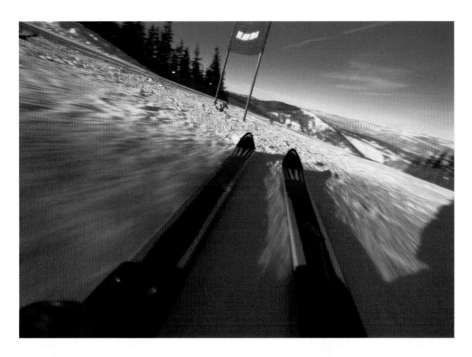

What did you do last weekend? You say that you jumped out of an airplane while videotaping your buddy doing air acrobatics on a surfboard? Well, we've identified the skysurfers in the group. There are at least a couple of other variations on hurling oneself from a plane. Style skydivers perform six maneuvers as fast as possible (without the surfboard or cameraperson) while accuracy skydivers attempt to land on silver dollar-sized targets.[1] Bungee jumping is nothing extraordinary these days. People even get married while taking the plunge, and the new freestyle bungee jumping involves going over the edge while sitting in a recliner or dumpster.[2] Another extreme sport, the street luge, involves plummeting downhill feet first on a wheeled sled. In snow mountain bike racing, pedal speeds of 65 mph are reached before crashing into the padded speed trap at the end of the course—*if* you don't fall off of your bike on the way downhill.[3]

If scaling a fifty-foot artificial frozen waterfall sounds like your thing, have somebody time you. After some practice, you may be the next Speed Ice Climbing Champion. If you haven't read about your favorite sport here yet, don't despair. A few of the other options are skateboarding, downhill or half-pipe snowboarding, indoor climbing, barefoot water ski jumping, aggressive in-line skating, supermodified shovel racing (likened to a soap box derby on snow), and the multisport endurance ecochallenge.[2,3,4,5] An ecochallenge involves 50 five-person teams that race twenty-four hours a day for seven days over 370 miles of rugged terrain. The team members take turns horseback riding and running alongside the horse for twenty-six miles, swimming with backpacks in cold mountain creeks, hiking a hundred miles across desert, navigating a 1,200-foot cliff face by rope, rafting over advanced-class rapids, and finishing with

a twelve-hour, fifty-mile canoe paddle across a lake.

How did this extreme sports phenomenon arise? Sports writer K. Hamilton puts it this way: "The world's always had daredevils; they're just more organized and obvious now."[2]

Origins and Growth

Extreme sports competition emerged in the mid-eighties as fun.[6] It was also about this time that in-line skates began replacing the old-style roller skates. Now more than 25 million Americans in-line skate at least once a year, which makes the sport more popular than tennis and about as popular as golf.[7] In addition, over 6.5 million mountain bikes were sold in 1995 alone and indoor climbing gyms are springing up across the country. There are 2 million snowboarders, that many rock climbers, and mountain climbers, thousands of extreme skiers, and over 25% more skydivers than there were a few years ago.[1]

Television has played a key role in the phenomenal growth of extreme sports. In 1992 *MTV Sports* premiered to cover this new generation of sport.[1] Three years later, ESPN 1997 launched the X Games, billed as "not your father's Olympics." The Summer X Games, now a weeklong annual event, draw athletes from around the world. More than four hundred athletes competed in nine sports for over $375,000 in prize money in the Summer 1996 version.[8,9] Not to be outdone, *MTV Sports* coverage may expand, and the News Corp. and Fox networks are planning extreme sports programs. Some of the events have gone mainstream; for example, halfpipe snowboarding is now included in the Olympic Games.[1,3]

Who Pays

Where there is public interest and televised coverage, there is advertising. Being associated with extreme sports reinforces Pepsico's active and cutting-edge ad campaign for its Mountain Dew product. Taco Bell, a Pepsico subsidiary, markets the free-spirited, outdoor, energetic attitude to its core group of customers, who are age eighteen to thirty-four. Some Chevy dealers offer trucks with X Game logos and include an extreme whitewater rafting trip or an extreme mountain bike with purchase.[4] Volkswagen offers K2 skis or a K2 snowboard with some of its car models.[10] Other extreme sports sponsors include the U.S. Marines, Visa, Pringles, Snickers, AT&T, and Nike.[3] HealthSouth Corp., a rehabilitation care provider, is a sport climbing sponsor, and some equipment manufacturers sponsor competitions or individual athletes by providing free gear or small stipends.[6]

As K. Hamilton writes: "extremists take the money because it's there. They take the risks for reasons of their own."[2]

Who Plays

Although much of the marketing is directed at twenty-somethings, extreme sports attract participants from teens to athletes in their seventies. Neither is it strictly an American craze. Indoor climbing events in Europe routinely draw more than five thousand spectators, and the roster of contestants at the 1997 Winter X Games revealed participants from the following countries: Austria, Switzerland, Norway, Finland, Italy, Canada, and the United States.[3,6]

Tim Fairfield is one of the nation's top indoor sport climbers. He identifies with the "packaged radicalism" of what he sees as an "anti-establishment" sport.[6] Cheryl Stearns, world champion style and accuracy skydiver, sees her sport as fun, exciting, and different, building self-assurance and openmindedness. Top U.S. in-line skater Anjie Walter, cites an addictive sense of accomplishment and empowerment, a feeling of heightened awareness, and a greater appreciation for living as benefits of the risks she takes.[1] Helen Klein, the great-grandmother and ultramarathoner who finished the ecochallenge, put it this way: "I'd rather wear out than rust out."[2]

The Risks

Despite the physical fitness peak and mental rushes that these sports provide, they can be very expensive and involve serious risks. These sports require specialized equipment, safety gear, and clothing. A pair of in-line skates costs between $40 and $299.[7] That's only the beginning—if you get really into a sport, the costs skyrocket. Mia Azon, the 1994 number two women's sport climber, spent more than her $10,000 sponsorship and prize money training and competing in her sport in one year.[6] Extreme sports can also cost some athletes their health and even their life. People get hurt; injuries range from broken bones to dehydration to exertional rhabdomyolysis (the body's digestion of its own muscle tissue from overwork). Extreme athletes put not only themselves in danger by their activity; rescue workers who rescue extreme skiers from avalanches and medical workers called on to helicopter-lift athletes in trouble out of the rugged terrain are also put at risk.

More Than a Passing Fancy

Risky or not, extreme sports have caught on. Yet as these events grow in popularity, they may lose some of their offbeat appeal. However, extreme sports are not likely to get boring since participants continue to add variety to their sports to keep the intensity of the experience fresh.

For those of you who want to check out the extreme scene from the safety of your computer, ICon CMT Corp. has a new online magazine, *Charged*, for extreme sport enthusiasts.[11] You can check out any of four sections in *Charged:* Tar (street sports), Wet (water sports), Dirt (biking, etc.), and Frost (snow sports) at www.charged.com. So what are you doing this weekend?

For Discussion . . .

Have you ever tried an extreme sport? If so, would you recommend the experience to a friend? Why or why not? Do you think that the benefits of participation outweigh the risks? Were you surprised to learn of the level of popularity of these sports?

References

1. Bower J. Going over the top. *Women's Sports & Fitness* 1995; 17(7):21–23.
2. Hamilton K. Outer limits. *Newsweek* 1995; 125(25):78–81.
3. ESPN. Televised Coverage of Day 2 of Winter X Games, 1997.
4. Elliott S. The X Games: going to extremes in an effort to tap a growing segment of sports. *The New York Times* 1996; 145:D6.
5. Fitzgerald K. Extreme-ly hot: ESPN leads charge into new, daring sports targeted to young people. *Advertising Age* 1996; 67(26):44–45.
6. Fatsis S. Rad sports give sponsors cheap thrills. *The Wall Street Journal* 1995 May 12:B12.
7. Consumer Reports. The best deal on street wheels. *Consumer Reports* 1996; 61(7):20–25.
8. Brown R. X marks the spot for ESPN; extreme sports competition has lined up over a dozen sponsors. *Broadcasting & Cable* 1996; 126(15):53.
9. Hoffer R. Down and way out. *Sports Illustrated* 1995; 83(1):42–49.
10. Volkswagen. Television commercial, 1996.
11. Wilson S. Electronically charged. *Folio: the Magazine for Magazine Management* 1996; 25(10):37.

InfoLinks

www.adventuresports.com
http://espn.go.com

personal assessment

what is your level of fitness?

You can determine your level of fitness in 30 minutes or less by completing this short group of tests based on the National Fitness Test developed by the President's Council on Physical Fitness and Sports. If you are over 40 years old or have chronic medical disorders such as diabetes or obesity, check with your physician before taking this or any other fitness test. You will need another person to monitor your test and keep time.

Three-minute Step Test

Aerobic capacity. Equipment: 12-inch bench, crate, block, or step ladder; stopwatch. Procedure: face bench. Complete 24 full steps (both feet on the bench, both feet on the ground) per minute for 3 minutes. After finishing, sit down, have your partner find your pulse within 5 seconds, and take your pulse for 1 minute. Your score is your pulse rate for 1 full minute.

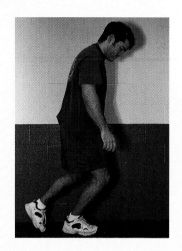

Scoring standards (heart rate for 1 minute)

Age	18–29		30–39		40–49		50–59		60+	
Gender	F	M	F	M	F	M	F	M	F	M
Excellent	<80	<75	<84	<78	<88	<80	<92	<85	<95	<90
Good	80–110	75–100	84–115	78–109	88–118	80–112	92–123	85–115	95–127	90–118
Average	>110	>100	>115	>109	>118	>112	>123	>115	>127	>118

Sit and Reach

Hamstring flexibility. Equipment: yardstick; tape. Between your legs, tape the yardstick to the floor. Sit with legs straight and heels about 5 inches apart, heels even with the 15-inch mark on the yardstick. While in a sitting position, slowly stretch forward as far as possible. Your score is the number of inches reached.

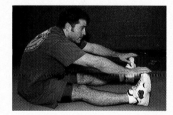

Scoring standards (inches)

Age	18–29		30–39		40–49		50–59		60+	
Gender	F	M	F	M	F	M	F	M	F	M
Excellent	>22	>21	>22	>21	>21	>20	>20	>19	>20	>19
Good	17–22	13–21	17–22	13–21	15–21	13–20	14–20	12–19	14–20	12–19
Average	<17	<13	<17	<13	<15	<13	<14	<12	<14	<12

Arm Hang

Upper body strength. Equipment: horizontal bar (high enough to prevent your feet from touching the floor); stopwatch. Procedure: hang with straight arms, palms facing forward. Start watch when subject is in position. Stop when subject lets go. Your score is the number of minutes and seconds spent hanging.

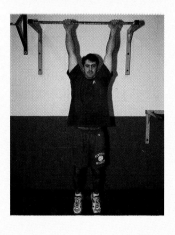

Scoring standards (hanging time)

Age	18–29		30–39		40–49		50–59		60+	
Gender	F	M	F	M	F	M	F	M	F	M
Excellent	>1:30	>2:00	>1:20	>1:50	>1:10	>1:35	>1:00	>1:20	>:50	>1:10
Good	:46–1:30	1:00–2:00	:40–1:20	:50–1:50	:30–1:10	:45–1:35	:30–1:00	:35–1:20	:21–:50	:30–1:10
Average	<:46	<1:00	<:40	<:50	<:30	<:45	<:30	<:35	<:21	<:30

Curl-ups

Abdominal and low back strength. Equipment: stopwatch. Procedure: Lie flat on upper back, knees bent, shoulders touching the floor, arms extended above your thighs or by your sides, palms down. Bend knees so that feet are flat and 12 inches from the buttocks. Curl up by lifting head and shoulders off the floor, sliding hands forward above your thighs or the floor. Curl down and repeat. Your score is the number of curl-ups in 1 minute.

Scoring standards (number in 1 minute)

Age	18–29		30–39		40–49		50–59		60+	
Gender	F	M	F	M	F	M	F	M	F	M
Excellent	>45	>50	>40	>45	>35	>40	>30	>35	>25	>30
Good	25–45	30–50	20–40	22–45	16–35	21–40	12–30	18–35	11–25	15–30
Average	<25	<30	<20	<22	<16	<21	<12	<18	<11	<15

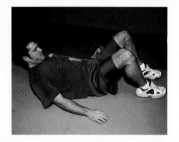

Push-ups (Men)

Upper body strength. Equipment: stopwatch. Assume a front-leaning position. Lower your body until chest touches the floor. Raise and repeat for 1 minute. Your score is the number of push-ups completed in 1 minute.

Scoring standards (number in 1 minute)

Age	18–29	30–39	40–49	50–59	60+
Excellent	>50	>45	>40	>35	>30
Good	25–50	22–45	19–40	15–35	10–30
Average	<25	<22	<19	<15	<10

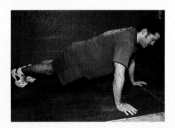

Modified Push-ups (Women)

Upper body strength. Equipment: stopwatch. Assume a front-leaning position with knees bent up, hands under shoulders. Lower your chest to the floor, raise, and repeat. Your score is the number of push-ups completed in 1 minute.

Scoring standards (number in 1 minute)

Age	18–29	30–39	40–49	50–59	60+
Excellent	>45	>40	>35	>30	>25
Good	17–45	12–40	8–35	6–30	5–25
Average	<17	<12	<8	<6	<5

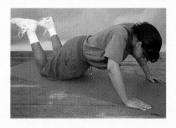

To Carry This Further . . .

Note your areas of strengths and weaknesses. To improve your fitness, become involved in a fitness program that reflects the concepts discussed in this chapter. Talking with fitness experts on your campus might be a good first step.

chapter five

Understanding nutrition and your diet

Chapter Objectives

After reading this chapter, you should be able to:

▌ name and describe the seven types of nutrients.

▌ describe saturated, monounsaturated, and polyunsaturated fats, and explain their effects on the human body.

▌ discuss the recent growth in fat-free foods and their possible advantages and disadvantages.

▌ define complete protein foods and incomplete protein foods, and give examples of each.

▌ describe three processes that vitamins help perform in the body.

▌ discuss the roles of minerals and water in the body.

▌ describe the benefits of soluble and insoluble fiber.

▌ describe the Food Guide Pyramid and the number of recommended servings for each food group in the pyramid.

▌ discuss seven recommendations in the *Dietary Guidelines for Americans*.

▌ describe foodbourne illnesses and strategies for preventing them.

▌ name three types of vegetarian diets and describe the advantages and disadvantages of each.

Online Learning Center Resources

www.mhhe.com/payne8e

Log on to our Online Learning Center (OLC) for access to these additional resources:

- Chapter key terms and definitions
- Learning objectives
- Student interactive question-and-answer sites

- Self-scoring chapter quiz
- Online assessments
- Key term flash cards

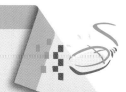

Talking It Over

Food Fiction vs. Food Fact

When it comes to food and nutrition, there are many myths that people believe are true. Here are some of the most popular ones:

FICTION: If I don't eat fat, I won't get fat.
FACT: Overeating—consuming more calories than you need or expend—can lead to storing any type of food as fat, even salad!

FICTION: Pasta is bad and should be avoided.
FACT: Pasta is a good source of carbohydrate, an important source of energy, and protein, the fundamental structural material for every cell in your body. Both are essential!

FICTION: Fat is bad and should be avoided.
FACT: Fat provides the body with slow-releasing energy and helps it carry and absorb vitamins and essential nutrients. It also provides the body with a sense of satisfaction, which helps us to avoid overeating.

FICTION: Eating certain foods—such as celery or grapefruit—makes your body burn extra calories and helps you to lose weight.
FACT: No matter what you've eaten, digestion only burns a small percentage of calories consumed—not nearly enough to affect your weight.

FICTION: Eating after 8 P.M. is bad and causes weight gain.
FACT: It's not what time you eat, but what time you go to sleep that's important. When you are sleeping, your metabolism tends to be lower than when you are active and awake. Researchers suggest limiting food intake 2 to 3 hours before going to sleep for this reason. So if you go to sleep at midnight, you certainly may want a nutritious snack at 8 P.M.!

The Truth About Food Addiction

There is a lot of debate about whether we can be addicted to food. Certainly some chocolate lovers will tell you that they are "chocoholics," and must have their dose of daily chocolate or suffer miserably. But even though there may be a psychological dependence or issue with food (as we'll discuss in Chapter 6 on Weight Management), there is no evidence that people can become physiologically addicted to particular foods. Yet many popular diets—including Overeaters Anonymous, Sugar Busters, and the Carbohydrate Addicts Diet among others—are based on the premise that we can become addicted to food in the same way that we can become addicted to alcohol or drugs. What is the truth about food addiction?

Diet programs that are based upon an addiction model lack sufficient scientific support for their claims. These diets suggest that there is a biological craving for carbohydrates—especially white flour and refined sugar—and that we need more and more of these foods in order to satisfy this craving. But it is important to recognize the difference between a physiological need and psychological craving. A craving is based on your thoughts and feelings, while hunger is a biological or physiological process. While individuals with eating disorders or problems with compulsive overeating may experience psychological cravings, their cravings are not physiologically based. Indeed, there are some similarities between overeating and substance abuse—such as obsessively thinking about the food or drug, having periods of fasting and bingeing, and experiencing problems in day-to-day functioning—but this is where the likeness ends. Because, while even an addict can live without alcohol or drugs, nobody can abstain from food. We don't build up tolerance to certain foods, nor do we go through physiological withdrawal when abstaining from certain foods similar to what is seen with drug or alcohol withdrawal and physical dependence.

A number of popular diets are predicated on the idea that you can be addicted to sugar or carbohydrates because of the insulin reaction that occurs in the body when you eat any food. The glycemic index measures how much a food provokes the body to release insulin into the blood, causing the body to convert blood sugar (glucose) into fat. A high level of insulin speeds up the conversion too quickly and the blood sugar level plummets, causing individuals to feel light-headed, tired, and hungry. The higher the glycemic index, the faster the insulin response.

Diets based on the addiction model (such as The Atkins' Diet, Sugar Busters, the Carbohydrate Addict's Diet, or The Zone diet) are based upon the theory that people who are addicted to carbohydrates are "insulin resistant," and have an insulin imbalance in which their bodies produce too much insulin, causing them to feel constantly hungry which in turn causes them to overeat. Foods high in sugar, corn syrup, and complex carbohydrates like potatoes and carrots have a high glycemic index, and this is the reason the food addiction diets suggest avoiding carbohydrates.

The premise behind these diets is problematic for a number of reasons. First, they fail to take into consideration that when these foods are eaten in combination with other foods, such as eating carrots or potatoes with meat, this insulin response is not provoked. Second, these diets treat all carbohydrates the same, but we know this is not the case. Simple carbohydrates such as refined sugar provoke an insulin release into the blood, but the complex carbohydrates such as whole grains, fruits, and vegetables do not, even though they too have a high glycemic index. Also problematic is these diets' reliance on high fat, high cholesterol meals that put you at risk for heart disease, colon cancer, and ketosis.

The best way to keep your insulin levels stable is to follow the food pyramid guide and avoid sugary foods and drinks. So don't be fooled by diets based on the myth of food addiction!

Sources: Hall R. *The Unofficial Guide to Smart Nutrition*. Foster City, CA: IDG Books Worldwide International, 2000.
Poston W and Haddock C. *Food as a Drug*. New York: The Haworth Press, Inc., 2000.

Healthy eating is important from the prenatal period throughout life, in order to prevent malnourishment and minimize the development of illnesses that may be worsened by poor dietary practices. Food supports growth and development by providing the body with the nutrients needed for the production of energy, repair of damaged tissue, growth of new tissue, and regulation of physiological processes, all of which support full participation in the activities that constitute our days, weeks, months, and years of living. But our diets are more than that. Our food selections reflect personal, familial, and cultural traditions. The preparation and serving of food at regular mealtimes and during holiday gatherings and other special occasions enhances all of the dimensions of health. For example, taking bread and wine during Communion supports the spiritual dimension of health, sharing popcorn at the movies with your friends enhances the social dimension of health, and learning about the cuisine of another culture develops the cultural dimension of health. As you read this chapter, keep in mind this balanced view of food as sustenance and food as a resource for the dimensions of health.

dietary alternatives study. *JAMA*; 278(18): 1509–1525, 1997.

9. National Institutes of Health. *Practical Guide to the Identification, Evaluation and Treatment of Overweight and Obesity in Adults,* 2001.

10. Cheskin LJ, et al. Gastrointestinal symptoms following consumption of Olestra or regular triglyceride potato chips score. *JAMA*; 279(2): 150–152, 1998.

11. Wardlaw GM. *Contemporary nutrition: issues and insights.* McGraw-Hill, 1999.

12. Young VR. Soy protein in relation to human protein and amino acid nutrition. *J Am Diet Assoc.* 91, 828–835, 1991.

13. Anderson J, Johnstone R, Cook-Newell M. Meta-analysis of the effects of soy protein intake on serum lipids. *N Engl J Med* 333, 276–282, 1995.

14. Kant AK. A prospective study of diet quality and mortality in women. *JAMA*; 283(16): 2109–2115, 2000.

15. Czeizel AE, Dudaz I. Prevention of the first occurrence of neural-tube defects by periconceptional vitamin supplementation. *N Engl J Med*; 327(26): 1832–1835, 1992.

16. Position of the American Dietetic Association: vitamin and mineral supplementation, 1998. **www.eatright.org/asupple.html**

17. In Yankelovich Partners for the Nutrition Information Center at The New York Hospital and the Bottled Water Association. April, 1998. **www.bottledwater.org/public/PressRel1.htm**

18. Garigan TP, Ristedt DE. Death from hyponatremia as a result of acute water intoxication in an Army basic trainee. *Mil Med*; 164(3):234–238, 1999.

19. Arieff AI, Kronlund BA. Fatal child abuse by forced water intoxication. *Pediatrics*; 103(6 Pt 1): 1292–1295, 1999.

20. Chandalia M et al. Beneficial effects of high dietary fiber intake in patients with type 2 diabetes mellitus. *N Engl J Med*; 342(19):1392–1398, 2000.

21. Schatzkin A et al. Lack of effect of a low-fat, high-fiber diet on the recurrence of colorectal adenomas. Polyp Prevention Trial Study Group. *N Engl J Med*; 342(16):1149–1115, 2000.

22. Sears W. and Sears M. *The Family Nutrition Book.* New York: Little, Brown and Co., 1999.

23. FDA allows whole oat foods to make health claim on reducing the risk of heart disease. *FDA Talk Paper,* January 1998.

24. American Cancer Society. *Cancer facts and figures—2000.* The Association, 2000.

25. Joseph JA et al. Long-term dietary strawberry, spinach, or vitamin E supplementation retards the onset of age-related neuronal signal-transduction and cognitive behavioral deficits. *J Neurosci*; 18(19):8047–8055, 1998.

26. Kaplan NM. The dietary guideline for sodium: should we shake it up? No. *Am J Clin Nutr*; 71(5): 1020–1026, 2000.

27. McCarron DA. The dietary guideline for sodium: should we shake it up? Yes. *Am J Clin Nutr*; 71(5): 1013–1019, 2000.

28. U.S. Department of Agriculture. *The healthy eating index* (executive summary). July 2000. **http://Warp.nal.usda.gov/fnic/HEI/execsum.html**

29. Willett W. *Eat, Drink and Be Healthy.* New York: Free Press, 2001.

30. Waladkhani AR, Clemens MR. Effect of dietary phytochemicals on cancer. *Int J Mol Med*; 1(4): 747–753, 1998.

31. Fransworth ER. What we are trying to do? *Medicinal Food News*; 1(1):1–6, 1999. **www.medicinalfoodnews.com/vol01/issue1.html**

32. U.S. Food and Drug Administration Center for Food Safety and Applied Nutrition. FDA approves new health claim for soy protein and coronary heart disease [FDA talk paper]. October 1999. **www.fda.gov/fdac/bbs/topics/ANSWERS/ANS00980.html**

33. Kurtzweil P. Staking a claim to good health. *FDA Consumer,* November–December 1998. **www.fda/gov/fdac/features/1998,689-labl.html**

34. A bug for what's bugging you. *USA Today,* July 9, 2003, D-1.

35. USDA Gives Bite to Organic Label. *USA Today,* October 16, 2002.

36. The Truth about Irradiated Meat. *Consumer Reports,* 34–37, August 2003.

37. Oppel RA, Jr. Infected Cow Old Enough to Have Eaten Now-Banned Feed. *The New York Times,* December 30, 2003.

38. Grady D. U.S. Imposes Stricter Safety Rules for Preventing Mad Cow Disease. *The New York Times,* December 31, 2003.

39. Corporate Website, **http://www.eggland.com**

40. Food Sellers Push Animal Welfare, *USA Today,* August 13, 2003.

41. Insel P, Turner E, Ross D. *Nutrition.* Sudbury, MA: Jones and Barlett Publishers, 2002.

42. Americans are iffy on Genetically Modified Foods, *USA Today,* September 18, 2003.

43. U.S. Department of Agriculture, U.S. Department of Health and Human Services. *Nutrition and your health: dietary guidelines for Americans,* 5th ed. 2000. **www.usda.gov/cnpp/DierGd.pdf.**

44. Williams S and Schlenker E. *Essentials of Nutrients and Diet Therapy,* 8th edition. St. Louis, MO: Mosby Inc., 2003.

How would you like to be part of an experiment in which all you eat for an entire month is McDonald's food? In our fast paced society, many people tend to eat out at fast-food restaurants much of the time, eating on the run. Thirty-three year old filmmaker Morgan Spurlock decided to make a documentary called, SuperSize Me, to look at the potential consequences of America's tendency to order bigger portion sizes.

Spurlock supersized all of his orders and eat three meals a day at McDonald's for an entire month and filmed his experiences. At 6′2″, Spurlock gained 25 lbs and his cholesterol went from 168 to 230 within the month. Typically 40–70% of the calories in fast-foods are from fat and so it is not hard to see how Spurlock had these results. After three weeks of this fast-food diet, he was complaining of "pounding headaches," his liver was at toxic levels, and his sex drive had dramatically decreased. Spurlock and his physicians were shocked at how rapidly he became dramatically ill.

Recently McDonald's announced it is phasing out SuperSize fries and drinks in its more than 13,000 U.S. restaurants and will stop selling them altogether by year's end, except in promotions. McDonald's denied that the award winning documentary "SuperSize Me" nor the two lawsuits claiming McDonald's hid the health risks associated with eating Big Macs and Chicken McNuggets had anything to do with this decision. They contend that the move is part of their "Eat Smart, Be Active" initiative in an attempt to revive sales.

With obesity on the rise and 35% of food consumed by Americans eaten away from home, it is more important than ever to make healthy choices in eating out such as those suggested in the "Changing for the Better" box on page 149.

Sources:
My Month at Mickey D's. *People Magazine,* February 9, 2004.
McDonald's Menu to Go on Diet in 2005. *ABC News,* March 3, 2004.

genetically modified food

Chances are you've had it for breakfast. And lunch. And dinner. It is now virtually impossible for Americans to avoid eating genetically modified (GM) foods, or what the British tabloids call "Frankenfood."

Britain's Prince Charles proclaims that he would never eat the stuff and won't stand for it being grown on his land.[1] In Britain and throughout Europe, public fears about GM foods are running high and have provoked a trade war with the United States. Americans, however, appear only dimly aware of GM foods, and Kraft's million taco-shell recall in September 2000 didn't prove to be the tide-turning cataclysm that some GM critics had hoped for. The taco shells contained traces of corn meal from StarLink, a genetically engineered variety of corn that hadn't been approved for human consumption, but no one suffered harm from eating the shells. Nevertheless, in the worst-case scenario, allergens or other harmful substances, added to food by design or accident, could have found their way into our stomachs.[2]

Since the mid 1990s, armed with new knowledge about DNA and how it functions, scientists have been able to manipulate the genetic code of organisms that are food sources and have created new strains of plants and animals capable of growing larger in less time on less suitable soil. Some new plant strains can do this while also resisting insect pests.

Farmers have long engaged in "traditional genetics," favoring seeds from plants with the most desirable characteristics or crossbreeding closely related species. Scientists have tried to speed things up by exposing plants to chemicals and radiation. These ongoing experiments produce hundreds of mutations among genes, some of which may be useful.

Genetic engineering, in contrast, is very specific. It allows scientists to select a single gene for a single characteristic and insert that stretch of DNA into another organism, or even another species. The ability to crossbreed diverse forms of life has had a profound effect on U.S. agriculture and on the food we purchase in the grocery store. An example is the Flavr-Savr tomato, developed by Calgene to soften more slowly, meaning it can stay on the vine longer and develop a fuller taste. Its longer shelf life also reduces waste.

The percentage of genetically modified seed is now estimated to approach 40% to 60% of all U.S. planting, designed either to make the crops resistant to weedkillers or to produce their own pesticides. Bioengineered corn and soybeans in particular are used as ingredients in a wide range of processed food, from soft drinks and beer to chips and breakfast cereal. Genetically modified organisms are fed to farm animals. Even health-food products like tofu and canola oil often contain genetically modified ingredients.

What Are the Potential Health Risks?

Genetically engineered crops hold down food production costs and reduce the need for pesticides and herbicides. Modified foods in the works are more nutritious and flavorful, and productive grains, drought-resistant crops, caffeine-free coffee beans, and even plants that produce drugs and vaccines have been developed.

While the potential benefits of higher-yielding GM food and a new revolution in agricultural practices appear indisputable, serious concerns have also arisen. Biotechnology foes warn that we do not know enough about the way genes operate and interact to be sure of the outcome of any modification. They worry that alterations could accidentally lead to substances that are poisonous or that trigger allergies.

Critics fear that the use of DNA from plant viruses and bacteria in the modification of crops may also somehow trigger disease. They also argue that antibiotic-resistant genes could be passed to the microorganisms that make us sick. If this happened, we might not have the drugs necessary to fight back.[3]

Environmental concerns are also an issue. The green lobby (that is, environmentalists working in the political arena) is worried about genes that confer herbicide and insect resistance. They believe some of these genes could "escape" and be transferred to other crops, resulting in the emergence of "superweeds." They fear this leakage could cause the disappearance of familiar species of insects and birds as food chains are damaged.

In addition, the corporations at the forefront of GM food production are also the world's biggest producers of agrochemicals. Critics claim these companies are trying to handcuff farmers by attempting to tie them into deals where they have little choice but to buy the GM seed and the designer chemicals to go with it.

How Do Bioengineers Counter These Objections?

The biotechnology industry claims that there is no evidence of any GM food causing serious ill effects. Proponents point out that many of our conventional food products have gotten to grocery stores only after their non-GM, raw ingredients have been treated to remove undesirable or toxic substances.[3]

While genetic modification may result in the emergence of new allergens, so too may conventional plant breeding, say GM defenders. The new technology holds out the possibility of engineering such problems out of food, however.

Use of DNA from plant viruses and bacteria presents minimal risk, precisely because we are not plants. Further, genetic modifications allow us to improve the flavor, texture, nutritional value, and shelf life of food. It could boost the vitamin content of fruits and vegetables, incorporate anticancer substances, and reduce our exposure to less healthy fats and oils. A recent example of genetically engineered food is "miracle" rice with higher levels of vitamin A, developed with the hope that rice with boosted nutritional value will stave off illness in developing countries.

Proponents also argue that GM technology offers a chance to recover biodiversity, since GM crops will require fewer chemicals that have low toxicity, are rapidly degraded, and stay in the soil rather than being washed into streams and rivers. At the same time these crops will produce higher yields, reducing pressure on remaining uncultivated habitats. Scientists also are investigating plants that may be modified to produce new plastics and biofuels that would be kinder to the environment than oil-based products.

Some companies are bowing to perceived consumer pressure by shying away from genetically modified ingredients. Baby food manufacturers Gerber and Heinz have removed themselves from the debate by saying no to genetically modified corn and soybeans, at least for now. Frito-Lay (owned by PepsiCo) stopped using engineered corn in its chips. McDonald's has asked suppliers to stop shipping genetically altered potatoes, as has McCain Foods, the world's largest producer of french fries.[4]

Many of these companies are not actually abandoning biotechnology, however. PepsiCo, Frito-Lay's parent company, still uses corn syrup made from GM crops for its soft drinks. And McDonald's still cooks its fries in oil made from genetically altered corn and soy.[4] According to big food producers, GM crops are so pervasive, there's simply no method to segregate them from other crops. In many instances, food manufacturers may not even know which genetically modified ingredients are contained in their products. As Pillsbury has noted in a written statement, "Many of our products contain food ingredients derived from soy (soy oil, soy protein, soy sauce) and corn (corn starch, corn oil, high fructose corn syrup), all of which could have been produced using genetic modification. Since soy and corn are managed as commodity ingredients in the United States, it is possible that traditional and genetically modified products could become commingled during harvest, storage, and processing."[1]

Nobody, from farmers to grain handlers to Kraft Foods executives, could explain how StarLink got mixed into corn meal meant for taco shells. And critics were more alarmed that the tests that detected its presence were administered not by Kraft or others along the production line, nor by government inspectors, but by a private company working for the Genetically Engineered Food Alert, a volunteer coalition of biotechnology skeptics and foes.[2]

Kraft now favors a more aggressive federal policy on testing GM foods and assuring their purity, including a requirement that developers of new crops provide an easy-to-use test for identifying GM material in food products. Since grain handlers claim it's not possible to fully segregate one type of corn from all others, Kraft also proposes that the government ban the planting of any food crop not certified for humans.[2] That a major food company is proposing such steps suggests that the food industry is realizing that growing public unease about GM food demands something more than companies' assurances about its safety.

Britain, Japan, Australia, Italy, and a dozen other nations currently require labels on foods containing genetically altered ingredients. U.S. regulators so far have rejected pressure for similar labeling requirements (with the exception of organic food products), saying the foods are no different from those grown with conventional crops. The Food and Drug Administration is expected to issue voluntary labeling guidelines for U.S. companies that wish to say a food does or does not contain GM ingredients. Critics, however, say that consumers need a clear choice at the grocery store. In response, Greenpeace has issued a "shopping list" that includes thousands of brand-name cereals, snacks, frozen dinners, and other foods that contain genetically altered corn, soybeans, and other ingredients. The "True Food Shopping List" is posted on the Internet (**www.truefoodnow.org**), along with a list of foods that do not contain gene-spliced ingredients, to help American consumers avoid genetically engineered food.

In Western society, our overriding concern is quality, safety, and consumers' rights to make informed choices about what they eat, yet Americans readily accept drugs and medicines that have been modified and rarely think twice about swallowing a pill for the slightest ailment, often seizing on new research before it has been proven. If foods can be modified to improve the quality of our lives, do you object to biotechnology being applied to agriculture?

For Discussion . . .

Should labeling of genetically modified foods be required? Why or why not? Do you think a moratorium should be imposed on GM crops until long-term studies prove them safe, or do you believe the potential nutritional and environmental benefits outweigh the risks?

References

1. Longman PJ. The curse of Frankenfood. *U.S. News & World Report,* 26 July 1999.
2. Editorial. Taco-shell recall—a mishap that could have been worse. *Minneapolis-St. Paul Star Tribune,* 29 September 2000.
3. Genetically-modified Q&A, *BBC News,* 6 April 1999. **http://news.bbc.co.uk**
4. Schueller G. Seeds of change: understanding the GM food revolution. *Environmental News Network* 29 September 2000. **http://enn.com**

personal assessment

rate your plate

Take a closer look at yourself—your current food decisions and your lifestyle. Think about your typical eating pattern and food decisions.

Do You . . .

	Usually	Sometimes	Never
Consider nutrition when you make food choices?	❑	❑	❑
Try to eat regular meals (including breakfast), rather than skip or skimp on some?	❑	❑	❑
Choose nutritious snacks?	❑	❑	❑
Try to eat a variety of foods?	❑	❑	❑
Include new-to-you foods in meals and snacks?	❑	❑	❑
Try to balance your energy (calorie) intake with your physical activity?	❑	❑	❑

Now for the Details

Do You . . .

	Usually	Sometimes	Never
Eat at least 6 servings* of grain products daily?	❑	❑	❑
Eat at least 3 servings* of vegetables daily?	❑	❑	❑
Eat at least 2 servings* of fruits daily?	❑	❑	❑
Consume at least 2 servings* of milk, yogurt, or cheese daily?	❑	❑	❑
Go easy on higher-fat foods?	❑	❑	❑
Go easy on sweets?	❑	❑	❑
Drink 8 or more cups of fluids daily?	❑	❑	❑
Limit alcoholic beverages (no more than 1 daily for a woman or 2 for a man)?	❑	❑	❑

Score Yourself

Usually = 2 points
Sometimes = 1 point
Never = 0 points

If You Scored . . .

24 or more points—Healthful eating seems to be your fitness habit already. Still, look for ways to stick to a healthful eating plan—and to make a "good thing" even better.

---

*Serving sizes vary depending on the food and food group.

16 to 23 points—You're on track. A few easy changes could help you make your overall eating plan healthier.
9 to 15 points—Sometimes you eat smart—but not often enough to be your "fitness best."
0 to 8 points—For your good health, you're wise to rethink your overall eating style. Take it gradually—step by step!

Whatever your score, make moves for healthful eating. Gradually turn your "nevers" into "sometimes" and your "sometimes" into "usually."

Adapted from *The American Dietetic Association's Monthly Nutrition Companion: 31 Days to a Healthier Lifestyle,* Chronimed Publishing, 1997.

Sample Serving Sizes
Bread, Cereals, Rice, and Pasta Group—6 to 11 Servings Daily:
1 slice (1 oz.) enriched or whole-grain bread
½ hamburger roll, bagel, English muffin, or pita
½ cup cooked rice or pasta
1 ounce (1 cup) ready-to-eat cereal

Vegetable Group—3 to 5 Servings Daily:
½ cup chopped raw, non-leafy vegetables
½ cup cooked vegetables
1 small baked potato (3 ounces)
¾ cup vegetable juice

Fruit Group—2 to 4 Servings Daily:
1 medium fruit (apple, orange, banana, peach)
¾ cup fruit juice
½ cup canned, frozen, or cooked fruit

Milk, Yogurt, and Cheese Group—2 to 3 Servings Daily:
1 cup milk, buttermilk, or yogurt
1 ½ ounces natural cheese (cheddar, mozzarella, Swiss)
1 cup frozen yogurt

Meat, Poultry, Fish, Beans, Eggs, and Nuts Group—2 to 3 Servings Daily:
2 to 3 ounces cooked lean meat, poultry, or fish
½ cup cooked legumes (equals 1 ounce meat)
1 egg (equals 1 ounce meat)

Fats, Oils, and Sweets—Use Sparingly:
sugars
salad dressings
oils
cream
butter
soft drinks

personal assessment

are you feeding your feelings?

Sometimes people use food as a way of coping with their emotions and problems. To identify how you might be using food as a coping strategy and what feelings you tend to associate with eating, complete the following inventory.

1 = Never

2 = Rarely

3 = Occasionally

4 = Often

5 = Always

1. _____ Do you eat when you are angry?
2. _____ When you feel annoyed, do you turn to food?
3. _____ If someone lets you down, do you eat to comfort yourself?
4. _____ When you are having a bad day, do you notice that you eat more?
5. _____ Do you eat to cheer yourself up?
6. _____ Do you use food as a way of avoiding tasks you don't want to do?
7. _____ Do you view food as your friend when you are feeling lonely?
8. _____ Is food a way for you to comfort yourself when your life seems empty?
9. _____ When you are feeling upset, do you turn to food to calm yourself down?
10. _____ Do you eat more when you are anxious, worried, or stressed?
11. _____ Does eating help you to cope with feeling overwhelmed?
12. _____ Do you eat more when you are going through big changes or transitions in your life?
13. _____ Do you reward yourself with food?
14. _____ When you think you have done something wrong, do you punish yourself by eating?
15. _____ When you are feeling badly about yourself, do you eat more?
16. _____ When you feel discouraged about your efforts to improve yourself, do you eat more, thinking "what's the use of trying"?

_____ TOTAL SCORE

Interpretation

If you scored between . . .

0–13   You don't eat to cope with your emotions. Your eating may not be related to your emotional state. However, you may avoid eating when you are upset or having trouble coping with your feelings. You may run away from food rather than running to food to cope.

14–66   Although you fall in the average range, you may use food to deal with specific situations or feelings such as anger, loneliness, or boredom. See the breakdown of scores below to identify how you may be using food to cope with particular feelings.

67 and above   You run to food to cope with your emotions, and you may want to consider developing other ways of appropriately expressing your feelings.

If you answered "4" or "5" to most of questions #1–#4, this can be indicative of eating when you are angry.

If you answered "4" or "5" to most of questions #5–#8, this can be indicative of eating when you are lonely or bored.

If you answered "4" or "5" to most of questions #9–#12, this can be an indication that you are a stress eater.

If you answered "4" or "5" to most of questions #13–#16, this can be an indication that you are using food to cope with feelings of low self-esteem and self-worth.

chapter six

maintaining a healthy weight

Chapter Objectives

After reading this chapter, you should be able to:

▌ describe the role of the media and entertainment industry in defining the ideal body image.

▌ define overweight and obesity.

▌ discuss how effective body mass index, electrical impedance, skin fold measurements, hydrostatic weighing, and appearance are as methods of assessing body weight.

▌ discuss the causes of obesity including genetics, metabolism, physiological and hormonal changes, environmental factors, dietary practices, sociocultural factors, and psychological factors.

▌ describe the body's use of food in activity requirements, in basal metabolism, and in the thermic effect.

▌ discuss the primary types of weight management techniques including dietary alterations, surgical interventions, medications, weight loss programs, and physical activity.

▌ provide evidence supporting physical exercise as the most important component of a weight loss program.

▌ define anorexia nervosa, bulimia nervosa, binge eating disorder, chewing and spitting food syndrome, and night-time eating syndrome.

▌ discuss the at-risk groups for eating disorders and factors to consider for males with eating disorders.

▌ discuss ways of treating eating disorders.

Online Learning Center Resources

www.mhhe.com/payne8e

Log on to our Online Learning Center (OLC) for access to these additional resources:

- Chapter key terms and definitions
- Learning objectives
- Student interactive question-and-answer sites
- Self-scoring chapter quiz
- Online assessments
- Key term flash cards

Talking It Over

Is Fat a Feeling?

Have you ever said or heard someone say, "I feel fat"? Is fat a feeling? Typically "fat" refers to our weight and body composition and is not a feeling such as anger, happiness, or sadness. However, we often say that we feel fat when we are feeling one of these emotions. When you are "feeling fat," think about how you felt the day before. If you felt better yesterday and your weight has not changed, why are you feeling fatter and worse today? Most likely, there is something bothering you other than your weight and appearance— sometimes it seems easier to focus on some-thing concrete and physical (such as weight) rather than on emotions that are less tangible and obvious. Perhaps you are really feeling unloved, hurt, angry, annoyed, bored, overwhelmed, or stressed.

When you are "feeling fat" or "having a fat day," you might ask yourself, "What is bothering me? What am I upset about?" It might be helpful to write in a journal about your feelings or talk with a trusted friend or family member about your feelings.

Eye on the Media

Bye or Buy to Quick and Easy Weight Loss

What's on TV tonight? A minute of channel surfing tells you that it's bodies—bodies conditioned through athletics, dance, or grueling training and drug enhancement, or bodies thinned to anorexic proportions to show off the latest fashions. Tune in to the cable medical channel and watch a liposuction procedure being done to remove excess fat. Or watch a program in which "ordinary people" volunteer to have their bodies made over to be "rock star bodies" in a 3-month period.

Commercials for weight loss products and procedures abound on television and in newspapers and magazines; people are further bom-barded with email offers and Internet pop-up ads promoting various weight loss products. With all of these ads, it's important to look carefully at the small print disclaimers that say "results may vary" or "results not typical." The Federal Trade Commission (FTC) has issued a warning to be wary of advertisements for weight loss products and services that make "grossly exaggerated claims" such as "I lost

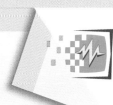

Weight management has become an obsession in American culture as well as a significant health problem. In the United States, obesity has risen at an epidemic rate during the past 20 years. One of the national health objectives for the year 2010 is to reduce the prevalence of obesity among adults to less than 15 percent. Research indicates that the situation is worsening rather than improving. According to the National Center for Chronic Disease Prevention and Health Promotion, an estimated 61% of U.S. adults are either overweight or obese. In 2000 38.8 million American adults met the criteria for obesity. Today, 27% of American adults are obese—nearly twice the figure for 1980. Children are affected as well. There are nearly twice as many overweight children and almost three times as many overweight adolescents as there were 20 years ago.[1, 2] These people face an increased risk of developing serious health problems, independent of other risk factors not directly related to weight. In a more recently reported study, the trend described above appears to have continued through the end of the 1990s.[3] Most likely the same trend is in evidence today.

What accounts for the high percentage of Americans defined as overweight or obese? Experts point to two salient factors: greater daily caloric consumption and a relatively low level of consistent physical activity. The average caloric intake for Americans has increased by 10% over the past two decades. Meanwhile, nearly two-thirds of Americans are not physically active on a regular basis and 25% are completely sedentary[4] (see Chapter 4).

The increase in weight just reported occurs, of course, when the body is supplied with more energy than it can use and the excess energy is stored in the form of adipose tissue, or fat. This is called a positive caloric balance. The continuous buildup of **adipose tissue** leads to excess weight and can eventually result in obesity. Obesity may account for as many as 280,000 to 325,000 deaths annually, depending on the smoking status of the persons within the sample being studied.[5]

Among the health problems caused by or complicated by excess body fat are increased surgical risk, hypertension, various forms of heart disease, stroke, type II diabetes, several forms of cancer, deterioration of joints, complications during pregnancy, gallbladder disease, and an overall increased risk of mortality (see the Star box on page 177 and Table 6.1). So closely is obesity associated with chronic conditions, such as those just mentioned, that medical experts now recommend that obesity itself be defined and treated as a chronic disease. In fact, the combination of type 2 diabetes, hypertension, and atherosclerosis (high triglycerides and low HDL cholesterol which fosters plaque build-up in the artery walls) along with obesity is now referred to as *Syndrome X* and can result in shortening your life span.[6]

Key Terms

adipose tissue tissue made up of fibrous strands around which specialized cells designed to store liquefied fat are arranged.

Table 6.1 Health Problems Associated with Excess Body Fat

Health Problems	Partially Attributed to:
Surgical risk	Increased anesthesia needs and greater risk of wound infections
Pulmonary disease	Excess weight over lungs
Type II diabetes mellitus (NIDDM)	Enlarged fat cells, which then poorly bind insulin and also poorly respond to the message insulin sends to the cell
Hypertension	Increased miles of blood vessels found in the fat tissue; however, no validated cause is yet known
Coronary heart disease	Increases in serum cholesterol and triglyceride levels, as well as a decrease in physical activity
Bone and joint disorders	Excess pressure put on knee, ankle, and hip joints
Gallbladder stones	An increase in the cholesterol content of bile
Skin disorders	The trapping of moisture and microbes in fat folds
Various cancers	Estrogen production by fat cells; animal studies suggest excess energy intake encourages tumor development
Shorter stature (in some forms of obesity)	An earlier onset of puberty
Pregnancy risk	More difficult delivery and increased anesthesia needs (if used)
Early death	A variety of risk factors for diseases listed above

The greater the degree of obesity, the more likely and the more serious these health problems generally become. They are much more likely to appear in people who are greater than twice their desirable body weight.

Body Image and Self-Concept

Although clinicians now have specific guidelines for the diagnosis and treatment of obesity, the general public has its own set of definitions and concerns regarding body weight. Principal among these is the issue of perceived physical attractiveness. This concern is caused (or reinforced) by the media, which tells people that being overweight does not conform to certain ideal **body images** (such as being tall, thin, and "cut" with muscular definition). The average actress or model, for example, is thinner than 95% of the female population and weighs 23% less than the average woman;[7] while the average American woman is 5′4″, 143 pounds, and wears a size 10–12, the average model is 5′10″ and 110 pounds.[8] Today's lean but muscular version of perfection is a very demanding standard for both women and men to meet. Men, in fact, make up approximately 10% of those with eating disorders, for which body image concerns is an important component. For both men and women, the demands of athletics seems to be a significant factor in the development of body image-related concerns, particularly in sports such as gymnastics, boxing, wrestling, dancing, track, swimming, and rowing, in which "making weight" is an important component.[9]

In light of this challenge, people may become dissatisfied and concerned about their inability to resemble ideal images. The scope of this dissatisfaction is evident in a study of more than 800 women, which revealed that nearly half were unhappy with their weight, muscle tone, hips, thighs, buttocks, and legs.[10] Not surprisingly, when this dissatisfaction exists, people can question their own attractiveness, and eventually, their self-concept and self-esteem declines.

Health Risks of Obesity

Each of the diseases listed below is followed by the percentage of cases that are caused by obesity:

Colon cancer	10%
Breast cancer	11%
Hypertension	33%
Heart disease	70%
Diabetes (type II, non-insulin-dependent)	90%

As these statistics show, being obese greatly increases your risk of many serious and even life-threatening diseases.

Key Terms

body image our subjective perception of how our body appears.

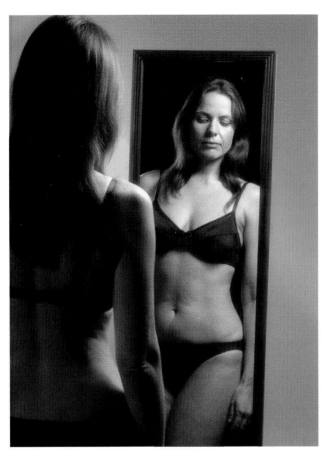

Studies show that mirrors make us more self-conscious, critical, and conforming.

In comparison with being overweight, little media attention has been paid to being underweight. However, the body image problems experienced by some extremely thin people can be equally distressing, particularly for males. Men tend to have the desire to be more muscular, more "cut," to be bigger and stronger.[11]

Defining Overweight and Obesity

The most prevalent forms of malnutrition in affluent countries are overweight and obesity. Most people think of malnourishment as a shortage of essential nutrients. In developing countries, food deprivation forms the basis of malnutrition. However, malnutrition can also be a disease of plenty. Because our food supply exceeds the needs of our population, people are able to eat more than is required for healthful living. They often consume more calories than they expend. They can then become overweight and may become obese.

How can people tell the difference between overweight and obesity? Doctors usually define **overweight** as a con-

dition in which a person's weight is 1% to 19 % higher than normal, as defined by a standard height/weight chart. **Obesity** is usually defined as a condition in which a person's weight is 20% or more above normal weight. *Morbid obesity* refers to being 50% to 100% above normal weight, more than 100 pounds over normal weight, or sufficiently overweight to interfere with health or normal functioning.[12] Of course, an exception to this relationship between overweight and obesity is excessive weight caused by extreme muscularity, such as that seen in many football players.

Being most familiar with the weight guidelines used in the past, most clinicians and the general public continue to use standard height/weight tables to determine the extent to which scale weight exceeds **desirable weight** and, thus, the existence of mild, moderate, or severe obesity. However, other techniques are now available that can be used to determine body composition. In the next section of this chapter, several of those techniques, including waist/hip ratio (*healthy body weight*), body mass index, hydrostatic weighing, "BOD POD" assessment, skinfold measurements, and electrical impedance, are described.

Most recently the scientific community has issued guidelines for determining obesity for purposes of medical intervention. Women with a BMI over 27.3 and men with a BMI above 27.8 are considered overweight. Individuals are considered obese when BMI is 30.0 or above. Severe or morbid obesity is when the BMI is greater than 40.[12] Aggressive medical intervention is necessary for people who, in addition to being obese, have a waist circumference of 40 or more inches (males) or 35 or more inches (females) and two or more of the following risk factors: diabetes, high blood pressure, high blood cholesterol, and **sleep apnea.**[13] For obese people who demonstrate fewer risk factors, less aggressive treatment may suffice.

Key Terms

overweight a condition in which a person's excess fat accumulation results in a body weight that exceeds desirable weight by 1% to 19%.

obesity a condition in which a person's body weight is 20% or more above desirable weight as determined by standard height/weight charts.

desirable weight the weight range deemed appropriate for people, taking into consideration gender, age, and frame size.

sleep apnea a condition in which abnormalities in the structure of the airways lead to periods of greatly restricted air flow during sleep, resulting in reduced levels of blood oxygen and placing greater strain on the heart to maintain adequate tissue oxygenation.

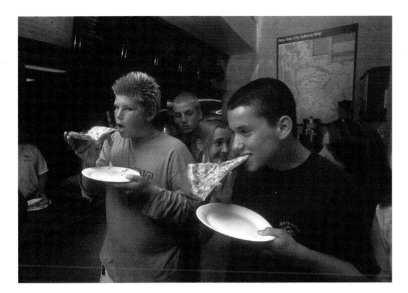

Childhood obesity, a condition that is increasing in incidence, is viewed as a precursor to the development of type 2 diabetes mellitus.

Obesity, although perhaps genetically and behaviorally determined early in life, often takes many years to develop fully. A daily caloric surplus of only ten calories yields ten unwanted pounds of fat in ten years; twenty or thirty years of consistent excess food intake or gradually declining activity can easily result in a **positive caloric balance** and, eventually, being overweight and even obese. Accordingly, to maintain a specific weight people must balance their energy intake with their energy expenditure. The key to losing weight and keeping it off is regular, aerobic exercise and a balanced diet that is consistent with the current nutritional recommendations described in Chapter 5; in other words, eat healthfully and exercise regularly.

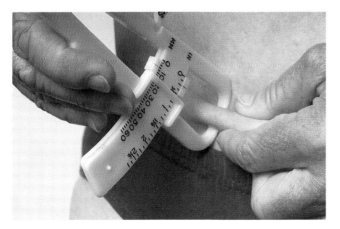

Body fat determination using skinfold calipers. Skinfold measurements are used in equations that calculate body fat density and percent body fat.

Determining Weight and Body Composition

A wide array of techniques exist to determine weight and body composition. Some techniques are, of course, much more accurate and more expensive than others. In the section that follows, a variety of these techniques are described.

Body Mass Index

One means of assessing healthy body weight is the **body mass index (BMI).** The BMI indicates the relationship of body weight (expressed in kilograms) to height (expressed in meters) for both men and women. The BMI does not reflect body composition (fat versus lean tissue) or consider the degree of fat accumulated within the central body cavity. It is, nevertheless, widely used in determining obesity (see Table 6.2). BMI is calculated metrically as weight divided by height squared (kg/m^2).

> **Key Terms**
>
> **positive caloric balance** caloric intake greater than caloric expenditure.
>
> **body mass index (BMI)** a mathematical calculation based on weight and height; used to determine desirable body weight.

Table 6.2 Charting Weight

Height

Weight

Height	100	105	110	115	120	125	130	135	140	145	150	155	160	165	170	175	180	185	190	195	200	205	210	215	220	225	230	235	240	245	250
5'0"	20	21	21	22	23	24	25	26	27	28	29	30	31	32	33	34	35	36	37	38	39	40	41	42	43	44	45	46	47	48	49
5'1"	19	20	21	22	23	24	25	26	26	27	28	29	30	31	32	33	34	35	36	37	38	39	40	41	42	43	43	44	45	46	47
5'2"	18	19	20	21	22	23	24	25	26	27	27	28	29	30	31	32	33	34	35	36	37	37	38	39	40	41	42	43	44	45	46
5'3"	18	19	19	20	21	22	23	24	25	26	27	27	28	29	30	31	32	33	34	35	35	36	37	38	39	40	41	42	43	43	44
5'4"	17	18	19	20	21	21	22	23	24	25	26	27	27	28	29	30	31	32	33	33	34	35	36	37	38	39	39	40	41	42	43
5'5"	17	17	18	19	20	21	22	22	23	24	25	26	27	27	28	29	30	31	32	32	33	34	35	36	37	37	38	39	40	41	42
5'6"	16	17	18	19	19	20	21	22	23	23	24	25	26	27	27	28	29	30	31	31	32	33	34	35	36	36	37	38	39	40	40
5'7"	16	16	17	18	19	20	20	21	22	23	23	24	25	26	27	27	28	29	30	31	31	32	33	34	34	35	36	37	38	38	39
5'8"	15	16	17	17	18	19	20	21	21	22	23	24	24	25	26	27	27	28	29	30	30	31	32	33	33	34	35	36	36	37	38
5'9"	15	16	16	17	18	18	19	20	21	21	22	23	24	24	25	26	27	27	28	29	30	30	31	32	32	33	34	35	35	36	37
5'10"	14	15	16	16	17	18	19	19	20	21	22	22	23	24	24	25	26	27	27	28	29	29	30	31	32	32	33	34	34	35	36
5'11"	14	15	15	16	17	17	18	19	20	20	21	22	22	23	24	24	25	26	26	27	28	29	29	30	31	31	32	33	33	34	35
6'0"	14	14	15	16	16	17	18	18	19	20	20	21	22	22	23	24	24	25	26	26	27	28	28	29	30	31	31	32	33	33	34
6'1"	13	14	15	15	16	16	17	18	18	19	20	20	21	22	22	23	24	24	25	26	26	27	28	28	29	30	30	31	32	32	33
6'2"	13	13	14	15	15	16	17	17	18	19	19	20	21	21	22	22	23	24	24	25	26	26	27	28	28	29	30	30	31	31	32
6'3"	12	13	14	14	15	16	16	17	17	18	19	19	20	21	21	22	22	23	24	24	25	26	26	27	27	28	29	29	30	31	31
6'4"	12	13	13	14	15	15	16	16	17	18	18	19	19	20	21	21	22	23	23	24	24	25	26	26	27	27	28	29	29	30	30

KEY: Healthy   Overweight   Obese

The starting point of what's considered overweight is now set at a body mass index of 25 to less than 30, say new guidelines from the National Institutes of Health. One previous definition set the starting point at a BMI of 27. The new and old guidelines define obese as a BMI of 30 or above.

Source: National Institutes of Health

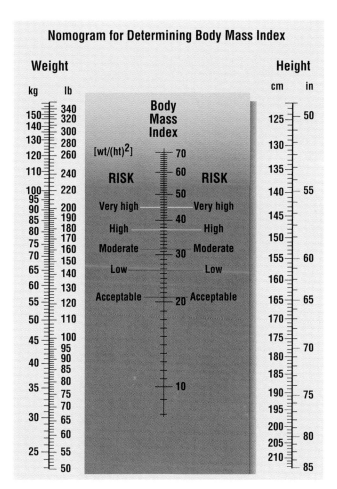

Nomogram for Determining Body Mass Index

Figure 6-1 To use this nomogram, place a ruler or other straightedge between the body weight in kilograms or pounds (without clothes) located on the left-hand column and the height in centimeters or in inches (without shoes) located on the right-hand column. The BMI is read from the middle of the scale and is in metric units.

An alternative method of determining the BMI is to use a **nomogram** such as that in Figure 6-1. Like the BMI, the nomogram requires information about both weight and height. Once you have determined your BMI, you can determine whether it falls within the acceptable range for your age group (see Table 6.3). Note that with aging, generally higher BMI values are found.[12] This reflects the gradual weight gain (and indirectly the changing body composition) seen in adults as they age. Table 6.4 on page 182 presents data on BMI related to age, gender and ethnicity.

The newest BMI chart to appear is the recently released BMI chart for children and adolescents. The importance of having a BMI chart appropriate for age 2 years through 20 years was stimulated by the increasing percent of children and adolescents who are now classified as being obese (20%). Because of the availability of this chart, pediatricians and parents will now have the ability to more quickly and more accurately determine the risk of potential obesity

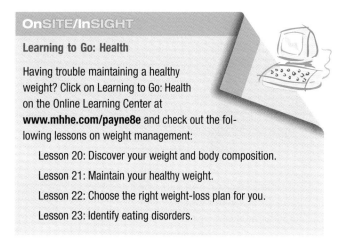
in children and take appropriate action to minimize its occurrence. Additional information on this newly released BMI chart can be obtained at **www.cdc.gov/growthcharts** or **www.cdc.gov/nccdphp/dnpa/bmi.**

Height/Weight Tables

Traditionally the 1983 Metropolitan Life Insurance Height and Weight Table has been the basis for determining the desirable or ideal weight for your gender, height, and frame size. However, the use of this table and others like it is no longer considered the best way to determine whether body weight is acceptable. It is now recognized that this table excludes uninsurable people, disregards the influence of age, fails to consider other causes of mortality (such as smoking), and relies on subjective determinations of frame size *to express the influence of body composition* on weight. In addition, people have failed to take into consideration that the Metropolitan Life Insurance Height and Weight Tables were based upon height that included 1-inch heel shoes and allowed 3 pounds of clothing. The tables were also designed for adults aged 25–59 years of age and were not intended for use with children.[14] Fortunately, newer tables intended for use with the guidelines describing healthy body weight (Table 6.2) and body mass index (BMI) (Table 6.3) appear on pages 180 and 182, respectively.

Healthy Body Weight

You can determine your healthy body weight by using the weight guidelines found in the 2000 *Dietary Guidelines for Americans* (Table 6.2).[15] This assessment involves converting two body measurements, the waist and the hip circumferences, into a waist-to-hip ratio (WHR) that can then be

---

Key Terms

nomogram a graphic means of finding an unknown value.

---

applied to weight ranges found in Table 6.2 for people of particular ages and heights. The size of your waist is a surprisingly accurate measure of your abdominal fat. Among people who have an acceptable WHR, female "healthy weight" is near the lower end of each weight range, whereas male "healthy weight" is at the higher end of each weight range.

To use these new weight ranges, the following procedure must be performed:

1. Measure around your waist near your navel while you stand relaxed, not pulling in your stomach.
2. Measure around your hips, over the buttocks where your hips are the largest.
3. Divide the waist measurement by the hip measurement.

Women with a WHR of .80 or less generally have a body weight that falls within the healthy range for their age and height as depicted in Table 6.2; men with a WHR of .90 or less will also probably fall within the range that is considered healthy for their age and height as seen in Table 6.5.

This assessment procedure was developed in response to the growing concern over the relationship between the amount of fat in the central abdominal cavity (upper body obesity) and the development of several serious health problems. The risk of health problems such as heart disease and diabetes increases at a waist measurement of 35 inches for women and 40 inches for men, regardless of height.[16]

In comparison with the "spare tire" pattern of fat distribution seen in men, women more often demonstrate an excessive accumulation of fat in the hips, thighs, and buttocks. This lower body obesity is less closely associated with chronic health problems.

As a point of interest, the guidelines found in the *Dietary Guidelines for Americans* do not use WHR as a clinical marker for the treatment of obesity, but rather use only waist circumference, believing it to be a better predictor of risk. Only time will tell about the continued use of healthy body weight in assessing risk for CVD and other chronic conditions.

The *Dietary Guidelines for Americans* assessment procedure recognizes increasing age as a factor that influences body weight.[15] For people older than 35 years of age, this alleviates some of the pressure to maintain an unrealistic weight. Some nutritionists, however, believe that the same weight standards should apply to both older adults and younger adults.

Table 6.3 Desirable Body Mass Index in Relation to Age

Age Group (years)	BMI (kg/m²)
19–24	19–24
25–34	20–25
35–44	21–26
45–54	22–27
55–65	23–28
>65	24–29

Table 6.4 Mean Body Mass Index and Percentage of Overweight and Obese U.S. Adults

	Men			Women		
	Mean BMI	Overweight (N = 15.4 Million)	Obese (N = 5.1 Million)	Mean BMI	Overweight (N = 18.6 Million)	Obese (N = 7.4 Million)
AGE						
20–24	23.5	12.1	4.2	22.6	11.4	3.5
25–34	25.2	20.4	6.7	24.1	20	8.8
35–44	26	28.9	8.9	25.3	27	12.1
45–54	26.3	31	10.7	26.1	32.5	12.9
55–64	26.1	28.1	9.2	26.5	37	14.2
All ages	25.3	24.2	8	25	27.1	10.6
ETHNICITY						
White	25.4	24.4	7.8	24.8	24.6	9.6
Black	25.3	26.3	10.4	27.1	45.1	19.7
Mexican	25.9	31.2	10.8	26.6	41.5	16.7
Cuban	26	28.5	10.3	25.8	31.9	6.9
Puerto Rican	25.5	25.7	7.9	26.1	39.8	15.2

Table 6.5 Healthy Weight: Recommended Guidelines

	Weight*	
Height⁺	19–34 years	35 years and over
5'	97–128	108–138
5'1"	101–132	111–143
5'2"	104–137	115–148
5'3"	107–141	119–152
5'4"	111–146	122–157
5'5"	114–150	126–162
5'6"	118–155	130–167
5'7"	121–160	134–172
5'8"	125–164	138–178
5'9"	129–169	142–183
5'10"	132–174	146–188
5'11"	136–179	151–194
6'	140–184	155–199
6'1"	144–189	159–205
6'2"	148–195	164–210
6'3"	152–200	168–216
6'4"	156–205	173–222
6'5"	160–211	177–228
6'6"	164–216	182–234

*Without clothes.
⁺Without shoes.

Note: The higher weights in the ranges generally apply to men, who tend to have more muscle and bone mass; the lower weights more often apply to women, who generally have less muscle and bone mass.

Electrical Impedance

Electrical impedance is a relatively new method to determine body composition. This assessment procedure measures the electrical impedance or resistance to a weak electrical flow directed through the body. Because adipose tissue resists the passage of the electrical current more than muscle tissue does, electrical impedance can be used to calculate the percentage of body fat. However, in addition to high cost and limited availability, psychological variables, such as fear or discomfort associated with the electrical current flow, can reduce the practicality of electrical impedance.

BOD POD (Body Composition System)

The newest method of determining body composition involves the use of the BOD POD, an egg-shaped chamber that uses computerized pressure sensors to determine the amount of air displaced by the person's body (larger people displace more air than smaller people). The person is allowed to breath normally during the test, and the amount of air in the lungs can either be measured directly in the BOD

POD or is estimated. A complete test, with printed results, can be achieved in less than 4.5 minutes.[17] Body density can itself be used to determine the percentage of the subject's body that is comprised of fat. Upon knowing the percent body fat, the percent of lean body mass can be calculated, again using a mathematical formula.[18] The BOD POD is highly accurate and much more comfortable for subjects than hydrostatic weighing, which is described on page 184.

Skinfold Measurements

A **skinfold measurement** provides another way to measure body fat percentage. Skinfold measurements rely on constant-pressure **calipers** to measure the thickness of the layer of fat beneath the skin's surface. Skinfold measurements of subcutaneous fat are taken at several key places on the body. Measurements of skinfold thickness can then be used to calculate the percentage of body fat, and then a relatively simple conversion can be made to determine desired body weight. It should be noted that there are some drawbacks to this type of measure. First, body fat calipers may require someone else to perform the test as it is sometimes difficult to get an accurate measurement on yourself. Second, skinfolds are notoriously hard to locate precisely, and just a few millimeters off can make a significant difference. Research recommends that 50–100 tests are needed before an examiner can be classified as "competent" with body fat calipers. Body fat calipers used correctly are accurate to within 4% at best.[12]

Young adult men normally have a body fat percentage of between 10% and 15%. The normal range for young adult women is 22% to 25%. When a man's body fat percentage exceeds 25% and a woman's body fat percentage exceeds 30%, they are classified as obese.

The relatively higher percentage of fat found in women is related to the female's capacity for pregnancy and lactation. Women require a sufficient amount of body fat in order to ovulate, menstruate, and become pregnant. In fact, some suggest that lack of sex drive can be related to the adverse changes in hormonal level due to insufficient

> **Key Terms**
>
> **electrical impedance** a method used to measure the percentage of body fat using a harmless electrical current.
>
> **skinfold measurement** a measurement to determine the thickness of the fat layer that lies immediately beneath the skin; used to calculate body composition.
>
> **calipers** a device used to measure the thickness of a skinfold from which percent of body fat can be calculated.

body fat. The danger zone begins when a woman's BMI is about 18 or below. Women tend to store fat in their pelvic region, around their hips and thighs. Not only does this fat help to protect vital reproductive organs, it also acts as a source of stored energy for pregnancy and breast-feeding. As women enter menopause, they produce less estrogen. This leads to a change in body shape and fat distribution. During a woman's fertile years, the female hormones estrogen and progesterone are responsible for maintaining the female shape of a narrow waist and rounded hips. During and after menopause, the female waist thickens and fat is deposited around the stomach area similar to the male's pattern of fat distribution. In addition, as in men, the metabolic rate slows and fewer calories are required. So if a woman continues to eat the same amount of food as she has throughout her fertile years, without increasing her exercise, weight and fat gain are likely to occur.[19]

Hydrostatic Weighing

Hydrostatic weighing (underwater weighing) is a precise method for determining the relative amounts of fat and lean body mass that make up body weight. A person's percentage of body fat is determined by comparing the underwater body weight with the body weight out of the water and dry. The necessity for expensive equipment and trained technicians makes the use of this method impractical for the average person. Traditionally hydrostatic weighing has been considered the most accurate or sensitive means of determining body composition, with a 97% accuracy rate. The BOD POD (see page 183) appears to be just as accurate and certainly more comfortable to use than underwater weighing.

Additional techniques used to determine body composition include computerized axial tomography (CAT) scans, magnetic resonance imaging (MRI), infrared light transmission, and neutron activation. These techniques have limited application because of cost and availability.

Appearance

While it may seem as though the simplest method of determining one's body size is to look in the mirror, for most people this is not an accurate measure. Research shows that most women are dissatisfied with their appearance or body image and perceive themselves as needing to lose an average of 10–15 pounds when in actuality they are in a healthy weight range. Body dissatisfaction is endemic to young women in Western culture as evidenced by the rate of dieting in the United States, starting at a young age. In fact, on any given day, 50% of 10-year-olds are on a diet, two-thirds of high school women and a third of all adult women are dieting.[20] There is also an important difference between one's internal concept of memory of one's body and actual body perception, and this is particularly problematic for people with eating disorders.

Most people use scales to determine their weight, but scales can be highly inaccurate, as evidenced by weighing yourself on a variety of scales and weighing different amounts. Also, you will probably weigh less in the morning when you first wake up and more in the evening, after having eaten during the day. So if you are using a scale to monitor your weight, you need to do so on the same scale, at the same time of day, and with approximately the same weight of clothing. Also, remember that muscle weighs more than fat, which explains why some toned and muscular athletes can weigh as much as someone who is sedentary and overweight. In general, risk of disease increases with a higher percentage of body fat, not weight.

For many people, it is important to appear physically attractive. This desired body image may or may not be compatible with their inherited body type or their ability to gain or lose weight. Nevertheless, they try to achieve the look that they have in mind (see the Discovering Your Spirituality box on page 185).

In the body image that appears popular for today's women, the hips, waist, and shoulders line up to suggest a vertical line. The once-popular emphasis on an "hourglass" figure has given way to a more angular, athletic appearance, somewhat similar to the body build of many young men. As is true for women, the weight and body composition of many men do not align with the body they wish to possess.

Whether the body image desired can realistically be achieved seems unimportant to many people. Some spend hours each week in weight rooms and reduce or increase their food intake dramatically in a quest to attain the desired body image. For those who are ultimately unsuccessful, disappointment, frustration, and serious medical problems can result.

In extreme cases, a clinical condition referred to as "body dysmorphic disorder" (BDD) may develop. BDD is a secret preoccupation with an imagined or slight flaw in one's appearance. Sometimes, people become almost completely fixated on concerns regarding body image, leading to repeatedly weighing themselves and checking in mirrors throughout the day, compulsively dieting, and exercising and undergoing cosmetic surgery.[21] These attempts to achieve the perfect body may lead to psychological dysfunction such as not wanting to leave the house because of imagined defects.

> **Key Terms**
>
> **hydrostatic weighing** weighing the body while it is submerged in water.

Causes of Obesity

There is still an ongoing debate as to the causes of obesity. Genetic, physiological, metabolic, environmental, psychological, and other factors may all play a part. In the past decade, the overall prevalence of obesity has increased so that currently one-third of all Americans are obese. Moreover, in the last 20 years, the number of obese children in the United States has doubled to one in five children.[22] Genetics, dietary practice, and activity level seem to all play a role in this dramatic increase.

There are four additional factors that seem to play a significant role in the prevalence of obesity: sex, age, socioeconomic status, and race. As biology only accounts for 33% of the variation in body weight, the environment can also exert an enormous influence. According to the Centers for Disease Control, prevalence rates for obesity in women is 35% and 31% among men and is found mainly in the 20–55 age group. Among women, obesity is strongly associated with socioeconomic status, being twice as common among those with lower socioeconomic status as it is among those with higher status.[23] Although prevalence among black and white men does not differ significantly, obesity is far more common among black than among white women, affecting 60% of middle-aged black women compared with 33% of white women.

While the precise cause of obesity remains unclear, we do know that obesity is a complex condition caused by a variety of factors. Until we are sure what causes obesity, it makes sense that it is difficult to develop effective ways of managing weight.

Genetic Factors

Through years of research, we do know that heredity plays a major role in the development of body size and obesity.[24] Based on studies comparing both identical and fraternal (nonidentical) twins raised together and separately, it's evident that both environment and genetics influence obesity. In fact, it is estimated that heredity accounts for 25% to 40% of the development of obesity.[12] Women have a higher percentage of body fat than do men and this seems stable across cultures and dietary habits.[24] While there is some scientific research exploring the role that the X chromosome may be linked to fat distribution, there has not been any conclusive evidence to substantiate this idea.

There is also some speculation about population differences and prevalence of obesity suggesting that some groups possess a "thrifty genotype".[25] For example, the differences in diabetes and obesity rates in Native Americans as compared with European Americans prompted some to consider that some groups of people have survived periods of feast and famine by increased efficiency in energy storage and expenditure through a particular genotype. However, no specific thrifty gene or genotype has been identified.

There is a complex interplay of genetic factors that very likely influence the development of obesity as more than 250 genes may play a role in obesity. There has been promising research exploring how the leptin gene influences obesity. The leptin gene, referred to as the "fat gene" was discovered in the mid 1990s to influence satiety or the feeling of fullness in mice.[26] When the leptin gene was faulty in mice, it produced lower leptin levels, and the mice experienced excessive weight gain. However, when the leptin gene was normal, the leptin levels were higher and the mice were able to maintain normal weight. It has been theorized that leptin resistance may be involved in weight gain and the maintenance of excessive weight, but much more research needs to be conducted in this area.[27] While we know that leptin helps to regulate fat storage and energy efficiency in humans, it still remains unclear as to how this research can be utilized in the treatment of obesity.

Physiological and Hormonal Factors

Building on this new information about the genetic and neuropsychological basis of obesity, researchers have identified centers for the control of eating within the hypothalamus of the central nervous system (CNS). These centers—the feeding center for hunger and the satiety center for fullness—tell the body when it should begin consuming food and when food consumption should stop. It takes 20 minutes on average for these signals to go from the stomach to the brain to relay the message "stop eating." These centers are thought to continuously monitor a variety of factors regarding food intake including smell, taste, visual cues, glucose levels, amino acids, the degree of stomach distention, and information regarding basal metabolic rate, gastrointestinal hormone level, orexin A, and orexin B that influence hunger in rats.[27]

There are also hormonal factors that influence obesity. Obesity can be caused by a condition called **hypothyroidism,** in which the thyroid gland produces an insufficient amount of thyroxin, a hormone that regulates metabolism. Over five million Americans have this common medical condition and as many as 10% of women may have some degree of thyroid hormone deficiency. In such individuals, the underactive thyroid makes burning up food difficult and so weight gain is common. As we acquire greater understanding of the hormones and neurotransmitters that influence hunger and satiety, drugs designed to influence their actions will be developed. Some of these drugs already exist and will be described later in this chapter.

The effects of hormonal changes on eating can be seen each month just before a woman's menstrual cycle, as many women say that they crave salty and sugary foods during this time. Pregnancy brings about another host of hormonal and metabolic changes. During a normal pregnancy, a woman requires an extra 300 calories a day to support the developing fetus and supportive tissues, and to fuel her elevated maternal metabolic rate. In addition, typically pregnant women will develop approximately 9 extra pounds of adipose tissue which will be used as an energy source during lactation. The average woman is expected to gain between 25 to 35 pounds during pregnancy.[12] Many women express concern about their ability to lose this weight following the birth of the child, and some women do gain much more than the recommended amount of weight. However, the majority of women lose their pregnancy weight within 6 months to a year after having a baby. Nevertheless, obesity is one of the most frequent causes for complications in pregnancy. The mother is considered obese if at the beginning of her pregnancy her BMI is over 25. Women who are obese during pregnancy have a much higher risk of hypertension and gestational diabetes. Obesity has also been associated with infertility, poor pregnancy outcomes and miscarriage.[28]

Typically, breast-feeding can help women to burn more calories and return to their prepregnancy weight, although extra fat may linger, as nature intended this to be a store of energy for breast-feeding. Breast-feeding requires an additional 500 calories a day.[29] Mothers who breast-feed tend to lose more weight when their babies are 3 to 6 months old than formula-feeding mothers who consume fewer calories. One study of mothers at 1 month postpartum found that mothers who breast-fed had slimmer hips and weighed less than women whose babies received formula.[29] Infants who are breast-fed also have a lower chance of developing obesity and asthma in childhood and adolescence.[30, 31, 32]

Metabolic Factors

Traditional theory has suggested that the energy expenditure and energy storage centers of the body possess a genetically programmed awareness of the body's most physiologically desirable weight, called **set point.**[33] However, the term *set point* is somewhat misleading in that it does not refer to a certain number or point but a weight range that the body is genetically programmed to maintain. When the body falls below its natural set point, one's metabolism reacts by slowing down the body's functioning in order to conserve energy. In other words, the body

---

Key Terms

hypothyroidism a condition in which the thyroid gland produces an insufficient amount of the hormone thyroxin.

set point a genetically programmed range of body weight, beyond which a person finds it difficult to gain or lose additional weight.

will sense that it is not receiving enough calories to maintain healthy functioning and so it will send calories to essential areas of the body and use the energy as efficiently as possible. Alternatively, when someone consumes more calories than are needed, the body will begin to increase the rate of metabolism in an effort not to gain weight above the set point. The process of storing or burning more energy to maintain the body's "best" weight is called **adaptive thermogenesis.** This process also explains the reason that 90% of people who go on any diet gain all their weight back plus more within a year of going off the diet. When dieting, people reduce their caloric intake which in turn lowers their metabolism. When they discontinue the diet, they typically eat more calories and foods with higher fat content on a lowered metabolism. This is a good formula for weight gain. In addition, dieters tend to lose muscle and regain their weight as fat.

There is a great deal of debate on how an individual's set point can be altered. The number of fat cells in the body, the blood level of insulin, and regions of the brain such as the hypothalamus all seem to play a role in determining set point. Certain drugs such as amphetamines and other diet pills and herbal supplements can act on the brain to temporarily lower the set point. However, once these drugs are discontinued, the set point returns to the previous level or perhaps an even higher level and weight increases as a result. Healthier and more permanent methods of changing one's set point are through regular exercise and healthy eating patterns. In fact, a recent study of 8,000 successful dieters found that the majority of them used "my own diet and exercise regimen" and did not follow any formal weight reduction program.[34]

The body's requirement for energy to maintain basic physiological processes decreases progressively with age. This change reflects the loss of muscle tissue as both men and women age. This loss of muscle mass eventually alters the ratio of lean body tissue to fat. As the proportion of fat increases, the energy needs of the body are more strongly influenced by the lower metabolic needs of the fat cells.[35] This excess energy is then stored in the fat cells of the body. A gradual decrease in caloric intake and a conscious effort to expend more calories can effectively prevent this gradual increase in weight leading to obesity.

Social and Cultural Factors

There are also ethnic differences related to the incidence of obesity and cultural differences regarding what is seen as a healthy weight. African American, American Indian, and Hispanic American women have the highest risk of becoming overweight, according to the Centers for Disease Control. In fact, the results of a national study showed that more than half of all African American and Hispanic women in the United States are above what is considered a healthy body weight. The statistics are startling: 66% of African American women are overweight and 33% are obese. For Caucasian women, 49% are considered overweight and 24% obese. Only one minority group, Asian Americans, has a lower rate of obesity than the general population.

Obesity is second only to tobacco as the leading cause of premature deaths and disproportionately affects women of color and women of lower socioeconomic classes. On the positive side, African American women report less pressure to be thin than their white counterparts and tend to be less self-conscious about their weight.[36] Acculturation also has a significant impact on the rates of obesity—the more an ethnic group has adapted to and absorbed Western culture, the higher the rate of obesity within that group.[37]

Socioeconomic status is also an important influence on obesity, particularly in women. Upper socioeconomic women tend to be thinner than lower socioeconomic women, while among men there is not such a pattern.[38] Interestingly, higher obesity levels are also related to marriage, parenthood, and geographical location as married men, parents, and people living in rural areas tend to have a higher incidence of obesity.[39]

Environmental Factors

Certainly environmental factors such as the smell or sight of freshly made cookies, or an advertisement for a candy bar can affect your eating habits. Even the clock signaling it is "time to eat" can encourage us to eat even when we aren't hungry. While this may seem adaptive and helpful in regulating our food intake, Dr. Kelly D. Brownell, a professor of psychology at Yale and an expert on eating disorders, has gone so far as to label American society a "toxic environment" when it comes to food. Researchers contend that the local environment has a powerful effect on eating. Factors such as portion size, price, advertising, the availability of food, and the number of food choices presented all can influence the amount the average person consumes. For example, moviegoers will eat 50% more popcorn if given an extra-large tub of popcorn instead of a container one size smaller, even if the popcorn is stale. If a tabletop in the office is stocked with cookies and candy, co-workers tend to nibble their way through the workday, even if they are not hungry. One study showed that when

---

Key Terms

adaptive thermogenesis the physiological response of the body to adjust its metabolic rate to the presence of food.

Declaring War on Overweight

With the majority of adult Americans being overweight, some experts have declared war on the food industry and advocate treating obesity in a similar way to smoking. The food industry produces 3,800 calories a day for every adult and child in the United States, which far exceeds the recommended caloric requirements[1]. Not only are people consuming too many calories each day, but they are also overfeeding their pets. Studies show that at least 25 percent of dogs and cats in the Western world are obese and are at greater risk for developing obesity-related health problems such as diabetes and heart disease[2]. It has been suggested that strategies used to decrease cigarette smoking be used to encourage healthier and smaller food choices. For example, a "fat tax" (also called the "Twinkie tax") on junk food has been suggested to subsidize the price of healthier foods so they cost less. Others suggest putting warning labels on the nutritional packaging for junk food similar to the warning labels on cigarettes. Legislators have discussed requiring fast-food and other restaurants to post calories and fat content on their menus. Some individuals are fighting back using the court system. McDonald's, Wendy's, Burger King, and Kentucky Fried Chicken were taken to court by a 270-pound maintenance worker who held them responsible for his obesity-related health problems; the suit, however, was dismissed.

Some companies are responding to this outcry by changing their packaging, pricing, and options. For example, McDonald's plans to test a Happy Meal with an option of a piece of fresh fruit instead of the French fries that usually accompanies it. Kraft Foods, the nation's largest food company, plans to reduce the portion sizes, fat, and calories of many of its foods. Frito Lay has set a goal of eliminating all trans fatty acids from its chips and snacks.

Some speculate that there may be an increasing movement against the food industry, particularly against unhealthy foods, in regulating television commercials and advertising, and even perhaps prohibiting children from being able to buy junk food, again similarly to what has been done in the past 30 years with the tobacco industry.

[1] Nestle M. *Food Politics: How the Food Industry Influences Nutrition and Health.* Los Angeles, California: University of California Press, 2002.
[2] Fatter Cats and Dogs Are a Sizeable Problem. *USA Today,* September 9, 2003.

the candy was in plain sight on workers' desks, they ate an average of nine pieces each. Storing the candy in a desk drawer reduced consumption to six pieces, as compared to putting the candy a couple of yards from the desk, cutting the number to three pieces per person.[40] In response to these and other findings, many public schools have begun offering only healthy foods in their cafeterias, replacing soft drinks, candy, and chips with juice, milk, fruit, and granola bars.

Packaging and price can also influence the amount people consume, a concept of which advertisers, restaurants, and grocery stores are well aware. Dropping the price of the low-fat snacks by even a nickel resulted in dramatically increased sales. In contrast, stickers signaling low-fat content or cartoons promoting the low-fat alternatives had little influence over which snacks were more popular. This is not only true of food but also with beverages, as people tend to drink *more* from short, wide glasses than from thinner, taller ones, thinking they are drinking less.[40]

Having more choices also appears to make people eat more. In one study, people ate more when offered sandwiches with four different fillings than they did when they were given sandwiches with their single favorite filling. In another study, participants who were served a four-course meal with meat, fruit, bread, and a pudding, ate 60% more food than those served an equivalent meal of only their favorite course. Even the cup holders in automobiles have grown larger to make room for giant drinks. It is important to note that these findings were seen in people of all body sizes, not just with people who are overweight or obese as is often the misconception. However, there does seem to be a difference in the age of the individuals studied. One study found that 3-year-olds who were served three different portion sizes of macaroni and cheese for lunch on three different days ate the same amount each time. Five-year-olds, however, ate more when more was put in front of them.[40]

TALKING POINTS Do you think there should be more regulation of the food industry? If so, what recommendations would you make? What food would you include for regulation and how should this be determined?

Psychological Factors

Psychological factors related to overeating refer to the reasons people eat rather than due to physiological hunger. Individuals with eating disorders often report that they don't know when they are hungry and often eat when they are not hungry and don't eat when they have a biological reason for doing so. Why do people eat if not in response to hunger? Frequently people eat in response to their emotions such as eating to comfort themselves, when bored, tired, stressed, or depressed. Some people say they use food as a way of coping with hurt, sadness, and anger, suppressing their feelings and putting food on top of them. Others eat out of habit, and associate food with certain activities such as eating popcorn at a movie, eating chips in front of the television, or having dessert after dinner. There are certainly many associations with chocolate when feeling down as a way of cheering yourself up. Food is also part of celebrations, holidays, family bonding, and a mainstay of socialization. It is difficult to think about social activities we engage in that don't involve food in some way.

Many people develop relationships with food that substitute for real human relationships. Comments like "Food is my best friend" or "A great meal is better than sex" are indicative to the degree to which many people rely on food to fill their needs. As we'll learn in our discussion of eating disorders later in the chapter, psychological issues with food can become serious, even life-threatening problems.

Dietary Practices

Many researchers believe that the number of fat cells a person has will be initially determined during the first 2 years of life. Babies who are overfed will develop a greater number of fat cells than babies who receive a balanced diet of appropriate, infant-sized portions. Overfed babies, especially those with a family history of obesity, will tend to develop **hypercellular obesity.** When these children reach adulthood, they will have more fat cells. An increase in fat cells during infancy and childhood can increase the chances of developing obesity. This increase can result in five times as many fat cells in obese people as in people of normal weight. Dieting only reduces the size of fat cells, not the number of fat cells. People who have hypercellular obesity have an abnormally high number of fat cells and are biologically limited in their ability to lose weight.[41]

Hypercellular obesity in adulthood can also result from excessive weight gain in late childhood and adolescence. If an individual's weight is 75% above the desirable weight, this can stimulate an increase in the number of fat cells, resulting in eventual obesity.

Hypertrophic obesity is the result of a pattern of overeating for a long period of time. Over a period of years, the existing fat cells increase in size to accommodate excess fat intake. It is important to note that after puberty, as your body stores more fat, the number of fat cells remains the same but each fat cell can get bigger. Hypertrophic obesity is generally associated with excessive fat around the waist and is thought to contribute to conditions such as type 2 diabetes, high levels of fat in the blood, high blood pressure, and heart disease. Hypertrophic obesity generally appears during middle age when physical activity tends to decline while caloric intake remains the same.[41]

The information, values, traditions, and messages you receive from your family also have a significant impact on your dietary habits. If an infant's cries for food are immediately responded to, that child will be more likely to learn what the sensation of hunger is and the appropriate response. If crying unrelated to hunger is responded to by offering a cookie or candy, that child will learn to soothe himself or herself with food. Studies show that children become confused about what hunger is and how to satisfy it if their hunger needs are neglected or overindulged in infancy.[42]

Some of the first power struggles between parents and their children revolve around issues of food. A child who has little power in her life can exert power and control through her refusal to eat certain foods and demanding other foods and when she wants to eat. Parents who use food as a reward for good behavior: "If you get an "A" on your test, I will treat you to ice cream," as punishment: "You weren't behaving so you can't have dessert," or as a guilt trip: "Don't waste food. Clean your plate. Children are starving in the world," may inadvertently be creating negative dietary practices that will continue on throughout the child's life. Interestingly, research has shown that children are extraordinarily adept at meeting their nutritional needs when left to their own devices. One study allowed children to eat whatever they wanted for a week. Did they always pick high-fat, high-sugar foods? No. Actually, when we look at each day's intake, they didn't eat a balanced diet. However, when one takes the full week into consideration, they met their nutritional needs perfectly.

Not only does what your parents say to you have a tremendous influence on your eating behavior, but what they do themselves, their own eating practices, can have even a greater impact. Children are exposed to different foods and model what their parents eat. If a parent makes comments such as "I shouldn't eat that because I will get fat" or doesn't eat fruits or vegetables, or sits down with a bag of chips in front of the television every night, the child will probably do the same. In the same vein, when parents exercise regularly, eat a balanced diet, and make positive comments about their weight, children tend to mimic this behavior.

Inactivity

When weight management experts are asked to identify the single most important reason that obesity is so high in today's society, they are most certain to point to inactivity. People of all ages tend to be less active and burn fewer calories than did their ancestors only a few generations ago (see Star box on page 193). Both adults and children

---

Key Terms
hypercellular obesity a form of obesity that results from having an abnormally high number of fat cells.
hypertrophic obesity a form of obesity in which there are a normal number of fat cells, but the individual fat cells are enlarged.

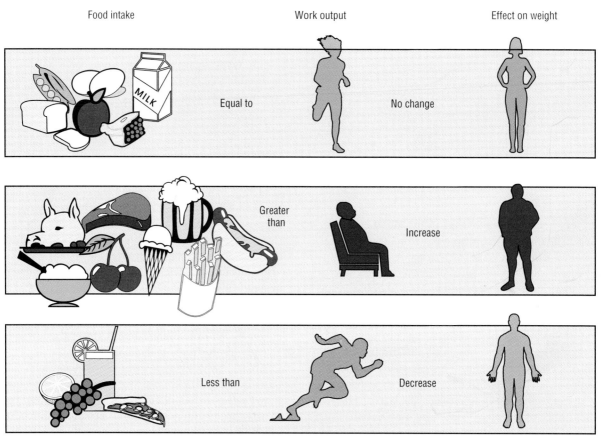

Food intake | Work output | Effect on weight

Equal to — No change

Greater than — Increase

Less than — Decrease

Figure 6-2 Caloric balance: energy input equals energy output, some of which comes from physical activity.

spend less time devoted to exercise as a result of longer work hours at sedentary jobs, a decline in physical education programs in school, and increased participation in sedentary recreational activities, such as browsing the Internet, playing video games, and watching television. In addition, many of the laborsaving devices and increased automation in the home and workplace have contributed to increased inactivity. According to some studies, nearly two-thirds of Americans are not physically active on a regular basis and 25% are completely sedentary.[44] It is not surprising that as inactivity becomes the norm, so does overweight.

 TALKING POINTS What were the messages you received in childhood regarding food? What positive and negative eating habits have you learned from your family?

Caloric Balance

As previously mentioned, any calories consumed beyond those that are used by the body are converted to fat stores. People gain weight when their energy input exceeds their energy output. Consuming about 3,500 calories more than is needed results in a weight gain of one pound of fat.[43] Conversely, they lose weight when their energy output exceeds their energy input (Figure 6-2). The basic formula is quite simple and can be analogous to a seesaw. Weight remains constant when caloric input and caloric output are equal. In such a situation, our bodies are said to be in *caloric balance.*

Energy Needs of the Body

What are our energy needs? How many calories should we consume (or expend) to achieve a healthy weight? There is no single answer for everyone. That said, however, the most recent Recommended Daily Allowances (RDA) envision that the average 19- to 24-year-old male requires 2900 calories to maintain weight, while females of the same age require 2200 calories.[44] Any one individual within this age group will need fewer or more than the RDA recommendation, depending on three factors: (1) the person's basal metabolism, (2) the person's activity requirements, and (3) the thermic effect of food. Of these factors, basal metabolism is the most important determinant of the total calories required by an individual.

Basal Metabolic Rate

Basal Metabolic Rate (BMR) is a measure of resting energy expenditure that is taken upon awakening, 10–12 hours after eating, or 12–18 hours after significant physical activity. A closely related construct, resting metabolic rate (RMR), is often used interchangeably with BMR. In comparison with the BMR, the RMR is measured at rest, without the stringent controls on physical activity required as with measuring BMR. RMR measures the calories needed for functioning such as blood circulation, respiration, brain activity, muscle function, body temperature, and heart beat.[45]

Basal metabolism changes as people age. For both males and females, the BMR is relatively high at birth and continues to increase until the age of two. Except for a slight rise at puberty, the BMR will gradually decline throughout the remainder of life. A variety of other variables also affect BMR, including body composition (muscular bodies are associated with higher BMRs), physical condition (fit people have higher BMRs), sex (males have 5% higher BMRs), hormone secretions (people with excessively active thyroid and adrenal glands have higher BMRs), sleep (BMRs are about 10% lower during sleep), pregnancy (a 20% increase in BMR is typical, especially in the last trimester), body temperature (a 1° rise in body temperature increases BMR about 7%), and environmental temperature (deviations above and below 78° F result in increased BMRs).[46]

The most important variables related to BMR are: age, body composition, activity level, and caloric intake. For example, if people fail to recognize that BMR declines with aging, they might fail to adjust food intake accordingly and weight gain will occur. Also, for those who are thinner, the presence of lean tissue favors a higher basal metabolic rate with greater resistance to weight gain. Finally, an increase in physical activity will foster a faster BMR that will contribute to weight loss. In contrast, in those people with above-average levels of body fat, BMR rates are lower, thus providing the body with excess calories that will be stored as fat. Use the formula in the Star box on this page to determine your BMR and the approximate number of calories you require.

Activity Requirements

Each person's caloric *activity requirements* vary directly according to the amount of daily physical work completed. For example, sedentary office workers will require a smaller daily caloric intake than will construction workers, letter carriers, or farm workers. Even within a given general job type, the amount of caloric expenditure will vary according to the physical effort required. A police officer who walks a neighborhood beat will usually expend many more calories than the typical police dispatcher, equestrian or motorcycle officer.

Calculating Basal Metabolic Rate

The basal metabolic rate (BMR) reflects the amount of energy in calories (C) that your body requires to sustain basic functions. The formula below can be used to calculate your approximate basal metabolic rate.

$$\text{BMR per day} = 1C \times \frac{\text{body weight (lb)}}{2.2} \times 24$$

Example: 150-lb person

$$\text{BMR per day} = 1\,C \times \frac{150}{2.2} \times 24$$
$$= 1\,C \times 6.82 \times 24$$
$$= 1636.8\,C$$

This person would need approximately 1,637 calories to sustain the body at rest for an entire day. Activity of any kind, of course, elevates the requirement for calories.

_____

Note: A woman's BMR would be approximately 5% lower than that of a man of the same age.

Physical activity that occurs outside the occupational setting also adds to caloric needs. Sedentary office workers may be quite active in their recreational pursuits, or active employees may spend their off-hours lounging in front of the television. You must closely examine the total amount of work or activity you perform to accurately estimate your caloric requirements. Physical activity uses between 20% and 40% of caloric intake. See Table 6.6 on page 192 for a breakdown of caloric expenditures for various activities.

Thermic Effect of Food

Thermic effect of food (TEF) refers to the amount of energy our bodies require for the digestion, absorption, and transportation of food. This energy breaks down the bonds that hold complex food molecules together, resulting in smaller nutritional units that can be distributed throughout the body. The amount of TEF burned

See Table 6.6 on page 192

> **Key Terms**
>
> **basal metabolic rate (BMR)** the amount of energy, expressed in calories, that the body requires to maintain basic functions.
>
> **thermic effect of food (TEF)** the amount of energy our bodies require for the digestion, absorption, and transportation of food.

Table 6.6 Calories Expended during Physical Activity

To determine the number of calories you have spent in an hour of activity, simply multiply the *calories per hour per pound* column by your weight (in pounds). For example, after an hour of archery, a 120-pound person will have expended 209 calories; a 160-pound person, 278 calories; and a 220-pound person, 383 calories.

Activity	Calories/Hour/Pound	Activity	Calories/Hour/Pound
Archery	1.74	Marching (rapid)	3.84
Baseball	1.86	Painting (outside)	2.10
Basketball	3.78	Playing music (sitting)	1.08
Boxing (sparring)	3.78	Racquetball	3.90
Canoeing (leisure)	1.20	Running (cross-country)	4.44
Cleaning	1.62	Running	
Climbing hills (no load)	3.30	11 min 30 sec per mile	3.66
Cooking	1.20	9 min per mile	5.28
Cycling		8 min per mile	5.64
5.5 mph	1.74	7 min per mile	6.24
9.4 mph	2.70	6 min per mile	6.84
Racing	4.62	5 min 30 sec per mile	7.86
Dance (modern)	2.28	Scrubbing floors	3.00
Eating (sitting)	0.60	Sailing	1.20
Field hockey	3.66	Skiing	
Fishing	1.68	Cross-country	4.43
Football	3.60	Snow, downhill	3.84
Gardening		Water	3.12
Digging	3.42	Skating (moderate)	2.28
Mowing	3.06	Soccer	3.54
Raking	1.44	Squash	5.76
Golf	2.34	Swimming	
Gymnastics	1.80	Backstroke	4.62
Handball	3.78	Breaststroke	4.44
Hiking	2.52	Free, fast	4.26
Horseback riding		Free, slow	3.48
Galloping	3.72	Butterfly	4.68
Trotting	3.00	Table tennis	1.86
Walking	1.14	Tennis	3.00
Ice hockey	5.70	Volleyball	1.32
Jogging	4.15	Walking (normal pace)	2.16
Judo	5.34	Weight training	1.90
Knitting (sewing)	0.60	Wrestling	5.10
Lacrosse	5.70	Writing (sitting)	0.78

varies for different types of food, with some food such as fat requiring less energy to convert to energy stores and others such as protein and carbohydrates requiring more. The TEF peaks in about 1 hour after eating and accounts for approximately 10% of total energy expenditure.[46]

Weight Management Techniques

Weight loss occurs when the calories consumed are less than the energy the body needs for physiological maintenance and activity. This may sound overly simplified and certainly the $50 billion-a-year weight loss industry would like us to think it is much more complicated than this.

Weight loss followed by weight gain may be less healthy and certainly more frustrating than maintaining body weight, even at weight above the desirable levels. When a diet or weight loss strategy fails, the person, not the diet, is blamed. This causes people to jump to another weight loss method and then another, and a vicious cycle has begun. However, a commitment to a lifestyle change of eating in healthy ways and engaging in regular exercise seems to be the most effective strategy for weight loss and weight maintenance. It is also important to set a goal to

American children expend significantly less energy on a daily basis than their parents and grandparents did at equivalent ages. This "couch potatoing" of today's children can be explained by several factors, including video games that involve endless hours of inactivity at home in front of a television or computer screen or in hand-held units that can be easily carried along on the ride to school. Schools have also contributed to children's decreased activity by reducing or eliminating once-required physical education classes. In some cases, elementary schools have further reduced opportunities for physical play by eliminating recess, either to increase instructional time or because of concerns over potential liability associated with inadequate supervision on the playground or maintenance of play equipment.

Adults often find that their job demands ten to fifteen more hours per week than the once-standard 40-hour work week. For them, the end of the workday signals a time for relaxation and emotional recovery rather than an opportunity to engage in planned physical activity that would improve their health. Additionally, the concept of "work" as it relates to employment, is often confused with the concept of "work" as it applies to planned physical activity. As a result, many American adults convince themselves that they do not need to take non-employment time for physical fitness because they "work hard" at their jobs. For some, this is an accurate assessment, but for the vast majority of Americans employment does not involve great physical demands.

For older adults, the situation is more complex. When fragility, chronic illnesses, unawareness of the value of physical activity, lack of social support, and limited access to facilities are in play, many older adults find their activity level limited to activities of daily living. The consequences of this situation are only now being recognized as a growing body of research shows that even limited increases in planned physical activity for older adults can make a significant contribution to overall health and continued independence and self-sufficiency.

Another group of Americans whose lives could be enhanced by increased physical activity is the disabled. For these individuals, access to necessary expertise and specialized equipment and facilities is often restricted in terms of availability or financial resources. On college campuses today, however, the situation is much better than it was a decade or two ago, and opportunities for individuals with disabilities to take part in planned physical activity are greater than those available outside the campus environment.

---

lose not more than 2 pounds a week because the body tends to lose muscle rather than fat if the weight loss occurs too rapidly. Many people also complain of "hanging skin" after a rapid, drastic weight loss, which can then require cosmetic surgery to rectify.

A number of approaches to weight loss can be pursued. How do dieters know when they have succeeded? Figure 6-3 shows how Americans measure their progress at losing weight.

Dietary Alterations

A diet that reduces caloric intake is the most common approach to what seems to be a national obsession with weight loss. The choice of foods included in the diet and the amount of food that can be consumed are the two factors that distinguish the wide range of diets currently available. Unfortunately, dieting alone usually does not result in long-term weight loss. Effective and lasting weight

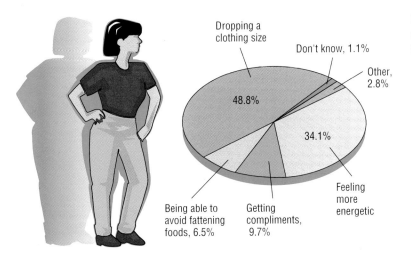

Figure 6-3 How do Americans measure success when it comes to losing weight? Most say dropping a clothing size is the best indicator that their diet is working.

pages 215–217 takes a look at the "portion distortion" so prevalent in America. It also suggests ways you can control serving sizes.

TALKING POINTS Have you ever tried to lose weight? What methods were effective for you? What is the longest time you have stuck to a particular weight management strategy?

A balanced diet-portion control approach to weight loss reflects a nutritionally sound program that offers some probability of success without the negative feature of forcing people to adapt to a restrictive approach to eating. People have extreme difficulty adjusting to a diet that presents them with uncommon foods. To people who need to lose weight, dieting is often bad enough without

loss requires a lifestyle change, not just going on a diet for a specific time period only to return to your old patterns of eating. This is the problem many people face, as they go on strict diets and overly restrict their calories. Because the diet is so restrictive and demanding, it is impossible to continue to follow it for very long and so people return to their previous eating patterns. In addition, people tend to overeat the foods they denied themselves while dieting because they feel deprived and the forbidden food seems even more alluring. This can also lead to binge eating. Thus diets tend not to work in the long run. The Changing for the Better box on this page provides suggestions for changing your eating patterns to increase your chances for long-term success (see also the Learning from Our Diversity box on page 200).

Balanced Diets Supported by Portion Control

For nutritional health, a logical approach to weight loss and subsequent management of that loss is to establish a nutritionally sound balanced diet (low fat, low saturated fat, and high complex carbohydrate) that controls portions. This approach is best undertaken with nutritionists and physicians who are knowledgeable in diet management. After a study of your day-to-day energy needs, they can establish a diet designed to produce a gradual loss. Diet scales or food models can assist in gaining an understanding of portion sizes. However, a simple way of measuring one serving size is to think of a serving as equal to the size of the palm of your hand or your fist. This is not to say that this is all you need to eat for a meal, as the food pyramid recommends that we eat six to eleven servings of grains, three to five servings of vegetables, two to four servings of fruit, two to three servings of milk, and two to three servings of meat each day. The Focus On article on

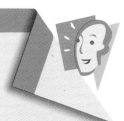

Changing for the Better

Tips for Losing Weight Successfully

I've tried all kinds of diets, and nothing seems to work for me. I've got to lose weight, but I can't face another failure. What should I do?

- Keep a log of the times, settings, reasons, and feelings associated with your eating.
- Set realistic long-term goals (for example, loss of 2 pounds per week instead of 5 pounds per week).
- Don't completely deprive yourself of enjoyable foods (occasionally reward yourself with a small treat).
- Realize that the sacrifices you're making are important for your health and happiness.
- Eat slowly. It takes about 20 minutes for your brain to recognize satiety signals from your body.
- Put more physical activity into your daily routine (take stairs instead of elevators or park in the distant part of a parking lot, for example).
- Reward yourself when you reach your goals (with new clothes, sporting equipment, a vacation trip).
- Share your commitment to weight loss with your family and friends so that they can support your efforts.
- Keep careful records of your daily food consumption and weekly weight change.
- Be prepared to deal with occasional plateaus and setbacks in your quest for weight loss.
- Remember that low-fat, low-saturated fat, and high-complex carbohydrate meals in combination with regular physical activity are the basis for these strategies.
- See this as a lifestyle change, not a diet. This is a lifelong commitment you are making in terms of your dietary patterns and activity level.

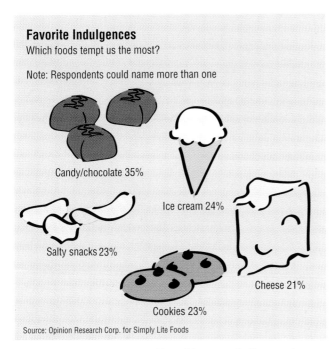

Favorite Indulgences
Which foods tempt us the most?

Note: Respondents could name more than one

Candy/chocolate 35%

Ice cream 24%

Salty snacks 23%

Cheese 21%

Cookies 23%

Source: Opinion Research Corp. for Simply Lite Foods

Figure 6-4 Late night kitchen raids and too many daytime snacks can compromise a healthy diet. Which foods are the most difficult for you to resist?

feeling that they must be deprived of foods that satisfy their emotional needs. Figure 6-4 depicts favorite foods that are the biggest hazards to a healthy diet.

Fad Diets

People use a variety of fad diets in an attempt to achieve rapid weight loss. Currently there are over 150 popular diets, often promoted by celebrities or people who claim to be nutrition experts. With few exceptions, these approaches are both ineffective and potentially dangerous. In addition, some require far greater expense than would be associated with weight loss or management techniques using portion control and regular physical activity. The pros and cons of a variety of popular diet plans are presented in Table 6.7 on page 196.

Currently, the most popular of the faddish diets are those that reduce carbohydrate intake to an extremely low level, while permitting an almost unlimited consumption of animal protein (meat), with its accompanying high fat content. As indicated in Table 6.7 on page 196, these diets, such as *Dr. Atkins' New Diet Revolution*, *Mastering the Zone*, and *Sugar Busters*, involve potential problems, particularly if followed for long periods.

The restriction of calories is the basis of all diets. Some suggest limiting the consumption of fat, others sugar, or the caloric intake is dangerously low for all food groups. Many diet plans, such as the Atkins' Diet, advocate the re-

striction of carbohydrates which can cause ketosis. When the carbohydrate calories are limited, intake of fat usually increases. This high fat diet can cause an increase in blood ketones from fat breakdown and too few carbohydrates. Ketosis can cause the blood to become too acidic and dehydration can occur. The body requires a minimum of 50–100 grams of carbohydrate per day to avoid ketosis.[46] Low-carbohydrate diets are characterized by initial rapid weight loss which is appealing to most people, but this loss is primarily due to water and not fat loss. Complications associated with low-carbohydrate, high-protein diets include dehydration, electrolyte loss, calcium depletion, weakness due to inadequate dietary carbohydrate, nausea due to ketosis, vitamin and mineral deficiencies, and possible kidney problems. Gout is another potential side effect since the uric acid increases in the blood and competes with ketones for excretion. This higher blood acid level can also increase the risk of kidney failure. The risk of coronary heart disease may be higher in those who stay on the diet a long time, due to the increased consumption of foods high in saturated fat and cholesterol.

Low-Calorie Foods and Controlled Serving Sizes

Recently a variety of familiar foods have been developed in a reduced-calorie form. By lowering the carbohydrate content with the use of nonnutritive sweeteners, reducing the portion size, reducing the fat content of the original formulations, or removing fat entirely (see the discussion of Olestra in Chapter 5), manufacturers have produced "lite" versions of many food products. For example, many frozen entrees, such as Healthy Choice Oriental Beef with Vegetables (290 calories), Weight Watchers Lasagna Florentine (210 calories), and Healthy Choice Fettucine with Turkey and Vegetables (350 calories), are attractively low in calories. Because fat helps us to feel satiated or not hungry, these low fat, low-calorie meals tend not to satisfy our hunger for very long and people may find themselves wanting to snack or binge by late afternoon.

 TALKING POINTS Your best friend is trying to follow a low-fat, low-calorie diet in order to lose weight, but is finding herself constantly hungry. What can you tell her about the diet plan she's chosen? What changes might she make to increase her chances of success?

Controlled Fasting

In cases of extreme obesity, some patients are placed on a complete fast in a hospital setting. The patient consumes only water, electrolytes, and vitamins. Weight loss is substantial because the body is quickly forced to begin

Table 6.7 Advantages and Disadvantages of Selected Diets

Type of Diet	Advantages	Disadvantages	Examples
Limited food choice diets	Reduce the number of food choices made by the users Limited opportunity to make mistakes Almost certainly low in calories after the first few days	Deficient in many nutrients, depending on the foods allowed Monotonous—difficult to adhere to Eating out and eating socially are difficult Do not retrain dieters in acceptable eating habits Low long-term success rates No scientific basis for these diets	Banana and milk diet Fitonics for Life diet Kempner rice diet The New Beverly Hills Diet Fit for Life Sommersizing
Restricted-calorie, balanced food plans	Sufficiently low in calories to permit steady weight loss Nutritionally balanced Palatable Include readily available foods Reasonable in cost Can be adapted from family meals Permit eating out and social eating Promote a new set of eating habits May employ a point system	Do not appeal to people who want a "unique diet" Do not produce immediate and large weight losses	Weight Watchers Diet Prudent Diet (American Heart Association) Eating Thin for Life Take Off Pounds Sensibly (TOPS) Overeaters Anonymous Jenny Craig
Fasting starvation diet	Rapid initial loss	Nutrient deficient Danger of ketosis $>$60% loss is muscle $<$40% loss is fat Low long-term success rate	ZIP Diet 5-Day Miracle Diet Hollywood Diet
High-carbohydrate diet	Emphasizes grains, fruits, and vegetables High in bulk Low in cholesterol	Limits milk, meat Nutritionally very inadequate for calcium, iron, and protein	Quick Weight Loss Diet Pritikin Diet Hilton Head Metabolism Diet
High-protein, low-carbohydrate diets	Rapid initial weight loss because of diuretic effect Very little hunger Usually include all the meat, fish, poultry, and eggs you can eat Occasionally permit milk and cheese in limited amounts Prohibit fruits, vegetables, and any bread or cereal products	Too low in carbohydrates Deficient in many nutrients— vitamin C, vitamin A (unless eggs are included), calcium, and several trace elements High in saturated fat, cholesterol, and total fat Extreme diets of this type could cause death Impossible to adhere to these diets long enough to lose any appreciable amount of weight Dangerous for people with kidney disease Weight lost, which is largely water, is rapidly regained Expensive Unpalatable after first few days Difficult for dieter to eat out Unattractive side effects (e.g., bad breath) May require potassium and calcium supplements	Dr. Stillman's Quick Weight Loss Diet Calories Don't Count by Dr. Taller Dr. Atkins' New Diet Revolution Scarsdale Diet Air Force Diet The Carbohydrate Addict's Life Span Program Mastering the Zone Diet The Carbohydrate Addict's Diet Sugar Busters Protein Power Get Skinny on Fabulous Food (with modifications) South Beach Diet

continued

Table 6.7 **Advantages and Disadvantages of Selected Diets**—*continued*

Type of Diet	Advantages	Disadvantages	Examples
Low-calorie, high-protein supplement diets	Usually a premeasured powder to be reconstituted with water or a prepared liquid formula Rapid initial weight loss Easy to prepare—already measured Palatable for first few days Usually fortified to provide recommended amount of micronutrients Must be labeled if >50% protein	Usually prescribed at dangerously low calorie intake of 300 to 500 cal Overpriced Low in fiber and bulk—constipating in short amount of time	Metracal Diet Cambridge Diet Liquid Protein Diet Last Chance Diet Oxford Diet Genesis New Direction
High-fiber, low-calorie diets	High satiety value Provide bulk	Irritating to the lower colon Decreases absorption of trace elements, especially iron Nutritionally deficient Low in protein	Pritikin Diet F Diet Zen Macrobiotic Diet
Protein-sparing modified fast <50% protein: 400 cal	Safe under supervision High-quality protein Minimize loss of lean body mass	Decreases BMR Monotonous Expensive	Optifast Medifast
Premeasured food plans	Provide prescribed portion sizes—little chance of too small or too large a portion Total food programs Some provide adequate calories (1200) Nutritionally balanced or supplemented	Expensive Do not retrain dieters in acceptable eating habits Preclude eating out or social eating Often low in bulk Monotonous Low long-term success rates	Nutri-System Carnation Plan

catabolizing its fat and muscle tissue. Complete fasting is such an extreme approach to weight loss that it must be done in an institutional setting so that the patient can be closely monitored. Sodium loss, a negative nitrogen balance, and potassium loss are particular concerns.

Today some people regularly practice short periods of modified fasting. Solid foods are removed from the diet for a number of days. Fruit juices, water, supplements, and vitamins are used to minimize the risks associated with total fasting. However, unsupervised short-term fasting can be dangerous and is not generally recommended.

In addition to the controlled fasting just discussed, a somewhat different version of this practice is appearing with the long-term use of readily available, low-calorie, nutrient-dense food supplementation products such as Ensure, Boost, SlimFast, and Sustical. Regardless of whether they are marketed as nutrient-dense supplements for older adults or as adjuncts to weight loss diets, these drinks should not be viewed, or used, as meal replacements. Because these products contain no more than

400 calories (and the lite versions contain as few as 200 calories), their routine use as meal replacements could move even a young, healthy adult dangerously close to caloric inadequacy in a short time. Perhaps if used in place of a high-calorie snack or as a very occasional substitute for lunch, these supplements may not present the dangers that their routine use does.

Weight Reduction Programs

In virtually every area of the country, at least one version of the popular weight reduction programs, such as TOPS

Key Terms

catabolizing the metabolic process of breaking down tissue for the purpose of converting it to energy.

(Take Off Pounds Sensibly), Jenny Craig, and Nutri-System Weight Loss Centers, can be found. Pioneered by Weight Watchers, these programs generally feature a format consisting of (1) a well-balanced diet emphasizing portion control and low-fat, low–saturated fat, and high–complex carbohydrate foods, (2) specific weight loss goals to be attained over a set period of time, (3) encouragement from supportive leaders and fellow group members, (4) emphasis on regular physical activity, and (5) a maintenance program (follow-up program). The Changing for the Better box on this page presents some guidelines for choosing a weight loss program.

Although in theory these programs offer an opportunity to lose weight for people who cannot or will not participate in a physical activity program, their effectiveness is very limited. The minimal success of these programs and the difficulty that working adults have in attending meetings has resulted in falling enrollment and the development of home-based programs, such as those developed by hospital-based wellness programs, many YMCAs and YWCAs, and even Weight Watchers. Further, these programs can be costly, especially when the program markets its own food products, when compared with self-directed approaches.

The Weight Loss Industry

In response to our nation's near obsession with thinness, a thriving weight loss industry exists to assist us in our attempts to lose weight. Americans are spending in excess of $50 billion each year in an attempt to achieve and maintain weight loss (see Table 6.8).

The weight loss industry has capitalized and profited on the meaning that thinness has in the American culture, including a bias against large people. These programs are not just promising weight loss, but happiness and success in life as well. Thinness is not only associated with beauty, but also with one's ability to have successful relationships, careers, and self-worth. A recent study was conducted asking 32,000 women if they could have a successful career, a

Changing for the Better

Choosing a Diet Plan

I've been trying to find a good diet plan, but I'm confused by all the promotional materials. How can I recognize a sensible approach to weight loss?

- Make sure the program incorporates a balanced diet, an exercise program, and behavior modification.
- Beware of inflexible plans, such as those that require you to eat certain foods on certain days.
- Avoid plans that allow fewer than 1200 calories a day, which is the minimum needed to get essential nutrients.
- Make sure the recommended rate of weight loss does not exceed 2 pounds per week.
- Avoid programs that promote vitamins, pills, shots, gimmicks, gadgets, or brand-name diet foods.
- Look for a statement of approval by a reputable nutrition expert or institution.
- Beware of diets that promise fast, easy, or effortless weight loss or "a new secret formula."
- Choose a plan that teaches you how to keep the weight off once you've lost it.

InfoLinks
www.shapeup.org

satisfying romantic relationship, or lose 10–15 pounds, what would they choose. The majority of these women chose to lose weight, believing that they would also have a successful career and relationship if they lost 10–15 pounds.[7] Another study showed that the winner of the Miss America Pageant, 5 years consecutively, was always the thinnest contestant, looking at height proportional to weight. Another study showed children pictures of a minority child, a disabled child, and an overweight child and asked them to choose who they would like to be their friend. Overwhelmingly, the overweight child was their last choice. The American Association of University Women conducted a study to examine the changing attitudes children and adolescents have of themselves in terms of their body image. While 60% of elementary school girls said, "I am always happy with the way I am," only 29% of high school girls said the same thing. For boys, 67% of elementary school boys liked how they looked and 46% of high school boys continued to feel this way. It is these messages that play into the measures to which individuals will go and the price they will pay to achieve the cultural ideal.

The financial success of the weight loss industry in this country has in part been due to its effective television advertising. Skillfully produced commercials featuring successful program members suggest likely success for the

Table 6.8 The Real Cost of Dieting

Plan	Annual Cost
Weight Watchers	$709
Over the counter diet pills	$500
Nutritional counseling	$450–$1200
Physician supervised weight loss program	$2,000–$3,5000
Prescription diet pills	$1,090–$1,343
Gastric bypass surgery	$20,000–$25,000

Source: Chatzky JS. The real costs of diets, *USA Weekend*, December 2002.

viewer willing to sign on. Before 1994, these commercials were regular fare on daytime television. Today, however, commercials for diet programs such as Jenny Craig, Nutri-System, Weight Watchers, and others are considerably more restrained in their messages about success. Under directives issued by the Federal Trade Commission (FTC), today's advertisements cannot misrepresent program performance. They must disclose that most weight loss is temporary, and they now inform the viewer that their loss will most likely not approximate that of the successful subjects featured in their commercials.

Most recently some nationally franchised weight loss programs have added a "medical" component to their format that involves prescribing medications. Consumers should inquire the extent to which their medical supervision will be a regular component of the program rather than a brief, one-time physician visit involving little more than basic screening.

Physical Intervention

A second approach to weight loss involves techniques and products designed to change basic eating patterns.

Hunger- and Satiety-Influencing Products

Many overweight people want to lessen their desire to eat or develop a stronger sense of when they have eaten enough. Today, many dieters are confused about the safety of pharmaceutical approaches to weight loss, including both over-the-counter (OTC) and prescription drugs.

Some OTC appetite suppressants containing **phenylpropanolamine (PPA)** may still be sold in drugstores and supermarkets. PPA can also be found in OTC and prescription cough and cold medications. The FDA recommends that consumers not use any products with PPA due to its association with higher risk for stroke.

The FDA also continues to advise against using OTC weight loss products containing the recently banned ephedrine (*ma huang* and Chinese ephedra) (see the Considering Complementary Care box on page 201).

In 1994 Congress passed the Dietary Supplement and Education Act (DSHEA) which regulated herbal agents to the category of "dietary supplements." Thus the FDA can't regulate these products to ensure that they meet certain standards or are safe and effective. Many people see these supplements as safe because they are "natural," and yet they can be more dangerous and deadly than prescription medications because they are not inspected as to the purity and accuracy of the contents or the potency of the ingredients. A recent review showed that the use of herbal supplements increased by 370% between 1990 and 1997. Ephedrine, found in most herbal diet pills, has been linked to heart attacks, strokes, hepatitis, headache, tremors, anxiety, extreme irritability, and insomnia in consumers of all

ages. Metabolife, an herbal diet supplement that contains ephedra which was recently banned by the FDA, has sold 50 million bottles in the last 5 years, about 101,000 pills an hour. In 2003 the death of 23-year-old Baltimore Orioles pitcher Steve Bechler was linked to an ephedra supplement, prompting the FDA to reexamine the supplement. Ephedra was banned by the FDA in late 2003 (see the Considering Complementary Care box on page 201).[47]

Another herb, Aristolochia fangchi, was used as a weight loss supplement until many people developed kidney damage or complete renal failure, as well as precancerous and cancerous lesions in the kidneys. There is also a danger in the potential interactions between prescription medications and herbal agents that people can be unaware of and physicians may overlook because 60 percent of patients do not disclose the use of herbal medicines to their physicians. Research shows that the average person taking a combination of ephedra and caffeine lost 8.8 pounds over 6 months compared to 1.8 pounds among those who took a placebo pill. This translates into one-third of a pound a week that the ephedra subjects lost over the control group, roughly the same a person might lose cutting out 146 calories a day.[48]

Some prescription medications have also been shown to produce serious side effects. Two such medications, *phentermine* and *fenfluramine*, have been prescribed for patients who wanted to lose weight. Both drugs affect levels of serotonin, the neurotransmitter associated with satiety. This popular combination, referred to as *phenfen*, gradually raised concern among health experts because of the side effects it produced in people with angina, glaucoma, and high blood pressure. In addition, reports began to surface that some patients had developed a rare but lethal condition called *pulmonary hypertension*.

During the mid-1990s, a new serotonin-specific weight loss drug, *dexfenfluramine* (Redux), was approved for use in the United States. Results among patients who used the drug, in combination with dietary modification and exercise, seemed impressive during the initial months of its widespread use. However, some patients began to take dexfenfluramine with fenfluramine in an attempt to find a new combination that would be even more effective than phen-fen or Redux used alone, and death resulted in some cases.

Thus, two combinations of three serotonin-specific drugs were in vogue in early 1997. However, by May of

---

Key Terms

phenylpropanolamine (PPA) (fen ill pro pan **ol** ah meen) the active chemical compound still found in some over-the-counter diet products.

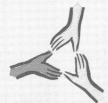

Learning from Our Diversity

Pyramid Power—Mediterranean Style

In Chapter 5 we explored the components of the USDA Food Guide Pyramid, which is designed to help Americans make healthful food choices in appropriate quantities. As you'll recall, we're encouraged to enjoy relatively more servings of bread, cereal, rice, pasta, fruits, and vegetables (located on the first and second levels of the pyramid), while eating fewer servings of meat and dairy products and restricting our intake of fats, oils, and sweets (which occupy the narrower top levels of the pyramid).

Did you know there's another food pyramid that points the way to nutritious food selections that are essential to successful weight control? It's called the Mediterranean Pyramid, and some nutritionists believe it offers the best diet for good health (see the illustration below). Like the USDA Food Guide Pyramid, the Mediterranean Pyramid emphasizes a diet based on grains, fruits, and vegetables. The Mediterranean Pyramid recommends eating red meat just a few times a month and allows generous amounts of olive oil. The USDA Pyramid likewise calls for limited consumption of lean red meat, but it urges sparing consumption of all fats, including olive oil. Another important difference between these two pyramids is that the Mediterranean Pyramid calls for limited consumption of alcohol, which may reduce the risk of coronary heart disease; the USDA Pyramid makes no such recommendation.

Here are some of the other reasons many nutritionists advocate a diet based on Mediterranean favorites:

Greens: Dark leafy greens are rich in antioxidant vitamins, which may help guard against cancer and heart disease and possibly prevent damage to the eyes. Greens are also excellent sources of calcium, iron, and the B vitamin folic acid, which research shows can reduce the risk of neural tube (spinal cord) defects in fetuses. Folic acid may also reduce the risk of heart disease and stroke.

Legumes: Like dark leafy greens, legumes such as garbanzo beans (chick peas), cannellini beans, and red kidney beans are rich in folic acid and iron. What's more, they're high in protein, making them low-fat, no-cholesterol alternatives to meat. And they're great sources of soluble fiber, which can help reduce levels of blood cholesterol.

Garlic: Also shown to be effective in lowering blood cholesterol even when eaten in small quantities, garlic is a traditional staple of Mediterranean cuisine that adds flavor without contributing either fat or sugar.

Olive oil: For centuries, olive oil has been the fat of choice in Mediterranean cooking. Unlike butter and lard, animal products that are loaded with saturated fat, olive oil is a monounsaturated fat, which some studies suggest may reduce the risk of atherosclerosis.

Do you know any students of Mediterranean descent, such as those of Italian, Greek, or Turkish ancestry, who follow a diet based on the Mediterranean Pyramid? If so, what foods do they typically eat? Using the pyramid structure, make a diagram of your current food choices, with those you consume the most at the bottom and those you eat least at the top. How close is your diet to that recommended by the USDA Food Guide Pyramid? The Mediterranean Pyramid?

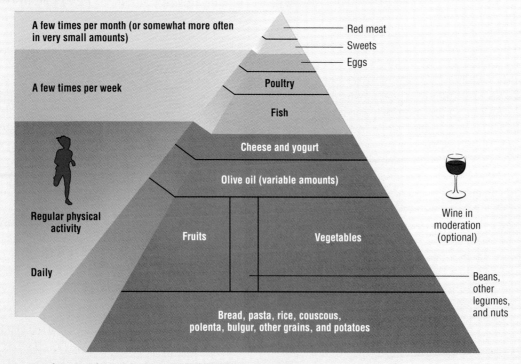

The Mediterranean Food Pyramid.

1997, there were reports of weight loss patients with newly diagnosed heart valve damage who had been using these drug combinations. In some cases, damage was correctable only by valve-replacement surgery. Accordingly, in September 1997, the FDA requested voluntary withdrawal of fenfluramine and dexfenfluramine from the market.[49] Manufacturers responded by ceasing all distribution of the drugs. In October 1999, a $4.8 billion class-action settlement was proposed, through which patients whose use of the drugs resulted in heart valve damage would receive monetary compensation and continuing medical care. Phentermine remains on the market and is used in combination with various antidepressants, such as Prozac, Zoloft, and Paxil. For those people whose use of the diet drug combinations led to heart valve damage, a study reported at the end of 1999 indicated that once medication use ceased, damage did not progress, and some indication of improvement was noted.[50]

At the same time that there was the initial concern over the use of phentermine and fenfluramine, the FDA approved yet another obesity drug, *sibutramine* (brand name Meridia), even though an advisory committee within the FDA recommended against approving it. Meridia acts on serotonin in the body similarly to how Phenfen and Redux functioned and, like its predecessors, has been linked to heart attacks, high blood pressure, strokes, and death; however, it still remains on the market in the United States. Italy recently pulled Meridia from the market following reports of death linked to this drug.

Nonhunger/Nonsatiety-Influencing Drugs

Currently a third approved medication, *orlistat* (brand name Xenical), is available for use in treating obesity. Unlike phentermine and sibutramine, which influence the neurotransmitter serotonin, orlistate reduces fat absorption in the small intestine by about 30%. The drug is intended for use among people who are 20% or more above their ideal weight. In persons who tolerate the drug's side effects, a 10% reduction of weight without significant dietary restriction is possible.

Some concerns related to the use of orlistat include: anal leakage, severe abdominal cramping, excessive flatulence, and inhibition of the absorption of vitamins and minerals in the body. Olestra has been used in fat-free chips such as "Wow!" potato chips and there have been complaints of stomach discomfort among people who ate them. In addition, people erroneously believe that they can eat as much as they want since it is fat free, but it is not calorie free and so they may end up gaining weight as a result.

Surgical Measures

When weight loss is critical and the initial level of obesity is great, surgical intervention may be considered. A *gastrointestinal* or *bariatric surgery* is a major operation in which a portion of the small intestine is bypassed in an attempt to decrease the body's ability to absorb nutrients. Candidates for this surgery include those with a BMI above 40 or about 100 pounds overweight for men and

80 pounds overweight for women. People with a BMI between 35–40 who suffer from type 2 diabetes or life-threatening cardiopulmonary problems may also be candidates for surgery. Although the procedure can produce substantial loss of body weight, it is associated with many unpleasant and dangerous side effects (including diarrhea and liver damage) and various nutritional deficiencies. Not only is surgery required for this approach, but lifetime medical management is also necessary.

Gastric Band Surgery

This is a surgical procedure in which a gastric band is implanted around the stomach, dividing the stomach into upper and lower parts. The band can be tightened or loosened by inflating or deflating the hollow connection tubing which is filled with liquid. After implantation, a small amount of food fills the top of the stomach and keeps the individual feeling full for longer periods of time, dramatically reducing food intake. The surgery takes around 2 hours and involves the risks associated with major surgery. The band is permanent and some potential side effects are vomiting and nausea, and excess food may back up into the esophagus. Typically, weight loss is somewhat slower with this type of surgery as compared to bypass surgery.

Gastroplasty, or stomach stapling, is a surgical procedure that involves sealing off about half of the stomach with surgical staples. Once the procedure has been completed, the reduced capacity of the stomach decreases the amount of food it can hold. As a result, patients feel full more quickly after eating a small meal. This procedure can sometimes be reversible but carries the risks associated with surgery and the costs of a major surgical procedure. Also it is possible to overeat and cause the staples to loosen, negating the effects of the surgery.

Liposuction, or *lipoplasty,* is another form of surgical weight loss management. During this surgical procedure, a physician inserts a small tube through the skin and vacuums away adipose tissue. Liposuction is more a cosmetic procedure than a general approach to weight loss. Along with unrealistic expectations, the risks of infection, pain and discomfort, bruising, swelling, discoloration, abscesses, and unattractive changes in body contours are possible outcomes of liposuction. Consequently, people considering this procedure should carefully investigate all aspects of it, including the training and experience of the surgeon, to determine whether it is appropriate for them.

There exists a growing concern regarding the safety of liposuction based on a comparison of surgery-related deaths during liposuction and the death rates for all surgery, including trauma-based cases. In the case of all types of surgery, the mortality rate is reported to be between 1 death for every 100,000 cases and 1 death for every 300,000 surgical cases, while for lipsosuction the rate may be 20 to 60 times higher (1 death per 5,000 cases between 1995 and 1998).[51] In spite of these figures, the Society of Plastic and Reconstructive Surgeons believes the procedure is still acceptably safe, explaining that an office-based procedure often carries a higher mortality rate than do procedures conducted in hospitals.

Although not a surgical procedure or weight loss technique, *body wrapping* is another form of body contouring. In this procedure, various areas of the body are tightly wrapped with 6-inch strips of material soaked in a solution of amino acids that are claimed to draw toxins out of the underlying tissue, shrink fatty deposits, diminish **cellulite,** lighten stretch marks, and eliminate inches of fat. Once the wrapping is removed, the newly contoured body area may remain this way for 4 to 10 weeks. Although the secret to the success of a particular spa's body wrapping approach is supposed to lie in its uniquely formulated soaking solution, the contouring effect probably results from dehydration of the underlying tissue and redistribution of extracellular fluids through pressure from the wrapping.

Regarding cellulite, readers should be aware that no product or noninvasive procedure currently in the marketplace has been shown to be effective in removing or reducing this tissue. Thus, the dimpled appearance of the buttocks, back of the arm, and upper leg seems destined to remain, despite cosmetic companies' advertisements of lotions and creams that claim to eliminate cellulite.

Acupuncture

Acupuncture is being used by an increasing number of American physicians as a treatment for obesity, as well as for a variety of other health problems. The appearance of acupuncture rings and earrings in drugstores, novelty shops, and in association with "one stop" weight loss/smoking abatement sessions advertised in the newspapers and held at local hotels suggests that the procedure has moved into the nonprofessional domain. Most people who receive acupuncture for the treatment of obesity are, fortunately, in the hands of fully trained practitioners. However, questions remain about its effectiveness, particularly in light of the difficulty of using double-blind studies to investigate techniques that employ the

---

Key Terms

cellulite tissue comprised of fat cells intertwined around strands of fibrous connective tissue.

acupuncture the insertion of fine needles into the body to alter electroenergy fields and treat disease.

surgery, and several musculoskeletal conditions. The effectiveness of acupuncture as a therapy for weight reduction has not yet been established.

Underweight

For some young adults, the lack of adequate body weight, called **underweight,** can be a serious concern, particularly for those who have inherited a tendency toward thinness (see the Changing for the Better box on this page). Males tend to be particularly concerned with too thin a body type, preferring a lean, muscular V-shape appearance.

Nutritionists believe that the healthiest way to gain weight is to increase the intake of "calorie-dense" food. These foods are characterized by high fat density resulting from high levels of vegetable fats (polyunsaturated fats). Particularly good foods in this regard are dried fruits, bananas, nuts, granola, and cheeses made from low-fat milk. The current recommendation is to eat three calorie-dense meals of moderate size per day, interspersed with two or three substantial snacks. Using the Food Guide Pyramid shown on page 143, one should eat the higher number of recommended servings for each group.[52]

A second component of weight gain for those who are underweight is an exercise program that uses weight training activities intended to increase muscle mass. For all the reasons detailed in Chapter 4, the use of anabolic drugs in the absence of highly competent medical supervision has no role in healthful weight gain. In addition,

insertion of needles. The National Center for Complementary and Alternative Medicine, on the basis of a carefully controlled study, has found acupuncture effective for the discomfort associated with chemotherapy, surgical anesthesia, the pain associated with pregnancy and

Key Terms

underweight a condition in which the body is below the desirable weight.

carefully monitored aerobic activity should be undertaken in sessions adequate to maintain heart-lung health, while at the same time one should restrict unnecessary activity that expends calories.

For those who cannot gain weight in spite of having tried the preceding approaches, a medical evaluation could supply an explanation for being underweight. If no medical explanation can be found, the person must begin to accept the reality of his or her unique body type.

Behavior Change Strategies

Several approaches designed to change learned eating patterns, such as *behavior modification,* aversive conditioning, and hypnosis, have been used by people who want to lose weight. Because of the relatively small number of people involved in many of these approaches and the limited extent to which they have been scientifically studied, it is difficult to assess their long-term effectiveness. Nevertheless, they remain as alternatives to the approaches already described.

Lifetime Weight Control

Obesity and frequent fluctuation in weight are clearly associated with higher levels of morbidity and mortality. Therefore, maintenance of weight and body composition at or near optimum levels is highly desirable. Although you may believe that this is a difficult goal to achieve, it is not unrealistic when practiced on a consistent basis. You will need to draw on resources from each dimension of your health to maintain a lifestyle that fosters the maintenance of optimum weight and body composition. Keys to your success will include:

- **Exercise** Caloric expenditure through regular exercise, including cardiovascular exercise and strength training, is a key to maintaining a healthy weight and body composition. For example, aerobic exercise is a particularly effective addition to a lifestyle of healthy eating patterns. This form of conditioning not only expends calories but also influences basal metabolic rate and trains the heart and lungs. The weight loss resulting from dieting alone, in comparison to dieting in combination with exercise, tends to be less effective and temporary at best.

- **Dietary modification** Plan your meals around foods low in total fat and saturated fat and high in complex carbohydrates. Choose fresh fruits, vegetables, pastas, and, occasionally, lean meat such as skinless chicken and baked fish (see the discussion of semivegetarianism in Chapter 5).

- **Lifestyle support** Not only do you need to be committed to a lifestyle of regular physical activity and healthy food choices, but you also need to build a sup-

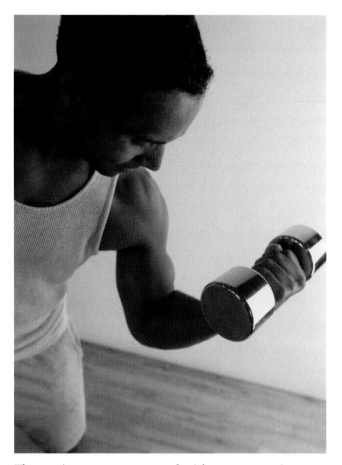

The most important component of weight management is regular exercise.

port group that will encourage you in these endeavors. Inform family, friends, classmates, and coworkers about your intent to rely on them for support and encouragement. Perhaps you will eventually serve as a role model for their involvement in a similar process.

- **Problem solving** Reevaluate your current approach to dealing with stressors. Replace any reliance on food as a coping mechanism with nonfood options, such as exercise or talking with friends or family members. Additionally, your personal reward system may need to be reviewed to decrease the use of food as a reward for a job well done.

- **Redefinition of health** Set your personal goals for your health and wellness in a manner that reinforces the importance of prevention and self-care (see Chapter 2) rather than waiting to become sick or incapacitated before attending to your diet and exercise.

The lifestyle choices just suggested will make a significant contribution to lessening the chances of developing a weight problem or weight-related health problems during your remaining adult years. Aging will exert its effects to some degree on weight and body composition, but you will avoid the damaging influences that poor dietary practices and a sedentary lifestyle present.

Physical Activity

The emphasis placed on physical activity in the model just described reflects our support of the many experts who now believe that the most important component of a weight-loss program is regular physical activity. Physical activity contributes to weight loss and the maintenance of weight loss because activity burns calories. It is important to remember that the need for calories decreases with age and with decreased activity.

An additional benefit derived from physical activity is that proportionately more fat is lost than is lost through dieting alone. Studies suggest that the weight loss achieved through physical activity is 95% fat and 5% lean tissue, such as muscle, in comparison with a loss of 75% fat and 25% lean tissue when dieting alone is used. Exercise also offers the benefits of increased heart and lung endurance, muscular strength, and flexibility.

How much exercise is enough? New studies suggest that Americans should engage in at least 45 minutes a day, 5 times a week, of moderately intense aerobic exercise. Also weight training has become a more important factor in weight management. As with most things, too much or too little exercise is not beneficial. As will be discussed in the next chapter, some people with eating disorders tend to overexercise which results in diminishing returns.

The importance of regular physical activity along with sound nutrition in the prevention of obesity is especially important for children. Today Americans are in the throes of an "epidemic" of diabetes type 2 (glucose intolerance) that begins in childhood, in comparison to the disease's traditional onset during adulthood.[53] When this form of diabetes develops and then cannot be adequately managed, the risks of heart attack, stroke, blindness, kidney failure, and inadequate wound healing leading to amputation increase significantly. Parents, educators, and society in general must place a greater emphasis on physical activity for children in order to lessen the likelihood of the obesity that fosters the development of this condition.

Eating Disorders

Perhaps it is not surprising that some people have medically identifiable, potentially serious difficulties with body image, body weight, and food selection. Among these disorders are two that are frequently seen among college students, anorexia nervosa and bulimia nervosa. In addition, binge eating, and disordered eating are also found in college populations. We have included these topics in the chapter

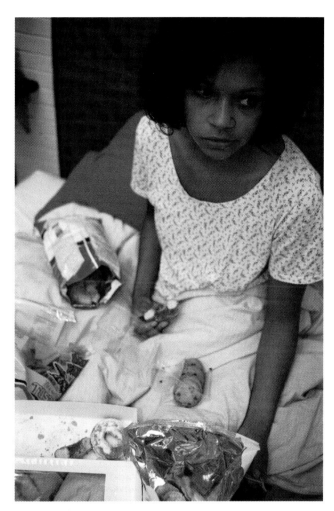

Using food to cope with feeling stressed, out of control, lonely, upset, or bored can lead to the development of an eating disorder.

on weight management because most eating disorders begin with dieting. However, most eating disorders also involve inappropriate food choices, as well as psychological issues. Those issues are discussed in Chapters 2 and 5.

A recent survey showed that dieting has become the norm for females starting at an early age. Fifty percent of 9-year-olds and 80% of 10-year-olds have reported dieting.[4] While eating disorders involve a preoccupation with food and weight, there are much deeper psychological issues underlying these conditions.

In the United States, conservative estimates indicate that after puberty 5 to 10 million females and 1 million males are struggling with eating disorders such as anorexia, bulimia, or binge eating disorder. It is estimated that approximately 8% of college women will develop an eating disorder, and the population most at risk for developing bulimia is college freshmen women. Ninety to 95% of people with eating disorders are women, although the prevalence of eating disorders in men is on the rise. Athletes such as dancers, gymnasts, swimmers, runners, and wrestlers are at risk for developing eating disorders because of the focus on weight and appearance for successful performance. In fact, any group in which success in influenced by weight or attractiveness is at risk for the development of an eating disorder, such as those involved in the performance arts, theatre, television, and modeling.

Anorexia Nervosa

Anorexia nervosa is an eating disorder in which a person denies his or her own feelings of hunger and avoids food, with marked weight loss occurring. Anorexics tend to run from food in the relentless pursuit of thinness although they never perceive themselves as thin enough. To meet the diagnostic criteria for anorexia nervosa, the individual has an intense fear of gaining weight, even though he or she weighs less than 85% of the expected weight for his/her age, gender, and height, and, in females, menstruation ceases for at least 3 consecutive months.[54] In addition, people with anorexia perceive themselves as overweight and much larger than what they look like in reality. Anorexics lose their ability to recognize when they are hungry and have difficulty eating even if they want to do so. Depression, irritability, withdrawal, perfectionism, and low self-esteem are some of the psychological problems associated with anorexia. In addition, anorexics tend to feel cold most of the time because they have very little body fat (2–10%) and also suffer from lightheadedness, dizziness, insomnia, hair loss, muscle cramps, stress fractures, fatigue, decreased memory and concentration, and gastrointestinal problems. More serious complications include heart and kidney failure, hypothermia, osteoporosis, infertility, and, in 25% of cases, death.

As with other eating disorders, anorexia nervosa also involves a sense of feeling out of control in one's life and attempting to find control through food and weight loss. It is not a coincidence that anorexia nervosa typically begins around puberty: Most individuals with anorexia have a fear of growing up and all that goes with being an adult, such as financial responsibility, sexual relationships, leaving one's family, and becoming more autonomous and independent.

Anorexia often begins with dieting, but may also begin as a result of an illness such as the stomach flu, a relationship that breaks up, or after dental surgery in which it might be expected that one would temporarily eat less. However, anorexics will tell you that the disorder begins to take on a life of its own after what started as wanting to lose a few pounds turns into losing 15% or more of body weight and still not feeling satisfied with one's appearance. Friends and family might initially encourage the person on his or her weight loss and say complimentary things about his or her appearance, but soon become concerned when the person's weight continues to dramatically decrease.

Anorexia has become more common as changing cultural ideals for beauty have changed. Our standards have gone from Marilyn Monroe who was a voluptuous 5'5", 128-pound woman to Kate Moss who has been reported to be 5'7" and 105 pounds.[7] Now the "lollipop look" is considered the "in look" in Hollywood, with actresses and models having stick-thin bodies, making their heads seem huge.

Denial of problems plays a major role in eating disorders in which the individual refuses to acknowledge that there is anything wrong, even though she is becoming thinner and wasting away, and family and friends are expressing great concern. While anorexia nervosa is considered a serious medical and psychological disorder, some anorexics argue that "Anorexia is a lifestyle not a disorder." These heated debates and discussions often occur through pro-anorexia websites. With names like "Thinspiration," "Stick Figures," and "Anorexic and Proud," these pro-anorexia forums have become very popular and deadly in the past few years. These websites show computer-enhanced pictures of models and actresses like Calista Flockhart and Lara Flynn Boyle, making them appear thinner and more skeletal than they really are.[55] Messages on these websites include tips for how to starve, how to purge, ways of hiding one's disorder and encouragement to lose more weight. There has been a push among health providers, educators, and health organizations to eliminate these types of websites, and they have been somewhat successful. However, these sites are purported to still exist, although more disguised and underground than in the past.[56]

Most recently, the three groups that have traditionally been overlooked in the incidence of anorexia are women of color, female athletes (see the Female Athlete Triad in Chapter 4), and men. The research shows a significant increase in the incidence of anorexia among these three groups. More focus has been given to anorexia among women of color, and it has been proposed that this group might be more vulnerable to developing eating disorders than Caucasian women because of ethno-cultural identity issues. It has been suggested that the more pressure women of color feel to fit into the dominant culture's standards of beauty and thinness, the more likely they are to develop eating disorders.

Key Terms

anorexia nervosa an eating disorder in which the individual weighs less than 85% of their expected weight for his or her age, gender, and height, has an intense fear of gaining weight, and in females, menstruation ceases for at least 3 consecutive months. People with anorexia perceive themselves as overweight, even though they are underweight.

Often female athletes are not diagnosed with eating disorders because the symptoms of anorexia, absence of menses, low body fat and weight, and osteoporosis, referred to as the "female athletic triad" are not uncommon among athletes and don't necessarily signify the presence of an eating disorder.

The prevalence of anorexia nervosa (as well as bulimia nervosa, which we'll cover later) has traditionally been very low in men as compared with women. Today, however, the incidence of both conditions is increasing in men as they begin to feel some of the same pressures that women feel to conform to the weight and body composition standards imposed by others. The "lean look" of young male models serves as a standard for more and more young men, whereas the requirements to "make weight" for various sports drives others. Runners, jockeys, swimmers, and gymnasts frequently must lose weight quickly to meet particular standards for competition or the expectations of coaches and trainers. Researchers report that men are less inclined than women to admit that they may have an eating disorder, thinking it is a "women's illness." Thus they are less likely to seek treatment. In addition, physicians tend not to suspect men as having eating disorders, and so they go untreated.

Fortunately, psychological treatment in combination with medical and dietary interventions can return the person with anorexia nervosa to a more life-sustaining pattern of eating. The person with anorexia needs to receive the care of professionals experienced in the treatment of this disorder. It is not uncommon for this treatment to take 3 to 5 years. If others, including friends, co-workers, roommates, and parents observe this condition, they should consult a health care provider for assistance.

 TALKING POINTS What would you do if you suspected a friend of yours had an eating disorder? Would you share your concern with him or her? If so, what would you say?

Bulimia Nervosa

While anorexics are underweight, people with **bulimia nervosa** often are of a normal weight. These individuals use food and weight as a way of coping with stress, boredom, conflict in relationships, and low self-esteem. It is not uncommon in our society to comfort ourselves with food, to have social activities based around food, and to eat as a way of procrastinating a dreaded activity. However, people with bulimia take this to the extreme, engaging in recurrent bingeing, consuming unusually large amounts of food, and feeling out of control with their eating.[54]

While anorexics run away from food, bulimics run to food to cope with their emotions, problems, and stress. Because they feel so guilty, ashamed, and anxious about the food they have consumed, people with bulimia **purge** by self-induced vomiting, taking an excessive number of laxatives and diuretics, excessively exercising or fasting. There is a strong preoccupation with weight, calories, and food among sufferers of bulimia. Most people with bulimia constantly count calories, weigh themselves throughout the day, and frequently make negative statements concerning different parts of their bodies, primarily focusing on the thighs, stomach, and waist. As with anorexia, bulimia is associated with depression, isolation, anxiety, perfectionism, and low self-esteem. Dental erosion, hair loss, esophageal lesions, blood in the vomit and stools, loss of voluntary gag reflex, kidney damage, heart failure, gastrointestinal problems, ketosis, edema, infertility, parotid gland swelling, depression, and insomnia are just some of the medical problems associated with bulimia nervosa.

As has been mentioned previously, bulimia often begins around age 17 to 18 years of age when young adults are separating from their families and are forging lives of their own. There may be some conflict around issues of independence, autonomy, and relationships with family. There is a higher incidence of bulimia than anorexia, although some bulimics may have had anorexia in the past. There is also a higher rate of bulimia among female college students as compared to their peers who are not attending colleges. Treatment for bulimia nervosa involves nutritional counseling, psychological treatment, and consultation with a physician. Often people with bulimia can recover from this disorder within a year of beginning treatment.

Binge Eating Disorder

Binge eating disorder is the newest term for what was previously referred to as compulsive overeating. Binge

Key Terms

bulimia nervosa an eating disorder in which individuals engage in episodes of bingeing, consuming unusually large amounts of food and feeling out of control, and engaging in some compensatory purging behavior to eliminate the food.

purging using vomiting, laxatives, diuretics, enemas, or other medications, or means such as excessive exercise or fasting to eliminate food.

binge eating disorder an eating disorder formerly referred to as compulsive overeating disorder; binge eaters use food to cope in the same way that bulimics do and also feel out of control, but do not engage in compensatory purging behavior.

Recognizing Anorexia Nervosa and Bulimia Nervosa

The American Psychological Association uses the following diagnostic criteria to identify anorexia nervosa and bulimia

Anorexia	Bulimia
• Body weight is 15% or more below desirable weight • Fear of weight gain • Distorted body image • In women, the absence of three or more menstrual periods (young girls may not start menstruating at the appropriate age); In men, sex hormones decrease	• Binge eating two or more times a week for at least 3 months • A lack of control over bingeing • Engaging in inappropriate compensatory behavior two or more times a week for at least 3 months to prevent weight gain • Overly concerned about body image

Characteristic symptoms include the following. Note that it is unlikely that all the symptoms will be evident in any one individual.

Anorexia	Bulimia
• Looks thin and keeps getting thinner • Skips meals, cuts food into small pieces, moves food around plate to appear to have eaten • Loss of menstrual periods and possible infertility • Wears baggy clothes in an attempt to disguise weight loss and to keep warm • Significant hair loss • Extreme sensitivity to cold • Dizziness, lightheadedness, headaches • Withdrawal, irritability, depression • Insomnia • Decreased sex drive • Dehydration, kidney dysfunction • Fatigue, loss of energy • Decreased concentration • Lanugo (fine downy body hair) • Heart irregularities, heart failure	• Bathroom use immediately after eating • Eating in secret • Excessive time (and money) spent food shopping • Shopping for food at several stores instead of one store • Menstrual irregularities and possible fertility problems • Excessive constipation • Swollen and/or infected salivary glands, sore throat • Bursting blood vessels in the eyes • Dental erosion in teeth and gums • Dehydration and kidney dysfunction • Significant hair loss; dry, brittle hair and nails • Increased acne and skin problems • Heart irregularities, heart failure

eaters use food to cope in the same way that bulimics do and also feel out of control and unable to stop eating during binges. People with this disorder report eating rapidly and in secret or may snack all day. They tend to eat until they feel uncomfortably full, sometimes hoarding food and eating when they aren't physically hungry.[54] Like people with bulimia, they feel guilty and ashamed of their eating habits and have a great deal of self-loathing and body hatred. People who have binge eating disorder do not engage in purging behavior and this is what differentiates it from bulimia nervosa. Typically, binge eaters have a long history of diet failures, feel anxious, are socially with-

drawn from others, and are overweight. Heart problems, high blood pressure, joint problems, abnormal blood sugar levels, fatigue, depression, and anxiety are associated with binge eating. The treatment of this eating disorder involves interventions similar to those described for treating bulimia nervosa.

Chewing and Spitting Out Food Syndrome

Chewing and spitting out one's food without swallowing it has also been used as a method for weight loss or weight management. This is a common eating disorder and falls

Resources for Anorexia and Bulimia Treatment

Local Resources

- College or university health centers
- College or university counseling centers
- Comprehensive mental health centers
- Crisis intervention centers
- Mental health associations

Organizations and Self-Help Groups

National Association of Anorexia Nervosa and Associated Disorders (ANAD)

ANAD is the oldest national nonprofit organization helping eating disorder victims and their families. In addition to its free hotline counseling, ANAD operates an international network of support groups for sufferers and their families, and it offers referrals to health care professionals who treat eating disorders across the U.S. and in fifteen other countries.

PO Box 7
Highland Park, IL 60035   Fax: 847-433-4632
Hotline: 847-831-3438   E-mail: *info@anad.org*

www://anad.org

American Psychological Association (APA) HelpCenter

The American Psychological Association is the largest professional organization comprised of health care professionals whose practices are limited to the diagnosis, treatment, and management of psychological health problems. The APA HelpCenter provides information concerning eating disorders and the treatment options that are available for both patients and their families. Links are provided to assist in finding psychological services in your local area.

www.helping.apa.org

Academy for Eating Disorders (AED)

The Academy for Eating Disorders' membership is comprised of academics and clinical professionals with demonstrated interest and expertise in the field of eating disorders. In addition to providing information to both professionals and the public regarding eating disorders, the AED also advocates on behalf of patients and the general public. The AED can provide guidelines to assist in the selection of a competent healthcare provider.

6728 Old McLean Village Drive
McLean, VA 22101
Telephone: 703-556-9222   Fax: 703-556-8729
E-mail: *aed@degnon.org*

Anorexia Nervosa and Related Eating Disorders, Inc. (ANRED)

ANRED is a nonprofit organization that provides information about anorexia, bulimia nervosa, compulsive eating, and other less well-known food and weight disorders. Printed and Web-based information regarding treatment, recovery, and prevention are available to the general public.

www.anred.com

American Anorexia/Bulimia Association, Inc. (AABA)

AABA is a national, nonprofit organization of concerned members of the public and health care industry dedicated to the prevention and treatment of eating disorders. General information related to eating disorders is provided to the general public, as well as more focused specific information for patients, families, and professionals. A list of upcoming events in various areas of the country is also provided.

(212) 501-8351

National Eating Disorder Association

The National Eating Disorders Association is the largest nonprofit organization in the United States dedicated to the elimination of eating disorders and body dissatisfaction. It disseminates information, offers prevention programs, publishes and distributes educational materials, and operates the nation's first toll-free eating disorders information and referral line. It states as part of its mission to "continually work to change the cultural, familial, and interpersonal factors which contribute to the development of eating disorders and body dissatisfaction."

www.NationalEatingDisorders.org

Additional Resources

www.eyeonwomen.com/eating.htm

www.noah-health.org/index.html

American Anorexia/Bulimia Association, Inc.
418 East 76th Street, New York, NY 10021
(212) 501-8351

Anorexia Nervosa and Associated Disorders, Inc.
P.O. Box 7, Highland Park, IL 60035
(708) 831-3438

Anorexia Nervosa and Related Eating Disorders, Inc.
P.O. Box 5102, Eugene, OR 97405
(503) 344-1144

This nonprofit organization, which collects information about eating and exercise disorders, distributes information through booklets and a monthly newsletter. Staff lead workshops, self-help groups, and training programs for professionals. They also provide speakers.

Bulimia Anorexia Nervosa Association
Windsor, Ontario (Canada)
(519) 253-7421 or 7545

National Eating Disorders Association (NEDO) at Laureatte Psychiatric Hospital
P.O. Box 470207, Tulsa, OK 74147
(918) 481-4092

This organization publishes a quarterly newsletter appropriate for professional and personal use.

within the "Eating Disorder Not Otherwise Specified" diagnosis. It differs from bulimia nervosa and researchers contend that chewing and spitting out food without swallowing may indicate a more severe eating disorder.[57]

Night Eating Syndrome

Night eating syndrome has not yet been formally defined as an eating disorder. The signs and symptoms of this syndrome include: eating more than half of one's daily food intake after dinner and before breakfast, feeling tense, anxious, and guilty while eating, difficulty falling or staying asleep at night, and having little to no appetite in the morning. Unlike binge eating, night eating involves eating throughout the evening hours rather than in short episodes. It is important to note that there is a strong preference for carbohydrates among night eaters. Some researchers speculate that night eating may be an unconscious attempt to self-medicate mood problems because eating carbohydrates can trigger the brain to produce so-called "feel good" neurochemicals. Research is underway in examining the underlying causes of this syndrome and developing subsequent treatment interventions. It seems likely that a combination of biological, genetic, and psychological factors contribute to this problem.

Treating Eating Disorders

The treatment for eating disorders is multimodal and multidimensional involving nutritionists, psychologists, physicians, family, and friends. There are different treatment modalities such as individual, group, and family counseling. Sometimes treatment requires in-patient hospitalization to medically stabilize the individual. In extreme cases, a feeding tube may be inserted to treat starvation, especially if the person refuses to eat. Behavioral modification and cognitive therapy are utilized in counseling people with eating problems. Medications such as antidepressants are often used to decrease obsessive-compulsive behavior, reduce anxiety, alleviate depression, and improve mood. Some medications can stimulate or reduce appetite as well. There is some debate over the efficacy of using an addictions model, similar to the twelve-step Alcoholics Anonymous philosophy, with eating disorders. Overeaters Anonymous utilizes this model in helping people with eating problems and many hospital programs employ this model in their treatment programs. While there seems to be some overlap with substance abuse problems such as denial of problems, feeling out of control of one's behavior, and using food or drugs or alcohol to cope with problems, this is where the similarities end as obviously one needs food to live which is not the case with drugs and alcohol.

A Final Thought about Health and Weight Management

Recognizing the attention placed on physical attractiveness and its relationship to thinness, it is important to ask yourself if you are healthy enough to accept your unique body even if it does not match the cultural ideal. As you recall from Chapter 1, it is important to develop every dimension of health, not simply the physical dimension. We hope that a high enough level of self-esteem grounded in your own respect for your feelings, beliefs, interpersonal skills, intellect, and sense of contribution to society will more than offset the absence of perfect alignment with a body image that is unrealistic and obtainable by only a few.

Taking Charge of Your Health

- Investigate the resources available on your campus that you could use to determine your healthy weight and body composition profile.
- Evaluate your eating behaviors to find out if you are using food to cope with stress. If you are, develop a plan to use nonfood options, such as exercise or interaction with friends or family members, to deal with stress.
- Formulate a realistic set of goals for changing your weight and body composition in a time frame that allows you to do so in a healthful way.

- Establish a daily schedule that lets you make any necessary dietary and physical activity adjustments.
- Keep a daily journal of your weight-management efforts.
- Monitor your progress toward meeting your weight-management goals.
- Design a reward system for reaching each goal.
- Learn to accept your body including the imperfections.
- Focus on other aspects of yourself that you like that are not related to appearance.

Summary

- Weight management has become an obsession in American culture as well as a significant health problem; an estimated 61% of U.S. adults are either overweight or obese.
- The average caloric intake for Americans has increased over the past two decades while the majority of Americans are not physically active on a regular basis.
- Doctors usually define "overweight" as a condition in which a person's weight is 1% to 19% higher than "normal," as defined by a standard height/weight chart. Obesity is usually defined as a condition in which a person's weight is 20% or more above normal weight. "Morbid obesity" refers to being 50% to 100% over normal weight, more than 100 pounds over normal weight, or sufficiently overweight to interfere with health or normal functioning.
- Some of the methods for assessing one's weight are: Body Mass Index, current height and weight tables, waist to hip ratios, electrical impedance, BOD POD, skinfold measurements, hydrostatic weighing, and medical scales.
- Body dysmorphic disorder (BDD) is a secret preoccupation with an imagined or slight flaw in one's appearance.
- Basal Metabolic Rate (BMR) is a measure of resting energy expenditure that is taken upon awakening, 10–12 hours after eating, or 12–18 hours after significant physical activity.
- Thermic effect of food (TEF) refers to the amount of energy our bodies require for the digestion, absorption, and transportation of food.
- There are four factors that seem to play a significant role in the prevalence of obesity: sex, age, socioeconomic status, and race.
- Hypothyroidism is a condition caused by an underactive thyroid gland, which produces an insufficient amount of metabolism-regulating hormone called thyroxin.
- The energy expenditure and energy storage centers of the body possess a genetically programmed awareness of the body's most physiologically desirable weight called set point.
- The process of storing or burning more energy to maintain the body's "best" weight is called adaptive thermogenesis.
- Lower socioeconomic status, married men, parents, and people living in rural areas are associated with a higher incidence of obesity.
- Environmental factors such as portion size, price, advertising, the availability of food, and the number of food choices presented all can influence the amount the average person consumes.
- Psychological reasons for eating refer to eating not out of hunger but as a way of coping with feelings, as a way of socializing and celebrating with others, and due to associating certain activities with eating.
- Weight management experts identify inactivity as the single most important reason that obesity is so high in today's society.
- Hypercellular obesity refers to having a greater number of fat cells than those of normal weight resulting in obesity.
- Hypertrophic obesity is a form of obesity in which there are a normal number of fat cells but the fat cells are enlarged.
- Weight loss occurs when the calories consumed are less than the energy the body needs for physiological maintenance and activity.
- The primary types of weight management techniques include dietary alterations, surgical interventions, medications, weight loss programs, and physical activity.
- A commitment to a lifestyle change of eating in healthy ways and engaging in regular aerobic exercise seems to be the most effective strategy for weight loss and weight maintenance.
- Anorexia nervosa is a psychological condition in which the individual weighs less than 85% of his/her expected weight for his/her age, gender, and height. In women menstruation ceases for at least 3 consecutive months, and there is an intense fear of gaining weight. People with anorexia perceive themselves as overweight, even though they are underweight.
- People with bulimia nervosa often are of a normal weight. These individuals use food and weight as a way of coping with stress, boredom, conflict in relationships, and low self-esteem. People with bulimia engage in recurrent bingeing, consuming unusually large amounts of food and feeling out of control with their eating. They engage in purging to eliminate the food from their bodies.
- Binge eaters use food to cope in the same way that bulimics do and also feel out of control and unable to stop eating during binges but do not engage in inappropriate compensatory purging behaviors.
- The treatment for eating disorders is multimodal and multidimensional involving nutritionists, psychologists, physicians, family, and friends.

Review Questions

1. What percentage of U.S. adults are either overweight or obese?
2. How has the average caloric intake and physical activity level for Americans changed over the past two decades?
3. Define overweight, obesity, and morbid obesity.
4. List at least four of the methods used for assessing weight.
5. Describe body dysmorphic disorder(BDD).
6. Define Basal Metabolic Rate (BMR).
7. Describe the thermic effect of food (TEF) and how it relates to the BMR.
8. What are four factors that seem to play a significant role in the prevalence of obesity?
9. Describe hypothyroidism and its impact on weight management.
10. Define set point.
11. The process of storing or burning more energy to maintain the body's "best" weight is called what?
12. What are two factors associated with a higher incidence of obesity?
13. Give four examples of how environmental factors can influence the amount the average person consumes.
14. Describe at least two psychological reasons for eating.
15. What is the single most important reason that obesity is so high in today's society, according to the experts?
16. Define hypercellular obesity.
17. Define hypertrophic obesity.
18. How does weight loss occur?
19. Give examples of four different types of weight management techniques.
20. What is the most effective strategy for weight loss and weight maintenance?
21. Describe the symptoms of anorexia nervosa.
22. Describe the symptoms of bulimia nervosa.
23. How is binge eating disorder different from bulimia nervosa?
24. Discuss some of the components for effective treatment for eating disorders.

References

1. National Center for Chronic Disease Prevention and Health Promotion. Defining Overweight and Obesity, September 2002.
2. National Research Council, *Diet and Health: Implications for Reducing Chronic Disease Risk,* Washington, D.C. National Academy Press; 1989.
3. Mokdad AH, et al. The spread of the obesity epidemic in the United States, 1991–1998. *JAMA* 1999; 282(16):1519–1522.
4. Harvard Women's Health Watch: Panel issues new guidelines for healthy eating. *Harvard Medical School,* November 2002, Volume 10(3).
5. Allison DB, et al. Annual deaths attributed to obesity in the United States. *JAMA* 2982, 16, 1530–1538, 1999.
6. Heart and Stroke Facts. *American Heart Association,* 2003.
7. Poulton T. *No Fat Chicks.* Secaucus, N.J. Carol Publishing Group, 1997.
8. Maine M. *Body Wars.* Carlsbad, CA: Gurze Books, 2000.
9. Andersen A, Cohn L, Holbrook T. *Making Weight: Men's Conflicts With Food, Weight, Shape and Appearance.* Carlsbad, CA: Gurze Books, 2000.
10. Cash T, Henry P. Women's body images: the results of a national survey in the U.S.A. *Sex Role Res* 33(1), 19–29, 1995.
11. Andersen A. Males With Eating Disorders. Philadelphia, PA: Brunner/Mazel Inc. 1990.
12. Brownell KD and Fairburn CG. *Eating Disorders and Obesity: A Comprehensive Handbook.* New York: Guilford Press. 1995.
13. National Institute of Health. *Clinical guidelines on the identification, evaluation, and treatment of overweight and obesity in adults.* As reported in First Federal Obesity Clinical Guidelines (NIH News Advisory). The National Institutes of Health, 17 June 1998.
14. Gaesser G. *Big Fat Lies.* Carlsbad, CA: Gurze Books, 2002.
15. U.S. Department of Agriculture/U.S. Department of Health and Human Services. Nutrition and your health: dietary guidelines for Americans. *Home and Garden Bulletin,* 232, 2000.
16. Waist Management, Gauging Your Risk. *Consumer Reports,* p. 48, August 2003.
17. International Health Racquet and Sportsclub Association. BOD POD Body Composition System to Descend on San Francisco's *IHRSA CONVENTION* as reported in the 29th Anniversary Exhibition in San Francisco's Moscone Convention Center, March 22–24, 2001.
18. Dempster P, Aitkens S. A new air displacement method for the determination of human body

composition. *Medical Science Sports Exercise* 27(2), 1692–1697, 1995.

19. Lindzey G, Thompson R and Spring B. *Psychology*, 3rd ed. New York: Worth Publishers, Inc. 1988.

20. Thelen MH, Powell AL, Lawrence C, and Kuhnent ME. Eating and body image concerns among children. *Journal of Consulting and Clinical Psychology* 21, 41, 46, 1992.

21. A Dangerous Duo: Body Dysmorphic Disorder with Anorexia Nervosa. *Eating Disorders Review*, November/December, 4–5, 2002.

22. Troiano RP, Flegal KM, Kuczmarski RJ, Campbell SM, and Johnson CL. Overweight prevalence and trends for children and adolescents. *Archives of Pediatrics and Adolescent Medicine* 149, 1085–1091, 1995.

23. Sobal J. Obesity and socioeconomic status: A framework for examining relationships between physical and social variables. *Medical Anthropology* 13, 231–247, 1991.

24. Wadden TA and Stunkard AJ. *Handbook of Obesity Treatment.* New York: Guilford Press, 2002.

25. Halaas J, et al. Weight-reducing effects on the plasma protein encoded by the obese gene. *Science* 269(5223), 543–546, 1995.

26. Folsom AR, Jensen MD, Jacobs DR, Hilner JE, Tsai AW, and Schreiner PJ. Serum leptin and weight gain over eight years in African American and Caucasian young adults. *Obesity Research* 7(1), 1–8, 1999.

27. Sakurai T, et al. Orexins and orexin receptors: a family of hypothalamic neuropeptides and G protein-coupled receptors that regulate feeding behavior. *Cell* 92(4), 573–585, 1998.

28. Pettigrew R and Hamilton FD. Obesity and female reproductive function. *Br Med Bull* 53:2, 341–358, 1997.

29. La Leche League International. *The Womanly Art of Breastfeeding.* 1997.

30. Dell S, To T. Breastfeeding and asthma in young children. *Archives of Pediatric and Adolescent Medicine* 155: 1261–1265, 2001.

31. Hediger ML, et al. Association between infant breastfeeding and overweight in young children. *JAMA* 285(19): 2453–2460, 2001.

32. Gillman MW, et al. Risk of overweight among adolescents who were breastfed as infants. *JAMA* 285(19): 2461–2467, 2001.

33. Set Point: What your body is trying to tell you. *National Eating Disorders Information Centre Bulletin*, 7(2), June, 1992.

34. The truth about dieting. *Consumer Reports*, 26–31 June, 2002.

35. Saladin KS. *Anatomy & Physiology: the unity of form and function.* Dubuque, IA: William C. Brown/McGraw-Hill, 1998.

36. Sorbara M and Geliebter A. Body image disturbance in obese outpatients before and after weight loss in relation to race, gender and age of onset of obesity. *Internal Journal of Eating Disorders*, 416–423, May, 2002.

37. Sobal J, and Stunkard AJ. Socioeconomic status and obesity: A review of the literature. *Psychological Bulletin* 105, 260–275, 1989.

38. Stunkard AJ and Wadden TA. *Obesity: Theory and Therapy.* New York: Raven Press, 1993.

39. Sobal J, Rauschenbach B, and Frongillo E. Marital status, fatness and obesity. *Social Science and Medicine* 35, 915–923, 1992.

40. Obesity in America: The Gorge Yourself Environment. *The New York Times,* August 19, 2003.

41. Shils, M, Olson, J. Shike, and Ross, A. Modern Nutrition in Health and Disease 9th edition. Philadelphia, Pennsylvania, 1999.

42. Weight Watchers. *Stop Stuffing Yourself: 7 Steps to Conquering Overeating.* New York: Wiley Publishing Inc., 1988.

43. Kirby, J. Dieting for Dummies. New York: Wiley Publishing Inc., 1998.

44. National Academy of Sciences. *Recommended Daily Allowances,* 10th ed. National Academy Press, 1998.

45. Insel P, Turner RE, Ross D. *Nutrition.* Sudbury, MA: Jones and Bartlett Publishers, 2002.

46. Wardlaw, GM. *Perspectives in Nutrition,* 4th ed. McGraw-Hill, 1999.

47. Ephedra Ban Puts Herb Industry on Notice. *The New York Times,* December 31, 2003.

48. Roering JL. Herbal agents used by eating disorder patients. *Eating Disorders Review,* 13(4), July/August 2002.

49. Center for Drug Evaluation and Research, U.S. Food and Drug Administration. FDA announces withdrawal of fenfluramine and dexfenfluramine. *News Release #97-32,* September 15, 1997.

50. Hensrud DD, et al. Echocardiographic improvement over time after cessation of use of fenfluramine and phentermine. *May Clin Pro* 74(12), 1191–1197, 1999.

51. Grazer FM, de Jong RH. Fatal outcomes from liposuction; census survey of cosmetic surgeons. *Plastic Reconstructive Surgery* 105(1) 436–446, 2000.

52. The American Dietetic Association. Gaining weight: a healthy plan for adding pounds. *Hot Topics,* www.eatright.org/nfs10html, 1998.

53. Young TK, et al. Childhood obesity in a population at high risk for type 2 diabetes. *Journal of Pediatrics* 136(3), 365–369, 2000.

54. *Diagnostic and Statistical Manual of Mental Disorders IV TR.* Washington, D.C., American Psychiatric Association, 2000.

55. Gotthelf M. The new anorexia outrage. *Self Magazine,* 82–84. August 2001.

56. Lilenfeld L. Academy members debate over pro-anorexia websites. *Academy of Eating Disorders Newsletter,* June 2001.

57. *Update:* Chewing and Spitting Out Food. *Eating Disorders Review,* July/August, 2002.

As We Go to Press

How healthy is the Atkins diet? There are some who argue that Robert Atkins, author of the book "*Dr. Atkins' New Diet Revolution,*" died from complications related to his diet. On April 8th, 2003, Atkins slipped on the ice, hit his head, and died on April 17th. The medical examiner's report stated that Atkins had a history of heart trouble, including congestive heart failure and high blood pressure. Dr. Atkins weighed 258 lbs and was 6 feet in height at the time of his death, which would put him in the obese category according to the Centers for Disease Control and Prevention. When he was admitted to the hospital, he weighed 195 lbs, which is considered overweight.

Atkins had suffered cardiac arrest in 2002, and there is speculation that this is a direct result of following his own diet which is high in fat and protein. In fact, the Atkins diet allows up to two-thirds of one's daily intake to be from fat, more than double the U.S. Department of Agriculture's Food Pyramid Guide. Critics of the Atkins diet have warned for years that following this diet can result in high cholesterol levels, cardiovascular problems, and hypertension.

However, Veronica Atkins, his widow, claims his death was "completely unrelated to his diet or any diet", and the weight gain had been attributed to retaining 60 lbs of fluid after he entered the hospital, while in a coma after his fall. Furthermore, some claim that Atkins suffered from cardiomyopathy, a disease of the heart muscle that may have been caused by a virus.

While the jury is out on how much Atkins's diet contributed to his own death, if at all, it remains to be seen if the renewed interest in the Atkins diet will produce an accompanying increase in the incidence of heart disease and hypertension in the years to come.

Sources: Did the Atkins Diet Fail Dr. Atkins?, *People Magazine,* February 23, 2004. Atkins obesity report sparks new round in diet fight, *The Seattle Times,* February 11, 2004.

are you a victim of portion distortion? learning to control serving sizes

Americans love to live large. According to social scientists, this is part of our national psyche that is directly traceable to our wide-spaced national boundaries, ample open space, and rags-to-riches dreams. Buying into this myth is beneficial when it motivates people to stretch themselves in areas of personal growth and achievement. When it comes to eating, however, the living-large philosophy puts Americans on a collision course with a variety of health risks and hinders their weight control efforts.[1]

A Supersized Trend

The trend toward supersized food portions is nothing new. Restaurants have long used large portions to lure value-seeking customers. The trend reversed for a while during the health-conscious 1980s, when meat consumption was coincidentally at an all-time high. Large serving sizes are enjoying a revival, however, as part of the current wellness backlash, which includes such risky behaviors as cigar smoking and increased consumption of hard liquor.

Fast-food chains target bargain-hungry consumers weary of wellness warnings. In an attempt to fend off competition within the industry as well as from new steak houses, ethnic eateries, full-service delis, and take-out restaurants, the fast-food industry is selling—and customers are buying—oversized portions of traditional favorites, such as burgers, fries, fried chicken, and pizza, in record numbers. Typically these supersized portions cost just pennies more than the standard-size serving. Another fattening sales strategy is to offer combo meals—essentially the addition of a large order of fries and a giant drink to popular menu items for under fifty cents.[1, 2, 3]

Serving Size Recommendations

As with many health-related issues, portion control embodies many contradictions. The USDA has standardized food portions, which are used to develop labeling laws and the Food Guide Pyramid (FGP) serving size recommendations. The average American, accustomed to gigantic servings when dining out, finds serving sizes on food labels surprisingly puny and, on the other hand, the number of servings of produce and grains suggested on the FGP surprisingly high (see the table comparing typical with recommended serving sizes).[4] Record numbers of low-fat and low-calorie foods are available, yet Americans are fatter than ever (average body weight has increased 7.5 pounds in the last decade).[1] Gourmets tend to favor small portions of fine food, whereas homestyle cooking enthusiasts prefer an abundance of food, especially meat and starch. Yet both groups are sporting wider waistlines.

Americans aren't entirely to blame for their ignorance of serving sizes. The USDA's standardization of serving sizes seems anything but standard to the average consumer. Food manufacturers and restaurant managers have been happy to ignore the USDA's advice and give cost-sensitive consumers the supersized servings they desire. According to USDA standards, the amount of food that constitutes a serving varies. Some serving sizes are based on volume and others on weight. For example, one-half of a three-inch-diameter bagel and one-half cup of cooked rice both constitute one serving from the grain, bread, and pasta group of the FGP. Three ounces of cooked chicken, one-half cup of cooked dried beans, or two tablespoons of peanut butter constitute one serving from the meat group. Even a single food, such as broccoli, can have different serving sizes depending on how it's prepared: According to the FGP, one serving of a fruit or vegetable equals one cup if eaten raw but only one-half cup if it's cooked.[4]

Despite pressure from the Nutrition Labeling and Education Act of 1990, food manufacturers continue to package foods in nonstandard sizes. They are simultaneously producing giant versions of trendy carbohydrate-rich foods, such as mega-muffins, behemoth bagels, and miniature versions of favorite high-fat snacks like mini-cheese-filled Ritz crackers and bite-sized Oreos.

Food companies also persist in packaging multiple servings of certain foods, particularly snack foods, in what appear to be single-serving containers. For instance, the USDA identifies a serving of soda as six ounces, but the typical soda can contains twelve ounces. This extra serving is inconsequential if you're drinking diet soda, but regular soda adds sixty-five calories, or roughly five teaspoons of sugar. Small packages of candy, chips, and cookies often exhibit this same deceptive packaging.[4]

The Portion-Distortion Trend Takes Shape

Well-meaning health care experts are partly to blame for this supersized servings trend. During the late 1980s and early 1990s, many of them urged people to eat less fat and more carbohydrates. The selling point for giving up favorite high-fat foods was that "you can eat more food for fewer calories." The underlying reasoning was sound—gram for gram, fat has twice as many calories as carbohydrates. Unfortunately, portion-ignorant Americans took this advice too literally and began devouring triple-sized tortillas, muffins, pretzels, bagels, and platters of pasta.

Letting someone else do the cooking doesn't make weight management any easier. Obesity experts identify dining out as a serious liability for diet-conscious diners. Presently, Americans spend more than 40% of every food dollar in restaurants.[5] Chic restaurants, featuring small portions of artistically prepared food, are blossoming on every corner in large cities, but in the suburbs and the heartland, the trend is fast-food chains, take-out shops, casual restaurants, and convenience foods, including frozen meals, packaged mixes, and full-service deli items.[3]

More than 80% of all dining-out dollars are spent at family-friendly eateries. Prices at these establishments are relatively low, but thanks to the supersized portions, calories tend to be high.[6]

Gourmets aren't faring any better when it comes to waist whittling. The small portions served in fine restaurants are no guarantee of low-calorie ingredients. Furthermore, just being in a restaurant, confronted with an overwhelming number of appealing food choices, causes many people to order more courses than they typically eat when dining at home. How often have you ordered an appetizer or felt overly full but still fallen prey to the dessert cart when it arrived at your table? Obesity experts believe this tendency to be seduced by the sight and smell of food partly explains the lack of healthy food choices on fast-food menus. Responding to consumer demand, McDonald's, Burger King, Taco Bell, and Kentucky Fried Chicken all added a variety of low-fat choices to their menus but found that, once on-site, their patrons were still ordering fries, burgers, full-fat burritos, or breaded and fried chicken. Paradoxically, the larger-portion items were selling better than the standard-sized versions of these foods. These chains have quietly been phasing out or significantly reducing their healthy menu options since early 1993.[7] For example, McDonald's replaced its McLean with a triple cheeseburger that has significantly more calories than the Big Mac. Kentucky Fried Chicken's skinless, roasted chicken was replaced by popcorn chicken, a breaded, deep-fried dish that has been breaking sales records.

Even diet-conscious diners who stick to heart-healthy menu choices can fall into calorie traps. A recent trip to an Olive Garden restaurant revealed that the pasta dishes on the heart healthy menu were large enough to feed three or four healthy hearts! Furthermore, they were accompanied by enough cheesy garlic breadsticks, soup or salad, to destroy anyone's best diet efforts. And Olive Garden is no exception. According to restaurant surveys conducted by the Center for Science in the Public Interest, most restaurants serve portions big enough for two to three people.[2]

Shrinking Your Serving Sizes

How can you make healthy choices when eating out? Putting into practice the American Dietetic Association's 1997 National Nutrition Month campaign theme "All Foods Can Fit" is one option.[7] This slogan is based on the idea that a balanced lifestyle can lead to a balanced body weight. Educating yourself about dietary balance and serving sizes is a first step. The FGP provides a pattern for overall dietary balance and even allows you to include small amounts of sweets and fatty

---

Typical Serving Sizes vs. USDA Food Guide Pyramid Official Serving Sizes

Food	Typical Serving Size and Number of Calories	Official Serving Size and Number of Calories
Popcorn	Movie theater serving (small) 7 cups—400 calories	3 cups—160 calories
Muffins	Restaurant serving ¼ lb. (4 oz)—430 calories	⅛ lb. (2 oz)—190 calories
French fries	McDonald's Super Size Fries 3 cups (6 oz)—540 calories	1½ cups (3 oz)—220 calories
Soft drinks	Can 1½ cups (12 oz)—140 calories 7-Eleven Double Gulp 8 cups (64 oz)—800 calories	1 cup (8 oz)—100 calories
Steak	Restaurant serving of sirloin steak About ½ lb. cooked 7 oz—410 calories	About ⅛ lb. cooked 3 oz—170 calories

A Rule of Thumb for Serving Sizes

Use the parts of your hand to estimate serving sizes when it's not possible or convenient to use a food scale or measuring cups and spoons.

1 thumb = 1 ounce of cheese

1 thumb tip = 1 teaspoon of foods such as mayonnaise, peanut butter, and sugar

3 thumb tips = 1 tablespoon

1 fist = 1 cup of pasta, rice, or vegetables

1 or 2 handfuls = 1 ounce of a snack food (1 handful of small foods, such as nuts, or 2 handfuls of larger foods, such as chips and pretzels)

1 palm (minus the fingers) = 3 ounces of meat, fish, or poultry

treats.[4] The FGP booklet supplies tables of food choices and serving size information. Learning to guesstimate sizes is also essential. You may need to use measuring cups and spoons and a food scale at home until you get the gist of it. A variety of mnemonic devices for estimating serving sizes are also available. The "Rule of Thumb for Serving Sizes" shown above is an easily learned, readily available approach. Other techniques include limiting meat servings to the size of a deck of cards or cassette tape, envisioning a tennis ball to estimate one-cup servings, and thinking of a one-half cup serving as the size of two Ping-Pong balls. Books featuring attractive photographs are available to assist parents and teachers in teaching children to recognize the sizes of portions of various types of food.[8]

Additional lifestyle changes may also be necessary. Learning to eat more slowly will allow you to feel satisfied with a smaller portion of food because your brain will have time to receive the signal that you have eaten. You should avoid other activities while eating so that you're fully aware of what and how much you're consuming. Dining out less frequently or dividing all restaurant portions in two and packaging up half before beginning to eat can also help. Accepting the fact that planned activity is an essential element of weight control and learning how much activity it takes to burn off a slice of cake is also important. Remember, there are 3,500 calories in a pound of body fat. Each mile you walk expends about 100 calories, so you would need to walk thirty-five miles to lose one pound of fat.

In essence, Americans can have their cake and eat it too, but it takes practice and persistence to become adept at balancing it all.

For Discussion . . .

What foods do you often consume in supersized portions? Would you be satisfied with smaller servings? Do you tend to order more courses and eat past the point of satiation when you dine in a restaurant because you're treating yourself or because you want to be sure to get your money's worth? What factors do you think are driving the "wellness backlash"?

References

1. Califano J. Nation's "supersize" trend leading to supersized people. *The New York Times* 1996 Nov 24: F8.
2. Liebman B, Hurley J. One size doesn't fit all. *Nutrition Action Healthletter* 1996; 23(9):10–12.
3. Mowma P. What will customers want in 1996 and beyond? *Restaurants USA* 1995 December: P35.
4. The Food Guide Pyramid. U.S. Department of Agriculture. *Home & Garden Bulletin* 1992; 232.
5. Critser, G. *Fat Land* New York: Houghton Mifflin Co. 2003.
6. National Restaurant Association. *Dining trends, 1996, quarterly reports.*
7. Woodburg R. The great fast-food pig-out. *Time* 1993; 141(26):51.
8. Hess MA. *Portion photos of popular foods.* Marketplace: The American Dietetic Association, 1997. **www .eatright.org/catalog**

personal assessment

how many calories do you need?

Resting Energy Requirement (RER)

Women

3–10 years 22.5 × weight (kg) + 499

10–18 years 12.2 × weight (kg) + 746

18–30 years 14.7 × weight (kg) + 496

30–60 years 08.7 × weight (kg) + 829

>60 years 10.5 × weight (kg) + 596

Men

3–10 years 22.7 × weight (kg) + 495

10–18 years 17.5 × weight (kg) + 651

18–30 years 15.3 × weight (kg) + 679

30–60 years 11.6 × weight (kg) + 879

>60 years 13.5 × weight (kg) + 487

Activity Energy Requirement (AER)

At bed rest: 1.20

Low activity (walking): 1.30

Average activity: 1.50–1.75

High activity: 2.0

Instructions: Calculate your resting energy requirement based on your sex, age, and weight. Then multiply your RER by your AER to determine how many calories you need each day to maintain your weight.

Example: Woman

    24 years

    120 lbs = 54.5 kg

    High activity

    (RER) × (AER) = Total Energy Requirement

    14.7 × 54.5 (kg) + 496 × 2.0 = 2594 calories/day

Note: 1 kg = 2.2 lbs.

Data from *Energy and protein requirements: report of a joint FAO/WHO/UNU expert consultation.* Technical Report Series 724. World Health Organization, 1985; Zeam FJ: *Clinical nutrition and dietetics,* 1991, Macmillan.

personal assessment

body love or body hate?

When you catch a glimpse of yourself in a mirror, do you smile at what you see or grimace? The following quiz will help you to assess your body self-esteem associated with your appearance. Please answer using the following rating scale:

1 = Rarely or never

2 = Sometimes

3 = Almost always or always

Add up your scores to determine your total score, and look at the summary below for an interpretation of your scores.

_____ 1. I worry about my weight and weighing "too much."

_____ 2. I prefer to eat by myself and not with other people.

_____ 3. My mood is determined by the scale and how I feel about my appearance.

_____ 4. I make negative comments about my appearance to myself and others.

_____ 5. I think I look less attractive on days that I haven't exercised.

_____ 6. I have a difficult time accepting compliments about my appearance from others.

_____ 7. I compare myself to other women and find myself lacking.

_____ 8. I ask other people how I look.

_____ 9. I avoid social situations, activities, and events involving food.

_____ 10. I feel more anxious about my body in the summertime because of the need to wear bathing suits and clothing suitable for warmer temperatures.

_____ **TOTAL SCORE**

Interpretation:

If you scored between 10 and 15, you have positive body self-esteem and are accepting of yourself and your appearance.

If you scored between 16 and 23, you scored in the average range. While you are in good company, feeling about your body the way most people do, you may want to reframe your body image and develop more of an appreciation for your body and appearance.

If your score was between 24 and 30, you have poor or low body self-esteem. Your self-esteem in general is probably driven by how you see yourself, and you may be putting too much emphasis on your appearance and are too self-critical. You may feel as though you never are thin enough or look good enough and can always find a flaw when looking in the mirror. In order to improve your body self-esteem, you need to focus on other aspects of yourself, focus on the positive aspects of your body, and be more accepting of yourself and less perfectionistic.

preventing drug abuse and dependence

Health educators have no doubt that the use, misuse, and abuse of many drugs can impair health. These substances not only alter the functioning of the body and mind but also affect the other dimensions of health. In Part Three, we take a look at addictive substances and their effects on the user.

1. **Physical Dimension**
   The effects of substance use, especially the long-term use of tobacco and alcohol, are well understood. These substances cause illness and death. Alcohol abuse can destroy the structure and function of many body systems. Tobacco use damages the cardiovascular system and the tissues of the respiratory tract and can cause cancer in many sites throughout the body. Chronic abuse of psychoactive drugs impairs many central nervous system functions. Even the experimental use of these drugs carries the danger of toxic overdose.

2. **Emotional Dimension**
   Because psychoactive drugs alter nervous system functioning, many users experience depression and mood swings. For people who are predisposed to enter dependent relationships, drug use can become an unhealthy way of relieving stress. When psychological dependence combines with physical dependence, the addict may begin to lose touch with reality.

3. **Social Dimension**
   Psychoactive drug use often takes place in social settings. For many people, drinking or using other drugs is a necessary first step toward enjoying the company of others. However, most people have little tolerance for inappropriate substance use, such as use of illegal drugs, excessive alcohol intake, and smoking in public places where tobacco use is banned.

4. **Intellectual Dimension**
   Intellectual impairment is one consequence of chemical abuse. People cannot perform well intellectually when they are feeling high or low or when their senses are dulled. Some people prefer to disregard information about the dangers of substance abuse, a choice that could prove extremely harmful to their health.

5. **Spiritual Dimension**
   Although drug use has long played a role in the religious practices of people throughout the world, the nonceremonial use of drugs conflicts with the principles of service to others. Substance abuse can hinder spiritual growth by turning a person's focus inward, making it impossible to develop the other-directedness that is essential to a rich spiritual life.

6. **Occupational Dimension**
   Use of both legal and illegal drugs clearly stands in the way of occupational health. Most workplaces are smoke-free, forcing smokers to stand outside or walk to the smoker's lounge to have a cigarette. These continual interruptions lower a worker's productivity. Illegal drug use can keep a job candidate from being hired, and use of illegal drugs or alcohol on the job can be dangerous and will certainly lower a worker's level of performance.

chapter seven

making decisions about drug use

Online Learning Center Resources

www.mhhe.com/payne8e

Log on to our Online Learning Center (OLC) for access to these additional resources:

- Chapter key terms and definitions
- Learning objectives
- Student interactive question-and-answer sites
- Self-scoring chapter quiz
- Online assessments
- Key term flash cards

Talking It Over

Legalization of Marijuana

Discussions about the legalization of marijuana frequently focus on the following points.

Pros:

1. Marijuana is a natural plant product.
2. People should be allowed to use or not use marijuana.
3. Many more harmful drugs than marijuana are available.
4. The government spends too much time, energy, and taxpayer money enforcing marijuana laws.
5. The "high" of marijuana is enjoyable, and harmless.

Cons:

1. The possession, use, and distribution of marijuana are illegal.
2. Marijuana use is related to several significant health concerns.
3. Marijuana is a gateway drug.
4. Marijuana use keeps certain users from undertaking productive activities.
5. In combination with other drugs or medicines, marijuana use is dangerous.

Where do you stand on this issue?

CommunicationLinks

www.samhsa.gov
www.drugfreeamerica.org

Eye on the Media

Do Media Scare Tactics Keep People from Using Drugs?

The media has tried to frighten people in many ways to keep them away from unhealthy behaviors. Bloody films showing the aftermath of a prom night car crash have been used to scare teenagers about dangerous drinking and driving behaviors. The late Frank Zappa, founder of the alternative music group the Mothers of Invention, warned young people in the early 1970s not to use stimulants (speed) because doing so would cause them "to turn out like your parents," a frightening thought for many counter-culture youth. More recently, television ads have featured celebrities speaking out against drug use.

Posters produced by both government and private health agencies have depicted cigarette smokers as filthy, wrinkled old men and women. Many of these posters are eye-catching in an almost humorous way. They grab the observer's attention and send the clear message that "this could happen to YOU." Advertisements for drug and alcohol rehabilitation facilities have shown alcoholics drowning in a sea of alcohol, drug users being confronted by their families, and employees caught by a drug screening test. The message is that miserable life situations can be changed if people are willing to get help.

It's difficult to measure the effectiveness of these approaches to drug prevention. Many people recall these media presentations, so they do make an impression. But, given the variables involved in drug-taking behavior—family influence, inherited predispositions, life events and situations, drug availability, and peer influence—it's impossible to pinpoint the influence of a single media event. These scare tactics seem to be especially effective among people who have already made the decision not to use drugs. They remind these people how dangerous it is to use drugs. For people who are thinking about starting

drug use, these messages may be beneficial, since they portray drug use in a negative light.

For hard-core drug users, though, it's unlikely that scare tactics will be effective. These people tend to lead chaotic lives, may never see the ads, and often remain in denial about their addiction. Nonusers and individuals leaning away from drug use are more likely to be influenced by this approach. Despite the fact that these ad campaigns are highly visible and costly, they seem to have only limited influence in drug prevention.

The use of psychoactive drugs can be tremendously disruptive in many people's lives, from causing tragic deaths to being the reason for the loss of employment opportunities (most Fortune 500 companies use preemployment drug testing), from promoting the deterioration of personal relationships to being the cause of babies born with profound birth defects. Perhaps realizing this, college students have generally moved away from using the most dangerous illegal drugs.

It is safe to say that drug use remains a significant problem for both college students and the general population. Alcohol is the most important problem drug for most college students (see Chapter 8), but other drugs pose risks for certain students (Table 7.1). Additionally, many nontraditional-age students see the destructive effects of drug use on their neighborhoods and worry about their children being exploited by drug dealers.

Prevention: The Best Solution

We combat the drug problem in the United States on two fronts: the demand side and the supply side. The United States government attempts to reduce the supply of illegal (illicit) drugs through drug interdiction efforts at our borders, through joint efforts with countries such as Mexico and Colombia, and through law-enforcement measures within our own borders.

However, the best way to avoid the immense costs of drug abuse is simply to reduce the demand. We do this by helping people develop the tools needed to avoid the use of illegal drugs (see the Changing for the Better box on page 226). Experts are currently mounting prevention efforts on three levels: primary, secondary, and tertiary. Take a look at each of these three levels. Which level is most familiar to you?

Primary Prevention

Primary prevention means reaching people who have not yet used drugs and reducing their desire to try drugs.

Table 7.1 Annual Prevalence among College Students: Alcohol and Other Drugs

Drug	% Students Using Drug 1 or More Times
Tobacco	46.5
Alcohol	85.3
Marijuana	36.4
Cocaine	5.1
Amphetamines	8.5
Sedatives	4.4
Hallucinogens	6.3
Opiates	2.7
Inhalants	2.2
Designer drugs	9.1
Steroids	0.9
Other	2.5

Note: Statistics were drawn from a sample of 54,444 college students from 131 two- and four-year colleges in the United States in 2001.
Source: CORE Institute: Center for Alcohol and Other Drug Studies. *American Campuses: 2001 Statistics on Alcohol and Other Drug Use.* Southern Illinois University at Carbondale (online). **www.siu.edu/departments/coreinst/public_html/2000.html** accessed 22 May 2003.

Key Terms

primary prevention measures intended to deter first-time drug use.

It's tempting to reach for a pill when I feel down, but I don't want to get into that habit. What can I do to improve my mood without using drugs?

Talk with a trusted friend. Confide your feelings to a close, trusted friend or family member. By opening up to another person, you'll gain insights into how you can get beyond your negative feelings without resorting to drug use.

Get moving. Go for a walk, ride your bike, or swim a few laps. Physical activity is a natural way to enhance your mood. Nearly every college provides recreation programs such as aerobics, swimming, dancing, or weight lifting.

Give yourself a break. If you're tired, take a quick power nap. If you're overworked, set aside some personal time—just for yourself. Read, watch TV, surf the net, or phone an old friend. Decide what you like to do, and then do it. You'll return to your responsibilities with renewed enthusiasm.

Do volunteer work. One way to feel good is to help others. Teach reading to adults, become a Big Brother or Big Sister, work in a soup kitchen, or drive a van for the elderly in your community.

Reexamine your spiritual health. Many people find comfort by making connections to their spiritual life. Through activities such as meditation, spiritual reflection, and renewal of faith, people often gain reassurance and a sense of calmness.

Restructure your daily activities. If you have one hectic day after another but feel as though you're not accomplishing anything, try reorganizing your daily activities. Experiment with new patterns. Plan to get sufficient sleep, eat regular meals, and set aside specific times for work, family activities, and pleasure. Find out what works best for you.

Seek professional guidance. If you've tried these strategies but your mood still isn't improving, consider seeking professional help. This important first step is up to you. Visit your college health center or counseling center, and talk with people who are trained to help you learn how to become a happier person.

Primary prevention programs can target individuals, families, peer groups, neighborhoods, schools, workplaces, colleges, and the community. The key to primary prevention is to keep potential users from starting to use drugs.[1]

Secondary Prevention

Secondary prevention targets those who are beginning to experiment with drugs and uses detection, screening, intervention, and treatment of early drug abuse to help avoid further drug use. These programs do not prevent initial drug use but instead involve detection and early treatment of drug problems before they become severe. Popular methods include crisis telephone hotlines, peer counseling, individual and family counseling, school and worksite drug screening programs, and student and employee assistance programs.[1]

Tertiary Prevention

Tertiary prevention (third-level prevention) targets drug-dependent people, such as cocaine abusers, heroin addicts, or alcoholics. These individuals require specialized, intensive help that includes rehabilitation and maintenance. Such intensive treatments may require temporary hospitalization. Additional treatment methods include intensive outpatient care, support groups, and after-care programs. Relapse prevention is designed to help people recovering from drug abuse maintain their drug-free lifestyles.[1]

Effects of Drugs on the Central Nervous System

To better understand the disruption caused by the actions of psychoactive drugs, a general knowledge of the normal functioning of the nervous system's basic unit, the **neuron,** is required.

Key Terms

secondary prevention measures aimed at early detection, intervention, and treatment of drug abuse before severe physical, psychological, emotional, or social consequences can occur.

tertiary prevention treatment and rehabilitation of drug-dependent people to limit physical, psychological, emotional, and social deterioration or prevent death.

neuron a nerve cell.

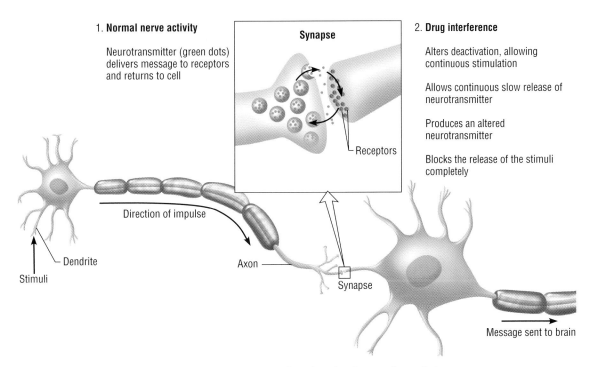

1. Normal nerve activity

Neurotransmitter (green dots) delivers message to receptors and returns to cell

Synapse

Receptors

2. Drug interference

Alters deactivation, allowing continuous stimulation

Allows continuous slow release of neurotransmitter

Produces an altered neurotransmitter

Blocks the release of the stimuli completely

Direction of impulse

Dendrite

Stimuli

Axon

Synapse

Message sent to brain

Figure 7-1 This illustration depicts the disruption caused by the action of psychoactive drugs on the central nervous system. Neurotransmitters are chemical messengers that transfer electrical impulses across the synapses between nerve cells. Psychoactive drugs interrupt this process, thus disrupting the normal functioning of the nervous system.

First, stimuli from the internal or external environment are received by the appropriate sensory receptor, perhaps an organ such as an eye or an ear. Once sensed, these stimuli are converted into electrical impulses. These impulses are then directed along the neuron's **dendrite,** through the cell body, and along the **axon** toward the synaptic junction near an adjacent neuron.[2] On arrival at the **synapse,** the electrical impulses stimulate the production and release of chemical messengers called **neurotransmitters.** These neurotransmitters transmit the electrical impulses from one neuron to the dendrites of adjoining neurons. Thus neurons function in a coordinated fashion to send information to the brain for interpretation and to relay appropriate response commands outward to the tissues of the body.

The role of neurotransmitters is critically important to the relay of information within the system. A substance that has the ability to alter some aspect of neurotransmitter function has the potential to seriously disrupt the otherwise normally functioning system. Psychoactive drugs are capable of exerting these disruptive influences on the neurotransmitters. Drugs "work" by changing the way neurotransmitters work, often by blocking the production of a neurotransmitter or forcing the continued release of a neurotransmitter (see Figure 7-1).

Addictive Behavior

This chapter explores the health consequences of drug use, misuse, and abuse. Before we talk about specific drugs, however, drug use should be put in the broader context of addictive behavior. Experts in human behavior

---

Key Terms

dendrite the portion of a neuron that receives electrical stimuli from adjacent neurons; neurons typically have several such branches or extensions.

axon the portion of a neuron that conducts electrical impulses to the dendrites of adjacent neurons; neurons typically have one axon.

synapse (**sinn** aps) the location at which an electrical impulse from one neuron is transmitted to an adjacent neuron; also referred to as a *synaptic junction.*

neurotransmitters chemical messengers that transfer electrical impulses across the synapses between nerve cells.

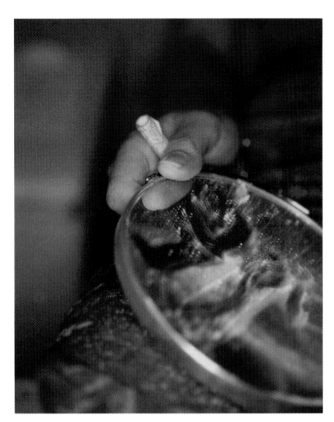

Drug use of all types remains a significant problem in our society today.

temporarily replaces an unpleasant feeling or sensation. This initial pleasure gradually (or in some cases quickly) becomes a focal point in the person's life.

Compulsion

Increasingly more energy, time, and money are spent pursuing the drug use or behavior. At this point in the addictive process, the person can be said to have a compulsion for the drug or behavior. Frequently, repeated exposure to the drug or behavior continues despite negative consequences, such as the gradual loss of family and friends, unpleasant physical symptoms after taking the drug, and problems at work.

During the compulsion phase of the addictive behavior, a person's "normal" life often degenerates while she or he searches for increased pleasures from the drug or the behavior. An addicted person's family life, circle of friends, work, or study patterns become less important than the search for more and better "highs." The development of tolerance and withdrawal are distinct possibilities. (These terms are discussed later in the chapter.)

Why some people develop compulsions and others do not is difficult to pinpoint, but addiction might be influenced by genetic makeup, family dynamics, physiological processes, personality type, peer groups, and available resources for help.

Loss of Control

Over time, the search for highs changes to a desire to avoid the effects of withdrawal from the drug or behavior. Addicted people lose their ability to control their behavior. Despite overwhelming negative consequences (for example, deterioration of health, alienation of family and friends, or loss of all financial resources), addicted people continue to behave in ways that make their lives worse. The person addicted to alcohol continues to drink heavily, the person addicted to shopping continues to run up heavy debts, and the person addicted to food continues to eat indiscriminately. This behavior reflects a loss of control over one's life. Frequently, a person has addictions to more than one drug or behavior.

view drug use and abuse as just one of the many forms of addictive behavior. Addictive behavior includes addictions to shopping, eating, gambling, sex, television, video games, Internet use, or work, as well as addictions to alcohol or other drugs.

 TALKING POINTS How would you approach a friend and tell him he has a gambling addiction that needs to be controlled?

The Process of Addiction

The process of developing an addiction has been a much-studied topic. Addictive behavior seems to have three common aspects: exposure, compulsion, and loss of control.

Exposure

An addiction can begin after a person is exposed to a drug (such as alcohol) or a behavior (such as gambling) that he or she finds pleasurable. Perhaps this drug or behavior

Intervention and Treatment

The good news for people with addictions is that help is available. Within the last two decades, much attention has been focused on intervention and treatment for addictive behavior. Many people can be helped through programs such as those described at the end of this chapter. These programs often include inpatient or outpatient treatment, family counseling, and long-term aftercare counseling.

It is common for people in aftercare treatment for addictive behavior to belong to a self-help support

Making Social Connections without Drugs

According to many college and university drug counselors, students who undergo drug counseling often say that they started (or continued) to use drugs because they felt inadequate in social situations. These students believed that they were not attractive, talented, wealthy, or socially skilled enough to start and maintain relationships. In a dating situation, the drug allowed them to be more relaxed and less conscious of their perceived shortcomings. Then, if they did something foolish while socializing, they had an instant excuse—the drug made them act inappropriately.

What are some drug-free strategies you can use to enhance your social relationships? Start by finding people and activities that are free of drug use. Contrary to popular opinion, most college students do not use illegal drugs. More students than ever are supportive of a drug-free lifestyle, so it shouldn't be difficult to find individuals and groups who will be a good match for you. Be aware of all the people around you. Don't get locked into one group too quickly. Keep your options open.

As you explore your inner self and try to connect with people at a deeper level, also consider these approaches:

Be true to yourself. Most people like someone who is genuine, so try to be the person you know yourself to be. Don't present a false image of yourself to others.

Be a good listener. One sure way to discourage a growing relationship is to talk more than you listen. Show others that you're interested in them by hearing what they have to say. Let the other person be the center of attention, at least early in the relationship. By listening carefully, you can evaluate the person or group better and see if you're a good fit.

Be open to new people and ideas. It's good to have firm opinions and ideas, but it's also important to be open to new people and ideas. Take the attitude that the next person you meet or the next group you interact with may change your life forever. Don't limit yourself to a particular group of people or friends. Flexibility can be a real asset to your social life.

Be willing to laugh at yourself. Most surveys indicate that people rate humor as an important quality in people they want to date. Try to find humor in everyday situations. Focusing on the lighter side will make things easier for you and the people around you. Most important—be willing to laugh at yourself sometimes.

Be prepared for setbacks. One sign of social maturity is to recognize that setbacks can happen. Don't be defeated by them. Sometimes it's best for everyone involved when things don't work out. You'll always have another opportunity. Focus on the attitude that things will get better. Don't give in to the idea that drugs will make up for an unsatisfying social life. Seek professional help if things do not improve after a reasonable time.

---

group, such as Alcoholics Anonymous, Gamblers Anonymous, or Sex Addicts Anonymous. These groups are often listed in the phone book or in the classified ads section of the newspaper.

Codependence

With all the focus placed on the person with a drug problem, often the families and loved ones of the addict do not receive the attention and help they need. You may already be familiar with the term *codependent,* but you might have assumed that this term applies only to those close to an alcoholic. In fact, this term can apply to anyone who is close to an individual addicted to any type of behavior, including addiction to drugs, sex, gambling, or other behaviors.

Codependent people typically become unaware of their own feelings, needs, and boundaries in their preoccupation with the addicted individual. They become focused on protecting or coping with the addict and often lose their own sense of identity. This stress often results in chaotic behaviors, addictions, and physical illnesses in the codependent person.

Private and public programs are also available to help the codependent person learn new behaviors. See Chapter 8 for more information about codependent behavior and resources.

Drug Terminology

Before examining drug actions or drug behavior, you must first be familiar with some basic terminology. Much of this terminology originates in the field of pharmacology, or the study of the interaction of chemical agents with living material.

What does the word **drug** mean? Each of us may have different ideas about what a drug is. Although a

> **Key Terms**
>
> **drug** any substance, natural or artificial, other than food, that by its chemical or physical nature alters structure or function in the living organism.

number of definitions are available, we will consider a drug to be "any substance, natural or artificial, other than food, that by its chemical or physical nature alters structure or function in the living organism."[3] Included in this broad definition is a variety of psychoactive drugs, medicines, and substances that many people do not usually consider to be drugs.

Psychoactive drugs alter the user's feelings, behavior, perceptions, or moods when using stimulants, depressants, hallucinogens, opiates, or inhalants. Prescribed medications function to heal unhealthy tissue as well as ease pain, prevent illness, and diagnose health conditions. Although some psychoactive drugs are used for medical reasons, as in the case of tranquilizers and some narcotics, the most commonly prescribed medicines are antibiotics, hormone replacement drugs, sulfa drugs, diuretics, oral contraceptives, and cardiovascular drugs. Legal substances not usually considered to be drugs (which certainly are drugs) include caffeine, tobacco, alcohol, aspirin, and other over-the-counter (OTC) drugs. These common substances are used so frequently in our society that they are rarely perceived as true drugs.

For organizational reasons, this chapter primarily deals with psychoactive drugs. Alcohol is covered in Chapter 8. The effects of tobacco are delineated in Chapter 9. Prescription and OTC drugs and medicines are discussed at length in Chapter 18. Anabolic steroids, drugs used primarily for increasing muscle growth, are discussed in Chapter 4.

Dependence

Psychoactive drugs have a strong potential for the development of **dependence.** In this chapter the term **addiction** is used interchangeably with physical dependence. When users take a psychoactive drug, the patterns of nervous system function are altered. If these altered functions provide perceived benefits for the user, drug use may continue, perhaps at increasingly larger dosages. If persistent use continues, the user can develop a dependence on the drug. Pharmacologists have identified two types of dependencies—physical and psychological.

A person can be said to have developed a *physical dependence* when the body cells have become reliant on a drug. Continued use of the drug is then required because body tissues have adapted to its presence.[4] The person's body needs the drug to maintain homeostasis, or dynamic balance. If the drug is not taken or is suddenly withdrawn, the user develops a characteristic **withdrawal illness.** The symptoms of withdrawal reflect the attempt by the body's cells to regain normality without the drug. Withdrawal symptoms are always unpleasant (ranging from mild to severe irritability, depression, nervousness, digestive difficulties, and abdominal pain) and can be life threatening, as in the case of abrupt withdrawal from barbiturates or alcohol.

Continued use of most drugs can lead to **tolerance.** Tolerance is an acquired reaction to a drug in which continued intake of the same dose has diminishing effects.[4] The user needs larger doses of the drug to receive previously felt sensations. The continued use of depressants, including alcohol, and opiates can cause users to quickly develop a tolerance to the drug.

 TALKING POINTS You're out with your friends and they decide to compete to see who can drink the most beer. How would you tell them that what they are doing is dangerous without sounding like a parent?

Tolerance developed for one drug may carry over to another drug within the same general category. This phenomenon is known as **cross-tolerance.** The heavy abuser of alcohol, for example, might require a larger dose of a preoperative sedative to become relaxed before surgery than the average person would. The tolerance to alcohol "crosses over" to the other depressant drugs.

A person who possesses a strong desire to continue using a particular drug is said to have developed *psychological dependence.* People who are psychologically dependent on a drug believe that they need to consume the drug to maintain a sense of well-being (see the Discovering Your Spirituality box on page 229). They crave the drug for emotional reasons despite having persistent or recurrent physical, social, psychological, or occupational problems that are caused or worsened by the drug use. Abrupt withdrawal from a drug by such a person would not trigger the fully expressed withdrawal illness, although some unpleasant symptoms of withdrawal might be felt. The term *habituation* is often used interchangeably with the term *psychological dependence.*

Drugs whose continued use can quickly lead to both physical and psychological dependence are depressants (barbiturates, tranquilizers, and alcohol), narcotics (the opiates, which are derivatives of the Oriental poppy: heroin, morphine, and codeine), and synthetic narcotics (Demerol and methadone). Drugs whose continued use can lead to various degrees of psychological dependence and occasionally to significant (but not life-threatening) physical dependence in some users are the stimulants (amphetamines, caffeine [see the Focus On article on pages 251–253], and cocaine), hallucinogens (LSD, peyote, mescaline, and marijuana), and inhalants (glues, gases, and petroleum products).

Drug Misuse and Abuse

So far in this chapter we have used the term *use* (or *user*) in association with the taking of psychoactive drugs. At this point, however, it is important to define *use* and to introduce the terms *misuse* and *abuse.*[3] By doing so, we can more accurately describe how drugs are used.

The term *use* is all-encompassing and describes drug-taking in the most general way. For example, Americans use drugs of many types. The term *use* can also refer more narrowly to misuse and abuse. We often use the word in this latter regard.

The term **misuse** refers to the inappropriate use of legal drugs intended to be medications. Misuse may occur when a patient misunderstands the directions for use of a prescription or OTC drug or when a patient shares a prescription with a friend or family member for whom the drug was not prescribed. Misuse also occurs when a patient takes the prescription or OTC drug for a purpose or condition other than that for which it was intended or at a dosage other than that recommended.

The term **abuse** applies to any use of an illegal drug or any use of a legal drug when it is detrimental to health and well-being. The costs of drug abuse to the individual are extensive and include absenteeism and underachievement, loss of job, marital instability, loss of self-esteem, serious illnesses, and even death. Complete the Personal Assessment on page 255 to test your drug awareness.

Dynamics of Drug Abuse

Many factors influence drug-taking behavior, including individual factors, immediate environmental factors, and societal factors. Specific aspects of each are discussed in the following sections.

Individual Factors

Genetic predisposition, personality traits, attitudes and beliefs, interpersonal skills, and unmet developmental needs can lead to drug use.

Genetic Predisposition

The importance of genetic predisposition (inherited vulnerability) to drug use has not been fully determined. However, studies of alcoholics have demonstrated that genetic factors do play some role in the development of alcoholism. Research on genetic predisposition to the abuse of other drugs is much farther behind than for alcohol abuse.

Personality Traits, Attitudes, and Beliefs

Although drug-taking behavior cannot be predicted strictly on the basis of personality type, correlations have

---

Key Terms

misuse the inappropriate use of legal drugs intended to be medications.

abuse any use of a legal or illegal drug in a way that is detrimental to health or well-being.

been noted with certain aspects of personality (or temperament). For example, children who are easily bored and need continual activity and challenge are more likely to take drugs when they are older. A similar tendency is seen in children who are driven to avoid negative consequences for their actions and who crave immediate external reward for their efforts. Clusters of traits (as measured by personality inventories), including rebelliousness, rejection of behavioral norms, resistance to authority, and high tolerance for deviance, are also reported in drug abusers.

However, a cause-and-effect relationship between personality profile and drug abuse is difficult to prove. Perhaps the abuse of drugs actually creates the personality traits, rather than the other way around.

Interpersonal Skills and Self-Esteem

Drug abusers are usually deficient in interpersonal skills. They are likely to score lower on tests that measure well-being, tolerance of others, and achievement. They also often have lower self-esteem than do those who do not abuse drugs. Again, the question of cause and effect must be raised.

Personal development results from success in daily living. When people lack positive experiences in school, employment, parenting, and varied aspects of community involvement, they may attempt to compensate through chronic heavy drug use. Of course, drug abuse removes them further from productive and satisfying growth and development, thus increasing the desire for the compensatory use of drugs.

Environmental Factors

Drug use can be fostered by factors within the immediate environment, which includes home and family, school, peers, and the community.

Home and Family

Drug abuse that begins in childhood is often associated with the home and family.[4] Children seem to be at greater risk when parents exhibit poor management skills, antisocial behavior, and even criminality. These families are often disorganized and have poorly defined roles for parenting and being a productive member of society. In many cases, adult family members abuse drugs themselves or tolerate those who do. As with tobacco use, parents can be the best or worst models children can have. The Star box above explores the family environment in greater detail.

School

Children from disorganized or socially maladjusted families often have difficulty adjusting to the organized environment of the school. The following chain of events has been suggested to explain the relationship of a poor home environment and weak academic performance to drug abuse: An undesirable home environment contributes to poor school performance and poor social development; failure at school leads to loss of self-esteem, aggressive behavior, and loss of interest in school; these factors in turn may foster truancy and drug experimentation.

Peers

A clear relationship exists between peer group drug abuse and drug abuse among individual members. It is unusual for a student to remain an active member of a peer group and abstain from drug use while other members abuse drugs. The pressure to "join in" is just too powerful to resist.

Community

Drug availability, drug education, and drug treatment and rehabilitation vary among communities. As a result, drug abuse rates differ from one community to another. Students who are parents may be interested in the degree to which their communities foster or deter drug abuse.

Societal Factors

Factors such as the existence of a youth subculture, modeling and advertising, and the self-care movement affect drug use.

Youth Subculture

For many reasons, a distinctive youth subculture exists in the United States. It comprises people from 12 to 17 years of age. This subculture has its own expectations, roles, and standards, and its own language, dress code, and behaviors.

Many people assume that the rate of drug abuse is higher in this group than in any other segment of American society. However, this belief is not supported by research. A recent study indicates that a higher rate of drug abuse occurs among 18- to 20-year-olds.[5] Nevertheless, the drug abuse that does occur among those in the younger age group is of concern because patterns that are established at an early age can carry over into later life. In fact, during this period, experimentation with a **gateway drug** (alcohol, nicotine, or marijuana) often begins, which may lead to heavier drug use later.[3]

Modeling and Advertising

The influence others have on us by example of their own behavior is called *modeling*. Modeling of drug use within the peer group and family has already been presented. However, movie stars, musicians, and athletes also serve as models of behavior. Their example exerts a powerful influence on children and adolescents.

When models are employed by the media to sell products, advertising becomes an important factor in fostering drug use. The marketing of tobacco and alcohol products is perhaps the best example. "Beautiful people" are depicted enjoying a social drug, such as alcohol, coffee, tea, or tobacco, in opulent surroundings that most viewers can only dream of being in. Celebrities participate in events sponsored by alcohol or tobacco companies.

The Self-Care Movement

People's ability to engage in medical self-care makes drug use easier and more socially acceptable than in the past. In a society conditioned by the effectiveness and availability of OTC and prescription medications, the use of other drugs, both legal and illegal, to make ourselves feel better seems more reasonable than ever before. This attitude, then, fosters drug misuse and, for some, drug abuse.

Combination Drug Effects

Drugs taken in various combinations and dosages can alter and perhaps intensify effects.

A **synergistic effect** is a dangerous consequence of taking different drugs in the same general category at the same time. The combination exaggerates each individual drug's effects. For example, the combined use of alcohol and tranquilizers produces a synergistic effect greater than the total effect of each of the two drugs taken separately. In this instance, a much-amplified, perhaps fatal sedation will occur. In a simplistic sense, "one plus one equals four or five."

When taken at or near the same time, drug combinations produce a variety of effects. Drug combinations have additive, potentiating, or antagonistic effects. When two or more drugs are taken and the result is merely a combined total effect of each drug, the result is an **additive effect.** The sum of the effects is not exaggerated. In a sense, "one plus one plus one equals three."

When one drug intensifies the action of a second drug, the first drug is said to have a **potentiated effect** on the second drug. One popular drug-taking practice during the 1970s was the consumption of Quaaludes and

---

Key Terms

gateway drug an easily obtainable legal or illegal drug that represents a user's first experience with a mind-altering drug; this drug can serve as the "gateway" to the use of other drugs.

synergistic effect a heightened, exaggerated effect produced by the concurrent use of two or more drugs.

additive effect the combined (but not exaggerated) effect produced by the concurrent use of two or more drugs.

potentiated effect a phenomenon whereby the use of one drug intensifies the effect of a second drug.

"Club Drugs"

Within the last decade, increasing numbers of so-called "club drugs" are being used by young adults at all-night dance parties called "trances" or "raves," bars, and dance clubs. Among these club drugs are ones already described in this chapter such as MDMA (Ecstasy), Rohypnol, methamphetamine, and LSD. According to research studies supported by the National Institute on Drug Abuse (NIDA), the use of club drugs can cause serious health problems and even death.* When club drugs are taken in combination with alcohol, dangerous consequences are even more likely to happen.

Two additional club drugs are GHB (gamma-hydroxybutyrate) and ketamine. GHB is a club drug frequently used in combination with alcohol. Also known as Grievous Bodily Harm, G, Liquid Ecstasy, or Georgia Home Boy, GHB comes in various forms: a clear liquid, a white powder, a tablet, or a capsule. GHB has become increasingly connected to poisonings, overdoses, date rapes, and fatalities. Frequently manufactured in homes with recipes and ingredients found on the Internet, GHB is usually abused for its intoxicating/sedative/euphoriant effects or for its ability to release growth hormone and help build muscles.

GHB is a central nervous system depressant. Like all depressants, GHB relieves anxiety and produces relaxation at low dosages. The intoxicating effects of GHB begin 10 to 20 minutes after the drug is ingested and last up to 4 hours, depending on the dose. At higher doses, GHB slows breathing and heart rate, produces sleep and eventually causes coma and death. GHB is cleared rather rapidly from the body, so it can be difficult to detect in treatment facilities and emergency rooms.

Ketamine (also known as Special K, K, Vitamin K, or Cat Valiums) is an injectable anesthetic that has been approved for use on animals and humans since 1970. Approximately 90 percent of the ketamine sold legally in the United States is for veterinary use. This drug is produced in liquid form or as a white powder. The powder can be snorted through the nostrils or smoked with tobacco products or marijuana. At low dosages, ketamine produces an intoxication that results in impaired attention, memory, and learning ability. At higher dosages, ketamine produces delirium, amnesia, and impaired motor functioning.

In the 1980s, ketamine rose in popularity because of its perceived ability to produce dreamlike states and hallucinations when used in high doses. The sensations were similar to those produced by phencylidine (PCP). However, ketamine is known to cause high blood pressure, depression, and potentially fatal respiratory problems. Clearly, ketamine is not a safe drug.

The National Institute on Drug Abuse (NIDA) has taken concerns about club drugs so seriously that it has started a website to provide the latest scientific findings on club drugs: **www.clubdrugs.org.** NIDA hopes that it can facilitate the development of treatment and prevention strategies that are specifically aimed at the populations of young persons who abuse club drugs.

*National Institute on Drug Abuse. *Club drugs: community drug alert bulletin: some facts about club drugs.* **www.clubdrugs.org** accessed 22 May 2003.

---

beer. Quaaludes potentiated the inhibition-releasing, sedative effects of alcohol. This particular drug combination produced an inexpensive but potentially fatal drunklike euphoria in the user. More recently, the combined use of various "**club drugs**" results in unpredictable potentiated drug effects (see the Star box above).

An **antagonistic effect,** on the other hand, is a drug's action in reducing another drug's effects. Knowledge of this principle has been useful in the medical treatment of certain drug overdoses, as in the use of tranquilizers to relieve the effects of LSD or other hallucinogenic drugs.

Because of these possible synergistic drug effects, patients should always inform their doctors and dentists of any illegal drugs they have taken.

Drug Classifications

Drugs can be categorized according to the nature of their physiological effects. Most psychoactive drugs fall into one of six general categories: stimulants, depressants, hallucinogens, cannabis, narcotics, and inhalants (Table 7.2).

Stimulants

In general, **stimulants** excite or increase the activity of the CNS. Also called "uppers," stimulants alert the CNS by increasing heart rate, blood pressure, and the rate of brain function. Users feel uplifted and less fatigued. Examples of stimulant drugs include caffeine, amphetamines, and cocaine. Most stimulants produce psychological dependence and tolerance relatively quickly, but they are unlikely

> ### Key Terms
>
> **club drug** one of a variety of psychoactive drugs typically used at raves, bars, and dance clubs.
>
> **antagonistic effect** the effect produced when one drug reduces or offsets the effects of a second drug.
>
> **stimulants** psychoactive drugs that stimulate the function of the central nervous system.

Table 7.2 Psychoactive Drug Categories

Drugs	Trade or Common Names	Medical Uses	Possible Effects
Stimulants			
Cocaine*	Coke, crack, gin, girlfriend, girl, double bubble, California cornflakes, caballo, bouncing powder, flake, snow	Local anesthetic	Increased alertness, excitation, euphoria, increased pulse rate and blood pressure, insomnia, loss of appetite
Amphetamines	Biphetamine, Delcobese, Desoxyn, Dexedrine, mediatric, methamphetamine (ice), black Mollies, aimies, amps, bam, beans, benz	Hyperactivity, narcolepsy, weight control	
Phendimetrazine	Prelu-2		
Methylphenidate	Ritalin, Methidate		
Other stimulants	Adipex, Bacarate, Cylert, Didrex, Ionamin, Plegine, PreSate, Sanorex, Tenuate, Tepanil, Voranil, ephedra		
Depressants			
Chloral hydrate	Noctec, Somnos	Hypnotic	Slurred speech, disorientation, drunken behavior without odor of alcohol
Barbiturates	Amobarbital, Butisol, phenobarbital, phenoxbarbital, secobarbital, Tuinal, blockbusters, black bombers, blue devils, blue dogs, blue tips, tombica	Anesthetic, anticonvulsant, sedative, hypnotic	
Glutethimide	Doriden	Sedative, hypnotic	
Methaqualone	Optimil, Parest, Quaalude, Somnafec, Sopor	Sedative, hypnotic	
Benzodiazepines	Ativan, Azene, Clonopin, Dalmane, diazepam, Librium, Serax, Tranxene, Valium, Verstran	Antianxiety, anticonvulsant, sedative, hypnotic	
GHB	Gamma-hydroxybutyrate (G, Liquid ecstacy, Georgia Home Boy)[1]	None	Unconsciousness, seizures, amnesia, vomiting, coma
Other depressants	Equanil, Miltown, Noludar, Placidyl, Valmid	Antianxiety, sedative, hypnotic	
Hallucinogens			
LSD	Acid, microdot, brown dot, cap, California sunshine, brown bomber	None	Delusions and hallucinations, poor perception of time and distance
Mescaline and peyote	Mesc, buttons, cactus, chief	None	
Amphetamine variants (designer drugs)	2,5-DMA, DOM, DOP, MDA, MDMA, PMA, STP, TMA, clarity, chocolate chips, booty juice	None	
Phencyclidine	Angel dust, hog, PCP, AD, boat, black whack, amoeba, angel hair, angel smoke	Veterinary anesthetic	
Phencyclidine analogs	PCE, PCPy, TCP	None	Euphoria, relaxed inhibitions, increased appetite, disorientation
Other hallucinogens	Bufotenin, DMT, DET, ibogaine, psilocybin, psilocyn	None	
Cannabis			
Marijuana	Acapulco gold, black Bart, black mote, blue sage, bobo, butterflowers, cannabis-T, cess, cheeba, grass, pot, sinsemilla, Thai sticks	Under investigation	Euphoria, relaxed inhibitions, increased appetite, disoriented behavior
Tetrahydrocannabinol	THC	Under investigation	
Hashish	Hash	None	
Hashish oil	Hash oil	None	
Narcotics			
Opium	Dover's powder, paregoric, Parapectolin, cruz, Chinese tobacco, China	Analgesic, antidiarrheal	Euphoria, drowsiness, respiratory depression, constricted pupils, nausea
Morphine	Morphine, Pectoal syrup, emsel, first line	Analgesic, antitussive	
Codeine	Codeine, Empirin compound with codeine, Robitussin A–C	Analgesic, antitussive	
Heroin	Diacetylmorphine, horse, smack, courage pills, dead on arrival (DOA)	Under investigation	
Hydromorphone	Dilaudid	Analgesic	Intoxication, excitation, disorientation, aggression, hallucination
Meperidine (pethidine)	Demerol, Pethadol	Analgesic	
Methadone	Dolophine, Methadone, Methadose	Analgesic, heroin substitute	
Other narcotics	Darvon,[†] Dromoran, Fentanyl, LAAM, Leitine, Levo-Dromoran, Percodan, Tussionex, Talwin,[†] Lomotil	Analgesic, antidiarrheal, antitussive	
Inhalants			
Anesthetic gases	Aerosols, petroleum products, solvents	Surgical anesthetic	Intoxication, excitation, disorientation, aggression, hallucination, variable effects
Vasodilators (amyl nitrile, butyl nitrite)	Aerosols, petroleum products, solvents	None	

*Designated a narcotic under the Controlled Substances Act.
[†]Not designated a narcotic under the Controlled Substances Act.
[1]Project GHB. What is GHB? **www.projectghb.org/what_is_ghb.htm** accessed 15 May 2003.

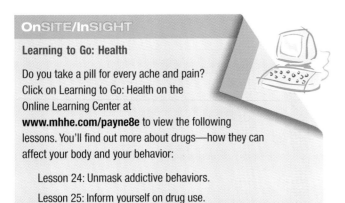
to produce significant physical dependence when judged by life-threatening withdrawal symptoms. The important exception is cocaine, which seems to be capable of producing psychological dependence and withdrawal so powerful that continued use of the drug is inevitable in some users.

Caffeine

The methylxanthines are a family of chemicals that includes three compounds: caffeine, theophylline, and theobromine. Of these, caffeine is the most heavily consumed.

Caffeine is a tasteless drug found in coffee, tea, chocolate, many soft drinks, and several groups of over-the-counter drugs. It is a relatively harmless CNS stimulant when consumed in moderate amounts. Many coffee drinkers believe that they cannot start the day successfully without the benefit of a cup or two of coffee.

The chronic effects of long-term caffeine use are less clear. Chronic users show evidence of tolerance and withdrawal, indicating that they are physically dependent. Researchers have attempted to link caffeine to coronary heart disease, pancreatic cancer, and fibrocystic breast disease. So far, the results have been inconclusive, or, in some cases, inconsistent with those of other studies.

For the average healthy adult, moderate consumption of caffeine is unlikely to pose any serious health threat. However, excessive consumption (equivalent to eight or more cups of coffee daily) could lead to anxiety, diarrhea, restlessness, delayed onset of sleep or frequent awakening, headache, and heart palpitations. Pregnant women are advised to use caffeine sparingly.

Do you use caffeine to help you meet the demands of your daily life? Are you overly dependent on caffeine? For a closer look at caffeine and tips on curtailing excessive use, see Focus On article on pages 251–253.

Ephedra

Health professionals are warning people about the dangers of using any over-the-counter herbal supplement containing ephedra. Also known as *ma huang,* ephedra is an amphetaminelike drug which provides benefits to consumers who need to lose weight but[6] can be especially dangerous for people with hypertension or other cardiovascular disease. Presently, ephedra is used in many over-the-counter decongestants and asthma drugs warning consumers with labels indicating possible harmful side effects and drug interactions. At the time of this writing some states were banning ephedra as a weight control aid.[7]

Amphetamines

Amphetamines produce increased activity and mood elevation in almost all users. The amphetamines include several closely related compounds: amphetamine, dextroamphetamine, and methamphetamine. These compounds do not have any natural sources and are completely manufactured in the laboratory. Medical use of amphetamines is limited primarily to the treatment of obesity, **narcolepsy,** and **attention deficit hyperactivity disorder (ADHD).**

Amphetamines can be ingested, injected, or snorted (inhaled). At low-to-moderate doses, amphetamines elevate mood and increase alertness and feelings of energy by stimulating receptor sites for two naturally occurring neurotransmitters. They also slow the activity of the stomach and intestine and decrease hunger. In the 1960s and 1970s, amphetamines were commonly prescribed for dieters, but when it was discovered that the appetite suppression effect of amphetamines lasted only a few weeks, most physicians stopped prescribing them. At high doses, amphetamines can increase heart rate and blood pressure to dangerous levels. As amphetamines are eliminated from the body, the user becomes tired.

When chronically abused, amphetamines produce rapid tolerance and strong psychological dependence. Other effects of chronic use include impotence and episodes of psychosis. When use is discontinued, periods of depression may develop.

Today the abuse of amphetamines is a more pressing concern than it has been in the recent past because of the

---

Key Terms

narcolepsy a sleep-related disorder in which a person has a recurrent, overwhelming, and uncontrollable desire to sleep, often at inappropriate times.

attention deficit hyperactivity disorder (ADHD) an above-normal rate of physical movement; often accompanied by an inability to concentrate well on a specified task; also called *hyperactivity.*

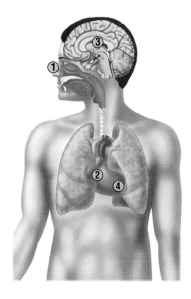

① **The nose:** as cocaine is snorted, nasal vessels immediately constrict and prohibit about 40% of the drug from entering the body. The remaining 60% enters the bloodstream.

② **The heart:** electrical impulses that regulate rhythmic pumping are impaired. Beating becomes irregular (arrhythmia). The heart can no longer supply itself with enough oxygenated blood.

③ **The brain:** dopamine and norepinephrine are released into the brain, producing a feeling of euphoria and confidence. Electrical signals to the heart are distorted, heart rate and pulse increase. A seizure may occur, causing coma and breathing stoppage.

④ **The heart:** blood circulation is out of control. The heart may simply flutter and stop, or it can be pumping so little oxygenated blood to the brain that the brain dies and the heart stops beating.

Figure 7-2 Cocaine's effects on the body.

sharp increase in the abuse of methamphetamine. Known by a variety of names and forms, including "crank," "ice," "crystal," "meth," "speed," "crystal meth," and "Zip," methamphetamine is produced in illegal home laboratories.[8]

Crystal Methamphetamine

Crystal methamphetamine, or ice, is among the most dangerous forms of methamphetamine. Ice is a very pure form of methamphetamine that looks like rock candy.[9] When smoked, the effects of ice are felt in about seven seconds as a wave of intense physical and psychological exhilaration. This effect lasts for several hours (much longer than the effects of crack), until the user becomes physically exhausted. The user experiences a rush of pleasure which is the result of the drug telling the brain to release large amounts of dopamine.[10]

Chronic use leads to nutritional difficulties, weight loss, reduced resistance to infection, and damage to the liver, lungs, and kidneys. Psychological dependence is quickly established. Withdrawal causes acute depression and fatigue but not significant physical discomfort.

Ritalin

Although Ritalin has not historically been considered a significant drug of abuse, the recent surge in the prescribing of Ritalin for children and teens has become a subject of debate. In a recent year, 8 million prescriptions were written for children and adolescents.

Ritalin is typically prescribed to children to help focus attention if they are hyperactive or cannot concentrate. Critics argue that the drug is being prescribed to treat a variety of problems. Studies suggest that access to health care may influence a diagnosis of ADHD, when the better course of treatment would be to identify and treat the root cause of the problems.[11] Supporters respond that Ritalin enables their children to succeed in school (see the Star box on page 225).

Cocaine

Cocaine, perhaps the strongest of the stimulant drugs, has received much media attention. Cocaine is the primary psychoactive substance found in the leaves of the South American coca plant.[12] The effects of cocaine last only briefly—from five to thirty minutes (Figure 7-2). Regardless of the form in which it is consumed, cocaine produces an immediate, near-orgasmic "rush," or feeling of exhilaration. This euphoria is quickly followed by a period of marked depression. Used only occasionally as a topical anesthetic, cocaine is usually inhaled (snorted), injected, or smoked (typically as crack). There is overwhelming scientific evidence that users quickly develop a strong psychological dependence on cocaine. Considerable evidence suggests that physical dependence also rapidly develops.

Key Terms

crystal methamphetamine a dangerous form of methamphetamine that quickly produces intense physical and psychological exhilaration when smoked.

Ritalin Abuse on College Campuses

Ritalin abuse on college campuses continues to rise. Studies have shown that one in every five college students has used Ritalin illegally.[1] Students who take Ritalin without a prescription are using this drug to help enhance concentration during late night study sessions, to snort it for a cocaine-like high or to suppress their appetites. However, students may not realize the serious side effects they can experience from taking Ritalin illegally.

These side effects can include nervousness, insomnia, loss of appetite and headaches,[2] increased heart and respiratory rates, dilated pupils, dry mouth, perspiration, and feeling of superiority.[1] Higher doses can result in tremors, convulsions, paranoia, and/or a crawling sensation of bugs under the skin. These health risks are considerably higher if Ritalin is snorted. Death can also occur from abusing Ritalin.[2]

[1]The Johns Hopkins News-Letter. *Ritalin abuse is increasing* (online). Available: **www.jhunewsletter.com/vnews/display.v/ART/2002/11/22/3ddd766faebeb** accessed 20 May 2003.
[2]Howard B. College 101: Getting in, getting through, getting out. *Ritalin Rampage* (online). Available: **www.journalism.indiana.edu/gallery/student/j201spring02/rabeam/health/blieberm/** accessed 20 May 2003.

Cocaine users risk a weakened immune system making them "more susceptible to infections, including HIV."[13] However, physical dependence on cocaine does not lead to death on withdrawal.

The status of cocaine as a substitute for amphetamines (during the 1960s), as a recreational drug for the wealthy (during the 1970s), and as a widely abused drug by many segments of society (during the 1980s) is well documented. During the 1990s, overall cocaine use decreased, although heavy use increased. In addition, the proportion of high school seniors who used cocaine at least once decreased from 9.8% in 1999 to 5.0% in 2000 and to 4.8% in 2001 according to the annual *Monitoring the Future Study* of drug use.[14] Studies have shown that the mean age of first cocaine use has declined from 23.6 years in 1992 to 20.6 years in 1998.[12]

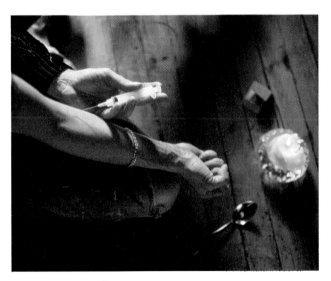

Intravenous injection of cocaine results in an almost immediate high for the user.

Crack Cocaine Crack is made by combining cocaine hydrochloride with common baking soda. When this paste-like mixture is allowed to dry, a small rocklike crystalline material remains. This crack is heated in the bowl of a small pipe, and the vapors are inhaled into the lungs.[12] Some crack users spend hundreds of dollars a day to maintain their habit.

The effect of crack is almost instantaneous. Within ten seconds after inhalation, cocaine reaches the CNS and influences the action of several neurotransmitters at specific sites in the brain. As with the use of other forms of cocaine, convulsions, seizures, respiratory distress, and cardiac failure have been reported with this sudden, extensive stimulation of the nervous system.

Within about six minutes, the stimulating effect of crack has been completely expended, and users frequently become depressed. Dependence develops within a few weeks, because users consume more crack in response to the short duration of stimulation and rapid onset of depression.

Intravenous administration has been the preferred route for cocaine users who are also regular users of heroin and other injectable drugs. Intravenous injection results in an almost immediate high, which lasts about ten minutes. A "smoother ride" is said to be obtained from a "speedball," the injectable mixture of heroin and cocaine (or methamphetamine).[4] However, such a mixture can be volatile and even fatal.

Freebasing Like inhaling crack, freebasing developed as a technique for maximizing the psychoactive effects of cocaine. Freebasing first requires that the common form of powdered cocaine (cocaine hydrochloride) be chemically altered (alkalized). This altered form is then dissolved in a solvent such as ether or benzene. This liquid solution is heated to evaporate the solvent. The heating process leaves the freebase cocaine in a powder form that can then be smoked, often through a water pipe.

Because of the large surface area of the lungs, smoking cocaine facilitates fast absorption into the bloodstream.

One danger of freebasing cocaine is the risk related to the solvents used. Ether is a highly volatile solvent capable of exploding and causing serious burns. Benzene is a known carcinogen associated with the development of leukemia. Clearly, neither solvent can be used without increasing the level of risk normally associated with cocaine use.

Depressants

Depressants (or sedatives) sedate the user, slowing down CNS function. Drugs included in this category are alcohol (see Chapter 8), barbiturates, and tranquilizers. Depressants produce tolerance in abusers, as well as strong psychological and physical dependence.

Barbiturates

Barbiturates are the so-called sleeping compounds that function by enhancing the effect of inhibitory neurotransmitters. They depress the CNS to the point where the user drops off to sleep or, as is the case with surgical anesthetics, the patient becomes anesthetized. Medically, barbiturates are used in widely varied dosages as anesthetics and for treatment of anxiety, insomnia, and epilepsy.[3] Regular use of a barbiturate quickly produces tolerance— eventually such a high dose is required that the user still

feels the effects of the drug throughout the next morning. Some abusers then begin to alternate barbiturates with stimulants, producing a vicious circle of dependence. Other misusers combine alcohol and barbiturates or tranquilizers, inadvertently producing toxic or even lethal results. Abrupt withdrawal from barbiturate use frequently produces a withdrawal syndrome that can involve seizures, delusions, hallucinations, and even death.

Methaqualone (Quaalude, "ludes," Sopor) was developed as a sedative that would not have the dependence properties of other barbiturates.[3] Although this did not happen, Quaaludes were occasionally prescribed for anxious patients. Today, compounds resembling Quaaludes are manufactured in home laboratories and sold illegally so that they can be combined with small amounts of alcohol for an inexpensive, drunklike effect.

Tranquilizers

Tranquilizers are depressants that are intended to reduce anxiety and to relax people who are having problems managing stress. They are not specifically designed to produce sleep but rather to help people cope with stress during their waking hours. Such tranquilizers are termed *minor tranquilizers*, of which diazepam (Valium) and chlordiazepoxide (Librium) may be the most commonly prescribed examples. Unfortunately, some people become addicted to these and other prescription drugs.[15]

Some tranquilizers are further designed to control hospitalized psychotic patients who may be suicidal or who are potential threats to others. These major *tranquilizers* subdue people physically but permit them to remain conscious. Their use is generally limited to institutional settings. All tranquilizers can produce physical and psychological dependence and tolerance.

"Date Rape" Depressants

"Date rape" drugs or club drugs are commonly used on college campuses. These drugs are usually slipped into the drink of an unsuspecting woman and can result in a coma or even death.

Common "date rape" drugs include GHB (gamma hydroxybutyrate), also known as G, liquid ecstasy, Easy Lay, and Georgia Home Boy, and Rohypnol ("roophies"). When these drugs are consumed they cause a drunklike or

> ### Key Terms
>
> **depressants** a category of drugs that sedate the user by slowing CNS function; they produce tolerance and strong psychological and physical addiction in users.

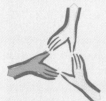

sleepy state that can last for hours. During this time is when unsuspecting individuals are taken advantage of, against their will and sometimes against their knowledge. For additional information see Club Drugs Star box on page 234.

High school and college students should not accept drinks from people they do not know. This recommendation extends to all parties where drinkers do not know what has been added to the punch or other drinks.[16]

Hallucinogens

As the name suggests, hallucinogenic drugs produce hallucinations—perceived distortions of reality. Also known as *psychedelic drugs,* or *phantasticants,* **hallucinogens** reached their height of popularity during the 1960s (see the Learning from Our Diversity box above). At that time, young people were encouraged to use hallucinogenic drugs to "expand the mind," "reach an altered state," or "discover reality." Not all of the reality distortions, or "trips," were pleasant. Many users reported "bummers," or trips during which they perceived negative, frightening distortions.

Hallucinogenic drugs include laboratory-produced lysergic acid diethylamide (LSD), mescaline (from the peyote cactus plant), and psilocybin (from a particular genus of mushroom). Consumption of hallucinogens seems to produce not physical dependence but mild levels of psychological dependence. The development of tolerance is questionable. **Synesthesia,** a sensation in which users report hearing a color, smelling music, or touching a taste, is sometimes produced with hallucinogen use.

The long-term effects of hallucinogenic drug use are not fully understood. Questions about genetic abnormalities in offspring, fertility, sex drive and performance, and the development of personality disorders have not been fully answered. One phenomenon that has been identified and documented is the development of flashbacks—the

unpredictable return to a psychedelic trip that occurred months or even years earlier. Flashbacks are thought to result from the accumulation of a drug within body cells.

LSD

The most well-known and powerful hallucinogen is lysergic acid diethylamide (LSD). LSD was first isolated in 1938 by Albert Hoffmann, who was studying a group of chemicals that were extracted from a fungus that infects rye and other cereal grains. Five years later, he accidentally discovered its hallucinogenic effects. Dr. Timothy Leary helped to spread the popularity of LSD in the 1960s by promoting the use of LSD in mind expansion and experimentation. LSD helped define the counterculture movement of the 1960s. During the 1970s and the 1980s, this drug lost considerable popularity. LSD use has made a comeback, with studies reporting that 6.6% of high school seniors in 2001[14] and 14.7% of young adults age 18–20[5] had experimented with LSD. Fear of cocaine and other powerful drugs, boredom, low cost, and an attempt to revisit the culture of the 1960s are thought to have increased LSD's attractiveness to today's young people.

LSD is manufactured in home laboratories and frequently distributed in blotter paper decorated with cartoon characters.[17] Users place the paper on their tongue

---

Key Terms

hallucinogens psychoactive drugs capable of producing hallucinations (distortions of reality).

synesthesia a sensation of combining of the senses, such as perceiving color by hearing it or perceiving taste by touching it.

or chew the paper to ingest the drug. LSD is similar in structure to the neurotransmitter serotonin and produces psychedelic effects by interfering with the normal activity of this neurotransmitter. The effects can include altered perception of shapes, images, time, sound, and body form. Synesthesia is common to LSD users. LSD is metabolized in the liver and excreted. Its effects last an average of six to nine hours.

Users may describe LSD experiences as positive and "mind-expanding," or negative and "mind-constricting," depending on the user's mood and the social setting in which the drug is taken. Positive sensations include feelings of creativity, deep understanding of oneself and the universe, and feelings of grandeur. Although LSD users report feelings of increased insight and creativity, a real increase in these skills has not been demonstrated. At the same time, some reports of bad trips on LSD are thought to have been caused by other substances, such as PCP, that were sold to the user as LSD. Deaths resulting from bizarre behavior after taking LSD have been reported. Dangerous side effects include panic attacks, flashbacks, and occasional prolonged psychosis.

Although the typical doses ("hits") today are about half as powerful as those in the 1960s, users still tend to develop high tolerance to LSD. Physical dependence does not occur.

Designer Drugs

In recent years, chemists who produce many of the illicit drugs in home laboratories have designed versions of drugs listed on **FDA Schedule 1.** These designer drugs are similar to the controlled drugs on the FDA Schedule 1 but are sufficiently different so that they escape governmental control. The designer drugs are either newly synthesized products that are similar to already outlawed drugs but against which no law yet exists, or they are reconstituted or renamed illegal substances. Designer drugs are said to produce effects similar to their controlled drug counterparts.

People who use designer drugs do so at great risk because the manufacturing of these drugs is unregulated. The neurophysiological effect of these homemade drugs can be quite dangerous. So far, a synthetic heroin product (MPPP) and several amphetamine derivatives with hallucinogenic properties have been designed for the unwary drug consumer.

DOM (STP), MDA (the "love drug"), and ecstacy ("MDMA" or "XTC") are examples of amphetamine-derivative, hallucinogenic designer drugs. These drugs produce mild LSD-like hallucinogenic experiences, positive feelings, and enhanced alertness. They also have a number of potentially dangerous effects. Experts are particularly concerned that MDMA can produce strong psychological dependence and can deplete serotonin, an important excitatory neurotransmitter associated with a state of alertness. Permanent brain damage is possible.[3] On a positive note, one recent major survey indicates that MDMA use is declining among teens.[18]

Phencyclidine

Phencyclidine (PCP, "angel dust") is unique because it not only produces hallucinogenic effects but also acts as an analgesic, a depressant, a stimulant, and an anesthetic. This makes the typical PCP experience impossible to predict or describe. The physical effects of PCP begin a few minutes after consumption and continue for four to six hours. PCP was studied for years during the 1950s and 1960s and was found to be an unsuitable animal and human anesthetic.[19]

Manufactured in tablet or powder form, PCP can be injected, inhaled, taken orally, or smoked. Some users report mild euphoria, although most report bizarre perceptions, paranoid feelings, and aggressive behavior. PCP overdose may cause convulsions, cardiovascular collapse, and damage to the brain's respiratory center.

In a number of cases the aggressive behavior caused by PCP has led users to commit brutal crimes against both friends and innocent strangers. PCP accumulates in cells and may stimulate bizarre behavior months after initial use.

PCP is an extremely unpredictable drug. Although PCP has been blamed in many reports of bizarre, even homicidal, behavior, it continues to be abused. Because PCP is easily and cheaply manufactured in home laboratories, authorities have difficulty limiting its availability.

Cannabis

Cannabis (marijuana) has been labeled a mild hallucinogen for a number of years. However, most experts now consider it to be a drug category in itself. Marijuana produces mild effects like those of stimulants and depressants. The recent implication of marijuana in a large number of traffic fatalities makes this drug one whose consumption should be carefully considered. Marijuana is actually a wild plant (*Cannabis sativa*) whose fibers were once used in the manufacture of hemp rope. When the leafy material and small stems are dried and crushed, users can smoke the mixture in rolled cigarettes ("joints"), cigars ("blunts"), or pipes. The resins collected from scraping the flowering tops of the plant yield a marijuana product called hashish, or hash, commonly smoked in a pipe.[17]

The potency of marijuana's hallucinogenic effect is determined by the percentage of the active ingredient,

---

Key Terms

FDA Schedule 1 a list of drugs that have a high potential for abuse but no medical use.

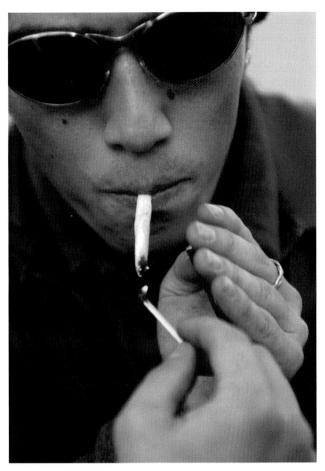

Marijuana is considered a gateway drug because its use often leads the user to heavier drug use.

ular foods, and a relaxed mood. There is widespread consensus that marijuana's behavioral effects include four probabilities: (1) Users must learn to recognize what a marijuana high is like, (2) marijuana impairs short-term memory, (3) users overestimate the passage of time, and (4) users lose the ability to maintain attention to a task.[3]

The long-term effects of marijuana use are still being studied. Chronic abuse may lead to an amotivational syndrome in some people. Heavy marijuana users have trouble paying attention and retaining new information for at least a day after last using the drug, according to a recent study.

The irritating effects of marijuana smoke on lung tissue are more pronounced than those of cigarette smoke, and some of the more than 400 chemicals in marijuana are now linked to lung cancer development. In fact, one of the most potent carcinogens, benzopyrene, is found in higher levels in marijuana smoke than in tobacco smoke. Marijuana smokers tend to inhale deeply and hold the smoke in the lungs for long periods. It is likely that at some point the lungs of chronic marijuana smokers will be damaged.

Long-term marijuana use is also associated with damage to the immune system and to the male and female reproductive systems and with an increase in birth defects in babies born to mothers who smoke marijuana. Chronic marijuana use lowers testosterone levels in men, but the effect of this change is not known. The effect of long-term marijuana use on a variety of types of sexual behavior is also not fully understood.

Because the drug can distort perceptions and thus perceptual ability (especially when combined with

tetrahydrocannabinol (THC), present in the product. The concentration of THC averages about 3.5% for regular grade marijuana, 7% to 9% for higher-quality marijuana (sinsemilla), 8% to 14% for hashish, and as high as 50% for hash oil.[3] Today's marijuana has THC levels that are higher than in past decades.

THC is a fat-soluble substance and thus is absorbed and retained in fat tissues within the body. Before being excreted, THC can remain in the body for up to a month. With the sophistication of today's drug tests, trace metabolites of THC can be detected for up to 30 days after consumption.[3] It is possible that the THC that comes from passive inhalation of high doses (for example, during an indoor rock concert) can also be detected for a short time after exposure.

Once marijuana is consumed, its effects vary from person to person (see Table 7.3). Being "high" or "stoned" means different things to different people. Many people report heightened sensitivity to music, cravings for partic-

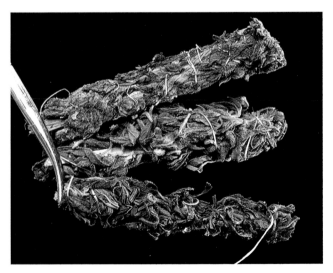

Thai sticks are a potent form of marijuana.

Table 7.3 Effects of Marijuana

Short-Term Effects	Long-Term Effects
• Increased heart rate and blood pressure	• Lung damage
• Feeling of elation	• Increased risk of bronchitis
• Drowsiness and sedation	• Emphysema
• Increased appetite	• Lung cancer
• Red eyes	• Heart attack[2]
• Food cravings	• Loss of motivation and short-term memory
• Slow reaction time	• Increased panic or anxiety
• Feelings of depression, excitement, paranoia, panic, and euphoria	• May become tolerant to marijuana
• Problems with attention span, memory, learning, problem-solving, and coordination	• Damage to lungs, immune system, and reproductive organs
• Sleeplessness[1]	• Can remain in the body for up to a month
	• Can cause birth defects
	• Five times more damaging to the lungs than tobacco products[3]

[1]Miller A. Campus Alcohol and Drug Resource Center, University of Florida; Health Education of Ball State University. 1 March 2002.
[2]Stronger Marijuana Is Major Health Risk. *The Independent,* 1 February 2001.
[3]Sternberg S. Pot smoking linked to sudden heart attacks. *USA Today,* 3 March 2000.

alcohol), its use by automobile drivers clearly jeopardizes the lives of many innocent people.

The only medical uses for marijuana are to relieve the nausea caused by chemotherapy, to improve appetite in AIDS patients, and to ease the pressure that builds up in the eyes of glaucoma patients. However, a variety of other drugs, many of which are nearly as effective, are also used for these purposes. The U.S. Supreme Court recently struck a blow to the proponents of the medical use of marijuana (see the Star box on page 244).

Narcotics

The **narcotics** are among the strongest dependence-producing drugs. Medically, narcotics are used to relieve pain and induce sleep. On the basis of origin, narcotics can be subgrouped into the natural, quasisynthetic, and synthetic narcotics.

Natural Narcotics

Naturally occurring substances derived from the Oriental poppy plant include opium (the primary psychoactive substance extracted from the Oriental poppy), morphine (the primary active ingredient in opium), and thebaine (a compound not used as a drug). Morphine and related compounds have medical use as analgesics in the treatment of mild to severe pain.

Quasisynthetic Narcotics

Quasisynthetic narcotics are compounds created by chemically altering morphine. These laboratory-produced drugs are intended to be used as analgesics, but their benefits are largely outweighed by a high dependence rate and a great risk of toxicity. The best known of the quasisynthetic narcotics is heroin. Although heroin is a fast-acting and very effective analgesic, it is extremely addictive. Heroin can be inhaled ("snorted"), smoked, injected into a vein, or "skin-popped" (injected beneath the skin surface). Heroin produces dreamlike euphoria and, like all narcotics, strong physical and psychological dependence and tolerance.

Most new heroin users are smoking or snorting heroin, rather than injecting the drug. Many new heroin users are also young, with one-quarter of the new users of heroin being under age 18, while nearly half are age 18 to 25.[20]

Key Terms

narcotics opiates; psychoactive drugs derived from the Oriental poppy plant; narcotics relieve pain and induce sleep.

Medical Marijuana Ruling

In May of 2001, the United States Supreme Court ruled that the distribution of marijuana for medicinal purposes to people in California must be stopped. The court decided in an 8–0 decision that there is no medical necessity exception to the federal laws prohibiting the manufacturing and distribution of marijuana. This Supreme Court ruling does not overturn similar state laws in Alaska, Arizona, Hawaii, Maine, Nevada, Oregon, and Washington where these laws have made it possible for seriously ill patients to grow (or purchase) marijuana for pain relief, when recommended by a physician. This ruling allows the federal government to prosecute individuals for the manufacturing and distribution of marijuana even though some state laws might have decriminalized medical marijuana use.* The government's position is that marijuana is not a safe product, has no medical purpose, and cannot be administered safely under medical supervision, and conflicts with the Controlled Substance Act.

Proponents of medical marijuana argue that marijuana can act as an appetite stimulant, muscle relaxant, and pain reliever, and that it can treat the following conditions:

- Nausea resulting from cancer treatment
- Appetite loss in persons with AIDS
- Pain from diseases such as multiple sclerosis
- Eye pressure and pain resulting from glaucoma

In 1985, the FDA approved the drug dronabinol (Marinol) for use by cancer chemotherapy patients who were experiencing nausea. Marinol is a capsule that contains a controlled amount of marijuana's active ingredient, THC. In 1993, the FDA approved Marinol for use as an appetite stimulant in persons with AIDS. Proponents of medical marijuana, however, believe that the THC dose is better controlled and more effective (and thus safer) when taken by smoking the raw plant material.

*The United States v. Oakland Cannabis Buyer's Co-op., (2001), 121 S. Ct. 1711.

Heroin users who inject the drug face an additional risk. As with the use of all other injectable illegal drugs, the practice of sharing needles increases the likelihood of transmission of various communicable diseases, including HIV (see Chapter 13). Abrupt withdrawal from heroin use is rarely fatal, but the discomfort during **cold turkey** withdrawal is reported to be overwhelming.

Synthetic Narcotics

Meperidine (Demerol) and propoxyphene (Darvon), common postsurgical painkillers, and methadone, the drug prescribed during the rehabilitation of heroin addicts, are synthetic narcotics. These opiatelike drugs are manufactured in medical laboratories. They are not natural narcotics or quasisynthetic narcotics because they do not originate from the Oriental poppy plant. Like true narcotics, however, these drugs can rapidly induce physical dependence. One important criticism of methadone rehabilitation programs is that they merely shift the addiction from heroin to methadone.

Inhalants

Inhalants are a class of drugs that includes a variety of volatile (quickly evaporating) compounds that generally produce unpredictable, drunklike effects in users and feelings of euphoria.[21] Users of inhalants may also have some delusions and hallucinations. Some users may become quite aggressive. Drugs in this category include anesthetic gases (chloroform, nitrous oxide, and ether), vasodilators (amyl nitrite and butyl nitrite), petroleum products and commercial solvents (gasoline, kerosene, plastic cement, glue, typewriter correction fluid, paint, and paint thinner), and certain aerosols (found in some propelled spray products, fertilizers, and insecticides).

Most of the danger in using inhalants lies in the damaging, sometimes fatal effects on the respiratory and cardiovascular systems.[21] Furthermore, users may unknowingly place themselves in dangerous situations because of the drunklike hallucinogenic effects. Aggressive behavior might also make users a threat to themselves and others.

For more information about inhalants, contact the National Inhalant Prevention Coalition at **www.inhalants.org.**

Society's Response to Drug Use

During the last 25 years, society has responded to illegal drug use with growing concern. Most adults see drug abuse as a clear danger to society. This position has been supported by the development of community, school, state, and national organizations interested in the reduction of illegal drug use. These organizations have included such diverse groups as Parents Against Drugs, Parents for a Drug-Free Youth, Drug Abuse Resistance Education (DARE), Mothers Against Drunk Driving (MADD), Narcotics Anonymous, and the federal Drug Enforcement Administration. Certain groups have concentrated

---

Key Terms

cold turkey immediate, total discontinuation of use of a drug; associated withdrawal discomfort.

inhalants psychoactive drugs that enter the body through inhalation.

OxyContin

OxyContin, also known as hillybilly heroin, Oxy, and Oxycotton, is a time-released legal prescription drug used to treat individuals with moderate to severe pain.[1] Illegal use of OxyContin brought national attention when individuals in rural areas of the country were found abusing this drug. Now abuse of OxyContin is continuing to spread across the country.[2] Classified as a narcotic drug, OxyContin is an addictive controlled substance with an addiction potential similar to morphine. This prescription drug is considered extremely dangerous as an illicit drug. Some methods of usage which increase the likelihood of dangerous effects, including death, are chewing the tablets, snorting crushed tablets, and dissolving the tablets in water then injecting the drug. When OxyContin is not taken in tablet form, the controlled-release dosage is defeated and the user has a high potential of receiving a lethal dose due to the drug being released immediately into one's system.[3] Many other long-term consequences of OxyContin abuse are physical dependence and severe respiratory depression that may lead to death. Common withdrawal symptoms include restlessness, muscle and bone pain, insomnia, diarrhea, vomiting, cold flashes with goose bumps, and involuntary leg movements.[2] The FDA continues to monitor the abuse of OxyContin and has approved the strongest warning labels for this drug with the intent of changing prescription practices as well as increasing the physician's focus on the potential for abuse.[3]

[1]OxyContin Questions and Answers. Drug Information. U.S. Food and Drug Administration, Center for Drug Evaluation and Research. 25 July 2001. **www.fda.gov/cder/drug/infopage/oxycontin/oxycontin-qa.htm**
[2]OxyContin. OxyContin Addiction and Treatment and Rapid Detox Services (online). Available: **www.oxycontin-detox.com/index-overture-kw-oxycontin.html** accessed 14 July 2003.
[3]FDA Strengthens Warnings for OxyContin. U.S. Food and Drug Adminstration. 25 July 2001. **www.fda.gov/bbs/topics/ANSWERS/2001/ANS01091.html**

their efforts on education, others on enforcement, and still others on the development of laws and public policy.

The personal and social issues related to drug abuse are very complex. Innovative solutions continue to be devised. Some believe that only through early childhood education will people learn alternatives to drug use. Starting drug education in the preschool years may have a more positive effect than waiting until the upper elementary or junior high school years. The focus on reducing young people's exposure to gateway drugs (especially tobacco, alcohol, and marijuana) may help slow down the move to other addictive drugs. Some people advocate much harsher penalties for drug use and drug trafficking, including extreme measures such as public executions.

Others support legalizing all drugs and making governmental agencies responsible for drug regulation and control, as is the case with alcohol. Advocates of this position believe that drug-related crime and violence would

virtually cease once the demand for illegal products is reduced. Sound arguments can be made on both sides of this issue. What is your opinion?

Unless significant changes in society's response to drug use take place soon, the disastrous effects of virtually uncontrolled drug abuse will continue to be felt. Families and communities will continue to be plagued by drug-related tragedies. Law enforcement officials will be pressed to the limits of their resources in their attempts to reduce drug flow. Our judicial system will be heavily burdened by thousands of court cases. Health care facilities could face overwhelming numbers of patients.

In comparison with other federally funded programs, the "war on drugs" is less expensive than farm support, food stamps, Medicare, and national defense. However, it remains to be seen whether any amount of money spent on enforcement, without adequate support for education, treatment, and poverty reduction, can reduce the illegal drug demand and supply. Currently, approximately $19.2 billion is spent to fight the drug war in the United States—$13 billion on law enforcement (supply reduction) and $6.2 billion on education, prevention, and treatment (demand reduction).[22, 23]

Drug Testing

Drug testing is one of society's responses to drug use and is becoming an increasingly popular prevention tool. In 1986 the federal government instituted drug testing policies for federal employees in safety-sensitive jobs. In 1988 the Drug Free Workplace Act extended the drug-free federal policy to include all federal grantees (including universities) and most federal contractors. Although this act did not mandate drug testing, it encouraged tougher approaches to prevent and deal with drug problems at the work site.

Private companies have developed drug-testing procedures similar to those used with federal agencies. Most Fortune 500 companies use drug testing to screen applicants or monitor employee drug use.

Drug tests commonly search for amphetamines, barbiturates, benzodiazepines (the chemical bases for prescription tranquilizers such as Valium and Librium), cannabinoids (THC, hashish, and marijuana), methaqualone, opiates (heroin, codeine, and morphine), and PCP. With the exception of marijuana, most traces of these drugs are eliminated by the body within a few days after use. Marijuana can remain detectable for up to 30 days after use.

How accurate are the results of drug testing? At typical cutoff standards, drug tests are likely to identify 90% of recent drug users. This means that about 10% of recent users will pass undetected. (These 10% are considered *false negatives.*) Nonusers whose drug tests indicate drug use (*false positives*) are quite rare. (Follow-up tests on these false positives would nearly always show negative

Drug abuse in the workplace is a growing concern. In factories, stores, and offices, employee drug use is suspected to be the cause of one-third to one-half of all absenteeism, accidents, medical claims, insubordination, thefts, and loss of productivity.

In response, more than half of Fortune 500 companies have instituted mandatory preemployment drug screening. Prospective employees of these firms are required to pass one or more drug tests to be considered for employment. Preemployment screening is also becoming more popular in the public employment sector. Such drug testing is controversial in several ways.

Supporters of mandatory preemployment drug screening argue that employers have an obligation to provide a safe and healthy work environment. They also contend that drug abuse is driving the cost of health care to ever-higher levels. Workers' compensation costs are also high, perhaps in part because of an increase in drug-related accidents and the chronic nature of drug-related illnesses. Employers also say that those who have taken drugs and have failed a drug screening have already broken the law and thus have forfeited their right to be considered for employment.

Opponents of preemployment screening express two concerns. First, they argue that the validity and reliability of screening tests are too low. If 1 million tests are performed in a year, a conservative estimate, and .05% of those tests yield false positives, also a conservative estimate, then 500 people may be fired from their jobs or not offered jobs for which they are qualified, according to the American Civil Liberties Union (ACLU).

The second concern is that employers invade the privacy of applicants by assuming them guilty until proved innocent by the testing laboratory. Privacy is invaded in two ways, says the ACLU. First, the specimen-collection process itself often involves direct or indirect observation to prevent tampering by the employee. Even indirect observation can be degrading. Typically, employees must remove all outer garments and urinate in a bathroom in which the water supply has been cut off. A second search takes place in the lab. Urinalysis can reveal not only the presence of illegal drugs, but also many other physical and medical conditions, such as medication for epilepsy, hypertension, or diabetes; a genetic predisposition to heart disease or cancer; and pregnancy. Employees are usually required to fill out forms listing all the medications they currently are taking, a clear invasion of privacy, says the ACLU.

Do you feel that mandatory preemployment drug screening is justified? Do you feel that it is an invasion of privacy? Would you agree to take a preemployment drug test as a condition of employment?

results.) Human errors are probably more responsible than technical errors for inaccuracies in drug tests.

Recently, scientists have been refining procedures that use hair samples to detect the presence of drugs. These procedures seem to hold much promise, although certain technical obstacles remain. Watch for refinements in hair-sample drug testing in the near future.

Do you think that the possibility of having to take a drug test would have any effect on college students' use of drugs? Do you think that drug testing is an acceptable method of prevention? See the Star box above for differing viewpoints.

College and Community Support Services for Drug Dependence

Students who have drug problems and realize they need assistance might select assistance based on the services available on campus or in the surrounding community and the costs they are willing to pay for treatment services.

One recently developed approach to convince drug-dependent people to enter treatment programs is the use of *confrontation*. People who live or work with chemically dependent people are being encouraged to confront them directly about their addiction. Direct confrontation helps chemically dependent people realize the effect their behavior has on others. Once chemically dependent people realize that others will no longer tolerate their behavior, the likelihood of their entering treatment programs is increased significantly. Although effective, this approach is very stressful for family members and friends and requires the assistance of professionals in the field of chemical dependence. These professionals can be contacted at a drug treatment center in your area.

Treatment

Comprehensive drug treatment programs are available in very few college or university health centers. College settings for drug dependence programs are more commonly found in the university counseling center. At such a center the emphasis will probably be not on the medical management of dependence but on the behavioral dimensions of drug abuse. Trained counselors and psychologists who specialize in chemical dependence counseling will work with students to (1) analyze their particular concerns, (2) establish constructive ways to cope

Using Acupuncture for Drug Treatment

Acupuncture involves the insertion of very fine needles on the body's surface to help influence the body's physiological functioning. Although many people in the Western world think of acupuncture as a new alternative type of medicine, the practice has been a part of Chinese medicine for thousands of years.

Acupuncture theory holds that there is an energy force that runs throughout the body on special pathways called meridians. When the meridians become unbalanced, perhaps through various obstructions, deficiencies, or excesses, the body can become sick. Acupuncture restores the balance in the energy forces and helps return the body to good health.

Acupuncture has been used to treat a number of health conditions. Among these are low back pain, headaches, arthritis, and relief of muscle spasms. According to the National Institutes of Health (NIH) 1997 Consensus Statement,[1] acupuncture may be helpful in treating musculoskeletal conditions, such as fibromyalgia, myofacial pain, and tennis elbow. Additionally, postoperative pain and low back pain seem to respond well to acupuncture. The NIH Consensus Panel reported that there is clear evidence that needle acupuncture reduces adult postoperative nausea and chemotherapy nausea and vomiting, and it may reduce the nausea of pregnancy.

However, the Consensus Statement indicated that there was insufficient evidence to demonstrate that acupuncture was significantly helpful in promoting the cessation of smoking and some other conditions. Studies suggest that acupuncture can help reduce drug cravings.[2] Certainly, interest in the practice of Eastern medicine is increasing in the United States, and studies are underway to examine the benefits of acupuncture in treating addictions. However, because there are so many factors that impact on a person's ability to be successfully treated, it will be difficult to isolate acupuncture as the sole reason for treatment success.

It is likely that acupuncture will eventually be viewed as one of a number of beneficial approaches used in a comprehensive drug treatment program. Acupuncture will probably be helpful to some people and not so helpful to others.

If you had a drug addiction, would you be willing to try acupuncture? Why or why not?

[1] *Acupuncture,* National Institutes of Health Consensus Statement Online, 3–5 November 1997; 15(5): 1–34.
[2] Leinwand D. Study: Acupuncture cuts cocaine cravings: Counseling, recovery programs also advised. *USA Today, 14 August 2000.*

---

with stress, and (3) search for alternative ways to achieve new "highs" (see the Personal Assessment on page 257).

Medical treatment for the management of drug problems may need to be obtained through the services of a community treatment facility administered by a local health department, community mental health center, private clinic, or local hospital. Treatment may be on an inpatient or outpatient basis. Medical management might include detoxification, treatment of secondary health complications and nutritional deficiencies, and therapeutic counseling related to chemical dependence (see the Considering Complementary Care box above).

Some communities have voluntary health agencies that deliver services and treatment programs for drug-dependent people. Check your telephone book for listings of drug treatment facilities. Some communities have drug hot lines that offer advice for people with questions about drugs (see the Changing for the Better box on page 248 for a list of anti-drug abuse organizations and hot line numbers).

TALKING POINTS Do you think that confronting a friend about her regular marijuana use will prompt her to seek treatment?

Costs of Treatment for Dependence

Drug treatment programs that are administered by colleges and universities for faculty and students usually require no fees. Local agencies may provide either free services or services based on a **sliding scale.** Private hospitals, physicians, and clinics are the most expensive forms of treatment. Inpatient treatment at a private facility may cost as much as $1,000 per day. Since the length of inpatient treatment averages three to four weeks, a patient can quickly accumulate a very large bill. However, with many types of health insurance policies now providing coverage for alcohol addiction and other types of drug dependence, even these services may not require additional out-of-pocket expenses.

Key Terms

sliding scale a method of payment by which patient fees are scaled according to income.

Finding Help for Drug Abuse

I have a college friend who may need help for drug abuse. Where can I find information about drug abuse and treatment options?

National Groups

Alcoholics Anonymous
(212) 870-3400
www.alcoholics-anonymous.org

Cocaine Anonymous
(800) 347-8998
www.ca.org

Drug Strategies
(202) 289-9070
www.drugstrategies.org

Go Ask Alice! Columbia University's Health Education Program
www.goaskalice.columbia.edu

The Higher Education National Center for Alcohol and Other Drug Prevention
(800) 676-1730
www.edc.org/hec

Narcotics Anonymous
(818) 773-9999
www.na.org

National Clearinghouse for Alcohol and Drug Information
(800) 729-6686
www.health.org

National Inhalant Prevention Coalition
(800) 269-4237
www.inhalants.org

National Institute on Drug Abuse
(301) 443-1124
www.nida.nih.gov

Partnership for a Drug-Free America
(212) 922-1560
www.drugfreeamerica.org

PRIDE (Parent's Resource Institute for Drug Education)
(800) 279-6361
www.pridesurveys.com

Substance Abuse and Mental Health Services Administration (SAMHSA)
(301) 443-4795
www.samhsa.gov

Toughlove International
(215) 348-7090
www.toughlove.org

Hot Lines

American Council for Drug Education
www.drughelp.org

Center for Substance Abuse Treatment
National Hotline
(800) 662-HELP

National Alcohol Hot Line
(800) ALCOHOL

National Cocaine Hot Line
(800) COCAINE

Taking Charge of Your Health

- Assess your knowledge of drug use by completing the Personal Assessment on page 255.
- Calculate the amount of caffeine you consume daily. If you're drinking more than three cups of caffeinated beverages per day, develop a plan to reduce your overall intake.
- Prepare a plan of action to use if someone you know needs professional assistance with a drug problem.

- Identify five activities that can provide you with a drug-free high.
- Analyze your drug use patterns (if any), and assess the likelihood that you might fail a pre-employment drug test.
- Assess your lifestyle for addictive behaviors that do not involve drugs, such as over-exercising or watching too much TV. Develop a plan to moderate these activities and achieve more balance in your life.

Summary

- Abuse of drugs takes a tremendous toll on human lives and has a devastating effect on society.

- Primary prevention of drug abuse targets individuals and groups to reach people who have not used illegal drugs and reduce their desire to try drugs.

- Secondary prevention targets people who are beginning to use drugs.
- Tertiary prevention (third-level prevention) targets people who are drug dependent, such as crack or heroin addicts, and their families.
- Drugs affect the CNS by altering neurotransmitter activity on neurons.
- The addiction process has three components: exposure, compulsion, and loss of control.
- A drug is any substance, natural or artificial, other than food, that by its chemical nature alters structure or function in the living organism.
- Psychoactive drugs alter the user's feelings, behavior, perceptions, or moods.
- Physical drug dependence occurs when body cells become reliant on a drug, causing withdrawal illness if the drug is not taken.
- Tolerance to a drug has developed when continued intake of the same dose has diminishing effects.
- Psychological drug dependence occurs when a user has a strong desire to continue using a particular drug and believes that he or she must use the drug to maintain a sense of well-being.

- Drug misuse is the inappropriate use of legal drugs intended to be medications.
- Drug abuse is any use of an illegal drug or use of a legal drug in a way that is detrimental to health and well-being.
- Individual, environmental, and societal factors influence drug taking behavior.
- Combination drug effects include synergistic, additive, potentiated, and antagonistic effects.
- Psychoactive drugs are classified as stimulants, depressants, hallucinogens, cannabis, narcotics, or inhalants.
- Society has responded to drug use with educational programs, law enforcement efforts, and legislation and public policy.
- Club drugs and the use of marijuana for medical reasons are current issues facing American society.
- Drug testing can be used as a means of primary, secondary, or tertiary prevention.
- College and community drug treatment services are available.

Review Questions

1. Explain the terms *primary prevention, secondary prevention,* and *tertiary prevention,* and give examples of each.
2. Describe how neurotransmitters work.
3. Identify and explain the three steps in the process of addiction.
4. How is the term *drug* defined in this chapter? What are psychoactive drugs? How do medicines differ from drugs?
5. Explain what *dependence* means. Identify and explain the two types of dependence.
6. Define the word *tolerance.* What does *cross-tolerance* mean? Give an example of cross-tolerance.
7. Differentiate between drug misuse and drug abuse.
8. Identify some individual, environmental, and societal factors that affect drug abuse.
9. Explain the terms *synergistic effect, additive effect, potentiated effect,* and *antagonistic effect.*

10. List the six general categories of drugs. For each category, give several examples of drugs and explain the effects they would have on the user. What are designer drugs?
11. What are the side effects and health risks of abusing Ritalin.
12. What is the active ingredient in marijuana? What are its common effects on the user? What are the long-term effects of marijuana use?
13. Identify three or four so-called "club-drugs" and describe how they can cause serious medical problems.
14. How accurate is drug testing?
15. Describe several drug treatment services that are available. Who administers these services and how do their approaches differ?

References

1. Tricker R. *Preventing Substance Use in Young Athletes.* **www.tpronline.org.** accessed 10 June 2003.
2. Shier D, Butler J, Lewis R. *Hole's Human Anatomy and Physiology,* 9th ed. McGraw-Hill, 2002.
3. Ray O, Ksir C. *Drugs, society, and human behavior,* 9th ed. McGraw-Hill, 2002.
4. Pinger RR, Payne WA, Hahn DB, Hahn EJ. *Drugs: issues for today,* 3rd ed. McGraw-Hill, 1998.
5. Substance Abuse and Mental Health Services Administration (SAMHSA). *2001 National Household Survey on Drug Abuse.* **www.samhsa.gov/oas/nhsda/2k1nhsda/vol1/toc.htm** accessed 22 May 2003.

6. Ephedra Education Council. *Ephedra Supported by Science—A Ban Is Not, Industry Tells FDA.* 8 April 2003.

7. Associated Press. Illinois becomes 1st state to ban ephedra. *Indianapolis Star,* 26 May 2003.

8. National Institute on Drug Abuse. National Institutes of Health. *Methamphetamine.* **www.nida.nih.gov/ Infofax/methamphetamine.html** accessed 17 March 2001.

9. U.S. Department of Justice. Drug Enforcement Administration. *Methamphetamine.* **www.usdoj.gov/ dea/concern/meth.htm,** 31 December 2001.

10. Frackelmann K. Breaking bonds of addiction: Compulsion traced to part of the brain. *USA Today,* 18 April 2002.

11. Attention Deficit Rate Tops Estimates. *Cox News Service,* 22 May 2002.

12. U.S. Department of Justice. *Drugs of Concern,* **www.dea.gov,** October 2000.

13. Cocaine Weakens Immune System. *Boston Herald,* 7 March 2003.

14. Johnston LD, O'Malley PM, Bachman JG. *Monitoring the Future: National Survey Results on Drug Use, 1975–2001.* University of Michigan Institute for Social Research (online). Available: **www. monitoringthefuture.org/pubs/monographs/ vol1_2001.pdf** accessed 22 May 2003.

15. Health-Nexus. *Depressants* (online). Available: **www.health-nexus.com/depressants.htm.** 10 June 2003.

16. National Institute on Drug Abuse. NIDA InfoFacts. *Rohypnol and GHB* (online). Available: **www.nida.nih.gov/InfoFax/RohypnolGHB.html.** 10 June 2003.

17. Leinwand, D. A strange new world of teenage drug use: the lowdown on the hippest highs. *USA Today,* 28 February 2001.

18. NIDA Press Office. *2002 Monitoring the Future Survey shows decrease in Use of Marijuana, Club Drugs, Cigarettes and Tobacco.* 16 December 2002.

19. National Institute on Drug Abuse. NIDA InfoFacts. *PCP (Phencyclidine).* **www.nida.nih.gov/InfoFax/pcp.html.** 10 June 2003.

20. Leinwand D. Heroin's resurgence closes drug's traditional gender gap: Teenage girls are increasingly falling prey to narcotic in purer, 'more mainstream', sniffable form. *USA Today,* 9 May 2000.

21. Frackelmann K. Inhalants' hidden treat: Access makes huffing popular but kids can recover with help. *USA Today,* 25 June 2002.

22. **www.whitehousedrugpolicy.gov/publications/ policy/04budget/exec_sum.pdf,** February 2003 accessed 21 May 2003.

23. Keen J. Bush plans hit on drug abuse: White House goal is to reduce 'crisis' by 25% in five years. *USA Today,* 13 February 2002.

As We Go to Press

In late December 2003 the Food and Drug Administration (FDA) announced its plans to soon ban the sale of dietary supplements containing ephedra. Until this date, Illinois and New York were the only states that had already banned the sale of ephedra.

This consumer alert was issued to notify consumers about the health risks of ephedra and to urge them not to purchase or consume ephedra products. Ephedra dietary supplements have been used to aid in weight control, to increase energy, and to enhance athletic performance. Health risks such as high blood pressure, heart problems, stroke, and stress on the circulatory system have been the result of consuming ephedra products.

As we go to press, on February 6, 2004, the FDA published its final rule banning ephedra. This ban becomes effective 60 days after the ruling. Once the ban is in effect, manufacturers and distributors may no longer market or sell ephedra products. Any violations of this rule will result in criminal prosecution.

Caffeine: america's most popular drug

Coffee is definitely hip again. On two popular television sitcoms, "Friends"hang out at Central Perk and Drs. Frasier and Niles Crane solve many of life's problems over cups of gourmet brew. Starbucks, a coffeehouse chain based in Seattle, has swept the West Coast and is becoming an international phenomenon. They're not the only ones jumping at the chance to serve you your favorite cup of espresso, cappuccino, or latte. Bookstores, fast-food restaurants, and even gas stations are beginning to offer these specialty brews. This is just the latest twist on a very old habit.

As the story goes, tea was discovered in 2737 B.C. by Chinese emperor Shen Nung when leaves from a local plant fell into water he was boiling.[1] Thousands of years later, around A.D. 600, coffee berries were discovered by a goat herder in Ethiopia after the goats consumed the red berries and stayed up all night. From there, coffee consumption spread to the Middle East and then to Europe in 1615.[2] Soft drinks and over-the-counter (OTC) medications are part of caffeine's more recent history, and the latest caffeinated product is caffeinated water, marketed under the brand name Water Joe. David Marcheschi, a 29 year-old Chicago mortgage banker, invented Water Joe while trying to stay awake in college. A 16.9-ounce bottle has the caffeine equivalent of an 8-ounce cup of coffee and retails for 99 cents.[3] It's coffee without the bitterness and a soft drink without the sweetness.

Economics

Coffee is one of the most widely consumed beverages in the world. An estimated 400 billion cups of coffee are consumed worldwide every year.[4] The coffee trade competes with wheat in global importance. Five million tons are produced annually in fifty countries. South American countries lead production, followed by Africa, Asia, and North and Central America. The larger producers ship most of their crop abroad to countries like the United States and

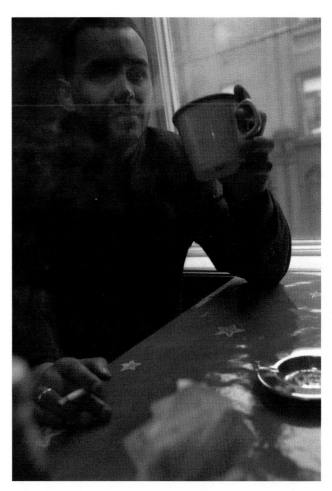

Combining coffee drinking and cigarette smoking may make it more difficult to decrease or eliminate either habit.

Europe. The United States consumes one-third of the world's coffee production.[4]

Social Issues

Coffee breaks are a time to socialize. Mid-morning or midafternoon caffeine, conversation, and company improve the rest of the workday for many people. Whether it's at work, a high style downtown brasserie, a homey neighborhood cafe, or a college hangout, coffee consumption is a social activity.

Historically, leaders in many countries have tried to ban coffeehouses for this very reason: being the meeting places that they are, coffeehouses tended to breed revolutionary political ideas.[5] There may be a few revolutionaries who frequent today's coffeehouses in the United States, but by and large the clientele is more mainstream. On a typical day at a Washington, D.C. coffeehouse, mothers and their babies gather after dropping older children at school. Later in the morning, retirees come in. In the afternoon, people who work at home stop in. After school, the same coffeehouse becomes a high school hangout. After dark, young professionals and couples on dates arrive. This is evidence that coffeehouses are nongenerational meeting places that everyone can enjoy.

The draw of the coffeehouse is varied. It provides a relaxing atmosphere, a refuge from unpaid bills and unmade beds, a place to work where you're not entirely alone, a place to engage in conversation, a place to watch the world go by, and a familiar place where you'll probably run into someone you know in the next 15 minutes.

Health Effects

Caffeine does have pharmacological effects on the function of cardiovascular, respiratory, renal, and nervous systems, but at the low, fixed pattern of consumption that most people enjoy, caffeine is merely a mild stimulant.[6] However, withdrawal from even a mild caffeine habit may cause headaches, fatigue, and difficulty concentrating. These symptoms peak in 18 to 24 hours, causing many weekday coffee drinkers to experience weekend withdrawal headaches.[7] In high doses, acute effects such as restlessness, agitation, tremors, cardiac dysrhythmias (irregular heartbeat), gastric disturbance, and diarrhea have been reported. Women who are trying to get pregnant or are pregnant are advised to avoid caffeine consumption.[8]

Caffeine is just one of the more than one hundred active substances present in coffee.[9] Even if caffeine does have certain effects on the body, they may not be apparent because other chemicals in the coffee counteract them or because the effects themselves may be short-lived. Study results of caffeine's effect on the cardiovascular system have not been consistent. It seems, though, that caffeine does trigger a rise in blood pressure and a lowering of heart rate. These effects last only for a matter of hours initially. After a few days of consumption, caffeine tolerance sets in, and these conditions no longer occur. It seems that the only permanent toll that coffee takes on the cardiovascular system is not even related to caffeine. If the coffee is unfiltered, fats from the coffee beans can raise cholesterol levels.[10]

Suspicion that caffeine causes cancer is undeserved as well. Research suggests no meaningful association of coffee with most common cancers, including those of the digestive tract, breast, and genital tract.[11] There is also no evidence of a dose-response relationship between coffee/caffeine consumption and delayed conception or persistent infertility.[12]

In children, caffeine causes inattentiveness, distraction, and impulsivity. Parents are wise to monitor the caffeine intake of their children. Pregnant women should avoid caffeine use. Three or more cups of coffee or tea a day during the first 4 months of pregnancy seems to increase the risk of miscarriage.[8] This finding may not be entirely attributable to caffeine because coffee consumption increases with age, and aging itself is a risk factor in pregnancy.

Breaking the Habit

You may want to break the caffeine habit because it generates dependence and you don't like the headache you get when you can't find a vending machine or when nobody at the office made coffee. You may want to set a good example for your children to avoid caffeine, or you may simply want to live as drug-free as possible. Whatever your reasons, the following list

offers suggestions that will help you to attain your goal.[13]

1. Keep a log of where, when, how much, and with whom you consume coffee, tea, caffeinated soda, or caffeinated pills.
2. To avoid withdrawal symptoms such as headaches, don't quit cold turkey. Instead, reduce your consumption slowly, by one cup, can, or pill per day.
3. If you are a coffee drinker, gradually switch from regular to decaffeinated coffee by mixing them before brewing, or substitute decaffeinated instant coffee for some of the caffeinated instant you drink. Increase the decaffeinated proportion each day. Choose a premium decaf to reward yourself and to keep your coffee routine enjoyable.
4. Substitute decaffeinated tea for your regular caffeinated tea, and replace caffeinated soda with a caffeine-free drink.
5. Drink from smaller cups instead of large mugs or glasses. Avoid the huge mugs made popular by the television show "Friends." If your favorite mug is a comfort to you, don't discard it, but fill it with a caffeine-free beverage. If, on the other hand, you find your coffee paraphernalia to be a temptation, get rid of those mugs, pots, filters, and grinders. Change your daily routine by taking a walk instead of your usual coffee break.
6. Use more low-fat milk in your coffee or tea to reduce the amount of caffeinated beverage you consume while increasing your calcium consumption.
7. Consider an alternative to a caffeinated beverage, such as bouillon, cider, herbal tea, or a grain-based beverage such as Postum.
8. Do not restructure your home and work routines to avoid caffeine so much that you lose the healthful aspects of a coffee break or an evening at your favorite hangout. Remember that noncaffeinated beverages are available; simply plan ahead.

9. When you find yourself getting sleepy while studying, driving, or working and feel tempted to drink a caffeinated beverage, take a break, open a window, breathe deeply and stretch, jog in place, go for a walk, get a cold drink, or take a short nap!

If you get enough sleep, exercise regularly, and follow a healthy diet, you'll be less reliant on the artificial "pep" that caffeine provides.

For Discussion . . .

Of the caffeinated beverages—coffee, tea, and soda—which do you prefer? Do you consume more than three cups or glasses a day? If so, have you thought about why you rely so heavily on caffeine? Would you like to reduce your consumption?

Are you part of the coffeehouse craze? What's special about your hangout?

References

1. The Great Idea Finder. *Fascinating facts about the invention of Tea by Chinese Emperor Shen Nung in 2737 B.C.* (online). Available: **http://www.ideafinder.com/history/inventions/story027.htm,** accessed 25 May 2003.

2. The Roast and Post Coffee Company. *The History of Coffee* (online). Available: **http://www.realcoffee.co.uk/Article.asp?Cat=History,** accessed 25 May 2003.

3. Water Joe. **www.waterjoe.com,** accessed 25 May 2003.

4. Coffee Universe: *A Brief History of Coffee* (online). Available: **http://www.coffeeuniverse.com/university_hist.html,** accessed 25 May 2003.

5. Morse M: Across the country, it's all happening at the coffeehouse. *Smithsonian* 27(6):10–13, 1996.

6. The Coffee Science Information Centre. *Caffeine* (online). Available: **http://www.cosic.org/caffeine/stimulanteffects/,** accessed 25 May 2003.

7. Alpha Nutrition Health Education. *Withdrawal Symptoms* (online). Available: **http://www.nutramed.com/symptoms/withdrawal.htm,** accessed 25 May 2003.

8. *Caffeine.* Johns Hopkins InteliHealth online newsletter, November 10, 1998. Available: **www.intelihealth.com,** accessed 25 May 2003.

9. Institute for Coffee Studies. *Chemical Composition of Coffee* (online). Available: **http://www.mc.vanderbilt.edu/coffee/chemical.html,** accessed 25 May 2003.

10. Jee SH, He J, Appel W, et al. Coffee consumption and serum lipids: meta-analysis of randomized controlled clinical trials. *American Journal of Epidemiology* 153, pp. 353–362, 2001.

11. Coffee Science Source. *Coffee and Caffeine Content* (online). Available: **http://www.coffeescience.org/other.html,** accessed 25 May 2003.

12. PregnancyMD.org. *Lifestyle Factors and Infertility* (online). Available: **http://www.pregnancymd.org/lifestyle-infertility-factors.htm,** accessed 25 May 2003.

13. Anonymous. *Tips for breaking the caffeine habit.* 1996.

InfoLinks

www.gardfoods.com/coffee/index.htm
www.roble.com/marquis/caffeine

personal assessment

test your drug awareness

1. What is the most commonly used drug in the United States?
   A. heroin
   B. cocaine
   C. alcohol
   D. marijuana
2. Name the three drugs most commonly used by children.
   A. alcohol, tobacco, and marijuana
   B. cocaine, crack, alcohol
   C. heroin, inhalants, marijuana
3. Which drug is associated with the most teenage deaths?
   A. heroin
   B. cocaine
   C. alcohol
   D. marijuana
4. By the eighth grade, how many kids have tried at least one inhalant?
   A. one in one hundred
   B. one in fifty
   C. one in twenty-five
   D. one in five
   E. one in two
5. "Crack" is a particularly dangerous drug because it is
   A. cheap.
   B. readily available.
   C. highly addictive.
   D. all of the above.
6. Fumes from which of the following can be inhaled to produce a high?
   A. spray paint
   B. model glue
   C. nail polish remover
   D. whipped cream canisters
   E. all of the above
7. People who have not used alcohol and other drugs before their 20th birthday:
   A. have no risk of becoming chemically dependent.
   B. are less likely to develop a drinking problem or use illicit drugs.
   C. have an increased risk of becoming chemically dependent.

8. A speedball is a combination of which two drugs?
   A. cocaine and heroin
   B. PCP and LSD
   C. valium and alcohol
   D. amphetamines and barbiturates
9. Methamphetamines are dangerous because their use can cause
   A. anxiety/nervousness/irritability.
   B. paranoia/psychosis.
   C. loss of appetite/malnutrition/anorexia.
   D. hallucinations.
   E. aggressive behavior.
   F. all of the above.
10. How is marijuana harmful?
   A. It hinders the user's short-term memory.
   B. Students may find it hard to study and learn while under the influence of marijuana.
   C. It affects timing and coordination.
   D. All of the above.

Answers to Personal Assessment
1. C
2. A
3. C
4. D
5. D
6. E
7. B
8. A
9. F
10. D

personal assessment

getting a drug-free high

Experts agree that drug use provides only short-term, ineffective, and often destructive solutions to problems. We hope that you have found (or will find) innovative, invigorating drug-free experiences that make your life more exciting. Circle the number for each activity that reflects your intention to try that activity. Use the following guide:

1	No intention of trying this activity
2	Intend to try this within 2 years
3	Intend to try this within 6 months
4	Already tried this activity
5	Regularly engage in this activity

1.	Learn to juggle	1	2	3	4	5
2.	Go backpacking	1	2	3	4	5
3.	Complete a marathon race	1	2	3	4	5
4.	Start a vegetable garden	1	2	3	4	5
5.	Ride in a hot air balloon	1	2	3	4	5
6.	Snow ski or water ski	1	2	3	4	5
7.	Donate blood	1	2	3	4	5
8.	Go river rafting	1	2	3	4	5
9.	Learn to play a musical instrument	1	2	3	4	5
10.	Cycle 100 miles	1	2	3	4	5
11.	Go skydiving	1	2	3	4	5
12.	Go rockclimbing	1	2	3	4	5
13.	Play a role in a theater production	1	2	3	4	5
14.	Build a piece of furniture	1	2	3	4	5
15.	Solicit funds for a worthy cause	1	2	3	4	5
16.	Learn to swim	1	2	3	4	5
17.	Overhaul a car engine	1	2	3	4	5
18.	Compose a song	1	2	3	4	5
19.	Travel to a foreign country	1	2	3	4	5
20.	Write the first chapter of a book	1	2	3	4	5

TOTAL POINTS _____

Interpretation

61–100	You participate in many challenging experiences
41–60	You are willing to try some challenging new experiences
20–40	You take few of the challenging risks described here

To Carry This Further . . .

Looking at your point total, were you surprised at the degree to which you are aware of alternative activities? What are the top five activities, and can you understand their importance? What activities would you add to this list?

chapter eight

taking Control of alcohol use

Talking It Over

Getting a Friend into Treatment

Someone close to you has a drinking problem. What can you do to help this person get professional help?

- Talk with an alcohol or drug treatment counselor to learn what to expect.
- Confront your friend when both of you are sober.
- Express genuine concern for your friend's life.
- Point out specific situations when your friend's alcohol-related behavior was dangerous to him or her and to other people.
- Tell your friend where he or she can go to find help. Have names, phone numbers, and addresses ready.
- Offer to accompany your friend to the counselor or treatment center.
- Tell your friend that "now—this minute—is the time to get into treatment." Be persistent. Also be ready to transport your friend immediately, before his or her denial begins.

CommunicationLinks

www.way2hope.org
www.aca-usa.org
www.health.org

Eye on the Media

TV Ads Target Drunk Driving

The first successful national campaign against drunk driving, "Designated Driver," began in 1998. Besides targeting specific audiences and using well-timed and strategically placed public service announcements, its developers convinced TV producers and writers to work references to the designated driver into the dialogue of their shows. Gradually, the message got through to young people. It does make sense to plan to have someone else drive if you're not going to be up to it. The designated-driver approach is still considered a good idea on college campuses today.

In contrast, the "Campaign for Alcohol Free Kids," relied heavily on dramatic graphics, such as grisly photos of car crash scenes on prom night.[1] Although the overall visual

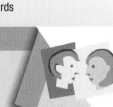

impact was powerful, the campaign lacked a practical element. Worse, the ads seemed to be preaching.

The Ad Council's "Friends Don't Let Friends Drive Drunk" is based on the idea that we all have responsibility for each other. If someone is your friend, you want to take care of that person. So don't let your friend do something dangerous.[2] Here the message is practical, not preachy.

The "You Drink & Drive, You Lose" campaign, a part of the National Public Education Campaign, targets two high-risk groups, 21- to 34-year-olds and repeat offenders. The message is simple: Make the right choice—don't drink and drive. The "Don't Lose It!" TV spot focuses on the fact that it's inconvenient to be stopped but the time spent at the checkpoint is for your own safety. It seems to be saying: "Sure, you're in a hurry, but this is important. So be patient." The graphics range from a serious-looking police officer talking to a motorist to hands locked in handcuffs.

What the successful campaigns have in common is a message that is simple, believable, and acceptable. Rather than scolding or preaching, the ads emphasize the fact that you have a choice and ask you to make the right choice.

"Road Predators," an American Public Television special that aired in December 1999, touched off strong controversy. Funded by the Century Council, a corporation backed by a group of U.S. distillers, the program used tragic accounts of alcohol-related accidents to dramatize the fact that innocent people lose their lives, families are shattered, and billions of dollars are spent because of drunk drivers. The contrast between the life of the featured victim (a good and caring school-teacher) and that of the drunk driver (an aimless man who spends most of his time drinking) was highlighted.

Beer manufacturers became angry. To them, the show suggested that drinking beer and driving is the problem, not drinking *any* type of alcohol and driving. Why, they wondered, was there no sign of hard liquor in the show? Other critics argued that by focusing on hard-core drinkers, the program implied that the problem of drunk driving is limited to a small group. What about bias? According to *The Wall Street Journal* ("Brewers Attack Drunken-Driving Special," Dec. 14, 1999, p. B8), the special's producer first claimed that the Century Group had had no input into its content but later conceded that it had supplied news clippings as background and had recommended that certain people be interviewed. As for accuracy, the deputy district attorney who tried the case said that it was not true that the drunk driver "very likely won't be required to complete" his 15-year sentence, as the program said. The producer responded that this was probably "a little dramatic license" on the writer's part. The sophisticated and expensive advertising for the special included an elaborate spread in *Newsweek* (Dec. 6, 1999), with an 8-page booklet featuring the drunk driver and the victim.

What is the motivation for an alcohol industry group to fund a campaign to discourage drunk driving? How do such campaigns compare with the tobacco industry's efforts to discourage smoking among teenagers? How effective do you think each kind of ad campaign is?

1. Campaign for Alcohol Free Kids: Who We Are (online). **www.alcoholfreekids.com/au_who_we_are.html** accessed 13 June 2003.
2. Website Information: Ad Council. **www.adcouncil.org/** accessed 13 June 2003.

The push for zero tolerance laws, the tightening of standards for determining legal intoxication, and the growing influence of national groups concerned with alcohol misuse show that our society is more sensitive than ever to the misuse of alcohol.

People are concerned about the consequences of drunk driving, alcohol-related crime, and lowered job productivity. Alcohol use remains quite high among young people in the United States and national data indicate that per capita, alcohol consumption has slowly decreased in the United States since the 1980s.[1] Alcohol use remains the preferred form of drug use for most adults (including college students), but as a society, we are increasingly uncomfortable with the ease with which alcohol can be misused.

is generally held in check is expressed (Figure 8-1). At least temporarily, drinkers become a different version of themselves—more outgoing, relaxed, and adventuresome.

 TALKING POINTS If alcohol did not make people more outgoing, relaxed, and adventuresome, then do you think they would consume as much?

Alcohol Use Patterns

From magazines to billboards to television, alcohol is one of the most heavily advertised consumer products in the country.[2] You cannot watch television, listen to the radio,

Choosing to Drink

Clearly, people drink for many different reasons. Most people drink because alcohol is an effective, affordable, and legal substance for altering the brain's chemistry. As **inhibitions** are removed by the influence of alcohol, behavior that

> **Key Terms**
>
> **inhibitions** inner controls that prevent a person from engaging in certain types of behavior.

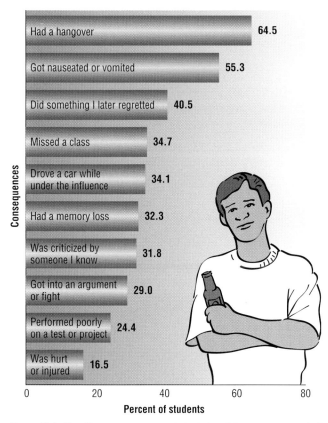

Figure 8-1 Negative consequences of alcohol and drug use as reported by college students. (*Occurred at least once in the past year.)

Source: Core Institute. 2001 Statistics on Alcohol and Other Drug Use on American College Campuses (online). Available: **www.siu.edu/departments/coreinst/public_html/recent.html** accessed 16 June 2003.

or read a newspaper without being encouraged to buy a particular brand of beer, wine, or liquor. The advertisements create a warm aura about the nature of alcohol use. The implications are clear: Alcohol use will bring you good times, handsome men or seductive women, exotic settings, and a chance to forget the hassles of hard work and study.

With many pressures to drink, it is not surprising that most adults drink alcoholic beverages. Two-thirds of all American adults are classified as drinkers. Yet one in three adults does not drink. In the college environment, where surveys indicate that 85% to 90% of all students drink, it is difficult for many students to imagine that every third adult is an abstainer. Complete the Personal Assessment on page 289 to rate your own alcohol use.

Alcohol consumption figures are reported in many different ways, depending on the researchers' criteria. Figures from various sources support the contention that about one-third of adults eighteen years of age and older are abstainers, about one-third are light drinkers, and one-third are moderate-to-heavy drinkers (see the Star box on page 262). As a single category, heavy drinkers make up about 10% of the adult drinking population.

Drinking on Campus

Students who drink in college tend to classify themselves as light-to-moderate drinkers. It comes as a shock to students, though, when they read the criteria for each drinking classification. Many students will find that they fall into the category of heavy drinkers. The criteria are

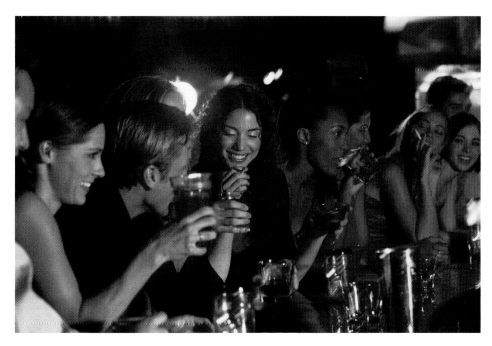

Two-thirds of American adults are classified as drinkers. Only one-third choose to abstain from using alcohol.

Table 8.1 Criteria for Drinking Classifications

Classification	Alcohol-Related Behavior
Abstainers	Do not drink or drink less often than once a year
Infrequent drinkers	Drink once a month at most and drink small amounts per typical drinking occasion
Light drinkers	Drink once a month at most and drink medium amounts per typical drinking occasion, or drink no more than three to four times a month and drink small amounts per typical drinking occasion
Moderate drinkers	Drink at least once a week and small amounts per typical drinking occasion or three to four times a month and medium amounts per typical drinking occasion or no more than once a month and large amounts per typical drinking occasion
Moderate/heavy drinkers	Drink at least once a week and medium amounts per typical drinking occasion or three to four times a month and large amounts per typical drinking occasion
Heavy drinkers	Drink at least once a week and large amounts per typical drinking occasion[1]

Note: Small amounts = One drink or less per drinking occasion
Medium amounts = Two to four drinks per drinking occasion
Large amounts = Five or more drinks per drinking occasion (binge drinking)
Drink = 12 fluid oz of beer, 5 fluid oz of wine, or 1.5 fluid oz of 80 proof distilled spirits[2]

[1]U.S. Department of Health and Human Services: *Fourth Special Report to the U.S. Congress, Washington, D.C.*, 1981, DHHS Pub No. ADM 81-1080.
[2]Dufour M. (1999). What is Moderate Drinking? Defining "Drinks" and Drinking Levels. *Alcohol Research and Health.* 23(1), 5–14.

based on a combination of quantity of alcohol consumed per occasion and the frequency of drinking, as shown in Table 8.1.

 TALKING POINTS How would you tell a friend you think she has a drinking problem?

Binge Drinking

Alcohol abuse by college students usually takes the form of a drinking pattern called **binge drinking.** Binge drinking refers to the consumption of five drinks in a row, at least once during the previous two-week period. One large study of more than seventeen thousand students on 131 campuses found that 49.7% of students binged.[3] The strongest predictors for bingeing were living in a fraternity or sorority, adopting a party-centered lifestyle, and engaging in other risky behavior. The study also suggested that many college students began binge drinking in high school.

By its very nature, binge drinking can be dangerous. Drunk driving, physical violence, property destruction, date rape, police arrest, and lowered academic performance are all highly associated with binge drinking. Besides the role that heavy drinking may play in the aggressor in date rape, a recent study found that more than half the victims in sexual assaults also were at least somewhat drunk.

The direct correlation between the amount of alcohol consumed and lowered academic performance results in impaired memory, verbal skill deficiencies, and altered

Moderate Drinking Redefined

Alcohol Research and Health defines moderate drinking as no more than two drinks each day for most men and one drink each day for women. A drink is defined as one 12-ounce regular beer, a 5-ounce glass of wine, or 1.5-ounces of 80 proof distilled spirits.* These cutoff levels are based on the amount of alcohol that can be consumed without causing problems, either for the drinker or society. (The gender difference is due primarily to the higher percentage of body fat in women and to the lower amount of an essential stomach enzyme in women.) Elderly people are limited to no more than one drink each day, again due to a higher percentage of body fat.

These consumption levels are applicable to most people. Indeed, people who plan to drive, women who are pregnant, people recovering from alcohol addiction, people under age twenty-one, people taking medications, and those with existing medical concerns should not consume alcohol at all. In addition, although some studies have shown that low levels of alcohol consumption may have minor psychological and cardiovascular benefits, nondrinkers are not advised to start drinking.

*Dufour M. (1999). What is Moderate Drinking? Defining "Drinks" and Drinking Levels. *Alcohol Research and Health* 23(1), 5–14.

Key Terms

binge drinking the consumption of five drinks or more on one drinking occasion.

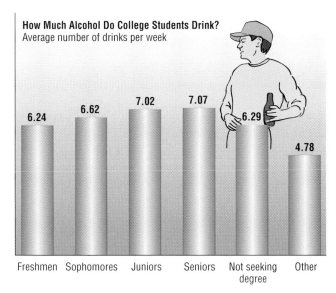

How Much Alcohol Do College Students Drink?
Average number of drinks per week

Freshmen: 6.24
Sophomores: 6.62
Juniors: 7.02
Seniors: 7.07
Not seeking degree: 6.29
Other: 4.78

Figure 8-2 Twenty-one- to twenty-four-year-olds drink more beer than any other age group. How many servings a month do you have?

perceptions.[4] Frequently, the social costs of binge drinking can be very high, especially when intoxicated people demonstrate their level of immaturity. How common is binge drinking on your campus?

For large numbers of students who drink, the college years are a time when they will drink more heavily than at any other period during their lifetime (Figure 8-2). Some will suffer serious consequences as a result. These years will also mark the entry into a lifetime of problem drinking for some.

Drinking Games

Drinking games are one form of binge drinking that seeks to make binge drinking socially acceptable.

Drinking games are especially risky for inexperienced drinkers who are unfamiliar with changes associated with heavy alcohol consumption. They place themselves at increased risk for drinking-related problems, such as alcohol poisoning, injuries, property destruction, legal problems, and sexual assaults.

Declining Alcohol Use

As you learned in Chapter 7, "Making Decisions about Drug Use," being able to decline drugs and alcohol when others around are using these substances is a challenge that you can learn to meet. For example, if you are fit, participating in a long bicycle ride or run, it can leave you with an excellent sense of well-being produced by endorphins, natural painkillers produced by the brain. Such a "high" is enhanced by the knowledge that you have earned the good feeling through your efforts (see the Discovering

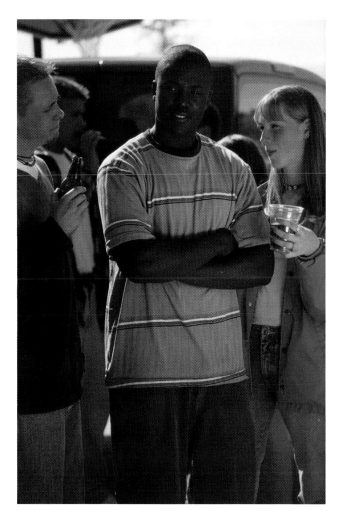

Mature adults know how to enjoy alcohol responsibly and understand how to decline alcohol use when they don't want to drink.

Your Spirituality box on page 264). Consider some additional techniques for avoiding alcohol:

- Avoid parties where you can logically expect heavy drinking.
- Avoid people who are drinking heavily or becoming erratic or threatening.

OnSITE/InSIGHT

Learning to Go: Health

Do you drink occasionally or on a daily basis? Click on Learning to Go: Health on the Online Learning Center at **www.mhhe. com/payne8e** to find these lessons, which will put your approach to alcohol use in perspective:

Lesson 26: Know your limits; drink responsibly.

Lesson 27: Recognize the signs of problem drinking.

What's a Social Life Without Alcohol?

When was the last time you went to a get-together where alcoholic drinks weren't served? It's probably been years. Socializing and drinking are connected in our consciousness in many ways. For instance, it's Friday night after a hard week and your friends ask you to join them for a beer. Why not? It'll be fun. Or you're invited to a party and want to bring something. How about a bottle of wine? That's easy and always appreciated.

Associating drinking with fun is something that many people, including college students, do. For various reasons, though, some college students are choosing to plan their fun around activities that don't involve drinking. Instead of going to a bar for a beer, they find a coffee shop and have a latte. Or they order soda with their pizza (not bad!). Others have discovered that they can get something that tastes great and is actually healthy at a juice bar.

What happens, though, when you go to a party and everyone else seems to be drinking? Choose something nonalcoholic—club soda, juice, soda, or water. (You probably won't be the only one doing this.) If someone gives you trouble about your choice, be firm. Just say that's what you want. You don't need to explain. And you don't have to say "yes" to be nice.

But maybe you want to drink at a party because it loosens you up and makes it easier to talk to people. How will you start a conversation without a drink to relax you? Think about how you talk easily and naturally with the people in your drama group or one of your favorite classes. You've got things in common, so it's easier to do. When you meet someone new at a party, look for common interests. You may feel self-conscious at first. But soon you'll forget about the fact that he or she is a stranger because you'll be involved in what you're talking about. Without that drink, you'll actually be more yourself.

Some students are making the commitment to be active instead of sitting around and drinking. They're going backpacking, joining a cycling group, taking an exercise class, or playing a team sport. What they're discovering is that it feels good—physically and mentally. They're socializing, doing something they enjoy, and getting in better shape. Think about something you've always wanted to try, and get going on it.

Making the choice to have fun without alcohol doesn't mean cutting yourself off from your friends. (If they're real friends, they'll respect your choice.) It's all about deciding what's right for you and making a commitment to that choice.

- Request a nonalcoholic beer, soft drink, or glass of water instead of alcohol.
- Participate in activities that can provide a nonchemical high. See the Personal Assessment on page 257 of Chapter 7 for a variety of suggestions.
- Cultivate friends who find their highs through natural, positive activities in which you share an interest.

Alcohol and the Family

The alcohol abuser hurts more than just himself or herself. Everyone around the addicted person suffers. Alcoholism is a family disease, and a family can be defined as a person, a family, a fraternity, a sorority, a dormitory floor, even a therapy group or a 12-step group. Eventually everyone around the alcoholic suffers, including the spouse, parents, children, siblings, friends, boyfriend/girlfriend, and roommates.

Following are some of the behaviors that the dysfunctional family typically experiences:[5]

- Lives in fear, teaching you to fear others different from yourself in race, religion, color, nationality, appearance, and so forth.

- Teaches that the family members should depend on each other to the exclusion of the outside world. An exception can be made for outsiders who are identical to the family members.
- Teaches that, to be successful, you must have money, make money or marry into money.
- Teaches that the authority figures in the family are right.
- Teaches every member of the family to adapt to the emotional sickness of the family and feels threatened when a member attempts to recover.
- Teaches conditional love.
- Teaches that, to have a worthwhile identity, you must gain the approval of the outside world, and especially the group itself.
- Feels threatened and abandoned at the death or departure of a loved member of the group.
- Tries to maintain the group through guilt and pity, which it calls "love."
- Expects all members to like the same things and people.
- Thrives on excitement, and teaches that if you are not excited, you are not alive.

As a result of these constant lessons, the person living with alcoholism can develop many of the following problems. The person living with alcoholism can tend to:

- Become isolated and afraid of people and authority figures.
- Become an approval-seeker and lose his or her identity in the process.
- Become frightened by angry people and any criticism.
- Become an alcoholic, marry one, or find another compulsive personality such as a workaholic to continue the sickness.
- Develop a victim mentality and be attracted by weakness in potential friends or loved ones.
- Have an extreme sense of responsibility and focus on others to the detriment of himself or herself.
- Feel guilty when being assertive or saying no.
- Become addicted to excitement.
- Confuse pity with love.
- Lose the ability to feel or express feelings.
- Be terrified of abandonment and be willing to tolerate abuse to hold on to a relationship.
- Develop all the symptoms of an alcoholic without actually drinking.

The good news is that many resources, such as recovery and support groups, have become available in the last few years for both the alcoholic and those who live with the alcoholic. See the sections on alcohol self-assessment, codependence, rehabilitation and recovery, and adult children of alcoholic parents beginning on page 275.

Those who have lived with an alcoholic will face their own issues as they work through their own recovery. They may find that they learned compulsions from the alcoholic, or they may transfer the compulsions to other behaviors, such as excessive eating, gambling, house cleaning, or taking up lost causes or people. Those who know, or are still living with, an active alcoholic also can consider intervention to urge the alcoholic to seek help.

The Nature of Alcoholic Beverages

Alcohol (also known as *ethyl alcohol* or *ethanol*) is the principal product of **fermentation.** In this process, yeast cells act on the sugar content of fruits and grains to produce alcohol and carbon dioxide.[6]

The alcohol concentration in beverages such as whiskey, gin, rum, and vodka is determined through a process called **distillation.** These distilled beverages are expressed by the term *proof,* a number that is twice the percentage of alcohol by volume in a beverage. Thus 70

percent of the fluid in a bottle of 140 proof gin is pure alcohol. Most proofs in distilled beverages range from 80 to 160. The pure grain alcohol that is often added to fruit punches and similar beverages has a proof of almost 200.

The nutritional value of alcohol is extremely limited. Alcoholic beverages produced today through modern processing methods contain nothing but empty calories—about 100 calories per fluid ounce of 100-proof distilled spirits and about 150 calories per each twelve-ounce bottle or can of beer. Alcohol consumption is a significant contributor to the additional pounds that many college students accumulate. Pure alcohol contains only simple carbohydrates; it has no vitamins and minerals, and no fats or protein.

Recently, some researchers have suggested that moderate consumption of alcoholic beverages can reduce the risk of coronary heart disease.[7] Alcohol appears to increase levels of HDL cholesterol (the good cholesterol) in the bloodstream and, perhaps, reduce LDL cholesterol levels. However, there are various other ways to alter a person's cholesterol profile. Doctors caution anyone against drinking merely because of this one possible health benefit.

"Light" beer and low-calorie wines have been introduced in response to concerns about the number of calories in alcoholic beverages. These light beverages are not low-alcohol beverages but merely low-calorie beverages. Only beverages marked "low alcohol" contain a lower concentration of alcohol than the usual beverages of that type. Recently, manufacturers have introduced a new form of beer called low carbohydrate beer. See Star box on page 266.

Ice beers actually contain a higher percentage of alcohol than do other types of beer. The term *ice* refers to the way in which this beer is processed. After brewing and fermentation, it is deep-chilled at 24 to 28 degrees Fahrenheit, which causes ice crystals to form in the mixture. When these ice crystals are removed, the remaining liquid contains a higher percentage of alcohol. Most regular and light beers contain less than 5% alcohol, whereas ice beer generally contains 5% to 6% alcohol. Do you think beer drinkers are choosing this beer for its reportedly rich flavor or simply because it contains more alcohol?

Key Terms

fermentation a chemical process whereby plant products are converted into alcohol by the action of yeast cells on carbohydrate materials.

distillation the process of heating an alcohol solution and collecting its vapors into a more concentrated solution.

Low Carbohydrate Beer

Many dieters in the United States consume low carbohydrate diets with the hope of shedding and keeping off unwanted pounds. Carbohydrates, which include a variety of sugars and starches, serve as a major dietary source of energy. Recently, beer brewers have launched low carbohydrate beers for the diet-conscious consumers. These beers contain as few as 2.6 grams of carbohydrates per 12-ounce bottle of beer. Most regular beers contain between 3.2 grams to 6.6 grams of carbohydrates per 12-ounce serving. Ice beers may contain as many as 32 grams of carbohydrates per 12-ounce serving. Although these new low carbohydrate beers are similar in alcohol and calorie content to other beers, the carbohydrate content is lower. The brewers do state that there has been no health or weight loss claims attributed to this new type of beer. These beers let the consumer drink, yet keep carbohydrate intake to a minimum.

The Physiological Effects of Alcohol

First and foremost, alcohol is classified as a drug—a very strong CNS depressant. The primary depressant effect of alcohol occurs in the brain and spinal cord. Many people think of alcohol as a stimulant because of the way most users feel after consuming a serving or two of their favorite drink. Any temporary sensations of jubilation, boldness, or relief are attributable to alcohol's ability as a depressant drug to release personal inhibitions and provide temporary relief from tension.

Factors That Influence the Absorption of Alcohol

The **absorption** of alcohol is influenced by several factors, most of which can be controlled by the individual. These factors include the following:

Strength of the Beverage

The stronger the beverage, the greater the amount of alcohol that will accumulate within the digestive tract.

Number of Drinks Consumed

As more drinks are consumed, more alcohol is absorbed.

Speed of Consumption

If consumed rapidly, even relatively few drinks will result in a large concentration gradient that will lead to high blood alcohol concentration.

Presence of Food

Food can compete with alcohol for absorption into the bloodstream, thus slowing the absorption of alcohol.

When you slow your alcohol absorption, your body can remove alcohol already in the bloodstream. Serving food at a party is a healthy idea.

Body Chemistry

Each person has an individual pattern of physiological functioning that may affect the ability to process alcohol. For example, in some conditions, such as that marked by "dumping syndrome," the stomach empties more rapidly than is normal, and alcohol seems to be absorbed more quickly. The emptying time may be either slowed or quickened by anger, fear, stress, nausea, and the condition of the stomach tissues.

Gender

Women produce much less alcohol dehydrogenase than do men.[8] This enzyme is responsible for breaking down alcohol in the stomach. With less alcohol dehydrogenase action, women absorb about 30% more alcohol into the bloodstream than men do, despite an identical number of drinks and equal body weight.

Three other reasons help explain why women tend to absorb alcohol more quickly than do men of the same body weight: (1) Women have proportionately more body fat than men. Since alcohol is not stored easily in fat, it enters the bloodstream relatively quickly. (2) Women's bodies have proportionately less water than men's bodies of equal weight. Thus consumed alcohol does not become as diluted as it does in men. (3) Alcohol absorption is influenced by a woman's menstrual cycle. Alcohol is more quickly absorbed during the premenstrual phase of a woman's cycle. Also, there is evidence that women using birth control pills absorb alcohol more quickly than usual.[8]

With the exception of a person's body chemistry and gender, all factors that influence absorption can be moderated by the alcohol user.

Blood Alcohol Concentration

A person's **blood alcohol concentration (BAC)** rises when alcohol is consumed faster than it can be removed (oxidized) by the liver.[9] As outlined in Figure 8-3, a fairly

---

Key Terms

absorption the passage of nutrients or alcohol through the walls of the stomach or intestinal tract into the bloodstream.

blood alcohol concentration (BAC) the percentage of alcohol in a measured quantity of blood; BAC can be determined directly, through the analysis of a blood sample, or indirectly, through the analysis of exhaled air.

Table 8.2 Blood Alcohol Concentration and the Effects of Alcohol

Blood Alcohol Concentration	Sporadic Drinker	Chronic Drinker	Hours for Alcohol to be Metabolized
.05%	Congenial euphoria; decreased tension	No observable effect	2–3
.075%	Talkative	Often no effect	
.10%	Uncoordinated; legally drunk (as in drunk driving) in most states; a level of 0.08% is legal drunkenness in 18 states	Minimal signs	4–6
.125%–.150%	Unrestrained behavior; episodic uncontrolled behavior	Pleasurable euphoria or beginning of uncoordination	6–10
.20%–.25%	Alertness lost; sluggish	Effort required to maintain emotional and motor control	10–24
.30%–.35%	Stupor to coma; death is possible	Drowsy and slow	
.40%–.50%	Death is likely	Coma; some will die	>24

predictable sequence of events takes place when a person drinks alcohol at a rate faster than one drink every hour. When the BAC reaches 0.05%, initial measurable changes in mood and behavior take place. Inhibitions and everyday tensions appear to be released, while judgment and critical thinking are somewhat impaired. This BAC would be achieved by a 160-pound person drinking about two drinks in an hour (see Table 8.2 above and Figure 8-3 on page 266).

At a level of 0.10% (one part alcohol to 1,000 parts blood), the drinker typically loses significant motor coordination. Voluntary motor function becomes quite clumsy. At this BAC, most states consider a drinker legally intoxicated and thus incapable of safely operating a vehicle. Although physiological changes associated with this BAC do occur, certain users do not feel drunk or appear impaired.

As a person continues to elevate the BAC from 0.20% to 0.50%, the health risk of **acute alcohol intoxication** increases rapidly. A BAC of 0.20% is characterized by the loud, boisterous, obnoxious drunk person who staggers. A 0.30% BAC produces further depression and stuporous behavior, during which time the drinker becomes so confused that he or she may not be capable of understanding anything. The 0.40% or 0.50% BAC produces unconsciousness. At this BAC a person can die, because brain centers that control body temperature, heartbeat, and respiration may virtually shut down.

An important factor influencing the BAC is the individual's blood volume. The larger the person, the greater the amount of blood into which alcohol can be distributed. Conversely, the smaller person has less blood into which alcohol can be distributed, and as a result, a higher BAC will develop.

Sobering Up

Alcohol is removed from the bloodstream principally through the process of **oxidation.** Oxidation occurs at a constant rate (about one-fourth to one-third ounce of pure alcohol per hour) that cannot be appreciably altered. Because each typical drink of beer, wine, or distilled spirits contains about one-half ounce of pure alcohol, it takes about two hours for the body to fully oxidize one typical alcoholic drink.[14]

After a night of drinking alcohol, the next morning people may experience uncomfortable symptoms such as a headache, nausea, fatigue, diarrhea, loss of appetite, or an overall feeling of being sick. These symptoms are commonly known as a *hangover* and are the result of the body reacting to too much alcohol in its system. These symptoms may also be attributed to dehydration, poor nutrition, an empty stomach, lack of sleep, poor health, or increased physical activity while drinking.

Although people have attempted to sober up by drinking hot coffee, taking cold showers, or exercising, the oxidation rate of alcohol is unaffected. Thus far the FDA has not approved any commercial product that can help people achieve sobriety. Passage of time remains the only effective way to sober up.

> **Key Terms**
>
> **acute alcohol intoxication** a potentially fatal elevation of BAC, often resulting from heavy, rapid consumption of alcohol.
>
> **oxidation** the process that removes alcohol from the bloodstream.

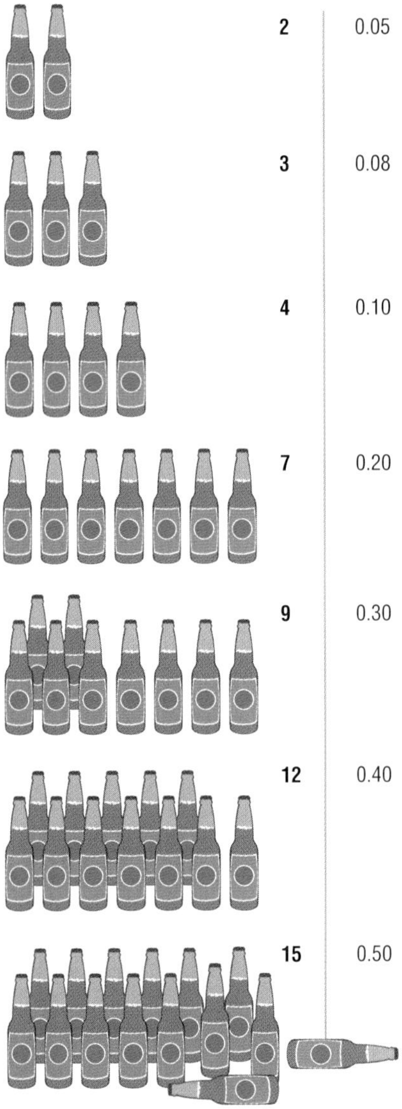

Number of drinks consumed in two hours	Alcohol in blood (percentage)	Typical effects
2	0.05	Judgment, thought, and restraint weakened; tension released, giving carefree sensation
3	0.08	Tensions of everyday life lessened; cheerfulness
4	0.10	Voluntary motor action affected, making hand and arm movements, walk, and speech clumsy
7	0.20	Severe impairment—staggering, loud, incoherent, emotionally unstable, 100 times greater traffic risk; exuberance and aggressive inclinations magnified
9	0.30	Deeper areas of brain affected, with stimulus-response and understanding confused; stuporous; blurred vision
12	0.40	Incapable of voluntary action; sleepy, difficult to arouse; equivalent of surgical anesthesia
15	0.50	Comatose; centers controlling breathing and heartbeat anesthetized; death increasingly probable

Note: A drink refers to a typical 12-ounce bottle of beer, a 1.5-ounce shot of hard liquor, or a 5-ounce glass of wine.

Figure 8-3 Effects of alcohol by number of drinks.

First Aid for Acute Alcohol Intoxication

Not everyone who goes to sleep, passes out, or even becomes unconscious after drinking has a high BAC. People who are already sleepy, have not eaten well, are sick, or are bored may drink a little alcohol and quickly fall asleep. However, people who drink heavily in a rather short time may be setting themselves up for an extremely unpleasant, toxic, potentially life-threatening experience because of their high BAC.

Although responsible drinking would prevent acute alcohol intoxication (poisoning), such responsible drinking will never be a reality for everyone. As caring adults,

what should we know about this health emergency that may help us save a life?

The first real danger sign we need to recognize is **shock** and its typical signs. By the time these signs are

---

Key Terms

shock profound collapse of many vital body functions; evident during acute alcohol intoxication and other serious health emergencies.

---

evident, a drinker will already have become unconscious. He or she cannot be aroused from a deep stupor. The person will probably have a weak, rapid pulse (over 100 beats per minute). The skin will be cool and damp, and breathing will be increased to once every three or four seconds. These breaths may be shallow or deep but will certainly occur in an irregular pattern. The skin will be pale or bluish. (In a person with dark skin, these color changes will be more evident in the fingernail beds or in the mucous membranes inside the mouth or under the eyelids.) Whenever any of these signs are present, seek emergency medical help immediately (see the Changing for the Better box above for a summary of these signs).

Involuntary regurgitation (vomiting) can be another potentially life-threatening emergency for a person who has drunk too much alcohol. When a drinker has consumed more alcohol than the liver can oxidize, the pyloric valve at the base of the stomach tends to close. Additional alcohol remains in the stomach. This alcohol irritates the lining of the stomach so much that involuntary muscle contractions force the stomach contents to flow back through the esophagus. By removing alcohol from the stomach, vomiting may be a life-saving mechanism for conscious drinkers.

An unconscious drinker who vomits, however, may be lying in such a position that the airway becomes obstructed with the vomitus from the stomach. This person is in great risk of dying from **asphyxiation.** As a first-aid measure, unconscious drinkers should always be rolled onto their sides to minimize the chance of airway obstruction. If you are with a person who is vomiting, make

certain that his or her head is positioned lower than the rest of the body. This position minimizes the chance that vomitus will obstruct the air passages.

It is also important to keep a close watch on anyone who passes out from heavy drinking. Unfortunately, partygoers sometimes make the mistake of carrying these people to bed and then forgetting about them. You should do your best to monitor the physical condition of anyone who becomes unconscious from heavy drinking because of the risk of death. If you really care about these people, you will observe them at regular intervals until they appear to be clearly out of danger. Although this may mean an evening of interrupted sleep for you, you might save a friend's life.

Alcohol-Related Health Problems

The relationship of chronic alcohol use to the structure and function of the body is reasonably well understood. Heavy alcohol use causes a variety of changes in the body that lead to an increase in morbidity and mortality. Figure 8-4 describes these changes.

Research shows that chronic alcohol use also damages the immune system and the nervous system. Thus chronic users are at high risk for a variety of infections and neurological complications.

Fetal Alcohol Syndrome and Fetal Alcohol Effects

A growing body of scientific evidence shows that alcohol use by pregnant women can cause birth defects in unborn children. When alcohol crosses the **placenta,** it enters the fetal bloodstream in a concentration equal to that in the mother's bloodstream. Because the fetal liver is underdeveloped, it oxidizes this alcohol much more slowly than the alcohol in the mother. During this time of slow detoxification, the developing fetus is certain to be overexposed to the toxic effects of alcohol. Mental retardation frequently develops.

Key Terms

asphyxiation death resulting from lack of oxygen to the brain.

placenta the structure through which nutrients, metabolic wastes, and drugs (including alcohol) pass from the bloodstream of the mother into the bloodstream of the developing fetus.

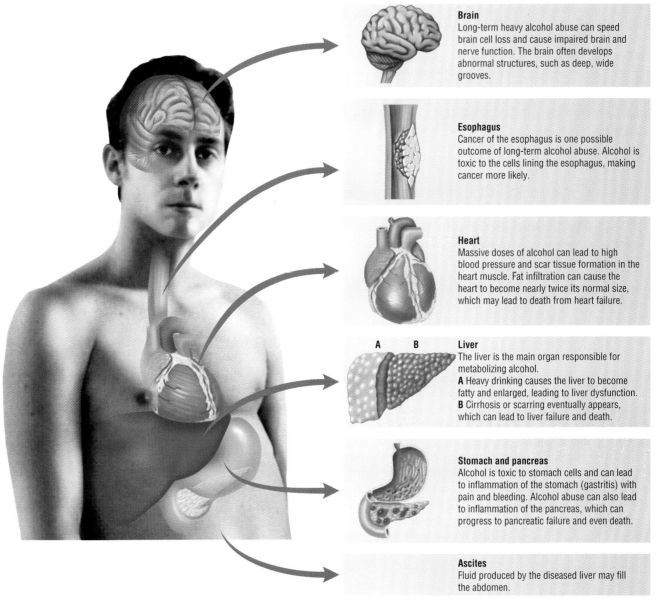

Figure 8-4 Effects of alcohol use on the body. The mind-altering effects of alcohol begin soon after it enters the bloodstream. Within minutes, alcohol numbs nerve cells in the brain. The heart muscle strains to cope with alcohol's depressive action. If drinking continues, the rising BAC causes impaired speech, vision, balance, and judgment. With an extremely high BAC, respiratory failure is possible. Over time, alcohol abuse increases the risk for certain forms of heart disease and cancer and makes liver and pancreas failure more likely.

This exposure has additional disastrous consequences for the developing fetus. Low birth weight, facial abnormalities, such as a small head and widely spaced eyes, and heart problems are often seen in such infants (Figure 8-5). This combination of effects is called **fetal alcohol syndrome (FAS).** Recent studies estimate that the full expression of this syndrome occurs at a rate of 1 to 3 per 1,000 births. Partial expression (*fetal alcohol effects, [FAE]*) can be seen in 3 to 9 per 1,000 live births. In addition, it is likely that many cases of FAE go undetected.[11]

Is there a safe limit to the number of drinks a woman can consume during pregnancy? Because no one can accurately predict the effect of drinking even small

Key Terms

fetal alcohol syndrome (FAS) characteristic birth defects noted in the children of some women who consume alcohol during their pregnancies.

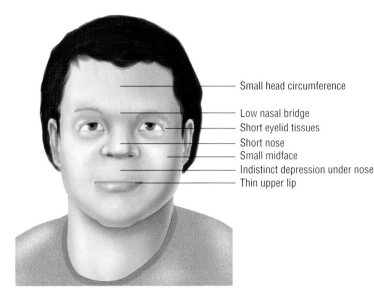

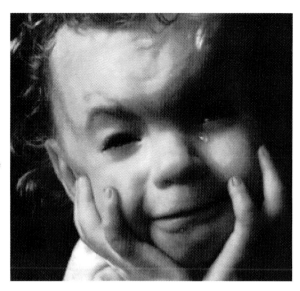

Figure 8-5 Fetal alcohol syndrome. The facial features shown are characteristic of affected children. Additional abnormalities in the brain and other internal organs accompany fetal alcohol syndrome but are not obvious in the child's appearance.

Labels on Figure 8-5:
- Small head circumference
- Low nasal bridge
- Short eyelid tissues
- Short nose
- Small midface
- Indistinct depression under nose
- Thin upper lip

amounts of alcohol during pregnancy, the wisest plan is to avoid alcohol altogether.

Because of the critical growth and development that occur during the first months of fetal life, women who have any reason to suspect they are pregnant should stop all alcohol consumption. Furthermore, women who are planning to become pregnant and women who are not practicing effective contraception should also keep their alcohol use to a minimum.

Alcohol-Related Social Problems

Alcohol abuse is related to a variety of social problems. These problems affect the quality of interpersonal relationships, employment stability, and the financial security of both the individual and the family. Clearly, alcohol's negative social consequences lower our quality of life. In financial terms the annual cost of alcohol abuse and dependence has been estimated at more than $185 billion.[12]

Accidents

The four leading causes of accidental deaths in the United States (motor vehicle collisions, falls, drownings, and fires and burns) have significant statistical connections to alcohol use.

Motor Vehicle Collisions

Data from the National Highway Traffic Safety Administration (NHTSA) indicate that in 2001 over seventeen

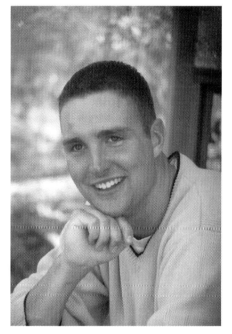

On August 4, 2000, 23-year-old Casey Ray Beaver was driving with two friends along U.S. Highway 71 near Goodman, Missouri, when an oncoming vehicle crossed the center line and collided with his car. Casey, a recent graduate of the University of Kansas, was pronounced dead at the scene, as was the driver of the other vehicle. The offender, who had seven prior convictions of driving under the influence and whose driver's license had been revoked seven years earlier, had a BAC above 10%. Casey was due to begin classes at the Illinois College of Optometry ten days after the accident occurred.

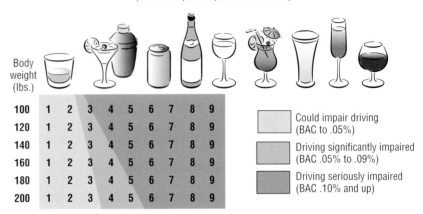

Figure 8-6 In most states, a BAC of 0.10% or .08% constitutes legal intoxication. However, a BAC as low as 0.05% can impair functioning enough to cause a serious accident.

Number of drinks in a 2-hour period
(1½-oz 86-proof liquor or 12-oz beer)

Body weight (lbs.)									
100	1	2	3	4	5	6	7	8	9
120	1	2	3	4	5	6	7	8	9
140	1	2	3	4	5	6	7	8	9
160	1	2	3	4	5	6	7	8	9
180	1	2	3	4	5	6	7	8	9
200	1	2	3	4	5	6	7	8	9

Could impair driving (BAC to .05%)

Driving significantly impaired (BAC .05% to .09%)

Driving seriously impaired (BAC .10% and up)

thousand alcohol-related vehicular crash deaths occurred. This figure represented 41% of the total traffic fatalities for 2001. Although seventeen thousand remains an unacceptably high figure, this total represented a 13% reduction from the twenty thousand alcohol-related fatalities reported in 1991.[13]

Presently in the United States, an alcohol-related car crash fatality occurs every 30 minutes. Every 2 minutes, an alcohol-related car crash injury happens. More than 275,000 people were injured in such crashes in 2001. In 2000, the NHTSA reported that approximately 1.5 million drivers were arrested for drunk driving, reflecting an arrest rate of 1 for every 130 licensed drivers in the United States.[13] (To find out what happens to people after they are arrested, read the Star box on page 273.)

One response to drunk driving has been for all states to raise the minimum legal drinking age to 21 years. This was accomplished in the mid-1980s. In October 2000, President Clinton signed into law a federal bill that requires all states to lower the legal BAC to .08% by the year 2003 or risk losing federal highway funds. Has your state enacted this .08% BAC limit? You can search the MADD website at **www.madd.org** to find out current .08% BAC law information (see Figure 8-6).

Other programs and policies are being implemented that are designed to prevent intoxicated people from driving. Many states have enacted **zero tolerance laws** to help prevent underage drinking and driving. Also included have been efforts to educate bartenders to recognize intoxicated customers, to use off-duty police officers as observers in bars, to place police roadblocks, to develop mechanical devices that prevent intoxicated drivers from starting their cars, and to encourage people to use designated drivers.

Falls

Many people are surprised to learn that falls are the second leading cause of accidental death in the United States. Alcohol use increases the risk for falls. Various studies suggest that alcohol is involved in between 21% and 77% of deadly falls and between 18% and 53% of nonfatal falls.[15]

Drownings

Drownings are the third leading cause of accidental death in the United States. Studies have shown that alcohol use is implicated in 21% to 47% of these deaths.[15] High percentages of recreational boaters have been found to drink alcohol while boating.[16]

Fires and Burns

Fires and burns are responsible for an estimated five thousand deaths each year in the United States, the fourth leading cause of accidental death. This cause is also connected to alcohol use: studies indicate that half of burn victims have BACs above the legal limit.[15]

Crime and Violence

Have you noticed that most of the violent behavior and vandalism on your campus is related to alcohol use? The

> **Key Terms**
>
> **zero tolerance laws** laws that severely restrict the right to operate motor vehicles for underage drinkers who have been convicted of driving under the influence of alcohol or any other drug.

Getting Arrested for Drinking and Driving: The Aftermath

Many college students will admit to having driven a car after drinking alcohol. Some will even admit that they have left a party after drinking and then driven to another location, but could not remember actually driving the car. This behavior reflects an alcoholic blackout. These dangerous activities are serious enough for the driver, the passengers, and anyone else on (or near) the road. For people who get arrested, another drama will unfold—the aftermath of an arrest for drinking and driving.

Although laws vary from state to state, here is the general sequence of events: If you are driving a car and are stopped by a police officer who suspects you may have been driving under the influence of alcohol, you will first be asked to show your driver's license and proof of your car's registration. You may be asked to get out of your car and undergo a field test for sobriety. This test could include tests of motor coordination, such as walking in a line in a heel-to-toe fashion. You may even be given an alcohol breath test on the spot.

If you appear to fail the field test, you could be arrested and frisked, read your Miranda rights, and taken to the local jail. There you will likely be fingerprinted and photographed. A more precise blood alcohol test may be given. Depending on local or state law, you will either spend some hours in jail (until your BAC is lowered) or be immediately eligible for bail (if you, a family member, or a friend can come up with the cash to get you released).

A date for your court appearance will be set. You will be required to face a judge and answer the charges against you. By this time, you probably will have hired an attorney to help you in this process. If you are convicted or decide to plead guilty to misdemeanor charges of driving while intoxicated (DWI) and this is your first offense, a typical scenario will follow. You will receive a fine (perhaps $200–$500) and be required to pay court costs (perhaps $125). You will probably be required to attend alcohol education classes and be placed on probation (for a year). Many states also require a person convicted of DWI to pay a probationer's fee of $50 plus $10 each month during the probation period. You will generally be required to see your probation officer once a month, and you may be required to take random drug tests.

Some communities require people convicted of DWI to pay a fee (perhaps $200) that goes to local drug prevention programs. Finally, some jurisdictions require judges to impose a term of community service hours that you must serve. You will likely lose points on your driver's license and have an official police and court record. The total cost for a simple, first-time conviction can easily reach $1,000 or more, depending on fines and legal fees.

For first-time offenders in jurisdictions in which the courts and jails are overcrowded, "pretrial diversionary programs" may exist.

In these programs, lawyers work with local prosecutors to help first-time offenders avoid facing a judge and having a court record. Those arrested agree to pay a set community drug program fine (perhaps $300–$500) and attend alcohol education classes. They typically must perform community service and meet with a probation office each month. (They must also pay the probationer's fees.) At the end of a year, after a positive probationary experience, the arrest record is removed from the police files. Again, the total cost can amount to over $1,000.

The preceding discussion applies to misdemeanor charges. However, if you are arrested and charged with a felony (such as operating a vehicle while intoxicated and you kill or injure someone), the whole ball game changes radically. You will be arrested and put in jail. You may not be able to be bailed out of jail. Almost certainly, you will need an attorney to assist you through a lengthy court process. If you are ultimately convicted of a felony, you are likely to pay a heavy fine and spend time in jail or prison. After a criminal trial, injured people can also pursue a civil suit against you. A civil suit can be quite expensive and time consuming. Indeed, the repercussions of a criminal DWI felony conviction will last for years and will have a significant impact on you, your family, and the lives of others.

Unfortunately, people who drink and drive fail to consider the aftermath of their behavior before it is too late.

connection of alcohol to crime has a long history. Prison populations have large percentages of alcohol abusers and alcoholics: People who commit crimes are more likely to have alcohol problems than are people in the general population. This is especially true for young criminals. Furthermore, alcohol use has been reported in 53% to 66% of all homicides, with the victim, the perpetrator, or both found to have been drinking. In rape situations, rapists are intoxicated 50% of the time and victims 30% of the time.[17]

Because of research methodological problems, pinpointing alcohol's connection to family violence is difficult.[18] However, it seems clear that among a large number of families, alcohol is associated with violence and other harmful behavior, including physical abuse, child abuse, psychological abuse, and abandonment.[17]

The difficult question that arises when discussing the relationship between alcohol use and violence is whether a cause-effect link can be proven. Obviously, not everyone who drinks becomes violent, but in many violent crimes, at least one person involved has been drinking. The answer perhaps is that alcohol use by itself is not enough to cause violence, but use of alcohol may be one of several factors that act in combination to cause violent behavior in some instances.

Partying 101: How to Party Responsibly

My friends and I are planning a big holiday party. We want to have fun, but we also want to be responsible about alcohol. What guidelines should we follow?

- Provide other social activities as a primary focus when alcohol is served.
- Respect an individual's decision about alcohol if that decision is either to abstain or to drink responsibly.
- Recognize the decision not to drink and the respect it warrants by providing equally attractive and accessible nonalcohol drinks when alcohol is served.
- Recognize that drunkenness is neither healthy nor safe. One should not excuse otherwise unacceptable behavior solely because of "too much to drink."
- Provide food when alcohol is served.
- Serve diluted drinks, and do not urge that glasses be constantly full.

- Keep the cocktail hour before dinner to a reasonable time and consumption limit.
- Recognize your responsibility for the health, safety, and pleasure of both the drinker and the nondrinker by avoiding intoxication and helping others do the same.
- Make contingency plans for intoxication. If it occurs in spite of efforts to prevent it, assume responsibility for the health and safety of guests—for example, by providing transportation home or overnight accommodations.
- Serve or use alcohol only in environments conducive to pleasant and relaxing behavior.
- Discard unattended drinks immediately. This reduces the possibility of someone consuming a drink containing Rohypnol, GHB, Ketamine (see Chapter 7), or other powerful intoxicants.

The Focus On article on pages 286–287 explores the connection between alcohol use and violence.

Suicide

Alcohol use has been related to large percentages of suicides. Alcoholism plays a large role in 30% of completed suicides.[19] Also, alcohol use is associated with impulsive suicides rather than with premeditated ones. Drinking is also connected with more violent and lethal means of suicide, such as the use of firearms.[17]

For many of these social problems, alcohol use impairs critical judgment and allows a person's behavior to quickly become reckless, antisocial, and deadly. Because most of us wish to minimize problems associated with alcohol use, acting responsibly when we host a party is a first step in this direction.

Hosting a Party Responsibly

Some people might say that no party is totally safe when alcohol is served. These people are probably right, considering the possibility of unexpected **drug synergism,** overconsumption, and the consequences of released inhibitions. Fortunately, an increasing awareness of the value of responsible party hosting seems to be spreading among college communities. The impetus for this awareness has come from various sources, including respect for an individual's right to choose not to drink alcohol, the growing recognition that many automobile crashes are alcohol related, and the legal threats posed by **host negligence.**

For whatever reasons, responsibly hosting parties at which alcohol is served is becoming a trend, especially among college-educated young adults. The Education Commission of the States' Task Force on Responsible Decisions about Alcohol has generated a list of guidelines for hosting a social event at which alcoholic beverages are served. The list includes the recommendations shown in the Changing for the Better box above.

In addition to these suggestions, the use of a **designated driver** is an important component of responsible alcohol use. By planning to abstain from alcohol or to carefully limit their own alcohol consumption, designated drivers are able to safely transport friends who have been drinking.

Designated drivers have indisputably saved many lives. However, there may be a down side. Some health

Key Terms

drug synergism (sin er jism) enhancement of a drug's effect as a result of the presence of additional drugs within the system.

host negligence a legal term that reflects the failure of a host to provide reasonable care and safety for people visiting the host's residence or business.

designated driver a person who abstains from or carefully limits alcohol consumption to be able to safely transport other people who have been drinking.

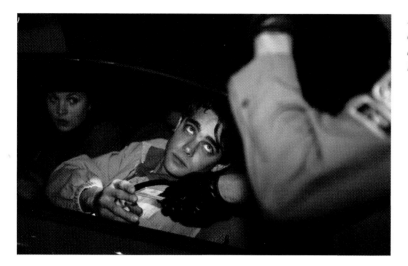

Police have stepped up their efforts to keep drunk drivers off the road by using sobriety checkpoints and roadside sobriety tests for people suspected of being intoxicated.

professionals are concerned that the use of designated drivers allows the nondrivers to drink more heavily than they might otherwise. In effect, designated drivers "enable" drinkers to be less responsible for their own behavior. This freedom from responsibility might eventually lead to further problems for the drinkers.

 TALKING POINTS Have you noticed an increased use of designated drivers in your community? Would you be willing to be a designated driver?

Organizations That Support Responsible Drinking

The serious consequences of the irresponsible use of alcohol have led to the formation of a number of concerned-citizen groups. Although each organization has a unique approach, all attempt to deal objectively with two indisputable facts: Alcohol use is part of our society, and irresponsible alcohol use can be deadly.

Mothers Against Drunk Driving

Mothers Against Drunk Driving (MADD) is a national network of over 600 local chapters in the United States and Canada. This organization attempts to educate people about alcohol's effects on driving and to influence legislation and enforcement of laws related to drunk drivers. For more information about MADD, visit its website at **www.madd.org.**[14]

Students Against Destructive Decisions

Many students have known the acronym *SADD* to stand for the youth group Students Against Driving Drunk or Students Against Destructive Decisions. Recently, the group has restructured itself to expand beyond drunk driving to include other high-risk activities that are detrimental to youth, such as underage drinking, drug use, drugged driving, and failure to use seat belts. Founded in 1981, this organization now has millions of members in thousands of chapters throughout the country. Remaining central to the drunk driving aspect of SADD is the "Contract for Life," a pact that encourages students and parents to provide safe transportation for each other if either is unable to drive safely after consuming alcohol. This contract also stipulates that no discussions about the incident are to be started until both can talk in a calm and caring manner. For more information about SADD, visit its website at **www.saddonline.com.**[20]

BACCHUS and GAMMA Peer Education Network

BACCHUS (Boost Alcohol Consciousness Concerning the Health of University Students) began in 1975 as an alcohol-awareness organization at the University of Florida. Run by student volunteers, this organization promoted responsible drinking among college students who chose to drink. It was not an anti-alcohol group, but a "harm reduction" group. Over the years, hundreds of chapters were formed on campuses across the country.

When supporters of BACCHUS realized that many students interested in alcohol awareness were from fraternities and sororities, they developed GAMMA (Greeks Advocating Mature Management of Alcohol) to join BACCHUS to form a peer education network. Campuses are now able to choose BACCHUS, GAMMA, or any other acronym or name of their groups.

With the broadening of the original BACCHUS organization has come an expansion of the health issues this group addresses. Originally, the focus was on alcohol abuse and prevention. Now the BACCHUS and GAMMA Peer Education Network confronts a variety of student health and safety issues. For additional information about this organization, check out its website at **www.bacchusgamma.org.**[21]

Other Approaches

Other responsible approaches to alcohol use are surfacing nearly every day. Even among college fraternity organizations, attitudes toward the indiscriminate use of alcohol are changing. Most fraternity rush functions are now conducted without the use of alcohol, and growing numbers of fraternities are alcohol-free.

Another encouraging sign on college campuses is the increasing number of alcohol use task forces. Although each of these groups has its own focus and title, many are meeting to discuss alcohol-related concerns on their particular campus. These task forces often try to formulate detailed, comprehensive policies for alcohol use across the entire campus community. Membership on these committees often includes students (on-campus and off-campus, graduate and undergraduate), faculty and staff members, academic administrators, residence hall advisors, university police, health center personnel, alumni, and local citizens. Does your college have such a committee?

Problem Drinking and Alcoholism

Problem Drinking

At times the line separating problem drinking from alcoholism is difficult to distinguish (see the Star box). There may be no true line, with the exception that an alcoholic is unable to stop drinking. **Problem drinking** is a pattern of alcohol use in which a drinker's behavior creates personal difficulties or difficulties for other people. What are some of these behaviors? Examples might be drinking to avoid life stressors, going to work intoxicated, drinking and driving, becoming injured or injuring others while drinking, solitary drinking, morning drinking, an occasional **blackout,** high-risk sexual activity, and being told by others that you drink too much. For college students, two clear indications of problem drinking are missing classes and lowered academic performance caused by alcohol involvement. The Changing for the Better box on page 277 offers suggestions that can help you keep drinking under control.

Problem drinkers are not always heavy drinkers; they might not be daily or even weekly drinkers. Unlike alcoholics, problem drinkers do not need to drink to maintain "normal" body functions. However, when they do drink,

Progressive Stages of Alcohol Dependence

Early

Escape drinking

Binge drinking

Guilt feelings

Sneaking drinks

Difficulty stopping after beginning to drink

Increased tolerance

Preoccupation with drinking

Occasional blackouts

Middle

Loss of control

Self-hate

Impaired social relationships

Changes in drinking patterns (more frequent binge drinking)

Temporary sobriety

Morning drinking

Dietary neglect

Increased blackouts

Late

Prolonged binges

Alcohol used to control withdrawal symptoms

Alcohol psychosis

Nutritional disease

Frequent blackouts

they (and others around them) experience problems . . . sometimes with tragic consequences. It is not surprising that problem drinkers are more likely than other drinkers to eventually develop alcoholism.

Key Terms

problem drinking an alcohol use pattern in which a drinker's behavior creates personal difficulties or difficulties for other people.

blackout a temporary state of amnesia experienced by an alcoholic; an inability to remember events that occurred during a period of alcohol use.

TALKING POINTS Do you know people who show signs of problem drinking?

Alcoholism

In the early 1990s, a revised definition of **alcoholism** was established by a joint committee of experts on alcohol dependence.[22] This committee defined alcoholism as follows: *Alcoholism is a primary, chronic disease with genetic, psychosocial, and environmental factors influencing its development and manifestations. The disease is often progressive and fatal. It is characterized by impaired control over drinking, preoccupation with the drug alcohol, use of alcohol despite adverse consequences, and distortions in thinking, most notably denial. Each of these symptoms may be continuous or periodic.*

This definition incorporates much of the knowledge gained from addiction research during the last two decades. It is well recognized that alcoholics do not drink for the pleasurable effects of alcohol but to escape being sober. For alcoholics, being sober is stressful.

Unlike problem drinking, alcoholism involves a physical addiction to alcohol. For the true alcoholic, when the body is deprived of alcohol, physical and mental withdrawal symptoms become evident. These withdrawal symptoms can be life threatening. Uncontrollable shaking can progress to nausea, vomiting, hallucinations, shock, and cardiac and pulmonary arrest. Uncontrollable shak-

ing combined with irrational hallucinations is called *delirium tremens (DTs),* an occasional manifestation of alcohol withdrawal.[23]

The complex reasons for the physical and emotional dependence of alcoholism have not been fully explained. Why, when more than 100 million adults use alcohol without becoming dependent on it, do 10 million or more others become unable to control its use?

Could alcoholism be an inherited disease? Studies in humans and animals have provided strong evidence that genetics plays a role in some cases of alcoholism. Two forms of alcoholism are thought to be inherited: type 1 and type 2. Type 1 is thought to take years to develop and may not surface until midlife. Type 2 is a more severe form and appears to be passed primarily from fathers to sons. This form of alcoholism frequently begins earlier in a person's life and may even start in adolescence.

Genetics may also help protect some Asians from developing alcoholism. About half of all Far East Asians produce low levels of an important enzyme that helps metabolize alcohol. These people cannot tolerate even small amounts of alcohol. In addition, genetic factors influencing the absorption rates of alcohol in the intestinal tract have been hypothesized to predispose some Native Americans to alcoholism. More research is needed about the role of genetic factors in all forms of chemical dependence.

The role of personality traits as conditioning factors in the development of alcoholism has received considerable

Key Terms

alcoholism a primary, chronic disease with genetic, psychosocial, and environmental factors influencing its development and manifestations.

attention. Factors ranging from unusually low self-esteem to an antisocial personality have been implicated. Additional factors making people susceptible to alcoholism may include excessive reliance on denial, hypervigilance, compulsiveness, and chronic levels of anxiety. Always complicating the study of personality traits is the uncertainty of whether the personality profile is a predisposing factor (perhaps from inheritance) or is caused by alcoholism.

Denial and Enabling

Problem drinkers and alcoholics frequently use the psychological defense mechanism of *denial* to maintain their drinking behavior. By convincing themselves that their lives are not affected by their drinking, problem drinkers and alcoholics are able to maintain their drinking patterns. A person's denial is an unconscious process that is apparent only to rational observers.

Formerly, alcoholics were required to admit that their denial was no longer effective before they could be admitted to a treatment program. This is not the case today. Currently, family members, friends, and coworkers of alcohol-dependent people are encouraged to intervene (with the help and supervision of a professional) and force an alcohol-dependent person into treatment.

During treatment, chemically dependent people must break through the security of denial and admit that alcohol controls their lives. This process is demanding and often time consuming, but there is no alternative path to recovery.

For family and friends of chemically dependent people, denial is part of a process known as *enabling.* In this process, people close to the problem drinker or alcoholic inadvertently support drinking behavior by denying that a problem really exists. Enablers unconsciously make excuses for the drinker, try to keep the drinker's work and family life intact, and in effect make the continued abuse of alcohol possible. For example, college students enable problem drinkers when they clean up a drinker's messy room, lie to professors about a student's class absences, and provide class notes or other assistance to a drinker who cannot perform academically. Even the use of designated drivers has been criticized as enabling behavior.

Alcohol counselors contend that enablers can significantly delay the onset of effective therapy. Do you know of a situation in which you or others have enabled a person with alcohol problems?

Codependence

A new term was coined in the 1980's to describe the relationship between drug-dependent people and those around

them—codependence. This term implies a kind of dual addiction. The alcoholic and the person close to the alcoholic are both addicted, one to alcohol and the other to the alcoholic. People who are codependent often find themselves denying the addiction and enabling the alcohol-dependent person.

Unfortunately, this kind of behavior damages both the alcoholic and the codependent. The alcoholic's intervention and treatment may be delayed for a considerable time. Codependent people often pay a heavy price as well. They often become drug or alcohol dependent themselves, or they may suffer a variety of psychological consequences related to guilt, loss of self-esteem, depression, and anxiety. Codependents may be at increased risk for physical and sexual abuse.

Fortunately, researchers continue to explore this dimension of alcoholism. Many students have found some of the sources listed at the end of this chapter to be especially helpful. To determine whether you could benefit from a support program such as Al-Anon or Alateen, answer the questions in the Personal Assessment on page 291.

Helping the Alcoholic: Rehabilitation and Recovery

When an alcoholic realizes that alcoholism is not a form of moral weakness but rather a clearly defined illness, the chances for recovery are remarkably good. It is estimated that as many as two-thirds of alcoholics can recover. Recovery is especially improved when the addicted person has a good emotional support system, including concerned family members, friends, and employer. When this support system is not well established, the alcoholic's chances for recovery are considerably lower. See the Star box on page 279 concerning older adults and alcohol.

Alcoholics Anonymous (AA) is a voluntary support group of recovering alcoholics who meet regularly to help each other get and stay sober. There are over 100,000 groups in 150 countries worldwide.[24] AA encourages alcoholics to admit their lack of power over alcohol and to turn their lives over to a higher power (although the organization is nonsectarian). Members of AA are encouraged not to be judgmental about the behavior of other members. They support anyone with a problem caused by alcohol.

Al-Anon and Alateen are parallel organizations that give support to people who live with alcoholics. Al-Anon is geared toward spouses and other relatives, whereas Alateen focuses on children of alcoholics. Both organizations help members realize that they are not alone and that successful adjustments can be made to nearly every situation. AA, Al-Anon, and Alateen chapter organizations are

Alcohol and Older Adults: A Hidden Problem

We know that children, adolescents, and adults all can succumb to the risks of alcohol abuse. Unfortunately, we should not assume that the risk goes away as we age.

As the body ages, everyone will experience the effects of alcohol differently. In older adults, the body becomes more sensitive to alcohol and the effects of alcohol can become greatly exaggerated.[1] Alcohol levels can rise 30 percent to 40 percent higher than in younger drinkers who consume the same amount.[2]

About 3 million people over the age of 60 are alcoholics. Alcohol abuse by widowers and older men is higher than for widows and older women. Twenty-one percent of hospitalized people 50 and older are alcoholics. Alcohol-related hospital care in the elderly costs over $60 billion per year.[3]

As the number of older adults is expected to grow over the next few decades as baby boomers begin retiring, we will see an increase in the number of older problem drinkers. Likewise, we can expect alcohol to continue to contribute to motor vehicle accidents involving older adults, as alcohol already appears at a relatively high frequency in crashes involving older adults, especially men.[4]

Health care professionals need to be aware of this growing problem and offer help to older people facing the risks of alcohol abuse. In particular, we need to realize that older adults have special needs:

- Older adults may experience problems even at lower levels of alcohol consumption.

- Signs and symptoms of alcohol problems in older adults may differ from those of younger problem drinkers.
- Those most at risk are men, especially those men in transition from work to retirement.
- Older alcoholics tend to do well in alcohol treatment.

Sources:
[1]Alcohol Use and Abuse. National Institute on Aging: Age Page. **www.nia.nih.gov/health/agepages/alcohol.htm** accessed 18 June 2003.
[2]Brody JE. Hidden Plague of Alcohol Abuse by the Elderly. *New York Times,* 2002 April 2.
[3]Campbell B. Elderly Drug and Alcohol Abuse Often Undetected. Available: **www.csindy.com/csindy/2000-02-02/news.html.** 2 February 2000.
[4]About Men's Health. Illinois Department on Aging. **www.state.il.us/aging/1news_pubs/onage05.htm,** 15 May 1999.

---

usually listed in the telephone book or in the classified sections of local newspapers. You can locate Al-Anon and Alateen on the web at **www.al-anon.alateen.org.**[25]

For people who feel uncomfortable with the concept that their lives are controlled by a higher power, secular recovery programs are becoming popular. These programs maintain that sobriety comes from within the alcoholic. Secular programs strongly emphasize self-reliance, self-determination, and rational thinking about one's drinking. Secular Organizations for Sobriety (SOS) and Rational Recovery are examples of secular recovery programs.

Medical Treatment for Alcoholism

Could there be a medical cure for alcoholism? For nearly fifty years, the only prescription drug physicians could use to help drinkers stop drinking was antabuse. Antabuse would cause drinkers to become extremely nauseated whenever they used alcohol.

In 1995 the Food and Drug Administration approved a drug called naltrexone that works by reducing the craving for alcohol and the pleasurable sensations felt when drinking. Combining naltrexone with conventional behavior modification has been shown to reduce alcohol relapse significantly. For a nontraditional approach to treatment of alcoholism, see the Considering Complementary Care box on page 280.

Current Alcohol Concerns

Adult Children of Alcoholic Parents

In recent years a new dimension of alcoholism has been identified—the unusually high prevalence of alcoholism among adult children of alcoholics (ACOAs). It is estimated that these people are about four times more likely to develop alcoholism than are persons whose parents are not alcoholics. Even the ACOAs who do not become alcoholics may have a difficult time adjusting to everyday living. Janet Geringer Woititz, author of the best-selling book *Adult Children of Alcoholics,*[26] describes thirteen traits that, to some degree, most ACOAs exhibit (see the Star box on page 281).

In response to this concern, support groups have been formed to prevent the adult sons and daughters of alcoholics from developing the condition that afflicted their parents (see the Star box on page 281). If a stronger link for an inherited genetic predisposition to alcoholism is found, these groups may play an even greater role in the prevention of alcoholism.

Women and Alcohol

For decades, women have consumed less alcohol and had fewer alcohol-related problems than men. Evidence is mounting that a greater percentage of women are choosing to drink and that some subgroups of women, especially young women, are drinking more heavily. A greater number of admissions of women to treatment centers may also reflect that alcohol consumption among women is on the rise. Special approaches for women to use for staying sober are discussed in the Learning from Our Diversity box on page 282.

Studies show that there are now almost as many female as male alcoholics. However, differences appear to exist between men and women when it comes to alcohol abuse.[17] Some of the more pronounced differences are: (1) More women than men can point to a specific triggering event, such as a divorce, death of a spouse, a career change, or children leaving home, that started them drinking heavily. (2) Alcoholism among women often starts later and progresses more quickly than alcoholism among men. (3) Women tend to be prescribed more mood-altering drugs than men. Thus women face a greater risk of drug interaction or cross-tolerance. (4) Nonalcoholic men tend to divorce their alcoholic spouses nine times more often than nonalcoholic women divorce their alcoholic spouses. Thus alcoholic women are not as likely to have a family support system to aid them in their recovery attempts. (5) Female alcoholics do not tend to receive as much social support as men in their treatment and recovery. (6) Although men outnumber women entering treatment programs by almost 4 to 1, women alcoholics tend to come into treatment earlier than men. (7) Women alcoholics are more likely than male alcholics to have medical complications. This may result from the differences in the metabolism of alcohol between men and women. Women are particularly susceptible to diseases of the liver. (8) Unmarried or divorced single-parent women often have economic problems that make entry into treatment programs especially difficult. In light of the generally recognized educational, occupational, and social gains made

Common Traits of Adult Children of Alcoholics

Adult children of alcoholics may:

- Have difficulty identifying normal behavior
- Have difficulty following a project from beginning to end
- Lie when it would be just as easy to tell the truth
- Judge themselves without mercy
- Have difficulty having fun
- Take themselves very seriously
- Have difficulty with intimate relationships
- Overreact to changes over which they have no control
- Constantly seek approval and affirmation
- Feel that they are different from other people
- Be super-responsible or super-irresponsible
- Be extremely loyal, even in the face of evidence that the loyalty is undeserved
- Tend to lock themselves into a course of action without considering the consequences*

Experts agree that adult children of alcoholics who believe they have come to terms with their feelings can sometimes face lingering problems. Support groups to contact include Al-Anon (**www.al-anon.alateen.org**). Adult Children of Alcoholics (**www.adultchildren.org**), and Children of Alcoholics Foundation (**www.coaf.org**).

Source: *Woititz JG. *Adult children of alcoholics*. Health Communications, Inc., 1990.

Health on the Web

Behavior Change Activities

Is Alateen for You?

Alateen is a support group for young people whose lives are affected by someone else's drinking (such as a parent or sibling). Visit its website at **www.al-anon.org** and scroll down to *Alateen*; then click to find out how this 12-step group works. Answer the twenty questions to decide whether Alateen is for you. What did you learn?

Estimating Your Blood Alcohol Content

You can instantly estimate your BAC at this website. The site's primary purpose is to provide useful information about the responsible use of alcohol. Go to **www.intox.com**, select "Drink Wheel," and complete the form. The information you provide is used to instantly estimate your BAC. Try entering different amounts of alcohol consumed over various time periods. Were you surprised that so few drinks could raise your BAC above the legal limit?

by women during the last two decades, it will be interesting to see whether these male-female differences continue. What's your best guess?

Alcohol Advertising

Every few years, careful observers can see subtle changes in the ways the alcoholic beverage industry markets its products. Recently, the marketing push appears to be directed toward minorities (through advertisements for malt liquor and fortified wines), women (through wine and wine cooler ads), and youth (through trendy, young adult-oriented commercials).

On the college campus, aggressive alcohol campaigns have used rock stars, beach party scenes, athletic event sponsorships, and colorful newspaper supplements to encourage the purchase of alcohol. Critics claim that most of the collegiate advertising is directed at minors and that the prevention messages are not strong enough to offset the potential health damage to this population. As a college student, how do you feel about alcohol advertising on your campus? If you are a nontraditional-age student, do you find the advertising campaigns amusing or potentially dangerous?

Some beer and liquor companies have begun using websites on the Internet to promote their products. Critics contend that the colorful graphics, hip language, games, chat rooms, and "virtual bars" are designed to recruit underage drinkers.

Alcohol Advertising in Ethnic Communities

A literature review by the Trauma Foundation at San Francisco General Hospital[27] reports some interesting facts concerning alcohol availability and alcohol advertising in ethnic communities. In the United States, low-income Latino and African American communities have a disproportionate number of alcohol outlets compared to white communities. This concentration of alcohol outlets seems to be related to an increase in traffic injuries and assaults. Additionally, as the number of alcohol outlets increases, the likelihood of increased crime and violence rises. Crime and violence drive out existing business establishments and discourage new businesses from locating in the area. Economic development can become thwarted.

The Trauma Foundation also reports that alcohol is more heavily advertised in low-income African American and Latino communities than in other neighborhoods. The advertisements are found on billboards as well as the displays inside and around the alcohol outlets. Advertising frequently exploits important cultural symbols, and promotions are targeted toward specific ethnic groups. For example, malt liquor is marketed especially to African Americans. Thus, rap singers are frequently featured in promotions and advertisements for malt liquor.

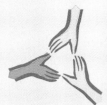

Learning from Our Diversity

Staying Sober: New Pathways for Women

Since 1935, when it was founded by two white American male alcoholics, Alcoholics Anonymous has expanded to encompass millions of members in virtually every region of the world who strive to achieve and maintain sobriety by adhering to AA's well-known 12-step program of recovery. With its strong spiritual orientation emphasizing the acknowledgment of a "higher power," AA offers safety, comfort, and structure to people of all ages and backgrounds, and both sexes. For decades, women as well as men have made AA the cornerstone of their efforts to get sober and stay sober.

Not all women, however, are comfortable with AA's focus on Christian spirituality and the perceived masculine orientation of its chief text, Alcoholics Anonymous (familiarly known as the "Big Book"), and other program literature. These women place an equally high value on sober living as do AA adherents, but they prefer to pursue that goal in other settings. In recent years, alternatives to AA have emerged that offer peer group acceptance and support for recovering alcoholic women, but do so in a nonspiritual, nonsexist context.

One such group, Women for Sobriety, is a mutual aid organization for women with alcohol problems that was founded in 1975 by Dr. Jean Kirkpatrick. The WFS program focuses on improving self-esteem; members achieve sobriety by taking responsibility for their actions and by learning not to dwell on negative thoughts. Another alternative, Rational Recovery, is open to both men and women. RR, which is based on the theories of psychologist Albert Ellis's Rational Emotive Therapy, also uses a cognitive, nonspiritual approach that fosters cohesiveness and provides the emotional support sought by people who seek to gain and maintain sobriety.

Particularly for "marginalized" alcoholic women such as lesbians, members of racial and ethnic minorities, and those of non-Christian religious backgrounds, alcoholism treatment professionals increasingly are being encouraged to present the full range of support-group options, including but not emphasizing the approach of Alcoholics Anonymous.

If you were seeking help to achieve and maintain sobriety, would you be more inclined to attend a program based on spirituality, or one that offers a rational, cognitive approach? Why?

Galanter M and others. Rational Recovery: alternative to AA for addiction? *American Journal of Drug and Alcohol Abuse,* 1993, vol. 19, p. 499.

Hall J. Lesbians' participation in Alcoholics Anonymous: experience of social, personal, and political tensions. *Contemporary Drug Problems,* Spring 1996, vol. 23, no. 1, p. 113.

Kaskutas L. A road less traveled: choosing the "Women for Sobriety" program. *Journal of Drug Issues.* Winter 1996, vol. 26, no. 1, p. 77.

Women for Sobriety, Inc. **www.womenforsobriety.org/** accessed 19 June 2003.

Taking Charge of Your Health

- Determine whether you are affected by someone's drinking by doing the Personal Assessment on page 291.
- Prepare for a possible alcohol-related emergency by reviewing the signs listed in the Changing for the Better box on page 264.
- Assess your level of social responsibility by using the Changing for the Better box on page 274.
- If you think that you are a problem drinker or an alcoholic, join a support group to get help.

- Enter into a "Contract for Life" with your parents or closest friends, a pact that says that you will provide safe transportation for each other if either of you is unable to drive safely after consuming alcohol.
- Make a commitment to responsible alcohol use by joining a campus group that works toward this goal.

Summary

- Alcohol is the drug of choice among college students and the rest of American society.
- Most people drink because alcohol is an effective, affordable, legal substance for altering the brain's chemistry.
- People are categorized as abstainers, light drinkers, moderate drinkers, or heavy drinkers, according to their alcohol use patterns.

- Binge drinking is dangerous and can lead to drunk driving, violence, lowered academic performance, and social problems.
- Alcohol is a product of fermentation, and its nutritional value is extremely limited.
- Alcohol is a drug that is a strong CNS depressant.
- Many factors affect the rate of absorption of alcohol into the bloodstream.

- As BAC rises, predictable depressant effects take place and the risk of acute alcohol intoxication increases; people with this condition are in danger and must receive first aid immediately.
- Federal legislation has pushed states to lower the legal BAC standard to .08%.
- Alcohol is removed from the bloodstream through the process of oxidation.
- Chronic alcohol use causes a variety of serious health problems for the drinker and can cause fetal alcohol syndrome in infants when a woman drinks during pregnancy.
- Alcohol-related social problems include accidents (motor vehicle crashes, falls, drownings, and fires and burns), crime and violence, and suicide.
- People who host events at which alcohol is served should follow certain guidelines, such as providing nonalcoholic alternative beverages, to help ensure the safety of their guests.
- Several groups of concerned citizens, such as MADD, SADD, BACCHUS, and GAMMA promote responsible alcohol use.
- Problem drinking is an alcohol use pattern in which a drinker's behavior creates personal difficulties or problems for others.

- Alcoholism is a primary, chronic disease characterized by addiction to alcohol; it has a variety of possible causes and manifestations.
- Problem drinkers and alcoholics often use the psychological defense mechanism of denial to maintain their drinking behavior.
- Enabling is a behavior pattern in which people close to the problem drinker or alcoholic make the continued use of alcohol possible by keeping the drinker's work and family life intact.
- An alcoholic's family members may unintentionally delay the alcoholic's intervention and treatment by becoming codependent.
- Alcoholics Anonymous and other support groups may help an alcoholic recover from the disease.
- The drugs antabuse and naltrexone are sometimes prescribed to discourage alcohol use.
- Children of alcoholic parents often have characteristic adjustment problems in adulthood.
- Women who abuse alcohol have unique problems and concerns.
- Alcohol advertising is often targeted at minorities, women, and youth.

Review Questions

1. What percentage of American adults consume alcohol? Approximately what percentage of adults are classified as abstainers? What percentage of college students drink?
2. What is binge drinking?
3. What is meant by the term *proof*?
4. What is the nutritional value of alcohol? How do "light" and low-alcohol beverages compare?
5. Identify and explain the various factors that influence the absorption of alcohol. Why is it important to be aware of these factors?
6. What is BAC? Describe the general sequence of physiological events that takes place when a person drinks alcohol at a rate faster than the liver can oxidize it.
7. What are the signs and symptoms of acute alcohol intoxication? What are the first-aid steps you should take to help a person with this problem?

8. Describe the characteristics of fetal alcohol syndrome and fetal alcohol effects.
9. Explain the differences between problem drinking and alcoholism.
10. What roles do denial and enabling play in alcoholism? What is codependence?
11. What are some common traits of ACOAs?
12. What unique alcohol-related problems do women face?
13. Describe the activities undertaken by SADD, MADD, BACCHUS, and GAMMA, and by AA, Al-Anon, and Alateen.
14. Describe the progressive stages of alcohol dependence.
15. List some ways you can keep alcohol consumption under control.

References

1. U.S. Department of Health and Human Services. *Alcohol and health: tenth special report to the U.S. Congress,* NIH Pub No 00-1583, 2000, U.S. Government Printing Office.

2. U.S. Bureau of the Census. *Statistical abstract of the United States, 1999,* 199th ed. Washington, D.C.: U.S. Government Printing Office, 1999.

3. Core Institute. 2001 Statistics on Alcohol and Other Drug Use on American College Campuses (online). Available: **www.siu.edu/departments/coreinst/public_html/recent.html** accessed 16 June 2003.

4. Brown SA, Tapert SF, Granholm E, et al. (2000). Neurocognitive functioning of adolescents: effects of protracted alcohol use. *Alcoholism, Clinical and Experimental Research* 24(2), 164–171.

5. Adult Children Educational Foundation Computer Bulletin Board. Sick families. 24 December 1997. **www.recovery.org/acoa/families.html**

6. Zest for Life. Alcohol and ethanol information page (online). Available: **www.anyvitamins.com/alcohol-ethanol-info.htm** accessed 16 June 2003.

7. Gaziano JM, et al. (2000). Light-to-moderate alcohol consumption and mortality in the Physicians' Health Study enrollment cohort. *Journal of the American College of Cardiology,* 35(1), 96–105.

8. Be Responsible About Drinking. Women and Alcohol (online). Available; **www.brad21.org/alcohol_and_women.html** accessed 16 June 2003.

9. Pinger RR, et al. *Drugs: issues for today,* 3rd ed. McGraw-Hill, 1998.

10. Ray O, Ksir C. *Drugs, society and human behavior,* 8th ed. McGraw-Hill, 1999.

11. ADA: Division of Drug and Alcohol Abuse. As a Matter of Fact . . . Fetal Alcohol Syndrome. **www.well.com/user/woa/fsfas.htm** accessed 16 June 2003.

12. National Institute on Alcohol Abuse and Alcoholism. *10th Special Report to the U.S. Congress on Alcohol and Health.* Chapter 6. NIH Publication No. 00-1583. Rockville, MD: U.S. Department of Health and Human Services, 2000.

13. *Traffic Safety Facts 2001: Alcohol.* U.S. Department of Transportation National Highway Traffic Safety Administration.

14. About Us. Mothers Against Drunk Driving. **www.madd.org** accessed 18 June 2003.

15. Alcohol and Unintentional Injury: A Brief Review of the Literature. The Trauma Foundation. **www.tf.org/tf/alcohol/ariv/reviews/injurev5.html** accessed 16 June 2003.

16. Training Guide for USLA Safety Tips: General Information on Drowning. USLA Lifeguards for Life. **www.usla.org/PublicInfo/Safety_guide.shtml** accessed 16 June 2003.

17. Kinney J. *Loosening the grip: a handbook of alcohol information,* 7th ed. McGraw-Hill, 2003.

18. Vaughn C. *Children of Alcoholics: At risk for family violence.* U.S. Department of Health and Human Services and SAMHSA's National Clearinghouse for Alcohol and Drug Information. 10 February 2003.

19. *Facts About Suicide.* CDC Prevention, National Center for Health Statistics, 1998.

20. SADD History. Students Against Drunk Driving. **www.saddonline.com** accessed 18 June 2003.

21. Organization History and Mission. The Baccus & Gamma Peer Education Network. **www.baccusgamma.org/** accessed 18 June 2003.

22. Morse RM, et al. The definition of alcoholism. *JAMA* 268(8): 1012–1014, 1992.

23. Gossman W. Delirium Tremens emedicine.com, Inc. 24 April 2001.

24. AA at a Glance. Alcoholics Anonymous. **www.alcoholics-anonymous.org** accessed 18 June 2003.

25. Website information: Al-Anon/Alateen. **www.al-anon.alateen.org/** accessed 19 June 2003.

26. Woititz JG. *Adult children of alcoholics.* Health Communications, Inc., 1990.

27. Trauma Foundation at San Francisco General Hospital. *The effects of alcohol on different ethnic communities: a brief review of the literature.* **www.tr.org/tf/alcohol/ariv/reviews** accessed 20 June 2003.

During the 2003–2004 academic year, Ball State University suffered the tragic deaths of two students in alcohol-related incidents. In November 2003, a student was fatally shot by a university police officer after a night of excessive drinking. The student allegedly lunged at the officer while he was investigating a reported break-in at a home near the campus. In March 2004, another student was robbed of two dollars and fatally shot after driving some local youths home from an off-campus party.

As we go to press, Ball State University has just launched an anti-alcohol campaign called "Police Yourself." This campaign will highlight the consequences of violating laws related to alcohol use and possible university consequences such as probation, suspension, or expulsion.

Alcohol misuse and abuse continues to be a major issue on most college campuses across the country. Many colleges and universities are using a variety of approaches to curb alcohol abuse on campus. What is your college doing to make your students more responsible in this area?

drinking and violence: a dangerous link

In recent years, there has been an increase in public service messages to raise awareness about driving under the influence of alcohol. In fact, the massive campaign against drinking and driving has been quite successful in reducing the number of drunk-driving accidents and fatalities. However, people may think that as long as a person doesn't get behind the wheel, it's okay to drink. But there are other potential dangers to the abuse of alcohol. One particular problem that perhaps has not been stressed enough in the media is the link between alcohol use and violence.

Obviously, not everyone who drinks becomes violent, but in many violent crimes at least one person involved has been drinking. It has been estimated that alcohol is involved as a factor in 63% of violent crimes.[1]

Alcohol and Types of Violent Crimes

The risk of a person becoming violent is higher among heavy drinkers than light drinkers. Heavy drinkers are also at higher risk of being victims of violent crime and are also more likely to inflict and to receive violent injuries. An environment where alcohol is prevalent is also a risk factor associated with gun injuries, particularly deaths among youths.[1] Alcohol plays a significant role in various types of violent crime. Substantial numbers of sexual-assault victims and offenders were drinking before their crime occurred. Spousal abuse by intoxicated men against women is the leading cause of nonfatal injury to women in the United States.[2]

Marital violence by husbands is common among men who abuse alcohol. Some researchers argue that spousal vio-

lence is the result of alcohol interfering with male power needs. Various consequences result from spousal violence which include miscarriage, depression, post-traumatic stress, substance abuse, and spousal homicide.[2] Spousal violence incurs societal costs including mental and physical health care, criminal justice interventions, child welfare, social services, and lost productivity at work.[3] A recent study suggests that in order to reduce marital violence, substance abuse needs to be a focal point during treatment for domestic violence.[2]

Campus Crime and the Effects of Alcohol

Of particular interest to college students is the data linking campus crimes to alcohol use. The CORE Institute conducted a 2001 survey of 54,444 undergraduate students that suggests that, when under the influence of alcohol or other drugs, the students experienced the following violent consequences:

- Argument or fight   31.8%
- Been hurt or injured   16.5%
- Threats of physical violence   58.8%
- Ethnic harassment   17.9%
- Actual physical violence   68.3%
- Forced sexual touching   76.0%
- Unwanted sexual intercourse   82.6%
- Theft involving force or
  threat of force   54.4%

Other violent consequences the students experienced include damaged property, driving under the influence, DWI/DUI arrests, and taking advantage of another person sexually. This survey reported that 85.3% of the students used alcohol within the last year and 74.4% used alcohol within the 30 days prior to taking the survey. This survey suggests

that alcohol and other drugs play a large role in violent acts among college age students.[4] College students tend to drink more heavily than the general population and therefore are at an increased risk of experiencing violence. When sexual assaults and rapes were reported, typically both the perpetrator and the victim had been drinking.[1]

Impact of Alcohol and Violent Behavior

So why is alcohol a contributing factor in violent crime? Alcohol acts as a depressant, which can reduce reaction time, impair cognition, and cloud judgment. Such impairment could decrease the chances of avoiding personal injury, once a physical altercation begins. Alcohol also decreases inhibitions and may increase aggressive behavior. It may increase the likelihood of inflicting or receiving a severe injury during a violent act and has been shown to increase the severity of injuries obtained in violent acts. Alcohol use interferes with attention and inhibits communication, both of which can drive aggressive behavior.

What Can You Do?

Although alcohol alone may not cause violence, when alcohol is introduced into a situation that has the potential to become violent, it can increase the chances that violence will occur. As the number of drunk drivers on the road has decreased, so has the number of drunk-driving accidents and fatalities. It seems logical to assume that if alcohol is kept out of the hands of people who are predisposed to violence, the number of alcohol-related crimes may also decrease.

You can choose to use good common sense when you are drinking or if you are with people who are drinking. Try to avoid potentially violent situations, and avoid people drinking around you who are acting in a reckless or violent manner. Drink in moderation, and help your friends recognize when they have had too much. Perhaps you or one of your friends can remain sober (a "designated thinker") to help avoid potentially dangerous situations and stay safe while partying. Finally, you can plan ahead by thinking carefully about an upcoming event before it happens. By "thinking before you drink," you can anticipate problems before they materialize and have solution strategies ready if they are needed.

For Discussion . . .

Have you ever encountered an angry drinker? Is there a safe way to handle a person who is drunk and intending to do harm to someone? If you have ever been drunk, do you feel that you could have controlled your actions in a confrontation while you were drunk?

References

1. Quigley BM, Corbett AB, and Tedeschi JT. Desired Image of Power, Alcohol Expectancies, and Alcohol-Related Agression. *Psychology of Addictive Behaviors,* 16(4), 318–324, 2002.

2. Smart GL, Moore TM, Kahler CW, and Ramsey SE. Substance Abuse and Relationship Violence Among Men Court-Referred to Batterers' Intervention Programs. *Substance Abuse,* 24(2), 107–122, 2003.

3. Schumacher JA, Fals-Stewart W, and Leonard KE. Domestic violence treatment referrals for men seeking alcohol treatment. *Journal of Substance Abuse Treatment,* 24, 279–283, 2003.

4. Core Institute. 2001 Statistics on Alcohol and Other Drug Use on American College Campuses (online). Available: **www.siu.edu/departments/ coreinst/public_html/recent.html** accessed 16 June 2003.

personal assessment

how do you use alcoholic beverages?

Answer the following questions about your own alcohol use. Record your number of "yes" and "no" responses at the end of the questionnaire.

Do you:

	Yes	No
1. Drink more often than you did a year ago?	_____	_____
2. Drink more heavily than you did a year ago?	_____	_____
3. Plan to drink, sometimes days in advance?	_____	_____
4. Gulp or "chug" your drinks, perhaps in a contest?	_____	_____
5. Set personal limits on the amount you plan to drink but then consistently disregard these limits?	_____	_____
6. Drink at a rate greater than two drinks per hour?	_____	_____
7. Encourage or even pressure others to drink with you?	_____	_____
8. Frequently want a nonalcoholic beverage but then end up drinking an alcoholic drink?	_____	_____
9. Drive your car while under the influence of alcohol or ride with another person who has been drinking?	_____	_____
10. Use alcoholic beverages while taking prescription or OTC medications?	_____	_____
11. Forget what happened while you were drinking?	_____	_____
12. Have a tendency to disregard information about the effects of drinking?	_____	_____
13. Find your reputation fading because of alcohol use?	_____	_____
TOTAL	_____	_____

Interpretation

If you answered yes to any of these questions, you may be using alcohol irresponsibly. Two or more yes responses indicate an unacceptable pattern of alcohol use and may reflect problem drinking behavior.

To Carry This Further . . .

Ask your friends or roommates to take this assessment. Are they willing to take this assessment and then talk about their results with you? Be prepared to discuss any follow-up questions they might have about their (or your) alcohol consumption patterns. Your willingness to talk about drinking behavior might help someone realize that this topic can and should be discussed openly. Finally, be aware of how people in your area can get professional help with drinking or other drug concerns.

Use the space below to write down important phone numbers where you can find alcohol-related assistance for you or your friends and relatives.

_____

_____

_____

_____

_____

_____

_____

_____

_____

personal assessment

does someone's drinking trouble you?

The following questions are designed to help you decide whether you are affected by someone's drinking and could benefit from a program such as Al-Anon. Record your number of yes and no responses in the boxes at the end of the questionnaire.

	Yes	No
1. Do you worry about how much someone else drinks?		
2. Do you have money problems because of someone else's drinking?		
3. Do you tell lies to cover up for someone else's drinking?		
4. Do you feel that if the drinker loved you, he or she would stop drinking to please you?		
5. Do you blame the drinker's behavior on his or her companions?		
6. Are plans frequently upset or meals delayed because of the drinker?		
7. Do you make threats, such as: "If you don't stop drinking, I'll leave you"?		
8. Do you secretly try to smell the drinker's breath?		
9. Are you afraid to upset someone for fear it will set off a drinking bout?		
10. Have you been hurt or embarrassed by a drinker's behavior?		
11. Are holidays and gatherings spoiled because of someone's drinking?		
12. Have you considered calling the police for help in fear of abuse?		
13. Do you search for hidden alcohol?		
14. Do you often ride in a car with a driver who has been drinking?		
15. Have you refused social invitations out of fear or anxiety that the drinker will cause a scene?		
16. Do you sometimes feel like a failure when you think of the lengths to which you have gone to control the drinker?		
17. Do you think that if the drinker stopped drinking, your other problems would be solved?		
18. Do you ever threaten to hurt yourself to scare the drinker?		
19. Do you feel angry, confused, or depressed most of the time?		
20. Do you feel there is no one who understands your problems?		
TOTAL		

Interpretation

If you answered yes to three or more of these questions, Al-Anon or Alateen may be able to help. You can contact Al-Anon or Alateen by looking in your local telephone directory or by writing to Al-Anon Family Group Headquarters, Inc., 1600 Corporate Landing Parkway, Virginia Beach, VA 23454–5617, or you may call (888) 4AL-ANON.

To Carry This Further . . .

Sometimes the decision to seek help from a support group is a difficult one. If you answered yes to any of the questions above, spend a few moments reflecting on your responses. How long have you been experiencing problems because of someone else's drinking? How would sharing your feelings with others—people who have dealt with very similar problems—help you cope with your own situation? Knowing you're not alone can often be a great relief; it's up to you to take the first step.

chapter nine

rejecting tobacco use

Chapter Objectives

After reading this chapter, you should be able to:

▌ examine smoking rates among demographic groups, student groups on your campus, and in different states, and speculate on the underlying reasons for these trends.

▌ identify techniques used by the tobacco industry to encourage people to smoke.

▌ critically evaluate tobacco advertisements to determine what audience particular ads target, and what messages they send to consumers.

▌ administer the ten-item Hooked on Nicotine Checklist (HONC) to friends who smoke to determine the existence and depth of dependence.

▌ explain the bolus theory, the adrenocorticotropic hormone (ACTH) theory, and the self-medication theory of nicotine addiction.

▌ explain the particulate phase and the gaseous phase of tobacco smoke and identify the primary components of each.

▌ describe the relationship between smoking and cardiovascular disease.

▌ trace the role of smoking in the development of respiratory-tract cancer.

▌ identify smoking-cessation aids, including various nicotine delivery techniques and describe steps that smokers can take to reduce or eliminate their use of tobacco.

▌ describe how parents of young children can discourage tobacco use in the future.

▌ explain the dangers of secondhand smoke and develop steps to reduce your exposure to it.

Online Learning Center Resources

www.mhhe.com/payne8e

Log on to our Online Learning Center (OLC) for access to these additional resources:

- Chapter key terms and definitions
- Learning objectives
- Student interactive question-and-answer sites
- Self-scoring chapter quiz
- Online assessments
- Key term flash cards

Talking It Over

Supporting a Smoker Who Wants to Quit

My roommate is trying to quit smoking, and I want to help. How can I do that without seeming judgmental?

- Help your friend get through stressful periods by being available for nonsmoking activities, such as walking or playing a sport.
- Establish an award system for "nonsmoking days completed," and participate in the "funding" of the rewards.
- Suggest going to places where nonsmoking is the norm, such as restaurants or coffee houses that are smoke-free.
- Continue being supportive even if your friend fails in her current attempt to stop smoking. Most persons are not successful in their first attempt. Just "being there" often communicates support and understanding better than words do.

CommunicationLinks

www.cancer.org/tobacco/index.html
www.lungusa.org/tobacco/index.html

Eye on the Media

Tobacco Industry Denies Ads Target Kids

On various occasions during the past 5 years the tobacco industry has run television commercials intended to "educate" the public about the fundamental changes that the industry has undertaken in terms of marketing, particularly in light of charges that the industry previously targeted children in an attempt to develop a new generation of smokers. In these commercials several changes were described, all of which were attributed to the 1998 settlement (formally signed in 1999) reached between the tobacco industry and the states' attorneys general stemming from a massive class action suit to recoup Medicaid money. There was no mention in the commercials that the original agreement reached between the states and the tobacco industry in June of 1997 was much more restrictive and closely reflective of the intent of the court in curbing the marketing

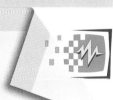

activities of the tobacco industry. The more permissive 1998 settlement, known as the Master Settlement Agreement (MSA), arose when the tobacco industry promised to vigorously fight the 1997 agreement in court. Thus, compromises favoring the tobacco industry were made by the states to save time and resources that would otherwise be lost to additional litigation.

The accompanying chart shows selected examples of the differences between the 1997 agreement and the final 1999 settlement. Because of the tobacco industry's ability to afford media exposure, the American public will continue to be led to believe that the tobacco industry complied completely with the intent of the courts.

Master Settlement Agreement (MSA)

Restriction	1997 Agreement	1999 (MSA)
Outdoor and Transit Ads	Bans all outdoor and transit ads	Allows signs of up to 14 sq feet on any building or property where tobacco products are sold, including those near schools and playgrounds. Bans other billboards and transit ads.
Cartoons and Human Images	Banned	Allows human images, such as the Marlboro man. Bans cartoons.
Brand Name Sponsorships	Banned	Each company allowed one brand name sponsorship of an event or series of events. Prohibits events in which contestants are under 18 years of age.
Free Samples	Banned	Free samples allowed in adult-only facilities.

In yet a more current example of the tobacco industry's relationship to media exposure, RJR withdrew its corporate sponsorship of NASCAR's premier racing series, the Winston Cup Series.[1] By finally complying with the 1999 Master Settlement Agreement RJR can redirect hundreds of millions of dollars once spent on NASCAR into other areas of media exposure, such as advertisements in magazines popular with teens (such as *Sports Illustrated* and *Hot Rod*) and point-of-purchase displays in convenience stores and drug stores.[2] In spite of RJR's absence, the name "Winston" will most likely remain in NASCAR fans' minds for years to come.

Tobacco Use in American Society

If you were to visit certain businesses, entertainment spots, or sporting events in your community, you might leave convinced that virtually every adult is a tobacco user. Certainly, for some segments of society, tobacco use is the rule rather than the exception. You may be quite surprised, however, to find out that the great majority of adults do not use tobacco products. Figure 9-1 shows the states with the highest and lowest smoking rates.[3]

Following the Surgeon General's 1964 report (the first official statement of concern by the federal government regarding the dangers of smoking),[4] the prevalence of smoking began a decline that lasted until 1991, when a leveling off was noted that lasted for the next three years.

Since 1994 the percentage of the population who smoke has declined slowly but progressively. Current statistics reveal that 22.5% of American adults smoke cigarettes on a daily or near-daily basis. Men are more likely to smoke (25.2%) than are women (20.0%).[5] When subsegments of

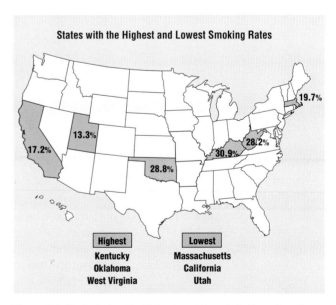

Figure 9-1 Kentucky has the highest smoking rate in the nation. Do you know what the rate is in your state?

Source: Prevalence of current cigarette smoking among adults and changes in prevalence of current and some day smoking—2001. *MMWR.* 52(14). April 2003.

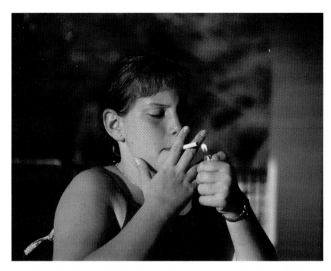

Smoking is a learned behavior and most smokers begin as kids.

the population, based on race and ethnicity, were studied it was found that whites and blacks were essentially smoking with the same prevalence (24.1% and 22.5%). At the same time, Hispanics were considerably less likely to smoke (15.9%), while American Indians and Alaska Natives (40.0%) were more likely to smoke. Persons of Asian or Pacific Island descent were the Americans least likely to smoke (13.7%) (see Table 9.1).[6]

Cigarette Smoking Among College Students

Until very recently, the rate of cigarette smoking among college graduates was lower than that reported for the population as a whole, and it was significantly lower than the rate for persons with very little formal education. In fact, the prevalence of smoking among college students decreased progressively from 21% in 1964 to 14% in 1995.[7] However, an upward trend in cigarette use by college students has been noted, with a recent study suggesting an incidence approaching 36% smoking within the past month.[8] In contrast, a downward trend in smoking by twelfth graders was reported in 2002.[9] Knowing that a segment of those twelfth graders (1998) are now undergraduates on college and university campuses, it is possible that the 35.8% prevalence of cigarette smoking among college students, as reported in 2000, is now experiencing a decline. This is, in fact, probable since among the 2002 twelfth graders with college aspirations, only 15.1% were cigarette smokers.[9]

TALKING POINTS Your 13-year-old brother inadvertently leaves a tin of smokeless tobacco on the desk in his room and you see it. Would you say anything to him about it? If so, what?

When a college community is viewed as a whole regarding which segments of the student body are most likely to smoke, there appears to be a direct relationship between the level of alcohol consumption and cigarette smoking, and between the importance that students assign to "partying" versus other aspects of the college experience.[10]

The historically predictable relationship between higher levels of completed education and the lessened likelihood of smoking remains clearly evident even today. For example, when comparing the percentage of heavy smokers (a pack or more per day) on the basis of education completed, the influence of education is evident— less than high school (37.5m/31.3f%), high school graduate (32.0m/26.2f%), some college (25.4m/21.9f%), and college graduate (11.0m/10.7f%).[11] Unfortunately, the most recently reported incidence of smoking among college students (2002) seems to indicate that the next college graduating class of 1998–2002 were much closer to the high school dropout rate of cigarette smoking.

The most disturbing aspect of the increase in reported smoking among college students, beyond the eventual influence it will have on health and life expectancy, is its negation of the traditional belief that the college and university experience "protected" this segment of the society from making some ill-informed choices. As recently as the mid-1990s it was still possible to believe that the college population was "too well informed" and "too future oriented" to engage widely in an addictive behavior that fosters dependence, compromises health, and eventually shortens life. Today that proposition seems to lack some of its former validity, but, hopefully, the corner is being turned.

Table 9.1 Patterns of Cigarette Smoking

Prevalence by Sex		
Total	Men	Women
22.5	25.2	20.0

Note: Subjects have smoked more than one hundred cigarettes and reported smoking every day or some days.

Percentage by Ethnicity and Race					
Total	White	Black	Hispanic	American Indian or Alaska Native	Asian or Pacific Islander
22.5	24.1	22.5	15.9	40.0	13.7

Note: Subjects have smoked more than 100 cigarettes and smoked at the time of the survey.

A Simple Dependency Test Regarding Your Relationships with Cigarettes

To nonsmokers it must seem that smokers would realize the existence of their dependency on cigarettes, however such might not be the case. The Hooked On Nicotine Checklist (HONC) appearing below is a simple way to determine whether a cigarette-based dependency exists. If you are a smoker, answer each question asked by the HONC in an honest manner. When completed, give careful consideration to your findings. If you are a nonsmoker, ask a smoker to complete the HONC and share responses to each item with you. In the latter case, a good discussion could ensue.

Nicotine Addiction's 10 Warning Signs

HONC - H ooked O n N icotine C hecklist

1.	Have you ever tried to quit but couldn't?
2.	Do you smoke now because it is really hard to quit?
3.	Have you ever felt like you were addicted to tobacco?
4.	Do you ever have strong cravings to smoke?
5.	Have you ever felt like you really needed a cigarette?
6.	Is it hard to keep from smoking in places where you are not supposed to, like school?

In answering the last four questions, when you tried to stop smoking, or when you have not used tobacco for a while. . . .

7.	Did you find it hard to concentrate?
8.	Did you feel more irritable?
9.	Did you feel a strong need or urge to smoke?
10.	Did you feel nervous, restless or anxious because you couldn't smoke?

Answering "yes" to any one of the above ten questions indicates that you may already be hooked on nicotine and are chemically dependent. Think about it! Your "yes" answer is your own honest self assessment that you have already lost the freedom and ability to simply and effortlessly walk away. Two-thirds of all teens who you see smoking regularly will spend their entire life as slaves to nicotine. If you HONC we'll help - www.WhyQuit.com

Source: HONC - (Hooked on Nicotine Checklist). Tobacco Control, Sept. 2002 Dr. JR Difranza, *Development of symptoms of tobacco dependency in youths. Reliability study of HONC factors* - July 2002
Created by www.WhyQuit.com - Join us for motivation, education and support!

Other Demographic Factors Influencing Tobacco Use

In addition to gender, race, ethnicity, and education level, other demographic facts appear to influence the extent to which smoking occurs. Included among these factors are the age groups into which persons fall, the region of the country in which they live, the size of their communities, and their employment status.

If age grouping is begun with 18- to 25-year-olds and progresses to 65 years of age and older, the general trend is for the percentage of persons smoking (during the past month) within each group to go down. For example, among the younger group (18–25), 28.5m/25.1f% report having smoked during the past month, while in the 26- to 34-year-olds, 29.0m/22.5f% smoked during the past month, and in the 65 plus group, only 10.2m/9.3f% did so.[5] Most likely over the course of time, both quitting and premature death serve to reduce the percentage of smokers.

Comparing smoking during the past month among people in different regions of the country reveals that persons living in the north central portion of the country are the most likely to smoke (26%). In contrast, persons living in the West are least likely to have smoked during the past month (20.0%). People in the South (25.4%) and the Northeast (23.9%) fall in between.[11] In terms of population density, one might be surprised to learn that persons living outside of metropolitan areas are more likely to have smoked during the past month (30.5%), while persons living in small metropolitan areas (27.2%) and large metropolitan areas (26.5%) are less likely to have smoked during the same period.[12]

Employment status too impacts on the likelihood of regular smoking. Persons who are employed part-time are more likely to have smoked during the past month (31.2%) than are people who are employed full-time (25.5%)—most likely reflecting the greater opportunity of the former group to smoke, since today's work place is increasingly a smoke-free environment. In stark contrast to those who have some degree of employment, the unemployed are by far the most likely to have smoked during the past month (50.1%).[12] This may reflect not only the lower level of education found among this group, but also the immediate gratification that smoking brings to persons who may have little opportunity to seriously pursue long-range goals and the postponed gratification that striving for such goals can often require.

Marketing of Tobacco Products

Shredded plant material, wrapped in paper or leaf, ignited with a flame, and then placed on or near the delicate tissues of the mouth . . . what other human behavior does this re- *semble?* If you answered *None!* to this question, then you appreciate that smoking is unique, and, therefore, that it must be learned. How it is learned is currently a less than fully understood process that most likely requires a variety of stimuli ranging from modeling to actual experimentation. The role of advertising as a source of models has long been suspected and intensely debated. Today, as in the past, controversy surrounds the intent of the tobacco industry's advertising. Are the familiar logos seen in a variety of media intended to challenge the brand loyalty of those who have already decided to smoke, as the industry claims? Or are the ads intended to entice new smokers, older children and young adolescents, in sufficient numbers to replace the 3,000 smokers who die each day from the consequences of tobacco use? This latter objective is now known, by admission of the tobacco industry, to have been pursued for decades. Its effectiveness has also been documented. The cartoon character Joe Camel was an especially successful tool for enticing children and teens to begin smoking.

Over the years the tobacco industry has used all aspects of mass media advertising, including radio, television, print, billboards, and sponsorship of televised athletic events and concerts, to sell its products. In addition, it has often distributed free samples and sold merchandise bearing the company or product logo.

Today the tobacco industry has been denied access to television and radio, and it can no longer distribute free samples to minors, but the industry continues to be active and innovative in other aspects of the media to which it has access. For example, Philip Morris has introduced an upscale lifestyle magazine called *Unlimited: Action, Adventure, Good Times,* to be provided free to over 1 million smokers. Interestingly, the magazine features articles about healthful activities that many long-time smokers would be unable to engage in because of the effects of smoking.

In the 9 months following the 1998 settlement, the tobacco industry increased their magazine advertising budget by 30% over presettlement levels in magazines with 15% or more youth (under 18 years of age) readership, even though they had agreed to discontinue advertising in youth-oriented publications.[13] Most recently, increased tobacco advertising has been noted in magazines that appeal specifically to younger women, working women, and women of color.

The development of nonmarket brands of cigarettes for free distribution to patrons of bars and restaurants who are attempting to "bum" cigarettes represents a second form of "advertising." This "premarketing" introduction of a prototype brand technically does not violate the law regarding the distribution of samples. To date, several hundred establishments in several major cities have participated.

Thanks, But No Cigar

If one were to judge on the basis of the number of newly opened cigar stores and clubs catering to cigar smokers, as well as the highly visible magazine *Cigar Aficionado*, one could conclude that cigar smoking was the hottest trend in tobacco use. To a degree this contention is true when one considers that in 1991 only 2.2% of the adult population smoked cigars on a regular basis,[14] while by 1998 the size of the cigar-smoking population had risen to 5.2%.[15] This said, however, a 2000 report demonstrates a decline to 4.5%, suggesting that the appeal of cigars has begun to wane.[16] However, for those cigar smokers who will apparently continue, and for those of you who might be increasingly interested in this form of tobacco use, the following information from the American Lung Association should be considered:

- *Secondhand (sidestream) cigar smoke is more poisonous than secondhand cigarette smoke.* The smoke from one cigar equals that of three cigarettes. Carbon monoxide emissions from one cigar are 30 times higher than for one cigarette.
- *Cigar smoking can cause cancer of the larynx (voice box), mouth, esophagus, and lungs.* Cancer death rates for cigar smokers are 34% higher than for nonsmokers.
- *Ninety-nine percent of cigar smokers have atypical cells found in the larynx.* These cells are the first step toward malignancy (cancer).

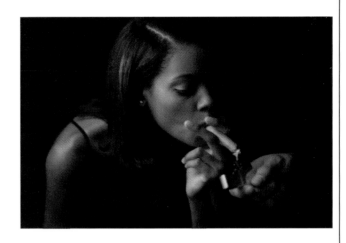

- *Cigar smokers are three to five times more likely to die of lung cancer than are nonsmokers.*
- *Cigar smokers have five times the risk of emphysema compared to nonsmokers.*
- *Nicotine does not have to be inhaled to damage the heart and blood vessels.* It is absorbed into the bloodstream through the mucous membranes of the mouth. Nicotine increases the heart rate and constricts the blood vessels, which reduces blood flow to the heart.

A final current example of the tobacco industry's subtle but effective presence in the mind of the public is that of tobacco use in motion pictures. In spite of a 1990 tobacco industry policy and the 1999 Master Settlement Agreement, both of which prohibit "brand placement" of tobacco products in films, cigarette and cigar smoking continue to be disproportionately represented in current films. Unfortunately, children and adolescents can easily identify with these characters (and their smoking), since they are generally depicted in a positive light. As an example, in a recent survey, two-thirds of the 43 movie stars most frequently named by 10- to 19-year-olds were seen smoking in their most recent films.[17]

Pipe and Cigar Smoking

Many people believe that pipe or cigar smoking is a safe alternative to cigarette smoking. Unfortunately, this is not the case. All forms of tobacco present users with a series of health threats (see the Star box above and Table 9.3 on page 308).

When compared with cigarette smokers, pipe and cigar smokers have cancer of the mouth, throat, larynx (voice box), and esophagus at the same frequency. Cigarette smokers are more likely than pipe and cigar smokers to have lung cancer, cancer of the larynx, chronic obstructive lung disease (COLD), also called chronic obstructive pulmonary disease (COPD), and heart disease. The cancer risk of death to smokers is four times greater from lung cancer and ten times greater from laryngeal cancer than for nonsmokers.[18]

In comparison to cigarette smokers, pipe and cigar smokers are considerably fewer in number. Interestingly, cigar smoking enjoyed a resurgence through much of the 1990s. However, during 1998–1999 a substantial decline in sales of premium cigars occurred. Whether this downturn represents an emerging dissatisfaction with cigars as an enjoyable use of tobacco or simply reflects adjustments in the import market remains uncertain. In 1995 cigars generated sales of $1 billion, mainly to younger adults, including a very small but growing percentage of women.

Perhaps because of the increase in cigar smoking noted above, the National Cancer Institute commissioned the first extensive study of regular cigar smoking. That report confirmed and expanded upon the health risks identified in earlier smaller studies.[19] A subsequent study reported that cigar smokers are nearly twice as likely as nonsmokers to develop oral, throat, and lung cancer, as well as heart disease and chronic obstructive pulmonary disease.[20] These rates are somewhat lower than those of cigarette smokers.

In response to the recognition of these risks, the FTC now requires that cigar manufacturers must disclose the tobacco content and additives in their products. Most recently the FTC announced its intention of requiring five rotating health warnings to appear on cigars, including two that have been currently agreed upon by the FTC and major cigar manufacturers: *Cigars Are Not a Safe Alternative to Cigarettes* and *Cigar Smoking Can Cause Cancer of the Mouth and Throat, Even If You Don't Inhale.*

The use of smokeless tobacco, a third alternative to cigarette smoking, is discussed later in the chapter.

Tobacco Use and the Development of Dependence

Although not true for every tobacco user (see the discussion of "chippers" later in this section), the vast majority of users, particularly cigarette smokers, will develop a dependency relationship with the nicotine contained in tobacco. This state of **dependence** causes users to consume greater quantities of nicotine over extended periods of time, further endangering their health.

Dependence can imply both a physical and psychological relationship. Particularly with cigarettes, *physical dependence* or *addiction,* with its associated *tolerance, withdrawal,* and **titration,** is strongly developed by 40% of all smokers. The development of addiction reflects a strong genetic predisposition to physical dependence.[21] Most of the remaining population of smokers will experience lesser degrees of physical dependence. Psychological *dependence* or *habituation,* with its accompanying psychological components of *compulsion* and *indulgence,* is almost universally seen.

Compulsion is a strong emotional desire to continue tobacco use despite restrictions on smoking and the awareness of health risks. Very likely, users are "compelled" to engage in continual tobacco use in fear of the unpleasant physical, emotional, and social effects that result from discontinuing use. In comparison to compulsion, indulgence is seen as "rewarding" oneself for aligning with a particular behavior pattern—in this case, smoking. Indulgence is made possible by the existence of various reward systems built around the use of tobacco, including a perceived image, group affiliation, and even appetite suppression intended to foster weight control.

Much to the benefit of the tobacco industry, dependence on tobacco is easily established. Many experts believe that physical dependence on tobacco is far more easily established than is physical dependence on alcohol, cocaine (other than crack), or heroin. Of all people who experiment with cigarettes, 85% develop various aspects of a dependence relationship.

A small percentage of smokers, known as "chippers," can smoke on occasion without becoming dependent.

Most likely, chippers respond differently to environmental cues than do more dependent smokers,[22] thus smoking less frequently. They may be truly "social smokers" in that they smoke with only a few selected friends or in a very limited number of places. Unfortunately, many inexperienced smokers feel that they too are only social smokers; however, a few months or even a few days, of this type of occasional smoking could be a transitional period into a dependence pattern of tobacco use.

Sandwiched between regular smokers and chippers is a newly emerging group of smokers—part-time smokers. Today these smokers constitute about 23% of all smokers.[3] The practice most likely reflects the reality of the high cost of cigarettes and restrictions in the workplace. The health effects of this form of smoking appear to be the same as seen in regular smokers.[3]

Theories of Nicotine Addiction

The establishment and maintenance of physical dependence or addiction is less than fully understood. Most experts, however, believe that for a specific individual, addiction has a multifaceted etiology, or cause, with increasing attention being directed toward a genetic basis for addiction. Accordingly, several theories have been proposed to explain the development of dependence. We will present a brief account of some of these theories. Readers are reminded that many of these theories are technically sophisticated and only a most basic description can be provided in a personal health textbook. The more emotional aspects of dependence formation will be discussed later in the chapter.

Genetic Influences

Although the specific genetic pathways that influence both the initiation and maintenance of smoking (or other forms of tobacco use) are less than fully understood, a role for genetic influence is evident. Applying new statistical techniques to earlier studies of smoking patterns in families and between identical twins, it is now believed that initiation and maintenance of initial smoking is 60% driven by genetic influences. Of course, the smoking of the first few cigarettes is a choice made by beginning smokers. The remaining influence needed for initiation

---

Key Terms

dependence a physical and/or psychological need to continue the use of a drug.

titration (tie **tray** shun) the particular level of a drug within the body; adjusting the level of nicotine by adjusting the rate of smoking.

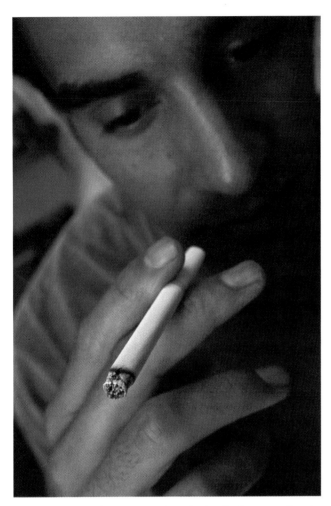

A smoker inhales about 70,000 times during the first year of smoking, resulting in a nicotine addiction that often lasts a lifetime.

and maintenance of initial smoking is 20% environmental and 20% the unique needs of individuals.[23]

Once the brief period of initial exposure is passed, the role of genetic influences may be even more powerful—providing 70% of the stimulus required over decades of smoking. Environmental and personality factors subside accordingly.[23]

Bolus Theory

In the **bolus theory** of nicotine addiction, one of the oldest and most general theories of addiction, each inhalation of smoke releases into the blood a concentrated quantity of nicotine (a ball or bolus) that reaches the brain and results in a period of neurohormonal excitement. The smoker perceives this period of stimulation as pleasurable but, unfortunately, short lived. Accordingly, the smoker attempts to reestablish this pleasurable feeling by again inhaling and sending another bolus of nicotine on its way to the brain. The 70,000 or more inhalations during the first year of smoking serve to condition the novice smoker, resulting in a lifelong pattern of cigarette dependence. The level needed for arousal is different for each individual smoker, depending on the length of addiction, the level of tolerance, genetic predisposition, and environmental and personal stimuli.

Recognition of two types of smokers emerges from an understanding of the bolus theory of smoking. *Peak smokers* are those smokers who become dependent on the arousal of pleasure centers in the brain (see page 301) that are stimulated by the rapid increase of nicotine levels following inhalation and distribution of nicotine within the CNS. In contrast, the *trough maintenance smokers* maintain an even consistently higher level of nicotine titration in order to avoid the negative consequences of withdrawal.[24] These feelings are experienced as unpleasant, and thus to be avoided.

Adrenocorticotropic Hormone (ACTH) Theory

Yet another theory of dependence suggests that nicotine stimulates the release of adrenocorticotropic hormone (ACTH) from the anterior pituitary, or "master gland" of the endocrine system (see Chapter 3) causing the release of **beta endorphins** (naturally occurring opiate-like chemicals) that produce mild feelings of euphoria. Perhaps this stresslike response mechanism involving ACTH accounts for the increased energy expenditure seen in smokers and thus their tendency to maintain a lower body weight. Others, however, have questioned the ability of nicotine to stimulate endorphin release.[25]

When these physiological responses are viewed collectively, nicotine may be seen as biochemically influencing brain activity by enhancing the extent and strength of various forms of "communication" between different brain areas and even glands of the endocrine system. If this is the case, it is apparent why, once addicted, the functioning of the smoker's control systems is much altered in comparison with that of nonsmokers.

Self-Medication Theory

Another explanation of the addiction to smoking, called self-medication, suggests that nicotine, through the effects

---

Key Terms

bolus theory a theory of nicotine addiction based on the body's response to the bolus (ball) of nicotine delivered to the brain with each inhalation of cigarette smoke.

beta endorphins mood-enhancing, pain-reducing, opiate-like chemicals produced within the smoker's body in response to the presence of nicotine.

of mood-enhancing dopamine, may allow smokers to "treat" feelings of tiredness, lack of motivation, or even depression.[26] In other words, a smoke lifts the spirits, if only briefly. Eventually, however, smokers become dependent on tobacco as a "medication" to make themselves feel better. Thus, because tobacco is a legal drug that is readily available, it becomes preferred to prescription medications and illegal drugs, such as cocaine and the stimulants, that elevate mood.

Regardless of the mechanism involved, as tolerance to nicotine develops, smoking behavior is adjusted to either maintain arousal or prevent the occurrence of withdrawal symptoms. At some point, however, the desire for constant arousal is probably superseded by the smoker's desire not to experience withdrawal.

The importance of nicotine as the primary factor in establishing dependence on tobacco is supported by research that demonstrates that smokers will not select a nontobacco cigarette if a tobacco cigarette is available. Even tobacco cigarettes with a very low level of nicotine seem to be unacceptable to most smokers, as do cigarettes with very low nicotine but with high tar content. Interestingly, users of low-nicotine cigarettes tend to inhale more frequently and deeply to obtain as much nicotine as possible.

Even more impressive (and alarming) regarding nicotine's dependency-producing power, is seen in conjunction with the small amount of time needed to become dependent. Using the HONC instruments described in the Star box on page 296, it is now established that beginning smokers (recall that most smokers begin during adolescence) become dependent on cigarettes within 3 weeks to 3 months of smoking on as little as two cigarettes per day. Males are more likely to be a bit more resistant to dependency, taking a month or 2, while females can become dependent in a matter of a very few days of initial experimentation.[27]

 TALKING POINTS A smoker says that she does not consider smoking to be a form of drug use. She becomes angry at the suggestion that cigarettes are part of a drug delivery system. How would you respond to her position?

Acute Effects of Nicotine on Nervous System Function

In comparison with the more chronic effects of nicotine on the central nervous system (CNS) that may eventually result in physical dependence or addiction, nicotine also produces changes of short duration. In the CNS, nicotine activates receptors within the nucleus accumbens (a reward center) and the locus caeruleus (a cortical activating center) of the brain. Stimulation of the brain is seen by changes in electroencephalogram (EEG) patterns, reflecting an increase in the frequency of electrical activity. This

is part of a general arousal pattern signaled by the release of the neurotransmitters **norepinephrine,** dopamine, acetylcholine, and serotonin. Heavy use of tobacco products, resulting in high levels of nicotine in the bloodstream, eventually produces a blocking effect as more and more receptor sites for these neurotransmitters are filled. The result is a generalized depression of the CNS.

The level of plasma nicotine associated with normal levels of heavy smoking (one to two packs per day) would not likely produce the depressive effect just described. However, in chain smokers (four to eight packs per day), plasma nicotine levels would be sufficient to have a depressive influence on nervous system function. In fact, it has been suggested that chain smoking is driven by the fruitless effort to counter the depressive influence of chronically excessively high levels of nicotine. In contrast to chain smokers, inexperienced smokers, lacking tolerance, can quickly reach a blood level of nicotine sufficient enough to activate the brain's vomiting centers. This response is a built-in protective mechanism against nicotine poisoning.

In carefully controlled studies involving both animals and humans, nicotine increased the ability of subjects to concentrate on a task. It must be noted, however, that the duration of this improvement was limited. Most would agree that this brief benefit is not enough to justify the health risks associated with chronic tobacco use.

Non–Nervous System Acute Effects of Nicotine

Outside the CNS, nicotine affects the transmission of nerve signals at the point where nerves innervate muscle tissue (called the *neuromuscular junction*) by mimicking the action of the neurotransmitter acetylcholine. Nicotine occupies receptor sites at the junction and prevents the transmission of nerve impulses from nerve cell to muscle cell.

Nicotine also causes the release of epinephrine from the adrenal medulla (see Chapter 3), which results in an increase in respiration rate, heart rate, blood pressure, and coronary blood flow. These changes are accompanied by the constriction of the blood vessels beneath the skin, a reduction in the motility in the bowel, loss of appetite, and changes in sleep patterns.

Although a lethal dose of nicotine could be obtained through the ingestion of a nicotine-containing insecticide,

---

Key Terms

norepinephrine (nor epp in **eff** rin) an adrenalin-like chemical produced within the nervous system.

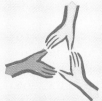
to "smoke oneself to death" in a single intense period of cigarette use would be highly improbable. In humans, 40 to 60 mg (.06–.09 mg/kg) is a lethal dose.[28] A typical cigarette supplies .05 to 2.5 mg of nicotine, and that nicotine is relatively quickly broken down for removal from the body.

Psychosocial Factors Related to Dependence

You will recall that a psychological aspect of dependence (habituation) exists and is important in maintaining the smoker's need for nicotine. Both research and general observation support many of the powerful influences this aspect of dependence possesses, especially for beginning smokers, prior to the onset of physical addiction. Consequently, in the remainder of this section, we will explore factors that may contribute to the development of this aspect of dependence.

Modeling

Because tobacco use is a learned behavior, it is reasonable to accept that modeling acts as a stimulus to experimental smoking. Modeling suggests that susceptible people smoke to emulate, or model their behavior after, smokers whom they admire or with whom they share other types of social or emotional bonds. Particularly for young adolescents (ages 14 to 17), smoking behavior correlates with the smoking behavior of slightly older peers and very young adults (ages 18 to 22), older siblings, and, most importantly, parents.[29] Negative parental influences on cigarette smoking by their own children include their own smoking in combination with their failure to clearly state their disapproval of smoking by children.[30] Further, for parents who smoke, it is important that they cease smoking before their children turn 8 years of age if they wish to maximize an antismoking message.

Modeling is particularly evident when smoking is a central factor in peer group formation and peer group association and can lead to a shared behavioral pattern that differentiates the group from others and from adults. Further, when risk-taking behavior and disregard for authority are common to the group, smoking becomes the behavioral pattern that most consistently identifies and bonds the group. Particularly for those young people who lack self-directedness or the ability to resist peer pressure, initial membership in a tobacco-using peer group may become inescapable. The ability to counter peer pressure is a salient component of successful anti-smoking programs for use with older children and younger adolescents.[31]

In addition, when adolescents have lower levels of self-esteem and are searching for an avenue to improve self-image, a role model who smokes is often seen as tough, sociable, and sexually attractive. These three traits have been played up by the tobacco industry in their carefully crafted advertisements. In fact, teens from any background may see the very young and attractive models used in tobacco (and beer) advertisements as being more peer-like in age than they really are. FCC regulations require that models for both products be 21 years of age or older, regardless of how youthful they might (and the advertisers hope they do) appear to older children and young adolescents. See the Learning from Our Diversity box on page 302 for a counterapproach to the acceptance of tobacco.

Manipulation

In addition to modeling as a psychosocial link with tobacco use, cigarette use may meet the beginning smoker's need to manipulate something and at the same time provide the manipulative "tool" necessary to offset boredom, feelings of depression, or social immaturity. Clearly the availability of affordable smoking paraphernalia provides smokers with ways to reward themselves. A new cigarette lighter, a status brand of tobacco, or a beach towel with a cigarette's logo are all reinforcements to some smokers. Fortunately, the latter will become increasingly harder to find as logos can no longer be placed on items such as beach towels. For others, the ability to take out a cigarette or fill a pipe adds a measure of structure and control to situations in which they might otherwise feel somewhat ill at ease. The cigarette becomes a readily available and dependable "friend" to turn to during stressful moments.

Susceptibility to Advertising

The images of the smoker's world portrayed by the media can be particularly attractive. For adolescents, women, minorities, and other carefully targeted groups of adults, the tobacco industry has paired suggestions of a better life with the use of its products. To these users and potential users, the self-reward of power, liberation, affluence, sophistication, or adult status is achieved by using the products that they are told are associated with these desired states. Thus the self-rewarding use of tobacco products becomes a means of achievement.

With this multiplicity of forces at work, it is possible to understand why so many who experiment with tobacco use find that they quickly become dependent on tobacco. Human needs, both physiological and psychosocial, are many and complex. Tobacco use meets the needs on a short-term basis, whereas dependence, once established, replaces these needs with a different, more immediate set of needs.

Despite the satisfaction of the dependency that continued smoking brings, approximately 80% of adult smokers have, on at least one occasion, expressed a desire to quit, and the majority of these have actually attempted to become nonsmokers. Today, with the over-the-counter availability of transdermal nicotine patches, nicotine-containing gum, prescription medications such as antidepressants, and nicotine inhalers, the number of smokers making

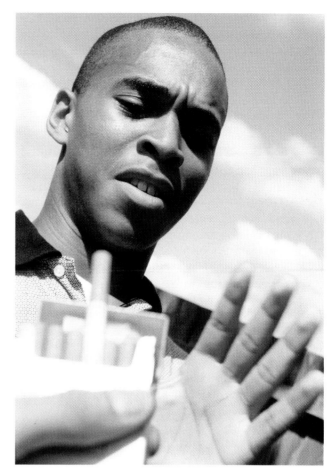

Not starting is much easier than quitting.

concerted and repeated attempts to stop smoking is up considerably over that seen in the past. It therefore seems apparent that tobacco use is a source of **dissonance.** This dissonance stems from the need to deal emotionally with a behavior that is both highly enjoyable and highly dangerous but known to be difficult to stop. The degree to which this dissonance exists probably varies from user to user.

Preventing Teen Smoking

Even before the 1997 release of tobacco industry documents confirming the targeting of young adolescents, the

---

Key Terms

dissonance (**dis** son ince) a feeling of uncertainty that occurs when a person believes two equally attractive but opposite ideas.

---

federal government stated its intention to curb these cigarette advertisements. In August 1995 the FDA described the specific actions that it hoped it would be given authority to implement. Collectively, the restrictions described in the following list were intended to discourage cigarette smoking among America's teens, resulting in 50% fewer adolescents beginning smoking in the year 2002 than in 1995.

1. Limit tobacco advertising in publications that appeal to teens and restrict billboards with tobacco-related content to no closer than 1,000 feet of schools and playgrounds. (An August 1995 study in California found that stores near schools displayed significantly more tobacco-related advertisements than those farther from schools.)

2. Restrict the use of logo and other tobacco-related images on nontobacco-related products, such as towels, T-shirts, and caps.

3. Bar certain sources of access to tobacco products, such as mail order sales, the distribution of free samples, and vending machines.

4. Halt sponsorship of high-visibility events, such as auto racing and athletic contests in which brand names appear on highly televised surfaces, including hoods, fenders, uniforms, and arena sign boards. (It is estimated that the Marlboro logo is seen 5,933 times during the course of a 90-minute televised Winston Cup auto race.)

5. Require merchants to obtain proof of age when selling tobacco products to adolescents. (This particular component of the initial plan became law in 1997. Merchants are required to validate the age of people whom they suspect to be younger than 27 years of age before selling cigarettes to those 18 years of age and older. If found in violation, both the salesperson and the store owner will be fined $500.)

By mid-1998 the federal government's desire to reduce youth smoking through implementation of the steps just described was mired in a larger package of tobacco-related policies being debated in Congress. This undertaking was related to the class action suit filed by all 50 (46 as a single large class and 4 as a smaller class) states against the tobacco industry in an attempt to recoup Medicaid expenditures for treating tobacco-related illnesses. As Congress attempted to construct a settlement that would be acceptable to all parties, the impasse fragmented attempts to reduce youth smoking. Unfortunately, this outcome diluted some restrictions on tobacco advertisements, as well as the FDA's ability to reduce smoking by defining cigarettes as drug delivery systems. In fact, in 2000 the United States Supreme Court ruled that the FDA lacked the regulatory authority to bring tobacco products under its control, unless Congress was willing to rescind laws that currently define tobacco as an agricultural product that can be freely marketed to persons 18 years of age or older. (If defined as a drug delivery system, cigarettes would be obtainable only with a physician's prescription, which would essentially prevent, or greatly limit, children's access to them.)

As noted earlier in the chapter, the Master Settlement Agreement (1999), that required the tobacco industry to pay the states 246 billion dollars, was able to restrict some forms of youth-oriented advertising and fund anti-smoking education, which may accomplish some of the changes initially proposed. Unfortunately, during the economic downturn, some states have used or borrowed against the funds to meet taxation shortfalls.

Early Childhood Intervention

Although significant concern centers on the onset of smoking behavior by adolescents in the 11- to 14-year-old age group and later teen years, the decision to smoke (or use other forms of tobacco) may be made at a much earlier age. Accordingly, parents (and other adults) who do not want their children to smoke or use tobacco in other forms should begin educating their children as preschoolers and certainly by school age. The following recommendations, and many additional ones as well, can be found in *A Parent's Guide to Prevention*, available from the National Clearinghouse for Alcohol and Drug Information.

When dealing with preschool children, it should be remembered that facts are unlikely to be comprehended. Accordingly, the following activities are suggested:

- Set aside regular time when you can give your child your full attention. Playing and reading together builds a strong parent-child bond.

- Point out poisonous and harmful substances that can be found in the home.

- Explain how medicines can be harmful if used incorrectly.

- Provide guidelines that teach the child what kind of behavior is expected.

- Encourage the child to follow instructions.

- Help the child learn decision-making skills; give positive feedback when appropriate decisions have been made.

For children in kindergarten through third grade, new skills and insights need to be developed to deal with drugs, including tobacco products. Adults should attempt to:

- Help the child recognize and understand family rules.

- Discuss how television advertisements try to persuade people to buy their products.

- Practice ways in which the child can say no to other people.
- Develop a "helper" file made up of the names and phone numbers of people the child can turn to when confronted by others who want them to try smoking or smokeless tobacco.

As children approach the preteen years, more focused presentations can be made regarding the dangers associated with smoking and the use of other substances. Adults working with children in grades four through six should focus on the following activities:

- Create special times when an adult is available to talk with the child about whatever he or she wants to talk about.
- Encourage participation in a variety of activities that are both fun and allow the child to meet new friends.
- Teach the child how drugs, including tobacco products, are promoted and how their messages can be "defused."
- Continue to assist the child in learning how to say no.
- Become acquainted with the parents of the child's friends so that you will be able to work with them in support of antismoking activities in the community.
- Participate in providing support for supervised activities for children of this age.

Although nothing is certain regarding the decision that older preadolescents or teens make about beginning to smoke, the activities just listed may be effective in countering the influences of the peer group and the mass media.

Tobacco: The Source of Physiologically Active Compounds

When burned, the tobacco in cigarettes, cigars, and pipe mixtures is the source of an array of physiologically active chemicals, many of which are closely linked to significant changes in normal body structure and function. At the burning tip of the cigarette, the 900° C (1,652° F) heat oxidizes tobacco (as well as paper, wrapper, filter, and additives). With each puff of smoke, the body is exposed to approximately 4,700 chemical compounds, hundreds of which are known to be physiologically active, toxic, and carcinogenic (see Table 9.2 for a partial listing[32]). These chemicals have their origins in the tobacco or have been introduced as additives, pesticides, and other agricultural chemicals. An annual 70,000 puffs taken in by the one-

pack-a-day cigarette smoker results in an environment that makes the most polluted urban environment seem clean by comparison.

Particulate Phase

Cigarette, cigar, and pipe smoke can be described on the basis of two phases. These phases include a particulate phase and a gaseous phase. The **particulate phase** includes **nicotine,** water, and a variety of powerful chemicals known collectively as tar. **Tar** includes phenol, cresol, pyrene, DDT, and a benzene-ring group of compounds that includes benzo[a]pyrene. Most of the carcinogenic compounds are found within the tar. A person who smokes one pack of cigarettes per day will collect four ounces of tar in his or her lungs in a year. Only the gases and the smallest particles reach the small sacs of the lungs, called the *alveoli*, where oxygen exchange occurs. The carcinogen-rich particles from the particulate phase are deposited somewhere along the air passage leading to the lungs.

Gaseous Phase

The **gaseous phase** of tobacco smoke, like the particulate phase, is composed of a variety of physiologically active compounds, including carbon monoxide, carbon dioxide, ammonia, hydrogen cyanide, isopyrene, acetaldehyde, and acetone. At least sixty of these compounds have been determined to be **carcinogens,** or co-carcinogenic promoters, thus capable of stimulating the development of

---

Key Terms

particulate phase portion of the tobacco smoke composed of small suspended particles.

nicotine physiologically active, dependence-producing drug found in tobacco.

tar a chemically rich, syrupy, blackish-brown material obtained from the particulate matter within cigarette smoke when nicotine and water are removed.

gaseous phase portion of the tobacco smoke containing carbon monoxide and many other physiologically active gaseous compounds.

carcinogens environmental agents, including chemical compounds within cigarette smoke, that stimulate the development of cancerous changes within cells.

Table 9.2 A Partial Listing of Toxic and Carcinogenic Components of Cigarette Smoke Including Vapor (Gaseous)-Phase and Particulate Phase Components

Agent	Toxic	Ciliotoxic	Carcinogenic
Carbon Monoxide	X		
Nitrogen Oxides (NO$_x$)	X		
Hydrogen Cyanide	X	X	
Formaldehyde		X	X
Acrolein		X	
Acetaldehyde		X	
Ammonia	X		
Hydrazine			X
Vinyl Chloride			X
Urethane			X
2-Nitropropane			X
Quinoline			X
Benzo[a]pyrene			X
Dibenz[a,h]anthracene			X
Benzo[b]fluoranthene			X
Benzo[j]fluoranthene			X
Dibenzo[a,h]pyrene			X
Dibenzo[a,i]pyrene			X
Dibenz[a,j]acridine			X
Indeno[1,2,3-cd]pyrene			X
Benz[a]anthracene			X
Benzo[e]pyrene			X
Chrysene			X
Methylchrysene			X
Methylfluoranthene			X
Dibenz[a,c]anthracene			X
Dibenz[a,h]acridine			X
Dibenzo[c,g]carbazole			X
Nitrosodimethylamine			X
Nitrosoethymethylamine			X
Nitrosodiethylamine			X
Nitrosodi-n-propylamine			X
Nitrosodi-n-butylamine			X
Nitrosopyrrolidine			X
Nitrosopiperidine			X
Nitrosomorpholine			X
N′-Nitrosonornicotine			X
4-(methylnitrosamino)-1-(3-pyridyl)-1-butanone			X
N′-Nitrosoanabasine			X
N′-Nitrosoanatabine			X
Aromatic Amines			X
Aromatic Nitrohydrocarbons			X
Polonium-210			X
Nickel			X
Arsenic			X
Cadmium			X

Source: Mulcahy S. *The toxicology of cigarette smoke and environmental tobacco smoke.* A Review of Cigarette Smoke and Its Toxicological Effects. **http://www.csn.ul.ie/-stephen/reports/bc4927.html**

cancer. Carbon monoxide is, however, the most damaging compound found in this component of tobacco smoke. Its impact is discussed next.

Carbon Monoxide

Like every inefficient engine, a cigarette, cigar, or pipe burns (oxidizes) its fuel with less than complete conversion into carbon dioxide, water, and heat. As a result of this incomplete oxidation, burning tobacco forms **carbon monoxide (CO)** gas. Carbon monoxide is one of the most harmful components of tobacco smoke.

Carbon monoxide is a colorless, odorless, tasteless gas that possesses a very strong physiological attraction for hemoglobin, the oxygen-carrying pigment on each red blood cell. When CO is inhaled, it quickly bonds with hemoglobin and forms a new compound, carboxy-hemoglobin. In this form, hemoglobin is unable to transport oxygen to the tissues and cells where it is needed.

Although it is true that normal body metabolism always keeps an irreducible minimum of CO in our blood (0.5% to 1%), the blood of smokers may have levels of 5% to 10% CO saturation.[33] We are exposed to additional CO from environmental sources such as automobiles and buses and other combustion of fossil fuels. By combining a smoker's CO with environmental CO, it is little wonder that smokers more easily become out of breath than nonsmokers. The half-life of CO combined with hemoglobin is approximately 4 to 6 hours.[34] Most smokers replenish their level of CO saturation at far shorter intervals than this.

As mentioned, the presence of excessive levels of carboxyhemoglobin in the blood of smokers leads to shortness of breath and lowered endurance. Because an adequate oxygen supply to all body tissues is critical for normal functioning, any oxygen reduction can have a serious impact on health. Brain function may be eventually reduced, reactions and judgment are dulled, and of course, cardiovascular function is impaired. Fetuses are especially at risk for this oxygen deprivation (hypoxia) because fetal development is so critically dependent on a sufficient oxygen supply from the mother.

Illness, Premature Death, and Tobacco Use

For people who begin tobacco use as adolescents or young adults, smoke heavily, and continue to smoke, the likelihood of premature death is virtually ensured. Two-pack-a-day cigarette smokers can expect to die 7 to 8 years earlier than their nonsmoking counterparts. (Only nonsmoking-related deaths that can afflict smokers and nonsmokers alike keep the difference at this level rather than much higher.) Not only will these people die sooner, but they will also probably be plagued with painful, debilitating illnesses for an extended time. Smoking is responsible for nearly 440,000 premature deaths each year.[35] An overview of illnesses known to be caused or worsened by tobacco use is presented in Table 9.3.[36]

Cardiovascular Disease

Cardiovascular disease is the leading cause of death among all adults, accounting for 945,836 deaths in the United States in 2000.[37] Tobacco use, and cigarette smoking in particular, is clearly one of the major factors contributing to this cause of death. Although overall progress is being made in reducing the incidence of cardiovascular-related deaths, tobacco use impedes these efforts. So important is tobacco use as a contributing factor in deaths from cardiovascular disease that the cigarette smoker more than doubles the risk of experiencing a **myocardial infarction,** the leading cause of death from cardiovascular disease. Smokers also increase their risk of **sudden cardiac death** by two to four times. Fully one-third of all cardiovascular disease can be traced to cigarette smoking.

The relationship between tobacco use and cardiovascular disease is centered on two major components of tobacco smoke: nicotine and carbon monoxide.

Nicotine and Cardiovascular Disease

The influence of nicotine on the cardiovascular system occurs when it stimulates the nervous system to release norepinephrine. This powerful stimulant increases the heart rate. In turn, an elevated heart rate increases cardiac output, thus increasing blood pressure. The extent to which this is dangerous depends in part on the coronary circulation's ability to supply blood to the rapidly contracting heart muscle. The development of **angina pectoris** and the possibility of sudden heart attack are heightened by this sustained elevation of heart rate,

---

Key Terms

carbon monoxide (CO) chemical compound that can "inactivate" red blood cells.

myocardial infarction heart attack; the death of heart muscle as a result of a blockage in one of the coronary arteries.

sudden cardiac death immediate death resulting from a sudden change in the rhythm of the heart.

angina pectoris (an **jie** nuh **peck** tor is) chest pain that results from impaired blood supply to the heart muscle.

Table 9.3 Selected Established and Suspected Health Effects of Cigarette Smoking

Category of Condition	Established and Suspected Effects
1 Lung Disease	lung cancer, chronic obstructive lung disease; increased severity of asthma; increased risk of developing various respiratory infections
2 Cancer Risk	esophageal, laryngeal, oral, bladder, kidney, stomach, pancreatic, vulvar, cervical, and colorectal cancers
3 Heart Disease	coronary heart disease; angina pectoris; heart attack; repeat heart attack; arrhythmia; aortic aneurysm; cardiomyopathy
4 Peripheral Vascular Disease	pain and discomfort in the legs and feet resulting from restricted blood flow into the extremities
5 Skin Changes	wrinkling; fingernail discoloration; psoriasis; palmoplantar pustulosis
6 Surgical Risk	need for more anesthesia; increased risk of postsurgical respiratory infection; increased need for supplemental oxygen following surgery; delayed wound healing
7 Orthopedic Problems	disc degeneration; less successful back surgery; musculoskeletal injury; delayed fracture healing
8 Rheumatologic Conditions	osteoporosis and osteoarthritis
9 Environmental Tobacco Smoke and Pediatric Illnesses	infections of the lower respiratory tract; more severe asthma; middle ear infections; Crohn's disease and ulcerative colitis; sudden infant death syndrome; impaired delivery of oxygen to body tissues
10 Complications in Obstetrics and Gynecology	infertility; miscarriage; fetal growth retardation; prematurity; stillbirth; transmission of HIV to the fetus from the infected biological mother; birth defects; intellectual impairment of offspring; sudden infant death syndrome; earlier menopause
11 Male Infertility and Sexuality Dysfunctions	decreased sperm motility; decreased sperm density; impotence
12 Neurological Disorders	transient ischemic attack; stroke; worsened multiple sclerosis
13 Brain and Behavior	depression
14 Abnormalities of the Ears, Nose, and Throat	snoring and hearing loss
15 Eyes	cataracts; complications from Graves' disease; macular degeneration; optic neuropathy
16 Oral Health	periodontal disease
17 Endocrine System	increased metabolic rate; blood-sugar abnormalities; increased waist-to-hip ratio; redistribution of body fat
18 Gastrointestinal Diseases	stomach and duodenal ulcers; Crohn's disease
19 Immune System	impaired humoral and cell-mediated immunity
20 Emergency Medicine	injuries from fires; occupational injuries

Source: Kapier KN, et al. *Cigarettes: What the warning label doesn't tell you.* American Council on Science and Health, 1997.

particularly in those individuals with existing coronary artery disease (see Chapter 10).

Nicotine is also a powerful vasoconstrictor of the peripheral blood vessels. As these vessels are constricted by the influence of nicotine, the pressure against their walls increases. Recent research shows that irreversible atherosclerotic damage to major arteries also occurs with smoking.

Nicotine also increases blood **platelet adhesiveness.**[38] As the platelets become more and more likely to "clump," a person will be more likely to develop a blood clot. In people already prone to cardiovascular disease, more rapidly clotting blood is an unwelcome liability. Heart attacks occur when clots form within the coronary arteries or are transported to the heart from other areas of the body.

In addition to other influences on the cardiovascular system, nicotine possesses the ability to decrease the proportion of high-density lipoproteins (HDLs) and to increase the proportion of low-density lipoproteins (LDLs) and very-low-density lipoproteins that constitute the

---

Key Terms

platelet adhesiveness tendency of platelets to clump together, thus enhancing the speed at which the blood clots.

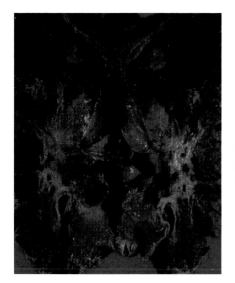
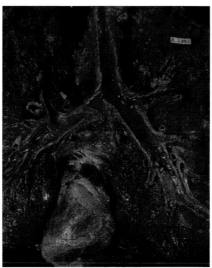

A healthy lung (right) vs. the lung of a smoker (left).

body's serum cholesterol. Low-density lipoproteins appear to support the development of atherosclerosis and are clearly increased in the bloodstreams of smokers. (See Chapter 10 for further information about cholesterol's role in cardiovascular disease.)

Carbon Monoxide and Cardiovascular Disease

A second substance contributed by tobacco influences the type and extent of cardiovascular disease found among tobacco users. Carbon monoxide interferes with oxygen transport within the circulatory system.

As described earlier in the chapter, carbon monoxide is a component of the gaseous phase of tobacco smoke and readily joins with the hemoglobin of the red blood cells. Carbon monoxide has an affinity for hemoglobin 206 times that of oxygen. Once the hemoglobin of a red cell has accepted carbon monoxide molecules, the hemoglobin is transformed into carboxyhemoglobin. Thereafter, the carboxyhemoglobin permanently weakens the red blood cell's ability to transport oxygen. So long as smoking continues, these red blood cells remain relatively useless during the remainder of their 120-day lives. Levels of carboxyhemoglobin in heavy smokers are associated with significant increases in the incidence of myocardial infarction.

When a person has impaired oxygen-transporting abilities, physical exertion becomes increasingly demanding on both the heart and the lungs. The cardiovascular system will attempt to respond to the body's demand for oxygen, but these responses are themselves impaired as a result of the influence of nicotine on the cardiovascular system. If tobacco does create the good life, as advertisers claim, it also unfortunately lessens the ability to participate actively in that life.

Cancer

Over the past 60 years, research from the most reputable institutions in this country and abroad has consistently concluded that tobacco use is a significant factor in the development of virtually all forms of cancer and the most significant factor in cancers involving the respiratory system.

In describing cancer development, the currently used reference is 20 pack-years, or an amount of smoking equal to smoking one pack of cigarettes a day for 20 years. Thus the two-pack-a-day smoker can anticipate cancer-related tissue changes in as few as 10 years, while the half-pack-a-day smoker may have 40 years to wait. Regardless, the opportunity is there for all smokers to confirm these data

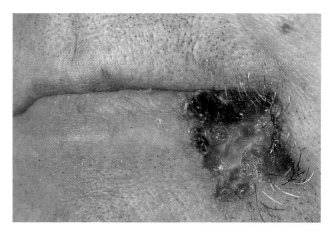

Oral cancer may appear near the edge of the mouth as well as inside the oral cavity.

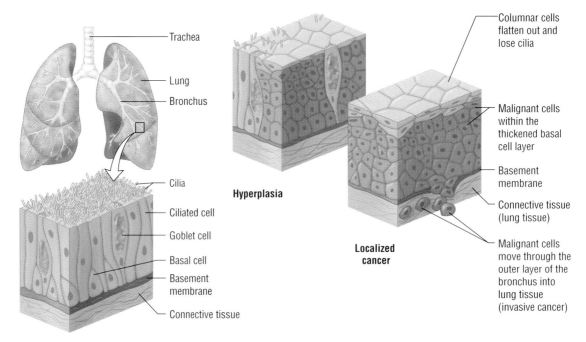

Figure 9-2 Tissue changes associated with bronchogenic carcinoma (lung cancer).

Labels in figure:
Trachea
Lung
Bronchus
Cilia
Ciliated cell
Goblet cell
Basal cell
Basement membrane
Connective tissue

Hyperplasia

Columnar cells flatten out and lose cilia
Malignant cells within the thickened basal cell layer
Basement membrane
Connective tissue (lung tissue)
Malignant cells move through the outer layer of the bronchus into lung tissue (invasive cancer)

Localized cancer

by developing cancer as predicted. It is hoped that most people will think twice before disregarding this evidence.

Data supplied by the American Cancer Society (ACS) indicate that during 2003 an estimated 1,334,000 Americans developed cancer.* These cases were nearly equally divided between the sexes and resulted in approximately 556,500 deaths.[35] In the opinion of the ACS, 30% of all cancer cases are heavily influenced by tobacco use.[35] Lung cancer alone accounted for about 171,900 of the new cancer cases and 157,200 deaths in 2003. Fully 87% of men with lung cancer were cigarette smokers.[35] A genetic "missing link" between smoking and lung cancer was established, when mutations to an important tumor suppressor gene were identified. If it was necessary to have a final "proof" that smoking causes lung cancer, that proof appears to be in hand.[39]

Cancer of the entire respiratory system, including lung cancer and cancers of the mouth and throat accounted for about 185,200 new cases of cancer and 163,700 deaths.[35] Despite these high figures, not all smokers develop cancer.

Respiratory Tract Cancer

Recall that tobacco smoke produces both a gaseous and a particulate phase. As noted, the particulate phase contains the tar fragment of tobacco smoke. This rich chemical environment contains more than four thousand known chemical compounds, hundreds of which are known to be carcinogens.

In the normally functioning respiratory system, particulate matter suspended in the inhaled air settles on the tissues lining the airways and is trapped in **mucus** produced by specialized *goblet cells*. This mucus, with its trapped impurities, is continuously swept upward by the beating action of hairlike **cilia** of the ciliated columnar epithelial cells lining the air passages (Figure 9-2). On reaching the throat, this mucus is swallowed and eventually removed through the digestive system.

When tobacco smoke is drawn into the respiratory system, however, its rapidly dropping temperature allows the particulate matter to accumulate. This brown, sticky tar contains compounds known to harm the ciliated cells, goblet cells, and the basal cells of the respiratory lining. As the damage from smoking increases, the cilia become

---

*Excluding cases of nonmelanoma skin cancer.

<table>
<tr><td colspan="2">Key Terms</td></tr>
<tr><td>mucus</td><td>clear, sticky material produced by specialized cells within the mucous membranes of the body; mucus traps much of the suspended particulate matter within tobacco smoke.</td></tr>
<tr><td>cilia</td><td>(sill ee uh) small, hairlike structures that extend from cells that line the air passages.</td></tr>
</table>

less effective in sweeping mucus upward to the throat. When cilia can no longer clean the airway, tar accumulates on the surfaces and brings carcinogenic compounds into direct contact with the tissues of the airway.

At the same time that the sweeping action of the lining cells is being slowed, substances in the tar are stimulating the goblet cells to increase the amount of mucus they normally produce. The "smoker's cough" is the body's attempt to remove this excess mucus.

With prolonged exposure to the carcinogenic materials in tar, predictable changes will begin to occur within the respiratory system's basal cell layer (Figure 9-2). The basal cells begin to display changes characteristic of all cancer cells. In addition, an abnormal accumulation of cells occurs. When a person stops smoking, preinvasive lesions do not repair themselves as quickly as once thought.[40]

By the time lung cancer is usually diagnosed, its development is so advanced that the chance for recovery is very poor. Still today, only 15% of all lung cancer victims survive for 5 years or more after diagnosis.[35] Most die in a very uncomfortable, painful way.

Cancerous activity in other areas of the respiratory system, including the larynx, and within the oral cavity (mouth) follows a similar course. In the case of oral cavity cancer, carcinogens found within the smoke and within the saliva are involved in the cancerous changes. Tobacco users, such as pipe smokers, cigar smokers, and users of smokeless tobacco, have a higher (4 to 10 times) rate of cancer of the mouth, tongue, and voice box.

In addition to drawing smoke into the lungs, tobacco users swallow saliva that contains an array of chemical compounds from tobacco. As this saliva is swallowed, carcinogens are absorbed into the circulatory system and transported to all areas of the body. The filtering of the blood by the liver, kidneys, and bladder may account for the higher-than-normal levels of cancer in these organs among smokers.

As reported earlier in the chapter, documents released in 1997 from within the tobacco industry clearly show that the major tobacco companies were aware of tobacco's role in the development of cancer and had made a concerted effort to deprive the American public access to such knowledge.

Chronic Obstructive Lung Disease

Chronic obstructive lung disease (COLD), also known as chronic obstructive pulmonary disease (COPD), is a disorder in which the amount of air that flows in and out of the lungs becomes progressively limited. COLD is a disease state that is made up of two separate but related diseases: **chronic bronchitis** and **pulmonary emphysema.**

With chronic bronchitis, excess mucus is produced in response to the effects of smoking on airway tissue, and the walls of the bronchi become inflamed and infected. This produces a characteristic narrowing of the air passages. Breathing becomes difficult, and activity can be severely restricted. With cessation of smoking, chronic bronchitis is reversible.

Emphysema causes irreversible damage to the tiny air sacs of the lungs, the **alveoli.** Chest pressure builds when air becomes trapped by narrowed air passages (chronic bronchitis) and the thin-walled sacs rupture. Emphysema patients lose the ability to ventilate fully. They feel as though they are suffocating. You may have seen people with this condition in malls and other locations as they walk slowly by, carrying or pulling their portable oxygen tanks.

More than 10 million Americans suffer from COLD. It is responsible for a greater limitation of physical activity than any other disease, including heart disease. COLD patients tend to die a very unpleasant, prolonged death, often from a general collapse of normal cardiorespiratory function that results in congestive heart failure (see Chapter 10).

Additional Health Concerns

In addition to the serious health problems stemming from tobacco use already described, other health-related changes are routinely seen. These include a generally poor state of nutrition, the gradual loss of the sense of smell, and premature wrinkling of the skin. Tobacco users are also more likely to experience strokes (a potentially fatal condition), lose bone mass leading to osteoporosis, experience more back pain and muscle injury, and find that fractures heal more slowly. Further, smokers who have surgery spend more time in the recovery room. Although not perceived as a health problem by people who continue smoking in order to control weight, smoking does appear to minimize weight gain. In studies using identical twins, twins who smoked were six to eight pounds lighter than their nonsmoking siblings. Current understanding about why smoking results in lower body weight is less than complete. One factor may be an increase in Basal Metabolic

> ### Key Terms
>
> **chronic bronchitis** persistent inflammation and infection of the smaller airways within the lungs.
>
> **pulmonary emphysema** an irreversible disease process in which the alveoli are destroyed.
>
> **alveoli** (al **vee** oh lie) thin, saclike terminal ends of the airways; the site at which gases are exchanged between the blood and inhaled air.

Rate (BMR) (see Chapter 6) brought about by the influence of nicotine on sympathetic nervous system function. Additionally, smokers have a fourfold greater risk of developing serious gum (periodontal) disease. Also, smokers may need supplementation for two important water-soluble vitamins, vitamin C and vitamin B.

Smoking and Reproduction

In all of its dimensions, the reproductive process is impaired by the use of tobacco, particularly cigarette smoking. Problems can be found in association with infertility, problem pregnancy, breastfeeding, and the health of the newborn. So broadly based are reproductive problems and smoking that the term *fetal tobacco syndrome* or *fetal smoking syndrome*[41] is regularly used in clinical medicine. Some physicians even define a fetus being carried by a smoker as a "smoker" and, upon birth, as a "former smoker."

Infertility

Recent research indicates that cigarette smoking by both men and women can reduce levels of fertility. Among men, smoking adversely affects blood flow to erectile tissue, reduces sperm motility, and alters sperm shape, and it causes an overall decrease in the number of viable sperm. Among women, the effects of smoking are seen in terms of abnormal ovum formation, including a lessened ability on the part of the egg to prevent polyspermia, or the fertilization by multiple sperm.[36] Smoking also negatively influences estrogen levels, resulting in underdevelopment of the uterine wall and ineffective implantation of the fertilized ovum. Lower levels of estrogen may also influence the rate of transit of the fertilized egg through the fallopian tube, making it arrive in the uterus too early for successful implantation or, in some cases, restricting movement to the point that an *ectopic,* or *tubal,* pregnancy may develop. Also, the early onset of menopause is associated with smoking.[36]

Problem Pregnancy

The harmful effects of tobacco smoke on the course of pregnancy are principally the result of the carbon monoxide and nicotine to which the mother and her fetus are exposed. Carbon monoxide from the incomplete oxidation of tobacco is carried in the maternal blood to the placenta, where it diffuses across the placental barrier and enters the fetal circulation. Once in the fetal blood, the carbon monoxide bonds with the fetal hemoglobin to form fetal carboxyhemoglobin. As a result of this exposure to carbon monoxide, the fetus is progressively deprived of normal oxygen transport and eventually becomes compromised by chronic **hypoxia.**[41]

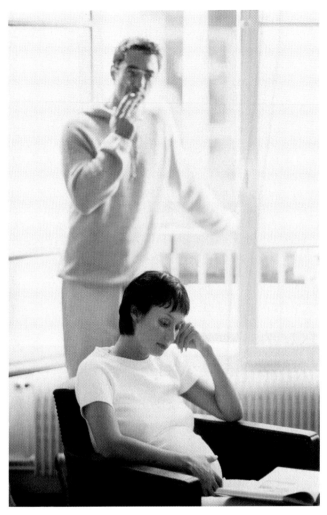

Pregnant women and those around them should refrain from smoking to protect the health of the developing fetus.

Nicotine also exerts its influence on the developing fetus. Thermographs of the placenta and fetus show signs of marked vasoconstriction within a few seconds after inhalation by the mother. This constriction further reduces the oxygen supply, resulting in hypoxia. In addition, nicotine stimulates the mother's stress response, placing the mother and fetus under the potentially harmful influence of elevated epinephrine and corticoid levels (see Chapter 3). Any fetus exposed to all of these agents is more likely to be miscarried, stillborn, or born prematurely.[36] Even when

> **Key Terms**
>
> **hypoxia** oxygenation deprivation at the cellular level.

carried to term, children born to mothers who smoked during pregnancy have lower birth weights and may show other signs of a stressful intrauterine life.[41]

Breastfeeding

For women who decide to breastfeed their infants, smoking during this period will continue to expose their children to the harmful effects of tobacco smoke. It is well recognized that nicotine appears in breast milk and thus is capable of exerting its vasoconstricting and stress-response influences on nursing infants. Mothers who stop smoking during pregnancy should be encouraged to continue to refrain from smoking while they are breastfeeding.

Neonatal Health Problems

Babies born to women who smoked during pregnancy will, on average, be shorter and have a lower birth weight than children born to nonsmoking mothers. During the earliest months of life, babies born to mothers who smoke experience an elevated rate of death caused by sudden infant death syndrome.[42] Statistics also show that infants are more likely to develop chronic respiratory problems, be hospitalized, and have poorer overall health during their early years of life. Problems such as those just mentioned may also be seen in children of nonsmoking mothers, when they were exposed prenatally to environmental tobacco smoke. In addition, environmental tobacco smoke exposure extending beyond the home and into the workplace may increase the probability of problem pregnancies and neonatal health problems.[43] Most recently, the interest in the effects of tobacco smoke on pregnancy has been extended to include behavioral differences in infants born to women who smoked during pregnancy.[44]

Parenting, in the sense of assuming responsibility for the well-being of children, does not begin at birth, but during the prenatal period. In the case of smoking, this is especially true. Pregnant women who continue smoking are disregarding the well-being of the children they are carrying. Other family members, friends, and coworkers who subject pregnant women to cigarette, pipe, or cigar smoke are, in a sense, exhibiting their own disregard for the health of the next generation.

Oral Contraceptives and Tobacco Use

Women who smoke and use oral contraceptives, particularly after age 35, are placing themselves at a much greater risk of experiencing a fatal cardiovascular accident (heart attack, stroke, or **embolism**) than oral contraceptive users who do not smoke. This risk of cardiovascular complications increases further for oral contraceptive users

40 years of age or older. Women who both smoke and use oral contraceptives are four times more likely to die from myocardial infarction (heart attack) than are women who only smoke. Because of this adverse relationship, *it is strongly recommended that women who smoke should not use oral contraceptives.*

Combining Tobacco and Alcohol Use

Although there are exceptions to every generalization, it is very common to see tobacco and alcohol being used by the same people, often at the same time. Younger people who use both tobacco and alcohol are also more likely to use additional drugs. Accordingly, both tobacco and alcohol are considered *gateway drugs* because they are often introductory drugs that "open the door" for a more broadly based polydrug use pattern (see Chapter 7).

Beyond the potential for polydrug use initiated by the use of tobacco and alcohol is the simple reality that the use of both tobacco products and alcoholic beverages is associated with a wide array of illnesses and with premature death. As you have seen in this chapter and in Chapter 8 regarding alcohol use, the negative health impact of using both is significant. When use is combined, of course, the risks of living less healthfully and dying prematurely are accentuated.

Smokeless Tobacco Use

As the term implies, smokeless tobacco, such as Skoal and Copenhagen, is not burned; rather, it is placed into the mouth. Once in place, the physiologically active nicotine and other soluble compounds are absorbed through the mucous membranes and into the blood. Within a few minutes, chewing tobacco and snuff generate blood levels of nicotine in amounts equivalent to those seen in cigarette smokers.

Chewing tobacco is taken from its foil pouch, formed into a small ball (called a "wad," "chaw," or "chew"), and placed into the mouth. Once in place, the bolus of tobacco is sucked and occasionally chewed, but not swallowed.

Snuff, a more finely shredded smokeless tobacco product, is marketed in small round cans. Snuff is formed into a small mass (or "quid") for dipping or used in prepackaged pouches. The quid or pouch is placed

---

Key Terms

embolism a potentially fatal condition in which a circulating blood clot lodges in a smaller vessel.

between the jaw and the cheek; the user sucks the quid or pouch, then spits out the brown liquid. Snuff, as once used, was actually a powdered form of tobacco that was inhaled through the nose.

Although smokeless tobacco would seem to free the tobacco user from many of the risks associated with smoking, chewing and dipping are not without their own substantial risks. The presence of *leukoplakia* (white spots) and *erythroplakia* (red spots) on the tissues of the mouth indicate precancerous changes. In addition, an increase in **periodontal disease** (with the pulling away of the gums from the teeth, resulting in later tooth loss), the abrasive damage to the enamel of the teeth, and the high concentration of sugar in processed tobacco all contribute to dental problems among users of smokeless tobacco. In those who develop oral cancer, the risk is dramatically heightened if the cancer metastasizes from the site of origin in the mouth to the brain. Clearly, it is important that users be aware of any signs of damage being done by their use of smokeless tobacco (see the Changing for the Better box below). The validity of this warning was made clear in 1998 when 59% of smokeless tobacco-using major league baseball players were found to have tobacco-related lesions when oral examinations were performed by team physicians on the first day of spring training.

In addition to the damage done to the tissues of the mouth, the need to process the inadvertently swallowed saliva that contains dissolved carcinogens places both the digestive and urinary systems at risk of cancer.

In the opinion of health experts, the use of smokeless tobacco and its potential for life-threatening disease is very real and should not be disregarded. Consequently,

television advertisements have been banned, and the following warnings have been placed in rotation on all smokeless tobacco products:

> WARNING: THIS PRODUCT MAY CAUSE MOUTH CANCER
> WARNING: THIS PRODUCT MAY CAUSE GUM DISEASE AND TOOTH LOSS
> WARNING: THIS PRODUCT IS NOT A SAFE ALTERNATIVE TO CIGARETTE SMOKING

Clearly, smokeless tobacco is a dangerous product, and little doubt exists that continued use of tobacco in this form is a serious problem to health in all of its dimensions.

The Risks of Involuntary (Passive) Smoking

The smoke generated by the burning of tobacco can be classified as either **mainstream smoke** (the smoke inhaled and then exhaled by the smoker) or **sidestream smoke** (the smoke that comes from the burning end of the cigarette, pipe, or cigar that simply disperses into the air without being inhaled by the smoker). When either form of tobacco smoke is diluted and stays within a common source of air, it can eventually be referred to as **environmental tobacco smoke.** All three forms of tobacco smoke lead to involuntary or passive smoking and can present health problems for both nonsmokers and smokers (see the Discovering Your Spirituality box on page 315).

Surprisingly, mainstream smoke makes up only 15% of our exposure to the harmful substances associated with involuntary smoking. Sidestream smoke is responsible for 85% of the harmful substances associated with secondhand smoke exposure. Because it is not filtered by the tobacco, the filter, or the smoker's body, sidestream smoke contains more free nicotine and produces higher yields of carbon dioxide and carbon monoxide. Much to the

Changing for the Better

Early Detection of Oral Cancer

I started using smokeless tobacco a few years ago, thinking it was safe. Recently, I read an article about it that was frightening. What are the real danger signs?

If you have any of the following signs, see your dentist or physician immediately:

- Lumps in the jaw or neck area
- Color changes or lumps inside the lips
- White, smooth, or scaly patches in the mouth or on the neck, lips, or tongue
- A red spot or sore on the lips or gums or inside the mouth that does not heal in 2 weeks
- Repeated bleeding in the mouth
- Difficulty or abnormality in speaking or swallowing

┌─ **Key Terms** ─────────────────────

periodontal disease destruction of soft tissue and bone that surround the teeth.

mainstream smoke smoke inhaled and then exhaled by a smoker.

sidestream smoke smoke that comes from the burning end of a cigarette, pipe, or cigar.

environmental tobacco smoke tobacco smoke, regardless of its source, that stays within a common source of air.

The Hidden Price Tag of Smoking

"I started to hug him but felt myself drawing back. It was almost like a reflex action." Those are the words of a young woman after greeting her brother when he returned home from his first semester at college. The young man had recently become a smoker, and his sister was reacting to the strong smell of smoke on his clothes and hair.

Dramatic as it may sound, smoking does set up barriers between people. First, there's the health issue. Some nonsmokers are adamant about not wanting people they care about to smoke. They also want to protect their children from this danger. And they certainly don't want to breathe in smoke themselves. So, at a family gathering, a smoker may want to have a cigarette after dinner, in the living room with everyone else. But the nonsmokers say no—go outside if you want to smoke. In the process, a birthday dinner or a special holiday is marred by this disagreement.

Whether the person is a family member or a friend, it's difficult to feel close to someone who's doing something you disapprove of—such as smoking. But, from the smoker's point of view, it's hard to feel good about someone who acts superior and doesn't accept you as you are. What do children think about all this? Does a "good" aunt or uncle smoke? If smoking is bad, as a little girl constantly hears at school and at home, why does her favorite uncle smoke?

The physical toll that smoking takes is apparent when the smoker finds himself sitting on the sidelines. A young man wants to play basketball with his buddies, but the last time he tried, he had a coughing fit—very embarrassing. A young woman meets some new people, and they ask her to join them for an "easy hike." Well, easy for them. She needs a break after only 10 minutes and sees what looks like pity in her friends' eyes.

On the job, smoking has gone the way of the three-martini lunch. It's just not politically correct. In fact, many companies have a no-smoking policy, or smoking is allowed in designated areas only. Ever drive by a big factory or office building and see a group of people standing outside, perhaps huddled under umbrellas? They're not organizing a strike—they're having a smoke (and being reminded of their high school days). Once again, the smoker feels isolated. Just as in the family group, the smoker feels the judgment of others—only now it's her boss or secretary who's frowning.

The price of smoking is hard to measure. The damage to the smoker's health is beyond dispute. But the spiritual and psychological costs are also real. How does it feel to always be the outsider? The unaccepted? Why does the smoker have to take the chance of missing an exciting play in the stadium to go smoke a cigarette? Or feel the resentment of others at work because he leaves to take a smoking break every hour? It's easy for nonsmokers to say: "Just quit." Smokers know it's not that simple. Many who have stopped smoking—often after several attempts—say that they thought about more than their health in deciding to quit. They thought about many situations—involving family, outdoor activities, and work—before they threw away the pack and said: "That was my last cigarette."

detriment of nonsmokers, sidestream smoke has a much higher quantity of highly carcinogenic compounds, called *N-nitrosamines,* than mainstream smoke has.

Current scientific opinion suggests that smokers and nonsmokers are exposed to very much the same smoke when tobacco is used within a common airspace. The important difference is the quantity of smoke inhaled by smokers and nonsmokers. It is likely that for each pack of cigarettes smoked by a smoker, nonsmokers who must share a common air supply with the smokers will involuntarily smoke the equivalent of three to five cigarettes per day. Even today, because of the small size of the particles produced by burning tobacco, environmental tobacco smoke cannot be completely removed from a workplace, restaurant, or shopping mall by the most effective ventilation system.

Recently reported research indicates that involuntary smoke exposure may be responsible for 35,000 to 40,000 premature deaths per year from heart disease among non-smokers in the United States.[35] Other estimates range upward to 53,000 premature deaths when lung cancer and COPD are included. In addition, large numbers of people exposed to involuntary smoke develop eye irritation, nasal symptoms, headaches, and a cough. Furthermore, most nonsmokers dislike the odor of tobacco smoke.

For these reasons, state, local, and private-sector initiatives to restrict smoking have been introduced. Most buildings in which people work, study, play, reside, eat, or shop now have some smoking restrictions. Some have complete smoking bans. Nowhere is smoking more noticeably prohibited than in the U.S. airline industry. Currently, smoking is banned on all domestic plane flights of less than six hours, and most American airlines have extended the ban on smoking to selected international flights as well.

Involuntary smoking poses major threats to nonsmokers within residential settings. Spouses and children of smokers are at greatest risk for involuntary smoking. Scientific studies suggest that nonsmokers married to smokers are three times more likely to experience heart attacks than nonsmoking spouses of nonsmokers, and the former have a 30% greater risk of lung cancer than do the latter. It should be noted, however, that a recent study of 35,561 nonsmoking spouses of smoking partners failed to show significantly higher death rates from heart disease, lung cancer, and COPD than did nonsmoking spouses in nonsmoking relationships.[45]

In spite of what may or may not be the effects of passive smoking on the nonsmoking partners of smokers, the effects of environmental tobacco smoke on the health of children seems well established. The children of parents who smoke are twice as likely as children of nonsmoking parents to experience bronchitis or pneumonia during the first year of life. In addition, throughout childhood these children will experience more wheezing, coughing, and sputum production than will children whose parents do not smoke. Otitis media (middle ear infection), one of the most frequently seen conditions in pediatric medicine, is also significantly more common in children under age 3 who reside with one or more adults who smoke.[35]

In July 1998, the tobacco industry challenged in court the salient 1993 EPA report that was the basis for restricting smoking in a wide array of public places and work sites. The federal judge who heard the case concluded that the principal study used in the report was flawed in its methodology and that its conclusions therefore were of questionable validity. Since this decision, the scientific community has documented to a very substantial degree the inherent dangers of passive or environmental tobacco smoke to the health of nonsmokers and smokers alike. Accordingly, restrictions on public smoking have been large scale and continue to be imposed. The states, cities, and work sites mentioned represent only a partial list of either smoking bans already imposed or bans on tobacco use being considered. Included in this list are statewide bans, including restrictions on all indoor smoking in Delaware; smoking in bars and restaurants in California, Indiana, New York, and Maine; smoking in cars with children under 4 in Georgia; all smoking on school properties in Pennsylvania; and the possession of tobacco products by all teens in Missouri. On a local level, Los Angeles may ban smoking in parks, Purdue University has banned smoking within 25 feet of all residence halls, while the Hartford, Connecticut, Police Department will no longer hire officers who smoke. Perhaps the most encompassing restriction was the March 2004 ban of smoking in all public buildings in Ireland, including pubs.

New Product Development

The development of new products by the tobacco industry also attests, in an interesting way, to the inherent dangers of tobacco use long known by the tobacco industry (and forcibly admitted to the public in the 1999 tobacco settlement). The products include the development of Eclipse (by R.J. Reynolds), a cigarette that heats rather than burns most of its tobacco. According to its manufacturer, Eclipse is the first cigarette that produces smoke so low in carcinogens

that it is the "next best choice" to quitting. This latter contention certainly states in a null manner something about cigarettes marketed before the development of Eclipse.

Unfortunately for customers who switched to Eclipse in search of a safe cigarette, the claims made by the company about the cigarette's low carcinogenic composition proved inaccurate (or purposefully false). In October 2000, the office of the Massachusetts state health commissioner reported that studies conducted by its laboratory found that two carcinogenic chemicals found in tobacco smoke, acetaldehyde and acrolein, were over seven times and four times more prevalent, respectively, in Eclipse than in leading low-tar brand cigarettes. Two additionally powerful carcinogens, benzo(a)pyrene and NNK, were found to be as prevalent in Eclipse as in low-tar brands. Most likely the end of the "safe cigarette" is in sight.

Another recently introduced cigarette, Accord, features a "smoking system" intended to reduce the production of sidestream smoke. This system uses a battery-powered device into which a special small cigarette is inserted. The smoker inhales through the device, and the cigarette is electrically ignited only when actively inhaled. The ability to release this product into the marketplace so quickly after the publication of documents revealing the tobacco industry's knowledge regarding the dangers of smoking attests to the industry having such knowledge and suggests that the industry was preparing for eventual worst-case scenarios.

Three additional new products appeared in 2003, including Advance, cigarettes with "Trionic" filters supposedly capable of extracting more toxins than any filter to date; Omni, a brand advertised to significantly reduce selected carcinogens, nitrosamines, and catechols, the "major causes of lung cancer" according to their advertisements; and Quest, a brand intended to lead smokers to "nicotine free smoking."[46] It should be noted that none of these new brands can deliver anything approaching a safe cigarette, nor are they intended to assist smokers in becoming nonsmokers.

Nontobacco Sources of Nicotine

Regardless of whether they are intended as aids to smoking cessation or only supplemental forms of nicotine for use when smoking is not permitted, numerous new forms of nicotine delivery systems have appeared in the marketplace in recent years. An area of growing concern is, of course, that these nontobacco delivery sources of nicotine could provide introductory exposure to nicotine, at a tragically early age, for the next generation of nicotine-dependent youth. Included among these nontobacco sources of nicotine are multiple flavors of nicotine suckers, nicotine-flavored gum, nicotine straws, nicotine-enhanced water (Nico Water), inhalers, sprays, drops, lozenges, and

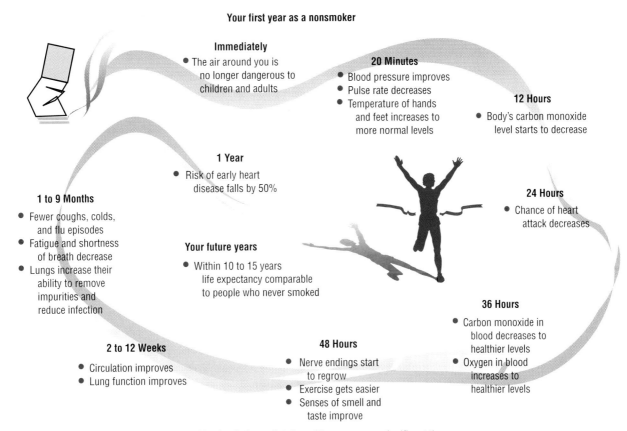

Your first year as a nonsmoker

Immediately
- The air around you is no longer dangerous to children and adults

20 Minutes
- Blood pressure improves
- Pulse rate decreases
- Temperature of hands and feet increases to more normal levels

12 Hours
- Body's carbon monoxide level starts to decrease

1 Year
- Risk of early heart disease falls by 50%

24 Hours
- Chance of heart attack decreases

1 to 9 Months
- Fewer coughs, colds, and flu episodes
- Fatigue and shortness of breath decrease
- Lungs increase their ability to remove impurities and reduce infection

Your future years
- Within 10 to 15 years life expectancy comparable to people who never smoked

36 Hours
- Carbon monoxide in blood decreases to healthier levels
- Oxygen in blood increases to healthier levels

2 to 12 Weeks
- Circulation improves
- Lung function improves

48 Hours
- Nerve endings start to regrow
- Exercise gets easier
- Senses of smell and taste improve

Figure 9-3 The health benefits of quitting smoking begin immediately and become more significant the longer you stay smoke-free.

transdermal patches. To date, only Nico Water has been formally addressed by the Food and Drug Administration, other than those that came into the marketplace as prescription-only or approved OTC products.

Stopping What You Started

Experts in health behavior contend that before people will discontinue harmful health behaviors, such as tobacco use, they must appreciate fully what they are expecting of themselves. This understanding grows in relationship to the following:

1. *Knowledge* about the health risks associated with tobacco use
2. *Recognition* that these health risks are applicable to all tobacco users
3. *Familiarity* with steps that can be taken to eliminate or reduce these risks
4. *Belief* that the benefits to be gained by no longer using tobacco will outweigh the pleasures gained through the use of tobacco
5. *Certainty* that one can start and maintain the behaviors required to stop or reduce the use of tobacco

On closer examination it is evident that these steps combine both knowledge and desire (or motivation). Being knowledgeable about risks, however, will not always stop behaviors that involve varying degrees of psychological and physical dependence. The 75% failure rate thought to be common among tobacco cessation programs suggests that the motivation is not easy to achieve or maintain. In fact, on the basis of information reported by the Hazelden Foundation, for persons who are successful in quitting, approximately 18.6 years elapse between the first attempt to stop and the actual time of quitting. The many health benefits of quitting smoking are shown in Figure 9-3.

A variety of smoking cessation programs exist, including those using highly organized formats, with or without the use of prescription or OTC nicotine replacement systems. In past years, most of the 1.3 million people who managed to quit smoking each year did so by throwing away their cigarettes (going cold turkey) and paying the physical and emotional price of waiting for their bodies to adjust to life without nicotine. Today, however, the use of nicotine replacement products in combination with external smoking cessation approaches, such as those described later in this chapter, or the use of prescription medication, such as antidepressants, is more common. The Changing for the Better box on page 319 provides a plan for smoking cessation that incorporates nicotine replacement products. For those who are concerned about weight gain following smoking cessation, the Changing for the Better box on page 320 offers some helpful weight management tips.

Programs to help people stop their tobacco use are available in a variety of formats, including educational programs, behavior modification, aversive conditioning, hypnosis, acupuncture, and various combinations of these approaches. See the Considering Complementary Care box on page 321. Programs are offered in both individual and group settings and are operated by hospitals, universities, health departments, voluntary health agencies, churches, and private practitioners. The better programs will have limited success rates—20% to 50% as measured over one year (with self-reporting), whereas the remainder will have even poorer results. If results are monitored using the assessment of nicotine breakdown products in the blood, the effectiveness rate of these programs falls even lower, as some "successful" self-reporters are not completely honest in their reporting of cessation.

Two methods for weaning smokers from cigarettes to a nontobacco source of nicotine are nicotine-containing chewing gum (Nicorette) and transdermal patches, in either prescription or OTC versions (Nicoderm, Nicotrol, Habitrol, Prostep), using either single-strength or step-

down formulas. A brief description of both gum and the transdermal patch is provided next, although subtle variations exist between prescription and OTC formulations and between brands.

Nicotine-Containing Chewing Gum Correct use of nicotine-containing chewing gum requires an immediate cessation of smoking, an initial determination of dosage (4 mg or 2 mg of nicotine per piece), knowledge of the appropriate manner of chewing each piece of gum, the appropriate time to chew each piece, the maximum number of pieces to be chewed each day, and time to begin withdrawal from the therapy. When used in combination with physician guidance or program support provided by the manufacturer, cessation using nicotine-containing gum may have a success rate of 40% or more, based on blood evaluation. Nicotine-containing chewing gum therapy ranges in cost from an initial $50 kit to weekly refills of approximately $30.

Transdermal Nicotine Patches The more recently developed transdermal (through the skin) nicotine patches appear to be less effective (25%) than the gum just described, but in many ways the patches are more easily used. If a step-down version (21 mg, 14 mg, 7 mg) is employed, determinations must be made as to the appropriate initial dosage (based on number of cigarettes smoked per day and body weight), the length of time at the initial dosage before stepping down, and the manner of withdrawal after a usual 8- to 12-week treatment period. The single-dose (15 mg) version, of course, eliminates the step-down component. Costs associated with transdermal nicotine replacement therapy are similar to those for the gum-based program.

In addition to the nicotine-replacement therapies already described, a nicotine inhaler and spray have been approved (in prescription form) by the FDA. Because of the large surface area of the lungs and rapid absorption into the blood, inhalation-based delivery of nicotine should become a very attractive alternative to transdermal and oral routes of replacement.

In all delivery forms and formulations, nicotine replacement therapy can be associated with contraindications and adverse reactions, including skin irritation, redness, and irregular heart rates.

A recently developed prescription medication, mecamylamine, used in combination with the transdermal nicotine patch improves the latter's effectiveness rate to somewhat above the 40% (perhaps approaching 50%) level reported for nicotine-containing chewing gum, according to a blood-based assessment. The drug affects receptors in the CNS, reducing the pleasurable effects of nicotine and thus decreasing dependency. An even more recently "discovered" prescription medication for smoking cessation is methoxsalen. Although intended for the treatment of psoriasis, a skin condition, this medication has been found to constructively alter the breakdown of nicotine in persons who have a particular genetic mutation that lessens their need for frequent cigarettes.[47] The most recently approved drug for use in smoking cessation is varenicline. On the basis of clinical trials, it is reported that nearly one-half of all persons receiving the drug were able to cease smoking.[48] Should this efficacy carry over into long-term trials, this medication would equal or most likely exceed the most effective approaches now available.

Several additional nicotine-free prescription medications to aid smoking cessation have now been approved or are nearing approval. These agents can be used alone or with nicotine replacement therapy. Zyban and Wellbutrin are antidepressant drugs that increase the production of dopamine, a neurotransmitter. Production of dopamine declines when a smoker quits, creating the craving to smoke. Prozac, the serotonin-reuptake inhibitor antidepressant approved for the treatment of depression, bulimia nervosa, PMS, and obsessive-compulsive disorder, has also shown promise as an adjunct to smoking cessation. See Figure 9-4 for a comparison of various cessation approaches.

Those who are concerned that nicotine-replacement therapies are simply a "trade-off" of addictions (from cigarettes to gum or patches) should remember that while using the therapy the former smoker is no longer being exposed to carbon monoxide and carcinogens, while the

step-down feature allows for a gradual return to a totally nicotine-free lifestyle. Therefore a short period of cross-addiction should be seen as simply a cost of recovery for those persons who will be successful.

In a recent meta-analysis of smoking cessation program success involving African Americans, it was found that there is no statistically significant difference between the success

How methods of smoking cessation stack up
Of the nation's estimated 48 million smokers, 70% want to quit, and 46% try each year. Only 1 in 40 succeeds. Federal guidelines, based on published studies, estimate varied success rates for a number of medications designed to help smokers quit.

Medications	Nicotine gum	Nicotine inhaler	Buproprion SR (Zyban)	Nicotine spray	Nicotine patch	Combination
Number of studies	13	4	2	3	27	3
Five-month quit rate	23.7%	22.8%	30.5%	30.5%	17.7%	28.6%
Advantage	Can be used to offset cravings	Mimics smoking	Non-nicotine, an antidepressant	Higher nicotine levels	Private, one/day	Combines benefits
Disadvantage	Poor taste	Low nicotine levels	Must screen for seizures	Irritation, sneezing	Skin irritation	Not FDA-approved
Over the counter (OTC) or prescription (Rx)	OTC	Rx	Rx	Rx	Both	Both

Figure 9-4

Source: Treating tobacco use and dependence. U.S. Public Health Service: John Hughes, University of Vermont.

of this racial group and others. Of interest, however, was a finding that church-based programs might be more successful for smoking cessation than previously recognized.[49]

Tobacco Use: A Question of Rights

For those readers who have found themselves involved (or nearly so) in confrontation situations involving smokers' versus nonsmokers' rights, we hope the section that follows will be helpful in allowing you to see more clearly the positions that you have taken. For those who have somehow remained removed from this discussion, consideration of these issues now may be good preparation for the future. Regardless, consider these two important questions:

1. To what extent should smokers be allowed to pollute the air and endanger the health of nonsmokers?
2. To what extent should nonsmokers be allowed to restrict the personal freedom of smokers, particularly since tobacco products are sold legally?

At this time, answers to these questions are only partially available, but one trend is developing: The tobacco user is being forced to give ground to the nonsmoker. Today, in fact, it is becoming more a matter of where the smoker will be allowed to smoke, rather than a matter of where smoking will be restricted. Smoking is currently becoming less and less tolerated. The health concerns of the majority are prevailing over the dependence needs of the minority.

TALKING POINTS You're having a discussion with a friend about life insurance and mention that you get a 10% reduction in your annual premium because you're a nonsmoker. Your friend, who is a smoker, becomes annoyed and says that this is just one example of how smokers are penalized. How would you respond?

OnSITE/InSIGHT

Learning to Go: Health

Is smoking a part of your everyday life? Click on Learning to Go: Health on the Online Learning Center at **www.mhhe.com/payne8e** to find more information about tobacco in these lessons:

Lesson 28: Adopt a no-smoking rule.

Lesson 29: Keep your lungs healthy.

Enhancing Communication Between Smokers and Nonsmokers

Exchanges between smokers and nonsmokers are sometimes strained and, in many cases, friendships are damaged beyond the point of repair. As you have probably observed, roommates are changed, dates are refused, and memberships in groups are withheld or rejected because of the opposing rights of these two groups.

Recognizing that social skills development is an important task for young adults, the following simple considerations or approaches for *smokers* can reduce some conflict presently associated with smoking:

- Before lighting up, ask whether smoking would bother others in close proximity to you.
- When in a neutral setting, seek physical space in which you will be able to smoke and in a reasonable way not interfere with nonsmokers' comfort.
- Accept the validity of the nonsmoker's statement that your smoke causes everything and everyone to smell of smoke.
- Respect stated prohibitions against smoking. If a nonsmoker requests that you refrain from smoking, respond with courtesy, regardless of whether you intend to comply.
- Practice "civil smoking" by applying a measure of restraint when you recognize that smoking is offensive to others. Particularly, respect the aesthetics that should accompany any act of smoking—placing ashes on dinner plates, leaving cigarette butts in flower pots, and emptying car ashtrays on shopping center parking lots are hardly popular with others.

The preceding suggestions can become skills for the social dimension of your health that can be applied to other social conflicts. Remember that as a smoker you are part of a statistical minority living in a society that often makes decisions and resolves conflict based on majority rule.

For *nonsmokers*, we suggest several approaches we believe will make you more sensitive and skilled in dealing with smoking behavior:

- Attempt to develop a sensitivity to the power of the dependence that smokers have on their cigarettes.
- Accept the reality of the smoker's sensory insensitivity—an insensitivity so profound that the odors you complain about are not even recognized by the smoker.
- When in a neutral setting, allow smokers their fair share of physical space in which to smoke. So long as the host does not object to smoking, you, as a guest, do not have the right to infringe on a person's right to smoke.
- When asking a person not to smoke, use a manner that reflects social consideration and skill. State your request clearly, and accept a refusal gracefully.
- Respond with honesty to inquiries from the smoker as to whether the smoke is bothering you.

If you are contemplating smoking, examine closely whether the social isolation that appears to be more and more common for smokers will be offset by the benefits you might receive from cigarettes. The ability to find satisfaction through social contact may be one of the most important avenues to a sense of well-being.

Final Thoughts about Tobacco and Health

Recalling the alternative definition of the role and composition of health presented in Chapter 1, we raise this question for readers who currently use tobacco in some form: "Are you healthy (resourceful) enough to continue your use of tobacco?" We ask you to think about the degree to which tobacco use functions as a resource in each of the multiple dimensions of your health. For example, to what degree does tobacco use enhance the structure and function of the physical body? To what degree does it increase the positive feelings that comprise the emotional dimension of health versus increase those more negative or uncomfortable feelings that all people feel to various degrees? How does smoking or smokeless tobacco use serve as a social lubricant, making its users more desirable people with whom to spend time? To what extent does tobacco use reflect the intellect's role in shaping important behavioral choices? How is tobacco use a contributing factor in workplace relationships and the effective use of time for which employees are financially compensated? Certainly, in our opinion, tobacco use decreases resourcefulness in each of health's six dimensions.

When the mastery of developmental tasks that compose each life cycle segment is assessed in terms of the contribution (or lack thereof) made by tobacco use, the picture seems no more positive. Simply stated, what are the positive contributions of tobacco use to a growing sense of responsibility for self and others, desired independence, intimacy with others, success in developing social skills, parenting, and making a statement about your adult identity? Again, we see little contribution to adult growth and development from the use of tobacco products. We believe the compromising of your resourcefulness caused by tobacco use and its detrimental effect on adult growth and development will quickly become evident.

Taking Charge of Your Health

- Commit yourself to establishing a smoke-free environment in the places where you live, work, study, and recreate.
- Support friends and acquaintances who are trying to become smoke-free.
- Support legislative efforts, at all levels of government, to reduce your exposure to environmental tobacco smoke.

- Be civil toward tobacco users in public spaces, but respond assertively if they infringe on smoke-free spaces.
- Support agencies and organizations committed to reducing tobacco use among young people through education and intervention.

Summary

- The percentage of American adults who smoke is continuing to decline.
- In spite of a reversal on the part of more recent college graduates, cigarette smoking has traditionally been inversely related to the level of formal education.
- A number of demographical variables influence the incidence of tobacco use.
- The tobacco industry continues to aggressively market its products to potential smokers.
- Multiple theories regarding nicotine's role in dependence have been advanced, including a better understanding of the proportional influences of genetics, environment, and personality.
- Nicotine exerts acute effects both within the central nervous system and on a variety of other tissues and organs.
- Tobacco smoke can be divided into gaseous and particulate phases. Each phase has its unique chemical composition.
- Thousands of chemical components and hundreds of carcinogenic agents are found in tobacco smoke.
- Nicotine and carbon monoxide have predictable effects on the function of the cardiovascular system.
- The development of nearly one-third of all cancers can be attributed to tobacco use, and virtually every

form of cancer is found more frequently in smokers than in nonsmokers.
- Chronic obstructive lung disease (COLD), also called chronic obstructive pulmonary disease (COPD), is a likely consequence of long-term cigarette smoking, with early symptoms appearing shortly after beginning regular smoking.
- Smoking alters normal structure and function of the body, as seen in a wide variety of noncardiovascular and noncancerous conditions, such as infertility, problem pregnancy, and neonatal health concerns. Additional health concerns include the diminished ability to smell, periodontal disease, vitamin inadequacies, and bone loss leading to osteoporosis.
- The use of smokeless tobacco carries its own health risks, including oral cancer.
- The presence of secondhand smoke results in involuntary (or passive) smoking by those who must share a common air source with smokers. This secondhand smoke threatens the health of the spouse, children, and coworkers of the smoker.
- Stopping smoking can be undertaken in any one of several ways, including within a group setting or on an individual basis. A variety of supportive medications are also available.

Review Questions

1. What percentage of the American adult population smoke? In what direction has change been occurring?
2. What is the current direction that adolescent smoking is taking?
3. What was the outcome of the class action suit brought by the forty-six states, and what was the effect of the Master Settlement Agreement (1999)

on the ability of the tobacco industry to market its products?
4. In comparison to cigarettes, what health risks are associated with pipe and cigar smoking?
5. What are the two principal dimensions of nicotine dependence? What are specific aspects seen within physical dependence? To which dimension does compulsion belong?

6. What percentage of smokers appear to be strongly addicted to nicotine?
7. Identify each of the theories of nicotine dependence discussed in the chapter.
8. How do modeling and manipulation explain the development of emotional dependence on tobacco?
9. In the amount consumed by the typical smoker, what is the effect of nicotine on central nervous system function? How does this differ in chain smokers?
10. What effects does nicotine have on the body outside of the central nervous system? How does the influence of nicotine resemble that associated with the stress response?
11. What is the principal effect of carbon monoxide on cardiac function?

12. What influences does passive smoking have on nonsmoking adult partners of smokers? On their children?
13. How is the federal government attempting to limit the exposure that children and adolescents currently have to tobacco products and tobacco advertisements?
14. How might concerned parents begin to "tobacco proof" their children to keep them from becoming smokers in the future?
15. What prescription and OTC products are now available to assist smokers in quitting?
16. What percentage of smokers are able to quit, and how many attempts to quit are generally required?
17. What are the rights of smokers and of nonsmokers? How can they be respected by both groups?

References

1. *Nextel to take wheel at NASCAR.* CNNMoney. June 18, 2003 (online service).
2. Wakefield MA, et al. Tobacco industry marketing of point of purchase after the 1999 MSA billboard ban. *AJPH* 9, No. 6. June 2002.
3. Prevalence of current cigarette smoking among adults and changes in prevalence of current and some day smoking—2001. *MMWR* 52(14). April 2003.
4. Smoking and Health: Report of the Advisory Committee to the Surgeon General of the Public Health Service. U.S. Department of Health and Human Services. Public Health Service. 1964.
5. U.S. National Center for Health Statistics. *Health, United States, 2002: Early release of selected estimates based on data from the 2002 National Health Interview Survey,* 2002.
6. *Cigarette smoking among adults—United States 1998.* Tobacco Information and Prevention Sources (TIPS).
7. National Center for Health Statistics. *Health, United States, 1998, with socioeconomic status and health chartbook.* NCHS, 1998.
8. *2000 Statistics on Alcohol and Other Drug Uses on College Campuses.* The Core Institute. Southern Illinois University. 2000 **http://www.siu/edu/ departments/coreinst/public_html/2000.html**
9. Johnston LD, O'Malley PM, Bachman JG. *Cigarettes: trends in thirty-day prevalence of use by subgroups for eighth and tenth graders.* Monitoring the Future Study-2002. The University of Michigan, 2003.
10. Rigotti NA, Lee JE, Weschler H. U.S. college use of tobacco products: results of a national survey. *JAMA* 284(6):699–705, 2000.

11. Schoenborn CA, Jackline VL, Barnes PM. *Cigarette smoking behavior of adults: United States, 1998.* Advanced Data from Vital and Health Statistics, No. 331. Division of Interview Statistics, National Center for Vital Statistics, February 2003.
12. *National household survey on drug abuse main findings 1998* (H-11) Substance Abuse and Mental Health Services. Department of Health and Human Services. March 2000.
13. Massachusetts Department of Health, as reported in *USA Today,* 8 May 2000.
14. Surveillance for selected tobacco-use behaviors— U.S. 1990–1994. *MMWR* 43(SS-3):1–43, 1995.
15. State-specific prevalence of current cigarette smoking and cigar smoking among adults—United States, 1998. *MMWR* 48(45):1034–1039, 1999.
16. U.S. Substance Abuse and Mental Health Services. *Summary of findings from the 2000 National Household Survey on Drug Abuse,* 2001.
17. Tickle JJ, et al. Favourite movie stars, their tobacco use in contemporary movies, and its association with adolescent smoking. *Tob Control* 10(1):16–22, March 2001.
18. Shapiro JA, Jacobs EJ, Thun MJ. Cigar smoking in men and the risk of death from tobacco-related cancers. *J Natl Cancer Inst* 92(4):333–337, 2000.
19. Burns DM, ed. *Cigars: health effects and trends.* Cancer Monograph Series (No. 9) National Cancer Institute, 1998.
20. Iribarren C, et al. Evidence of cigar smoking on the risk of cardiovascular disease, chronic obstructive pulmonary disease, and cancer in men. *N Engl J Med* 340(23):1173–1180, 1999.

21. Zickler P. Evidence builds that genes influence cigarette smoking. *NIDA Notes* 15(3):1–15, 2000.

22. Sayette MA, et al. A multi-dimensional analysis of cue-elicited craving in heavy smokers and tobacco chippers. *Addiction* 96(10):1419–1432, 2001.

23. Sullivan PK, Kendler KS. The genetic epidemiology of smoking. *Nicotine Tob Res, Suppl.* 2:S51–7, 1999.

24. Longnecker GL. *How drugs work: drug abuse and the human body.* Ziff-Davis Press. 1994.

25. Olive MF, et al. Stimulation of endorphin neurotransmission in the nucleus accumbens by ethanol, cocaine, and amphetamine. *J of Neurosci* 21(23):RC 184, December 2001.

26. Balfour DJ, Ridley DL, The effects of nicotine on neural pathways implicated in depression. *Pharmacol Biochem Behav* 66(1):79–85, 2000.

27. DiFranza JR, et al. Development of symptoms of tobacco dependence in youth: 30-month follow-up from the DANDY study. *Tob Control* 11(3):228–235, 2002.

28. *17. Tobacco.* School of Veterinary Medicine. Purdue University. **http://www.vet.purdue/edu/depts/addl/toxic/plant17.htm**

29. Simons-Morton BG. Prospective analysis of peer and parental influences on smoking initiation among early adolescents. *Prev Sci* 3(4):275–283, December 2002.

30. Bricker JB, et al. Nine-year prospective relationship between parental smoking cessation and children's daily smoking. *Addiction* 98(5):585–593, May 2003.

31. Pechmann C, Reibling RT. Anti-smoking advertising campaigns targeting youth: case studies from USA and Canada. *Tob Control* 9 Suppl: 118–131, 2000.

32. Mulcahy S. *The toxicology of cigarette smoke and environmental tobacco smoke.* A Review of Cigarette Smoke and Its Toxicological Effects. **http://www.csn.ul.ie/-stephen/reports/bc4927.html**

33. Saladin KS. *Anatomy and physiology: the unit of form and function,* 3rd ed. McGraw-Hill, 2004.

34. Hecht MI. Smoking cessation: pre-operative. *University of Wisconsin anesthesia topics.* November 1998.

35. *Cancer facts and figures—2003.* Atlanta: Cancer Society, 2003.

36. Kapier KN, et al. *Cigarettes: What the warning label doesn't tell you.* American Council on Science and Health, 1997.

37. American Heart Association. *Heart disease and stroke statistics—2003 update.* 2002.

38. Lilienberg G, Venge P. Platelet adhesion in patients prone to arterial and venous thrombosis: the impact of gender, smoking and heredity. *Scand J Clin Lab Invest* 58(4):279–284. 1998.

39. Campling B, El-Deiry W. Clinical implications of p53 mutation in lung cancer. *Mol Biotechnol* 24(2):141–156, June 2003.

40. Lam S, et al. Sex-related differences in bronchial epithelial changes associated with tobacco smoking. *J Natl Cancer Inst* 91(8):691–696, April 1999.

41. Habek D, et al. Fetal tobacco syndrome and perinatal outcome. *Fetal Diagn Ther* 17(6):367–371, November–December 2002.

42. Fleming PJ, et al. Sudden infant death syndrome and social deprivation: assessing epidemiological factors after post-matching for deprivation. *Paediatr Perinat Epidemiol* 17(3):272–280. July 2003.

43. Misra DP, Nguyen RH. Environmental tobacco smoke and low birth weight: a hazard in the workplace? *Enviro Health Perspect* 107 (suppl) (6):897–904. 1999.

44. Keknabson IA, et al. Maternal smoking during pregnancy and behavioral characteristics in 2–4-month infants. *Klin Padiatr* 214(6):359–364. 2002.

45. Enstrom JE, Kabat GC. Environmental tobacco smoke and tobacco related mortality in a prospective study of Californians, 1990–1998. *BMJ* 326(7398):1048–1049, May 2003.

46. Information taken from advertisements appearing in multiple issues of *USA Today* and major news magazines, including *Time* and *Newsweek.*

47. Sellers EM, Kaplan HL, Tyndale RF. Inhibition of cytochrome P450 2A6 increases nicotine's oral bioavailability and decreases smoking. *Clin Pharmacol Ther* 68(1):35–43. 2000.

48. Pfizer unveils anti-smoking drug. *CNN Money.* June 17, 2003. **http://www.money.cnn.com/2003/06/17/news/companies/Pfizer/index.htm**

49. Pederson LL, et al. Smoking cessation among African Americans: what we know and do not know about interventions and self-quitting. *Prev Med* 31(1): 23–38. 2000.

On Page 321 your textbook discusses the growing displeasure with smoking that results in the inclusion of environmental tobacco smoke into the lives of nonsmokers. Two recent events lend further credence to the continuing efforts to ban all public smoking.

The first report stems from an initial follow-up study of a small group of New York city bar and restaurant workers three months following the introduction (July 2004) of laws prohibiting smoking in virtually all of the city's public buildings, including their places of employment. Using as a baseline the blood levels of a nicotine break-down product, cotinine, taken just before the ban went into effect, the researchers found that by the end of three months an 85% decrease in cotinine levels had occurred. On the basis of this significant drop in cotinine in such a relative short period of time, a clearer picture of the negative influences associated with environmental tobacco smoke exposure can be more fully appreciated.

A second aspect of the ongoing movement to protect nonsmokers from the harmful effects of environmental tobacco smoke, is the recent recommendation of the state of Maine's Health and Human Services Committee to ban smoking in the homes and cars of foster parents when foster children are present. If approved by the state's House and Senate and signed into law by the governor, this ban will most likely serve as a model for other states who hold concerns about the wellbeing of foster children—whose care is paid for through state funds.

smokers vs. nonsmokers: a question of rights

A quiet battle is being waged in the United States over smoking, an activity that was once universally accepted. Within the last decade, regulations restricting smoking have affected stores, restaurants, offices, and public buildings. It is difficult these days to find a place of business in the United States where smoking is totally unrestricted. Some of these restrictions are put in place by law or municipal ordinances; some are placed voluntarily by business management. However, it is clear that the voices of nonsmokers, long silent and largely ignored by society, are finally being heard and are behind the recent increase in restrictions on smoking.

Changing Attitudes

For decades, people smoked whenever and wherever they wished. Smoking was glamorized in the movies, on television, and in print throughout most of the twentieth century. Famous athletes and movie stars were found in cigarette advertisements. Some ads even promoted the "health benefits" of smoking. Although a few people felt that smoking was dangerous, their voices had little effect on society's acceptance of tobacco use. Gradually, these attitudes began to change. As data from medical studies began to accumulate on the dangers of tobacco, antismoking advocates started to achieve some victories in society and in public policy.

Restrictions on Tobacco Use

In the 1980s, restrictions on smoking greatly increased. In 1987, smoking was banned on all domestic airplane flights of less than 2 hours;[1] in 1990, this ban was increased to include all domestic flights of less than 6 hours. Now most international flights ban smoking as well. A growing number of state and local laws curtailing or banning smoking in places of business have been enacted. Many businesses that were not forced by law to restrict smoking did so anyway. Smoking is prohibited on over 80% of Amtrak trains, and 1400 company-owned McDonald's restaurants are now smoke-free.[2] In fact, entire states have banned smoking in certain public buildings and facilities. Most recently a sixth state, Maryland, may join five other states. Delaware, New York, Maine, Connecticut, and California in prohibiting smoking inside restaurants and bars. If the "Clean Indoor Air Act of 2004" introduced into the Maryland legislature is passed and signed by the governor, Maryland would extend the ban to include sports arenas, gyms, the majority of hotel rooms, and bowling alleys.[3] Outside the United States, Ireland has banned smoking in pubs (public places) throughout the entire country.

As a result of these restrictions, smoking areas in places of business are shrinking in size or are being eliminated. Congregations of smokers outside office buildings have become a common sight. Some smokers have taken the changes in stride. Others have cut back on smoking or have quit altogether. Many, however, are not happy about having to go outside in all kinds of weather to smoke. They feel ostracized and are speaking out against what they perceive as an outright attack on their personal freedoms.

The Prosmoker Defence

Smokers have started to become organized on a worldwide level and within individual communities and workplaces. They are clearly worried that this trend of restricting tobacco use will not stop until smoking is eliminated everywhere or at least the regulation over the manufacturing and sales of tobacco products is brought under the control of the Food and Drug Administration where restrictions on availability might be significantly greater than currently exists.

Groups such as the British-based Freedom Organisation for the Right to Enjoy Smoking Tobacco (FOREST) have actively pushed smokers' rights and have exposed the "benefits" of smoking.[4] They cite controversial scientific studies demonstrating that smokers are less likely to develop Alzheimer's disease and Parkinson's disease. Of course, having now read the chapter, you know that the life expectancy of smokers is reduced to the point that late adulthood-onset diseases such as Alzheimer's and Parkinson disease may not have time to be clearly expressed.

Smokers are also worried about how their smoking activities are perceived by employers and insurers. Companies are growing less tolerant of unhealthy activities by their employees, since they must pay increased insurance costs for treatment. Many fear that insurance companies will begin to refuse treatment to smokers who continue to smoke.

The worst-case scenario for smokers is that their smoking will even be restricted at home. "What if the government starts keeping us from having kids because we smoke?" worries a two-pack-a-day smoker. "I've heard tell that we could have our kids taken away because we smoke at home. Do we have to step outside of our own homes to smoke?"

Fighting for Clean Air

Many nonsmokers are just as adamant about their position, saying that smokers have been subjecting them to cancer-causing agents for decades and that the restrictions are long overdue. They are tired of having smoke blown in their faces in public. Antismoking activists find the "individual freedom" argument of smokers objectionable. "What about my right to breathe?" asks an office worker who is subjected to smoke from nearby cubicles. "The management, most of whom smoke, have decided that since we don't deal directly with the public, smoking is okay," he complains.

Many nonsmoking activists feel that it is in the public's best interest to restrict exposure to tobacco smoke and cut back on overall tobacco use. They are angered not only because they have to be exposed to smoke, but also because a good portion of their insurance premiums is going toward health care costs from smoking. Additionally, as the data accumulate on the hazards of smoking, many non-smokers are becoming concerned about their exposure to secondhand smoke. They are also worried about the addictive properties of nicotine and are concerned that their children may get hooked.

Although they have had much success in getting restrictions adopted, antismoking activists have also faced defeat in the legislatures. Municipalities in North Carolina can no longer pass local laws restricting smoking, thanks to a preemptive state law passed on July 15, 1993. As a result, the majority of workers in North Carolina have no legal protection at all from exposure to tobacco smoke.[5]

Even without the health problems posed by tobacco smoke, many nonsmokers feel that smoking should be curtailed simply because of its unpleasant smell. Since smoking is not a self-contained activity, smoke diffuses far away from the smoker, often offending people many feet away. "What good does it do to seat a nonsmoker next to the smoking section in a restaurant?" notes an avid antismoking activist. "The smoke just drifts over anyway. It stinks, and not just during the meal. It gets into your clothes and hair and stays with you all day. Why must we tolerate smoke?"

What the Future May Hold

Such arguments may open the door to more restrictions on smoking, a possibility that makes smokers' rights advocates angry. Many are convinced that antismoking forces want nothing less than a total ban on tobacco use—or at least want these bans to be used more aggressively. This might occur, according to smokers' rights advocates, by allowing the courts to use smoking as a factor in determining child custody cases or in defining parental smoking as a form of child endangerment.

Antismoking advocates do not see these regulations as restrictions on individual freedom. They view them as a means of liberation from decades of exposure to smoke with little or no form of legal recourse. Many nonsmokers feel that they should not be forced to breathe in smoke simply because someone wants to light up. Advocates for these regulations claim that tobacco-related illnesses increase health care costs for everyone. They also complain that their tax dollars are being used to subsidize the tobacco industry—in effect, they are paying to be exposed to the smoke of others.

Since smoking, by its very nature, is not a self-contained activity, conflicts are bound to happen. Perhaps some acceptable middle ground can be reached between smokers and nonsmokers, both in law and in society.

For Discussion . . .

Have you ever asked someone not to smoke near you or been asked not to smoke around someone? Should taxpayers be responsible for taking on the burden of those being treated for smoking-related diseases? Are the individual freedoms of smokers being infringed on by smoking regulations? Are the individual freedoms of nonsmokers being violated by smokers? Is smoking at home around your children a form of child endangerment?

References

1. The tyranny of the majority, *The Economist* 313:7626, 1989.
2. Farley CJ. Toufexis A: The butt stops here, *Time* 143(16), Apr 18, 1994.
3. Johnson D. Smoking ban urged for all of Maryland. December 19, 2003. **www.washingtonpost.com**
4. Platt S: Ashes to ashes, *New Statesman and Society* 7(289), Feb 11, 1994.
5. Conlisk E. et al. The status of local smoking preemption bill, *JAMA* 273(10), 1995.

personal assessment

how much do you know about cigarette smoking?

Are the following assumptions about smoking true or false? Take your best guess, and then read the answer to the right of each statement.

Assumption

1. There are now safe cigarettes on the market.

2. A small number of cigarettes can be smoked without risk.

3. Most early changes in the body resulting from cigarette smoking are temporary.
4. Filters provide a measure of safety to cigarette smokers.
5. Low-tar, low-nicotine cigarettes are safer than high-tar, high-nicotine brands.
6. Mentholated cigarettes are better for the smoker than are non-mentholated brands.

7. It has been scientifically proven that cigarette smoking causes cancer.
8. No specific agent capable of causing cancer has ever been identified in the tobacco used in smokeless tobacco.

9. The cure rate for lung cancer is so good that no one should fear developing this form of cancer.
10. Smoking is not harmful as long as the smoke is not inhaled.

11. The "smoker's cough" reflects underlying damage to the tissue of the airways.

12. Cigarette smoking does not appear to be associated with damage to the heart and blood vessels.
13. Because of the design of the placenta, smoking does not present a major risk to the developing fetus.

14. Women who smoke cigarettes and use an oral contraceptive should decide which they wish to continue because there is a risk in using both.
15. Air pollution is a greater risk to our respiratory health than is cigarette smoking.

16. Addiction, in the sense of physical addiction, is found in conjunction with cigarette smoking.

Discussion

F   Depending on the brand, some cigarettes contain less tar and nicotine; none are safe, however.
F   Even a low level of smoking exposes the body to harmful substances in tobacco smoke.
T   Some changes, however, cannot be reversed—particularly changes associated with emphysema.
T   However, the protection is far from adequate.
T   Many people, however, smoke low-tar, low-nicotine cigarettes in a manner that makes them just as dangerous as stronger cigarettes.
F   Menthol simply makes cigarette smoke feel cooler. The smoke contains all of the harmful agents found in the smoke from regular cigarettes.
T   Particularly lung cancer and cancers of the larynx, esophagus, oral cavity, and urinary bladder.
F   Unfortunately, smokeless tobacco is no safer than the tobacco that is burned. The user of smokeless tobacco swallows much of what the smoker inhales.
F   Approximately 14% of people who have lung cancer will live the 5 years required to meet the medical definition of "cured."
F   Because of the toxic material in smoke, even its contact with the tissue of the oral cavity introduces a measure of risk in this form of cigarette use.
T   The cough occurs in response to an inability to clear the airway of mucus as a result of changes in the cells that normally keep the air passages clear.
F   Cigarette smoking is in fact the single most important risk factor in the development of cardiovascular disease.
F   Children born to women who smoked during pregnancy show a variety of health impairments, including smaller birth size, premature birth, and more illnesses during the first year of life. Smoking women also have more stillbirths than do nonsmokers.
T   Women over 35 years of age, in particular, are at risk of experiencing serious heart disease should they continue using both cigarettes and an oral contraceptive.
F   Although air pollution does expose the body to potentially serious problems, the risk is considerably less than that associated with smoking.
T   Dependence, including true physical addiction, is widely recognized in cigarette smokers.

preventing diseases

Part Four consists of four chapters that focus on disease prevention. Each illness you contract or develop can harm your health in each of its dimensions; therefore, prevention should be a high priority.

1. Physical Dimension

We usually associate illness with pain, fear, discomfort, and limitations. But paradoxically, health problems can also improve the physical dimension of health. For example, exposure to certain infectious diseases may allow your body to develop immunity. Illness can also force you to rest, reduce your workload, and reconsider your health behavior. Weight loss, smoking cessation, improved dietary practices, genetic counseling, or a renewed commitment to fitness may follow your recovery from an illness.

2. Emotional Dimension

Emotionally healthy people feel good about themselves and others and are able to cope with most of life's demands. Being diagnosed with an illness or disease can jeopardize your emotional resources. You may feel anxious, isolated, and vulnerable. Fortunately, many diseases can be prevented or at least managed or treated successfully.

3. Social Dimension

People rarely face an illness or manage a chronic health condition alone. People who have heart disease, cancer, diabetes, or HIV infection often join support groups or establish friendships with others who have the same condition. In addition, you probably interact with people during activities aimed at preventing diseases. For example, you might exercise with a partner or meet people at a weight loss group.

4. Intellectual Dimension

We can best use our intellect when we are free from health problems. In some cases, diseases or medications can impair our intellectual functioning. However, managing a condition or recovering from an illness can allow you to learn about your body, your personality, and the health care system. Learning how to reduce your risk of certain diseases will also require you to draw on your intellectual resources.

5. Spiritual Dimension

Your ability to serve others can be hindered by an illness or chronic condition. In addition, your faith can be shaken when a family member falls ill or when you are diagnosed with a serious disease. For most people, however, this initial questioning leads to an even stronger faith or spirituality than they had before the experience.

6. Occupational Dimension

Diseases and your efforts to prevent them can have a significant effect on your job performance. If you have an acute illness, you probably will not be able to work temporarily. If you have a chronic condition or disease, you must try to manage it well enough that you are still able to work. Some conditions are so severe that employment becomes impossible. On the other hand, your efforts to prevent illness, such as fitness activities, will enhance your job performance.

chapter ten

enhanCing your cardiovascular health

Chapter Objectives

Upon completing this chapter, you will be able to:

▌ describe the prevalence of cardiovascular disease compared to other diseases.

▌ list the cardiovascular disease risk factors and distinguish between those that can vs. cannot be modified.

▌ explain how each of the modifiable cardiovascular disease risk factors can be changed.

▌ explain atherosclerosis and the factors that are involved in causing it.

▌ list and describe the different forms of cardiovascular disease.

▌ explain the different forms of treatment for coronary heart disease.

▌ distinguish between the different types of stroke.

▌ explain the recommendations for prevention and treatment of hypertension.

Online Learning Center Resources

www.mhhe.com/payne8e

Log on to our Online Learning Center (OLC) for access to these additional resources:

- Chapter key terms and definitions
- Learning objectives
- Student interactive question-and-answer sites
- Self-scoring chapter quiz
- Online assessments
- Key term flash cards

Talking It Over

Encouraging Children to Be Active

You understand the value of being physically active. The challenge is to communicate this message to your kids—kids who are avalanched by video games, fast foods, rented movies, big screen TV, and hundreds of television channels!

- *Be a positive role model.* By your actions, show children that physical activity is fun.
- *Play with your kids.* Ask if they want to shoot baskets or teach you dance steps.
- *Don't preach.* Lectures just aren't as interesting as TV.

- *Support efforts at physical activity.* Praise kids when they're active. Help them get involved in activities they enjoy and help them be successful at them.
- *Limit passive activities.* Set time limits on TV watching and video-game playing.

CommunicationLinks

www.a1.com/ncppa
www.kidshealth.org
www.fantasyfit.com

Eye on the Media

How Credible Are Online Health Sites?

If you're looking for accurate health information on the Internet, make the site's credibility your first priority. Since just about anyone can post information on the Web (within legal limits), what you find there ranges from opinion to balanced, carefully researched information. Your challenge is to distinguish between reliable and dubious information.

According to health professionals Kotecki and Chamness,* certain key information can help you determine a health information website's credibility.

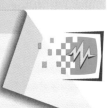

This section of the book contains four chapters that deal with diseases. Although uninformed people claim that "there is nothing you can do to avoid disease," ample evidence indicates that positive personal health choices can help reduce your risk of developing many diseases, from cardiovascular disease to cancer to sexually transmitted diseases, including HIV and AIDS.

In this chapter we will explain what you can do to reduce your risk of developing cardiovascular disease. Prevention efforts are most effective when started in childhood, but it is never too late to adopt a wellness lifestyle. Quitting smoking, becoming physically active, following a nutritious, low-fat diet, and controlling your blood pressure are important ways of reducing your risk of heart disease and improving your overall health.

Great progress has been made with respect to **cardiovascular** disease (CVD), the focus of this chapter. Although heart disease continues to be the number one killer of Americans, between 1990 and 2000 the death rates from CVD declined 17 percent.[1] Still, CVD claimed 1.4 million lives in 2001.[1] (American Heart Association, *Heart Disease and Stroke Statistics.* 2004 update.) By comparison, cancer caused about 554,000 deaths, accidents caused about 102,000, and HIV/AIDS caused about 14,000. This means CVD caused 38.5 percent of all deaths, or one out of every 2.6 deaths in 2001. Today, more than 2,600 Americans die each day of CVD, an average of one death every 34 seconds. Cardiovascular diseases claim more lives each year than the next five leading causes of death combined.

This chapter provides material to help you understand how the heart works. Beyond this, it will help you identify your CVD risk factors and suggest ways you can alter certain lifestyle behaviors to reduce your risk of developing heart disease.

Prevalence of Cardiovascular Disease

Cardiovascular diseases were directly related to 38.5 percent of deaths in the United States in 2001 and indirectly related to a large percentage of additional deaths.[1] Fortunately, the rate of deaths from coronary heart disease has been falling. If all major forms of CVD were eliminated, life expectancy in the United States would increase by almost 7 years (see Figure 10-1 and Table 10.1).[1]

OnSITE/InSIGHT

Learning to Go: Health

Want to keep your heart in good condition? Click on Learning to Go: Health on the Online Learning Center at **www.mhhe.com/payne8e** to find this lesson, which will guide you in how to do just that:

Lesson 33: Plan for a healthy heart.

Key Terms

cardiovascular pertaining to the heart (cardio) and blood vessels (vascular).

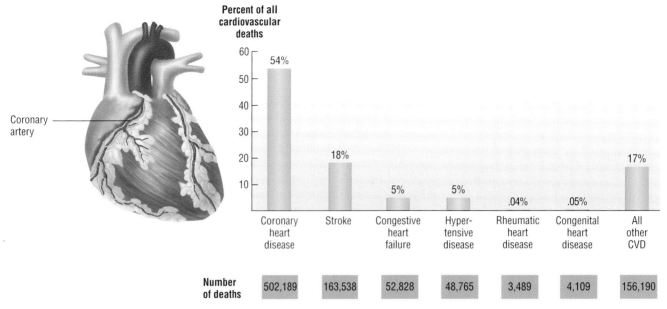

Percent of all cardiovascular deaths

	Coronary heart disease	Stroke	Congestive heart failure	Hyper-tensive disease	Rheumatic heart disease	Congenital heart disease	All other CVD
Percent	54%	18%	5%	5%	.04%	.05%	17%
Number of deaths	502,189	163,538	52,828	48,765	3,489	4,109	156,190

Coronary artery

Figure 10-1 Of the 931,108 deaths in the United States in 2001* resulting from cardiovascular diseases, nearly half were attributable to heart attack.[1] (*The most recent year for which statistics are available.*)

Normal Cardiovascular Function

The cardiovascular system, also called the circulatory system, uses a muscular pump to send a complex fluid on a continuous trip through a closed system of tubes. The pump is the heart, the fluid is blood, and the closed system of tubes is the network of blood vessels.

The Vascular System

The term *vascular system* refers to the body's blood vessels. Although we might be familiar with the arteries (vessels that carry blood away from the heart) and the veins (vessels that carry blood to the heart), arterioles, capillar- ies, and venules are also part of the vascular system. Arterioles are the smaller-diameter extensions of arteries. These arterioles lead eventually to capillaries, the smallest extensions of the vascular system. At the capillary level, oxygen, food, and waste are exchanged between cells and the blood.

After the blood leaves the capillaries and begins its return to the heart, it drains into small veins, or venules. The blood in the venules flows into increasingly larger vessels called *veins*. Blood pressure is highest in arteries and lowest in veins, especially the largest veins, which empty into the right atrium of the heart.

The Heart

The heart is a four-chambered pump designed to create the pressure required to circulate blood throughout the body. Usually considered to be about the size of a person's clenched fist, this organ lies slightly tilted between the lungs in the central portion of the **thorax.** The heart does not lie completely in the center of the chest. Rather, approximately two-thirds of the heart is to the left of the body midline and one third is to the right.[2]

Table 10.1 Estimated Prevalence of Major Cardiovascular Diseases*[1]

Hypertension	58,000,000
Coronary heart disease	12,900,000
Stroke	4,700,000
Rheumatic heart disease	1,800,000
Congenital heart disease	1,000,000
Congestive heart failure	4,900,000
TOTAL	83,300,000

*61,800,000 people total. The sum of the individual estimates exceeds 61,800,000 because so many people have more than one cardiovascular disorder.

Key Terms

thorax the chest; portion of the torso above the diaphragm and within the rib cage.

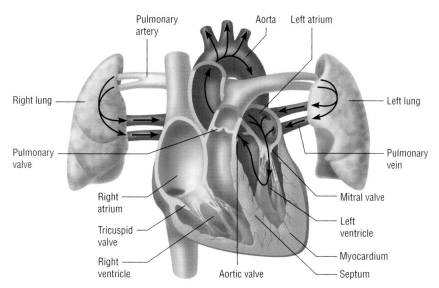

Pulmonary artery
Aorta
Left atrium
Right lung
Left lung
Pulmonary valve
Pulmonary vein
Right atrium
Mitral valve
Tricuspid valve
Left ventricle
Right ventricle
Myocardium
Aortic valve
Septum

Figure 10-2 The heart functions like a complex double pump. The right side of the heart pumps deoxygenated blood to the lungs. The left side of the heart pumps oxygenated blood through the aorta to all parts of the body. Note the thickness of the walls of the ventricles. These are the primary pumping chambers.

Two upper chambers, called *atria,* and two lower chambers, called *ventricles,* form the heart. The thin-walled atrial chambers are considered collecting chambers, whereas the thick-walled muscular ventricles are considered the pumping chambers. The right and left sides of the heart are divided by a partition called the *septum.* Study Figure 10-2 and follow the flow of blood through the heart's four chambers.

To function well, the heart muscle must receive adequate amounts of oxygen. The two main **coronary arteries** (and their many branches) accomplish this. These arteries are located outside of the heart. If the coronary arteries are diseased, a heart attack (myocardial infarction) is possible.

Heart Stimulation

The heart contracts and relaxes through the delicate interplay of **cardiac muscle** tissue and cardiac electrical centers, called *nodes.* Nodal tissue generates the electrical impulses necessary to contract heart muscle.[3] The heart's electrical activity is measured by an instrument called an *electrocardiograph (ECG or EKG),* which provides a printout called an *electrocardiogram* that can be evaluated to determine cardiac electrical functioning.

Blood

The average-sized adult has approximately five quarts of blood in his or her circulatory system. Blood's functions, which are performed continuously, are quite similar to the overall functions of the circulatory system and include the following:

- Transportation of nutrients, oxygen, wastes, hormones, and enzymes
- Regulation of water content of body cells and fluids

- Buffering to help maintain appropriate pH balance of body fluids
- Regulation of body temperature; the water component in the blood absorbs heat and transfers it
- Prevention of blood loss; by coagulating or clotting, the blood can alter its form to prevent blood loss through injured vessels
- Protection against toxins and microorganisms, accomplished by chemical substances called *antibodies* and specialized cellular elements circulating in the bloodstream.

Cardiovascular Disease Risk Factors

As you have just read, the heart and blood vessels are among the most important structures in the human body. By protecting your cardiovascular system, you lay the groundwork for a more exciting, productive, and energetic life. The best time to start protecting and improving your cardiovascular system is early in life, when lifestyle patterns are developed and reinforced (see the Learning from Our Diversity box on page 336). Of course, it is difficult to move backward through time, so the second-best

---

Key Terms

coronary arteries vessels that supply oxygenated blood to heart muscle tissues.

cardiac muscle specialized muscle tissue that forms the middle (muscular) layer of the heart wall.

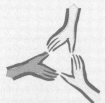

Learning from Our Diversity

Prevention of Heart Disease Begins in Childhood

Youth is one aspect of diversity that is sometimes overlooked. Yet age is important, especially when adults have influence over children's health behavior. Many adults never seriously consider that their health behaviors are imitated by the children around them. When adults care little about their own health, they can also be contributing to serious health consequences in young people. Nowhere is this age diversity issue more pronounced than in the area of cardiovascular health.

For many aspects of wellness, preventive behaviors are often best learned in childhood, when they can be repeated and reinforced by family members and caregivers. This is especially true for preventive actions concerning heart disease. Although many problems related to heart disease appear at midlife and later, the roots of heart disease start early in life.

The most serious childhood health behaviors associated with heart disease are poor dietary practices, lack of physical activity, and cigarette smoking. Unfortunately, the current state of health for America's youth shows severe deficiencies in all three areas. Children's diets lack

nutrient density and remain far too high in overall fat. Teenage children are becoming increasingly overweight and obese. Studies consistently show a decline in the amount of physical activity by today's youth, since television and video games have become the after-school companions for many children. In addition, cigarette smoking continues to rise among schoolchildren, especially teenagers.

These unhealthy behaviors are laying the foundation for coronary artery disease, hypertension, stroke, and other diseases in the future. The focus should be on health measures in childhood that prevent cardiovascular problems rather than treatment of older, already affected people. Parents must make efforts to encourage children to eat more nutritiously and be physically active. Adults should discourage cigarette use by young people. Perhaps the best approach for adults is to set a good example by adopting heart-healthy behaviors themselves. Following the Food Guide Pyramid (page 143) and exercising regularly are excellent strategies that can be started early in life.

---

time to start protecting your heart is today. Improvements in certain lifestyle activities can pay significant dividends as your life unfolds. Complete the Personal Assessment on pages 359–360 to estimate your risk for heart disease.

The American Heart Association encourages people to protect and enhance their heart health by examining the ten cardiovascular risk factors that are related to various forms of heart disease. A *cardiovascular risk factor* is an attribute that a person has or is exposed to that increases the likelihood that he or she will develop some form of heart disease. Three risk factors are those you will be unable to change. An additional six risk factors are those you can clearly change. One final risk factor is thought to be a contributing factor to heart disease. These risk factors are summarized in the adjacent Star box. Let's look at these three groups of risk factors separately.

Risk Factors That Cannot Be Changed

The three risk factors that you cannot change are increasing age, male gender, and heredity. Despite the fact that these risk factors cannot be changed, your knowledge that they might be an influence in your life should encourage you to make a more serious commitment to the risk factors you *can* change.

Increasing Age

Heart disease tends to develop gradually over the course of one's life. Although we may know of a person or two who experienced a heart attack in their twenties or thir-

ties, most of the serious consequences of heart disease become evident as we age. For example, nearly 84% of people who die from heart disease are aged 65 and older.

Male Gender

Men have a greater risk of heart disease than do women prior to age 55. Yet when women move through menopause

Risk Factors for Cardiovascular Disease

Factors You Cannot Change

- Increasing age
- Male gender
- Heredity

Factors You Can Change ("Big Six" Risk Factors)

- Tobacco smoke
- Physical inactivity
- High blood cholesterol level
- High blood pressure
- Diabetes mellitus
- Obesity and overweight

Contributing Factor

- Individual response to stress

Women and Heart Disease

Is heart disease mainly a problem for men? According to the American Heart Association, the answer is no. In fact, data indicate that 53% of all cardiovascular disease deaths occur in women. Sixty-three percent of women who died suddenly of coronary heart disease had no previous symptoms. Also, 38% of women who have a heart attack will die within 1 year, compared with 25% of men. A total of 60% of the deaths from stroke and high blood pressure are in women, compared with 40% in men. Coronary heart disease is the leading cause of death of American women (254,630 deaths in 2000).[1]

For many years, it was thought that men were at much greater risk than women for the development of cardiovascular problems. Today it is known that young men are more prone to heart disease than young women, but once women reach menopause (usually in

their early to middle 50s), their rates of heart-related problems quickly equal those of men.

The protective mechanism for young women seems to be the female hormone estrogen. Estrogen appears to help women maintain a beneficial profile of blood fats. When the production of estrogen is severely reduced at menopause, this protective factor no longer exists. Prescribing estrogen replacement therapy (ERT) was a common practice by many physicians in treating a number of factors in postmenopausal women. One of the benefits of ERT was considered to be prevention of cardiovascular diseases. However, in 2002 a major clinical research trial was stopped due to the finding that more women on ERT were experiencing heart attacks and strokes. Thus, the American Heart Association now recommends that ERT should not be used for the purpose of preventing cardiovascular

diseases. Certainly, ERT may still be utilized for other purposes (i.e., relief of menopausal symptoms or osteoporosis prevention). Women prescribed ERT need to be aware of the increased risk for cardiovascular disease in evaluating its value. Certainly, much more research is underway that may influence the use of ERT in the future.[2]

Young women should not rely solely on naturally produced estrogen to prevent heart disease. The general recommendations for maintaining heart health—good diet, adequate physical activity, monitoring blood pressure and cholesterol levels, controlling weight, avoiding smoking, and managing stress—will benefit women at every stage of life.

[1]American Heart Association, Statistical Fact Sheet: Women and Cardiovascular Diseases, 2003.
[2]**www.americanheart.org/presenter.jhtml? identifer=4536** 21 July 2003.

(typically in their fifties), their rates of heart disease become similar to men's rates (see the Star box above). It is thought that women have a degree of protection from heart disease because of their natural production of the hormone estrogen during their fertile years.

Heredity

Obviously, you have no input in determining who your biological parents are. Like increasing age and male gender, this risk factor cannot be changed. By the luck of the draw, some people are born into families where heart disease has never been a serious problem, whereas others are born into families where heart disease is quite prevalent. In this latter case, children are said to have a genetic predisposition (tendency) to develop heart disease as they grow and develop throughout their lives. These people have every reason to be highly motivated to reduce the risk factors they can control.

Race is also a consideration related to heart disease. The prevalence of hypertension among African Americans is among the highest in the United States.[1] More than one in every three African Americans has hypertension (two out of every three over age 65).[4] (For a detailed discussion of this topic, see the Focus On article on pages 356–358.) Hypertension significantly increases the risk of heart disease, stroke, and kidney disease. Fortunately, as you will soon read, hypertension can be controlled through a variety of methods. It is especially important for African

Americans to take advantage of every opportunity to have their blood pressure measured so that preventive actions can be started immediately if necessary.

Risk Factors That Can Be Changed

Six cardiovascular risk factors are influenced, in large part, by our lifestyle choices. These risk factors are tobacco smoke, physical inactivity, high blood cholesterol level, high blood pressure, diabetes mellitus, and obesity and overweight.[3] Healthful behavior changes you make concerning these "big six" risk factors can help you protect and strengthen your cardiovascular system.

Tobacco Smoke

Approximately, 46.5 million adults in the United States smoke cigarettes and 28.5% of high school students are smokers.[5] Smokers have a heart attack risk that is more than twice that of nonsmokers. Smoking cigarettes is the major risk factor associated with sudden cardiac death. In fact, smokers have two to four times the risk of dying from sudden cardiac arrest than do nonsmokers. Smokers who experience a heart attack are more likely to die suddenly (within an hour) than are those who don't smoke.

Smoking also adversely affects nonsmokers who are exposed to environmental tobacco smoke. Studies suggest that the risk of death caused by heart disease is increased about 30% in people exposed to secondhand smoke in the home. The risk of death caused by heart disease may even be higher in people exposed to environmental tobacco smoke in work settings (for example, bars, casinos, enclosed offices, some bowling alleys and restaurants), since higher levels of smoke may be present at work than at home. Because of the health threat to nonsmokers, restrictions on indoor smoking in public areas and business settings are increasing tremendously in every part of the country.

For years it was commonly believed that if you had smoked for many years, it was pointless to try to quit; the damage to one's health could never be reversed. However, the American Heart Association now indicates that by quitting smoking, regardless of how long or how much you have smoked, your risk of heart disease declines rapidly.

This news is exciting and should encourage people to quit smoking, regardless of how long they have smoked. Of course, if you have started to smoke, the healthy approach would be to quit now . . . before the nicotine controls your life and leads to heart disease or damages your lungs or leads to lung cancer. (For additional information about the health effects of tobacco, see Chapter 9.)

 TALKING POINTS A friend complains of not being able to quit smoking after several serious attempts. How could you direct this person toward a new approach?

Physical Inactivity

Lack of regular physical activity is a significant risk factor for heart disease. Regular aerobic exercise (discussed in Chapter 4) helps strengthen the heart muscle, maintain healthy blood vessels, and improve the ability of the vascular system to transfer blood and oxygen to all parts of the body. In addition, physical activity helps lower overall blood cholesterol levels for most people, encourages weight loss and retention of lean muscle mass, and allows people to moderate the stress in their lives.

With all the benefits that come with physical activity, it amazes health professionals that so many Americans refuse to become regularly active. The Centers for Disease Control and Prevention[6] reports that 60% or more of American adults do not achieve the recommended amount of physical activity each week and that 25% of Americans age 18 or older report no leisure-time physical activity. In terms of relative risk for developing CVD, physical inactivity is comparable to high blood pressure, high blood cholesterol, and cigarette smoking.

Critical findings reported in the year 2000 from the highly respected Harvard Alumni Health Study[7,8] support the contention that physical activity is closely associated with decreased risk of coronary heart disease. After monitoring Harvard alumni for nearly twenty years in a variety of epidemiological studies, researchers confirmed that sustained, vigorous physical activity produces the strongest reductions in CVD. Light and moderate physical activities such as golf, gardening, and walking are helpful in reducing CVD, but more vigorous activities (such as jogging, swimming, tennis, stair climbing, or aerobics) produce greater reductions in CVD.[7] Additionally, Harvard researchers found that physical activity produced reductions in CVD whether the daily activity comes in one long session or in two shorter sessions of activity.[8] The "bottom line" is this: to reduce your chances of experiencing

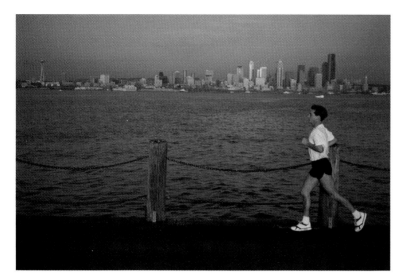

Regular physical activity helps prevent heart disease and also has many other health and functional benefits.

CVD, you must engage in some form of regular, sustained, physical activity (see the Discovering Your Spirituality box below).

If you are middle-aged or older and have been inactive, you should consult with a physician before starting an exercise program. Also, if you have any known health condition that could be aggravated by physical activity, check with a physician first (see Chapter 4 for more information).

TALKING POINTS You've started exercising many times by yourself, but you can't seem to stick to it. How would you convince a new friend that you can help each other get started on regular physical activity and keep it up?

High Blood Cholesterol Level

The third controllable risk factor for heart disease is high blood cholesterol level. Approximately 102 million

---

Discovering Your Spirituality

Getting a Spiritual Lift through Physical Activity

Pick up almost any book on exercise, and you'll read about the "feel good" effect. It's what happens when you start doing any type of aerobic activity, such as walking, running, or swimming. First you'll notice physical changes. You've got more energy. You're sleeping better. Maybe you're even a little less grouchy.

But something else is happening, too. Gradually, your outlook seems more positive. Things you couldn't even think about doing a few weeks ago seem possible. You find yourself thinking about starting to write poetry, figuring out what you want to do with your life, improving your grades, or making new friends. That's the feel-good effect spilling over into all areas of your life.

After a few weeks of starting your exercise program, you've dropped a few pounds and your clothes feel more comfortable. But how you think about yourself is changing, too. Maybe you're paying more attention to your appearance. Or you're eating in a healthier way—almost without thinking about it. What's happening is that your self-image is improving. The idea of taking care of yourself is starting to grow, so how you look, what you eat, and how you spend your time are becoming important.

Joining in physical activities with family or friends offers more than the obvious physical and social benefits. Canoeing, playing volleyball in the back yard, or backpacking builds connections. You see others in a new way, relate to them differently, gain new insights, and find ways to help others. People and experiences you may have taken for granted take on a new dimension, and you appreciate them more.

Some people get a spiritual lift from the great outdoors. Wilderness hiking, for example, transports you to a different setting. The quietness, beauty, and solitude can be soothing to the soul. You're looking at the sky, trees, and water. You're enjoying a very peaceful time. This feeling may seem to disappear as soon as you get back to your dorm, but it may make the things you need to deal with there a little easier.

To experience this type of spiritual lift, you don't have to become a marathon runner or climb a mountain. Start going for long walks—alone or with a friend. Start a group that plays games, such as basketball, tennis, or volleyball. Try going for an early morning swim. Get into bicycling. The spiritual effects may be hard to measure, but they'll surprise and reward you.

Table 10.2 Classification of Total Cholesterol Levels

Total Cholesterol Level	Classification
< 200 mg/dl	Desirable blood cholesterol level
200–239 mg/dl	Borderline-high blood cholesterol level
≥ 240 mg/dl	High blood cholesterol level

InfoLinks

www.nhlbi.nih.gov/guidelines/cholesterol/index.htm

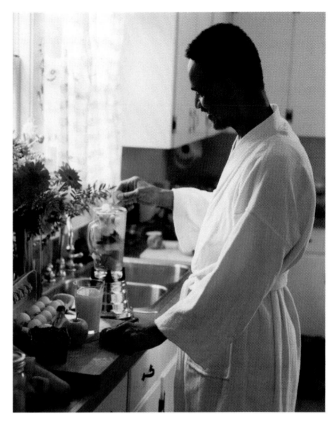

Preparing healthy food can be an enjoyable activity.

American adults have a total cholesterol level of greater than 200 mg/dl (about 41 million have levels great than 240 mg/dl). Generally speaking, the higher the blood cholesterol level, the greater the risk for heart disease. Table 10.2 shows ranges for cholesterol levels. When high blood cholesterol levels are combined with other important risk factors, the risks become much greater.

Fortunately, blood cholesterol levels are relatively easy to measure. Many campus health and wellness centers provide cholesterol screenings for employees and students. These screenings help identify people whose cholesterol levels (or profiles) may be dangerous. Medical professionals have linked people's diets with their cholesterol levels. People with high blood cholesterol levels are encouraged to consume a heart-healthy diet (see Chapter 5) and to become physically active. In recent years, researchers have developed a variety of drugs that are very effective at lowering cholesterol levels. In a later section in this chapter, you will read more about cholesterol, particularly the cholesterol carrying compounds—lipoproteins.

High Blood Pressure

The fourth of the six cardiovascular risk factors that can be changed is high blood pressure, or hypertension. Approximately 58 million Americans have hypertension, one-third of whom have not been diagnosed. High blood pressure can seriously damage a person's heart and blood vessels. High blood pressure causes the heart to work much harder, eventually causing the heart to enlarge and weaken. High blood pressure increases the risk of stroke, heart attack, congestive heart failure, and kidney disease.

When high blood pressure is seen with other risk factors, the risk for stroke or heart attack is increased tremendously. As you will soon see, this "silent killer" is easy to monitor and can be effectively controlled through a variety of approaches.

Diabetes Mellitus

Diabetes mellitus (discussed in detail in Chapter 12) is a debilitating chronic disease that has a significant effect on the human body. Approximately 17 million Americans have diabetes, one-third of whom have not been diagnosed. In addition to increasing the risk of developing kidney disease, blindness, and nerve damage, diabetes increases the likelihood of developing heart and blood vessel diseases. More than 65% of people with diabetes die of some type of heart or blood vessel disease. The cardiovascular damage is thought to occur due to the abnormal levels of cholesterol and blood fat found in individuals with diabetes. With weight management, exercise, dietary changes, and drug therapy, diabetes can be relatively well controlled in most people. Despite careful management of this disease, diabetic patients remain quite susceptible to eventual heart and blood vessel damage.[9]

 TALKING POINTS How would you show support for a friend who is struggling with the dietary requirements of diabetes?

Obesity and Overweight

According to the 1999 National Health and Nutrition Survey, approximately 61% of American adults are overweight and 26% are obese. Even if they have no other risk factors, obese people are more likely than are nonobese people to develop heart disease and stroke. Obesity, particularly if of the abdominal form, places considerable strain on the heart, and it tends to worsen both blood pressure and blood cholesterol levels. Obese men and women can expect a greater risk of heart disease, diabetes, gallbladder disease, osteoarthritis, respiratory problems, and certain cancers.[10] Maintaining body weight within a desirable range minimizes the chances of obesity ever happening. To accomplish this, you can elect to make a commitment to a reasonably sound diet and an active lifestyle.

 TALKING POINTS How could you tactfully bring up a friend's weight problem to show concern for his or her health?

Another Risk Factor That Contributes to Heart Disease

The American Heart Association identifies one other risk factor that is associated with an increased risk of heart disease. This risk factor is one's individual response to stress.

Individual Response to Stress

Unresolved stress over a long period may be a contributing factor to the development of heart disease. Certainly, people who are unable to cope with stressful life experiences are more likely to develop negative dependence behaviors (for example, smoking, underactivity, poor dietary practices), which can then lead to cardiovascular problems through changes in blood fat profiles, blood pressure, and heart workload. To discover ways of coping with stress, you might wish to return to the discussion in Chapter 3.

Forms of Cardiovascular Disease

The American Heart Association describes six major forms of CVD as coronary heart disease, hypertension, stroke, congenital heart disease, rheumatic heart disease, and congestive heart failure. These six diseases account for over 75% of the deaths due to CVD. Additionally many other diseases influence the heart and blood vessels, such as peripheral vascular disease and arrhythmias. (These CVDs will be discussed later in the chapter.)

A person may have just one of these diseases or a combination of forms at the same time. Each form exists in varying degrees of severity. All forms are capable of causing secondary damage to other body organs and systems.

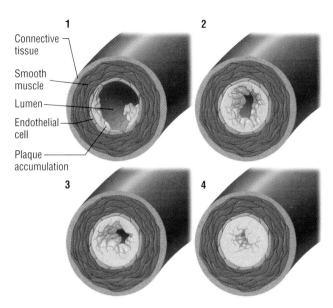

Figure 10-3 Progression of atherosclerosis. This diagram shows how plaque deposits gradually accumulate to narrow the lumen (interior space) of an artery. Shown enlarged here, coronary arteries are only as wide as a pencil lead.

Coronary Heart Disease

This form of CVD, also known as *coronary artery disease,* involves damage to the vessels that supply blood to the heart muscle. The bulk of this blood is supplied by the coronary arteries. Any damage to these important vessels can cause a reduction of blood flow (with its vital oxygen and nutrients) to specific areas of heart muscle. The ultimate result of an inadequate blood supply is a heart attack.

Atherosclerosis

The principal cause of coronary heart disease is **atherosclerosis** (Figure 10-3). Atherosclerosis produces a narrowing of the coronary arteries. This narrowing stems from the long-term buildup of fatty deposits, called *plaque,* on the inner walls of the arteries. This buildup reduces the blood supply to specific portions of the heart. Often arteries of the heart can become totally blocked (occluded) due to a clot so that all blood supply is stopped. Heart muscle tissue begins to die when it is deprived of oxygen

---

Key Terms

atherosclerosis the buildup of plaque on the inner walls of arteries.

---

and nutrients. This damage is known as **myocardial infarction.** In lay terms, this event is called a heart attack. The Changing for the Better box above explains how to recognize the signs of a heart attack and what to do next.

Within the past five years, researchers have found that a high blood level of the amino acid **homocysteine** may be related to an increased risk of CHD. It is thought that high concentrations of homosysteine may accelerate the atherosclerotic plaque formation process which will clog the artery passageways.[11] For persons who did not exhibit any of the traditional CHD risk factors (perhaps as many as 50% of the people who get heart attacks), the possibility that a blood test might identify this marker for heart disease was seen as good news.[11] If a person has a high homocysteine level, the theory is that he or she could probably lower the level by taking a multivitamin or by increasing the intake of certain B vitamins, especially B6, B12, and folic acid (folate). At the time of this writing, however, physicians and scientists are not fully convinced that this is a sound strategy.

While the jury remains undecided regarding the benefits of lowering homocysteine levels, a second possible marker for heart disease has emerged. This marker is a compound called **C-reactive protein.**[12] This protein is a byproduct of the inflammation process. Persons who have elevated levels of C-reactive protein appear to be at greater risk of CHD than those with low levels. Research is presently underway to determine what causes C-reactive protein to reach high levels and for potential treatments. Some promising reports have emerged suggesting that statin medications (used to treat blood cholesterol abnormalities) may help reduce C-reactive protein levels.

Cholesterol and Lipoproteins For many years, scientists have known that atherosclerosis is a complicated disease that has many causes. Some of these causes are not well understood, but others are clearly understood. Cholesterol, a

Key Terms

myocardial infarction heart attack; the death of part of the heart muscle as a result of a blockage in one or more of the coronary arteries.

homocysteine an amino acid found in the bloodstream; high levels of homocysteine are thought to be related to an increased risk of coronary heart disease.

C-reactive protein a chemical compound found in the blood that is associated with inflammation; high levels are related to increased risk of coronary heart disease.

soft, fatlike material, is manufactured in the liver and small intestine and is necessary in the formation of sex hormones, cell membranes, bile salts, and nerve fibers. Elevated levels of serum cholesterol (200 mg/dl or more for adults aged 20 and older, and 170 mg/dl or more for young people under age 20) are associated with an increased risk of developing atherosclerosis.

Initially, most people can help lower their serum cholesterol level by adopting three dietary changes: lowering their intake of saturated fats, lowering their intake of dietary cholesterol, and lowering caloric intake to a level that does not exceed body requirements. The aim is to reduce excess fat, cholesterol, and calories in our diet while promoting sound nutrition. By carefully following such a diet, people with high serum cholesterol levels may be able to reduce their cholesterol levels by 30 to 55 mg/dl. However, dietary changes do not affect people equally; some will experience greater reductions than others. Some will not respond at all to dietary changes and may need to take cholesterol-lowering medications and increase physical activity.

Cholesterol is attached to structures called *lipoproteins.* Lipoproteins are particles that circulate in the blood and transport lipids (including cholesterol).[3] The two major classes of lipoproteins are **low-density lipoproteins (LDLs)** and **high-density lipoproteins (HDLs).** A person's total cholesterol level is essentially determined by the amount of the LDLs and HDLs in a measured sample of blood. For example, a person's total cholesterol level of 200 mg/dl could be represented by an LDL level of 130 and an HDL level of 40, or an LDL level of 120 and an HDL level of 60. (Note that additional forms of lipoproteins do exist and carry some of the cholesterol in the blood, thus, the total cholesterol value is greater than the sum of LDL and HDL.)

After much study, researchers have determined that high levels of LDL are a significant cause of atherosclerosis. This makes sense, because LDLs carry the greatest percentage of cholesterol in the bloodstream. LDLs are more likely to deposit excess cholesterol into the artery walls. This contributes to plaque formation. For this reason, LDLs are often called the "bad cholesterol."[1] Borderline-high LDL levels (above 130 mg/dl) and high LDL levels (above 160 mg/dl) are determined partly by inheritance, but they are also clearly associated with smoking, poor dietary patterns, obesity, and lack of exercise.

On the other hand, high levels of HDLs (60 mg/dl or higher) are related to a decrease in the development of atherosclerosis. HDLs are thought to transport cholesterol out of the bloodstream. Thus HDLs have been called the "good cholesterol." Certain lifestyle alterations, such as quitting smoking, reducing obesity, regular aerobic-type exercise, and consumption of monounsaturated dietary fats, help many people increase their level of HDLs.

Improving cholesterol levels is a significant step in reducing the risk of death from coronary heart disease. Since 1980 the percentage of American adults with high cholesterol has dropped from 27.8% to 18%. The main reason for this decrease was the introduction of the National Cholesterol Education Program in the mid-1980s. Prior to this program, measurement of blood cholesterol was not a routine part of health screenings. The recommendations from this program were updated in 1993 and then most recently in 2001. It is now recommended that all Americans over the age 19 be tested for LDL, HDL, and triglycerides. Although identification and treatment of those with high total and LDL cholesterol levels remain important, the most recent report recommends more intensive therapy for individuals with multiple-risk factors for coronary artery disease. For people with elevated cholesterol levels, a 1% reduction in serum cholesterol level yields about a 2% reduction in the risk of death from heart disease. Thus a 10% to 15% cholesterol reduction can reduce risk by 20% to 30%.[13] The National Cholesterol Education Program has specific recommendations for improving your blood cholesterol concentration. The recommendations begin with what we call "therapeutic lifestyle changes," which include dietary modification, weight reduction for those overweight or obese, and regular physical activity. If the therapeutic lifestyle changes are not completely effective or if the individual is at increased risk for coronary artery disease, then lipid-lowering medications are recommended. Among the most potent of these is a group of drugs called "statins." These medications have been shown to lower the risk of death from heart disease.

Angina Pectoris When coronary arteries become narrowed, chest pain, or angina pectoris, is often felt. This pain is caused by a reduced supply of oxygen to heart muscle tissue. Usually, a coronary artery disease patient feels angina when he or she becomes stressed or exercises too strenuously. Angina reportedly can range from a feeling of

---

Key Terms

low-density lipoprotein (LDL) the type of lipoprotein that transports the largest amount of cholesterol in the bloodstream; high levels of LDL are related to heart disease.

high-density lipoprotein (HDL) the type of lipoprotein that transports cholesterol from the bloodstream to the liver, where it is eventually removed from the body; high levels of HDL are related to a reduction in heart disease.

Heart Disease: A Family Affair

When it comes to cardiovascular health, arming yourself with information is the first step. As with most health conditions, learning your family's medical history is a great way to start. Talk to parents, grandparents, aunts, and uncles to find out if there's a history of heart attack, stroke, or other cardiovascular disease in your family.

HealthQuest Activities

What would you do if the person you were with collapsed and stopped breathing? Would you know how to perform CPR? CPR is an important skill to have—it could save someone's life. Go to the *CPR Exploration* in the Cardiovascular module. Complete the tutorial, and then complete the exploration. It could mean the difference between life and death. (The materials found in this tutorial originated at "Learn CPR: You Can Do It." Learn CPR is a free public service supported by the University of Washington School of Medicine. Source: **http://depts.washington.edu/learncpr/index.html**)

mild indigestion to a severe viselike pressure in the chest. The pain may extend from the center of the chest to the arms and even up to the jaw. Generally, the more severe the blockage, the more pain is felt.

Some cardiac patients relieve angina with the drug nitroglycerin, a powerful blood vessel dilator. This prescription drug, available in slow-release transdermal (through the skin) patches or small pills that are placed under the patient's tongue, causes a major reduction in the workload of the heart muscle. Other cardiac patients may be prescribed drugs such as **calcium channel blockers** or **beta blockers.**

Emergency Response to Heart Crises

Heart attacks need not be fatal. The consequences of any heart attack depend on the location of the damage to the heart, the extent to which heart muscle is damaged, and the speed with which adequate circulation is restored. Injury to the ventricles may very well prove fatal unless medical countermeasures are immediately undertaken. Recognizing a heart attack is critically important (see the Changing for the Better box on page 342).

Cardiopulmonary resuscitation (CPR) is one of the most important immediate countermeasures that trained people can use when confronted with a person having a heart attack. Public education programs sponsored by the American Red Cross and the American Heart Association teach people how to recognize, evaluate, and manage heart attack emergencies. CPR trainees are taught how to restore breathing (through mouth-to-mouth resuscitation) and circulation (through external chest compression) in people who require such emergency countermeasures. Frequently, colleges offer CPR classes through health science or physical education departments. We encourage each student to enroll in a CPR course. Additionally, automated external defibrillators are now located in many public buildings. Studies have reported that survival rates of those in cardiac arrest is greater than 90% when defibrillation is provided within the first minute.[14]

Diagnosis

A blood test, measuring cardiac muscle enzymes (markers of damage to the heart muscle), is usually performed initially. After a person's vital signs have stabilized, further diagnostic examinations can reveal the type and extent of damage to heart muscle. Initially an ECG might be taken, which may be able to identify if areas of ischemia (insufficient blood flow) or damage has occurred to the heart muscle. Another test which may be used is echocardiography. This procedure can also detect ischemia. The diagnostic ability of both of these tests is improved if used in conjunction with exercise (i.e., stress ECG or stress echocardiography). This test analyzes the electrical activity of the heart. Heart catheterization, also called *coronary arteriography,* is a minor surgical procedure that starts by placing a thin plastic tube into an arm or leg artery. This tube, called a *catheter,* is guided through the artery until it reaches the coronary circulation, where a radiopaque dye is then released. X-ray pictures called *angiograms* then record the progress of the dye through the coronary arteries. Areas of blockage are relatively easily identified.

Some newer techniques for noninvasive diagnosis of coronary artery disease are positron emission tomography (PET), electron beam computed tomography (EBCT), and

---

Key Terms

calcium channel blockers drugs that reduce the workload of the heart; used in the treatment of blood pressure and the long-term management of angina pectoris.

beta blockers drugs that reduce the workload of the heart, which will reduce blood pressure and decrease the occurrence of angina pectoris.

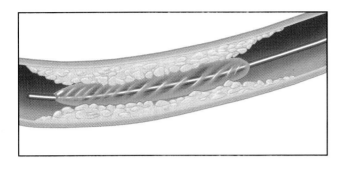 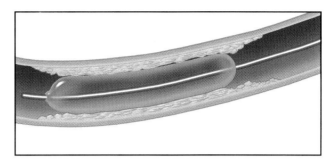

A   **B**

Figure 10-4 Angioplasty. A, A "balloon" is surgically inserted into the narrowed coronary artery.
B, The balloon is inflated, compressing plaque and fatty deposits against the artery walls.

magnetic resonance imaging (MRI). Now PET, EBCT, and MRI can be used to illustrate the anatomy of coronary arteries and the function of the heart, enabling physicians to evaluate such problems as valvular disease and cardiac shunts.

Nuclear medicine is another important tool in the diagnosis of cardiac disease. Nuclear medicine uses radiopharmaceuticals such as thallium-201 and technetium-99m sestamibi to evaluate perfusion of the heart muscle. Physicians use such tools to study the function of the heart and diagnose cardiac problems.

Treatment

After the extent of damage has been determined, a physician or team of physicians can decide on a medical course of action. Treatments can be divided into two broad categories: surgical and nonsurgical.

Surgical Treatments Currently popular is an extensive form of surgery called **coronary artery bypass surgery.** An estimated 316,000 bypass surgeries were performed in 2001. The purpose of such surgery is to detour (bypass) areas of coronary artery obstruction by usually using a section of an artery from the patient's chest (the internal mammary artery) and grafting it from the aorta to a location just beyond the area of obstruction. Multiple areas of obstruction result in double, triple, or quadruple bypasses.

Surgeons have recently begun performing heart bypass surgery through a three-inch incision in the rib cage, along with two to four small incisions in the patient's chest, rather than the traditional large, twelve- to fifteen-inch incision. Physicians manipulate the coronary arteries through the small ports, and they view their work through a fiber-optic camera called a *thoracoscope.* This new technique results in much less pain and blood loss, a shorter hospital stay, and a quicker recovery for the patient. This method has been nicknamed "keyhole" surgery and is still considered to be somewhat experimental.

Angioplasty

In 2001, about 1,050,000 people with heart disease had an angioplasty. Angioplasty is an alternative to bypass surgery, involving the use of a coronary catheter (described earlier) to place a doughnut-shaped "balloon" directly into the narrowed coronary artery (Figure 10-4). When this balloon is inflated, plaque and fatty deposits are compressed against the artery walls, widening the space through which blood flows. These balloons usually remain within the artery for less than a minute. Renarrowing of the artery will occur in about one-quarter of angioplasty patients. Many patients are now having a stent (small mesh tube) inserted in the region where the coronary artery was enlarged by the balloon. Recently, these stents were being coated with drugs to prevent blood clotting at this site.

Balloon angioplasty can be used for blockages in the heart, kidneys, arms, and legs. The decision whether to have angioplasty or bypass surgery can be a difficult one to make.

In the past 10 years, a number of devices have been developed to remove the diseased material inside a coronary artery. These are called atherectomy devices. Inserted through a leg artery and held in place by a tiny inflated balloon, these motor-driven cutters shave off plaque deposits from inside the artery. A nose cone in the scraper unit stores the plaque until the device is removed.

The use of laser beams to dissolve plaque that blocks arteries has been slowly evolving. The FDA has approved

> **Key Terms**
>
> **coronary artery bypass surgery** a surgical procedure designed to improve blood flow to the heart by providing alternative routes for blood to take around points of blockage.

three laser devices for use in clogged leg arteries. In 1992 the FDA approved the use of an excimer laser for use in coronary arteries. Other devices used to open coronary arteries are being researched. These techniques include thermal, photochemical, or acoustical energy to reduce the plaque.

Heart Transplants and Artificial Hearts

For approximately 30 years, surgeons have been able to surgically replace a person's damaged heart with that of another human being. Although very risky, these transplant operations have added years to the lives of a number of patients who otherwise would have lived only a short time. In 2001, doctors performed 2,202 heart transplants in the United States.[1]

Artificial hearts have also been developed and implanted in humans. These mechanical devices have extended the lives of patients and have also served as temporary hearts while patients wait for a suitable donor heart. One of the important difficulties with artificial heart implantation has been the control of blood clots that may form, especially around the artificial valves. Blood clots can cause heart attacks or strokes that can be fatal.

Nonsurgical Treatments

Platelet Inhibitors

Platelets are part of the physiological pathway that produces blood clots. This new class of drugs has been shown to prevent the formation of blood clots, a major cause of heart attacks, chest pain, and artery tightening after angioplasty. It is well established that platelet inhibitors reduce heart attacks in patients with unstable angina, or severe chest pain, by about half.[3] Observers say this new class of drugs will have a tremendous effect on the treatment of heart problems.

Aspirin

Studies released in the late 1980s highlighted the role of aspirin in reducing the risk of heart attack in men who had no history of previous attacks. Specifically, the studies concluded that for men with hypertension, elevated cholesterol levels, or both, taking one aspirin per day was a significant factor in reducing their risk of heart attack. Aspirin works by making the blood less able to clot, which reduces the likelihood of blood vessel blockages. Experts currently disagree about the age at which this preventive action should begin. The safest advice is to check with your physician before starting aspirin therapy.

Likewise, it now appears that women who take aspirin on a regular basis are less likely to have a heart attack than women who do not take aspirin. However, it is important that women first consult with their physicians about the correct dosage and the best way to use aspirin to protect their cardiovascular health.[15]

Can Alcohol Be Good for Your Heart?

You have probably seen the controversial headlines over the past couple of years, stating that moderate consumption of alcohol may actually reduce your risk of coronary heart disease. Such research is controversial because experts fear this may encourage problem drinkers or turn abstainers into problem drinkers.

Nevertheless, the evidence is strong that drinking alcohol in moderate amounts indeed reduces the risk of heart attack and death from coronary heart disease. The best evidence comes from population studies that show a reduction in coronary risk among moderate drinkers when compared with abstainers. The results are similar in both men and women, and among various ethnic groups. Moderate drinking is typically defined as one or two daily drinks for men and one for women.

Three possible explanations for the cardiovascular benefits are: (1) that alcohol raises the level of protective high-density lipoprotein (HDL) cholesterol in the blood, making atherosclerosis less likely, (2) that alcohol inhibits blood clotting by helping to dissolve clots in blood vessels, and (3) other substances in the alcoholic beverage may have antioxidant properties.

Researchers are looking at specific types of alcohol, such as red wine, but the results are not yet strong enough to justify recommending that people switch to wine from beer or liquor. It appears that the benefits come from any type of alcohol product.

The American Heart Association* makes the following recommendations:

- The beneficial effects of alcohol are limited to one or two drinks a day.
- Heavier consumption is related to many health problems, including alcoholism, high blood pressure, obesity, stroke, breast cancer, suicide, and accidents.
- Pregnant women should not use alcohol.
- Do not drink alcohol if you take aspirin on a regular basis. Check with your physician.

*American Heart Association, Alcohol and Heart Disease. *Circulation* 94:3023–3025, 1996.

InfoLinks

www.americanheart.org/Heart_and_Stroke_A_Z_Guide/ alcohol.html

Alcohol

For years, scientists have been uncertain about the extent to which alcohol consumption is related to a reduced risk of heart disease. The current thinking is that moderate drinking (defined as no more than two drinks per day for men and one drink per day for women) is related to a lower heart disease risk (see the Star box above). However, the benefit is much smaller than proven risk reduction behavior, such as stopping smoking, reducing cholesterol level, lowering blood pressure, and increasing physical activity. Experts caution that heavy drinking increases cardiovascular risks and that nondrinkers should not start to drink just to reduce heart disease risk.

Hypertension

Just as your car's water pump recirculates water and maintains water pressure, your heart recirculates blood and maintains blood pressure. When the heart contracts, blood is forced through your arteries and veins. Your blood pressure is a measure of the force that your circulating blood exerts against the interior walls of your arteries and veins.

Blood pressure is measured with a *sphygmomanometer*. A sphygmomanometer is attached to an arm-cuff device that can be inflated to stop the flow of blood temporarily in the brachial artery. This artery is a major supplier of blood to the lower arm. It is located on the inside of the upper arm, just above the elbow.

A health professional using a stethoscope listens for blood flow while the pressure in the cuff is released. Two pressure measurements are recorded: The **systolic pressure** is the highest blood pressure against the vessel walls during the heart contraction, and the **diastolic pressure** is the lowest blood pressure against the vessel walls when the heart relaxes (between heartbeats). Expressed in units of millimeters of mercury, blood pressure is recorded as the systolic pressure over the diastolic pressure, for example, 115/82.

Although a blood pressure of less than 120/80 is considered "normal" for adults, lower values do not necessarily indicate a medical problem. In fact, many young college women of average weight display blood pressures that seem to be relatively low (100/60, for example), yet these lowered blood pressures are quite "normal" for them.

Hypertension refers to a consistently elevated blood pressure. Generally, concern for high blood pressure begins when a person has a systolic reading of 140 or above or a diastolic reading of 90 or above, although now one is considered to have prehypertension if their systolic pressure is between 120–139 or their diastolic pressure is between 80–89. Table 10.3 shows the classifications for blood pressure.

Based on data from 1999–2000, approximately one in every three adults has hypertension.[16] In the United States, more men have hypertension than women until age 55, when women surpass men. In terms of prevalence for United States adults age 20 and older, non-Hispanic black females have the highest rate (38%) of hypertension. Thirty percent of non-Hispanic white males and 27% of non-Hispanic white females have high blood pressure. Among Hispanic males in the United States, 23% have hypertension; 20% of Hispanic females have high blood pressure.[1]

Table 10.3 Blood Pressure Classification

Blood Pressure (mm Hg)	Normal	Prehypertension	Hypertension
Systolic (top number)	less than 120	120–139	140 or higher
Diastolic (bottom number)	less than 80	80–89	90 or higher

High blood pressure, or hypertension, is defined in an adult as a systolic pressure of 140 mm Hg or higher and/or a diastolic pressure of 90 mm Hg or higher. Blood pressure is measured in millimeters of mercury (mm Hg).

InfoLinks

www.nhlbi.nih.gov/guidelines/hypertension/index.htm

The causes of 90 to 95% of the cases of hypertension are unknown, called essential hypertension. However, the health risks are real. Throughout the body, long-term hypertension makes arteries and arterioles become less elastic and thus incapable of dilating under a heavy workload. Brittle, calcified blood vessels can burst unexpectedly and produce serious strokes (brain accidents), kidney failure (renal accidents), or eye damage **(retinal hemorrhage).** Furthermore, it appears that blood clots are more easily formed and dislodged in a vascular system affected by hypertension. Thus hypertension can be a cause of heart attacks. Clearly, hypertension is a potential killer.

Hypertension is referred to as "the silent killer" because people with hypertension often are not aware that they have the condition. People with this disorder cannot feel the sensation of high blood pressure. The condition does not produce dizziness, headaches, or memory loss unless one is experiencing a medical crisis. Because it is a silent killer, it is estimated that 30% of the people who have hypertension do not realize they have it. Eleven percent know they have hypertension but are not taking any measures to reduce it. Twenty-six percent are on medication but do not

Key Terms

systolic pressure (sis **tol** ick) blood pressure against blood vessel walls when the heart contracts.

diastolic pressure (**dye** uh stol ick) blood pressure against blood vessel walls when the heart relaxes.

retinal hemorrhage uncontrolled bleeding from arteries within the eye's retina.

In the practice of Western medicine, the most frequently used methods for reducing hypertension are medical approaches (taking various drugs that lower blood pressure) and lifestyle changes (losing excess weight, reducing sodium intake, increasing exercise, and drinking less alcohol). Practitioners of Eastern medicine might employ some of the lifestyle changes used in the West, but they would also be likely to recommend some form of meditation to help reduce blood pressure.

Meditation refers to an activity that produces a mental state of alert relaxation. While the body rests, the mind remains active. As it is practiced in the West, meditation is usually employed twice a day for 15–20 minutes at a time. The person sits still with eyes closed and repeats a soothing sound (mantra). This permits the body to relax and release stressful sensations, allowing the body and mind to exist in a state of balance.[1]

Meditation is taught in its various forms through noncredit courses at universities, local mental health centers, health clubs, or commercial stress management or relaxation centers. Students can take classes in the movement forms of meditation, such as the Chinese martial art tai chi, the Japanese martial art aikido, yoga, and the walking meditation of Zen Buddhism. There are many books, audiotapes, and videotapes available that promise to teach meditation. One of the most well-known books (*The Relaxation Response,* Avon Books) is by Harvard cardiologist Herbert Benson.

The important question remains: How successful is meditation in reducing hypertension? The answer is that meditation can be helpful and should be used in combination with other therapeutic approaches. A particular benefit of meditation is that it does not come with any of the side effects of drugs. One study, conducted at California's West Oakland Health Center,[1] found that people age 55 and over who learned transcendental meditation and practiced it every day for 3 months lowered their systolic blood pressure by 11 points and their diastolic pressure by 6 points. This drop in blood pressure was thought to reduce the likelihood of stroke by 35 to 40 percent and the risk of congestive heart failure by 20 to 45 percent. Similar drops in blood pressure have been found in other controlled studies.

How meditation works to control hypertension is not fully understood. It may be that meditation alters the stress response (see Chapter 3) and that this lowers blood pressure. It may be that meditation causes people to curb many of their unhealthy behaviors, and the reduction in lifestyle excesses (overeating, overdrinking, underactivity) may cause the blood pressure to drop.

The National Institutes of Health is currently supporting research to further study the impact of meditation on hypertension. Increasingly, researchers are finding major connections between the mind and the heart.[2] Certainly, meditation won't effectively control every case of hypertension, but it may be a very useful approach for many people with hypertension.

[1]Meditation lowers blood pressure as well as drugs. *Tufts University Diet and Nutrition Letter,* January 1997; Vol. 14: No. 11, p. 3
[2]The mind and the heart: they really are connected. *Tufts University Health and Nutrition Letter,* August 2000; Vol. 18: No. 6, pp. 1–5.

keep their hypertension under control. Just 34% of people with hypertension are aware that they have high blood pressure *and* have it under control with medication.[17]

Hypertension is not thought of as a curable disease; rather, it is a controllable disease. When therapy is stopped, the condition returns. As a responsible adult, you should use every opportunity you can to measure your blood pressure regularly.

Prevention and Treatment

Weight reduction, physical activity, moderation in alcohol use, and the dietary approaches to stop hypertension (DASH eating plan) are all recommended to reduce hypertension. These lifestyle modifications are now recommended therapy for individuals classified as prehypertensive. For overweight or obese people, a reduction in body weight may produce a significant drop in blood pressure. Physical activity helps lower blood pressure by expending calories (which may lead to weight loss in those who are overweight or obese) and through other physiological changes that affect the circulation. Moderation in alcohol consumption helps reduce blood pressure in some people.

The restriction of sodium (salt) in the diet also helps some people reduce hypertension. Interestingly, this strategy is effective only for those who are **salt sensitive**—estimated to be about 25% of the population. Reducing salt intake would have little effect on the blood pressure of the rest of the population. Nevertheless, because our daily intake of salt vastly exceeds our need for salt, the general recommendation to curb salt intake still makes good sense. The DASH eating plan also recommends foods that are rich in potassium and calcium.

Many of the stress reduction activities we discuss in Chapter 3 are receiving increased attention in the struggle

Key Terms

salt sensitive term used to describe people whose bodies overreact to the presence of sodium by retaining fluid, thus increasing blood pressure.

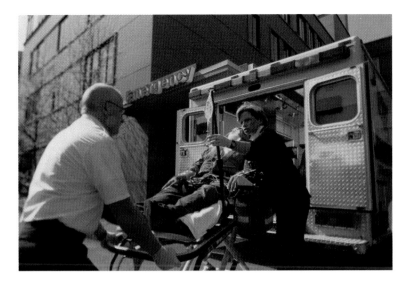

to reduce hypertension. In recent years, behavioral scientists have reported the success of meditation, biofeedback, controlled breathing, and muscle relaxation exercises in reducing hypertension (see the Considering Complementary Care box on page 348). Look for further research findings in these areas in the years to come.

Drugs used to lower high blood pressure are called *antihypertensives. Diuretic drugs* work by stimulating the kidneys to eliminate more fluid, thereby reducing blood volume. *Vasodilators* relax the smooth muscle in the walls of blood vessels (especially the arterioles), allowing the vessels to dilate (widen). Also used are calcium channel blockers, beta blockers, angiotension converting enzyme (ACE) inhibitors, and other drugs that work in various ways to relax blood vessels. The most disturbing aspect of drug therapy for hypertension is that many patients refuse to take their medication on a consistent basis, probably because of the mistaken notion that "you must feel sick to be sick."

Some people taking these medications report uncomfortable side effects, including depression, reduced libido (sex drive), muscle weakness, impotence, dizziness, and fainting. Thus the medication's side effects may seem worse than the disease. This is all the more reason to emphasize the lifestyle modifications described earlier. Because of the poor record of patient compliance with hypertension drug therapy, many television and radio public service announcements are geared to the hypertensive patient. Nutritional supplements, such as calcium, magnesium, potassium, and fish oil, have not proven to be effective and reliable in lowering blood pressure.

Stroke

A third major CVD is stroke. *Stroke* is a general term for a wide variety of crises (sometimes called cerebrovascular accidents [CVAs] or brain attacks) that result from blood vessel damage in the brain. African Americans have a 60% greater risk of stroke than white Americans do, probably because African Americans have a greater likelihood of having hypertension than do white Americans. About 700,000 (200,000 of which are recurrent events) people suffer a stroke in the United States each year, and of these, about a quarter die. A total of 163,538 Americans died of stroke in 2001.[1] Just as the heart muscle needs an adequate blood supply, so does the brain. Any disturbance in the proper supply of oxygen and nutrients to the brain can pose a threat.

Cerebrovascular Occlusions

Perhaps the most common form of stroke results from the blockage of a cerebral (brain) artery. Similar to coronary occlusions, **cerebrovascular occlusions** can be started by a clot that forms within an artery, called a *thrombus,* or by a clot that travels from another part of the body to the brain, called an *embolus* (Figure 10-5 A and B). The resultant accidents (cerebral thrombosis or cerebral embolism) cause more than 60% of all strokes. The portion of the brain deprived of oxygen and nutrients can literally die.

Cerebral Hemorrhage

A third type of stroke can result from an artery that bursts to produce a crisis called *cerebral hemorrhage* (Figure 10-5 C).

Key Terms

cerebrovascular occlusions (ser ee bro **vas** kyou lar) blockages to arteries supplying blood to the cerebral cortex of the brain; the most common type of stroke.

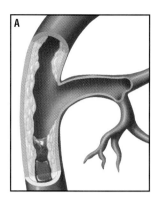

Thrombus
A clot that forms within a narrowed section of a blood vessel and remains at its place of origin.

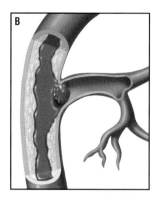

Embolus
A clot that moves through the circulatory system and becomes lodged at a narrowed point within a vessel.

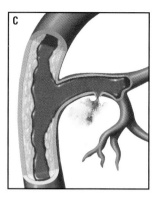

Hemorrhage
The sudden bursting of a blood vessel.

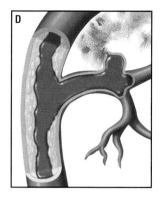

Aneurysm
A sac formed when a section of a blood vessel thins and balloons; the weakened wall of the sac can burst, or rupture, as shown here.

Figure 10-5 Causes of stroke.

Damaged, brittle arteries can be especially susceptible to bursting when a person has hypertension.

Cerebral Aneurysm

A fourth form of stroke is a *cerebral aneurysm.* An aneurysm is a ballooning or outpouching on a weakened area of an artery (Figure 10-5 D). Aneurysms may occur in various locations of the body and are not always life threatening. The development of aneurysms is not fully understood, although there seems to be a relationship between aneurysms and hypertension. It is quite possible that many aneurysms are congenital defects. In any case, when a cerebral aneurysm bursts, a stroke results. See the adjacent Changing for the Better box to learn the warning signs of stroke.

Diagnosis

A person who reports any warning signs of stroke or periods of temporary lack of bloodflow to a region of the brain, called a **transient ischemic attack (TIA),** is given a battery of diagnostic tests, which could include a physical examination, a search for possible brain tumors, tests to identify areas of the brain affected, electroencephalogram, cerebral arteriography, and a **CAT** (computerized axial tomography) **scan** or **MRI** (magnetic resonance imaging) **scan.** Many other tests can also be used.

Treatment

Researchers recently made a breakthrough in the treatment of stroke, with the discovery that the clot-dissolving drug

---

Changing for the Better

Recognizing Warning Signs of Stroke

Although many stroke victims have little warning of an impending crisis, there are some warning signals of stroke that you should recognize. The American Heart Association encourages everyone to be aware of the following signs:

- Sudden, temporary weakness or numbness of the face, arm, and leg on one side of the body
- Temporary loss of speech or trouble in speaking or understanding speech
- Temporary dimness or loss of vision, particularly in one eye
- Unexplained dizziness, unsteadiness, or sudden falls

Many severe strokes are preceded by "mini strokes," warning signals like the above, experienced days, weeks, or months before the more severe event. Prompt medical or surgical attention to these symptoms may prevent a fatal or disabling stroke.

InfoLinks

www.americanheart.org

Key Terms

transient ischemic attack (TIA) (**tran** see ent iss **key** mick) strokelike symptoms caused by temporary spasm of cerebral blood vessels.

CAT scan computerized axial tomography scan; an x-ray procedure designed to illustrate structures within the body that would not normally be seen through conventional x-ray procedures.

MRI scan magnetic resonance imaging scan; an imaging procedure that uses a giant magnet to generate an image of body tissue.

tissue plasminogen activators (TPA) and the cell-rebuilding drug citicoline could reduce the severity of strokes.

In the past, physicians essentially waited for a stroke to end before assessing damage and beginning rehabilitation. Now, experts find that TPA can actually reduce the severity of a stroke as it is occurring. TPA was previously used to dissolve clots in the treatment of heart attacks. This same effect, applied during a stroke, can help prevent brain cells from "starving" to death because of a lack of blood supply. TPA is useful only for strokes caused by clots (embolism or thrombosis).

As a result, experts are reclassifying stroke as a medical emergency that must be treated as quickly as possible. To be effective, TPA must be administered in the first 3 hours of the stroke. After that time, brain cells have been damaged and TPA can worsen the damage. Because 700,000 people suffer strokes and about one-quarter of these die each year, TPA has the potential to save thousands of lives a year.

Other treatment after a stroke depends on the nature and extent of the damage the patient has suffered. Some patients require surgery (to repair vessels and relieve pressure) and acute care in the hospital.

The advances made in the rehabilitation of stroke patients are amazing. Although some severely affected patients have little hope of improvement, our continuing advances in the application of computer technology to such disciplines as speech and physical therapy offer encouraging signs for stroke patients and their families.

Congenital Heart Disease

A congenital defect is one that is present at birth. About thirty-two thousand babies are born each year with one of at least thirty-five recognized congenital heart defects. In 2001, a total of 4,109 infants died from congenital heart disease.[1]

A variety of abnormalities may be produced by congenital heart disease, including valve damage, holes in the walls of the septum, blood vessel transposition, and an underdevelopment of the left side of the heart. All of these problems ultimately prevent a newborn baby from receiving adequate oxygenation of tissues throughout the body. A bluish skin color (cyanosis) is seen in some infants with such congenital heart defects.

The cause of congenital heart defects is not clearly understood, although one cause, rubella, has been identified. The fetuses of mothers who contract the rubella virus during the first three months of pregnancy are at great risk of developing congenital rubella syndrome (CRS), a catch-all term for a wide variety of congenital defects, including heart defects, deafness, cataracts, and mental retardation. Other hypotheses about the development of congenital heart disease implicate environmental

pollutants, maternal use of drugs, including alcohol, during pregnancy, and unknown genetic factors (see the Star box above).

Treatment of congenital defects usually requires surgery, although some conditions may respond well to drug therapy. Defective blood vessels and certain malformations of the heart can be surgically repaired. This surgery is so successful that many children respond quickly to the increased circulation and oxygenation. Many are able to lead normal, active lives.

Rheumatic Heart Disease

Rheumatic heart disease is the final stage in a series of complications started by a streptococcal infection of the throat (strep throat). The Star box above lists common symptoms of strep throat. This bacterial infection, if untreated, can result in an inflammatory disease called rheumatic fever (and a related condition, scarlet fever). Rheumatic fever is a whole-body (systemic) reaction that can produce fever, joint pain, skin rashes, and possible brain and heart damage. A person who has had rheumatic fever is more susceptible to subsequent attacks. Rheumatic

Key Terms

rheumatic heart disease chronic damage to the heart (especially the heart valves) resulting from a streptococcal infection within the heart; a complication of rheumatic fever.

fever tends to run in families. About 1.8 million Americans suffer from various stages of rheumatic heart disease. In 2001, this disease killed 3,489 people.

Damage from rheumatic fever centers on the heart's valves. For some reason the bacteria tend to proliferate in the heart valves. Defective heart valves may fail either to open fully (stenosis) or to close fully (insufficiency). A physician initially might diagnose valve damage when she hears a backwashing or backflow of blood (a **murmur**). Further tests, including chest X rays, cardiac catheterization, and echocardiography, can reveal the extent of valve damage. After it is identified, a faulty valve can be replaced surgically with a metal or plastic artificial valve or a valve taken from an animal's heart.

Congestive Heart Failure

Congestive heart failure is a condition in which the heart lacks the strength to continue to circulate blood normally throughout the body. During congestive heart failure, the heart continues to work, but it cannot function well enough to maintain appropriate circulation. Venous blood flow starts to "back up." Swelling occurs, especially in the legs and ankles. Fluid can collect in the lungs and cause breathing difficulties and shortness of breath, and kidney function may be damaged. In 2001, congestive heart failure led to 52,828 deaths in the United States.[1]

Congestive heart failure can result from heart damage caused by congenital heart defects, lung disease, rheumatic fever, heart attack, atherosclerosis, or high blood pressure. Generally, congestive heart failure is treatable through a combined program of rest, proper diet, modified daily activities, and the use of appropriate drugs. Without medical care, congestive heart failure can be fatal.

Other Heart Diseases

Peripheral Artery Disease

Peripheral artery disease (PAD), also called peripheral vascular disease (PVD), is a blood vessel disease characterized by pathological changes to the arteries and arterioles in the extremities (primarily the legs and feet but sometimes the hands). PAD affects approximately 10 million Americans. These changes result from years of damage to the peripheral blood vessels. Important causes of PAD are cigarette smoking, a high-fat diet, obesity, and sedentary occupations. In some cases, PAD is aggravated by blood vessel changes resulting from diabetes.

PAD severely restricts blood flow to the extremities. The reduction in blood flow is responsible for leg pain or cramping during exercise, numbness, tingling, coldness, and loss of hair on the affected limb. The most serious consequence of PAD is the increased likelihood of developing ulcerations and tissue death. These conditions can lead to gangrene and may eventually necessitate amputation.

PAD is treated in multiple ways, including efforts to improve blood lipid levels (through diet, exercise, or drug therapy), to reduce hypertension, to reduce body weight, and to eliminate smoking. Blood vessel surgery may be a possibility.

Arrhythmias

Arrhythmias are disorders of the heart's normal sequence of electrical activity that are experienced by more than 2 million Americans. They result in an irregular beating pattern of the heart. Arrhythmias can be so brief that they do not affect the overall heart rate. Some arrhythmias, however, can last for long periods of time and cause the heart to beat either too slowly or too fast. A slow beating pattern is called a **bradycardia** (fewer than 60 beats per minute) and a fast beating pattern is called a **tachycardia** (more than 100 beats per minute).

Hearts that beat too slowly may be unable to pump a sufficient amount of blood throughout the body. The body becomes starved of oxygen, and loss of consciousness and even death can occur. Hearts that beat too rapidly do not allow the ventricles to fill sufficiently. When this happens, the heart cannot pump enough blood

---

Key Terms

murmur an atypical heart sound that suggests a backflow of blood into a chamber of the heart from which it has just left.

congestive heart failure inability of the heart to pump out all the blood that returns to it; can lead to dangerous fluid accumulations in veins, lungs, and kidneys.

peripheral artery disease (PAD) atherosclerotic blockages that occur in arteries that supply blood to the legs and arms.

bradycardia slowness of the heartbeat, as evidenced by a resting pulse rate of less than 60.

tachycardia excessively rapid heartbeat, as evidenced by a resting pulse rate of greater than 100.

throughout the body. The heart becomes, in effect, a very inefficient machine. It beats rapidly but cannot pump much blood from its ventricles. This pattern may lead to fibrillation, which is the life-threatening, rapid uncoordinated contractions of the heart. Interestingly, whether the heart pumps too slowly or too rapidly, the result is the same: inadequate blood flow throughout the body.

The person most prone to arrhythmia is a person with some form of heart disease, including atherosclerosis, hypertension, or inflammatory or degenerative conditions. The prevalence of arrhythmia tends to increase with age. Certain congenital defects may make a person more likely to have an arrhythmia. Some chemical agents, including high or low levels of minerals (potassium, magnesium, and calcium) in the blood, addictive substances (caffeine, tobacco, other drugs), and various cardiac medications, can all provoke arrhythmias.

Arrhythmias are most frequently diagnosed through an ECG (electrocardiogram), which records electrical activity of the heart. After diagnosis, a range of therapeutic approaches can be used, including simple monitoring (if the problem is relatively minor), drug therapy, use of a pacemaker, or the use of implantable defibrillators.

Related Cardiovascular Conditions

Besides the cardiovascular diseases already discussed, the heart and blood vessels are also subject to other pathological conditions. Tumors of the heart, although rare, occur. Infectious conditions involving the pericardial sac that surrounds the heart (*pericarditis*) and the innermost layer of the heart (*endocarditis*) are more commonly seen. Some people develop serious diseases of the heart valves. In addition, inflammation of the veins (*phlebitis*) is troublesome to some people.

Taking Charge of Your Health

- Complete the Personal Assessment on pages 359–360 to determine your risk for heart attack and stroke.
- Review the Food Guide Pyramid in Chapter 5 (page 143), and make changes to your diet so that it is more "heart healthy."
- Begin or continue an aerobic exercise program that is appropriate for your current fitness level.
- If you are a smoker, resolve to quit smoking. Visit your physician to talk about safe and effective approaches. Begin putting your plan into action.

- Develop a plan to lower your dietary intake of fat to keep your blood cholesterol level low.
- Have your blood pressure checked, and review your weight, physical activity, alcohol intake, and salt intake to determine whether you can make changes in any of these areas.
- If you are overweight or obese, develop a plan to combine dietary changes and increased physical activity to lose weight gradually but steadily.

Summary

- Cardiovascular diseases are responsible for more disabilities and deaths than any other disease.
- The vascular system refers to the body's blood vessels, including arteries, veins, arterioles, capillaries, and venules.
- A cardiovascular risk factor is an attribute that a person has or is exposed to that increases the likelihood of heart disease.
- The "big six" risk factors are tobacco smoke, physical inactivity, high blood cholesterol level, high blood pressure, diabetes mellitus, and obesity and overweight. These are risk factors that can be changed.
- Smokers have a heart attack risk that is more than twice that of nonsmokers. However, the risk of heart disease declines rapidly if the smoker quits.

- Regular aerobic exercise helps strengthen the heart muscle, maintain healthy blood vessels, and improve the vascular system's ability to transport blood and oxygen to the body.
- People with high blood cholesterol should eat a heart-healthy diet and become physically active.
- The six major forms of cardiovascular disease are coronary artery disease, hypertension, stroke, congenital heart disease, rheumatic heart disease, and congestive heart failure.
- Each form of heart disease develops in a unique way and requires specialized treatment.
- Moderate alcohol consumption may be related to a lower risk of heart disease. However, heavy drinking increases cardiovascular disease risk.

- Weight reduction, physical activity, lowering alcohol use, sodium restriction, meditation, and antihypertensive drugs are often used to control hypertension.

- Other heart diseases include peripheral artery disease and heart arrhythmias.

Review Questions

1. Identify the principal components of the cardiovascular system. Trace the path of blood through the heart and cardiovascular system.
2. How much blood does the average adult have? What are some of the important functions of blood?
3. Define *cardiovascular risk factor*. What relationship do risk factors have to cardiovascular disease?
4. Identify the risk factors for cardiovascular disease that cannot be changed. Identify the risk factors that can be changed. Identify the risk factor that is a contributing factor.
5. Describe the relationship between smoking and heart disease, including the role of environmental tobacco smoke. Explain the cardiovascular benefits of quitting smoking.
6. What is C-reactive protein? What role might it play regarding cardiovascular disease?

7. What are the six major forms of cardiovascular disease? For each of these diseases, describe the disease, its cause (if known), and its treatment. Describe some additional CVDs.
8. Describe how high-density lipoproteins differ from low-density lipoproteins.
9. What problems does atherosclerosis produce?
10. Why is hypertension called the "silent killer"? What serious health problems can hypertension cause?
11. What are the warning signals of stroke? Identify and describe each of the four types of stroke.
12. What is a heart arrhythmia and what are its consequences? Identify the two main heart arrhythmia patterns.

References

1. American Heart Association. *Heart disease and stroke statistical update.* AHA, 2004.
2. Thibodeau GA, Patton KT. *Structure and function of the human body,* 11th ed. Mosby-Year Book, 2000.
3. Brubaker PH, Kaminsky LA, Whaley MH. *Coronary Artery Disease,* Human Kinetics, 2002.
4. American Heart Association: **www.americanheart. org/hbp/risk_afam.html,** 21 July 2003.
5. Centers for Disease Control and Prevention. **www.cdc. gov/tobacco/oshsummary02.htm,** 16 July, 2003.
6. Centers for Disease Control and Prevention. *CDC's National Physical Activity Initiative Fact Sheet.* 17 November 1999.
7. Sesso HD, Paffenbarger RS, Lee I. Physical activity and coronary heart disease in men: the Harvard alumni health study. *Circulation,* 2000; Vol 102, pp. 975–980.
8. Lee I, Sesso HD, Paffenbarger RS. Physical activity and coronary heart disease in men: does the duration of exercise episodes predict risk? *Circulation,* 2000; Vol. 102, pp. 981–986.
9. Diabetes and heart disease: new strategies emerge. *Harvard Heart Letter,* July 2000; Vol. 10: No. 11. pp. 1–4.
10. National Institutes of Health. *Clinical Guidelines on the Identification, Evaluation, and Treatment of Overweight and Obesity in Adults.* 1998.
11. American Heart Association. Homocyst(e)ine, diet, and cardiovascular diseases. *Circulation* 99:178–82, 1999.
12. American Heart Association. Markers of Inflammation and Cardiovascular Disease. *Circulation,* 2003; Vol. 107, pp. 499–511.
13. Cholesterol: up with the good. *Harvard Health Letter,* July 1995; Vol. 5; No. 11, pp. 3–4.
14. American Heart Association/American College of Sports Medicine. Automated external defibrillators in health/fitness facilities. *Circulation* 105:1147–1150, 2002.
15. Women and heart disease. *Harvard Heart Letter,* February 2000; Vol 10: No. 5, pp. 1–4.
16. National Center for Health Statistics. *Health, United States,* 2002.
17. National Heart, Lung, and Blood Institute. *The Seventh Report of the Joint National Committee on Prevention, Detection, Evaluation, and Treatment of High Blood Pressure (JNC 7).* **www.nhlbi.nih.gov/ guidelines/hypertension/index.htm,** 21 July 2003.

The 2004 meeting of the American College of Cardiology included up-to-date research on heart disease. Among the many notable findings presented were information about the value of newer markers for heart disease that can be obtained from blood tests. These tests, which include C-reactive protein and subfractions of LDL and HDL cholesterol, are becoming increasingly available and are especially important for those with a family history of heart disease.

focus on

hypertension in african americans: targeting prevention

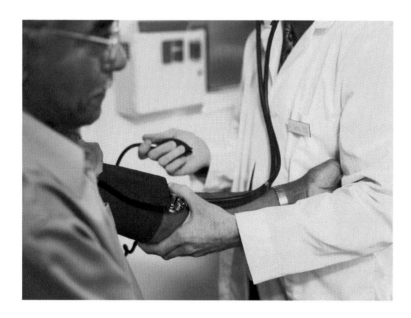

Development of disease is an area in which each societal group is disadvantaged in one way or another. Practically every group has a tendency to develop one or more afflictions at a higher rate than the general population. For the African American community, one particular problem is hypertension.

The existing data show that hypertension is more common in African Americans[1,2] and is more aggressive and less well managed in African Americans than in whites. African Americans also have higher rates of morbidity and mortality from diseases related to high blood pressure, such as stroke and renal failure. The natural nocturnal fall in blood pressure is less pronounced in African Americans, and their systolic blood pressure while awake is higher than in people of other races.[1]

The exact causes of these differences have not been pinpointed, but research

seems to be focused in two general areas. Some research suggests that certain physical and genetic factors contribute to increased incidence of hypertension in African Americans, whereas other studies have shown that hypertension in African Americans is related to environmental stress. This debate involves not just medical data but socioeconomic factors as well. In short, it is a nature vs. nurture debate, and there are supporting data for both arguments.

Nature vs. Nurture

Studies have shown that environmental stress may contribute to increased hypertension in African Americans. A study conducted by Dr. Norman Anderson of Duke University[3] shows that chronic stress may lead to an increase in the release of the hormone norepinephrine to the bloodstream. Norepinephrine reduces the amount of salt eliminated from the

kidneys, and the resulting increase in blood volume can lead to increased blood pressure. This chain reaction has been shown to occur in animal studies. The high rate of chronic exposure to stress in many African American communities has been well documented.[3] If these studies hold true for humans, it would lend credence to the idea that certain stressful factors found in some African American communities could cause hypertension. Stressors such as poverty, unemployment, the threat of violence, and racial discrimination could be shown to cause kidneys to reduce elimination of salt and thus may also increase the risk of hypertension.[3]

Anger in response to racism may be a significant contributing factor in increased hypertension in African Americans. A study conducted jointly at the University of Tennessee and Saint Louis University showed that blood pressure in African Americans increased significantly when they were shown film clips of racially motivated violence.[6] The responses of African Americans to these scenes of racial discrimination were more pronounced than their responses to viewing scenes that were anger-provoking but had no racial component. The increases in blood pressure were not into the hypertension range, but researchers believe that over time, such continued elevation of blood pressure could become dangerous.

Such conclusions seem to suggest that socioeconomic factors are the main cause of hypertension among African Americans. A study performed on twenty-six African American women on strict low-fat diets seems to support this. The data showed that women of higher socioeconomic

Suggested Lifestyle Modifications to Control or Reduce the Risk of Hypertension[4,5]

Stop smoking	A first heart attack convinces many people to quit smoking, but don't wait—you may not get a second chance.
Lose weight if you are overweight or obese	Losing 5% to 10% of your body weight drastically reduces your disease risk factors.
Reduce sodium intake	Consume < 2,400 mg of sodium per day. Excess sodium raises blood pressure in salt-sensitive people.
Moderate alcohol intake	Intake of alcohol above moderate levels increases blood pressure. Men should have no more than two drinks a day, and women should have no more than one drink a day.
Exercise regularly	Sedentary people have a 50% greater chance of developing hypertension. One simple plan for increasing your physical activity is to walk briskly 30 to 45 minutes three to five times per week.
Increase potassium intake	Potassium works to control blood volume and therefore blood pressure. Eat at least five servings of fruits and vegetables a day. Good sources of potassium are potatoes, tomatoes, bananas, and orange juice.
Maintain an adequate intake of calcium and magnesium	These minerals are important to blood pressure regulation. Eat two to three portions of low-fat milk or cheese per day and consider a calcium supplement.
Seek appropriate prenatal care during pregnancy	Prenatal visits help to ensure delivery of healthy babies whose kidneys are adequately developed. Follow your doctor's recommendations.
Consult your physician regularly	He or she can help you comply with and personalize your hypertension control program.

Note: If blood pressure cannot be controlled with these lifestyle changes, then medication is necessary. It is critical that individuals with hypertension take their medication no matter how good they feel.

status had more excretion of salt than those of lower status.[3] Since proportionately more African Americans are in lower socioeconomic classes than whites, increased stress from lower status could be the main factor behind the inflated rate of hypertension among the African American population.

But is it all due to environment? Perhaps not. Other groups of traditionally lower socioeconomic status, such as Hispanics, Asians, and Native Americans, have been found to have the same incidence of hypertension as whites.[1] African American children have been found to have higher blood pressure in general than white children;[1] it is not known whether stress plays a significant role in affecting the blood pressure of these children so early in life.

There is also evidence that African Americans may be predisposed to hypertension at the cellular level. Microscopic studies of blood vessels in African Americans with severe hypertension revealed that renal arterioles were thickened and had reduced flow. This thickening, not found in the renal arterioles of hypertensive whites, was caused by hypertrophy (excess growth) of smooth muscle cells in the

muscle walls of the arterioles. This thickening reduced the size of the lumen (inside opening) of the vessels, and the resulting reduced blood flow may have caused increased blood pressure. The smooth muscle cells were thought to be responding abnormally to growth factors, which caused the hypertrophy to occur.[2] The reason behind this abnormal reaction was not determined, however.

The best explanation of why African Americans are more prone to develop hypertension may not involve environment or genetics alone, but a combination of the two. Stress factors unique to the African American community may serve to aggravate or intensify an existing physical predisposition toward hypertension. It has already been shown that the tendency toward developing hypertension can be passed from parents to their children. Add several unique stress factors to a population already predisposed to high blood pressure, and the potential exists for high numbers of people to develop hypertension. Commenting on the UT-SLU study, Dr. Elijah Saunders agreed that "racism and Black rage are emotional stressors that could worsen a physiological tendency toward hypertension."[6]

Treatment of Hypertension in African Americans

The good news is that African Americans respond to medical treatment in a similar manner to whites. The treatment regimen for African Americans may have to be altered somewhat, however, since they do not respond as well to some hypertension medications as people of other races. For unknown reasons, drugs such as beta blockers and ACE (angiotensin converting enzyme) inhibitors do not work as well in African Americans and may need to be supplemented by other medications, such as diuretics.[1]

Lifestyle changes may also be needed and may be a more effective tool in lowering blood pressure in African Americans than in people of other races.[1] Effort should be made to exercise and lose weight if needed, since excess weight can be a contributing factor in hypertension. Hypertensive African Americans tend to have lower intakes of potassium and calcium, so diet changes should be made that ensure that these minerals are in adequate supply. A reduction in sodium may also be desirable, since research suggests that African Americans may be more sensitive to the effects of sodium on the cardiovascular system.[1]

Although African Americans are more likely to develop high blood pressure, prevention and treatment can help keep hypertension from becoming a deadly affliction. Proper diagnosis is essential, so people at risk should see their doctors to determine whether they have hypertension or are at risk for developing it. Through recommending lifestyle modifications, prescribing medications, or both, a physician can help manage this condition or help prevent its onset.[7]

For Discussion . . .

Do you feel that people in lower (or higher) socioeconomic groups suffer more from everyday stress? Do you believe physiological or genetic differences may exist between different ethnic or racial groups?

References

1. Kaplan NM. Ethnic aspects of hypertension. *Lancet* 1994; 344(8920).
2. Dustan HP. Growth factors and racial differences in severity of hypertension and renal diseases. *Lancet* 1992; 339:(8805).
3. Haywood RI. Why Black Americans suffer with more high blood pressure than Whites. *Jet* 5 December 1994; 87(5).
4. Kaplan NM. High blood pressure— why do we have it? And what are we doing about it? *Saturday Evening Post* 1997; 269(1): 48–52.
5. Alkinson RL Jr., Calloway CW, St. Jeor S, Wolf-Novak L. A sane approach to weight loss. *Patient Care* 1995; 29(18): 152–55.
6. Study reveals anger over racism causes high blood pressure in Blacks. *Jet* 14 May 1990; 78(5).
7. Too little attention paid to high blood pressure. *Tufts University Health and Nutrition Letter* January 1998; (15:11) p. 1.

Infolinks

www.libov.com
www.womensheartinstitute.com

personal assessment

what is your risk for heart disease?

Cholesterol

Your serum cholesterol level is:

0	190 or below
+ 2	191 to 230
+ 6	231 to 289
+12	290 to 319
+16	Over 320

Your HDL cholesterol is:

− 2	Over 60
0	45 to 60
+ 2	35 to 44
+ 6	29 to 34
+12	23 to 28
+16	Below 23

Smoking

You smoke now or have in the past:

0	Never smoked, or quit more than 5 years ago
+1	Quit 2 to 4 years ago
+3	Quit about 1 year ago
+6	Quit during the past year

You now smoke:

+ 9	½ to 1 pack a day
+12	1 to 2 packs a day
+15	More than 2 packs a day

The quality of the air you breathe is:

0	Unpolluted by smoke, exhaust, or industry at home and at work
+2	Live or work with smokers in unpolluted area
+4	Live and work with smokers in unpolluted area
+6	Live or work with smokers **and** live or work in air-polluted area
+8	Live **and** work with smokers **and** live and work in air-polluted area

Blood Pressure

Your blood pressure is:

0	120/75 or below
+ 2	120/75 to 140/85
+ 6	140/85 to 150/90
+ 8	150/90 to 175/100
+10	175/100 to 190/110
+12	190/110 or above

Exercise

Your exercise habits are:

0	Exercise vigorously 4 or 5 times a week
+2	Exercise moderately 4 or 5 times a week
+4	Exercise only on weekends
+6	Exercise occasionally
+8	Little or no exercise

Weight

Your weight is:

0	Always at or near ideal weight
+1	Now 10% overweight
+2	Now 20% overweight
+3	Now 30% or more overweight
+4	Now 20% or more overweight and have been since before age 30

Stress

You feel overstressed:

0	Rarely at work or at home
+ 3	Somewhat at home but not at work
+ 5	Somewhat at work but not at home
+ 7	Somewhat at work **and** at home
+ 9	Usually at work **or** at home
+12	Usually at work **and** at home

Diabetes

Your diabetic history is:

0	Blood sugar always normal
+2	Blood glucose slightly high (prediabetic) or slightly low (hypoglycemic)
+4	Diabetic beginning after age 40 requiring strict dietary or insulin control
+5	Diabetic beginning before age 30 requiring strict dietary or insulin control

Alcohol

You drink alcoholic beverages:

0	Never or only socially, about once or twice a month, or only one 5-ounce glass of wine or 12-ounce glass of beer or 1½ ounces of hard liquor about 5 times a week
+2	Two to three 5-ounce glasses of wine or 12-ounce glasses of beer or 1½-ounce cocktails about 5 times a week
+4	More than three 1½-ounce cocktails or more than three 5-ounce glasses of wine or 12-ounce glasses of beer almost every day

Interpretation

Add all sources and check below.

0 to 20:   **Low risk.** Excellent family history and lifestyle habits.

21 to 50:   **Moderate risk.** Family history or lifestyle habits put you at some risk. You might lower your risks and minimize your genetic predisposition if you change any poor habits.

51 to 74: **High risk.** Habits and family history indicate high risk of heart disease. Change your habits now.

Above 75: **Very high risk.** Family history and a lifetime of poor habits put you at very high risk of heart disease. Eliminate as many of the risk factors as you can.

To Carry This Further . . .

Were you surprised with your score on this assessment? What were your most significant risk factors? Do you plan to make any changes in your lifestyle to reduce your cardiovascular risks? Why or why not?

chapter eleven

living with cancer

Chapter Objectives

Upon completing this chapter, you will be able to:

■ describe cancer statistics and identify groups who are at high risk for developing particular forms of cancer.

■ explain the role of cell regulation in the development of cancer, and discuss the relationship of genetic mutations, viral infections, and carcinogens to the loss of cell regulation.

■ name specific steps that individuals can take to aid in early detection of specific cancers.

■ explain and discuss the role of self-examination in detecting certain cancers, including breast cancer, melanoma, and testicular cancer.

■ discuss the importance of medical screening for specific cancers, and identify several procedures used to screen for particular forms of cancer.

■ offer several lifestyle changes that effectively reduce your cancer risk.

■ summarize the status of our current "War on Cancer."

Online Learning Center Resources

www.mhhe.com/payne8e

Log on to our Online Learning Center (OLC) for access to these additional resources:

- Chapter key terms and definitions
- Learning objectives
- Student interactive question-and-answer sites

- Online assessments
- Key term flash cards
- Self-scoring chapter quiz

Talking It Over

Telling Coworkers about Your Cancer

When you decide it's time to tell your boss and coworkers that you have cancer, you'll have many things to consider—how much information to give, how this news will affect other people's perception of you, and how your condition will affect your ability to do your job.

- Tell people what they need to know.
- Ask for help when you need it, but remember that your coworkers have their own responsibilities.

- Consider how you want to present yourself—as a victim or a fighter—because your coworkers are likely to reinforce your attitude.

CommunicationLinks

Living With It www.livingwithit.org
Prostate Info www.prostateinfo.com

Eye on the Media

Support Is Just a Click Away

Support groups are composed of people who come together to help each other through the demands of a chronic health condition. These groups have traditionally been organized by institutions in the local health care community, such as hospitals, by the local affiliates of national organizations, such as the American Cancer Society, or by citizens who have the same chronic condition. Increasingly common today, however, we find support groups whose members are connected, not by physical proximity, but by the Internet.

Health self-help groups on the Internet develop in one of two ways. The first occurs when a brick-and-mortar organization, such as a national agency or health care institution, develops a support group for its homepage. The second way is for a person with the condition (or a family member of that person) to organize an online group.

You can find a health support group simply by surfing the net. Or you can be referred to a site by a health care professional, friend, family member, colleague, or someone with a similar condition. You can also go to the

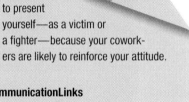

Eye on the Media *continued*
homepage of a medical institution or a national agency to find out if it provides a support group link.

For someone with a newly diagnosed chronic condition, the initial contact with a support group may be made to get information about the condition and its treatment. For others, it is a way of connecting with other people who have the condition. Web support groups provide windows to the outside world, particularly for those whose conditions limit their mobility and social contacts. The Internet support group transcends the restrictions of various diseases to make new connections possible.

It's important to realize that the online support group's members are rarely physicians or other highly trained health professionals, so you shouldn't rely on this source for specific technical information. Instead, your main sources of information about medical management of a chronic condition should be your health care providers. Seasoned members of support groups need to remind themselves that newly diagnosed members are inexperienced and vulnerable. It will take them time to adjust to the frankness and clinical sophistication demonstrated by some group members in addressing their health problems.

Some hospitals provide laptop computers to patients so they can maintain contact with their support groups. In this way, health care institutions are encouraging patients to support their efforts and, perhaps, helping them recover more quickly.

Most people can attest to the disruptive influence an illness can have on their ability to participate in day-to-day activities. When we are ill, school, employment, and leisure activities are replaced by periods of lessened activity and even periods of bed rest or hospitalization. When an illness is chronic, the effect of being ill may extend over long periods, perhaps even an entire lifetime. People with chronic illness must eventually find a balance between day-to-day function and the continuous presence of their condition. Cancer is usually a chronic illness.

In spite of our understanding of its relationship to human health and our ceaseless attempts to prevent and cure it, progress in "the war on cancer" has been relatively limited. In this regard, cancer is clearly an "expensive" condition, both in terms of its human consequences and its monetary costs. It is estimated that 1,334,100 people developed cancer in 2003 and that, since 1990, nearly 17 million new cases of cancer have developed in this country. Once diagnosed, approximately 62% (adjusted for other causes of death) of this group will be alive 5 years later.[1] The 5-year period that defines *relative survivability* encompasses "persons who are living 5 years after diagnosis, whether disease free, in remission, or under treatment with evidence of cancer."[1] Understandably, the use of the term *cured* is guarded since an initially diagnosed case of cancer can impact on survivability beyond the end of the 5-year time period. Regardless of survivability, for those who develop cancer, the physical, emotional, and social costs will be substantial.

The financial cost of cancer to society is also troublesome. The National Institutes of Health (NIH) estimates that in 2001 alone cancer cost the American economy 171.6 billion dollars, including 95.2 billion for loss of productivity due to death, 60.9 billion for direct medical costs, and 15.5 billion for indirect costs due to loss of productivity during treatment and recovery.[1] Not reflected in this total is the sizable amount of money spent on primary cancer prevention, such as school-based programs, public

Chemotherapy is a treatment for many types of cancer.

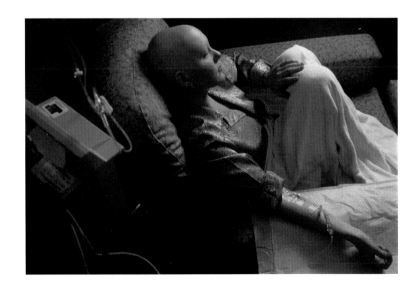

education efforts, and lobbying efforts intended to remove harmful products and pollutants from the environment.

No single explanation can be given for why progress in eliminating cancer has been so limited. It is a combination of factors, including the aging of the population, continued use of tobacco, the high-fat American diet, the continuing urbanization and pollution of our environment, the lack of health insurance for an estimated 41.2 million Americans to pay for early diagnosis and proper treatment,[2] or simply our recognition of cancer's true role in deaths once ascribed to other causes. Regardless, we continue to be challenged to control this array of abnormal conditions that we collectively call cancer. There is, however, increasing optimism that with new pharmacological agents and the completion of the Human Genome Project real progress will finally be made.

 TALKING POINTS A close friend justifies her high cancer–risk lifestyle by saying that "Everyone will die of something." How would you counter this point?

Cancer: A Problem of Cell Regulation

Just as a corporation depends on individuals to staff its various departments, the body depends on its basic units of function, the cells. Cells band together as tissues, such as muscle tissue, to perform a prescribed function. Tissues in turn join to form organs, such as the heart, and organs are assembled into the body's several organ systems, such as the cardiovascular system. Such is the "corporate structure" of the body.

If individuals and cells are the basic units of function for their respective organizations, the failure of either to perform in a prescribed, dependable manner can erode the overall organization to the extent that it might not be able to continue. Cancer, the second leading cause of death among adults, is a condition reflecting cell dysfunction in its most extreme form. In cancer, the normal behavior of cells ceases.

Cell Regulation

Most of the body's tissues lose cells over time. This continual loss requires that replacement cells come from areas of young and less specialized cells. The process of specialization required to turn the less specialized cells into mature cells is controlled by genes within the cells. On becoming specialized, these newest cells copy, or replicate, themselves. These two processes are carefully monitored by the cells' **regulatory genes.** Failure to regulate specialization and replication results in abnormal, or potentially cancerous, cells.

In addition to genes that regulate specialization and replication, cells also have genes designed to repair mistakes in the copying of genetic material (the basis of replication) and genes to suppress the growth of abnormal cells should it occur. Thus, repair genes and tumor suppressor genes, such as the *p53* gene (altered or missing in half of all cancers), can also be considered regulatory genes in place to prevent the development of abnormal cells. Should these genes fail to function properly, resulting in the development of malignant (cancerous) cells, the immune system (see Chapter 13) will ideally recognize their presence and remove them before a clinical (diagnosable) case of cancer can develop.

Because specialization, replication, repair, and suppressor genes can become cancer-causing genes, or **oncogenes,** when not working properly, these four types of genes could also be referred to as **proto-oncogenes,** or potential oncogenes.[3] How proto-oncogenes become oncogenes is a question that cannot be completely answered at this time. Regardless, abnormal cells produce abnormal proteins, and the absence of normal proteins alters the body's ability to function appropriately, from the molecular to the organ system level.

Oncogene Formation

Recognizing that all cells have proto-oncogenes, what events alter otherwise normal regulatory genes so that they become cancer-causing genes? Three mechanisms, genetic mutations, viral infections, and carcinogens, have received much attention.

Genetic mutations develop when dividing cells miscopy genetic information. If the gene that is miscopied is a gene that controls specialization, replication, repair, or tumor suppression (a proto-oncogene), the oncogene that results will allow the formation of cancerous cells. A variety of factors, including aging, free radical formation, and radiation, are associated with the miscopying of the complex genetic information that comprises the genes found within the cell, including those intended to prevent cancer.

In both animals and humans, cancer-producing viruses, such as the feline leukemia virus in cats and the

---

Key Terms

regulatory genes genes that control cell specialization, replication, DNA repair, and tumor suppression.

oncogenes faulty regulatory genes that are believed to activate the development of cancer.

proto-oncogenes (pro toe **on** co genes) normal regulatory genes that may become oncogenes.

human immunodeficiency virus (HIV) and multiple forms of the human papilloma virus (HPV) in humans (see Chapter 13), have been identified. These viruses seek out cells of a particular type, such as cells of the immune system or the lining of the cervix, and substitute some of their genetic material for some of the cells' thus converting them into virus-producing cells. In so doing, however, they change the makeup of the specialization, replication, repair, or suppressor genes, converting the proto-oncogenes into oncogenes. Once converted into oncogenes, the altered genes are passed on through cell division.

A third possible explanation for the conversion of proto-oncogenes into oncogenes involves the presence of environmental agents known as *carcinogens.* Over an extended period, carcinogens, such as chemicals found in tobacco smoke, polluted air and water, toxic wastes, and even high-fat foods, may convert proto-oncogenes into oncogenes. These carcinogens may work alone or in combination with co-carcinogenic promoters (see Chapter 9, Table 9.2) to alter the genetic material, including regulatory genes, within cells. Thus people might develop lung cancer only if they are exposed to the right combination of carcinogens over an extended period.

You may already see that some of the specific risk factors in each area—such as radiation in the development of mutations, sexually transmitted viruses in cancers of the reproductive tract, and smoking introduced carcinogens in the development of lung cancer—can be moderated by adopting health-promoting behaviors.

Our understanding of the role of genes in the development of cancer is expanding rapidly. Through ongoing research, including the Human Genome Project, the scientific community has now identified over three dozen genes that function as oncogenes in a variety of cancers. On occasion the public learns the identity of selected oncogenes. Very likely many readers have heard of the *BRCA1* and *BRCA2* genes associated with breast and ovarian cancer, the RAS oncogene thought to influence 30% of all cancers, and the *p53* suppressor oncogene that may be involved in more cancers than any other single oncogene. As geneticists continue to build on the base established by the recently completed Human Genome Project and in doing so discover additional genetic links to cancer, the possibility of some form of oncogene suppressor technology becomes a more realistic possibility in the war against cancer.

In light of the complexity of cancer, some in the scientific community believe that cancer can never be truly prevented. Rather, they feel that the ability to stop and then reverse cancerous changes at an early stage of their development is more likely than prevention of this complex disease process. However, this text will address the concepts of prevention in the belief that prevention-based practices reflect our personal contribution to the "war on cancer."[4]

The Cancerous Cell

Compared with noncancerous cells, cancer cells function in similar and dissimilar ways. It is the dissimilar aspects that often make them unpredictable and difficult to manage.

Perhaps the most unusual aspect of cancerous cells is their infinite life expectancy. Specifically, it appears that cancerous cells can produce an enzyme, *telomerase,* that blocks the cellular biological clock that informs normal cells that it is time to die.[5] In spite of this ability to live forever, cancer cells do not necessarily divide more quickly than normal cells. In fact, they can divide at the same rate or even on occasion at a slower rate.

In addition, cancerous cells do not possess the *contact inhibition*[6] (a mechanism that influences the number of cells that can occupy a particular space at a particular time) of normal cells. In the absence of this property, cancer cells accumulate, altering the functional capacity of the tissue or organ they occupy. Further, the absence of *cellular cohesiveness*[6] (a property seen in normal cells that "keeps them at home") allows cancer cells to spread through the circulatory or lymphatic system to distant points via **metastasis** (Figure 11-1). Interestingly, once migrating cancer cells arrive at a new area of the body, they "rediscover" their cellular cohesive capabilities. A final unique characteristic of cancerous cells is their ability to command the circulatory system to send them additional blood supply to meet their metabolic needs and to provide additional routes for metastasis. This *angiogenesis*[6] capability of cancer cells makes them extremely hardy compared with noncancerous cells.

Staging Cancer

In light of the interesting capabilities of malignant cells just described, it is critically important in the diagnosis and treatment of cancer that *oncologists* (physicians who have specialized in the care of cancer patients) know not only the type of cancer, but also its extent. This latter determination is reflected in the concept of "staging" cancer.

For purposes of effective communication regarding the staging of cancer, the international medical community has adopted the *TNS* staging system.[1] This system

---

Key Terms

metastasis (muh **tas** ta sis) the spread of cancerous cells from their site of origin to other areas of the body.

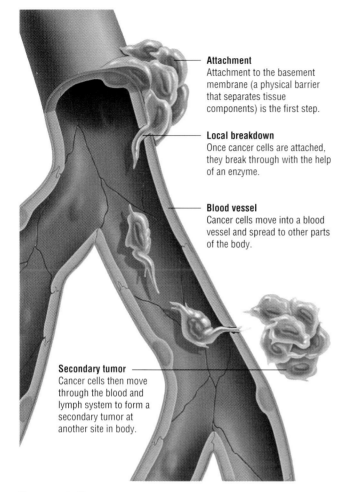

Attachment
Attachment to the basement membrane (a physical barrier that separates tissue components) is the first step.

Local breakdown
Once cancer cells are attached, they break through with the help of an enzyme.

Blood vessel
Cancer cells move into a blood vessel and spread to other parts of the body.

Secondary tumor
Cancer cells then move through the blood and lymph system to form a secondary tumor at another site in body.

Figure 11-1 How cancer spreads. Locomotion (movement) is essential to the process of metastasis (spread of cancer). Scientists have identified a protein that causes cancer cells to grow arms, or pseudopodia, enabling them to move to other parts of the body.

first identifies the extent of a malignancy as to whether it is primary (T), whether it has or has not progressed to regional lymph node involvement (N), and the presence or absence of metastasis (S). Upon establishing a TNS profile of the tumor, a numerical stage (I, II, III, or IV) is determined. This categorization reflects: (I) *in situ* or "at the point of origin", (II) *Local*—an invasive cancer confined to the organ of origin, (III) *Regional*—cancer extended into the immediately neighboring tissue or into regional lymph nodes, and (IV) *Distant*—cancer extended to distant parts of the body, either by discontinuous metastasis or through the lymphatic drainage to distant nodes.

On the basis of the system described above, important decisions regarding treatment, management, and prognosis (survivability) of the cancer are made—information important to all persons involved in the medical care to be received.

Benign Tumors

Noncancerous, or **benign,** tumors can also form in the body. These **tumors** are usually enclosed by a membrane and do not spread from their point of origin. Benign tumors can be dangerous when they crowd out normal tissue within a confined space.

Types of Cancer

Again, for the purposes of effective diagnosis and appropriate treatment, cancers can be named or labeled on the basis of their cell type of origin (such as hepatoma) and/or the organ in which they are located (such as the liver). To the medical community, the name of cancers, based on the cell type of origin, is most often used in making determination regarding diagnosis and treatment, while for the general public, the labeling of cancer on the basis of the organ of origin is more familiar and understandable. In this section the labeling based on the cell type of origin will be given brief consideration, while the body of the chapter will describe cancer based on its organ of origin. In some cases labeling may also be extended back to embryonic germ layer of origin, but this is beyond the scope of your textbook.

For the majority of physicians and the patients with whom they must communicate, descriptions of cancer based on the organ of origin are technically adequate and, with explanation to patients, understandable. In the list that follows, several cell- or tissue-based cancers are discussed.[7]

carcinoma—Found most frequently in the skin, nose, mouth, throat, stomach, intestinal tract, glands, nerves, breasts, urinary and genital structures, lungs, kidneys, and liver; approximately 85% of all malignant tumors are classified as carcinomas

sarcoma—Formed in the connective tissues of the body; bone, cartilage, and tendons are the sites of sarcoma development; only 2% of all malignancies are of this type

melanoma—Arises from the melanin-containing cells of skin; found most often in people who have had extensive sun exposure, particularly a deep, penetrating sunburn; although once rare, the amount of this cancer has increased markedly in recent years; remains among the most deadly forms of cancer

Key Terms

benign noncancerous; tumors that do not spread.

tumor mass of cells; may be cancerous (malignant) or noncancerous (benign).

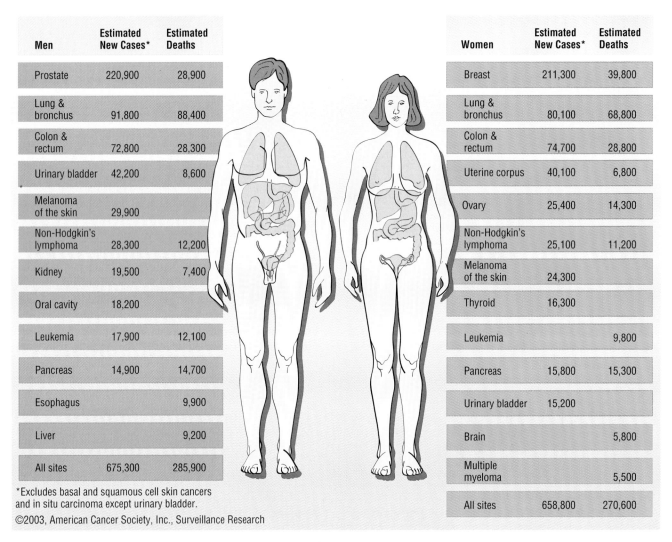

Men	Estimated New Cases*	Estimated Deaths
Prostate	220,900	28,900
Lung & bronchus	91,800	88,400
Colon & rectum	72,800	28,300
Urinary bladder	42,200	8,600
Melanoma of the skin	29,900	
Non-Hodgkin's lymphoma	28,300	12,200
Kidney	19,500	7,400
Oral cavity	18,200	
Leukemia	17,900	12,100
Pancreas	14,900	14,700
Esophagus		9,900
Liver		9,200
All sites	675,300	285,900

*Excludes basal and squamous cell skin cancers and in situ carcinoma except urinary bladder.

©2003, American Cancer Society, Inc., Surveillance Research

Women	Estimated New Cases*	Estimated Deaths
Breast	211,300	39,800
Lung & bronchus	80,100	68,800
Colon & rectum	74,700	28,800
Uterine corpus	40,100	6,800
Ovary	25,400	14,300
Non-Hodgkin's lymphoma	25,100	11,200
Melanoma of the skin	24,300	
Thyroid	16,300	
Leukemia		9,800
Pancreas	15,800	15,300
Urinary bladder	15,200	
Brain		5,800
Multiple myeloma		5,500
All sites	658,800	270,600

Figure 11-2 These 2003 estimates of new cases of cancer and deaths from cancer revealed some significant similarities between men and women. Note that lung cancer is the leading cause of cancer deaths for both genders.

neuroblastoma—Originates in the immature cells found within the central nervous system; neuroblastomas are rare; usually found in children

adenocarcinoma—Derived from cells of the endocrine glands

hepatoma—Originates in cells of the liver; although not thought to be directly caused by alcohol use, seen more frequently in people who have experienced **sclerotic changes** in the liver

leukemia—Found in cells of the blood and blood-forming tissues; characterized by abnormal, immature white blood cell formation; several forms are found in children and adults

lymphoma—Arises in cells of the lymphatic tissues or other immune system tissues; includes lymphosarco-

mas and Hodgkin's disease; characterized by abnormal white cell production and decreased resistance

Figure 11-2 presents information about the estimated new cases of cancer and deaths from cancer at various sites in both men and women.[1] Table 11.1 shows that cancer incidence and mortality rates vary among different racial and ethnic groups.

Key Terms

sclerotic changes (skluh **rot** ick) thickening or hardening of tissues.

Table 11.1 Incidence and Mortality Rates* by Site, Race, and Ethnicity, US, 1992–1999

Incidence	White	African American	Asian/ Pacific Islander	American Indian/ Alaskan Native	Hispanic[†]
All Sites					
Males	568.2	703.6	408.9	277.7	393.1
Females	424.4	404.8	306.5	224.2	290.5
Total	480.4	526.6	348.6	244.6	329.6
Breast (female)	137.0	120.7	93.4	59.4	82.6
Colon & rectum					
Males	64.4	70.7	58.7	40.7	43.9
Females	46.1	55.8	39.5	30.8	29.7
Total	53.9	61.9	47.9	35.2	35.7
Lung & bronchus					
Males	82.9	124.1	63.8	51.4	44.1
Females	51.1	53.2	28.5	23.3	22.8
Total	64.3	82.6	44.0	35.4	31.5
Prostate	172.9	275.3	107.2	60.7	127.6

Mortality	White	African American	Asian/ Pacific Islander	American Indian/ Alaskan Native	Hispanic[†]
All Sites					
Males	258.1	369.0	160.6	154.5	163.7
Females	171.2	204.5	104.4	110.4	105.7
Total	205.1	267.3	128.6	128.6	129.2
Breast (female)	29.3	37.3	13.1	14.8	17.5
Colon & rectum					
Males	26.7	34.8	16.5	14.6	16.6
Females	18.4	25.4	11.6	11.3	10.6
Total	21.9	29.1	13.7	12.8	13.2
Lung & bronchus					
Males	81.7	113.0	42.3	49.3	38.2
Females	41.1	39.6	19.3	24.9	13.8
Total	57.9	68.9	29.3	35.5	24.1
Prostate	32.9	75.1	15.1	18.8	22.6

*Per 100,000, age-adjusted to the 2000 US standard population. Incidence rates obtained from SEER registries covering 10%–15% of the US population. Mortality data are from all states.
[†]Hispanics are not mutually exclusive from whites, African Americans, Asian/Pacific Islanders, and American Indian/Alaskan Natives.
Source: Surveillance, Epidemiology, and End Results Program, 1973–99, Division of Cancer Control and Population Sciences, National Cancer Institute, Bethesda, MD, 2002.
American Cancer Society, Surveillance Research, 2003

Cancer at Selected Sites in the Body

A second and more familiar way to describe cancer is on the basis of the organ site at which it occurs. The following discussion relates to some of these more familiar sites. A lack of space, in combination with the wide arrays of human cancers, limits the number of specific malignancies that can be described. Remember also that regular screening procedures can lead to early identification of cancer at these sites (see the Changing for the Better box on page 369).

Lung Cancer

Lung cancer is one of the most lethal and frequently diagnosed forms of cancer. Primarily because of the advanced stage of the disease at the time symptoms first appear, only 15% of all people with lung cancer (all stages) survive 5 years beyond diagnosis.[1] By the time a person is sufficiently concerned about having a persistent cough, blood-streaked sputum, and chest pain, it is often too late for treatment to be effective. This failure to be able to diagnose lung cancer in its earlier stages could, however, begin to change. Currently the National Cancer Institute is studying the efficacy of *spiral CT scans* in detecting lung tumors earlier than can be done by conventional chest x-rays. However, an initial assessment of the technology questions its cost-effectiveness and potential for excessive false-positive findings.[8]

Risk Factors

Today it is known that a genetic predisposition is important in the development of lung cancer. Perhaps, in fact, the majority of people who develop this form of cancer have an inherited "head start." When people who are genetically at risk also smoke, their level of risk for developing lung cancer is significantly greater than it is for nonsmokers. Of particular interest at this time are multiple genes on chromosome 3. Damage to three tumor suppressors on this chromosome is found in virtually every case of small-cell lung cancer and 90% of nonsmall-cell lung cancer.[9] Most of the remaining lung cancer cases appear in people who smoke but are not genetically predisposed.

Cigarette smoking is the single most important behavioral factor in the development of lung cancer. For men who smoke, the rate of lung cancer is twenty-three times higher than for men who do not smoke. For women who smoke, the rate is eleven times higher than for women who do not smoke. Smokers account for nearly 90% of all cases of lung cancer, and lung cancer itself produces at least 30% of all cancer-caused deaths.[1] An earlier study also links smoking marijuana and crack cocaine with the same precancerous cellular changes to airway tissues seen in cigarette smoking. It is assumed that, like tobacco, the smoke generated by marijuana and crack contains compounds capable of damaging the important *p53* tumor suppressor gene.[10]

Since 1987, lung cancer has exceeded breast cancer as the leading cause of cancer deaths in women. The incidence of lung cancer has shown an encouraging decline in men that parallels their declining use of tobacco products, although it remains the leading cause of cancer deaths in men as well. Environmental agents, such as radon, asbestos, and air pollutants, make a smaller contribution to the development of lung cancer. Radon alone may be the principal causative agent in most lung cancer found in nonsmokers.

Prevention

The preceding information clearly suggests that not smoking or quitting smoking (see page 317) and avoidance of environmental tobacco smoke (see page 314) are the most important factors in the prevention of lung cancer. In addition, place of residence, particularly as it relates to air pollution, is a long-suspected risk factor for lung cancer.[11] Nonsmokers who are considering living with a smoker or working in a confined area where environmental tobacco smoke is prevalent should carefully consider the risk of developing lung cancer. A recent study does, however, lessen concern over moderate alcohol use and the risk of developing lung cancer.[12]

Treatment

The prognosis for surviving lung cancer remains extremely guarded. Depending on the type of lung cancer, its extent, and factors related to the patient's overall health, various combinations of surgery, radiation, and chemotherapy remain the physicians' primary approach to treatment. Today, for persons with early-stage lung cancer, chemotherapy, following surgery, has increased survivability slightly.[13] Additionally, new medications that primarily shrink tumors are also available. Although

Health on the Web

Behavior Change Activities

Learning about Cancer

The American Cancer Society is a nationwide, community-based, voluntary health organization dedicated to preventing cancer, saving lives, and diminishing suffering from cancer through research, education, advocacy, and service. Visit the American Cancer Society website at **www.cancer.org** and click on one of the many choices you are offered.

Doing Something about Breast Cancer

Breast cancer is a health issue, a family issue, and a woman's issue, and breast cancer is a political issue. Every day politicians make important decisions about breast cancer, including how much funding will be devoted to research, what resources will be allocated to the prevention of the disease, and what quality of care will be acceptable. Breast cancer policies made in the White House, Congress, and state governments can mean life or death to someone in your house. Click on **www.natlbcc.org/bin/index.htm** to learn how you can influence these decisions.

For the Early Detection of Cancer in Asymptomatic People

Site	Recommendation
Breast	Women 40 and older should have an annual mammogram, an annual clinical breast examination (CBE) by a health care professional, and should perform monthly breast self-examinations (BSE). Ideally the CBE should occur before the scheduled mammogram. Women ages 20–39 should have a CBE by a health care professional every three years and should perform BSE monthly.
Colon & rectum	Beginning at age 50, men and women should follow one of the examination schedules below: • A fecal occult blood test (FOBT) every year • A flexible sigmoidoscopy (FSIG) every five years • Annual fecal occult blood test and flexible sigmoidoscopy every five years[*] • A double-contrast barium enema every five years • A colonoscopy every 10 years *Combined testing is preferred over either annual FOBT, or FSIG every 5 years, alone. People who are at moderate or high risk for colorectal cancer should talk with a doctor about a different testing schedule.*
Prostate	The PSA test and the digital rectal examination should be offered annually, beginning at age 50, to men who have a life expectancy of at least 10 years. Men at high risk (African American men and men with a strong family history of one or more first-degree relatives diagnosed with prostate cancer at an early age) should begin testing at age 45. For both men at average risk and high risk, information should be provided about what is known and what is uncertain about the benefits and limitations of early detection and treatment of prostate cancer so that they can make an informed decision about testing.
Uterus	**Cervix:** Screening should begin approximately three years after a woman begins having vaginal intercourse, but no later than 21 years of age. Screening should be done every year with regular Pap tests or every two years using liquid-based tests. At or after age 30, women who have had three normal test results in a row may get screened every 2–3 years. However, doctors may suggest a woman get screened more often if she has certain risk factors, such as HIV infection or a weak immune system. Women 70 years and older who have had three or more consecutive normal Pap tests in the last 10 years may choose to stop cervical cancer screening. Screening after total hysterectomy (with removal of the cervix) is not necessary unless the surgery was done as a treatment for cervical cancer. **Endometrium:** The American Cancer Society recommends that all women should be informed about the risks and symptoms of endometrial cancer, and strongly encouraged to report any unexpected bleeding or spotting to their physicians. Annual screening for endometrial cancer with endometrial biopsy beginning at age 35 should be offered to women with or at risk for hereditary nonpolyposis colon cancer (HNPCC).
Cancer-related checkup	For individuals undergoing periodic health examinations, a cancer-related checkup should include health counseling, and depending on a person's age, might include examinations for cancers of the thyroid, oral cavity, skin, lymph nodes, testes, and ovaries, as well as for some nonmalignant diseases.

American Cancer Society guidelines for early cancer detection are assessed annually in order to identify whether there is new scientific evidence sufficient to warrant a re-evaluation of current recommendations. If evidence is sufficiently compelling to consider a change or clarification in a current guideline or the development of a new guideline, a formal procedure is initiated. Guidelines are formally evaluated every 5 years regardless of whether new evidence suggests a change in the existing recommendations. There are nine steps in this procedure, and these "guidelines for guideline development" were formally established to provide a specific methodology for science and expert judgment to form the underpinnings of specific statements and recommendations from the Society. These procedures constitute a deliberate process to insure that all Society recommendations have the same methodological and evidence-based process at their core. This process also employs a system for rating strength and consistency of evidence that is similar to that employed by the Agency for Health Care Research and Quality (AHCRQ) and the US Preventive Services Task Force (USPSTF).

these newer therapies have improved short-term survival, full recovery remains unlikely in all but a small percentages of cases.

Breast Cancer

Surpassed only by lung cancer, breast cancer is the second leading cause of death from cancer in women. It is the third leading cause of cancer deaths overall. Nearly one in eight women will develop breast cancer in her lifetime, resulting in an estimated 211,300 new invasive cases and 40,200 deaths in 2003.[1] In men, an estimated 1,500 new cases and 400 deaths occurred in 2003[1] (see the Learning from Our Diversity box on page 370). As they age, women's risk of developing breast cancer increases. Regardless of age, however, waiting to learn whether a suspicious lump is benign or is a

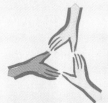

Learning from Our Diversity

Breast Cancer: A Rare Diagnosis in Men

With all the attention given to breast cancer in women—in the news, by physicians, and by research foundations—you may be surprised to learn that men can also be diagnosed with this condition. For every 100 women who develop breast cancer, however, only one case will be reported among men. Estimates for the year 2003 suggest that no more than 1,300 American men will develop breast cancer. When compared to the 211,300 cases anticipated in women during the same year, the rarity of breast cancer in men becomes apparent.

The typical male breast cancer victim is usually older than 60 and often has a family history of the disease. The *BRCA2* tumor suppressor gene mutation is also found within the victim's genetic linage. In some cases, the male breast cancer victim has the inherited condition of Klinefelter's syndrome, in which a second X (or female) sex chromosome is present. The presence of the extra sex chromosome produces enhanced estrogen within the male body, resulting in adolescent development of prominent breasts and a higher risk of breast cancer later in life. Other

conditions, such as various forms of liver disease, also result in higher levels of estrogen and, eventually, a greater risk of male breast cancer.

In most ways male breast cancer is very similar in type to that seen in women. Infiltrating ductal cancer, ductal carcinoma in situ, and a form of cancer arising from the ducts immediately beneath the nipple (Paget's disease) have been reported. Because of this close similarity to female breast cancer, medical management of male breast cancer closely parallels that seen in women. Surgery (a modified radical mastectomy), chemotherapy, external radiation, and hormonal therapy are used alone or in combination. The latter therapy may include not only drugs to block the influence of estrogen on estrogen-sensitive cancer cells, but removal of testicles as well. As with virtually all forms of cancer, early diagnosis and treatment are of critical importance.

InfoLinks

www.cancernet.nci.nih.gov

---

relatively harmless fluid-filled cyst will be stressful. Early detection is the key to complete recovery. Ninety-seven percent of women who discover their breast cancer before it has spread (metastasized) will survive more than 5 years.[1]

Risk Factors

Although all women and men are at some risk of developing breast cancer, the following groups of women have a higher risk.

- Women whose menstrual periods began at an early age, or whose menopause occurred late (although the former may be more powerful than the latter)[14]

- Women who had no children, had their first child later in life, or did not nurse[15]

- Women who have used hormone replacement therapy[16]

- Women whose diets are high in saturated fats, those who are sedentary, and those with excessive central body cavity fat[17] (see Chapter 6)

- Women with a family history of breast cancer

As presented in the bulleted list, significant concerns exist regarding the long-term use of hormone replacement therapy and the development of breast cancer in postmenopausal women. In fact, in a government-sponsored study (Women's Health Initiative Study) the link appeared so strongly and early that the study was terminated much earlier than had been planned. Researchers found that tumor development in women taking HRT versus those on a placebo was more common, that tumors were larger at diagnosis, and that tumors were more often invasive.[16] Physicians are now advising that HRT be used only on a very short-term basis to relieve the symptoms of menopause, rather than the much longer period of time previously deemed appropriate.

The effects of environmental pollutants and regional influences have also been investigated as causative factors in the development of breast cancer.[18] Environmental pollutants vary from region to region and are influenced by a number of factors, including the type of industrial and agricultural activity in a particular area. A wide array of regional factors may be involved, including genetic background of people in a given area and lifestyle differences involving diet, alcohol consumption, and exercise patterns.

The role of genetic predisposition in the development of breast cancer has also received considerable attention. For example, a small percentage (perhaps 5%) of women with breast cancer have inherited or developed mutations in one or both of two tumor suppressor genes (proto-oncogenes), *BRCA1* and *BRCA2*. Discovered in 1994 and 1995, respectively, and currently the focus of extensive research, more than two hundred mutations in these genes have been identified. In a recent study involving 5,000 Ashkenazi Jews (Jews of Central and Eastern European descent) living in the Washington, D.C., area, mutation in the *BRCA1* gene resulted in a 56% greater chance of developing breast cancer by age 70 (versus a 13% greater risk for people without a mutated version of the gene).[19] A more recent study suggests a role not only for mutations to *BRCA1* but to genetic material nearby on the same chromosome.[20] A mutation in the *BRCA2* gene has been found to be less likely to foster the development of breast cancer than the *BRCA1* mutation.[19] Both of these genes are also associated with increased risk of developing ovarian cancer (see page 376) and, perhaps, prostate cancer in men.

Uncertainty exists regarding the use of screening tests to determine the status of the *BRCA1* and *BRCA2* oncogenes. Central to this concern is that a complex set of circumstances must accompany the genetic mutation for breast or ovarian cancer to actually develop. Therefore, it cannot be definitively determined whether a given carrier of a mutated gene will actually develop cancer.

Other genetic links to breast cancer have been identified. One of these is a mutation of the gene that codes for a protein called *MAP kinase*. This protein functions as a "chemical switch" that controls cell replication. Another genetic link to breast cancer is a gene (*CYP17*) that codes for an enzyme that helps synthesize estrogen from cholesterol. This gene has three variations, two of which are associated with higher levels of estrogen production and probably a higher incidence of breast cancer, particularly in older women. Recently a mutation in the APC tumor suppressor gene, thought to be associated with an increased risk of several cancers, including breast cancer, was identified in a population of Ashkenazi Jews. More recently, additional genetic links to breast cancer development have been postulated, including one involving an increased risk for breast cancer development in black women.[21] The gene in question is *BPI*, a gene that, if shut off, allows cancer cells to establish cellular immortality. Factors that influence this gene to become dysfunctional have not been identified. The Personal Assessment on page 393 may be helpful in determining your relative level of risk for developing breast cancer.

Prevention

As already discussed, a variety of risk factors are thought to be important in the development of most cases of breast cancer. Accordingly, some degree of prevention is possible when factors such as diet; alcohol use; physical activity level; decisions about contraception, pregnancy, and breastfeeding; occupational exposure to toxins; and even place of residence are considered.

For women who have a primary family history of breast cancer (sisters, mother, or grandmothers with the disease) and who have been found to carry one or both of the mutated suppressor genes discussed, an extreme form of prevention is also possible— **prophylactic mastectomy.** In this surgical procedure, both noncancerous breasts are removed, in an attempt to eliminate the possibility of future cancer development. When carefully planned, breast reconstruction surgery can be undertaken immediately, with satisfactory results. A high level of satisfaction was found among women who had undergone this procedure. Accordingly some physicians, however, recommend against the surgery, preferring to monitor susceptible women very carefully and frequently.

One important consideration related to this procedure is that not every person who carries a mutated tumor suppressor gene will develop cancer, making the surgery unnecessary.

At the present time pharmacological prevention represents the newest approach to reducing the incidence of breast cancer. Two medications, Evista, or raloxifene (a drug developed for use in osteoporosis prevention), and tamoxifen (an estrogen-receptor blocker developed for use in the treatment of cancer) have been found to be effective in lowering the risk of cancer in high-risk women. However, a warning (August 2000) from the FDA reminds physicians that tamoxifen can have serious side effects, including the development of uterine cancer and potentially fatal blood clots. That said, however, it is now believed that 2.47 million women could benefit by using tamoxifen for breast cancer protection.[22]

Early Detection: Breast Self-Examination

For several decades a fundamental component of early detection of breast cancer has been breast self-examination (BSE). Generally recommended for women 20 years of age and older, the procedure was to be performed during the menstrual period or during the day immediately following the end of the menstrual period, when estrogen levels are at their lowest and cystic activity in breast tissue is minimal (or on the same day of each month by postmenopausal women). The proper technique is illustrated

Breast Self-Examination

I've never felt confident about doing a breast self-exam. What is the proper technique?

The following explains how to do a breast self-examination:

1. In the shower: Examine your breasts during a bath or shower; hands glide more easily over wet skin. With your fingers flat, move gently over every part of each breast. Use right hand to examine left breast, left hand for right breast. Check for any lump, hard knot, or thickening. This self-examination should be done monthly, preferably a day or two after the end of the menstrual period.

2. Before a mirror: Inspect your breasts with arms at your sides. Next, raise your arms high overhead. Look for any changes in contour of each breast, a swelling, dimpling of skin, changes in the nipple. Then rest palms on hips, and press down firmly to flex your chest muscles. Left and right breast will not exactly match—few women's breasts do.

3. Lying down: To examine your right breast, put a pillow or folded towel under your right shoulder. Place right hand behind your head—this distributes breast tissue more evenly on the chest. With left hand, fingers flat, press gently in small circular motions around an imaginary clock face. Begin at outermost top of your right breast for 12 o'clock, then move to 1 o'clock, and so on around the circle back to 12 o'clock. A ridge of firm tissue in the lower curve of each breast is normal. Then move in an inch toward the nipple; keep circling to examine every part of your breast, including the nipple. This requires at least three more circles. Now slowly repeat the procedure on your left breast with a pillow under your left shoulder and left hand behind head. Notice how your breast structure feels. Finally, squeeze the nipple of each breast gently between thumb and index finger. Any discharge, clear or bloody, should be reported to your doctor immediately.

Breast cancer can occur in men too. Therefore this examination should be performed monthly by men. Regular inspection shows what is normal for you and will give you confidence in your examination.

InfoLinks

www.mskcc.org

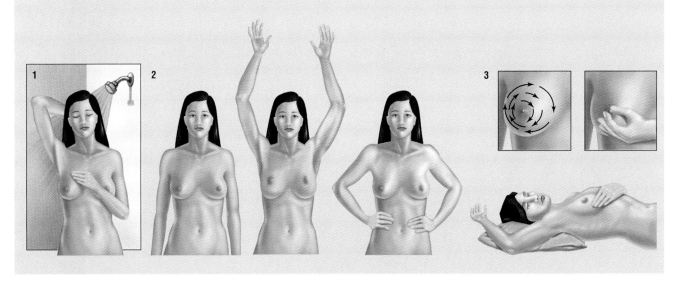

in the Changing for the Better box above. Although breast self-examination is an easily learned technique, today its value is being strongly challenged by researchers in both this country and in China.[23] It has, in fact, become the contention of some that teaching BSE to another generation of women is a misuse of time and money that could be better spent on other screening techniques. Others, however, feel that women who know the technique should not be discouraged from using BSE, but they also should be regularly reminded of its significant limitations in finding tumors. In 2003, the American Cancer Society revised its recommendation for breast cancer screening to better address the doubts regarding BSE's limitations. Specific to BSE the following statement summarizes the ACS's current position.[24]

> Previously, the guidelines (for BSE) recommended women perform breast self-exam every month. Now, (we) recommend that, beginning in their 20s, women should be told about the benefits and limitations of BSE, and that it is acceptable for women to choose not to do BSE, or to do it occasionally. The importance of promptly reporting changes to a physician is emphasized

The reason for this change is that research has shown that BSE plays a very small role in detecting breast cancer compared with self-awareness.

Regardless, monthly BSE can be viewed as an adjunct to regularly scheduled breast examination conducted by a physician and to the routine use of mammography. Breast self-examination also reinforces the importance of breast health, and thus the importance of regularly scheduled comprehensive breast cancer screening.

Early Detection: Mammography

Although researchers once disagreed about the age at which women should begin routine mammography and the extent to which mammography is effective in finding masses in dense breast tissue, today mammograms are physicians' best tool for the early detection of breast cancer. Accordingly, the American Cancer society recommends that mammography begin at age 40.

Whether women begin routine mammography at 40, as advised by the ACS, or as early as 35 years of age, particularly for women with earlier symptoms or a family history of breast disease, women should continue these examinations on an annual basis. Recommendations re-

garding mammography for older women (65+) are, however, a bit more individually determined and should be discussed annually with physicians. For older women, overall health status and expectations for reaching a normal life expectance will be weighed relative to the lowering cost-effectiveness of mammography.

Because of the important role routine mammography plays in the early identification of breast lesions, the Mammography Quality Standards Act (MQSA), formulated by the FDA (April 1998), is a valuable step toward ensuring that mammography is performed by experienced technicians, using correctly calibrated equipment, and interpreted by skilled radiologists. Every woman should be certain that her mammography is being performed in a MQSA-certified facility. However, even when interpreted by experienced radiologists, mammograms are at times difficult to read, and tumors will therefore be missed. In fact, misinterpreted mammograms represent the most common basis for medical malpractice suits in radiology and perhaps in all aspects of medicine as practiced in the United States.

To secure the highest quality images for interpretation, the soft-tissue X-ray-based mammography of the past is increasingly supplemented by newer technologies, including MRI, contrast media-based MRI, ultrasound, and the Image-Checker, in which MRI images are quickly checked against a computerized library of normal breast images and any suspicious areas are "tagged" for further evaluation, including biopsy. Magnetic Resonance Imaging (MRI) technology just mentioned is, however, very experienced and is generally used with women who have already had breast cancer or have strong family history (occurring in a mother or sister) of the disease. Ideally these newer approaches will identify tumors in their earliest stages of development and reduce the percentage of false-positive results associated with traditional mammography procedures.

Treatment

Regardless of the method of detection, if a lump is found, a breast biopsy can determine whether the lump is cancerous. If the lump is cancerous but localized, treatment is highly effective, with cure rates at nearly 100 percent. The most frequently used treatments are **lumpectomy**

Key Terms

lumpectomy a surgical treatment for breast cancer in which a minimal amount of breast tissue is removed; when appropriate, this procedure is an alternative to mastectomy, in which the entire breast and underlying tissue are removed.

combined with radiation, lumpectomy without radiation, and mastectomy. The use of chemotherapy following surgery is strongly advocated as well.[25] Today the injection of a radioactive "tag" prior to surgery allows identification of the nearest lymph node (the *sentinel node*) to which breast cancer cells may have spread, thus allowing the surgeon to spare noncancerous nodes. When the cancer is invasive or has metastasized, more radical surgery (mastectomy with lymph node removal) combined with chemotherapy and/or various forms of radiation may be the most effective course of treatment.

When drug therapy is deemed desirable in treating breast cancer, oncologists may consider two drugs that have recently become available or whose earlier protocols have been redefined. The first, tamoxifen, discussed earlier in terms of breast cancer prevention, is a hormonelike drug that prevents estrogen from stimulating cancer cell growth. The use of tamoxifen has proven highly effective in women who have the type of breast cancer stimulated by the presence of estrogen. Used for many years for more localized tumors, today the use of tamoxifen has been extended to the treatment of highly metastasized breast cancers. Tamoxifen's ability to stimulate uterine cancer development, blood clots, strokes, and cataracts, however, is a potentially serious side effect of the drug's use and must be closely monitored. That said, it is estimated that 2.4 million women could benefit from the drug's use in reducing the risk of future breast cancer.[26]

The second drug, herceptin, is an antibodylike agent used in combination with other chemotherapeutic drugs in highly advanced breast cancer. This newly approved drug interferes with the activity of a protein produced by the HER-2 oncogene that normally fosters tumor cell division. In initial studies, the use of herceptin extended life by approximately three months. Both of these drugs gained FDA approval in 1998.

Cervical Cancer

In 2002 an estimated 13,000 new cases of cancer of the cervix (the anatomical neck of the uterus) occurred in the United States.[1] Fortunately, the death rate from cervical cancer has dropped greatly since 1950, largely because of the **Pap test.** This test screens for precancerous cellular changes (called *cervical intraepithelial neoplasia,* or *CIN*) and malignant cells. If malignant cells are found, it is hoped that they represent only cancer in situ (at the site of origin), rather than a more advanced invasive stage of the disease. Unfortunately, this simple and relatively inexpensive screening test is still underused, particularly in women over age 60, the group in which cervical cancer is most frequently found.

Risk Factors

Because of the clear association between sexually transmitted infections and cervical cancer, risk factors for this form of cancer include early age of first intercourse, large number of sexual partners, history of infertility (which may indicate chronic pelvic inflammatory disease), and clinical evidence of *human papillomavirus* infections (see page 457 in Chapter 13). For patients with previous HPV infections or whose sexual history suggests a higher risk for HPV, a ThinPrep Pap test has been shown effective in detecting the DNA from four HPVs that are known to be cancer causing, while being as easy to use as the more widely used Pap smear. Today the test is only approved for identifying HPV infection, but it is also capable of detecting both chlamydia and gonorrhea. At the time of writing, human trials (Stage 1) are underway on a vaccine designed to protect against some HPV infections. Initial human studies have been highly effective in preventing infections from the most virulent of the HPVs, type 16.[27] Cigarette smoking and socioeconomic factors are also risk factors for cervical cancer. The latter most likely relates to less frequent medical assessment, including infrequent Pap tests. The Personal Assessment on page 393 will help women evaluate their risk of developing cervical cancer.

 TALKING POINTS Three risk factors are associated with HPV-induced cervical cancer: early age of first sexual intercourse, higher-than-average number of partners, and lack of protection against sexually transmitted diseases (e.g., condoms). How would you introduce this topic to a teenage daughter, sister, or niece?

Prevention

Sexual abstinence would be the most effective way of reducing the risk of developing cervical cancer (for example, Catholic nuns have extremely low rates of cervical cancer). However, since this is unlikely to be the choice for most women, other alternatives include fewer sexual partners, more careful selection of partners to minimize those at high risk, the use of condoms, and the use of spermicides. In addition, of course, regular medical assessment, including annual Pap tests (and the ThinPrep Pap test), represents prevention through early detection. Of course, when widely available, the HPV vaccine will further increase prevention.

> **Key Terms**
>
> **Pap test** a cancer screening procedure in which cells are removed from the cervix and examined for precancerous changes.

Early Detection

At this time, the importance of women having Pap tests for cervical cancer performed on a regular basis cannot be overemphasized. However, the specific scheduling of cervical screening is undergoing adjustment. For young sexually active women, initial screening using the Pap smear (preferably in combination with the ThinPrep) should be undertaken within 3 years of first exposure. For young women not sexually at risk, or for women who have had a hysterectomy, the initial screening with the Pap smear can be determined in consultation with health care providers. Once initiated, however, following three consecutive annual negative tests, the interval between tests may be increased upon discussion with health care providers. With screening, a 20-year-old woman of average risk has a 35 in 10,000 chance of developing this form of cancer and only an 11 in 10,000 chance of dying from it.[28] The American Cancer Society estimates that cervical cancer claimed the lives of 4,100 women in 2003.

The Pap test is not perfect, however. When tests are read in laboratories highly experienced in interpreting Pap slides, about 7% will be false negatives, resulting in a 93% accuracy rate. In less-experienced laboratories, false negatives may be as high as 20%. (The Star box above explains what the possible Pap smear results mean.) In addition, not all women whose test results are accurately assessed as abnormal receive adequate follow-up care, nor do they have subsequent Pap tests regularly enough. On a more positive note, potentially more effective tests have been developed and are gaining acceptance. AutoPap and PAP-NET are automated tests, while ThinPrep represents a new technology that identifies DNA from important cancer-causing HPV. Some, however, fear that ThinPrep and the automated Pap tests are too expensive and lack data from large-scale studies of effectiveness.

In addition to changes discovered by a Pap test, symptoms that suggest potential cervical cancer include abnormal vaginal bleeding between periods and frequent spotting.

Treatment

Should precancerous cellular changes (CIN) be identified, treatment can include one of several alternatives. Physicians can destroy areas of abnormal cellular change using cryotherapy (freezing), electrocoagulation, laser destruction, or surgical removal of abnormal tissue. More advanced (invasive) cancer of the cervix can be treated with a hysterectomy combined with other established cancer therapies. A combination of radiation and chemotherapy is the most effective treatment for cervical cancer.

Uterine (Endometrial) Cancer

The American Cancer Society estimates that in 2002, 39,300 cases of uterine cancer (cancer within the inner wall of the body of the uterus, rather than within the cervix or neck of the uterus) were diagnosed in American women. In addition, 6,800 women died of the disease.[1] Although African Americans have a lower incidence of uterine cancer than white women, their death rate is nearly twice as high.[1]

Risk Factors

Unlike cervical cancer, in which a strong viral link has been identified, the principal risk factor related to the development of endometrial cancer is a high estrogen level. Accordingly, the following factors are related to higher levels of estrogen and, thus, to the development of endometrial cancer:

- Early menarche (early onset of menstruation)
- Late menopause
- Lack of ovulation
- Never having given birth
- Estrogen replacement therapy (ERT not moderated with progesterone)
- Use of tamoxifen (a drug used in breast cancer therapy)

To some degree, endometrial cancer is seen more frequently in people who are diabetic, obese, or hypertensive or who have gallbladder disease and a family history of colon cancer.[1]

Prevention

The risk factors associated with high levels of estrogen are areas in which prevention might be targeted. In addition, the need for regular gynecological care that includes pelvic examination is a principal factor in minimizing the risk of uterine cancer. Pregnancy and the use of oral contraceptives both provide some protection from endometrial cancer.[1]

Early Detection

Compared with cervical cancer, which is routinely identified through Pap tests, endometrial cancer is much more likely to be suspected on the basis of symptoms (irregular or postmenopausal bleeding) and confirmed by biopsy. Although more invasive, biopsy is a more effective method than ultrasound to diagnose uterine cancer.

Treatment

The treatment for early or localized endometrial cancer is generally surgical removal of the uterus (hysterectomy). Other therapies, such as radiation, chemotherapy, and hormonal therapy, may then be added to the treatment regimen. However, in terms of hormone replacement therapy (HRT), in which estrogen is combined with a synthetic progesterone, the FDA, The National Institute on Aging, and various medical associations now advise that no women 65 or older should take HRT due to several concerns, including an increased risk for endometrial cancer. For women who are undergoing menopause and experiencing troublesome symptoms such as night sweats and hot flashes, HRT should be used in the smallest doses that provide relief and for the shortest duration of time possible.

Vaginal Cancer

Although rare, cancer of the vagina (the passage leading to the uterus) is of concern to a particular group of women: the daughters of more than 3 million mothers who were given the drug DES (diethylstilbestrol) to prevent miscarriages. Because of the effects of DES on the development of the fetal reproductive system, these daughters now face the risk of developing a form of vaginal (and cervical) cancer called *clear cell cancer*. The medical community has been following large groups of daughters to better assess their level of risk. In a longitudinal study that followed 5,421 such women, the risk of developing vaginal cancer was three to five times higher than that in women whose mothers were not given DES.[29]

Outside of this unique group of women, vaginal cancer is a relatively rare form of cancer. The American Cancer Society estimates that in 2003, there were 2000 new cases diagnosed and 800 women died as the result of vaginal cancer.[1] Early detection can be accomplished using a Pap test when vaginal wall cell samples are taken. Treat-

ment centers on surgical removal of the vagina and associated lymph nodes. Other supportive therapies may also be included in the treatment regimen.

Ovarian Cancer

Since the death in 1989 of actress Gilda Radner, a star in the early years of *Saturday Night Live,* public awareness of ovarian cancer has increased in the United States. The American Cancer Society estimates that in 2003, there were 25,400 new cases diagnosed and 14,300 women died of the disease.[1] Most cases develop in women over age 40 who have not had children or began menstruation at an early age. The highest rate is in women over age 60. Today ovarian cancer causes more deaths than any other form of female reproductive system cancer.

For a relatively small percentage of all women (10%), the inheritance of either the *BRCA1* or *BRCA2* suppressor gene mutation (see page 371) significantly increases the risk of developing both breast and ovarian cancer. Today it is estimated that about 20% of all cases of ovarian cancer stem from these genetic mutations.

Beyond the 20% of cases attributed to genetic mutations, what might account for the majority of ovarian cancers? Today, the accumulation of evidence points to the several decades during which millions of menopausal and postmenopausal women were placed on estrogen replacement therapy (ERT), often for years to counter the symptoms of menopause, maintain bone mass, and continue hormonal protection from cardiovascular disease.[30] As mentioned in conjunction with endometrial cancer, today hormone replacement therapy (HRT) is used, and then for only the briefest period of time.

Prevention

Methods of preventing or lowering the risk of developing ovarian cancer are very similar to those recommended for breast cancer. These include using oral contraceptives, giving birth and breastfeeding (for at least three months), reducing dietary fat intake, abstaining from alcohol use, and performing regular physical activity.

For the small group of women with a strong family history of ovarian cancer, a **prophylactic oophorectomy** should be seriously considered. In this surgical procedure, both ovaries are removed. Carefully monitored hormone

---

Key Terms

prophylactic oophorectomy surgical removal of the ovaries to prevent ovarian cancer in women at high risk of developing the disease.

replacement therapy is then used to provide the protective advantages of estrogen in maintaining cardiovascular health and bone density.

Early Detection

Because of its vague symptoms, ovarian cancer has been referred to as a *silent cancer*. Women in whom ovarian cancer has been diagnosed often report that the only symptoms of their cancer's presence were digestive disturbances, gas, and stomach distention. For this reason, annual pelvic examinations are important.

For women with a strong family history of ovarian cancer (four primary family members who have had breast or ovarian cancer, with two or more cases occurring before age 50) or women of Ashkenazi Jewish descent (see page 371), genetic screening and transvaginal ultrasound screening are likely to be recommended. These women may also be referred for participation in one of several prevention trials now under way.

Treatment

At this time, treatment of ovarian cancer requires surgical removal of the ovary, followed by aggressive use of chemotherapy. Use of the chemotherapeutic drug Taxol, obtained from the bark and needles of the Pacific yew tree, results in a 50% survival rate 19 months after the completion of therapy. Most recently, use of an experimental three-drug combination—cyclophosphamide, paclitaxel, and cisplatin—has resulted in a 70% survival rate 22 months after chemotherapy.

Prostate Cancer

If the names Bob Dole, General Norman Schwarzkopf, Jerry Lewis, and Colin Powell are familiar, then you know four older men who have been diagnosed with and treated for prostate cancer. In fact, prostate cancer is so common that in 2003 an estimated 220,900 new cases were diagnosed and 28,900 men died of the disease.[1] Prostate cancer is the second leading cause of cancer deaths in American men, exceeded only by lung cancer deaths. Cancer of the prostate is the third most common form of cancer in men and a leading cause of death from cancer in older men.

The prostate gland is a walnut-size gland located near the base of the penis. It surrounds the neck of the bladder and the urethra. The prostate secretes a number of components of semen, such as nutrients used to fuel sperm motility.

Risk Factors

Compared with other cancers, the risk factors for prostate cancer are less clearly defined. The most predictable risk factor is age. Nearly 80% of all prostate cancer cases are diagnosed in men over 65 years of age, while cases in men

Symptoms of Prostate Disease

- Difficulty urinating
- Frequent urination, particularly at night
- Continued wetness for a short time after urination
- Blood in the urine
- Low back pain
- Ache in the upper thighs

under age 50 are infrequent. African American men and men with a family history of prostate cancer are at greater risk of developing this form of cancer. A link between prostate cancer and dietary fat intake, including excessive red meat and dairy product consumption, has also been suggested. With the discovery of the *BRCA1* and *BRCA2* genes related to breast and ovarian cancer, a genetic link with prostate cancer was also established. Men with one of these genetic mutations have an increased risk of developing prostate cancer.

Prevention

Although the American Cancer Society does not specifically address prevention of prostate cancer, prevention is not an unrealistic goal. Clearly, moderation of dietary fat intake is a preventive step.[31] Increased dietary intake levels of vitamin E and the micronutrient selenium have been shown to play a preventive role in prostate cancer.[32] In addition, effective treatment of benign prostatic hyperplasia (BPH) (prostate enlargement) with the drug Proscar (finasteride) has proven effective in preventing low-grade tumors in clinical trials.[33]

Early Detection

The symptoms of prostate disease, including prostate cancer, are listed in the Star box above. A physician should be consulted if any of these symptoms appear, particularly in men aged 50 or older. Screening for prostate cancer should begin by age 40. This screening consists of an annual rectal examination performed by a physician and a blood test, the **prostate-specific antigen (PSA) test,**

Key Terms

prostate-specific antigen (PSA) test a blood test used to identify prostate-specific antigen, an early indicator that the immune system has recognized and mounted a defense against prostate cancer.

administered every 2 years. Although the initial version of the PSA test was very successful in diagnosing prostate cancer, new, age-specific test values are now employed. These new interpretive standards allow increased specificity in determining risk. This said, however, the PSA test continues to deliver both false negative and false positive results. Another version of the PSA test has also been developed. This test can identify the "free" antigen most closely associated with the more aggressive forms of prostate cancer, thus cutting down on the false positives and extensive use of biopsies. In addition, an ultrasound rectal examination is used in men whose PSA scores are abnormally high. In spite of the important contribution made by the PSA test, concern is being expressed about the possibility of overtreating 30% of men in the 60–84 age group, particularly in light of the side effects of treatment described below.[34]

Treatment

Today prostate cancer is treated surgically, or through the use of external radiation or the implantation of radioactive seeds (brachytherapy) into the gland. Of course, each form of treatment carries the potential for side effects, including an 80% chance of impotence over a 10-year period;[34] incontinence with surgery; diarrhea and tiredness with external radiation; and some anal discomfort in association with the implantation of radioactive seeds

into the prostate with internal radiation. The latter form of radiation therapy is highly effective for early-stage disease. One form of prostate cancer grows so slowly that men whose cancer is of this type, whose tumors are very localized, and whose life expectancy is less than 10 years at the time of diagnosis will not receive treatment but rather will be closely monitored for any progression of the cancer. For men who have the more aggressive form of the cancer, or whose tumor is no longer localized, physicians can employ a range of therapies, including surgery, radiation, chemotherapy, and hormonal therapy. In addition, an experimental vaccine has recently been tested on humans. The 5-year survival rate for men with localized prostate cancer is very high. In terms of treatment type, the choice of treatment to be employed can be influenced by the physician being consulted. A recent survey of urologists and radiation oncologists found the urologists (who are surgeons) strongly favor a surgical approach, while radiologists favor radiation. Accordingly, second opinions and/or enrollment in clinical trials are highly recommended.

Testicular Cancer

Cancer of the testicle is among the least common forms of cancer; however, it is the most common solid tumor in men ages 15 to 34. Awareness of this type of cancer was raised in 1996 and 1997, when five-time winner of the

---

Changing for the Better

Testicular Self-Examination

I feel unsure about how to perform a testicular self-exam. What is the correct method?

Your best hope for early detection of testicular cancer is a simple 3-minute monthly self-examination. The following explains how to do a testicular self-examination. The best time is after a warm bath or shower, when the scrotal skin is most relaxed.

1. Roll each testicle gently between the thumb and fingers of both hands.
2. If you find any hard lumps or nodules, you should see your doctor promptly. They may not be malignant, but only your doctor can make the diagnosis.

After a thorough physical examination, your doctor may perform certain x-ray studies to make the most accurate diagnosis possible.

Monthly testicular self-examinations are as important for men as breast self-examinations are for women.

InfoLinks

www.mskcc.org/document/WICTEST.htm

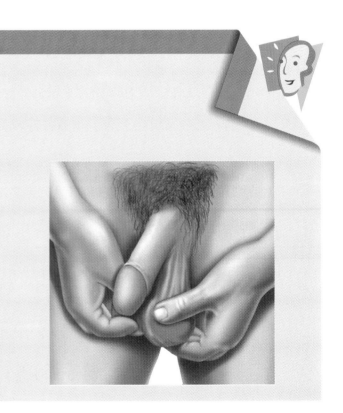

Tour de France Lance Armstrong and champion figure skater Scott Hamilton were diagnosed with testicular cancer. In both men, chronic fatigue and abdominal discomfort were the first symptoms of the disease. The American Cancer Society estimates that in 2003 testicular cancer was diagnosed in 7,600 men and caused the deaths of 400.[1]

Four forms of testicular cancer have been described: seminoma, teratoma, carcinoma, and choriocarcinoma. The most prevalent, seminoma, forms in the seminiferous tubules (where sperm originate) and is generally first observed during testicular self-examination as a small, hard mass on the side (or near the front) of the testicle. Fortunately, this form of testicular cancer is now highly curable.

Risk Factors

Risk factors for testicular cancer are variable, ranging from family history to environmental factors. The disease is more frequently seen in African Americans and in men whose testicles were undescended during childhood. Additional risk factors, such as difficulty during the mother's pregnancy, elevated temperature in the groin, and mumps during childhood, have been reported. The incidence of this cancer has been increasing in recent decades, while a corresponding drop in sperm levels has also been observed. Although no single explanation can be given for these changes, environmental factors such as agricultural pesticide toxicity may be involved. Once pesticides are concentrated in the tissues of the human body, during pregnancy they mimic estrogen. This, in turn, leads to testicular dysgenesis syndrome, or the failure of the testicles to develop normally.[35]

Testicular cancer is more frequently seen among white-collar workers than among people in blue-collar occupations. The suspicion that testicular cancer is linked to vasectomies appears to be unfounded.[36]

Prevention

Because risk factors for testicular cancer are so variable, prevention is limited to regular self-examination of the testicles. Symptoms such as fatigue, abdominal discomfort, and enlargement of the testicle should be reported to a physician, since these can be associated with other disease processes. A male infant with one or both testicles in the undescended position (resulting in an empty scrotum) should be seen promptly by a physician so that corrective procedures can be undertaken.

Early Detection

In addition to the fatigue and abdominal distress reported by both Armstrong and Hamilton, other symptoms of testicular cancer include a small, painless lump on the side or near the front of the testicle, a swollen or enlarged testicle, and a heaviness or dragging sensation in the groin or scrotum. The importance of testicular self-examination, as well as early diagnosis and prompt treatment, cannot be overemphasized for men in the at-risk age group of 15 to 34 years. The Changing for the Better box on page 378 explains how to perform a testicular self-examination.

Treatment

Depending on the type, stage, and degree of localization of the tumor, surgical intervention generally includes removal of the testicle, spermatic cord, and regional lymph nodes. Chemotherapy and radiation might also be used. Today, treatment is very effective, with 95% of all testicular cancer patients surviving 5 years and 99% surviving 5 years when the cancer was localized at the time of diagnosis. It should be noted, however, that concern exists regarding the development of other forms of cancer, such as leukemia, later in life.[37]

Colorectal Cancer

Cancer of the colon and rectum (colorectal cancer) has a death rate second only to that of lung cancer. In the most general sense, two types of tumors, carcinoma and lymphoma, can be found in both the colon and rectum. However, even within the most common form of colorectal cancer, there may subtle difference in type of tumors (or their origins) which influence the degree of potential spread and, thus, the nature of treatment itself. Fortunately, when diagnosed in a localized state, colorectal cancer has a relatively high survival rate (90% when localized and 65% for all stages).[1]

Risk Factors

Underlying the development of colorectal cancer are at least two potentially important areas of risk: genetic susceptibility and dietary patterns. Genes have recently been discovered that lead to familial colon cancer and familial polyposis (abnormal tissue growth that occurs before the formation of cancer) and are believed to be responsible for the tendency of colorectal cancer to run in families. Dietary risk factors include diets that are high in saturated fat from red meat and low in fruits and vegetables, which contain antioxidant vitamins and fiber. In regard to fiber's ability to prevent colorectal cancer, however, the ability of dietary fiber, when taken in supplement form, is in question. In addition, an association between colorectal polyps and smoking has been identified.[38]

Prevention

Small outpouchings in the lower intestinal tract wall, called *polyps,* are frequently important in the eventual development of colorectal cancer. Prompt removal of polyps has been shown to lower the risk of colorectal cancer. Further, some evidence indicates that the development of colorectal cancer may be prevented or slowed through regular exercise, the regular use of aspirin, an increase in dietary calcium intake, and long-term folic acid supplementation. Additionally, oral contraceptive use may be protective for women.

Again, routine screening for colorectal cancer should be considered a form of prevention, much as PSA testing is for prostate cancer and mammography is for breast cancer.

Early Detection

Symptoms of colorectal cancer include bleeding from the rectum, blood in the stool, and a change in bowel habits. In addition, a family history of inflammatory bowel disease, polyp formation, or colorectal cancer should make one more alert to symptoms.[1] In people over age 50, any sudden change in bowel habits that lasts 10 days or longer should be evaluated by a physician. The American Cancer Society recommends preventive health care that includes digital (manual) rectal examination after age 40, a stool blood test after age 50, and sigmoidoscopy every 3 to 5 years and **colonoscopy** every 10 years after age 50. At this time some experts are questioning the advisability of using sigmoidoscopy as the routine screening procedure for colorectal cancer in comparison to using colonoscopy, which can more effectively find distal (higher up in the colon) cancerous changes.[39]

Although colonoscopy is currently the "gold standard" in the screening for colorectal cancer, new technologies are on the horizon. Three alternatives include the Pre-Gen-Plus test that identifies cancer-indicating DNA mutations appearing in stool samples; a yet-named blood test capable of identifying "loss of imprinting" (LOI) factor associated with a high risk for colorectal cancer; and the CT colonography (CTC) that uses serial tomography to visualize the colon, thus eliminating the need to scope the colon.

Treatment

When one or more of these screening procedures suggests the possibility of disease within the lower intestinal tract, a careful visual evaluation of the entire length of the colon will be undertaken. During colonoscopy, areas of concern can be biopsied and the presence of a malignancy confirmed. Upon diagnosis, a localized and noninvasive malignancy will be removed surgically. When an invasive tumor is identified, supportive treatment with radiation or chemotherapy is necessary. Metastatic cancer requires chemotherapy. New guidelines regarding screening for metastatic tumors arising from a primary colorectal cancer are being formulated. These guidelines are meant to remind physicians that metastatic tumors are unlikely to be found through use of colonoscopy, as was the initial colorectal cancer.

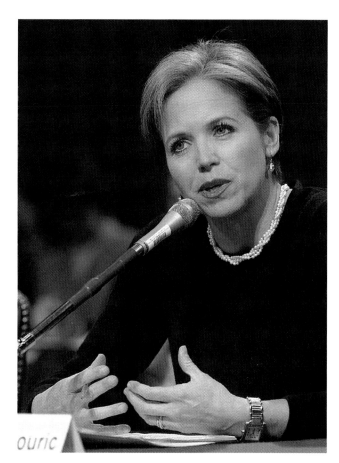

NBC Today Show *host Katie Couric, whose husband died of colon cancer, testified on Capitol Hill March 6, 2000, before a Senate Special Committee on Aging hearing that focused on the importance of colorectal cancer screening tests. (AP Photo/Dennis Cook)*

Pancreatic Cancer

Pancreatic cancer is one of the most lethal forms of cancer, with a survival rate of only 4% 5 years after diagnosis.[1] Because of this gland's important functions in both digestion and metabolic processes related to glucose utilization, its destruction by a malignancy leaves the body in a state incompatible with living.

In 2003 an estimated 30,700 new cases of pancreatic cancer were diagnosed and 30,000 deaths occurred.[1]

Key Terms
colonoscopy (co lun **os** ko py) examination of the entire length of the colon, using a flexible fiberoptic scope to inspect the structure's inner lining.

Risk Factors

Pancreatic cancer is more common in men than women, occurs more frequently with age, and develops most often in African American men. Smoking is clearly a risk factor for this form of cancer, with smokers more than twice as likely to develop the disease. Other risk factors have been tentatively suggested, such as chronic inflammation of the pancreas (pancreatitis), diabetes mellitus, alcohol-induced liver deterioration (cirrhosis), obesity, and high-fat diets.[1] Relatively little else is known about risk factors and, thus, prevention.

Prevention

Not smoking and abstaining from alcohol use are the most effective steps toward preventing this form of cancer. Further, reducing the risk of type 2 diabetes mellitus, through weight loss and exercise, would also make an important contribution to prevention. Annual medical examinations are, of course, associated with overall cancer prevention.

Early Detection

Early detection of this cancer is difficult because of the absence of symptoms until late in its course. Perhaps for people with a history of chronic pancreatitis, physicians might consider routine ultrasound assessment or computerized axial tomography scans (CAT scans). Once symptoms appear, a biopsy will be performed.

Treatment

At this time there is no effective treatment for pancreatic cancer. Surgical removal of malignant sites within the gland, in addition to radiation and chemotherapy, is usually tried. Certainly, if a particular patient with pancreatic cancer qualifies, enrollment in a clinical trial would be worth consideration.

Lymphatic Cancer

In 1996 sports fans were saddened by the news that National Hockey League great Mario Lemieux had been diagnosed with cancer of the lymphatic system, the basis of the body's immune capabilities. Lemieux's cancer was Hodgkin's disease, a form of lymphoma. Following treatment in 1996, he appears to be in complete remission. In fact, in 2001 he resumed his playing career, but has since retired.

An estimated 61,000 new cases of lymphoma (7,600 cases of Hodgkin's disease and 53,400 cases of non-Hodgkin's lymphoma) were diagnosed in 2003. The number of deaths from both forms of lymphoma was near 24,700.[1] The incidence of Hodgkin's disease has declined over the last 25 years, while the incidence of non-Hodgkin's disease has nearly doubled.[1]

Risk Factors

Risk factors for lymphoma are difficult to determine. Some possible factors are a general reduction in immune protection, exposure to toxic environmental chemicals such as pesticides and herbicides, and viral infections.[1] As you will learn in Chapter 13, the virus that causes AIDS (HIV) is a leukemia/lymphoma virus that was initially called HTLV-III (human T-cell leukemia/lymphoma virus-type III). A related leukemia/lymphoma virus, HTLV-I, is also suspected in the development of lymphatic cancer.

Prevention

Beyond limiting exposure to toxic chemicals and sexually transmitted viruses, few recommendations can be made about prevention. Again, early detection and diagnosis can serve as a form of prevention, since early-stage cancer is more survivable than advanced disease.

Early Detection

Unlike other cancers, the early symptoms of lymphoma are diverse and similar to symptoms of other illnesses, most of which are not serious. These symptoms include enlarged lymph nodes (frequently a sign of any infection that the immune system is fighting), fever, itching, weight loss, and anemia.

Treatment

Although surgery (beyond a biopsy) is usually not associated with the treatment of lymphoma, a variety of other therapies are employed. Depending on the stage and type of lymphoma, therapy may involve only radiation treatment of localized lymph nodes, as is seen in non-Hodgkin's lymphoma. Radiation combined with chemotherapy is generally used in the treatment of late-stage non-Hodgkin's lymphoma. More recently, other therapies, including more aggressive chemotherapy, monoclonal antibody therapy, and bone marrow and stem cell transplantation, have been employed.

After completion of therapy, one-year survival rates for Hodgkin's disease are near 95% and near 77% for non-Hodgkin's lymphoma. By the end of 5 years, these rates have dropped to 84% and 55%, respectively.[1] Lower rates of survival are seen at 10 years and beyond.

Skin Cancer

Thanks largely to our desire for a fashionable tan, many teens and adults have spent more time in the sun (and in tanning booths) than their skin can tolerate. As a result, skin cancer, once common only among people who had to work in the sun, is occurring with alarming frequency. In 2003, more than 1 million Americans developed basal or squamous cell skin cancer and 54,200 cases of highly dangerous malignant melanoma were diagnosed.[1]

Deaths from skin cancer do occur, with 9,800 estimated in 2003. More than 80% of these deaths were the result of malignant melanoma.

Risk Factors

Severe sunburning during childhood and chronic sun exposure during adolescence and younger adulthood are largely responsible for the "epidemic" of skin cancer being reported. The current emphasis on screening for skin cancer may also be increasing the incidence of early-stage cancer being reported. Progress is being made in deterring people from pursuing the perfect tan. The American Academy of Dermatology reports that the incidence of deliberate tanning is down, and the use of sunscreens has increased. Occupational exposure to some hydrocarbon compounds can also cause skin cancer.

Prevention

Prevention of skin cancer should be a high priority for people who enjoy the sun or must work outdoors. The use of sunscreen with a sun protection factor (SPF) of 15 or greater is very important. In addition, parents can help their children prevent skin cancer later in life by restricting their outdoor play from 11:00 A.M. to 2:00 P.M., requiring them to wear hats that shade their faces, and applying a sunscreen with an SPF of 15 on them regardless of skin tone. A recent evaluation of sunscreen effectiveness studies by Sloan-Kettering Cancer Center, however, suggests that sunscreens provide little protection against the deeply penetrating UV-A rays associated with the development of melanoma in susceptible people, and less protection than once thought against the UV-B rays associated with burning and wrinkling of the skin. Practicing dermatologists nonetheless continue to recommend their use. Regardless of the extent to which sunscreens provide protection, users are reminded that the level of protection provided is not doubled by simply doubling the SPF—for example, a sunscreen carrying an SPF of 30 does not provide twice the protection provided by a product with an SPF of 15. Therefore, the compliant use of a SPF-15 product is deemed not only appropriate, but may also save money over the more expensive products with a higher SPF rating.

A further rationale for preventing the development of skin cancer is the recently described relationship between skin cancer and the heightened probability of developing other forms of cancer later in life. Research conducted in the late 1990s suggests that people who have had skin cancer carry a 20% to 30% greater risk of developing other types of cancer than do people who have never developed skin cancer.[40] The Personal Assessment on page 393 will help you determine your own risk of developing this kind of cancer.

Early Detection

Although many doctors do not emphasize this point enough, the key to the successful treatment of skin cancer is early detection. For basal cell or squamous cell cancer, a pale, waxlike, pearly nodule or red, scaly patch may be the first symptom. Other types of skin cancer may be indicated by a gradual change in the appearance of an existing mole. A physician should be consulted if such a change is noted. Melanoma usually begins as a small, molelike growth that increases progressively in size, changes color, ulcerates, and bleeds easily. To help detect melanoma, the American Cancer Society recommends using the guidelines below:

A is for asymmetry.

B is for border irregularity.

C is for color (change).

D is for a diameter greater than 6 mm.

E is for elevation (raised margins).

Figure 11-3 shows a mole that would be considered harmless and one that clearly demonstrates the ABCDE characteristics just described. The Changing for the Better box on page 383 shows how to make a regular inspection of the skin.

Most recently, a relationship between the presence of abnormal moles, called *dysplastic nevi* (flat, irregularly shaped, mottled in color, with irregular edges), and the

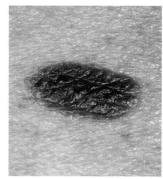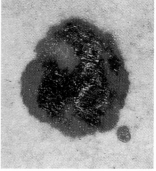

A   B

Figure 11-3 A, Normal mole. This type of lesion is often seen in large numbers on the skin of young adults and may affect any body site. Note its symmetrical shape, regular borders, uniform color, and relatively small size (about 6 millimeters). **B,** Malignant melanoma. Note its asymmetrical shape, irregular borders, uneven color, and relatively large size (about 2 centimeters).

Self-Examination for Melanoma

Through a routine physical exam, my brother found out he has melanoma. How should I check myself for this condition?

How to look for melanoma

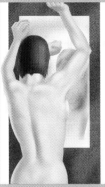 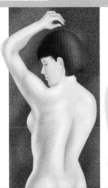 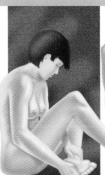 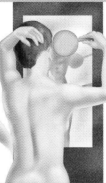 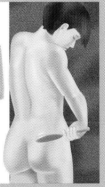

1. Examine your body front and back in the mirror, then right and left sides with arms raised.

2. Bend your elbows and carefully look at your palms, forearms, and under your upper arms.

3. Look at the backs of your legs and feet, the spaces between your toes, and the soles of your feet.

4. Examine the back of your neck and scalp with a hand mirror. Part your hair for a closer look.

5. Finally, check your back and buttocks with a mirror.

What to look for
Potential signs of malignancy in moles or pigmented spots:

Asymmetry

One half unlike the other half

Irregularity

Border irregular or poorly defined

Color

Color varies from one area to another; shades of tan, brown, or black

Size

Diameter larger than 6 mm, as a rule (diameter of a pencil eraser)

risk of developing malignant melanoma has been established.[41] By counting these "indicator moles," physicians can judge the relative risk of developing this serious form of skin cancer before it first appears.

Treatment

When nonmelanoma skin cancer is found, an almost 100 percent cure rate can be expected. Treatment of these skin cancers can involve surgical removal by traditional excising or laser vaporization, destruction by burning or freezing, or destruction using x-ray therapy. When the more serious melanomas are found at an early stage, a high cure rate (95%) is accomplished using the same techniques. However, when malignant melanomas are more advanced, extensive surgery and chemotherapy will be necessary. The 5-year survival rate for regionalized forms of the disease drops to 60%, and, unfortunately, long-term disease recovery is uncommon (14%).[1]

However, a new treatment for malignant melanoma offers a ray of hope to people with the disease. Among the more promising of these is a combination therapy using interleukin-2, an immune system chemical that stimulates various "killer cells" within the immune system, and histamine dihydrochloride, a drug that activates phagocyctic cells within the immune system. Additionally, a vaccine has been developed that stimulates the immune system to attack the melanoma cells more aggressively. This treatment-centered (rather than prevention-centered) vaccine uses components of the patient's own cancer cells to mobilize more white blood cells and produce more antibodies to fight the cancer.

The Future of Cancer Prevention, Diagnosis, and Treatment

It has been nearly 35 years since President Nixon declared a national "War On Cancer," and today the results are both encouraging and discouraging. On the positive side impressive technological advances have been and continue to be made in the diagnosis and treatment of cancer. As mentioned throughout the chapter, new screening procedures as well as treatment protocols seem to appear at a consistent rate. Additionally, the death rates from a variety of cancers have fallen, including a 70% decrease in the rate for Hodgkin's disease and a 14% decline in the death rate for breast cancer. Death rates for cervical, stomach, uterine, colon, bladder, and thyroid cancers have also fallen. Particularly important is a general increase in the public's awareness of cancer prevention and early detection.[42]

On the negative side is the reality that cancer is not only a biological disease, but also a disease (or more than 100 diseases) with strong sociopolitical implications. Central to this area are factors such as the inability of the majority of Americans to make needed changes in lifestyle, in regards to smoking, alcohol use, exercise, weight management, and dietary practices. Also impeding progress is the absence of health care insurance for 41.4 million Americans that prevents early diagnosis and treatment of cancer. In fact, virtually every cancer in adults is impacted negatively by one or more of these largely modifiable complicating factors. This said, the

federal government continues funding research in biological, behavioral, and education aspects of the war on cancer.[43]

In the final analysis, the "war" remains very challenging: progress is being made, setbacks occur, and the victory remains far from being in hand. The "Big C" remains.[42]

Prevention Through Risk Reduction

Because cancer will probably continue to be the second most common cause of death among adults, it is important that you explore ways to reduce your risk of developing cancer. The following factors, which could make you vulnerable to cancer, can be controlled or at least recognized.

- *Know your family history.* You are the recipient of the genetic strengths and weaknesses of your biological parents and your more distant relatives. If you are able

Cancer's Seven Warning Signals

Listed below are the seven warning signs of cancer, which the acronym CAUTION will help you remember:

1. **C**hange in bowel or bladder habits
2. **A** sore that does not heal
3. **U**nusual bleeding or discharge
4. **T**hickening or lump in the breast or elsewhere
5. **I**ndigestion or difficulty in swallowing
6. **O**bvious change in a wart or mole
7. **N**agging cough or hoarseness

If you have a warning signal for more than 5 days, see your doctor!

to determine that cancer is prevalent in your family medical history, you cannot afford to disregard this fact. It may be appropriate for you to be screened for certain types of cancer more often or at a young age. The importance of family history was clearly seen in our discussion of the *BRCA1/BRCA2* inheritance pattern and related decisions about prophylactic mastectomy and prophylactic oophorectomy.

- *Select and monitor your occupation carefully.* Because of recently discovered relationships between cancer and occupations that bring employees into contact with carcinogenic agents, you must be aware of the risks posed by certain job selections and assignments. Worksites where you will come into frequent contact with pesticides, strong solvents, volatile hydrocarbons, and airborne fibers could pay well but also shorten your life. The importance of this point is evident in reviewing the current list of environmental carcinogens studies funded by the National Cancer Institute. Included are studies that focus on indoor air pollution (tobacco smoke and cooking oils), dust (cotton, grain, plastic, and wood), organic solvents (benzene, carbon tetrachloride, toluene, xylene, and chlordane), organophosphates (diazinon, dichlorvos, malathion, triazines, and cyaniazine), polybrominated biphenyls, polychlorinated biphenyls, fumigants (ethylene), water pollution (chloride, phosphene, and fluoride), petroleum products (diesel fuel, gasoline, jet fuel), radiation (radon, neutron therapy, and reactor accidents), biological agents (chlamydia, HIV/HPV, helicobacter, hepatitis B and C) and radioisotopes (iodine and radium).

- *Do not use tobacco products.* You may want to review Chapter 9 on the overwhelming evidence linking all forms of tobacco use (including smokeless tobacco) to the development of cancer. Smoking is so detrimental to health that it is considered the number one preventable cause of death.

- *Monitor environmental exposure to carcinogens.* When carcinogenic concerns related to types of employment, residential radon levels, ozone depletion leading to increased exposure to solar radiation, and environmental tobacco smoke (Chapter 9) are seen in totality, it is apparent that the environment holds great potential as a source of carcinogenic exposure. To the extent to which it is possible to select the environment in which you will reside, work, and recreate, you should add selecting a low-risk environment to your list of cancer-prevention activities.

- *Follow a sound diet.* As mentioned in conjunction with folic acid and colorectal cancer and high-fat diets and prostate cancer, dietary patterns are known to play both a causative and a preventive role in cancer. Review

Chapter 5 for information about dietary practices and the incidence of various diseases, including cancer. In that chapter, the role of fruits and vegetables known to be sources of cancer-preventing phytochemicals is introduced. Good sources include a wide variety of fruits and vegetables, particularly the cruciferous vegetables, including cauliflower, broccoli, and brussels sprouts, and fruits high in beta-carotene, vitamin C, and fiber. Should research demonstrate an even clearer role for nutrients, **chemoprevention** may become an even more widely practiced component of cancer prevention (see the Considering Complementary Care box on page 387). Chemoprevention is not limited to food items and dietary supplements but can also involve pharmaceutical agents, such as aspirin, estrogen replacement therapy, and hormone replacement therapy.

- *Control your body weight.* For women, obesity is related to a higher incidence of cancer of the uterus, ovary, and breast because obesity correlates with high estrogen levels. Maintaining a desirable body weight could improve overall health and lead to more successful management of cancer should it develop. Additionally, consider carefully whether you want to follow the currently popular high-protein, high-fat diets (Chapter 6), given their recognized carcinogenic potential.

- *Exercise regularly.* Chapter 4 discusses in detail the importance of regular moderate exercise to all aspects of health, including reducing the risk of chronic illnesses. Moderate exercise increases the body's ability to deliver oxygen to its tissues and thus to reduce the formation of cancer-enhancing free radicals formed during incomplete oxidation of nutrients. Moderate exercise also stimulates the production of enzymes that remove free radicals.

- *Limit your exposure to the sun.* It is important to heed this message even if you enjoy many outdoor activities. Particularly for people with light complexions, the radiation received through chronic exposure to the sun may foster the development of skin cancer.

- *Consume alcohol in moderation if at all.* Heavier users of alcohol have an increased prevalence of several types of cancer, including cancer of the oral cavity,

---

Key Terms

chemoprevention cancer prevention using food, food supplements, or medications thought to bolster the immune system or reduce the damage caused by carcinogens.

Resources from the Home Front

Although we typically envision the treatment and management of cancer as being conducted in or near the confines of a medical center, certain aspects of our personal "war on cancer" can be conducted from home.

Social Support

One particularly useful component in managing the pain and discomfort often associated with cancer is social involvement and the support of family, friends, and coworkers. Studies now suggest that many cancer victims who maintain active involvement in the community and who maintain contact with other people demonstrate less pain and discomfort than those who cannot or choose not to be so involved. Unknown at this time, however, is whether less than average amounts of pain and discomfort have allowed these people to remain involved, or whether their decision to remain connected has helped lessen their level of discomfort.

Music Therapy

Another potential home front aid in dealing with cancer is music therapy. Using the professional expertise of a certified music therapist, cancer victims have been helped in reducing their level of discomfort by listening to carefully selected music recorded for their use. The home offers a wonderful environment in which musical selections can be enjoyed at little or no cost.

Stress Management

A final area of low-tech assistance for improving the long-term management of cancer is the use of stress management to enhance the function of the immune system. Experts in the field of psychoneuroimmunology (PNI) have contended, on the basis of both animal and human subject research and anecdotal reports, that reduction of stress enhances immune system function. Accordingly, oncological treatment plans increasingly involve stress management instruction that can be routinely used in the home and community.

Resources for People Living with Cancer

For people with cancer and their families, many telephone hot lines and Internet websites have been set up offering information and referrals:

- American Cancer Society National Hotline: (800) ACS-2345. Also, the ACS recommends calling local ACS chapters for support group information.

  www.cancer.org

- National Cancer Institute Cancer Information Service: (800) 4-CANCER.

  www.nci.nih.gov

- National Coalition for Cancer Survivorship (an umbrella group for cancer survivor units nationwide): (301) 650-8868.

  www.cansearch.org

- Candlelighters Childhood Cancer Foundation: Information on support groups for children with cancer and their families: (301) 657–8401 and (800) 366–2223.

  www.candlelightersaustin.org

- Surviving: Support group. Publishes a newsletter for Hodgkin's disease survivors. Stanford University Medical Center, Radiology Dept, Room C050, 300 Pasteur Dr., Stanford, CA 94305.

  www-radiology.stanford.edu

- Vital Options: Support group for people 17 to 40 who are cancer survivors: (818) 508-5657.

  www.vitaloptions.org

- The Resource Center: American College of Obstetricians and Gynecologists, 409 12th St. S.W., Washington, DC 20224-2188. Send a self-addressed, business-size envelope to receive the brochure *Detecting and Treating Breast Problems.*

  www.acog.org

- American College of Radiology, for accredited mammography centers, (800) ACR-LINE (members only) or (703) 648–8900, ask for mammography.

  www.acr.org

larynx, and esophagus. Whether this results directly from the presence of carcinogens in alcohol or is more closely related to the alcohol user's tendency to smoke has not yet been established.

Cancer and Wellness

When you carefully consider the preceding suggestions, it should be obvious that you can do a great deal to prevent or at least minimize the development of cancer. A wellness-oriented lifestyle is the best weapon in your "personal war against cancer." However, all risk factor reduction is relative. Observation and experience tell us that life cannot be totally structured around the desire to achieve maximum longevity or reduce morbidity at all costs. Most people need to strike a balance between life that is emotionally, socially, and spiritually satisfying and life that is structured solely for the purpose of living a long time and minimizing exposure to illness. Regardless of our personal lifestyle, however, we can educate others, provide comfort and support to those who are living with cancer, and support the funding of continuing and innovative new cancer research. Resources available for people with cancer and their families are listed in the Star boxes above.

The Macrobiotic Diet

As common and potentially serious as cancer is, it is not a condition likely to be treated exclusively with alternative therapies. However, the use of a *macrobiotic diet* has been used by some cancer patients with anecdotal reports of success.

When the macrobiotic diet was introduced into the United States from Asia in the 1960s, it was first viewed as nutritionally deficient in comparison to all recognized forms of dietary intake, including the more restrictive forms of vegan vegetarianism. Central to the diet was the extensive (if not total) reliance on brown rice, seaweed, and a fish-based gruel. It also involved restrictions regarding food preparation, such as the type of cookware to be used.

Today the typical macrobiotic diet has been nutritionally enhanced to derive 50% of its calories from whole grains, 25 to 30% from vegetables, 5 to 10% from soups of various types, and 5 to 10% from beans and sea vegetables. It also features highly specific "macrobiotic" lifestyle guidelines, such as when eating is to occur, the rate at which food is to be chewed, hours of sleep required, and restrictions on the types of clothing materials and cosmetics to be used. This complex program must be learned through careful study at an organization such as the Kushi Institute, established by Michio Kushi, who introduced macrobiotics into this country from Japan.

In an attempt to evaluate the merits of the macrobiotic diet, studies of macrobiotic-based cancer treatment plans were funded by the National Center for Complementary and Alternative Medicine (NCCAM) in 1993—one at the University of Minnesota (directed by Michio Kushi's son) and a second at the University of Colorado (Denver). On February 25, 2002, the NCCAM Advisory Committee and researchers met for an initial assessment of the macrobiotic diet study. During the meeting, nine Best Case Series (BCS) participant reports from an initial group of eighteen participants were reviewed, and six participants gave personal accounts to the review panel. From these sources of information, serious methodological flaws were noted, including a virtual absence of medical records and X-rays on any of the nine participants, the variety of ways in which diets were composed and prepared, and the absence of any oncology-based assessment prior to or during the study period. Of six participants that addressed the committee, all six reported (and demonstrated on assessments) an improved quality of life, while two had apparently lived longer than generally expected for persons with their forms of cancer. For the remaining four participants, survivability expectations could not be determined.

In light of the use of the Best Case Series format and the absence of various controls, the conclusion reached by the advisory committee was for continuation of the study using a prospective model involving approximately thirty subjects, including a methodology that minimized the concerns regarding medical assessment, standardization of the diet, assessment of compliance, medical assessment of the patients' malignancy status at selected time intervals, and each participant's final outcome.

InfoLinks

www.macrobiotics.org/whatmacro.html

Taking Charge of Your Health

- Stay attuned to media reports about chronic conditions so that you can make informed choices.
- Support agencies devoted to the prevention of chronic health conditions.
- Monitor your work, home, and recreational environments to determine whether they are placing you at risk for cancer.

- Perform regular self-examinations for forms of cancer that can be detected through these techniques.
- Undergo the recommended cancer screening procedures for your age and sex.
- If you have cancer or a chronic condition, participate actively in your own treatment.

Summary

- More than one and a quarter million people in the United States develop cancer each year.
- Cancer is a condition in which the body is unable to control the specialization, replication, and repair of cells or the suppression of abnormal cell formation.

- Genes that control the replication, specialization, and repair of cells and the suppression of abnormal cellular activity have the potential to become oncogenes and thus can be considered proto-oncogenes.

- A variety of agents, including genetic mutations, viruses, and carcinogens, stimulate the conversion of regulatory genes (proto-oncogenes) into oncogenes.
- Cancer cells demonstrate unique characteristics in comparison to normal cells.
- Cancer can be described on the basis of the type of tissue from which it originates, such as carcinoma, sarcoma, and melanoma.
- Cancer can be described on the basis of its location within the body, such as lung, breast, and prostate cancer.
- Cigarette smoking and genetic predisposition are both related to the development of lung cancer.
- Spiral CT scans may allow for earlier diagnosis of lung cancer.
- Most cases of breast cancer do not demonstrate a clear familial pattern that suggests a genetic predisposition, although some do.
- Long-term exposure to high levels of estrogen is an important risk factor for breast cancer.
- Mammograms are an important component of breast cancer identification. Drugs capable of preventing breast cancer are available; however, their use is being carefully studied.
- The screening role of BSE has been reduced in favor of it becoming a part of more comprehensive breast awareness.
- Regular use of Pap tests is related to the early detection of cervical cancer. Sexually transmitted viral infections are strongly suspected of causing cervical cancer.
- For women at high risk of HPV infections, screening for infections may be as effective in cervical cancer detection as the Pap test.
- Uterine (endometrial) cancer is more common than cervical cancer. High levels of estrogen are strongly associated with this form of cancer.
- A group of women who are the daughters of mothers given the drug DES during pregnancy have a high incidence of vaginal cancer.
- Ovarian cancer is often "silent" in its presentation of symptoms.

- The excessively long use of HRT is a strongly suspected cause of uterine cancer.
- Prostate cancer is the second leading cause of cancer deaths in men.
- The PSA test improves the ability to diagnose prostate cancer. Age, high-fat diets, and inheritance of a mutated suppressor gene are known risk factors.
- Regular self-examination of the testicles leads to early detection of testicular cancer. Environmental factors may be associated with an increasing rate of testicular cancer.
- Colorectal cancer has a strong familial link and is seen in populations that consume diets high in fat and low in fruits and vegetables. Polyp formation is associated with an increased risk of this form of cancer.
- Colonoscopy is the most effective method of detecting polyps and colorectal cancers.
- Pancreatic cancer is very difficult to survive, in part because of the absence of symptoms early in the disease's course.
- Lymphatic cancers display a wide array of initial symptoms that reflect failure of the immune system to function fully. Viral infections and environmental toxins are suspected causative agents.
- Basal cell and squamous cell carcinomas are highly curable forms of skin cancer when detected early. Malignant melanoma is life threatening if not detected early.
- Vaccine development for use in treating malignant melanoma has progressed significantly.
- Skin cancer prevention requires protection from excessive sun exposure.
- Early detection based on self-examination and screening is the basis for the identification and successful treatment of many cancers.
- The "War on Cancer" is experiencing both successes and failures.
- Risk reduction, through living a wellness lifestyle, remains at the heart of cancer prevention.

Review Questions

1. What is the relationship between regulatory genes and tumor suppressor genes in the development of cancer? Why are regulatory genes called both proto-oncogenes and oncogenes?
2. What properties do cancer cells possess that are lacking in normal cells?
3. What are some of the major types of cancer, based on the tissue from which they originate? What are some of the more familiar cancers based on organ of origin?
4. What are the principal factors that contribute to the development of lung cancer? Of breast cancer? What is prophylactic mastectomy and who might consider its use?
5. When should regular use of mammography begin, and which women should begin using it earliest?

6. What important information can be obtained with the use of Pap tests? What innovations are associated with the ThinPrep Pap Test?

7. Why is ovarian cancer described as a "silent" cancer?

8. How does the PSA test contribute to the early detection of prostate cancer?

9. What are the steps for effective self-examination of the breasts and testicles? What is the new status of Breast Self-Examination?

10. What signs indicate the possibility that a skin lesion has become cancerous?

11. Why is pancreatic cancer among the most lethal of all cancers?

12. What is now known about the effectiveness of the macrobiotic diet as a cancer treatment?

13. What are the risk reduction activities identified in this chapter?

References

1. American Cancer Society. *Cancer facts & figures 2003.* The Society, 2003.

2. *Number of Americans with and without health insurance rise.* Census Bureau Reports. United States Department of Commerce News. U.S. Census Bureau Public Information Office, 2002. **http://www.census.gov/press-release/www/2002/cb02-127.html**

3. Clark DP, Russell LD. *Molecular biology made simple and fun.* Cache River Press, 1997.

4. Hoover RN. Cancer—nature, nurture, or both. *N Engl J Med* 343(2):135–136, 2000.

5. Schwab M. (ed) *Encyclopedic reference of cancer.* Springer, 2001.

6. Bertino JR. (ed) *Encyclopedia of cancer, 2nd ed.* (Vols. 1–4.) Academic Press, 2002.

7. Hamann B. *Disease: identification, prevention, & control,* 2nd ed. McGraw-Hill, 2001.

8. Mahadevia PJ, et al. Lung cancer screening with helical computed tomography in older adult smokers: a decision and cost-effectiveness analysis. *JAMA* 289(3): 313–322, 2003.

9. Zabarovsky ER, Lerman MI, Minna JD. Tumor suppressor genes on chromosome 3p involved in the pathogenesis of lung and other cancers. *Oncogene* 21(45): 6915–6935, 2003.

10. Barsky SH, et al. Histopathologic and molecular alterations in bronchial expthelium in habitual smokers of marijuana, cocaine, and/or tobacco. *J Natl Cancer Inst* 90(16); 1198–1205, 1998.

11. Pope CA III, et al. Lung cancer, cardiopulmonary mortality, and long-term exposure to fine particulate air pollution. *JAMA* 287(9):1132–1141, 2002.

12. Djousse L, et al. Alcohol consumption and risk of lung cancer; the Framingham Study. *J Natl Cancer Inst* 94(24):1877–1882, 2002.

13. Massarelli E, et al. A retrospective analysis of the outcome of patients who have received two prior chemotherapy regimens including platinum and docetaxel for recurrent non-small cell lung cancer. *Lung Cancer* 39(1):55–61, 2003.

14. Hamilton AS, Mack TM. Puberty and genetic susceptibility to breast cancer in a case control study of twins. *N Engl J Med* 348(23):2313–2322, 2003.

15. Collaborative Group on Hormonal Factors in Breast Cancer. Breast cancer and breastfeeding reanalysis of individual data from 47 epidemiological studies in 30 countries, including 50302 women with breast cancer and 96973 women without the disease. *Lancet* 360(9328):203–210, 2002.

16. Chlebowski RT. Influence of estrogen plus progestin on breast cancer and mammography in healthy postmenopausal women: the Women's Health Initiative Randomized Trial. *JAMA* 289(24):3243–3253, 2003.

17. Folsom AR, et al. Association of general and abdominal obesity with multiple health outcomes in older women: the Iowa Women's Health Study. *Arch Intern Med* 160(14):2117–2128, 2000.

18. Blot WJ, McLaughlin JK. Geographic patterns of breast cancer among American women. *J Natl Cancer Inst* 87(24):1819–1820, 1995.

19. Krainer M, et al. Differential contributions of BRCA1 and BRCA2 to early on-set breast cancer. *N Engl J Med* 336(20):1416–1421, 1997

20. Thompson JA, et al. BRCA1 susceptibility markers and postmenopausal breast cancer: the Iowa Women's Health Study. *Cancer Epidemiol Biomarkers Prev* 9(5):507–511, 2000.

21. Fu SW, et al. Correlation of expression of BP1, a homeobox gene, with estrogen receptor status in breast cancer. *Breast Cancer Res* 5(4):R82–87. Epub 2003.

22. Freedman AN, et al. Estimates of the number of US women who could benefit from tamoxifen for breast cancer chemoprevention. *J Natl Cancer Inst* 95(7):526–532, 2003.

23. Thomas DB, et al. Randomized trial of breast self-examination in Shanghai: final results. *J Natl Cancer Inst* 94(19):1454–1457, 2002.

24. ACS News Center. *Updated breast cancer screening guidelines released.* American Cancer Society.

http://www.cancer.org/updated_breast_cancer_
screening_guidelines_released.

25. Du XL. Re: trends in use of adjuvant multi-agent chemotherapy and tamoxifen for breast cancer in the United States: 1975–1999. *J Natl Cancer Inst* 95(9):683, 2003.

26. Freedman AN, et al. Estimates of the number of US women who could benefit from tamoxifen for breast cancer chemoprevention. *J Natl Cancer Inst* 95(7):525–532, 2003.

27. Crum CP. The beginning of the end of cervical cancer? *N Engl J Med* 347(21):1703–1705, 2002.

28. American Cancer Society. *Cancer facts & figures–2000.* The Society, 2000.

29. Verloop J, Rookus MA, van Leeuwen FE. Prevalence of gynecologic cancer in women exposed to diethylstilbesterol in utero. *N Engl J Med* 342(24):1838–1839, 2000.

30. Lacey JV Jr, et al. Menopausal hormone replacement therapy and risk of ovarian cancer. *JAMA* 288(3):2544, 2002

31. Kushi L, Giovannucci E. Dietary fat and cancer. *Am J Med* 113 Suppl 9B:63S–70S, 2002.

32. Klein EA, et al. The selenium and vitamin e cancer prevention trial. *World J Urol* 21(1):21–27, 2003.

33. Thompson IM, et al. The influence of finasteride on the development of prostate cancer. *N Engl J Med* 349(3):215–224, 2003.

34. Etzioni R, et al. Overdiagnosis due to prostate-specific antigen screening: lessons from U.S. prostate cancer incidence trends. *J Natl Cancer Inst* 94(3): 981–990, 2002.

35. Skakkebaek NE. Endocrine disrupters and testicular dysgenesis syndrome. *Horm Res* 57 Suppl 2:43. 2002.

36. Schwingle PJ, Guess HA. Safety and effectiveness of vasectomy. *Fertil Steril* 73(5):923–936, 2000.

37. Travis LB, et al. Treatment-associated leukemia following testicular cancer. *J Natl Cancer Inst* 92(14):1165–1171, 2000.

38. Lieberman DA, et al. Risk factors for advanced colonic neoplasia and hyperplastic polyps in asymptomatic individuals. *JAMA* 290(22):2959–2967, 2003.

39. Lieberman DA, et al. Use of colonoscopy to screen asymptomatic adults for colorectal cancer. Veterans Affairs Cooperative Study 380. *N Engl J Med* 343(3):162–168, 2000.

40. Kahn, HS, et al. Increased cancer mortality following a history of non-melanoma skin cancer. *JAMA* 280(10):910–912, 1998.

41. Hussein MR, et al. Identification of novel deletion Loci at 1p36 and 9p22−21 in melanocytic dysplastic nevi and cutaneous malignant melanomas. *Arch Dermatol* 139(6):816–817, 2003.

42. *30 years of war on cancer.* Americans for Medical Progress. **http://www.amprogress.org/files/files. ctm?=136&c=68**

43. Halpern IM, Waters B. Fiscal year 2003 appropriations essential step forward in war against cancer. *ONS News* 18(4):11, 2003.

As We Go to Press

In the early 1990s a few small studies conducted in this country suggested a link between abortions and an increased risk for the development of breast cancer. In the politically charged atmosphere that generally surrounds the abortion issue, this information was frequently used to substantiate larger claims regarding the need to appeal the 1974 Supreme Court ruling legalizing abortions. However, upon review of these studies, the U.S. National Cancer Institute, in 1995, found the studies too flawed to be considered valid.

The most recent return of the question regarding the link between breast cancer and abortion appeared near the end of March 2004, when 53 separate studies, involving 44,000 women who had abortions and 39,000 women who had been diagnosed with breast cancer, were subjected to a meta-analysis. The new data analysis, conducted by the Collaborative Group on Hormonal Factors in Breast Cancer of Oxford University, found that no link between abortion or miscarriage and the increased risk of developing breast cancer could be found. Findings were reported in *The Lancet,* England's most prestigious medical journal.

stem cells: tomorrow's treatment for human diseases?

Researchers often must delve into murky ethical and moral waters in their ongoing quest for more effective technologies to prevent and cure human diseases, including cancer. Nowhere is this more apparent than in one of today's most controversial areas of medical research, the study of human stem cells.

All human life begins with stem cells. These are the basic, unspecialized cells that form the 3 to 5 day old blastocyst, which over time will yield the specialized cells that create all the tissue and organs of the human embryo. Each stem cell is pluripotent—that is, each stem cell can develop into many different cell types.[1] Stem cells are special for three reasons: they are capable of dividing and renewing themselves for long periods; they are entirely unspecialized; and they can give rise to specialized cells.[1] For these reasons, stem cells are of particular interest to medical researchers, who envision important new discoveries and therapies, from treating diseases like cancer and Parkinson's disease to replacing diseased organs with replacement organs generated from stem cells.

Already, the technology to move stem cells in the direction needed exists, but its application is the focus of great debate, depending on the source of cells being used.

The first and perhaps best source of stem cells in terms of minimum initial specialization is very early human embryos. These cells are obtained from frozen embryos—embryos that were created from eggs that have been fertilized in vitro at fertilization clinics, which have been donated with the consent of their donors. Embryos used for stem cell research are not obtained from embryos that have been fertilized or implanted inside a woman's uterus.[1]

In 2001, President Bush limited the use of Federal funding for stem cell research to only 60 existing stem cell lines. Citing the ethical dilemmas involved in using human embryos for research, Bush explained "Embryonic stem cell research is at the leading edge of a series of moral hazards.[2] For this reason, very little research using human embryonic stem cells is occurring in the United States. Some scientists believe that the current restrictions will place the United States at an extreme disadvantage in terms of potential application, and thus do a disservice to the American public.

Because harvesting the stem cells destroys the embryo, using human embryos for stem cell research is extremely controversial in the U.S., where the entire issue has become entangled in debates over abortion and cloning.[2] Voices on both sides of the issue have spoken out on it. One one hand, religious leaders argue that embryos destroyed in the process of harvesting stem cells are denied their basic human rights. On the other hand, those suffering from conditions who might benefit from the results of stem cell research plead for increased funding in hopes of finding new treatments and cures. Many celebrity advocates, including actor Michael J. Fox and boxer Muhammad Ali, both of whom suffer from Parkinson's disease, and paralyzed actor Christopher Reeve have spoken out before the public and before Congress on the importance of restoring funding for stem cell research.

A second source of human stem cells is the pluripotent cells located in various tissues of the human body, such as in the bone marrow. These adult stem cells too can be chemically directed to specialize in a desired direction, but some scientists believe that these stem cells are less unspecialized than their embryonic counterparts and, thus, not as useable. That said, the use of adult stem cells is largely free of the restrictions placed on embryonic stem cell research—unless the goal of the research is to clone a human. Stem cells might also be obtained from human placentas and umbilical cord blood, both of which are natural byproducts of childbirth, usually discarded after birth.

Despite the controversy and funding limitations, stem cell research has already made great strides. In July 2002, scientists at the University of Wisconsin medical school turned human embryonic stem cells into blood cells.[3] Stem cell research has also shown promise in treatments for neurological disorders and spinal cord injuries.

For Discussion . . .

How do you feel about stem cell research? If you had conceived a child in vitro and had additional embryos frozen at your fertilization clinic, but did not wish to have more children, would you donate them to science? Who has the right to make that decision? Is the value of the potential research worth more than the potential life of a frozen embryo?

References

[1] National Institutes of Health, Stem Cell Information Center, **http://stemcells. nih.gov**

[2] Remarks by the President on Stem Cell Research, George W. Bush, August 9, 2001.

[3] "Blood cells made from stem cells." CNN/Health, July 17, 2002. **http:// www.cnn.com/2001/HEALTH/09/03/ stem.cells/index.html**

personal assessment

are you at risk for skin, breast, or cervical cancer?

Some people may have more than an average risk of developing particular types of cancer. These people can be identified by certain risk factors.

This simple self-testing method is designed by the American Cancer Society to help you assess your risk factors for three common types of cancer. These are the major risk factors but by no means represent the only ones that might be involved.

Check your response to each risk factor. Add the numbers in the parentheses to arrive at a total score for each cancer type. Find out what your score means by reading the information in the "Interpretation" section. You are advised to discuss the information with your physician if you are at a higher risk.

Skin Cancer

1. Frequent work or play in the sun
   A. Yes (10)
   B. No (1)
2. Work in mines, around coal tars, or around radioactivity
   A. Yes (10)
   B. No (1)
3. Complexion—fair skin or light skin
   A. Yes (10)
   B. No (1)

Your total points _____

Explanation

1. Excessive ultraviolet light causes skin cancer. Protect yourself with a sunscreen.
2. These materials can cause skin cancer.
3. Light complexions need more protection than others.

Interpretation

Numerical risks for skin cancer are difficult to state. For instance, a person with a dark complexion can work longer in the sun and be less likely to develop cancer than can a light-complected person. Furthermore, a person wearing a long-sleeved shirt and a wide-brimmed hat may work in the sun and be less at risk than a person who wears a bathing suit and stays in the sun for only a short period. The risk increases greatly with age.

The key here is if you answered "yes" to any question, you need to realize that you have above-average risk.

Breast Cancer

1. Age group
   A. 20–34 (10)
   B. 35–49 (40)
   C. 50 and over (90)
2. Race/nationality
   A. Asian American (5)
   B. African American (20)
   C. White (25)
   D. Mexican American (10)
3. Family history of breast cancer
   A. Mother, sister, or grandmother (30)
   B. None or unknown (10)
4. Your history
   A. No breast disease (10)
   B. Previous noncancerous lumps or cysts (25)
   C. Previous breast cancer (100)
5. Maternity
   A. First pregnancy before age 25 (10)
   B. First pregnancy after age 25 (15)
   C. No pregnancies (20)

Your total points _____

Interpretation

Under 100   Low-risk women should follow the 2003 ACS cancer screening guidelines. Note that the role of BSE has been redefined. Consult your physician's possible modifications to this protocol.

100–199   Moderate-risk women should consult their physicians to determine whether the ACS guideline should be followed as stated or, possibly, be modified in terms of scheduling or procedures employed. Note that the role of BSE has been redefined.

200 or more   High-risk women should consult their physicians to determine whether the ACS guidelines should be followed as stated or, very likely, be modified in terms of scheduling or procedures employed. Note that the role of BSE has been redefined.

Cervical Cancer*

1. Age group
   A. Less than 25 (10)
   B. 25–39 (20)
   C. 40–54 (30)
   D. 55 and over (30)
2. Race/nationality
   A. Asian American (10)
   B. Puerto Rican (20)
   C. African American (20)
   D. White (10)
   E. Mexican American (20)
3. Number of pregnancies
   A. 0 (10)
   B. 1 to 3 (20)
   C. 4 and over (30)

*Lower portion of uterus. These questions would not apply to a woman who has had a complete hysterectomy.

4. Viral infections
   A. Herpes and other viral infections or ulcer formations on the vagina (10)
   B. Never (1)
5. Age at first intercourse
   A. Before 15 (40)
   B. 15–19 (30)
   C. 20–24 (20)
   D. 25 and over (10)
6. Bleeding between periods or after intercourse
   A. Yes (40)
   B. No (1)

Your total points _____

Explanations

1. The highest occurrence is in the 40-and-over age group. The numbers represent the relative rates of cancer for different age groups. A 45-year-old woman has a risk three times higher than that of a 20-year-old.
2. Puerto Ricans, African Americans, and Mexican Americans have higher rates of cervical cancer.
3. Women who have delivered more children have a higher occurrence.
4. Viral infections of the cervix and vagina are associated with cervical cancer.
5. Women with earlier intercourse and with more sexual partners are at a higher risk.
6. Irregular bleeding may be a sign of uterine cancer.

Interpretation/To Carry This Further . . .

40–69	This is a low-risk group. Ask your doctor for a Pap test. You will be advised how often you should be tested after your first test.
70–99	In this moderate-risk group, more frequent Pap tests may be required.
100 or higher	You are in a high-risk group and should have a Pap test (and pelvic examination) as advised by your doctor.

Regardless of score, you should discuss with your physician the desirability of the ThinPrep Pap test (or one similar to it), as it is designed to identify the presence of DNA from one or more of the HPV strains associated with cervical cancer.

chapter twelve

managing Chronic Conditions

Online Learning Center Resources

www.mhhe.com/payne8e

Log on to our Online Learning Center (OLC) for access to these additional resources:

- Chapter key terms and definitions
- Learning objectives
- Student interactive question-and-answer sites

- Self-scoring chapter quiz
- Online assessments
- Key term flash cards

Talking It Over

Chronic Condition vs. Disability

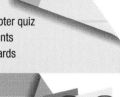

The federal government defines disability in conjunction with the Americans with Disabilities Act. Yet in a real sense a disability may only be disabling when the affected person defines it as such. Should a condition that is defined as a disability be treated as one when, according to the person with the condition, it does not interfere with his or her daily activities or distract from his or her quality of life? Should assistance of various kinds, including financial aid and access to special services, be made available to a person defined as disabled, even when the services are not asked for and appear unneeded? These questions may apply to chronic conditions that are routinely treatable or involve prolonged periods of remission, such as diabetes or hypoglycemia. What are your thoughts on these issues?

CommunicationLinks

http://www.simplystated.com
http://diseases-explained.com

Eye on the Media

Fibromyalgia: More Questions Than Answers

"Is it a real illness?" is a frequently asked question in media reports on fibromyalgia, a chronic disorder characterized by widespread musculoskeletal pain. Because there is not yet convincing physiological evidence for the symptoms suffered by people with fibromyalgia, even some physicians question its existence. But experts who have spent years studying this controversial illness say that 3 to 6 million Americans suffer from fibromyalgia syndrome, or FMS. Media coverage on internet sites, in journals, and in newspapers currently reflects our better understanding of underlying problems that trigger fibromyalgia symptoms and the medication and nondrug approaches, such as exercise, that can help many patients feel better.

FMS, which has no known cause or cure, is a frustrating and perplexing illness. It includes pain involving the tender points at the junctures between muscles and tendons.

The spectrum of symptoms may also include chronic fatigue, headaches, flulike symptoms, nonrestorative sleep, morning stiffness, impaired memory and concentration, and depression. It is called a syndrome rather than a disease, because the symptoms vary from person to person.

One frustrating aspect of the disorder stems from the perception among the general public (and some health care providers) that fibromyalgia is a psychosomatic problem, an emotional problem that manifests as a physical one. This perception can add to patients' emotional suffering. Although people with FMS often are anxious and depressed, most authorities believe that those feelings are the result rather than the cause of the problem.

According to coverage in *The New York Times* and **cnn.com,** environmental influences such as stress may play a part in FMS. Patients often report that their chronic pain is preceded by a mental or physical trauma, such as an auto accident, or a serious infection, such as Lyme disease. Despite considerable investigation, researchers have been unable to identity any infectious organism as a cause of fibromyalgia.

Increasingly, serious media coverage has helped develop a more comprehensive understanding of this disorder as well as competence to manage the illness over the long term. Information and support for those who suffer from FMS are available through websites such as **http://www.niams.nih. gov, www.arthritis.org, www.drlowe.com,** and **http://www.mdadvise.com.**

In clinical medicine, thousands of diseases, illnesses, and conditions can be diagnosed and treated. For ease of communication among health care professionals and between professionals and laypeople, these diseases and illnesses have been individually named and categorized. We have chosen a set of categories—*genetic/inherited, congenital, metabolic, autoimmune, degenerative,* and *infectious*—with which to organize a sample of conditions that we believe you will be interested in learning about. Knowledge of these conditions will increase your understanding of chronic disease processes and how they differ from infectious diseases. Where appropriate, you will also find useful information about risk factors and lifestyle changes you can make to reduce your risk of developing a chronic condition.[*][†]

The first five categories of conditions—genetic/inherited, congenital, metabolic, autoimmune, and **degenerative** —are discussed in the sections that follow. They have in common a slow, gradual course of development and remain a part of people's lives for long periods of time; thus they are said to be **chronic** conditions. Conversely, the infectious diseases are often quickly contracted and, once treatment has begun, stay active for a limited amount of time. These are referred to as the **acute** conditions (although HIV/AIDS is now defined as a chronic condition because of its extended duration). This sixth category, the infectious conditions, comprises illnesses caused by pathogenic organisms often transmitted from person to person. These conditions are discussed separately, in Chapter 13. The worldwide HIV/AIDS epidemic, the increasing threat of infectious diseases contracted from animals from distant areas of the world, and the comeback of familiar infections that are now resistant to antibiotics makes this separate coverage necessary.

Two types of chronic diseases, cardiovascular disease and cancer, are also addressed separately (in Chapters 10 and 11, respectively) because of their importance to so many families and to the health of the nation. Many other chronic conditions are addressed in appropriate chapters throughout the book. For example, low back pain is discussed in Chapter 4, osteoporosis in Chapter 4, and chronic obstructive lung disease in Chapter 9, as well as many others. Even though these conditions are not discussed in this chapter, they too fit into one or more of the categories described and are either chronic or acute in nature.

Chronic Disease Prevention

With the well-deserved emphasis placed on the prevention of heart disease and cancer, you might expect that virtually all diseases are preventable if you follow a wellness lifestyle. While it is true that many diseases are strongly linked to the lifestyle choices you make, we know little about how to prevent most of the chronic diseases described in this chapter. Learning about these conditions reminds us that even the most carefully tended human body is vulnerable

---

[*]Only a clinician can diagnose and treat these conditions. The information contained in this chapter is intended only to inform.
[†]We have placed each condition into its most appropriate category. However, the characteristics of a given condition may overlap with those in a second group. We will point this out when it occurs.

> **Key Terms**
>
> **degenerative** a slow but progressive deterioration of the body's structure or function.
>
> **chronic** develops slowly and persists for an extended period of time.
>
> **acute** has a sudden onset and a prompt resolution.

Chronic Illness—The End or a Turning Point?

Most people diagnosed with a chronic illness go through a period of serious adjustment. For college students, the necessary adaptations feel particularly burdensome because so few of their peers are faced with equal demands. Not only must self-care routines be changed, but the help of others may be necessary to carry out that care. The limitations imposed by a chronic illness can restrict the activities and behavior of the affected individual and his or her family and friends. Financial matters (including the ability to afford medications), the need to see physicians frequently, and insurance issues add to the person's stress. When young people's lives change so profoundly, they can feel isolated and singled out in a negative way.

People respond to the diagnosis of a chronic illness in various ways. Frequently, their first reaction is denial. When this occurs, care may be delayed. At the same time, school and work performance and relationships begin to suffer from the internalized stress. Eventually, though, denial gives way to anger, which is often directed at others. Common targets of this anger are people close to the ill person, such as family and friends. Then anger broadens to include the world or God (for "letting these things happen"). Eventually, the demands of the illness, combined with a sense of futility, give way to acceptance. At this stage, the individual's resourcefulness surfaces as he or she looks within for untapped sources of strength. Gradually, the person becomes open to the assistance offered by others, begins to discover new interests and abilities, and realizes that life is not over—just different.

The decision to accept the chronic condition often brings a sense of inner peace and allows for a new approach to living. People who believe that they will not be given a burden too great for them to bear may rise to the challenge and find a level of strength that they—and others—didn't know they had. With acceptance come new learning experiences. The person begins to understand the limitations of the body, to appreciate what true friendships are, and to recognize the importance of emotional resources once taken for granted. Even more significant is the realization that the spiritual dimension of health is bountiful. As the daily challenges of the illness continue, the person realizes that his or her personal beliefs and values have not only survived but are even stronger.

to the effects of aging and the array of diseases that, in many cases, we do not yet understand. Accordingly, we are challenged to move beyond our perception of health as the absence of disease and illness. Only then can we see that the value of health is not what it prevents, but rather what it makes possible—a life characterized by growth and development through each stage of the life cycle (see the Discovering Your Spirituality box above).

Genetic/Inherited Conditions

Genetic or inherited conditions can occur in any of three ways: (1) abnormal genetic material (genes) are transmitted from one or both biological parents at conception; (2) abnormal genetic material is formed by mutation of normal genetic material at a very early stage of cellular replication and, subsequently, passed on with each cell doubling; or (3) an abnormal number of chromosomes—more or fewer than the normal number of forty-six—is inherited or formed. We will present several conditions from this broad category, including Klinefelter's syndrome, Turner's syndrome, cystic fibrosis, and Duchenne muscular dystrophy.

In discussing chronic diseases, other than the more prominent ones such as cardiovascular disease, cancer, and diabetes mellitus, it is important to note that few requirements for reporting the incidence of such diseases exist (unlike infectious diseases). For example, only four states keep records of autoimmune diseases such as lupus, only seven monitor developmental disabilities, while fewer than one-half of the states report on asthma. Because of these inadequacies it is likely that many chronic diseases are underestimated, and emerging trends are difficult to determine, and environmental factors associated with their development remain unrecognized.

Abnormal Number of Sex Chromosomes

At the time of conception (fertilization) an ovum (egg) from the biological mother containing twenty-three chromosomes is penetrated by a sperm from the biological father that also contains twenty-three chromosomes. This fusion of genetic material results in an initial human cell that contains forty-six chromosomes, the number found in virtually every human cell. Of these 46 chromosomes, two are **sex chromosomes** (an X from the biological mother and an X or Y from the biological father). A normal male would thus possess a 44XY (44 nonsex

Key Terms

sex chromosomes the X and Y chromosomes that determine sex, chromosomes other than the autosomes.

chromosomes plus an X chromosome and a Y chromosome) chromosomal profile, and a normal female would be depicted as 44XX.[1] Occasionally people are born who possess more or fewer than the normal forty-six chromosomes because they have more than or fewer than the normal two sex chromosomes.

Klinefelter's Syndrome

Klinefelter's syndrome is one condition in which an abnormal number of sex chromosomes is present. It occurs in males and is a relatively rare (1 in 1,000 male births)[2] condition in which a Y sex chromosome from the biological father is combined with two X sex chromosomes. Klinefelter's syndrome would be graphically depicted as 44XXY, for a total of forty-seven chromosomes.[3] Advanced maternal age is thought to be related to the development of this syndrome.

Although they look normal at birth, male children with Klinefelter's syndrome gradually show signs of the condition by the time they reach puberty. Men with Klinefelter's syndrome are often tall, very thin, and have gynecomastia (breast enlargement).[3] In addition, a small penis, small testicles, and underdeveloped secondary sexual characteristics are typical. Men with Klinefelter's syndrome are generally infertile and have some impairment in learning ability and personality adjustment. The unique components of Klinefelter's syndrome are thought to reflect the feminizing influence of the additional X chromosome.

Prevention, Diagnosis, and Management Klinefelter's syndrome cannot, of course, be cured. Testosterone therapy is often used to minimize feminization. Since some males with Klinefelter's syndrome have minimal symptoms and are capable of spermatogenesis (sperm production), genetic counseling regarding reproduction is strongly advised.

Turner's Syndrome

Another genetic condition caused by an altered sex chromosome number is Turner's syndrome. It occurs in females (1 in 5,000 female births)[2] when one of the two X chromosomes is missing, resulting in a chromosomal number of forty-five. This pattern is graphically depicted as 44X0, with 0 reflecting the absence of the second X chromosome. Women with Turner's syndrome have equivalent versions of many of the problems seen in men with Klinefelter's syndrome: infertility, a characteristic body type, and diminished secondary sex characteristics. Treatment of Turner's syndrome involves the carefully coordinated use of growth hormone (GH), to stimulate growth in height and well-being in adulthood, and estrogen therapy to feminize the body.[4]

Inherited Genetic Mutations

Cystic Fibrosis

No inherited condition claims more children's and young adults' lives than cystic fibrosis (CF). In the United States, in about 1 of every 2,000 live births an infant is born with this inherited condition. In past decades, life expectancy for children with cystic fibrosis was only about 8 years. Today, however, with a fuller understanding of the disease and with more effective forms of treatment, life expectancy has increased significantly, to about 30 years. Unfortunately, the disease is very demanding, and effective management requires daily intervention.

Cystic fibrosis causes a profound disruption in the function of the **exocrine glands** in several areas of the body. This impaired function is due to the body's inability to produce a protein that helps regulate chloride content within the secretory cells of various exocrine glands. In the absence of this protein, the glands cannot produce certain enzymes needed to carry out important bodily functions.

For example, CF impairs the ability of the pancreas, an exocrine gland, to produce digestive enzymes. CF is known to affect other exocrine glands as well. It reduces the ability of sweat glands to conserve electrolytes, the ability of mucous glands lining the airway to control mucus production, and the ability of secretory glands within the digestive tract to produce digestive enzymes. These impairments of normal function underlie significant problems in respiration and digestion.[5]

Prevention, Diagnosis, and Management Although CF is sometimes not identified until later in life, the diagnosis is usually made during childhood. Infants and young children with CF present a combination of the following symptoms:

- Poor growth
- Frequent, foul-smelling stools
- Chronic coughing and wheezing
- Recurrent pneumonia
- Nasal polyps
- Enlarged fingertips
- Skin that has a salty taste

When CF is suspected on the basis of these symptoms, a diagnosis is made using a blood or saliva test. Today over 1,000 mutations to the CFTR gene on chromosome 7 have

---

Key Terms

exocrine glands glands whose secretions are released through tubes or ducts, such as sweat glands.

been identified as being potentially capable of causing cystic fibrosis. Of these 1,000 or more mutations, approximately 35 are clearly related to the classic expression of the disease. The remaining, in various pairings, recall that there are two number 7 chromosomes on which mutations could occur, are more likely related to "nonclassic cystic fibrosis" and other cystic fibrosis-like conditions, but not the absence of the protein that is missing in classic CF.[6]

The management of CF has improved dramatically in recent years. Diets designed to maintain weight and support growth, respiratory therapy to maintain the health of the airways, a newly approved inhaled antibiotic, a vaccine effective against CF's principal pneumonia-causing bacterium, and new drugs have improved the quality of life and increased the life expectancy of people with CF. Recently, **gene replacement therapy** through inhalation of virus-containing microscopic beads of genetic material has been attempted, but the existence of lung disease is a major obstacle to the effective delivery of the beads.[7] Accordingly, CF remains an incurable, life-shortening disease process.

Like sickle-cell disease which is described later, CF shows a **recessive inheritance pattern.** Genetic testing can determine whether a person who is apparently free from CF might, in fact, carry a copy of the recessive gene. In addition, if an at-risk pregnancy has occurred, chorionic villus sampling or amniocentesis can be performed, although this carries a risk of miscarriage. When the embryo is positive for CF, parents can seek counseling regarding their options, including whether to continue the pregnancy.

Sickle-Cell Trait and Sickle-Cell Disease

Of all the chemical compounds found within the body, few occur in as many forms as hemoglobin, which helps bind oxygen to red blood cells. Two forms of hemoglobin are associated with *sickle-cell trait* and *sickle-cell disease.* African Americans can possess either form of this abnormal hemoglobin. Those who inherit the trait form do not develop the disease but are capable of transmitting the gene for abnormal hemoglobin to their offspring. Those who inherit the disease form face a shortened life characterized by periods of pain and impairment called *crises.*

Approximately 8% of African Americans carry the recessive gene for sickle-cell trait; they experience little impairment, and they can transmit the gene to their children. For approximately 1.5% of African Americans, however, sickle-cell disease is a painful, incapacitating, and life-shortening condition.[3] Red blood cells are elongated, crescent-shaped (or sickled), and unable to pass through the body's minute capillaries (Figure 12-1). The body responds to the presence of these abnormal red blood cells by removing them very quickly. This sets the stage for

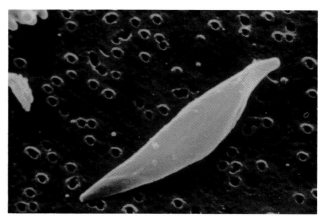

Figure 12-1 A sickled (crescent-shaped) red blood cell in a person with sickle-cell disease. The red blood cells are elongated and thus cannot pass through the body's minute capillaries, causing periods of pain and impairment called *crises.*

anemia—thus the condition is often called *sickle-cell anemia.* In addition to anemia, this form of the condition is associated with many serious medical problems, including impaired lung function, congestive heart failure, gallbladder infections, bone changes, and abnormalities of the eyes and skin. Living beyond early adulthood was until recently not possible. Today, however, with effective screening and new medications, people with sickle-cell disease may live to reach 50 years of age.[5]

Prevention, Diagnosis, and Management In about 1% of people with sickle-cell disease, a bone marrow or stem cell transplant may be able to give the body the ability to produce a normal form of hemoglobin. Early results are promising and raise hope of a "cure" of sorts, although the number of patients who might be helped by this therapy is small.[8] In addition, a newly introduced drug, hydroxyurea, has provided some relief from the pain caused by the clogging of vessels and the discomfort of acute chest congestion. The drug also reduces the number of blood transfusions normally needed to relieve pain.

Key Terms

gene replacement therapy an experimental therapy in which a healthy human gene is incorporated into a harmless virus to be delivered to cells that have an abnormal version of the gene.

recessive inheritance pattern the inheritance of traits whose expression requires that they be carried by both biological parents.

Screening to determine whether a woman or her partner carries the recessive gene may be the only key for preventing sickle-cell trait and disease. Genetic counseling can then help couples weigh the risk of passing on the gene to their children. Today, for couples at risk for passing on the gene, an ovum can be fertilized in vitro, the resulting embryo can then be tested, and if the ovum is found to be free of the condition it can be implanted in the uterus. This eliminates the need for any decision regarding a therapeutic abortion.[9] The adjacent Star box provides useful information about genetic counseling.

Sex Chromosome–Linked Inherited Genetic Mutations

Duchenne Muscular Dystrophy

Genetic mutations located on a maternal sex chromosome (which is always an X chromosome) present a unique problem for male offspring. The crux of the problem lies in the male's inability to "offset" or "override" the mutated gene's influence because he lacks a second X chromosome containing a normal version of the mutated gene. Females can carry the mutated gene but may not be affected by the abnormal trait because they have a normal second X chromosome.

Duchenne muscular dystrophy (DMD) is an inherited condition in which muscle fibers lack the ability to produce a protein called *dystrophin,* which is necessary for normal muscular function. In the absence of this protein, skeletal muscles deteriorate, impairing the ability to stand, walk, and, eventually, even breathe. Death occurs prematurely, generally due to respiratory collapse. Some people with DMD die during their teen years and some live to reach their thirties, but most die in their twenties.

Prevention, Diagnosis, and Management Muscular dystrophy can be relatively easily diagnosed by an experienced physician, but the symptoms are usually not apparent until after the age of 2. Before this age the signs of the disease are unlikely to be recognized, unless parents' concern about delayed walking prompts them to have the child seen by a physician. After age 2, however, falls, changes in gait, the development of distinct scoliosis (spinal curvature), and the appearance of muscle wasting become obvious, and the disease is identified. The diagnosis is generally made using a blood test that assesses the level of creatine kinase, an enzyme that leaks out of the muscle in response to the inadequate presence of dystrophin. Abnormally high levels of creatine kinase confirm the diagnosis.

The medical management of DMD centers on the prompt and effective use of physical therapy and occupational therapy to maintain the highest level of function possible. By the teen years, people with DMD usually can no longer walk and have begun to use a wheelchair. Scoliosis can be surgically corrected to provide relief from chest compression caused by the increasing rotation of the spine. Some people choose to use mechanical ventilation when breathing is no longer possible. Even with the best care, however, the course of the disease is irreversible. That said, however, gene therapy to correct the genetic error responsible for muscular dystrophy was attempted in 1999. Three years later some evidence of the stem cells' nuclei could be found within the muscle; however, the number of nuclei was deemed insufficient enough to be responsible for the limited improvement found in the patient's MD status.[10]

Several other forms of MD exist, including Becker, limb girdle, and a rare adult-onset form (Miyoshi myopathy). In very rare cases, muscular dystrophy is seen in females. The occurrence of the disease in females is almost certainly caused by a mutation in the person's genetic makeup that takes place during an early stage of development, rather than by inheritance.

Congenital Abnormalities

The second group of conditions, congenital abnormalities, refers to abnormalities that are present at birth. These conditions are caused by inappropriate changes in tissues (and thus in organs and organ systems) during embryonic development. Although both inherited (genetic) and congenital conditions are present at birth, congenital abnormalities differ in that they do not involve an atypical number of chromosomes, or an inherited chromosomal abnormality.

During the first 3 months of pregnancy (the first trimester), the embryo is "constructed" within the protective confines of the uterus. Tissues, organs, and organ systems are formed and take their proper positions according to the complex genetic blueprint established at conception. The embryo will be fully formed by the end of this 3-month period. Subsequent enlargement (growth) and refinement (maturation) will occur during the fetal period, which comprises the second and third trimesters.[11]

A congenital abnormality is a condition caused by the inappropriate or incomplete development of a particular embryonic structure or the failure of a structure to function properly at birth. In the section that follows, we will describe selected types of congenital abnormalities. Some congenital abnormalities are so severe that they are incompatible with life, even within the uterus. Thus the embryo is spontaneously aborted by the body (this event is commonly known as a *miscarriage*). Some other congenital abnormalities are life threatening, but the pregnancy can

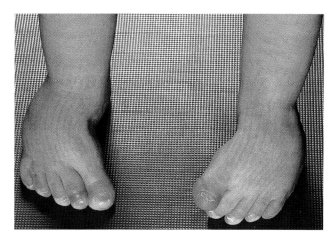

Figure 12-2 An infant with talipes (clubfoot). Treatment for this common congenital abnormality usually begins soon after birth, using plaster casts and manipulation of the foot. Surgery can be performed to give the foot a more normal appearance.

be carried to full term. And in many other cases the abnormality is recognized early in the child's life and can be corrected, or may even be so minor that it is not problematic.

No single factor is responsible for causing congenital abnormalities. They generally form early in pregnancy, during the critical weeks when the embryo's organs are being formed. They may be the result of genetic mutation or environmental factors, such as infections and drugs. Most congenital abnormalities, however, are caused by a complex interplay of factors, some genetic and some environmental. Thus their cause is considered to be **multifactorial.**

Talipes (Clubfoot)

Talipes (clubfoot) is among the most common congenital abnormalities, affecting 1 of every 1,000 infants (Figure 12-2).[12] A clubfoot is turned so that the heel points inward while the rest of the foot points inward and downward. The arch of the foot is prominent, and the muscles of the lower leg appear atrophied. This form of talipes is the most common form of the abnormality. Although there appears to be a genetic predisposition for talipes, the specific cause or causes are unknown. Early amniocentesis (at 11 to 12 weeks) also may foster the formation of talipes.[13]

Key Terms

multifactorial requiring the interplay of many factors; refers to the cause of a disease or condition.

Prevention, Diagnosis, and Management

Treatment of talipes begins soon after birth, with a combination of manipulation of the foot followed by a series of plaster casts. You may have seen infants in lower leg casts that contain a spacer board between one leg and the other. When the foot is profoundly deformed, tendon reassignment surgery can be performed to give the foot a more normal appearance. Some forms of talipes have responded well to stretching exercises performed regularly, combined with splinting or casting if necessary.

Cleft Palate and Cleft Lip

In the early weeks of embryonic life, the structures of the face, including the lips and roof of the mouth, form as separate halves on each side of the midline. Failure of the upper lip to fuse results in a split or cleft lip. Failure of the roof of the mouth to fuse causes cleft palate.[14] One of these conditions (or both) occurs in about 1 of every 800 live births.

Although a genetic predisposition may be a factor in some cases of cleft lip and palate, the cause of these conditions is unknown. Environmental factors, such as the use of certain medications during pregnancy, alcohol use, and smoking, may contribute to varying degrees.[14]

If a child's cleft lip or cleft palate is not corrected, he or she may have trouble eating or speaking clearly. In addition, cosmetic concerns may be at issue, an adequate bone foundation for tooth stability may not be established, and significant hearing loss may occur.[14] For these reasons, surgery is recommended to correct both conditions and prevent these difficulties. Figure 12-3 shows a child with cleft lip and cleft palate before surgery.

Prevention, Diagnosis, and Management

Cleft lip and cleft palate are diagnosed at delivery, when the newborn is screened for the presence of these and other abnormalities. A diverse team of health care specialists then assists parents in understanding the condition(s) and in planning the infant's presurgical and postsurgical care. This medical team would include a plastic surgeon, pediatrician, otolaryngologist (nose/throat specialist), speech pathologist, audiologist (hearing specialist), dentist, dietitian, and nurse. These health care professionals will collectively determine the child's treatment plan.

Surgery to repair a cleft lip is usually performed when the infant is three to four months old, while surgery to repair a cleft palate is usually completed before the child reaches his or her second birthday. If the nasal passages and throat structures are involved, additional surgeries may be required to achieve the high level of success that characterizes today's medical care of these facial abnormalities.[15]

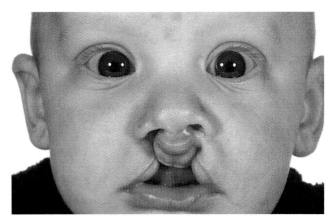

Figure 12-3 An infant with cleft lip and cleft palate. This common congenital abnormality is repaired before the child is two years old. Surgical correction is usually quite successful, both cosmetically and functionally.

Patent Foramen Ovale (PFO)

During intrauterine life, blood flow in the fetal heart by-passes the right ventricle, the chamber that normally pumps unoxygenated blood to the lungs for oxygenation (see Chapter 10). The lungs are bypassed because the fetus is in effect "under water" and, thus, cannot use its lungs. A hole (the foramen ovale) in the interatrial septum, the wall that divides the upper right chamber of the heart from the upper left chamber, provides the necessary passageway around the lungs. At the time of birth, however, when the fetus begins to breathe air, this hole is normally closed by a small flap of tissue. The blood is then redirected from the right atrium into the right ventricle to be sent to the lungs.[16]

In about one in five live births, the foramen ovale fails to close completely, without any apparent leakage of blood. In the absence of other cardiac abnormalities, this patent foramen ovale does not cause any problems, is rarely identified, and, thus, prompts no medical attention. In some infants or children, however, a patent foramen ovale may leak, allowing unoxygenated blood to flow into the left atrium and then into the left ventricle of the heart and out into the general circulation. This leakage may result in some **cyanosis** and cause a heart murmur to develop.[12]

> **Key Terms**
>
> **cyanosis** blue coloration of the lips, skin, and nail beds caused by inadequate oxygenation of the blood.

Prevention, Diagnosis, and Management

Patent foramen ovale is usually diagnosed by the child's primary care physician. No treatment is needed unless other heart abnormalities exist or the volume of unoxygenated blood reaching the left side of the heart is too great. Interestingly, recent treatment for patent ductus arteriosus, an abnormality similar in function and consequence, has been successfully treated with ibuprofen.[13] Perhaps ibuprofen, the active ingredient in OTC pain-relievers such as Motrin, will have a role in correcting patent foramen ovale.

The possible worsening of the leakage of PFO (both diagnosed and undiagnosed) in adults who regularly scuba dive has recently caused concern. Researchers speculate that pressure changes on the chest wall during descents may not only increase the right-to-left movement of blood but also reduce to a dangerous level the amount of oxygenated blood reaching the brain.[17] Experts disagree somewhat about whether scuba divers should undergo an echocardiogram to test for the presence of a patent foramen ovale.[18] If you are concerned, discuss the issue with your physician.

Scoliosis

Most cases of scoliosis (abnormal lateral spinal curvatures) have no known cause and are thus classified as *idiopathic*. For a small percentage, particularly when present at birth, a genetic basis is thought to exist. In general, curvatures that are less than 10 degrees (or 20 degrees and nonprogressive) are considered postural malalignments and do not require treatment.

Most spinal curvatures begin as a lateral deviation of the spine (curvature to the side) in either the thoracic (upper back) or lumbar (lower back) region (Figure 12-4). The normally aligned spine above or below the initial curvature then begins to curve in the opposite direction to offset the original curvature. This eventually gives the spine an "S" shape. If it is not corrected, the increasing curvature of the spine causes the vertebrae that form the spinal column to rotate. As the vertebrae rotate forward, the ribs follow accordingly, eventually altering the entire architecture of the chest cavity. This causes noticeable postural problems, including uneven positioning of the shoulder blades and a "rib hump" deformity. In addition, the changing shape of the chest compresses the heart, lungs, and related structures that pass through the middle of the chest. Increasing disfiguration and discomfort accompany each degree of additional curvature and rotation.

Prevention, Diagnosis, and Management

For most people with scoliosis, the curvature that initially develops during the preteen years progressively worsens until the spine stops growing after puberty. Since treatment

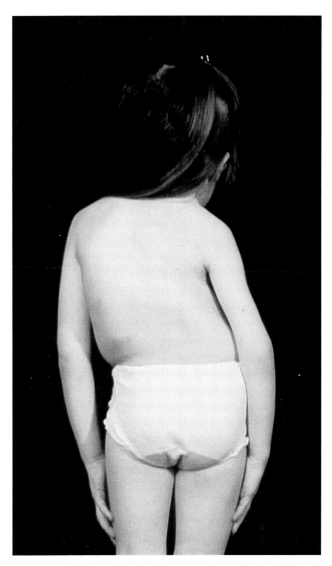

Figure 12-4 Evidence of scoliosis is commonly noted in late childhood or early adolescence.

is the key to preventing these problems, most American elementary schools screen students between the fourth and sixth grades to identify children who need additional evaluation. Children should be screened every 6 to 9 months until growth of the spine slows and then stops. Curvatures of 20 degrees but less than 30 degrees when initially found may require treatment but will generally not progress after skeletal growth stops. Curvatures greater than 30 degrees will, however, usually continue to increase well after skeletal growth has stopped and into adulthood unless effective treatment is undertaken. The Changing for the Better box on page 404 lists several signs of scoliosis.

In this country, scoliosis is treated by orthopedic surgeons. Once the spine has been radiographically evaluated and the precise nature of the condition determined, one of the following three treatment options is chosen:[19]

- *Do nothing.* Depending on the patient's age and the degree of curvature, it may be appropriate to do nothing and simply monitor the condition to see whether further change occurs.

- *Use a brace.* In children and adolescents, a curve in the mild range (between 25 and 35 degrees) is most effectively treated by bracing the back with a specially fitted metal brace for 23 hours per day. This treatment continues until the spine has moved into acceptable alignment.

- *Undergo surgery.* When a curvature in a preteen or adolescent is near or beyond 45 degrees, the treatment of choice may well be surgical realignment of several vertebrae within and beyond the curvature.

A recently completed longitudinal study could significantly alter both the role of the school in screening for scoliosis and aspects of the treatment. This study involved three groups of school students: one comprised of children with untreated scoliosis; a second group with treated scoliosis; and a third group without scoliosis. At the end of a half-century of periodic assessments, no significant differences were found between the treated and untreated scoliosis groups in terms of functionality, both physically and emotionally. Nor did either scoliosis group differ sig-

nificantly from their non-scoliosis classmates, using the same criteria. The non-scoliosis group members did, however, show somewhat less impairment than their scoliosis counterparts.[20] The authors concluded that the routine screening by schools might well be curtailed. Others, however, have questioned whether today's children would accept the deformities that were apparently acceptable to the children of 50 years ago.

Only about 2% of females and 1% of males have scoliosis. For those who do, however, new options regarding treatment could be forthcoming.

Metabolic Disorders

The third category of chronic conditions is metabolic. Metabolic disorders are caused by the body's inability to control chemical processes that regulate the building up (anabolism) and tearing down (catabolism) of tissue. Diabetes mellitus type 2 and diabetes mellitus type 1 are, perhaps, the most familiar of the metabolic disorders.

Congenital abnormalities, which you learned about in the last section, are caused by abnormal structure that leads to abnormal function. The metabolic disorders, on the other hand, are caused directly by abnormal function. The body is unable to normally utilize various nutrients in the growth and repair of tissues and in the regulation of body processes. The conditions described in this section have clear metabolic components. They may also have some characteristics that overlap with other categories of conditions. For example, a genetic predisposition is associated with non-insulin-dependent diabetes mellitus (type 2), and an autoimmune response with type 1.[21]

Non-Insulin-Dependent Diabetes Mellitus (Type 2)

In people who do not have diabetes mellitus, the body's need for energy is met through the "burning" of glucose (blood sugar) within the cells. Glucose is absorbed from the digestive tract and carried to the cells by the blood or stored in the liver as glycogen for later conversion back to glucose.[22] Glucose passes into the cell through a transport system that moves the glucose molecule across the cell's membrane. Activation of this glucose transport mechanism requires the hormone **insulin** (Figure 12-5).

Key Terms

insulin a hormone produced by the islet cells of the pancreas that is necessary for the normal utilization of glucose.

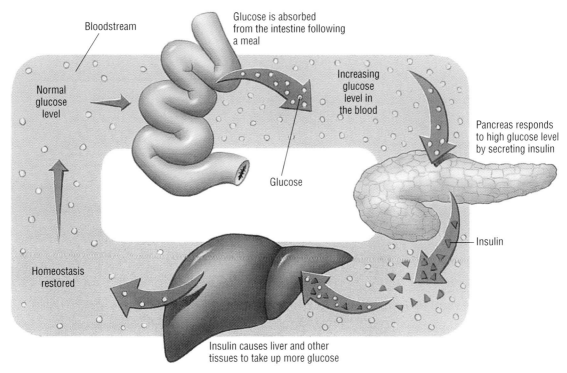

Bloodstream

Normal glucose level

Glucose is absorbed from the intestine following a meal

Increasing glucose level in the blood

Pancreas responds to high glucose level by secreting insulin

Glucose

Insulin

Homeostasis restored

Insulin causes liver and other tissues to take up more glucose

Figure 12-5 Normal blood glucose regulation. The secretion of insulin is regulated by a mechanism that tends to reverse any deviation from normal. Thus an increase in blood glucose level triggers secretion of insulin. Since insulin promotes glucose uptake by cells, blood glucose level is restored to its lower, normal level.

Specific receptor sites for insulin can be found on the cell membrane. Insulin is also required for the conversion of glucose into glycogen in the liver and for the formation of fatty acids in adipose cells. Insulin is produced in the islet cells of the pancreas. The release of insulin from the pancreas corresponds to the changing levels of glucose within the blood.[22]

In adults with a genetic predisposition for developing non-insulin-dependent diabetes mellitus (type 2), trigger mechanisms (most likely obesity and inactivity) begin a process through which the body cells become in-creasingly less sensitive to the presence of insulin.[23] The growing ineffectiveness of insulin in moving glucose into cells causes the buildup of glucose in the blood. Elevated levels of glucose in the blood give rise to **hyperglycemia,** a hallmark symptom of non-insulin-dependent diabetes mellitus.

In response to this buildup, the kidneys begin the process of filtering glucose from the blood. Excess glucose then spills over into the urine. This removal of glucose in the urine is a second important symptom of adult onset diabetes. Increased thirst, a third symptom of developing diabetes, occurs in response to the movement of fluid from extracellular spaces into the circulatory system to maintain homeostasis.[24]

Prevention, Diagnosis, and Management

For many adults with diabetes, dietary modification (with an emphasis on monitoring total carbohydrate intake, not

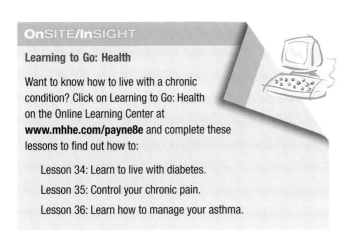

OnSITE/InSIGHT

Learning to Go: Health

Want to know how to live with a chronic condition? Click on Learning to Go: Health on the Online Learning Center at **www.mhhe.com/payne8e** and complete these lessons to find out how to:

Lesson 34: Learn to live with diabetes.

Lesson 35: Control your chronic pain.

Lesson 36: Learn how to manage your asthma.

> **Key Terms**
>
> **hyperglycemia** the condition of having an abnormally high blood glucose level.

just sugar) and regular exercise is the only treatment required to maintain an acceptable level of glucose. Weight loss improves the condition by "releasing" more insulin receptors, and exercise increases the actual number of receptor sites. With better insulin recognition, the person can return to a more normal state of functioning.

For people whose condition is more advanced, dietary modification and weight loss alone will not be effective in managing the condition, and oral drugs that stimulate insulin output, called hypoglycemic agents, will be required. Increasingly, very aggressive management, including drugs and insulin, is successfully reducing risks associated with the disease. Many persons, however, have difficulty controlling blood sugar levels even with the use of insulin.

In addition to genetic predisposition and obesity as important factors in non-insulin-dependent diabetes mellitus, unresolved stress appears to play a role in the development of hyperglycemic states. Although stress alone probably cannot produce a diabetic condition, it is likely that stress can induce a series of endocrine changes that can lead to a state of hyperglycemia. Depression too can elevate blood glucose levels and thus increase the risk of expressing type 2 diabetes.

Diabetes can cause serious damage to several important body structures. The extent to which people with diabetes develop these pathological changes can be markedly influenced by the nature of their particular condition and the type of management with which they comply. Today, in addition to the 17 million persons known to have type 2 diabetes, there may be another 16 million persons who are affected but not yet diagnosed. Particularly distressing is the rate of increase noted among Hispanic Americans, especially those of Mexican decent. Their rate of increase (double that of the population as a whole) may be explained on the basis of a unique genetic marker recently discovered. Once fully understood, this genetic uniqueness may add further insight into the pathology of diabetes mellitus type 2.

Because of the increased incidence in diabetes mellitus type 2, the medical community is now recommending routine blood glucose screening for persons age 25 and older and is urging the establishment of a more rigorous standard for defining normal blood glucose levels. Of course, prevention is always the best solution. Currently the American Diabetes Association (ADA) recommends a blood glucose of 90–130 mg/dl between meals and a level less than 180 mg/dl at 2 hours after beginning a meal.[25] (See Table 12.1 for a variation on these recommendations.)

A second important biomedical index to maintain, in addition to blood glucose, in the prevention type 2 is that of blood pressure. Today, for persons of susceptibility, it is now advised that pressure readings be 135 or less over 80 of less.[26] The Changing for the Better box on page 407 presents a wellness plan for preventing this type of diabetes.

Table 12.1 Normal and Target Blood Glucose Ranges (mg/dL)

Normal blood glucose levels in people who do not have diabetes

Upon waking (fasting)	70 to 110
After meals	70 to 140

Target blood glucose levels in people who have diabetes

Before meals	90 to 130
1 to 2 hours after the start of a meal	less than 180
Hypoglycemia (low blood glucose)	70 or below

Source: National Diabetes Information Clearinghouse (NIDC). Hypoglycemia. 2003. http://www.diabetes.niddk.nih.gov/dm/pubs/hypoglycemia/index.htm

Insulin-Dependent Diabetes Mellitus (Type 1)

A second type of diabetes mellitus is insulin-dependent diabetes mellitus (type 1). The onset of this type of diabetes usually occurs before age 35, most often during childhood. In contrast to type 2 diabetes, in which insulin is produced but is ineffective because of insensitivity, in type 1 diabetes the body produces no insulin at all. Destruction of the insulin-producing cells of the pancreas by the immune system (possibly in search of a viral infection within the islet cells of the pancreas) accounts for this sudden and irreversible loss of insulin production.[27]

Prevention, Diagnosis, and Management

In most ways the two forms of diabetes are similar, with the important exception that insulin-dependent diabetes mellitus always requires the use of insulin from an outside source (see the Star box on page 408). Today this insulin is obtained from either animals or genetically engineered bacteria. It is taken by injection (one to four times per day) or through the use of an insulin pump, which provides a constant supply of insulin. Delivery of insulin by inhalation has recently been introduced. Transdermal delivery of insulin (by a patch) is also an option. Development of the glucometer, a highly accurate device for measuring the amount of glucose in the blood, allows better management of this condition. Progress toward development of an immunization for type 1 diabetes mellitus and in vitro pancreas cell transplantation also has occurred. In the latter cases cells taken from the pancreatic duct, a tube leading from the pancreas to the small intestine, were cultured in a medium, enzymatically regressed back into a more youthful state, and then

A Wellness Plan for Preventing Type 2 Diabetes Mellitus

I've recently been diagnosed with type 2 diabetes. How can I live well with this condition?

The rate at which Americans develop non-insulin-dependent diabetes mellitus (type 2) is on the rise, partly because the population is aging. The disease typically affects older people and thus is sometimes called *adult-onset diabetes*. African Americans, Hispanic Americans, and Native Americans are at greater risk than are members of other ethnic groups, but anyone can develop the disease. There is no foolproof way to prevent diabetes, but you can take steps to lower your risk.

- Obesity and Overweight
  Not all obese people become diabetic, but 90 percent of people with diabetes are overweight. In addition, body fat distribution is important—those who are heavy around the middle ("apple shaped") are more susceptible to the disease than those whose fat is stored in the buttocks and thighs ("pear shaped"). Evidence indicates that both men and women who gain weight in adulthood increase their risk of diabetes. A recent study conducted at Harvard University showed that women who had gained 11 to 17 pounds since age 18 doubled their risk of diabetes; those who had gained between 18 and 24 pounds tripled their risk.

  If diabetes runs in your family and you are overweight, you are four times as likely to become diabetic as a person with neither risk factor and twice as likely as a person with only one of these risk factors. Whatever your family history, staying within a healthy weight range and losing weight if you are overweight (see Chapter 6) will lower your risk of diabetes. If you tend to weight-cycle (repeatedly lose weight and then gain it back), keep trying. It is not true, as was once believed, that weight-cycling (yo-yo dieting) is in itself harmful to health.

- Genetics
  Some progress has been made in identifying the genes that predispose a person to become obese or develop diabetes, but many more years of research will undoubtedly be required before this knowledge is of any practical use. As already mentioned, a family history of diabetes puts you at increased risk. This does not mean that people with a family history are certain to develop diabetes. But if the disease runs in your family, you should try to reduce other risk factors.

- Diet
  Following a sound diet is a worthwhile step toward preventing diabetes. A semivegetarian diet (see Chapter 5) is known to lower the risk of heart disease and cancer and may also lower the risk of diabetes. It is low in fat, especially animal fat, and rich in fruits, grains, vegetables, and low-fat or nonfat dairy products. Such a diet is unlikely to promote weight gain and often promotes weight loss. It also provides the vitamins, minerals, and other nutrients you need to help prevent chronic diseases.

- Exercise
  Direct evidence shows that regular physical activity helps prevent diabetes. In one study, researchers from the University of California at Berkeley and Stanford University found that men who were very active—expending 3,500 calories in exercise per week—were only half as likely to develop diabetes as men who were sedentary, expending less than 500 calories per week in leisure-time activity. In fact, those who benefited most from exercise were those at highest risk for diabetes.

  Other strong evidence indicates that vigorous exercise, even if done only once a week, has a protective effect against diabetes in both women and men. This is not just because exercise can promote weight loss—physical activity lowers blood sugar whether or not you lose weight.

- Vitamin and Mineral Supplements
  There is no evidence that any supplement can prevent diabetes, despite manufacturers' claims for chromium and other supplements. People with diabetes are often deficient in some vitamins and minerals, such as vitamin E, zinc, magnesium, and occasionally chromium. But these deficiencies may be caused in part by a reduced ability to absorb and utilize these nutrients. Thus they may be a result of the disease, not the cause.

- Smoking
  Smoking boosts your risk of diabetes and exacerbates the disease if you already have it. If you are a smoker, do whatever it takes to quit (see Chapter 9). Diabetes is just one of the many serious threats to your health that will be greatly reduced if you stop smoking now.

- Stress
  Stress negatively influences type 2 diabetes mellitus in two ways. First, with regard to physiological function, the body's natural response to stress (see Chapter 3) increases the level of glucose and free fatty acids in the blood, thus placing greater than normal demands on the diabetic's already compromised insulin response (see pages 64–66). Second, during periods of stress a person with diabetes may not maintain the level of control over their condition that is normally in place. This can occur in different ways. For example, while stressed, they may be too occupied to monitor blood glucose levels on a regular basis, they may alter their dietary patterns in a less than healthful manner, or they may decrease their level of physical activity and thus lower their level of insulin sensitivity.

  When taken in combination, the detrimental influence of stress and the control of type 2 diabetes mellitus demand advanced coping capabilities on the part of the person with this form of diabetes. Chapter 3 of your textbook discusses at length ways in which persons can increase their ability to prevent stress, moderate its intensity, or expend the high blood glucose levels found in association with the stress response.

stimulated to transform themselves into islet cells capable of producing insulin.[28]

An even more recently introduced variation of a transplant-based treatment (or cure) of diabetes mellitus type 1 is the use of cadaver islet cells. These cells are harvested from the pancreas of a non-diabetic deceased donor and implanted into the pancreas of a person with diabetes mellitus type 1. This highly experimental procedure is under refinement.[29]

With both forms of diabetes mellitus, sound dietary practices, planned activity, and control of stress are important for keeping blood glucose levels within a normal range. When diabetes mellitus is not properly managed, several serious problems can result, including blindness, gangrene of the extremities, kidney disease, and heart attack. These and other common complications of diabetes are listed in the Star box above. People who cannot establish good control of the disease are likely to die prematurely.

Hypoglycemia (Reactive and Functional)

When people with insulin-dependent diabetes mellitus do not eat enough, exercise too much, or take too much insulin, they may develop excessively low levels of blood sugar (blood glucose), resulting in a state of **hypoglycemia.** In nondiabetic people, difficulty maintaining high enough blood glucose levels may also be associated with drug use, liver damage, partial removal of the stomach, fasting, pancreatic tumors, and rare forms of adrenal and breast tumors, or as a prediabetic symptom.[30] People who have hypoglycemia experience headaches, mild confusion, low energy levels, anxiety, sweating, and tremors. They may look pale and behave somewhat abnormally. The blood glucose ranges shown in Table 12.1 are applicable to both the diagnosis of hypoglycemia and the management of diabetes.

A rare form of hypoglycemia called *reactive hypoglycemia* is seen in people who are hypersensitive to the presence of sugar in the blood. In these people, a meal that is high in simple carbohydrates (sugars) stimulates excessive insulin production. This insulin removes blood sugar too quickly, leading to a state of hypoglycemia. People with reactive hypoglycemia have the same symptoms seen in hypoglycemia caused by other factors.

Prevention, Diagnosis, and Management

Before reactive hypoglycemia can be definitively diagnosed, the many other causes of low blood sugar (including diabetes mellitus) must first be ruled out. Treatment of reactive hypoglycemia involves dietary modification centered on the consumption of frequent, small meals that contain high levels of complex carbohydrates and few simple carbohydrates. These dietary modifications make the movement of glucose into the bloodstream more gradual, thus eliminating high glucose loads. This

---

Key Terms

hypoglycemia the condition of having an abnormally low blood glucose level.

"spacing out" of glucose delivery to the blood reduces the body's tendency to over-produce insulin.

In the 1970s the diagnosis of hypoglycemia was made by some physicians to placate patients who complained of vague symptoms of anxiety, moodiness, fatigue, and a loss of interest in normal activities. Once clinical conditions such as depression were ruled out, patients were told that they "must be experiencing hypoglycemia." Patients were then put on a special diet and assured that they would begin to feel better "now that the problem was known." In many cases, patients reported dramatic improvement. Thus hypoglycemia was, for the better part of a decade, much more "common" than it is now believed to be. Today, this less frequently seen, yet still controversial, hypoglycemia is referred to as *functional hypoglycemia* by

some. Central to its clear substantiation is a normal blood glucose reading at the time of symptoms (which can be difficult to obtain) and suggestions of a psychiatric illness on a valid mental health inventory.[31, 32]

Autoimmune/Hypersensitivity Disorders

In Chapter 13 you'll learn more about the immune system. Until that time, the immune system can be described as an integrated collection of tissues, organs, and specific areas of endocrine (ductless) cells working to protect the body from foreign protein. On occasion, however, the immune system fails to recognize the body's own protein as being familiar (self) and mistakenly identifies its own protein as foreign (other) and begins attacking it in an attempt to "protect" the body. When this begins, an **autoimmune disorder** has begun. In this section of the chapter, examples of the autoimmune response will be described.

Fibromyalgia

Fibromyalgia syndrome (FMS) is a chronic condition with symptoms that are so complex an affected person might never be diagnosed and treated despite years of discomfort. For the 2% of the adult population believed to have FMS, intermittent periods of morning stiffness, muscle pain, fatigue, numbness and tingling, poor sleep, chronic headaches, jaw discomfort, and many other problems are often seen simply as signs of aging or stress. To trained physicians (often rheumatologists), however, these symptoms may indicate FMS. Accordingly, this syndrome can be diagnosed and effectively treated. Of course, other chronic conditions can coexist with FMS.

The cause of fibromyalgia is unclear at this time. Theories focus on immune system dysfunction (autoimmunity), altered neurotransmitter regulation, hormonal abnormalities (cortisol and HGH), and subtle brain dysfunction. Additionally, certain trigger events—infections, emotional stress, physical trauma such as a fall—thyroid dysfunction, and connective tissue disorders, such as lupus (see page 413), may cause or exacerbate FMS.[33]

Key Terms

autoimmune disorders disorders caused by the immune system's failure to recognize the body as "self"; thus the body mounts an attack against its own cells and tissues.

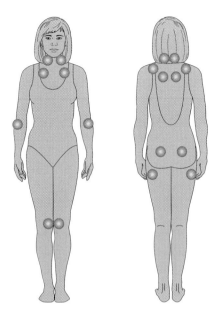

Figure 12-6 Tenderpoint locations Persons with fibromyalgia experience tenderness in at least eleven of the eighteen tenderpoint locations.

Prevention, Diagnosis, and Management

Preventive measures for fibromyalgia syndrome might be to reduce stress, avoid infections, and maintain a high level of overall health. Another preventive strategy is the appropriate diagnosis and treatment of associated conditions, such as lupus, rheumatoid arthritis, and thyroid disease.

The diagnosis of FMS is based on medical history and the assessment of discomfort in 18 so-called *tenderpoint locations* (see Figure 12-6). For research purposes, people who experience pain in at least 11 of the 18 tender points are diagnosed with FMS.[34] A lower number of "hits" is considered to be diagnostic in a nonresearch setting. Most people with chronic discomfort will be found to have several tender points during the examination. People who lack tender points and morning stiffness, but have other symptoms of FMS, may have chronic fatigue syndrome (CFS).[34]

The treatment of fibromyalgia centers on improving sleep and reducing pain. Physicians can prescribe medications to enhance the effectiveness of sleep-inducing neurotransmitters (such as serotonin and norepinephrine). Nonsteroidal anti-inflammatory drugs (NSAIDs), such as ibuprofen, are used for pain relief. Mild sedatives and muscle relaxants are also employed. Other therapies include synthetic narcotics or transdermal patches for pain relief, acupuncture, and therapeutic massage.

The prognosis for people with FMS is unclear, since few long-term studies have been carried out. For most patients, the condition will remain chronic, with periods of remission and active discomfort occurring intermittently. Whether daily functioning will be significantly impaired later in life remains to be seen.

Asthma

Bronchial asthma is a chronic respiratory disease characterized by acute attacks of breathlessness and wheezing caused by chronic airway inflammation with episodes of narrowing of the bronchioles. Although the mechanisms associated with asthmatic attacks are understood, the reason that some people develop a high level of immune system hypersensitivity is not fully known. The identification of a gene (which may be one of several) related to asthma suggests a genetic predisposition that is expressed during exposure to one or more triggering agents, or allergens.

Two main types of asthma have been identified: extrinsic and intrinsic. In extrinsic asthma, allergens such as pollen, dust mites, mold spores, animal fur or dander, and feathers produce sudden and severe bronchoconstriction that narrows the airways. Increased sputum production further narrows the bronchioles and restricts the passage of air. This narrowing fosters the development of chronic inflammation of the airways, which is the most damaging aspect of asthma. Wheezing is most pronounced when the person attempts to exhale air through the narrowed air passages. For many people with asthma, exercise, cigarette smoke, and certain foods or drugs can cause an asthma attack (Figure 12-7). Physicians once suspected that immunizations (for measles, mumps, and rubella) predisposed people to extrinsic asthmatic attacks by hypersensitizing the immune system, but this view currently finds lessened support.

The incidence of extrinsic asthma increased within the general population and particularly among children during the 1980s and 1990s. Today that increase has leveled. That said, however, asthmatic attacks account for nearly one-fifth of the pediatric emergency room visits in this country. Minority children, in particular, are most at risk of developing asthma and dying from its complications. Underlying this increased risk for asthma among minority children is a combination of factors. Among the environmental factors potentially causing this increase are the diminished quality of both outdoor and indoor urban air quality (acidic particles), high levels of urban violence (stress), and overexposure to ozone in high-density traffic areas. However, genetic predisposition may also play an important role in this increase, as studies comparing asthma levels among children of different races who share the same environment consistently find higher rates among minority children than their non-minority classmates. A final environmental factor that may account for some of the reported increase is the more complete reporting of acute asthmatic attacks and

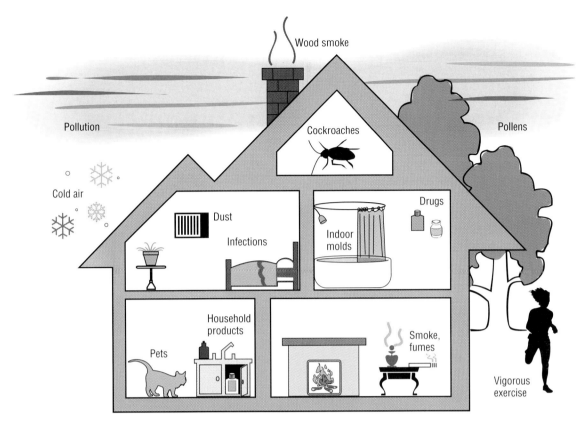

Figure 12-7 Common asthma triggers. If you have asthma, do you know which triggers are troublesome for you?

deaths (by hospital ERs) without, unfortunately, the much-needed increase in initial diagnosis and medical management that would have prevented the acute attacks and death.

Intrinsic asthma, the less common form, has similar symptoms but is caused by stress, frequent respiratory tract infections, or possibly by the aftereffects of maternal antibiotic during pregnancy.[35] Allergens play a lesser role in this form of asthma, which may be more strongly influenced by genetic predisposition for a hypersensitive immune response to foreign protein (allergens).

Prevention, Diagnosis, and Management

Prevention or effective management of asthma is often possible using a combination of approaches. Most important, of course, is the maintenance of high-level wellness through a healthful lifestyle that includes a sound diet, regular exercise, and effective stress management. Each person who has asthma should work with his or her physician to develop a sound, individually tailored management plan. The goals of such a plan are listed in the Star box on page 412. If you have asthma, complete the Personal Assessment on page 425 to determine whether you are doing all you can to manage your condition effectively.

A number of components can be included in an asthma management plan. Exercises that are well tolerated, such as swimming, can help maintain a more normal level of respiratory function. Immunotherapy, in which the patient with extrinsic asthma is desensitized through injections of weakened allergens, is often attempted. In addition, the careful use of corticosteroid drugs several times per day by inhalation reduces inflammation. Additional drugs have recently been introduced. Among these are *antileukotrienes* that reduce the immune system's ability to foster inflammation, a new class of engineered antibodies that bind to natural antibodies, thus preventing the activation of mast cells that trigger the asthmatic response,[36] and others that reduce the effects of exercise and cold air that frequently trigger asthma attacks.

Despite the use of older drugs, such as the bronchodilators that open constricted airways, and the newer drugs that counter specific allergens or immune system–based inflammation, asthma remains a serious and potentially fatal condition. Each year in this country, several thousand people die as the result of asthma attacks. Some experts believe that this number could be reduced if physicians were more aggressive in their treatment of the bronchial inflammation component of the condition.

Goals of an Effective Asthma Management Plan

The key to effective management of asthma is developing and following a management plan that is appropriate for your condition and fits your lifestyle. According to the *Guidelines for Diagnosis and Management of Asthma,* published by the National Heart, Lung, and Blood Institute of the National Institutes of Health, the goals of a successful asthma management plan are the following:

- To maintain normal activity levels (including exercise)
- To maintain near-normal pulmonary function rates
- To prevent chronic and troublesome symptoms, such as coughing or breathlessness at night, in the morning, or after exertion
- To prevent recurrent asthma attacks
- To avoid adverse effects from asthma medications
- To avoid emergency room visits and hospitalizations

People with exercise-induced asthma (EIA), a common type of extrinsic asthma, should take several important steps when attempting to exercise (see the Changing for the Better box below).

Many children who have asthma manage well with the proper use of exercise and medication. They may experience less asthma, or none at all, when they reach adulthood.

Changing for the Better

Tips for Controlling Exercise-Induced Asthma

I've been jogging every day for the past 3 years and recently found out that I have asthma. How can I keep jogging without triggering asthma attacks?

- Obtain a treatment and prevention plan from your physician.
- Alert instructors and coaches about the existence of any treatment plan.
- Medicate before exercising according to your physician's instruction.
- Warm up slowly to increase heart rate gradually and cool down slowly after exercise.
- Carry your bronchodilator with you at all times if one was prescribed.
- Wear a scarf or mask over your mouth and nose during cold weather to warm and moisten the air you breathe.
- Wear an allergy mask over the mouth and nose when exercising during pollen season.

Crohn's Disease

A wide array of chronic conditions that involve the gastrointestinal system are collectively referred to as *inflammatory bowel disease (IBD)*. One type of IBD is Crohn's disease, an erosive deterioration of the inner surface and muscular layer of the intestinal wall that affects nearly 500,000 Americans, many of whom are of traditional college age. The disease most often affects the terminal end of the small intestine and the beginning of the large intestine, or colon. When the disease is active (it frequently has long periods of remission), symptoms include abdominal pain in the lower right quadrant, fever, diarrhea, weight loss, and rectal bleeding that leads to anemia.

Although the cause of Crohn's disease is not fully understood, an autoimmune response, a genetic predisposition, and a history of emotional stress may be the principal factors. Multiple forms of Crohn's disease are thought to exist, with each reflecting different genetic components. Genes located on chromosomes 4, 12, and 16 are under investigation.[37,38] Because of the array of conditions that constitute IBD and the complex etiology

Changing for the Better

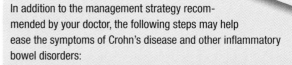

Managing Inflammatory Bowel Disease

What are the most important steps I should take to control my inflammatory bowel disease?

In addition to the management strategy recommended by your doctor, the following steps may help ease the symptoms of Crohn's disease and other inflammatory bowel disorders:

- Eat a low-fat diet. Avoid cream, butter, whole milk, and high-fat salad dressings, cheeses, and meats.
- Eat more high-fiber foods, such as fruits, grains, and vegetables. This should help if you are constipated. But take a gradual approach. Sudden increases in fiber may cause gas and diarrhea.
- Avoid sorbitol, a sugar substitute used in many products; it can cause diarrhea. Fructose, found in fruits and often in processed foods, may also be a problem.
- Try switching to lactose-free milk in case you have trouble digesting milk sugar.
- Cut down on or eliminate alcohol and caffeine.
- If you are taking medications, particularly antibiotics, ask your doctor if they could exacerbate the disease.
- Try eating several small meals a day rather than two or three large ones.
- If emotional stress is involved, try dealing with it directly by talking with a counselor.
- Regular exercise and other lifestyle alterations may help.

of each condition, it is difficult to account for the disproportionate incidence of Crohn's (and IBD) among women, and particularly among minority women. Within the latter, younger Jewish women are disproportionately represented.

Prevention, Diagnosis, and Management

When a patient reports the symptoms just described, the physician quickly suspects some form of IBD, such as Crohn's disease. Accordingly, blood tests are ordered and a complete series of gastrointestinal (GI) X-rays is taken. Additional diagnostic procedures could include a CT scan of the GI tract, endoscopic examination of the colon, and a biopsy of the intestinal wall. Positive results of these tests confirm the diagnosis of Crohn's disease.[5]

Today an array of pharmacological agents is available or in development for use in the management of Crohn's disease. Sulfasalazine, a widely used medication, is now available in new forms. In addition, a variety of monoclonal antibodies and proteins will soon be available to reduce the impact of tumor necrosis factor in some forms of the disease, as will other immunosuppressive drugs and a variety of newer steroids with fewer side effects. A medication (Lotronex) found effective in minimizing the diarrhea that often accompanies Crohn's and IBD was returned to the market in 2003 following its removal in 2000 by the FDA.

Currently the most promising trreatment for Crohn's and rheumatoid arthritis is the use of remicade, an antibody to tumor necrosis factor (TNF). TNF is an immune system component that, in Crohn's disease, attacks the lining of the intestinal tract.

Although Crohn's disease can often be well managed, intestinal obstructions can occur due to the progressive thickening of the intestinal wall in the area of inflammation. Surgery may be necessary to remove the obstruction. However, obstructions may form in neighboring areas of the intestinal tract, requiring additional surgery. **Fistulas** can develop between the intestinal tract wall and adjacent structures, such as the vagina or urinary bladder. These, too, will be corrected surgically. People with Crohn's disease may encounter further complications, including gallstones, arthritis, and chronic irritation of the skin. The Changing for the Better box on page 412 offers suggestions for managing Crohn's disease and other inflammatory bowel diseases.

Systemic Lupus Erythematosus (SLE)

Systemic lupus erythematosus, or simply *lupus,* is one of the most familiar autoimmune disorders or connective tissue disorders. These conditions are caused by an extensive and inappropriate attack by the body's immune system on its own tissues, which then serve as **self-antigens** (see Chapter 13 for a discussion of the immune response).

Considering Complementary Care

Symptomatic Irritable Bowel Disease

Gastrointestinal disorders in general, and irritable bowel disease (IBD) specifically, including irritable bowel syndrome (IBS), are treated through a wide array of conventional therapies. Recently, however, a less conventional therapy, hypnotherapy, was used with adequate success in three different studies.

In the three carefully controlled studies reported since 1996 (in the Netherlands, United States, and England) patients with symptomatic IBD were first judged suitable for hypnosis on the basis of psychiatric assessment. Once identified, experimental groups receiving hypnotherapy were matched to control groups receiving more conventional treatment protocols. In each study, members of the experimental group received gut-targeted hypnosis designed to reduce pain and flatulence as well as normalize bowel habits.

At the conclusion of each study, all three experimental groups demonstrated symptomatic relief comparable to that obtained by control group members. Additionally, the experimental groups were found to have experienced a level of attrition no greater that that experienced by the control groups. The study authors, understandably, concluded that hypnotherapy is as effective as more traditional medical protocols in the treatment of irritable bowel syndrome.

On the basis of these studies, and earlier anecdotal reports also suggesting positive results, hypnotherapy appears to be moving slowly in gaining acceptance as a conventional treatment for the symptomatic relief of IBS.

The word **systemic** refers to the widespread destruction of fibrous connective tissue and other tissues. *Erythematosus* (*erythema-* means "red") refers to the reddish rash that imparts a characteristic "mask" to the face of a person with SLE. The disease is seen in women twenty-five times more often than in men and first appears during young adulthood (see the Learning from Our Diversity box on page 414). Particularly interesting within this gender inequity is the higher incidence of lupus reported

Key Terms

fistula a fissure, break, or hole in the wall of an organ.

self-antigens the cells and tissues that stimulate the immune system's autoimmune response.

systemic (sis **tem** ic) distributed or occurring throughout the entire body system.

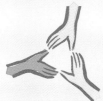
among African American women and women of Hispanic and Asian origin than among other women.

The course of systemic lupus erythematosus is gradual, with intermittent periods of inflammation, stiffness, fatigue, pleurisy (chest pain), and discomfort over wide areas of the body, including muscles, joints, and skin. Similar changes may take place in the tissues of the nervous system, kidneys, and heart.[5]

Researchers do not know why the immune system attacks the body in such an extensive and aggressive way. It is likely, however, that a combination of genetic predisposition, hormones (estrogen), chronic emotional stress (see Chapter 3), ultraviolet radiation (including sunlight), and an earlier viral infection may be involved in its development.

TALKING POINTS You learn that two young women who are your co-workers have recently been diagnosed with lupus and Crohn's disease, respectively. How can you be supportive of them? What would you say to them about their conditions, particularly on days when it is obvious that they are not feeling well?

Prevention, Diagnosis, and Management

A physician may suspect lupus based on the patient's description of her symptoms and make a diagnosis using a number of laboratory tests, including the identification of an SLE factor in the blood. A skin biopsy may be taken to confirm structural changes in the connective tissue layer below the skin.

Management of lupus generally involves the occasional or long-term use of nonsteroidal anti-inflammatory drugs (NSAIDs), malarial drugs for the skin rash, and a low dose of prednisone (a corticosteroid) to reduce fever, treat episodes of pleurisy, and minimize certain neurological symptoms. The immune system itself may be medically suppressed as well. These treatments must be carefully monitored because they have serious side effects. *Plasmapheresis,* a plasma exchange procedure, in which various immune system components are filtered from the blood, has also been employed in the treatment of SLE.[39]

Management of lupus centers on the prevention of episodes of the disease called *flares.* These periods of active lupus are often triggered by exposure to the sun, periods of fatigue, or an infectious disease, all of which should be avoided as much as possible.

Multiple Sclerosis (MS)

For proper nerve conduction to occur within portions of the brain and spinal cord, an insulating sheath of myelin must surround the neurons (nerve cells). In the progressive disease multiple sclerosis (MS), the cells that produce myelin are destroyed, myelin production ceases, and the underlying nerves are badly damaged. Neurological functioning eventually becomes so disrupted that vital functions are significantly impaired. The cause of MS is not known. Research continues to focus on multiple virus-induced autoimmune mechanisms in which T cells attack viral-infected myelin-producing cells.

Prevention, Diagnosis, and Management

Multiple sclerosis usually appears for the first time during the young adult years. It may take one of four forms, depending on the interplay of periods of stabilization (remitting), renewed deterioration (relapsing), and continuous deterioration (progressive) combinations of the above. The initial symptoms of the condition are often visual impairment, prickling and burning in the extremities, and an altered gait. In its most advanced stages, movement is greatly impaired and mental deterioration may be present.

Treatment of MS is aimed at reducing the severity of symptoms and extending the periods of remission. Today a variety of therapies are used, including immune system–targeted drugs, steroid drugs, drugs to relieve muscle spasms, a medication to fight fatigue, injections of nerve blockers, and physical therapy.

The development of immune system-related medications is at the center of the fight against MS. Four interferon-based medications, Avonex, Betaserone, Copaxone, and Novantrone, are currently at the forefront of treating MS. Depending on the specific form of MS being addressed, these medications are generally able to slow the progression of the illness, thus delaying the occurrence of the most debilitating symptoms, or to reduce the duration of relapses. In addition to these medications, other interferon-based medications, such as Rebif and Antegren, await full-scale entry into the marketplace. Additional medications are available to address complications of MS, such as spasticity. Also, initial studies involving the implantation of human adult stem cells into MS patients has proven promising in reducing the number of brain lesions,[40] as has the use of statins (cholesterol-lowering drugs) in MS-developing laboratory mice. To date, this represents the closest approximation of "prevention" that has been obtained in the field of MS treatment. In addition to the interferon-based drugs just described, monoclonal antibodies designed to prevent the movement of immune cells from the blood into the nerve tissue are under study.

Psychotherapy is an important adjunct to the treatment of MS. Profound periods of depression often accompany the initial diagnosis of this condition. Emotional support is helpful in dealing with the progressive impairment associated with the condition.

Degenerative Diseases

A fifth category of chronic conditions is that of degenerative diseases. Conditions within this category are among the most debilitating of all chronic conditions in that they generally appear late in life, in conjunction with the overall frailty of advanced age, and thus put great demand on caregivers. Eventually, expensive institutional care is required when the level of debilitation prevents the afflicted persons from meeting the activities of daily living (ADL) or even maintaining a sense of self and of the world in which they live. Paramount among these degenerative conditions are Parkinson's disease and Alzheimer's disease.

Parkinson's Disease

Once called "shaking palsy," Parkinson's disease is now recognized as a specific neurological disorder belonging to a family of conditions called *motor system disorders.* Parkinson's disease involves the chronic progressive loss of dopamine production within specific areas of the brain. These areas, called the substantia nigra and striatum, transmit signals required to produce purposeful muscle activity that leads to more highly coordinated movement. The four primary signs of the disease reflect this loss of muscular coordination: (1) tremor or trembling in the hands, arms, legs, jaw, and face; (2) rigidity or stiffness of the limbs or trunk; (3) slowness of movement; and (4) postural instability and impaired balance. As these symptoms worsen, people with Parkinson's disease become progressively less able to talk, walk, and perform simple tasks associated with daily living.[5]

Parkinson's-like symptoms are associated with other conditions, such as head injury, tumors, prolonged use of tranquilizers, and manganese and carbon monoxide poisoning. The labels *Parkinson's syndrome* and *atypical Parkinson's* are used to describe these conditions. It is

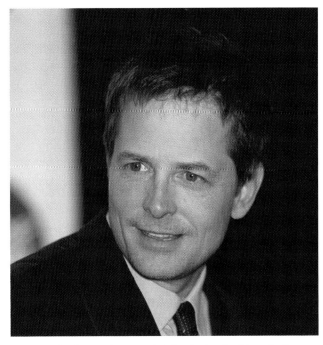

Actor Michael J. Fox has revealed that he has Parkinson's disease, and is supporting research for a cure.

believed that as many as one in five elderly Americans shows some Parkinsonian signs.

About five hundred thousand Americans have been diagnosed with primary Parkinson's disease, and about fifty thousand new cases are diagnosed annually. The exact number of people with this condition has always been difficult to establish with certainty, since some people assume that these changes are the result of aging and thus do not seek medical evaluation. The incidence of Parkinson's disease is the same in men and women. The condition is usually first seen in people over age 50, with 60 being the average age at first diagnosis. Compared with African Americans and Asian Americans, whites are more likely to be diagnosed with Parkinson's disease. A relatively small percentage of people develop the disease as early as age 40. Slightly fewer cases of Parkinson's disease are seen among smokers than among nonsmokers (the risks of smoking, however, greatly outweigh the slightly lower risk of Parkinson's disease among smokers). Additionally, for women, less Parkinson's disease is seen in those who consume little or no caffeine, but at the same time use hormone replacement therapy (HRT). However, a higher incidence of the disease is seen in women who both consume caffeine and use HRT, thus suggesting a caffeine-estrogen interplay.[41]

Three explanations of the cause of Parkinson's disease have been proposed. The first involves the formation of highly excited unstable chemical compounds known as *free radicals*. These compounds are formed in greater and greater quantities with age, as the body gradually loses its ability to completely oxidize substrates. These free radicals seek stability by physically altering the chemical structure of tissues with which they have contact, including the cells of the substantia nigra. Once damaged, the cells of the substantia nigra and striatum die; thus their dopamine production is lost and the symptoms of Parkinson's appear.

The second possible explanation relates to environmental toxins that are known to produce Parkinson's-like symptoms in humans. However, no widely occurring environmental toxins of this nature have been discovered that could account for the large number of cases of Parkinson's disease in this country and around the world. This theory was, however, given considerable support by a recent identical twin study that found Parkinson's disease usually occurs in only one twin, even though both have the same genetic makeup.[42]

The third theory about the cause of Parkinson's disease suggests an inherited predisposition associated with genetic material found within the mitochondria of cells. Mitochondria are cell structures in which energy is produced to fuel specific cellular tasks, such as the production of dopamine. In 1997 a mutated gene was identified within the mitochondrial DNA of members of a family with a long history of Parkinson's disease. Currently, however, a genetic basis for Parkinson's is thought most likely only in those cases of the disease that occur in persons considerably younger than typical victims and often with a substantial family history of the condition—perhaps 10% of all cases of Parkinson's disease.

Prevention, Diagnosis, and Management

Parkinson's disease is usually diagnosed by a neurologist after the patient is referred by a primary care physician. Although there is no single test for diagnosing Parkinson's disease, medical imaging, such as CT scans and MRI scans, may be helpful in ruling out conditions that mimic the disease.

Several medications are used to delay the progression of the disease. Most of these drugs affect dopamine production. Two drugs, carbidopa/levodopa, an older medication, and tolcapone (Tasmar), a newer drug, enhance the conversion of levodopa into dopamine. A third drug, Requip, a dopamine agonist, is available for use in combination with older levodopa-enhancing medications. This combination appears to delay the onset of the more severe symptoms of Parkinson's disease. As helpful as these medications are, however, their influence is temporary and at best only slows the progress of the disease.

Although only in the earliest stage of human trials, a compound derived from glial cells, called GDNF, has shown a remarkable ability to increase dopamine production, while at the same time reducing the limitations in the loss of motor control initially present.[43] Considerable research and development remains to be done on this new medication.

 TALKING POINTS Your grandmother seems increasingly frustrated by your grandfather's "clumsiness," and has complained that he is becoming increasingly unsteady and nervous. What might you say to her about his condition? What would you suggest she say to him?

At this time a radically different form of treatment for Parkinson's disease is under refinement. A **xenotransplant**-based technique has been developed through which fetal pig

Key Terms

xenotransplant a transplant of tissue from an animal, such as a pig, to a human recipient.

cells are transplanted into the brains of Parkinson's patients for the purpose of reestablishing functional dopamine-producing cells in the areas of the brain deprived of this ability by the disease. In the limited number of persons having had this procedure, approximately one-third had symptoms of the disease clearly reduced or disappear.[44] Additionally, initial concerns about the introduction to humans of viruses common to pigs appear to be unfounded.

Additionally, in some cases electrodes have been surgically implanted into the brain. This procedure appears to reduce tremors to the extent that affected people can achieve and maintain a more functional level of activity for as long as 2 years.

Alzheimer's Disease (AD)

Although it affects only 1% to 2% of elderly people, organic brain syndrome, in either its acute or chronic form, is a collection of incapacitating, heart-rending, and costly afflictions. Alzheimer's disease is the best known of these conditions, affecting approximately 4 to 5 million adults in this country and perhaps as many as 10 million worldwide. Today, more than ever before, it is the disease associated with longevity.

The initial signs of Alzheimer's disease are often subtle and may be confused with mild depression. At this stage of the disease process, however, the person might have some difficulty answering questions like these:

- Where are we now?
- What month is it?
- What is today's date?
- When is your birthday?
- Who is the president?

During the ensuing months, people with this condition experience greater memory loss, confusion, and **dementia.** In the most advanced stage, people with Alzheimer's disease are incontinent (unable to control bladder and bowel function), display infantile behavior, and finally become totally incapacitated as a result of the destruction of brain tissue. Patients with advanced Alzheimer's disease usually must be institutionalized.

Several theories have been advanced about the cause of Alzheimer's disease. Increasing evidence indicates that genetic mutations on chromosomes 10, 14, 19, or 21 may encourage the development of the disease. Other theories suggest links between Alzheimer's disease and abnormal protein development, deficiencies in acetylcholine (a neurotransmitter) production, loss of nicotine receptors in specific areas of the brain, abnormal blood flow, or exposure to infectious agents or toxins.

Prevention, Diagnosis, and Management

The precise diagnosis of Alzheimer's disease and similar disorders is difficult to make before the patient dies. Only during an autopsy can the characteristic signs of the disease—*neurofibrillary tangles* (twisted strands of neuronal material) and *senile plaque* (compressed masses of cellular material, badly damaged nerve fibers, and a core composed of *beta amyloid protein*)—be identified to confirm the diagnosis. Before death, all other conditions capable of causing dementia must be individually ruled out. Thus, tentative or probable diagnosis of Alzheimer's disease is made by a process of elimination. Newer medical imaging technologies, such as MRIs and PET scans, have become so refined that it is now *nearly* possible to confirm the diagnosis of Alzheimer's disease before death. Today these technologies have been combined with the application of selected memory tests allowing clinicians to clearly view subtle signs of diminished functional activity in specific areas of the brain. Using this approach, the ability to predict the development of Alzheimer's disease, particularly in persons with a known genetic marker for the condition, may be at hand.[45]

Effective drugs to treat Alzheimer's disease have not yet been developed. That said, four drugs (tacrine, donepezil, rivastigmine, and galantamine) are currently available that provide temporary improvement in intellectual function by inhibiting the enzyme that breaks down the neurotransmitter *acetylcholine,* whose diminished availability is the basis of Alzheimer's disease, or by blocking glutamate, a substance capable of damaging neurons. At least six additional drugs are in various clinical trials, including metrifonate and physostigmine.[46]

A number of studies have attempted to link behavioral patterns with the incidence of Alzheimer's disease. Among the prevention studies now ongoing or recently completed is a study to assess the role fish consumption in the prevention of AD.[47] This study found that persons who ate a fish meal (specific fish not defined) once a week were 60% less likely to have developed AD than those who did not. Fish, nuts, and flax seeds contain rich supplies of omega-3 fatty acid needed by the nervous system to maintain normal levels of function. In a second area of investigation, daily consumption of light to moderate amounts of alcohol is being studied.[48] The relationship of modest alcohol consumption to Alzheimer's disease focuses on the potential

> ### Key Terms
>
> **dementia** the loss of cognitive abilities, including memory and reason.

Resources for Selected Chronic Conditions

For additional information about the common chronic conditions described in this chapter, visit the following websites listed. Although each site is different, most provide information regarding the condition, identify ongoing clinical trials, suggest current books, and provide links to support groups. Keep in mind that information gleaned from these sites should not be used as a substitute for medical consultation.

Turner's Syndrome *The Turner's Syndrome Society of the United States*

www.turner-syndrome-us.org

Sickle Cell Trait/Disease *Sickle Cell Information Center*

www.emory.edu/PEDS/SICKLE

Duchenne Muscular Dystrophy *Muscular Dystrophy Association*

www.mdausa.org/research/index.html

Diabetes Mellitus Types 1 and 2 *American Diabetes Association*

www.diabetes.org/default.asp

Fibromyalgia *Fibromyalgia Network*

www.fmnetnews.com

Asthma *American Academy of Allergy, Asthma & Immunology*

www.aaaai.org

Systemic Lupus Erythematosus *Lupus Foundation of America*

www.lupus.org

Talipes/Cleft Palate/Cleft Lip *March of Dimes Birth Defects Foundation*

www.modimes.org

Parkinson's Disease *Parkinson's Disease Foundation*

www.pdf.org

Crohn's Disease *Crohn's & Colitis Foundation of America*

www.ccfa.org

Alzheimer's Disease *The Alzheimer's Page* (Washington University of St. Louis)

www.biostat.wustl.edu/alzheimer

Multiple Sclerosis *National Multiple Sclerosis Society*

www.nmss.org

---

for daily small amounts of alcohol to improve the health of blood vessels within the brain. A third study tested the effectiveness of two nonsteroidal anti-inflammatory drugs (NSAID) on the prevention of inflammation within the brain that, should it occur, could damage neurons.[49] No positive contribution by these OTC drugs was found. A fourth prevention-oriented study centers on the use of mental stimulation to determine its role in keeping the brain structurally younger, thus less susceptible to age-related decline and the onset of AD.[50] A fifth study involving diets high in antioxidant vitamins, including carotenes, vitamin C, and vitamin E, failed to find evidence supportive of previous assumptions that AD might be slowed by foods (or supplements) that provided antioxidants, thus decreasing the presence of free radicals within the body.[51] Finally, a study designed to determine the role of HRT in preventing or slowing memory decline with age demonstrated the absence of a positive contribution.[52]

In addition to the speculative preventive approaches just described, two vaccines for the prevention of Alzheimer's disease are now in clinical trials. These vaccines utilize a synthetic version of the beta-amyloid protein to stimulate an immune response against the beta-amyloid that occurs in conjunction with the disease. On the basis of the initial human trials, immunizations appear safe, but their effectiveness remains to be proven.

A Final Thought About Health and Chronic Conditions

In this chapter your authors have addressed different types of chronic conditions, many of which have their onset in younger adulthood. Recall the definitions of health, both traditionally and developmentally oriented, that were introduced in Chapter 1. For persons diagnosed with any of the illnesses presented here, the traditional definitions of health could easily label them as being "sick," "ill," or "unhealthy." From a developmental perspective, however, these persons almost certainly hold aspirations of living the fullest life possible, in light of the limitations imposed by their medical conditions. In order to do this, they must reassess the aspirations held for them by society and the life experiences they envisioned for themselves. Once having made these reassessments, and not always easily, they begin applying resources less dependent on the structure and function of the body, but more in tune with the resources of the mind, intellect, spirit, and the supportive presence of other people. As these alternative centers of resourcefulness become more easily recognizable and skillfully and comfortably called upon, the ability to engage more and more fully in life increases. Thus, they experience an increasing number of "good days" and a greater sense of being healthy—even though the body (and perhaps society) may disagree.

Taking Charge of Your Health

- Stay attuned to media reports about chronic conditions so that you can make informed choices.
- Support agencies devoted to the prevention of chronic health conditions.
- Monitor your work, home, and recreational environments to determine whether they are enhancing your risk for developing a chronic health condition.

- Undergo the recommended screening procedures and other preventive procedures related to chronic conditions for your age and sex.
- If you have a chronic condition, participate actively in your own treatment.

Summary

- Chronic conditions can be classified into several categories: genetic/inherited, congenital, metabolic, autoimmune, and degenerative.
- Chronic conditions are those that develop slowly and last a long time, while acute conditions are those that develop quickly and are generally resolved in a short period of time.
- Most chronic conditions cannot, at this time, be prevented.
- Klinefelter's syndrome is a genetic condition caused by the presence of one or more additional X chromosomes; it results in feminization of the male body.
- Turner's syndrome occurs in females who lack one of the normal two X chromosomes, resulting in a total of forty-five chromosomes, rather than forty-six.
- Cystic fibrosis is caused by the inheritance of a recessive gene that prevents the body from producing a protein required for the normal function of exocrine glands.
- Sickle-cell disease results from inheriting a gene for an abnormal form of hemoglobin associated with crescent-shaped red blood cells that have limited oxygen transport capabilities. People with sickle-cell trait are carriers of the abnormal hemoglobin gene.
- Duchenne muscular dystrophy is an X-linked recessive trait, thus seen almost exclusively in males, in which the body lacks the ability to produce dystrophin. The disease causes a progressive loss of muscular control and premature death.
- Talipes (clubfoot) is a common congenital abnormality in which, during embryonic formation of the lower extremity, the foot is turned inward and tipped into a clearly abnormal position.
- Cleft palate and cleft lip are caused by lack of fusion in the bones of the face during embryonic formation of the mouth and nasal cavity.
- Patent foramen ovale is a congenital heart abnormality in which a hole linking the right atrium to the left atrium fails to close completely at birth, allowing unoxygenated blood to enter the systemic circulation.

- Scoliosis, an abnormal lateral curvature of the spine, can begin to develop before birth; thus it is classified as a congenital abnormality, although most cases develop during later childhood and adolescence.
- Diabetes mellitus type 2, or non-insulin-dependent diabetes mellitus, occurs when the body's cells lose the ability to recognize insulin and thus are unable to utilize blood glucose normally. Hispanic Americans appear particularly susceptible to the development of diabetes mellitus type 2.
- Diabetes mellitus type 1, or insulin-dependent diabetes mellitus, occurs when the cells of the pancreas are destroyed, thus depriving the body of insulin, the hormone needed for the normal utilization of blood glucose.
- Reactive hypoglycemia is a relatively rare condition in which a high level of glucose in the blood after a meal stimulates the overproduction of insulin; thus glucose is removed from the blood too quickly, and the amount of glucose in the blood falls to an abnormally low level.
- Functional hypoglycemia is a more complicated form of "hypoglycemia" to substantiate because of emotional dynamics.
- Fibromyalgia is characterized by stiffness, poor sleep, chronic headaches, and other symptoms. Diagnosis is based on soreness in specific tender-point locations. Treatment is primarily aimed at reducing discomfort and enhancing sleep.
- Asthma is a chronic respiratory disease characterized by acute attacks of respiratory hypersensitivity caused by abnormal narrowing of the airways. Minority children experience asthma more frequently than do other children, even those living under similar environmental conditions.
- Crohn's disease, a type of inflammatory bowel disease, results from the erosion of the inner and middle layers of the intestinal tract wall, leading to pain, fever, weight loss, and rectal bleeding that causes anemia.

- Systemic lupus erythematosus is an autoimmune disorder in which the body's own immune system attacks connective tissue in the skin, muscles, nervous system, kidneys, and other areas. Minority women are particularly susceptible to the development of SLE.
- Multiple sclerosis is thought to be an autoimmune disorder in which the body loses the ability to produce myelin, an insulation material needed for proper conduction of nerve impulses.
- Parkinson's disease is characterized by loss of fine muscular control caused by the gradual cessation of dopamine production within the brain. A new medication and xenotransplantation hold promise for better management and/or prevention of PD.
- Alzheimer's disease is a form of dementia (or loss of cognitive ability) caused by the gradual loss of the brain's ability to produce acetylcholine, a neurotransmitter essential for normal mental functioning. A vaccine against AD has proven safe in early human trials, though its effectiveness has been seriously questioned.

Review Questions

1. Identify and describe the five categories of chronic conditions presented in this chapter.
2. Compare and contrast the terms *chronic* and *acute* in terms of the onset and duration of each type of illness.
3. What is the genetic basis of Klinefelter's syndrome? What physical characteristics would a person with Klinefelter's syndrome have?
4. What is the genetic basis of Turner's syndrome? What physical features characterize the person with Turner's syndrome?
5. Cystic fibrosis is a *recessive genetic disorder;* explain this term. What functional difficulties are experienced by people with cystic fibrosis? What is the condition's long-term prognosis? Why are genetic screening and counseling important for this condition?
6. What complex protein structure is present in an abnormal form in people with sickle-cell disease? What shape are the red blood cells in people with this condition? Why are genetic screening and counseling considered important for sickle-cell disease and trait? What medical procedure appears to hold the potential for cure in some persons with sickle-cell disease?
7. Duchenne muscular dystrophy is an *X-linked recessive disorder;* explain this term. Which gender carries this trait, and which is affected by it?
8. Describe the appearance of talipes. What is this condition's more common name? How and when is this condition generally treated?
9. What medical complications could arise if cleft palate and cleft lip are not corrected?
10. What is the function of the foramen ovale in the fetal heart? What recreational pursuit may be compromised by the presence of a patent foramen ovale?
11. What structures in the upper body are at risk if scoliosis is not corrected? What are the principal methods of treating scoliosis? How could the role of the school be changing?
12. What are the differences between non-insulin-dependent diabetes mellitus (type 2) and insulin-dependent diabetes mellitus (type 1)? How does treatment for each condition differ? How important is genetic predisposition in each form of diabetes? Which minority group appears particularly susceptible to the development of diabetes mellitus type 2, and on what basis?
13. How does a person with reactive hypoglycemia respond physiologically to a large blood glucose load? How is dietary management used to treat this condition?
14. How does functional hypoglycemia differ from reactive hypoglycemia?
15. Identify three symptoms that characterize fibromyalgia. What role do tender points play in the diagnosis and treatment of fibromyalgia?
16. How are intrinsic asthma and extrinsic asthma similar? In what important way are they different? How is exercise-induced asthma treated differently today than in the past? In what population group is this increase most noticeable and distressful? What factors might account for this increase?
17. How is Crohn's disease different from other forms of inflammatory bowel disease? What is currently believed to be the cause of Crohn's disease? What are some of the potentially serious consequences of this condition? How is the condition managed?
18. Systemic lupus erythematosus is an *autoimmune disorder;* explain this term. What environmental factors seem to trigger outbreaks or "flares" of SLE? In what gender is SLE most prevalent, and to what extent is it seen among members of minorities?
19. In multiple sclerosis, what important material associated with nervous system function cannot be produced? Why does the body lose its ability to produce this important material? To what important immune system chemical are several of the more effective MS drugs related?

20. What neurotransmitter is inadequately produced in people with Parkinson's disease? In which specific area of the brain is the production of this neurotransmitter lost? How do drugs used to manage the condition work?

21. Alzheimer's disease is classified as a form of *dementia;* explain this term. Which neurotransmitter is involved in Alzheimer's disease? How effective is drug treatment? What are the long-term consequences of Alzheimer's disease? What is the current status of vaccine development that might prevent the development of AD?

References

1. Nader S. *Human biology,* 8th ed. McGraw-Hill. 2004.
2. Griffiths AJF, et al. *An introduction to genetic analysis,* 7th ed. W.H. Freeman & Co. 2000.
3. Mange EJ, Mange AP. *Basic Human Genetics,* 2nd ed. Sinauer Assoc. 1998.
4. Bertelloni S, et al. Growth and puberty in Turner's syndrome. *J Pediatr Endocrinol Metab,* Suppl 2:307–313, March 2003.
5. Fauci AS, et al. *Harrison's principles of internal medicine,* 15th ed. McGraw-Hill, 2001.
6. Groman JD, et al. Variant cystic fibrosis phenotypes in the absence of CFTR mutations. *N Engl J Med* 347(6): 401–407. 2002.
7. Lim M, Zeitlin PL. Therapeutic strategies to correct malfunction of CFTR. *Paediatr Respir Rev* 2(2): 159–164. 2001.
8. Locatelli F, et al. Related umbilical cord blood transplantation in patients with thalassemia and sickle cell disease. *Blood* 101(6): 2137–2143, 2003.
9. XU K, et al. First unaffected pregnancy using preimplantation genetic diagnosis for sickle cell anemia. *JAMA* 281(18): 1701–1706. 1999.
10. Gussoni E, et al. Long-term persistence of donor nuclei in a Duchenne muscular dystrophy patient receiving bone marrow transplantation. *J Clin Invest* 110(6): 807–814, 2002.
11. Van De Graaff KM. *Human anatomy,* 6th ed. McGraw-Hill, 2002.
12. Bellenir K (editor). *Congenital disorders sourcebook: basic information about disorders acquired during gestation.* Omnigraphics, Inc., 1997.
13. Eisenberg B, Wapner RJ. Clinical procedures in prenatal diagnosis. *Best Pract Res Clin Obstet Gynaecol* 16(5): 611–627. 2002.
14. Kummer AW, Lourinia K. *Cleft palate and Craniofacial abnormalities.* Delmar Publishers, 2000.
15. Sargent L. *The carniofacial surgery book.* Tennessee Craniofacial Center. 2000. **http://www.erlanger.org/carniofacialsurgerybook.html**
16. Marieb EN, Mallatt J. *Human anatomy-updated.* Benjamin Cummings. 2003.
17. Buttinelli C, et al. Stroke in a scuba diver with patent foramen ovale. *Eur J Neurol* 9(1); 89–91. 2002.
18. Bove AA. Risk of decompression sickness with patent foramen ovale. *Undersea Hyperb Med* 25(3):175–178. 1998.
19. *The scoliosis treatment recovery system (STRS).* The Scoliosis Treatment Recovery Center. 2000. **http://www.scoliosis.com**
20. Weinstein SL, et al. Health and function of patients with untreated idiopathic scoliosis: a 50-year natural history. *JAMA* 289(5): 559–567. 2003.
21. Hamann B. *Disease identification, prevention, & control,* 2nd ed. McGraw-Hill, 2001.
22. Fox SI. *Human physiology,* 8th ed. McGraw-Hill, 2004.
23. Altschuler D, et al. The common PPARgamma Pro 12Ala polymorphism is associated with decreased risk of type 2 diabetes. *Nat Genetic* 26(1): 76–80. 2000.
24. Sherwood L. *Human physiology: from cells to systems* 5th ed. Thomson-Brooks/Cole, 2004.
25. *ADA-type 2 medical information: tight diabetes control,* 2003. **http://www.diabetes.org/main/type2/medical/blood_sugar/default3.jsp**
26. Vijan S, Hawward RA. Treatment of hypertension in type 2 diabetes: blood pressure goals, choice of agents, and setting priorities in diabetes care. *Ann Intern Med* 138(7):593–602. 2003.
27. Honeyman MC, et al. Association between rotavirus infection and pancreatic islet autoimmunity in children at risk of developing type 1 diabetes. *Diabetes* 49(8):1319–1324, 2000.
28. Bonner-Weir S, et al. In vitro cultivation of human islets from expanded ductal tissue. *Proc Natl Acad Sci USA* 97(14):7999–8004. 2000.
29. Markmann JF, et al. The use of non-heart-beating donors for isolated pancreatic islet transplantation. *Transplantation* 75(9):1423–1429, 2003.
30. National Diabetes Information Clearinghouse (NIDC). Hypoglycemia, 2003. **http://www.diabetes/niddk.nih.gov/dm/pubs/hypoglycemia/index.htm**
31. Snorgaard O. Functional hypoglycemia. Fancy or fact? *Ugeskr Laeger* 154(36):2406–2409, 1992
32. Hofeldt FD. Reactive hypoglycemia. *Endocrinol Metab Clin North Am* 18(1): 185–201, 1989.

33. Arthritis Foundation. *Fibromyalgia,* 2000. **http://www.arthritis.org/Answers/DiseaseCenter/fibromyalgia.asp**

34. *Diagnostic criteria for fibromyalgia and CFS,* 2000 **http://www.fmnetnews.com/pages/criteria.html**

35. McKeever TM, et al. The importance of prenatal exposures on the development of allergic disease: a birth cohort study using the West Midlands General Practice Database. *Am J Respir Crit Care Med* 166(6): 827–832. 2002.

36. Finegold I, et al. Immunotherapy for asthma. *Am J Crit Care Med* 165(10):1453–1454. 2002.

37. Satsagi J. Genetics of inflammatory bowel disease: from bench to bedside? *Acta Odonol Scand* 59(3):187–192. 2001.

38. Cho JH. The Nod2 gene in Crohn's disease: implication for future research into the genetic and immunology of Crohn's disease. *Inflamm Bowel Dis* 7(3):271–275, 2001.

39. *The state of lupus research.* The Lupus Foundation of American, 2002. **http://www.lupus.org**

40. Fassas A, et al. Hematopoietic stem cells transplantation for multiple sclerosis. A retrospective multicenter study. *J Neurol* 249(8):1088–1097. 2002.

41. Ascherio A, et al. Caffeine, postmenopausal estrogen, and the risk of Parkinson's disease. *Neurology* 60(5): 790–795, 2003.

42. Tanner CM, et al. Parkinson's disease in twins: an etiologic study. *JAMA* 281(4):342–346, 2000.

43. Gill SS, et al. Direct brain infusion of glial cell-line derived neurotrophic factor in Parkinson disease. *Nat Med* 9(5): 589–595, 2003.

44. Schumacher JM, et al. Transplantation of embryonic porcine mesencephalic tissue in patients with PD. *Neurology* 54(5):1042–1050, 2000.

45. Burggren AC, Bookheimer SY. Structural and functional neuroimaging in Alzheimer's disease: an update. *Curr Top Med Chem* 2(4):385–393, 2002.

46. Reichman WE. Current pharmacologic options for patients with Alzheimer's disease. *Ann Gen Hosp Psychiatry* 2(1):1, 2003.

47. Morris MC, et al. Consumption and n-3 fatty acids and risk of incident Alzheimer disease. *Arch Neurol* 60(7):923–924. 2003.

48. Mukamal KJ, et al. Prospective study of alcohol consumption and risk of dementia in older adults. *JAMA* 289(11):1405–1413, 2003.

49. Aisen PS, et al. Effects of rofecoxib or naproxen vs placebo on Alzheimer disease progression: a randomized controlled trial. *JAMA* 289(21): 2819–2826, 2003.

50. Verghese J, et al. Leisure activities and the risk of dementia in the elderly. *N Engl J Med* 348(25): 2508–2516, 2003.

51. Luchsinger JA, et al. Antioxidant vitamin intake and risk of Alzheimer disease. *Arch Neurol* 60(2): 203–208, 2003.

52. Hays J, et al. Effects of estrogen plus progestin on health-related quality of life. *N Engl J Med* 348(19):1835–1837, 2003.

As We Go to Press

A "cure" for multiple sclerosis (MS) may, for the first time, be on the distant horizon. Of course as is true for all medical research, an initial study must be repeated numerous times, using increasingly larger numbers of persons with the condition to be studied, and continually evaluated for both short- and long-term negative consequences. Researchers at Drexel University have begun this process with an initial study presented in Philadelphia in early 2004.

The MS-related study in question involved the use of a potent chemotherapy drug, cyclophosphamide, that is capable of quickly and completely killing the immune system cells that are destroying myelin production within the brain, spinal cord, and motor nerve fibers of the peripheral nervous system. Once all autoimmune recognition of the myelin producing cells was removed from the now devastated immune system, the immune system was reprogrammed using stem cells from the bone marrow that had remained protected from the chemotherapeutical drug's effect. This allowed newly forming lymphocytes to begin reestablishing a mature immune system, without the faulty autoimmune capability seen in the old immune system.

Although patients taking part in the initial study experienced severe nausea and lost all of their hair, most showed clear improvement in their movement and cognitive abilities. In the words of one patient undergoing this highly invasive and experimental procedure, "The chemo was rough but it was well worth it. I can walk unassisted. There are no words to described how dramatically this treatment has affected the quality of my life, physically and mentally."

Chronic illness and the demands of Caregiving

In the chapter you have just read, your textbook focused on several representative chronic illnesses. With what you have learned about these conditions, you should be able to imagine that a person whose ability to care for him- or herself has been gravely compromised by the ravages of Alzheimer's or Parkinson disease would have great difficulty meeting the specific demands of their illness, as well as the activities of daily living that are required for even minimal independence. If they hope to remain in a non-institutional setting, they will, most assuredly, need the assistance of a caregiver at some point, perhaps around the clock.

The need for caregivers is not limited to those suffering from Alzheimer's and Parkinsons. Many forms of cancer, stroke, epilepsy, brain injuries, rheumatoid arthritis, spinal cord injuries, chronic obstructive pulmonary disease, asthma, diabetes mellitus, glaucoma, hemophilia, renal failure, cleft lip and palate, and systemic lupus erythematosis are but a few of the other chronic conditions that at some point in their progression will require the afflicted person to receive care from others.[1]

Sixty-five percent of older persons requiring long-term care rely on family and friends as caregivers; an additional 30% make use of paid providers in addition to family and friends.[2] The average caregiver is 46 years old and female, and has the added responsibilities of being married and working outside the home.[3] Our nation has come to rely on families, rather than social service agencies, nursing homes, or other health care providers, to provide long-term care for the chronically ill. It is estimated that the combined economic value of these unpaid caregivers exceeds $257 billion each year.[4]

It is particularly important to recognize that under the law, few persons other than health care professionals, parents of dependent children, legally defined guardians, and specified public servants are required to meet the needs of the chronically ill. But when it comes to our aging and infirm population, it is most often those who are not required to do so who take care of their elderly parents, other family members, friends and neighbors. More than 22.4 million Americans are informal caregivers who provide some degree of assistance to older persons or persons with some limitations on their ability to care for themselves[4]

So, the decision to become the primary caregiver for a parent, grandparent, relative or friend who is chronically ill is a personal one. Thus, a person considering becoming a voluntary caregiver of a chronically ill person must carefully consider many issues related to the endeavor. Among the most pressing of these are:

- *What are both the present and future needs of the chronically ill person whose care you are assuming? Are you able to manage their care now? Will you be able to take on more responsibilities and difficulties should their condition worsen?*
- *Whose needs are most fundamentally at stake in this venture? In other words, are you stepping forward in the role of caregiver in order to meet your own unfulfilled needs, or are your genuinely focused on the person whole illness-related needs you are trying to meet?*
- *What resources are available to assist you in meeting the needs of this chronically ill person? Are there private, state or federal programs and/or facilities available that might provide you with assistance? Are you capable of accessing the agencies whose expertise and assistance would be beneficial?*
- *Can you remain above feelings of resentment once you have accepted the role of caregiver, knowing that others apparently have been comfortable setting aside the same ethical obligations? In other words, will you find yourself feeling bitter toward a sibling who did not volunteer to help you care for a parent?[5]*

It is crucial that you ask yourself these questions, and honestly deal with your feelings, before taking on the role of caregiver. If you are able to resolve these issues in a healthy manner, then you may be entering into one of the most demanding but rewarding undertakings that a person can experience.

For Discussion

Would you be willing to take on the full-time care of a parent if he or she became chronically ill? Should those in need of assistance be entitled to some level of government-funded at home care? How might employers be able to help workers who are struggling to balance work with the responsibilities of caregiving?

References

1. Chui, D. Occupational therapy in Community Rehabilitation Network. Hong Kong Occupational Association. 2003.
2. U.S Administration on Aging. *America's Families Care: A report on the needs of America's family caregivers.* Fall 2000.

[3] National Alliance for Caregiving (1997). *Family Caregiving in the Unied States: Findings from a national survey.* **http://www.caregiving.org/finalreport.pdf**

[4] The U.S. Department of Health and Human Services, Administration on Aging. *What We Do Makes A Difference: Fact Sheet on Family Caregiving.* **http://www.aoa.gov/prof/aoaprog/caregiver/carefam/taking_care_of_others/taking_care.asp**

[5] Pressing worldwide challenge of long-term care for ill and disabled presents difficult ethical questions. World Health Organization. 2003. **http://www.who.int/mediacentre/notes/2003/np3/en**

personal assessment

are you managing your asthma effectively?

Place a check mark next to each statement that applies to you.

Reducing or Avoiding Asthma Triggers

_____ I have identified my asthma triggers.

_____ I do not smoke, and I avoid environmental tobacco smoke as much as possible.

_____ I use and properly maintain an air filter and an air conditioner to keep my home cleaner and more comfortable.

_____ I avoid vacuuming or I use a dust mask.

_____ I avoid mowing the lawn or I use a dust mask.

_____ I avoid wood stoves and fireplaces.

_____ I use dustproof encasings on my pillows, mattress, and box spring.

_____ I use a dehumidifier as necessary in my home to reduce indoor mold.

_____ I use window shades or curtains made of plastic or other washable material for easy cleaning.

_____ My closets contain only needed clothing; clothing I do not currently wear is stored in plastic garment bags.

_____ I do not sleep or lie down on upholstered furniture.

_____ If I have a pet, it does not sleep in or go into the bedroom.

_____ I avoid perfume and cologne, cleaning chemicals, paint, and talcum powder as much as possible.

Preventing and Managing Asthma Attacks

_____ I have learned everything I can about asthma.

_____ I take medications as prescribed by my physician whether or not I am having an attack.

_____ I carry my inhaler with me at all times.

_____ I have asked my physician to help me develop a crisis plan for managing a severe asthma attack.

_____ I keep emergency numbers by the phone.

_____ I have learned about my asthma medications and know how quickly they should work.

_____ I use a peak flow meter to anticipate and respond quickly to asthma attacks.

Interpretation

17 or more items checked: You are doing a great job avoiding asthma triggers and preventing and managing asthma attacks.

14 to 16 items checked: In many ways you are doing a good job of managing your asthma. However, you may be unnecessarily exposing yourself to common asthma triggers, or your plan for preventing and managing asthma attacks may need some work.

13 or fewer items checked: You could be managing your asthma much more effectively. Modify your home and activities as necessary to avoid common asthma triggers. Talk to your physician right away about establishing an asthma management plan and an emergency plan. Remember, asthma can be fatal, and poor preventive asthma management is an important contributing factor. Don't let it happen to you!

To Carry This Further . . .

Discuss this assessment with other members of your family or your roommates. Secure their cooperation in helping you maintain a clean home free of dust, pet hair, smoke, and other asthma triggers. Make sure they know what to do to help you in case of a severe asthma attack.

chapter thirteen

preventing infectious diseases

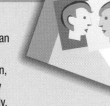

Talking It Over

Chronic Fatigue Syndrome: Real or Imaginary?

Communication with a friend who has chronic fatigue syndrome can sometimes be strained. You may think that the person is just being lazy. Or, because the person doesn't look sick, you may wonder if he is faking it.

- Show respect for your friend by letting him talk about it—just as you would behave if he had any other illness.
- Acknowledge the fact that your friend has a recognized medical condition. Don't suggest that he can "snap out of it."

- Do what you can to support the affected person, both physically and emotionally.

CommunicationLinks

www.cdc.gov/ncidod/diseases/cfs/index-htm
www.cfids.org/csn.html
www.chronicfatiguenews.com

Eye on the Media

From Fear to Hope—AIDS in the News

In the early days of news coverage about AIDS, magazines like *Time* and *Newsweek* ran articles called: "The AIDS Epidemic," "Epidemic of Fear," "Plague Mentality," "Fear of Sex," "The Growing Threat," "A Spreading Scourge," "The New Untouchables," "AIDS Spreading Panic Worldwide," "A Grim Race Against the Clock," and "The Lost Generation." The titles reflected fear of the unknown, a new killer disease.

When the case of Kimberley Bergalis broke into the news in 1991, a routine visit to the dentist was suddenly fraught with risk.

Bergalis was the first American to die of AIDS after being infected by her dentist, Dr. David Acer. Four of Acer's other patients became infected with AIDS—all traced back to Acer. The public's reaction was near-hysteria. *Time* ran an article called "Should You Worry About Getting AIDS from Your Dentist?" People started asking their dentists (and other doctors) about their use of sterile precautions and even whether they had been tested for HIV.

By 1996, when the "cocktail" approach to AIDS treatment started showing remarkably good results, Magic Johnson was on the cover of both *Time* and *Newsweek* the same week. After more than 4 years of retirement from pro basketball—and the announcement that he had tested positive for HIV—he was back in the game. The secret to his survival? New drug treatments, a healthy diet, regular exercise, support from family and friends, and a positive attitude.

By the late 1990s, many news articles reflected a more hopeful tone: "Living Longer with AIDS," "Hope with an Asterisk," "Are Some People Immune?" and "What—I'm Gonna Live?" Doctors, too, are feeling more positive about the disease. As one AIDS specialist said: "I go to work feeling like there's something I can do for my patients."

For people with HIV/AIDS in the most highly developed countries, the future holds different things. For some, who can't afford or tolerate the new drugs, it's still a matter of waiting to die. Others feel that they've been given a second chance. They can think about having relationships again—something many put on hold when they learned they were HIV positive. They can make plans for what they want to do with the rest of their lives— however long that may be.

Most people with HIV/AIDS are buying time—hoping for the big breakthrough, the cure for AIDS. They're trying new drug treatments, hoping that one treatment won't disqualify them from the next one. They're watching TV news, reading the newspapers, and using the Internet with greater attention. Will protease-inhibiting drugs be the answer? Are the even newer antiviral medications the breakthrough hoped for? Is a vaccine on the horizon?

Today, the media are calling our attention to yet other aspects of the AIDS pandemic. For the more developed countries, the failure of younger gays and bisexuals to protect themselves from exposure to HIV has led to a reversal in the progress made over the last 20 years. In ways all too familiar to public health professionals, a younger generation can too easily forget the progress against disease and premature death made by those who came before, and in doing so, unravel the threads of progress.

Increasingly, media attention has also been focused on the plight of the millions of HIV/AIDS victims in third world countries, particularly in Africa and areas of Asia. Television increasingly exposes the suffering in countries where diagnosis is inadequately undertaken and, once done, virtually no effective treatment exists for those infected. Beyond the suffering and limited hope for those infected, the media has also publicized the plights of the tens of thousands of orphaned children in these areas whose parents have died from AIDS. Our federal government and pharmaceutical industry has been exposed to this suffering as well, and initial responses are being mustered.

Sources: Gayle HD. Curbing the global AIDS epidemic. *N Engl J Med* 348(18):1802–1805, 2003. Klausner RD, et al. Medicine. The need for a global HIV vaccine enterprise. *Science* 300(5628): 2036–2039, 2003.

In the nineteenth century, infectious diseases were the leading cause of death. These deaths came after exposure to the organisms that produced such diseases as smallpox, tuberculosis (TB), influenza, whooping cough (pertussis), typhoid, diphtheria, and tetanus. However, since the early 1900s, improvements in public sanitation, the widespread use of antibiotic drugs, and vaccinations have considerably reduced the number of people who die from infectious diseases. People now die more often from chronic disease processes.

Today, however, we have a new respect for infectious diseases. We have learned that AIDS threatens 70 million people in many areas of the world. We are witnessing the resurgence of TB. We recognize the role of pelvic infections in infertility. We also know that failure to fully immunize children has laid the groundwork for a return of whooping cough, polio, and other serious childhood diseases. In fact, some experts suggest that because of HIV/AIDS and the emergence and re-emergence of infectious diseases, today's young adults may have a lower life expectancy than the generation immediately ahead of them.

Several new types of infectious disease have appeared, and new concerns have been raised about the spread of familiar infectious diseases. These include the following:

- The extremely virulent viruses, such as the Ebola virus in Zaire, which is fatal to 75% of those who contract it, for which we do not have an immunization (although one is being tested), and whose transmission we do not fully understand

- The increasing resistance of bacteria such as *Staphylococcus aureus, Enterococcus,* and *Mycobacterium* (which causes tuberculosis) to antibiotics as the result of overuse, improper use, and biological "redesign" of the organisms themselves

- The progressive cross-country march of the mosquito-borne West Nile virus, and the importation of SARS (sudden acute respiratory syndrome) into Canada and the United States from Asia

- The growing concern over transmission of infectious organisms through contaminated food, improper preparation of food, and contamination of water

Table 13.1 Pathogens and Common Infectious Diseases

Pathogen	Description	Representative Disease Processes
Viruses	Smallest common pathogens; nonliving particles of genetic material (DNA) surrounded by a protein coat	Rubeola, mumps, chicken pox, rubella, influenza, warts, colds, oral and genital herpes, shingles, AIDS, genital warts
Prion	Potentially self-replicating protein, lacking both DNA and RNA, viruslike in size, clinically called TSE (transmissible spongiform encephalopathies)	Creutzfeldt-Jakob disease, Gerstmann-Straussler-Scheinker syndrome, "mad cow" disease
Bacteria	One-celled microorganisms with sturdy, well-defined cell walls; three distinctive forms: spherical (cocci), rod shaped (bacilli), and spiral shaped (spirilla)	Tetanus, strep throat, scarlet fever, gonorrhea, syphilis, chlamydia, toxic shock syndrome, Legionnaires' disease, bacterial pneumonia, meningitis, diphtheria, food poisoning, Lyme disease
Fungi	Plant-like microorganisms; molds and yeasts	Athlete's foot, ringworm, histoplasmosis, San Joaquin Valley fever, candidiasis
Protozoa	Simplest animal form, generally one-celled organisms	Malaria, amebic dysentery, trichomoniasis, vaginitis
Rickettsia	Viruslike organisms that require a host's living cells for growth and replication	Typhus, Rocky Mountain spotted fever, rickettsialpox
Parasitic worms	Many-celled organisms; represented by tapeworms, leeches, and roundworms	Dirofilariasis (dog heartworm), elephantiasis, onchocerciasis

Infectious Disease Transmission

Infectious diseases can generally be transmitted from person to person, although the transfer is not always direct. Infectious diseases can be especially dangerous because they can spread to large numbers of people, producing epidemics or pandemics. The following sections explain the process of disease transmission and the stages of infection.

Pathogens

For a disease to be transferred, a person must come into contact with the disease-producing agent, or **pathogen,** such as a virus, bacterium, or fungus. When pathogens enter our bodies, the pathogens can sometimes resist body defense systems, flourish, and produce an illness. We commonly call this an *infection.* Because of their small size, pathogens are sometimes called *microorganisms,* or *microbes.* Table 13.1 describes infectious disease agents and some of the illnesses they produce.[1]

Chain of Infection

The movement of a pathogenic agent through the various links in the chain of infection (Figure 13-1 on page 430) explains how diseases spread.[1] Not every pathogenic agent moves all the way through the chain of infection, because various links in the chain can be broken. Therefore, the presence of a pathogen creates only the potential for causing disease.

Agent

The first link in the chain of infection is the disease-causing **agent.** Whereas some agents are very **virulent** and lead to serious infectious illnesses such as HIV, which causes AIDS, others produce far less serious infections, such as the common cold. Through mutation, some pathogenic agents, particularly viruses, can become more virulent.

Reservoir

Infectious agents require the support and protection of a favorable environment to survive. This environment forms the second link in the chain of infection and is called the *reservoir.* For many of the most common infectious diseases, the reservoirs are the bodies of people who are already infected. Here the agents thrive before being spread to others. These infected people are, accordingly, the hosts for particular disease agents. In some infectious illnesses a person's reservoir status may be restored after treatment and apparent recovery from the original infection.

Key Terms

pathogen a disease-causing agent.

agent the causal pathogen of a particular disease.

virulent (**veer** yuh lent) capable of causing disease.

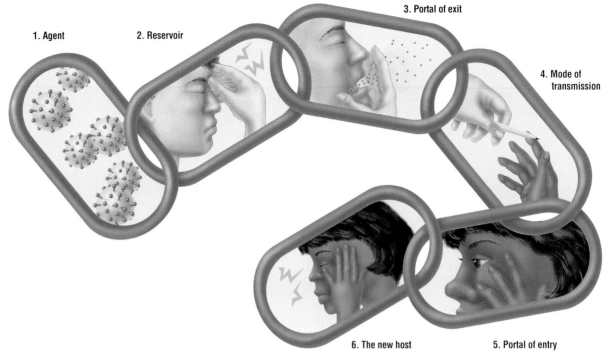

Figure 13-1 The six links in the chain of infection. The example above shows a rhinovirus, which causes the common cold, being passed from one person to another. l. the *agent* (pathogen) is a rhinovirus; 2. the *reservoir* is the infected person; 3. the *portal of exit* is the respiratory system (coughing); 4. the *mode of transmission* is indirect hand contact; 5. the *portal of entry* is the mucous membranes of the uninfected person's eye; 6. the virus now has a *new host.*

The labels in the figure read: 1. Agent; 2. Reservoir; 3. Portal of exit; 4. Mode of transmission; 5. Portal of entry; 6. The new host

This is because some pathogens, particularly viruses, can remain sequestered (hidden), emerging later to give rise to another infection. The herpes viruses are often sequestered.

For other infectious diseases, however, the reservoirs are the bodies of animals. Rabies is a well-known animal-reservoir disease. The infected animals are not always sick and do not always show symptoms similar to those seen in infected people.

The third type of reservoir in which disease-causing agents can live is in a nonliving environment, such as the soil. The spores of the tetanus bacterium, for example, can survive in soil for up to fifty years, entering the human body in a puncture wound.

Portal of Exit

For pathogenic agents to cause diseases and illnesses in others, they must leave their reservoirs. Thus the third link in the chain of infection is the portal of exit, or the point at which agents leave their reservoirs.

The principal portals of exit are familiar—the digestive system, urinary system, respiratory system, reproductive system, and the blood, especially with infectious diseases that infect humans.

Mode of Transmission

The fourth link in the chain of infection is the mode of transmission, or the way in which pathogens move from reservoirs to susceptible hosts. Two principal methods are direct transmission and indirect transmission.

We see three types of direct transmission in human-to-human transmission. These include contact between body surfaces (such as kissing, touching, and sexual intercourse), droplet spread (inhalation of contaminated air droplets), and fecal-oral spread (feces on the host's hands are brought into contact with the new host's mouth), as could occur when changing the diaper of an infected infant.

Indirect transmission between infected and uninfected people occurs when infectious agents travel by means of nonhuman materials. Vehicles of transmission include inanimate objects (known as *fomites*), such as water, food, soil, towels, clothing, and eating utensils.

Infectious agents can also be indirectly transmitted through vectors. The term *vector* describes living things, such as insects, birds, and other animals, that carry diseases from human to human. An example of a vector is the deer tick, which transmits Lyme disease.

Airborne indirect transmission includes the inhalation of infected particles that have been suspended in an air source for an extended time. Unlike droplet transmission, in which both infected and uninfected people must be in close physical proximity, noninfected people can become infected through airborne transmission by sharing air with infected people who were in the same room hours earlier. Viral infections such as German measles can be spread this way.

Portal of Entry

The fifth link in the chain of infection is the portal of entry. As with the portals of exit, portals of entry have three primary methods that allow pathogenic agents to enter the bodies of uninfected people. These are through the digestive system, respiratory system, and reproductive system. In addition, a break in the skin provides another portal of entry. In most infectious conditions, the portals of entry are the same systems that served as the portals of exit from the infected people. In HIV, however, we see cross-system transmission. Oral and anal sex allow infectious agents to pass between the warm, moist tissues of the reproductive and digestive systems.

The New Host

All people are, in theory, at risk for contracting infectious diseases and thus could be called susceptible hosts. In practice, however, factors such as overall health, acquired immunity, health care services, and health-related behavior can affect susceptibility to infectious diseases.

Stages of Infection

When a pathogenic agent assaults a new host, a reasonably predictable sequence of events begins. That is, the disease moves through five distinctive stages.[1] You may be able to recognize these stages of infection each time you catch a cold.

1. *The incubation stage.* This stage lasts from the time a pathogen enters the body until it multiplies enough to produce signs and symptoms of the disease. The duration of this stage can vary from a few hours to many months, depending on the virulence of the organisms, the concentration of organisms, the host's level of immune responsiveness, and other health problems. This stage has been called a *silent stage.* The pathogen can be transmitted to a new host during this stage, but this is not likely. A host may be infected during this stage but not infectious. HIV infection is an exception to this rule.

2. *The prodromal stage.* After the incubation stage, the host may experience a variety of general signs and symptoms, including watery eyes, runny nose, slight fever, and overall tiredness for a brief time. These symptoms are nonspecific and may not be severe enough to force the host to rest. During this stage the pathogenic agent continues to multiply. Now the host is capable of transferring pathogens to a new host,

but this is not yet the most infectious stage of an infectious disease. One should practice self-imposed isolation during this stage to protect others. Again, HIV infection is different in this stage.

3. *The clinical stage.* This stage, also called the *acme* or *acute stage,* is often the most unpleasant stage for the host. At this time the disease reaches its highest point of development. Laboratory tests can identify or analyze all of the clinical (observable) signs and symptoms of the particular disease. The likelihood of transmitting the disease to others is highest during this peak stage; all of our available defense mechanisms are in the process of resisting further damage from the pathogen.

4. *The decline stage.* The first signs of recovery appear during this stage. The infection is ending or, in some cases, falling to a subclinical level. People may suffer a relapse if they overextend themselves.

5. *The recovery stage.* Also called the *convalescence stage,* this stage is characterized by apparent recovery from the invading agent. The disease can be transmitted during this stage, but this is not probable. Until the host's overall health has been strengthened, he or she may be especially susceptible to another (perhaps different) disease pathogen. Fortunately, after the recovery stage, further susceptibility to the pathogenic agent is typically lower because the body has built up immunity. This buildup of immunity is not always permanent; for example, many sexually transmitted diseases can be contracted repeatedly.

Later in the chapter HIV/AIDS will be discussed, however, prior to that time, it may be helpful to state that this critically important pandemic infectious disease does not easily fit into the five-step model of infectious diseases just presented. In individuals infected with HIV there is an initial asymptomatic *incubation stage,* followed by a *prodromal stage* characterized by generalized signs of immune system inadequacy. However, once the level of specific protective cells of the immune system declines to the point that the body cannot be protected from opportunistic diseases, and the label AIDS is assigned, the five stage model becomes less easily applied.

Body Defenses: Mechanical and Cellular-Chemical Immune Systems

Much as a series of defensive alignments protect a military installation, so too is the body protected by sets of defenses. These defenses can be classified as either mechanical or cellular-chemical (Figure 13-2). Mechanical defenses are first-line defenses, because they physically separate the internal body from the external environment. Examples include the skin, the mucous membranes of the respiratory and gastrointestinal tracts, earwax, the hairs and cilia

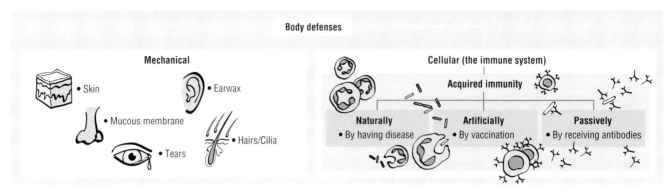

Figure 13-2 The body has a variety of defenses against invading organisms. Mechanical defenses are the first line of protection, since they separate the internal body from the external environment. Cellular defenses include chemicals and specialized cells that provide immunity to subsequent infections.

that filter incoming air, and even tears. These defenses serve primarily as a shield against foreign materials that may contain pathogenic agents. These defenses can, however, be disarmed, such as when tobacco smoke kills the cilia that protect the airway, resulting in chronic bronchitis, or when contact lenses reduce tearing, leading to irritation and eye infection.

The second component of the body's protective defenses is the cellular-chemical system or, more commonly, the **immune system.** The cellular-chemical component is far more specific than the mechanical defenses. Its primary mission is to eliminate microorganisms, foreign protein, and abnormal cells from the body. A wellness-oriented lifestyle, including sound nutrition, effective stress management, and regular exercise, supports this important division of the immune system. The microorganisms, foreign proteins, or abnormal cells that activate this cellular component are collectively called *antigens.*[2]

Divisions of the Immune System

Closer examination of the immune system, or cellular-chemical defenses, reveals two separate but highly cooperative groups of cells. One group of cells originates in the fetal thymus gland and thus has become known as *T cell-mediated immunity,* or simply *cell-mediated immunity.* The second group of cells that makes up cellular immunity are the B cells (bursa of Fabricius), which are the working units of *humoral immunity.*[3] Cellular elements of both cell-mediated and humoral immunity can be found within the bloodstream, the lymphatic tissues of the body, and the fluid that surrounds body cells.

Although we are born with the structural elements of both cell-mediated and humoral immunity, developing an immune response requires that components of these cellular systems encounter and successfully defend against specific antigens. When the immune system has done this

once, it is, in most cases, primed to respond quickly and effectively if the same antigens appear again. This confrontation produces a state of **acquired immunity (AI).**[1] Acquired immunity develops in different ways, as seen in Figure 13-2 above.

· **Naturally acquired immunity (NAI)** develops when the body is exposed to infectious agents. Thus when we catch an infectious disease, we fight the infection and in the process become immune (protected) from developing that illness if we encounter these agents again. Before the advent of immunizations, this was the only way of developing immunity.

· **Artificially acquired immunity (AAI)** occurs when the body is exposed to weakened or killed infectious agents introduced through vaccination or immunization. As in NAI, the body fights the infectious agents and records the method of fighting the agents. Young children, older adults, and adults in high-risk occupations

---

Key Terms

immune system the system of cellular and chemical elements that protects the body from pathogens, abnormal cells, and foreign protein.

acquired immunity (AI) the major component of the immune system; forms antibodies and specialized blood cells capable of destroying pathogens.

naturally acquired immunity (NAI) a type of acquired immunity resulting from the body's response to naturally occurring pathogens.

artificially acquired immunity (AAI) a type of acquired immunity resulting from the body's response to pathogens introduced into the body through immunizations.

Are Americans Too Clean?

Infectious disease specialists are increasingly concerned about the widespread popularity and availability of antimicrobial cleaning products and the contribution they may be making to the development of antibiotic-resistant "super bugs." In fact, it is estimated that approximately 75% of all liquid hand soaps and nearly 30% of all bar soaps contain either triclocarban or triclosan, antibacterial chemicals to which pathogenic agents are already showing resistance.

As concern about our increasing reliance on antimicrobial products grows, we are reminded of the first personal hygiene rule that most Americans were taught as children at home and in school: Wash your hands thoroughly with soap and *hot water!* Even today, microbiologists remind us that nothing is more effective in cleaning our bodies, our homes, and our work places than "old-fashioned" soap and hot water.

should consult their physicians about immunizations. See Table 13.2 on page 436 for a schedule.

- **Passively acquired immunity (PAI),** a third form of immunity, results when antibodies are introduced into the body. These extrinsic antibodies are for a variety of specific infections, and they are produced outside the body (either in animals or by the genetic manipulation of microorganisms). When introduced into the human body, they provide immediate protection until the body can develop a more natural form of immunity. Note that in PAI no actual pathogenic agents are introduced into the body—only the antibodies against various forms of disease-causing agents.

Regardless of how infectious agents are acquired, either through naturally acquired immunity (NAI) or through artificially acquired immunity (AAI), the result is an "arming" of the body's own immune system. This process is frequently labeled as *active immunity.* This contrasts to passively acquired immunity (PAI) in which the body "borrows" another's immune elements without actual involvement of the body's own immune system. This latter case is called *passive immunity.*[4]

In addition to the forms of immunity just described, infants are also provided with a period of short-term immunity via the biological mothers' immune system elements crossing the placental barrier (see Chapter 17) and following birth via breast milk. This *maternal immunity,* however, gradually deteriorates but is concurrently being replaced by the child's own increasingly functional immune system.

Collectively, these forms of immunity can provide important protection against infectious disease.

The Immune Response

Fully understanding the function of the immune system requires a substantial understanding of human biology and is beyond the scope of this text. Figure 13-3 on page 434 presents a simplified view of the immune response.

When antigens (whether microorganisms, foreign protein, or abnormal cells) are discovered within the body, various types of white blood cells confront and destroy some of these antigens. Principal among these blood cells are the *macrophages* (very large white blood cells) that begin ingesting antigens as they are encountered. In conjunction with this "eating" of antigens, macrophages display segments of the antigen's unique protein coat on their outer surface. Now in the form of macrophage/antigen complexes, macrophages transport their captured antigen identifiers to awaiting helper T cells whose recognition of the antigen will initiate the full expression of the cell-mediated immune response. This involves the specialization of "basic" T cells into four specialized forms: helper T cells, killer T cells, suppressor T cells, and memory T cells.

Once helper T cells have been derived from "parent" T cells by the presence of the macrophage/antigen complex, they notify a second component of cellular immunity, the killer T cells. Killer T cells produce powerful chemical messengers that activate specific white blood cells that destroy antigens through the production of caustic chemicals called cytotoxins, or "cell poisons." In addition to the helper T cells' activation of killer T cells, helper T cells also play a critical role in the activation of B cells, principal players in the expression of humoral immunity.

Activation of the humoral immunity component of the overall immune response involves the helper T cells' ability to construct a working relationship between themselves, the macrophage/antigen complexes (mentioned earlier), and the small B cells. Once these three elements have been constituted into working units, the B cells are transformed into a new version of themselves called *plasma cells.* Plasma cells then utilize the information about the antigen's identity to produce massive numbers of "locks" called **antibodies.** Upon release from the plasma cells, these antibodies then circulate throughout the body and "lock-up" or capture free antigens in the form of *antigen/antibody complexes.*[4]

Key Terms

passively acquired immunity (PAI) a temporary immunity achieved by providing extrinsic antibodies to a person exposed to a particular pathogen.

antibodies chemical compounds produced by the body's immune system to destroy antigens and their toxins.

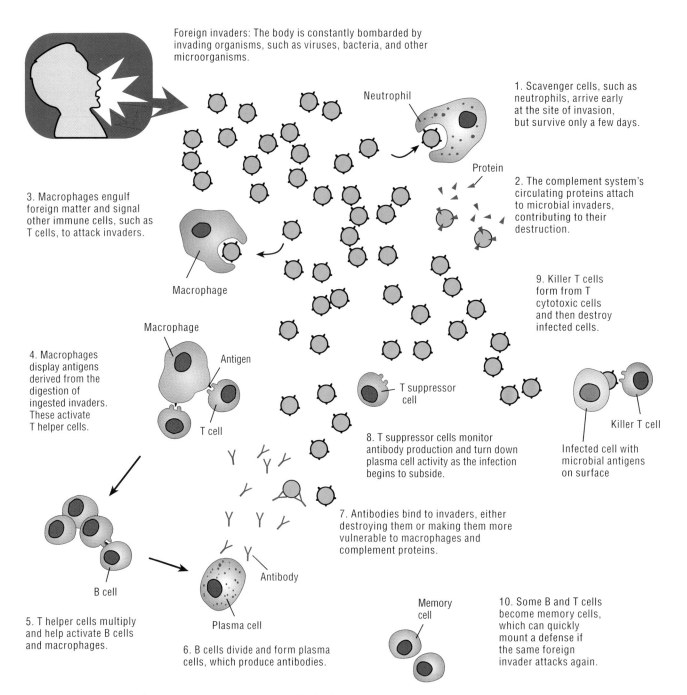

Foreign invaders: The body is constantly bombarded by invading organisms, such as viruses, bacteria, and other microorganisms.

Neutrophil

1. Scavenger cells, such as neutrophils, arrive early at the site of invasion, but survive only a few days.

Protein

2. The complement system's circulating proteins attach to microbial invaders, contributing to their destruction.

3. Macrophages engulf foreign matter and signal other immune cells, such as T cells, to attack invaders.

Macrophage

Macrophage

Antigen

T cell

9. Killer T cells form from T cytotoxic cells and then destroy infected cells.

4. Macrophages display antigens derived from the digestion of ingested invaders. These activate T helper cells.

T suppressor cell

Killer T cell

8. T suppressor cells monitor antibody production and turn down plasma cell activity as the infection begins to subside.

Infected cell with microbial antigens on surface

B cell

Antibody

Plasma cell

7. Antibodies bind to invaders, either destroying them or making them more vulnerable to macrophages and complement proteins.

5. T helper cells multiply and help activate B cells and macrophages.

6. B cells divide and form plasma cells, which produce antibodies.

Memory cell

10. Some B and T cells become memory cells, which can quickly mount a defense if the same foreign invader attacks again.

Figure 13-3 Biological warfare. The body commands an army of defenders to reduce the danger of infection and guard against repeat infections. Antigens are the ultimate targets of all immune responses.

The "captured" antigens are now highly susceptible to a variety of white blood cells that ingest or chemically destroy these infectious agents.

To assure that the initial response to the presence of the antigen can be appropriately controlled, a third group of T cells, the suppressor T cells, have been formed by the initial activation of parent T cells. These suppressor T cells monitor the outcome of the humoral response (antibody

formation) and when comfortable with the number of antibodies produced, turn off further plasma cell activity. The fourth group of specialized T cells, the memory T cells, record this initial recognition-based game plan for fighting the original antigen invasion so that any subsequent similar antigen appearance will be quickly mounted.

An additional group of cells that operates independently from the T cell/B cell interplay just described are the

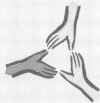

Learning from Our Diversity

Infectious Disease: A Challenge for Older Adults

It's not always easy for young adults in excellent health to recover quickly and completely from some infectious diseases. Later in life the recovery often becomes much more difficult and in some cases impossible. For a variety of reasons older adults do not respond to infectious conditions with the same resiliency as they once did.

Central to this issue is the gradual degradation of the immune system over time. For reasons not fully understood, the immune system loses both its ability to recognize the presence of pathogens that have entered the body and its ability to mount an effective response against them. Particularly important in this regard are the decreased prevalence of active immune system cells and the inability of existing immune cells to respond effectively. Whether this reduced level of immune protection is a "programmed" aspect of aging (all human life does end at some point in time) or whether it reflects a process that is preventable (perhaps through lifestyle modifications) remains hotly debated. Perhaps no group of older adults is at greater risk because of a compromised immune system than are those with AIDS. The nearly eighty thousand persons over age 50 with this immune system–destroying disease have a decreased ability to resist all infectious conditions, even when their HIV levels are suppressed through drug therapy.

In addition to the normal aging of their immune systems, older adults are generally afflicted with a variety of chronic conditions. The presence of multiple chronic illnesses (known as comorbidity) places the body under great stress, which also undermines the immune system. The combined effects of these conditions result in damage to different organ systems of the body—most importantly, the cardiovascular system, the respiratory system, and the renal system. Any time these systems are compromised by the effects of illness, either chronic or acute, the body becomes particularly vulnerable to infectious agents that routinely exist in our environment.

Compounding this situation is the inability of many older adults to understand the potential seriousness of infections at this stage of their lives. They may even have a false sense of confidence that their bodies are just as "good" at warding off infections as they once were. In addition, a lack of social support, isolation from health care facilities, and the inability to afford expensive prescription medication together make important medical care less available at a time when it could be effective.

When these factors are combined, as they are for many older adults, serious and even fatal infectious conditions become a reality. Therefore, anyone who is responsible for the health and well-being of older persons needs to understand their susceptibility to infectious conditions and recognize the fact that timely and competent care is of critical importance.

---

natural killer (NK) cells. These immune cells continuously patrol the blood and intracellular fluids looking for abnormal cells, including cancer cells and viral-infected cells. When these are found, the NK cells attack them with destructive cytotoxins in a process called *lysing*.[4]

Clearly, without a normal immune system employing both cellular and humoral elements, we would quickly fall victim to serious and life-shortening infections and malignancies. As you will see later, this is exactly what occurs in many people infected with HIV (see the Learning from Our Diversity box above).

Emerging medical technology holds promise for repairing damaged immune systems. In a current form of treatment, *adult stem cells* are harvested from nondiseased tissues of a person's body or from a biologically related family member and used to replace damaged or diseased cells within the immune system.[5, 6] A second form of immune system repair involves harvesting *cord blood (stem) cells* taken from the umbilical cord blood collected and "banked" at birth. After careful matching, these cells can be transplanted into a recipient in anticipation that they will specialize into the cell type needed by the damaged or diseased immune system.[7] The virtual absence of any specialization in stem cells at the time of harvesting provides an opportunity for the highly generic stem cells to develop into immune system cells once transplanted into the recipient's body. Perhaps the most interesting use of this technology occurred in October 2000, when a young cancer victim's immune system was restarted via a stem cell transplant obtained from her newborn brother, who was himself conceived for the purpose of being a stem cell donor. It should be noted, however, that this was a highly unusual procedure to follow. It is important to note that considerable controversy now surrounds the use of stem cells obtained from embryonic or fetal tissue sources. Even though these are considered to be the "best" stem cells, restrictions by the federal government (and several states) on their collection and use have forced clinicians to use stem cells from the sources mentioned earlier, as well as from cadavers.[8, 9]

Immunizations

Although the incidence of several childhood communicable diseases is at or near the lowest level ever, we are risking a resurgence of diseases such as measles, polio, diphtheria, and rubella. This possible increase in childhood infectious

Table 13.2 Recommended Childhood and Adolescent Immunization Schedule—United States, 2003

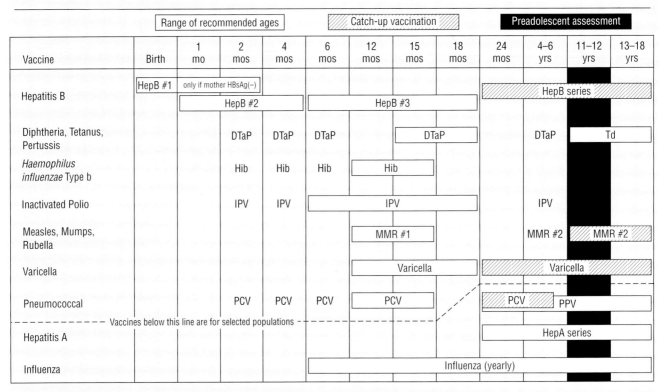

Vaccine	Birth	1 mo	2 mos	4 mos	6 mos	12 mos	15 mos	18 mos	24 mos	4–6 yrs	11–12 yrs	13–18 yrs
Hepatitis B	HepB #1	only if mother HBsAg(–)								HepB series		
		HepB #2			HepB #3							
Diphtheria, Tetanus, Pertussis		DTaP	DTaP	DTaP		DTaP			DTaP		Td	
Haemophilus influenzae Type b		Hib	Hib	Hib	Hib							
Inactivated Polio		IPV	IPV		IPV				IPV			
Measles, Mumps, Rubella						MMR #1			MMR #2		MMR #2	
Varicella						Varicella			Varicella			
Pneumococcal		PCV	PCV	PCV	PCV				PCV	PPV		
Hepatitis A									HepA series			
Influenza					Influenza (yearly)							

Range of recommended ages / Catch-up vaccination / Preadolescent assessment

Vaccines below this line are for selected populations

Note: Indicates the recommended ages for routine administration of currently licensed childhood vaccines, as of December 1, 2002, for children through age 18 years. Any dose not given at the recommended age should be given at any subsequent visit when indicated and feasible. ▨ Indicates age groups that warrant special effort to administer those vaccines not given previously. Additional vaccines may be licensed and recommended during the year. Licensed combination vaccines may be used whenever any components of the combination are indicated and the vaccine's other components are not contraindicated. Providers should consult the manufacturer's package inserts for detailed recommendations.
Recommended Childhood and Adolescent Immunization Schedule. *MMWR* 52(04):Q1–Q4, 2003.

illnesses is based on the disturbing finding that fewer than half of American preschoolers are adequately immunized, which is principally due to the failure of many parents to complete their children's immunization programs. Today health professionals are attempting to raise the level of immunization to 90 percent of all children under the age of 2 years.

Vaccinations against several potentially serious infectious conditions are available and should be given. These include the following:

- *Diphtheria:* A potentially fatal illness that leads to inflammation of the membranes that line the throat, to swollen lymph nodes, and to heart and kidney failure
- *Whooping cough:* A bacterial infection of the airways and lungs that results in deep, noisy breathing and coughing

- *Hepatitis B:* A viral infection that can be transmitted sexually or through the exchange of blood or bodily fluids; seriously damages the liver
- *Haemophilus influenzae type B:* A bacterial infection that can damage the heart and brain, resulting in meningitis, and can produce profound hearing loss
- *Tetanus:* A fatal infection that damages the central nervous system; caused by bacteria found in the soil
- *Rubella (German measles):* A viral infection of the upper respiratory tract that can cause damage to a developing fetus when the mother contracts the infection during the first trimester of pregnancy
- *Measles (red measles):* A highly contagious viral infection leading to a rash, high fever, and upper respiratory tract symptoms
- *Polio:* A viral infection capable of causing paralysis of the large muscles of the extremities

- *Mumps:* A viral infection of the salivary glands
- *Chicken pox:* A varicella zoster virus spread by airborne droplets, leading to a sore throat, rash, and fluid-filled blisters
- *Pneumococcal infection:* A bacterium capable of causing infections, including pneumonia, heart, kidney, and middle ear infections

Parents of newborns should take their infants to their family-care physicians, pediatricians, or well-baby clinics operated by county health departments to begin the immunization process. The schedule shown in Table 13.2 on page 436 is recommended by the American Academy of Pediatrics, the American Academy of Family Physicians, and the Centers for Disease Control and Prevention (CDC). The new chicken pox vaccine, VariVax, is now available. Currently the vaccine is recommended for the child 1 year of age or older who does not have a reliable history of having had chicken pox as determined by the health care provider. For children at high risk for pneumococcal infections of the upper respiratory system (including resultant middle ear infections), a vaccine is now available. For these children, including Native American children, African American children, and children with congenital immunodeficiency, chronic cardiopulmonary disease, immunosuppressive neoplastic disease, chronic renal insufficiency, and those on chemotherapy, immunization with pneumococcal conjugate and pneumococcal polysaccharide vaccines is recommended. Early studies regarding a decrease in middle ear infections (otitis media) in children having received the pneumococcal vaccine was encouraging. More recent reviews of previous studies, however, suggest that the reduction is very small, and should not be viewed as the basis on which this immunization is advised.[10] Researchers are also attempting to develop a single immunization that would combine many individual vaccines now used. In addition, research is being conducted on new delivery systems, including a skin patch, nasal spray, and vaccine-enriched foods, such as potatoes.

 TALKING POINTS Through community service work, you meet a couple that say that they have not had their children immunized and don't see the reason for doing so. How would you explain the importance of having this done?

In recent years concern has arisen regarding the role of childhood immunizations in the development of other serious childhood physical and emotional health problems, such as type 1 diabetes mellitus,[11] asthma,[12] autism,[13] and SIDS.[14] At this time studies investigating the possible relationship between recommended immu-

nizations and conditions mentioned above have found no demonstrable cause-and-effect relationships.

Although immunization is universally viewed as important for infants and children, adults have immunization needs that can be unmet. Accordingly, CDC's National Immunization Program has just released its first immunization schedule for adults. Table 13.4 lists the eight immunizations that should be updated or initially received by adults. Adults are particularly underprotected in regard to diphtheria and tetanus (see page 436).[15]

Causes and Management of Selected Infectious Diseases

This section focuses on some of the common infectious diseases and some diseases that are less common but serious. You can use this information as a basis for judging your own disease susceptibility.

The Common Cold

The common cold, an acute upper-respiratory-tract infection, must reign as humankind's supreme infectious

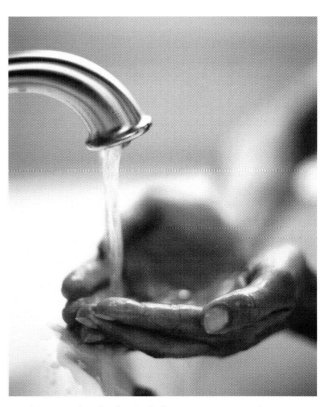

Washing your hands often is the best way to prevent the common cold.

Table 13.3 Is It a Cold or the Flu?

	Cold	Flu
Symptoms		
Fever	Rare	Characteristic, high (102°–104° + F); lasts 3–4 days
Headache	Rare	Prominent
General aches, pains	Slight	Usual; often severe
Fatigue, weakness	Quite mild	Can last up to 2–3 weeks
Extreme exhaustion	Never	Early and prominent
Stuffy nose	Common	Sometimes
Sneezing	Usual	Sometimes
Sore throat	Common	Sometimes
Chest discomfort, cough	Mild to moderate; hacking cough	Common; can become severe
Complications	Sinus congestion, earache	Pneumonia, bronchitis; can be life threatening
Prevention	Avoidance of infected people	Annual vaccination; amantadine or rimantadine (antiviral drugs)
Treatment	OTC products for symptom relief	Amantadine or rimantadine within 24–48 hours after onset of symptoms

Note: The need to consult a physician as the result of complications that might arise during the course of a cold or flu is not unknown. During the course of a cold any of the following should be called to the attention of a physician: (1) when a cold fails to resolve within 5 to 7 days, (2) when an elevated temperature develops (above 103°F), or (3) when a "deep chest" cough develops that produces either a brownish-tinged sputum or does not respond to OTC cough medication. Similar complications can occur in conjunction with the flu and require consultation with a physician. In addition, prolonged vomiting and diarrhea also should be called to the attention of a physician. Upon contracting the flu, children, older adults, pregnant women, and all persons with chronic conditions such as diabetes mellitus, cardiovascular diseases, and malignancies should be carefully monitored and complications should be promptly reported to a physician.

disease. Also known as **acute rhinitis,** this highly contagious viral infection can be caused by any of the nearly 200 known rhinoviruses. Colds are particularly common when people spend time in crowded indoor environments, such as classrooms.

The signs and symptoms of a cold are fairly predictable. Runny nose, watery eyes, general aches and pains, a listless feeling, and a slight fever all may accompany a cold in its early stages. Eventually the nasal passages swell, and the inflammation may spread to the throat. Stuffy nose, sore throat, and coughing may follow (Table 13.3 above). The senses of taste and smell are blocked, and appetite declines.

When you notice the onset of symptoms, you should begin managing the cold promptly. After a few days, most of the cold's symptoms subside. In the meantime, you should isolate yourself from others, drink plenty of fluids, eat moderately, and rest.

In addition to the unpleasantness of the symptoms associated with colds, these nearly universal respiratory infections are also expensive. Collectively, colds cost the American economy 40 billion dollars annually, due to lost work and out of pocket expenditures on cold medications, including 2.19 billion for cold remedies and 1.88 billion for cough drops.[16]

At this time there is no effective way to prevent colds. In 1999 a medication, pleconaril, appeared to be effective in reducing the extent and duration of colds once initial symptoms had developed. However, in 2002 the FDA denied approval of pleconaril (brand name Picovir) due, in part, to adverse reactions in some women using the drug and oral contraceptives; and the possibility of developing resistance to the drug within the family of viruses for which it is intended.

Some of the many OTC cold remedies can help you manage a cold. These remedies will not cure your cold but may lessen the discomfort associated with it. Nasal decongestants, expectorants, cough syrups, and aspirin or acetaminophen can give some temporary relief. Follow label directions carefully. (For herbal and homeopathic remedies, see the Considering Complementary Care box on page 439).

If a cold persists, as evidenced by prolonged chills, fever above 103 degrees Fahrenheit, chest heaviness or

Key Terms

acute rhinitis the common cold; the sudden onset of nasal inflammation.

Table 13.4 Recommended Adult Immunization Schedule—United States • 2002–2003

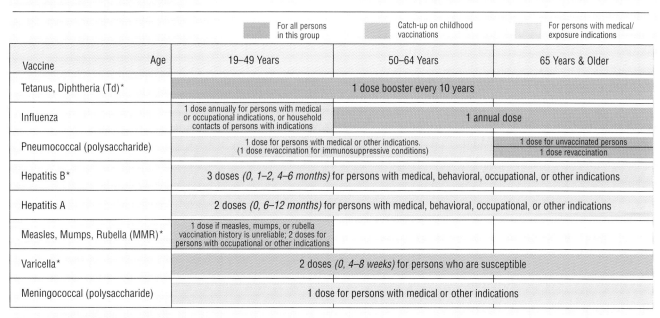

	For all persons in this group	Catch-up on childhood vaccinations	For persons with medical/exposure indications

Vaccine / Age	19–49 Years	50–64 Years	65 Years & Older
Tetanus, Diphtheria (Td)*	1 dose booster every 10 years		
Influenza	1 dose annually for persons with medical or occupational indications, or household contacts of persons with indications	1 annual dose	
Pneumococcal (polysaccharide)	1 dose for persons with medical or other indications. (1 dose revaccination for immunosuppressive conditions)		1 dose for unvaccinated persons / 1 dose revaccination
Hepatitis B*	3 doses *(0, 1–2, 4–6 months)* for persons with medical, behavioral, occupational, or other indications		
Hepatitis A	2 doses *(0, 6–12 months)* for persons with medical, behavioral, occupational, or other indications		
Measles, Mumps, Rubella (MMR)*	1 dose if measles, mumps, or rubella vaccination history is unreliable; 2 doses for persons with occupational or other indications		
Varicella*	2 doses *(0, 4–8 weeks)* for persons who are susceptible		
Meningococcal (polysaccharide)	1 dose for persons with medical or other indications		

Source: www.cdc.gov/nip/recs/adultschedule.htm

Considering Complementary Care

Fighting the Common Cold

Everyone, at one time or another, thinks about how to prevent a cold or how to recover from one. For many people the use of herbal or homeopathic products seems worthy of consideration. Four such products are routinely suggested as being effective in the prevention and/or recovery from colds (and in some cases the flu).

Echinacea, a dietary supplement derived from the roots of the purple cone flower *(Echinacea purpursa),* is purported to be effective in strengthening the immune system and in so doing reducing the number of colds typically contracted during the course of a year. A supportive effect, shortening the duration of symptoms, has also been reported when an echinacea liquid extract (in alcohol) was taken at the first appearance of a cold or the flu.

Elderberry, in extract form, represents a second herbal product whose ability to prevent the development of colds and influenza has been reported. Additionally, elderberry extract has been reported to be effective in reducing the duration of flu-related symptoms from the usual 6 days to as few as 2 days. Mild gastrointestinal complications have also been reported in conjunction with elderberry extract use if taken without food in the stomach.

Goldenseal, an herbal product, is generally taken in combination with echinacea. It is believed that goldenseal has some antibacterial efficacy, as well as the ability to stimulate the production of mucus within the respiratory track. To date no antiviral capabilities have been demonstrated with goldenseal, so a direct influence on cold and flu agents seems unlikely. Herbalists suggest that goldenseal detoxifies the body in some fashion.

Oscillococcinum, a nonherbal homeopathic flu medication popular in Europe, contains small quantities of duck liver (see the discussion of homeopathic medication in Chapter 18). Underlying the purported effectiveness of oscillococcinum is its vaccine-like protection resulting from a heightened immune system response to the minuscule amount of flu virus contained in the infected duck liver.

Remember that neither dietary supplements nor homeopathic medications must undergo the rigorous clinical trials required by the FDA for prescriptions medications. Nor do they need to meet the standards for safety and effectiveness required by the FDA for OTC products. Anecdotal information and studies conducted in other countries are the primary basis for the claims made for these products.

aches, shortness of breath, coughing up rust-colored mucus, or persistent sore throat or hoarseness, you should contact a physician. Because we now consider colds to be transmitted most readily by hand contact, you should wash your hands frequently.

Two factors seem predictable in terms of "preventing" colds. The first involves the less than average number of colds seen in children between 6 and 11 years of age, who had attended larger preschool programs (more than six other children).[17] The second factor involved a lower than average number of colds in adults (average age of 48) who exercised at the higher levels of intensity (based on current exercise guidelines from the U.S. Surgeon General).[18]

Influenza

Influenza is also an acute contagious disease caused by viruses. Some influenza outbreaks have killed many people, such as the influenza pandemics of 1889 to 1890, 1918 to 1919, 1957 and 2003/2004. The viral strains that produce this infectious disease have the potential for more severe complications than the viral strains that produce the common cold. The viral strain for a particular form of influenza enters the body through the respiratory tract. After brief incubation and prodromal stages, the host develops signs and symptoms not just in the upper respiratory tract but throughout the entire body. These symptoms include fever, chills, cough, sore throat, headache, gastrointestinal disturbances, and muscular pain. (See Table 13.3 on page 438.)

Antibiotics are generally not prescribed for people with influenza, except when the patient has a possible secondary bacterial infection. Physicians may recommend only aspirin, fluids, and rest. Parents are reminded not to give aspirin to children because of the danger of Reye's syndrome. Reye's syndrome is an aspirin-enhanced complication of influenza in which central nervous system changes can occur, including brain swelling. For a person seeking a quicker resolution to the debilitating symptoms of flu, four antiviral medications are currently available; two are intended for influenza virus type A and two for both virus types A and B. Specific recommendations regarding use of these prescription medications, including age limitations, also exist.[19]

Most young adults can cope with the milder strains of influenza that appear each winter or spring. However, pregnant women and older people—especially older people with additional health complications, such as heart disease, kidney disease, emphysema, and chronic bronchitis—are not as capable of handling this viral attack. People who regularly come into contact with the general public, such as teachers, should also consider annual flu shots.

Today approximately 70 million Americans receive annual "flu shots." In past years, these annual immunizations, tailored to work against the flu viruses anticipated for the coming flu season, were principally received by adults over 50 years of age and others with special needs. During the flu epidemic of 2003/2004 younger adults moved into the recipient population. Today, CDC is extending flu shot recommendations to include all children 6 to 23 months of age and youth between 6 months to 18 years of age who are residing with adults at greatest risk for contracting influenza due to illness or occupational exposure. This recommendation should increase the immunized pool to near 100 million.[19] It should be noted, however, that in the near future the term *flu shot* may be less frequently heard. In June of 2003, the FDA approved the sale of Flumist, a noninvasive nasal spray inhalation delivery system for influenza vaccine. Its use is approved for people ages 5 to 49. Its use is not, at this time, recommended for persons most in need of the highest level of protection.

The flu season generally runs from November through February, with nearly 115,000 persons developing clear symptoms of influenza, and 36,000 dying from its complications.[19]

Tuberculosis

Experts considered TB, a bacterial infection of the lungs resulting in chronic coughing, weight loss, and even death, to be under control in this country until the mid-1980s. The number of cases surged then, however, with a peak of 26,283 cases in 1992. The number has declined since then, with 15,989 cases reported in 2001, a 2% decline from 2000.[20] However, public health officials must continually watch this infectious disease, as people immigrate to the United States from areas of the world in which TB is considerably more common and drug-resistant strains of the bacterium emerge. As an example, it is estimated that 60% of all cases of TB in New York City are among foreign-born residents; and that 10 to 15 million U.S. residents have latent tuberculosis, from which 10% will develop active cases of TB.[21]

Tuberculosis thrives in crowded places where infected people are in constant contact with others, since TB is spread by coughing. This includes prisons, hospitals, public housing units, and even college residence halls. In such settings, a single infected person can spread the TB agents to many others.

When healthy people are exposed to TB agents, their immune systems can usually suppress the bacteria enough to prevent symptoms from developing and to reduce the likelihood of infecting others. When the immune system is damaged, however, such as in some older adults, malnourished people, and those who are infected with HIV, the disease can become established and eventually be transmitted to other people at risk.

As previously mentioned, multiple drug-resistant (MDR) TB has appeared. Increasingly prevalent in this country, MDR tuberculosis is the result of patients' inability to follow their physicians' instructions when initially treated (for whatever reason), inadequate treatment by physicians, and increased exposure of HIV-infected people to TB. Only 50% of people with this form of TB can be cured. Some believe that MDR tuberculosis will be the next epidemic in this country.

Health officials are again requesting that TB testing programs be implemented and that infected people be identified, isolated, and brought into treatment. A new serum-based TB screening test, ELISPOT, has been developed.[22] Similar to the screening test used to detect HIV infection, this test identifies T cells that have been sensitized to an antigen component of the principal tuberculosis bacterium, mycobacterium. This test is more accurate in identifying infected persons than the older and more familiar skin tests.

Pneumonia

Pneumonia is a general term that describes a variety of infectious respiratory conditions. There are bacterial, viral, fungal, rickettsial, mycoplasmal, and parasitic forms of pneumonia. However, bacterial pneumonia is the most common form and is often seen with other illnesses that weaken the body's immune system. In fact, pneumonia is so common in the frail older adult that it is often the specific condition causing death. *Pneumocystis carinii* pneumonia, a parasitic form, is important today because it is a principal opportunistic infection associated with AIDS in HIV-infected people.

Older adults with a history of chronic obstructive lung disease, cardiovascular disease, diabetes, or alcoholism often encounter a potentially serious midwinter form of pneumonia known as *acute (severe)community-acquired pneumonia*.[23] Characteristics of this condition are the sudden onset of chills, chest pain, and a cough producing sputum. In addition, a symptom-free form of pneumonia known as *walking pneumonia* is also commonly seen in adults and can become serious without warning.

As the number of older Americans grows, recommendations regarding immunization against pneumococcal pneumonia have been established and vaccination programs undertaken. Today, these recommendations encourage vaccination beginning at 50 years of age. The cost effectiveness of pneumonia immunizations for older adults, and particularly for minority older adults, is well established.[24] The first known drug-resistant strains of pneumonia have been identified in this country. As a result, some experts are calling for an even more comprehensive vaccination plan for older adults.

Mononucleosis

College students who contract **mononucleosis ("mono")** can be forced into a long period of bed rest during a semester when they can least afford it. Other common diseases can be managed with minimal disruption, but the overall weakness and fatigue seen in many people with mono sometimes require a month or two of rest and recuperation.

Mono is a viral infection in which the body produces an excess of mononuclear leukocytes (a type of white blood cell). After uncertain, perhaps long, incubation and prodromal stages, the acute symptoms of mono can appear, including weakness, headache, low-grade fever, swollen lymph glands (especially in the neck), and sore throat. Mental fatigue and depression are sometimes reported as side effects of mononucleosis. After the acute symptoms disappear, the weakness and fatigue usually persist—perhaps for a few months.

Mono is diagnosed by its characteristic symptoms. The Monospot blood smear can also be used to identify the prevalence of abnormal white blood cells. In addition, an antibody test can detect activity of the immune system that is characteristic of the illness.

This disease is most often caused by an Epstein-Barr virus, so antibiotic therapy is not recommended. Treatment usually includes bed rest and the use of OTC remedies for fever (aspirin or acetaminophen) and lozenges for sore throat. Corticosteroid drugs can be used in extreme cases. Rupture of the spleen is an occasional, but serious, consequence of the condition, particularly in persons who are too physically active during their recovery.[25] Adequate fluid intake and a well-balanced diet are also important in the recovery stages of mono. Fortunately, the body tends to develop NAI (naturally acquired immunity) to the mono virus, so repeat infections of mono are unusual.

For years, mono has been labeled the "kissing disease"; however, mono is not highly contagious and is known to be spread by direct transmission in ways other than kissing. No vaccine has been developed to confer AAI for mononucleosis. The best preventive measures are the steps that you can take to increase your resistance to most infectious diseases: (1) eat a well-balanced diet, (2) exercise regularly, (3) sleep sufficiently, (4) use health care services appropriately, (5) live in a reasonably healthful environment, and (6) avoid direct contact with infected people.

Key Terms

mononucleosis ("mono") a viral infection characterized by weakness, fatigue, swollen glands, sore throat, and low-grade fever.

Living with an Infectious Disease—Life Is Not Over, Just Different

A chronic infectious disease can wear down your body and your spirit. First, you've got to deal with the pain, fatigue, and medicinal side effects associated with the condition. But you also need to learn to adapt everything—your routine, your relationships, and your work—to the illness. As the quality of your life changes dramatically, you may feel depressed, frustrated, and alone. What is the best way to handle the different aspects of your life as you learn to cope with a long-term illness such as chronic fatigue syndrome, hepatitis, or HIV? Will it ever be possible to enjoy a full life again?

Your workplace may present the first big challenge. Since your energy level will be decreased by your illness, you may have trouble completing tasks on time and handling your normal workload. Your allotted sick time and vacation days may be used up quickly for doctor's appointments, hospitalizations, and those days when you are simply too exhausted to go to work. Your coworkers and your supervisor may discriminate against you in subtle ways, making you feel that you're not doing your fair share. The best way to handle these challenges is to maintain a positive and friendly attitude, carefully manage your time off, promote open communication with your employer, and do your best to produce quality work even when you're not feeling well.

Your intimate relationships may also be strained. Your partner may not understand the new limits your illness places on your activities, especially if you were very active before. The best approach is open and honest communication. Try to dispel (or come to terms with) any fears your partner may have about your illness. Take all necessary precautions to avoid infecting your partner if the disease is transmissible. Also, reassure your partner that you're taking these precautions so that he or she won't become ill. Make a point of including your partner in your daily routines. Keep him or her informed of all doctor's appointments, procedures you must undergo, and any news of progress or setbacks. Share your feelings as a way of reducing anxiety for both of you. Create adaptations so that you can still enjoy a romantic relationship. Make the most of your time together, and find new ways to enjoy each other's company.

If you have children, they will also be affected by your illness. Young children may not understand why you can't take them for a sled ride when you feel sick or why you can't go to a school play because of a doctor's appointment. It's best to let children know that their fears and anxieties are valid and that you want them to share

them with you. Tell them about your prognosis, taking care not to make any false promises of recovery if that is not expected. Spend time with each child—helping with homework, reading a story, or doing light chores around the house. Always allow the child to ask questions.

From your home to your workplace, your life will change along with your condition. As you adapt to your new situation, it is important to:

- *Be your own best friend.* Eat well, exercise as much as you can, rest when you need to, and follow the treatments prescribed by your physician.
- *Know and understand your limits.* Don't feel guilty about not doing things you used to do before you got sick. Instead, set goals and handle responsibilities as your condition allows.
- *Find new things to do for fun.* This is a good time to start a new hobby that's relaxing. You can also make adaptations so that you can continue activities you've always enjoyed. Maybe you can't run 3 miles a day, but an after-dinner walk might be a pleasant substitute.
- *Communicate openly with others.* Share your feelings respectfully, and allow others around you to share theirs. Together, you can calm your fears, instill hope in each other, and foster a sense of belonging.
- *Remain positive.* Remember, life is not over—just different. Look forward to the good days, when you feel well, and take advantage of them. Create new ways to fulfill your needs and desires. Remain positive about the future and your treatment. New discoveries do occur, and treatments are always evolving. However, be realistic about your situation. Joining a support group may be one of the best things you can do for yourself.

What you learn about yourself throughout your illness may surprise you. You may discover a strength of spirit you never knew you had. Some days may be very hard, but somehow you get through them. You may see life in a new way—slowing down and taking pleasure in a job well done, enjoying friendships more, listening to your inner voice, spending time with your children, taking a second look at nature, and being thankful for today and tomorrow.

Chronic Fatigue Syndrome

Chronic fatigue syndrome (CFS) may be the most perplexing "infectious" condition physicians see. First identified in 1985, this mononucleosis-like condition is most often seen in women in their thirties and forties. People with CFS, often busy professional people, report flulike symptoms, including severe exhaustion, fatigue, headaches, muscle aches, fever, inability to concentrate, allergies,

Key Terms

chronic fatigue syndrome (CFS) an illness that causes severe exhaustion, fatigue, aches, and depression; mostly affects women in their thirties and forties.

intolerance to exercise, and depression. Examinations of the first people with CFS revealed antibodies to the Epstein-Barr virus (EBV). Thus observers assumed CFS to be an infectious viral disease (and initially called it *chronic Epstein-Barr syndrome*).

In the years since its first appearance, the condition has received great attention that has produced considerable confusion over its exact nature. In fact, several theories have been advanced to identify the cause (or causes) of CFS. As suggested above, some experts believe an infectious agent may be partially responsible, possibly a virus such as EBV, cytomegalovirus, herpes simplex 1 and 2, or human herpes virus 6. To date no specific virus has been isolated. A second explanation involves an extended challenge to the immune system, possibly activated by an initial viral infection and resulting in the overproduction of immune system chemicals that produce flulike symptoms. A final CFS model suggests the involvement of one or more factors, including emotional, environmental, genetic, and infectious factors. In this model, a stresslike response is believed to disrupt the appropriate interplay among the pituitary, hypothalamus, and adrenal glands (see Chapter 3), thus reducing cortisol production.[26] On the basis of this explanation, other conditions, such as fibromyalgia (see Chapter 12), are related to CFS.

Regardless of its cause or causes, CFS is extremely unpleasant for people who have it. Those experiencing the symptoms over an extended time need to see a physician experienced in dealing with CFS (see the Discovering Your Spirituality box on page 442).

Bacterial Meningitis

Since approximately 1995, a formerly infrequently seen but potentially fatal infectious disease, meningococcal meningitis, has appeared on college campuses, suggesting that college students are currently at greater risk of contracting the disease than are their noncollege peers. Particularly interesting is the fact that among college students, the risk of contracting this infection on campus is highest for those students living in residence halls, suggesting that close living quarters, as well as sharing cigarettes and beverages, kissing (exchanging infectious oral fluids), and contact with students from other areas of the world favor transmission of the bacteria. Since many colleges and universities require that first-year students reside in residence halls, it is in this group that the incidence of meningococcal meningitis is highest.[27] Additionally, this group of students is most likely to be in large section lecture classes and take meals in large dining facilities. Since 1997 the American College Health Association has strongly suggested that parents have incoming students vaccinated against this condition—a $75 investment that could save a life. Annually, about 150 cases of meningococcal meningitis occur on American college campuses, resulting in 15 deaths per year. Understandably, more and more colleges and universities are requiring, as a condition of admission, documentation of immunization against bacterial meningitis, as well as chickenpox, hepatitis B, and tetanus/diphtheria. Additionally, a growing number of states are requiring that health care providers provide clearly stated information regarding the value of meningococcal meningitis immunization. Fortunately, new vaccines, initially used in Canada and Europe, are now available for use in this country.

Meningococcal meningitis is a bacterial infection of the thin membranous coverings of the brain. In its earliest stages, this disease can easily be confused with the flu. Symptoms usually include a high fever, severe headache, stiff neck, nausea with vomiting, extreme tiredness, and the formation of a progressive rash. For about 10% of people who develop this condition, the infection is fatal, often within 24 hours. Therefore the mere presence of the symptoms described above signals the need for immediate medical evaluation. If done promptly, treatment is highly effective.[28]

Lyme Disease

Lyme disease is an infectious disease that is becoming increasingly common in eastern, southeastern, upper midwestern, and West Coast states, with 23,763 cases in 2002. The significant increase in the number of cases of Lyme disease since 1992 (when 9,909 cases were reported) most likely reflects a wider geographical distribution of the disease, a greater awareness of its symptoms by the general public, and more consistent reporting by physicians. This bacterial disease results when infected deer ticks, usually in the nymph (immature) stage, attach to the skin and inject the infectious agent as they feed on a host's blood. Deer ticks become infected by feeding on infected white-tailed deer or white-footed mice.

The symptoms of Lyme disease vary but typically appear within 30 days as small red bumps surrounded by a circular red rash at the site of bites. The red rash, traditionally described as being "bulls eye" in shape, with a whitish center, may also be circular with redness through out. Flulike symptoms may accompany this phase 1 stage, including chills, headaches, muscle and joint aches, and low-grade fever. A phase II stage develops in about 20% of infected people. This phase may produce

Key Terms

Lyme disease a bacterial infection transmitted by deer ticks.

disorders of the nervous system or heart. Those who remain untreated even to this stage can develop a phase III stage, which can include chronic arthritis, lasting up to 2 years. Fortunately, Lyme disease can be treated with antibiotics.[29] Unfortunately, however, no immunity develops, so infection can recur. Because some physicians order tests and begin antibiotic therapy too quickly, however, the basis of concern should be the appearance of phase I symptoms, not simply having been bitten by a tick. Lyme disease may be more difficult to diagnose in children than in adults.

People who live in susceptible areas, including near small urban/suburban wood lots,[30] and participate in outdoor activities can encounter the nearly invisible tick nymphs that have fallen from deer or infected mice into the grass. Thus these people should check themselves frequently to be sure that they are tick-free. They should tuck shirts into pants, tuck pants into socks, and wear gloves and hats when possible. They should also shower after coming inside from outdoors and check clothing for evidence of ticks. Pets can carry infected ticks into the house. If you find ticks, they should be carefully removed from the skin with tweezers and the affected area washed. A vaccine, once available and reasonably effective, has been removed from the marketplace due to declining sales.

The tick that carries Lyme disease has also been found to be responsible for a potentially fatal bacterial infection called *human granulocytic ehrlichiosis (HGE)*. This disease is associated with high fever, headache, muscle aches, and chills. Fortunately, HGE is successfully treated with doxycycline, an antibiotic that can also be used in the treatment of Lyme disease. People with these symptoms who live in areas of the country where Lyme disease is reported should make certain that their physician considers HGE in the diagnosis and treatment of their symptoms.

Hantavirus Pulmonary Syndrome

Since 1993 a small but rapidly growing number of people have been dying of extreme pulmonary distress caused by the leakage of plasma into the lungs. In the initial cases, the people lived in the Southwest, had been well until they began developing flulike symptoms over one or two days, then quickly experienced difficulty breathing, and died only hours later. Epidemiologists quickly suspected a viral agent such as the hantavirus, known to exist in Asia and, to a lesser degree, in Europe. Exhaustive laboratory work led to the culturing of the virus and confirmed that all of these patients had been infected with an American version of the hantavirus. Researchers identified this latest infectious condition as *hantavirus pulmonary syndrome.*

Today hantavirus pulmonary syndrome has been reported in areas beyond the Southwest, including most of the western states and some of the eastern states. The common denominator in all these areas is the presence of deer mice. We now know that this common rodent serves as the reservoir for the virus. In fact, so common is the mouse that in 2000 the National Park Service began warning hikers, campers, and off-road bikers that hantavirus probably existed in every national park and that caution should be taken to avoid high-risk sites.

The virus moves from deer mice to humans when people inhale dust contaminated with dried virus-rich rodent urine or saliva-contaminated materials, such as nests. Health experts now warn people who live in areas with deer mouse populations (most of the United States) to be extremely careful when cleaning houses and barns in which deer mouse droppings are likely to be found. If you must remove rodent nests, wear rubber gloves, pour a disinfectant or bleach on the nests and soak them thoroughly, and finally, pick up the nests with shovels and burn them or bury them in holes that are several feet deep. These procedures should greatly reduce the airborne spread of the viral particles.

Because there is no vaccine for hantavirus pulmonary syndrome, people who are likely to be exposed to the infected excrement of deer mice should seek early evaluation of flulike symptoms.

West Nile Virus

First detected in New York City in 1999, the West Nile virus was, by the summer of 2000, identified in six eastern states—New York, Connecticut, New Jersey, Maryland, Rhode Island, and Massachusetts. By the end of 2002 the West Nile virus had spread westward and to include 34 states, with a reported 4,156 cases and 284 deaths. Incomplete data for 2003 (through August) report 1,442 cases and 21 deaths, with anticipation of weekly doubling to occur through September 2003. The West Nile virus was found in all but 2 of the 48 contiguous states by the end of 2003.

This vector-borne infectious virus is transmitted from a reservoir, most often birds, by mosquitoes that in turn infect humans.[1] Human to human transmission (via mosquitoes) apparently does not occur. West Nile virus infection involves flulike symptoms, including fever, headache, muscle ache, fatigue, and joint pain. In young children, persons with immune systems weakened by HIV, and older adults, West Nile virus infection may involve encephalitis, a potentially fatal inflammation of the brain that closely resembles St. Louis encephalitis. Physicians recommend that any unusual neurological symptoms be considered as a possible West Nile infection. The West Nile virus deaths that have occurred since the infection's initial appearance in 1999 have been the result of encephalitis.

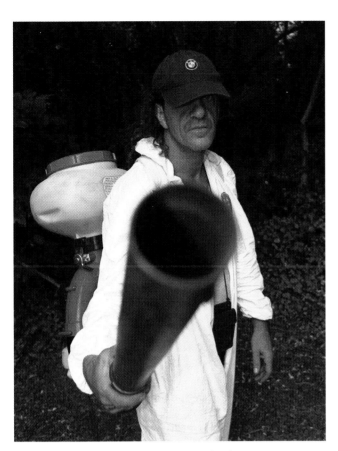

West Nile virus control efforts in Staten Island.

In an attempt to determine the extent of the West Nile virus range, public health officials throughout the eastern United States have tested mosquitoes, sentinel chickens, crows, other birds, cows, and other animals, including humans. Additionally, mosquito habitats are being treated in an attempt to reduce the vector population. Public service announcements focusing on protection against mosquito bites are routinely made in high-risk areas. Additionally, a newly developed immunization that protects birds is being field tested.

In the period 1999–2003, additional aspects of the disease were reported to CDC; these include transmission of the virus through blood transfusions, a possible case of prenatal transmission, and the presence of the virus in breast milk. Additionally, a new test to accurately screen for infected blood has been developed, as has a new diagnostic test, developed in Australia, that significantly reduced the time needed to obtain confirmation of the West Nile virus.

Toxic Shock Syndrome

Toxic shock syndrome (TSS) made front-page headlines in 1980, when the CDC reported a connection

Signs and Symptoms of Toxic Shock Syndrome

- Fever (102°F or above)
- Headache
- Vomiting
- Sore throat
- Diarrhea
- Muscle aches
- Sunburnlike rash
- Low blood pressure
- Bloodshot eyes
- Disorientation
- Reduced urination
- Peeling of skin on the palms of the hands and soles of the feet

between TSS and the presence of a specific bacterial agent *(Staphylococcus aureus)* in the vagina associated with the use of tampons. In addition to tampon misuse-induced TSS, the condition can be caused in conjunction with nasal packing following surgery, infected burns, and subcutaneous abscesses.

TSS causes the signs and symptoms listed in the Star box above. Superabsorbent tampons can irritate the vaginal lining three times more quickly than regular tampons. This vaginal irritation is aggravated when the tampon remains in the vagina for a long time (more than five hours). When this irritation begins, the staphylococcal bacteria (which are usually present in the vagina) have relatively easy access to the bloodstream. When these bacteria proliferate in the circulatory system, their resultant toxins produce a massive T cell response (see pages 433–435), in which powerful cytotoxins and other immune system chemicals, including tumor necrosis factor and interleukins, are produced.[31] These immune system products exacerbate the effects of the bacterial toxin on body tissues. A woman with TSS can die, usually as a result of cardiovascular failure, if left untreated. Fortunately, less than 10% of women diagnosed as having TSS die.

In comparison to other infectious diseases, the extent of TSS is limited. In 1998, the last year for which data are

Key Terms

toxic shock syndrome (TSS) a potentially fatal condition caused by the proliferation of certain bacteria in the vagina that enter the general blood circulation.

available, 133 cases were reported. More recently only about 10 cases have been reported annually. However, because of a tendency of many physicians to not report this condition, it may be far more prevalent than recent data suggest. Accordingly, every woman should exercise reasonable caution in the use of tampons. Consider these recommendations: (1) tampons should not be the sole form of sanitary protection used, and (2) tampons should not remain in place for too long. Women should change tampons every few hours and intermittently use sanitary napkins. Tampons should not be used during sleep. Some physicians recommend that tampons not be used at all if a woman wants to be extraordinarily safe from TSS.

 TALKING POINTS As a parent you are preparing yourself to discuss menstruation with your rapidly maturing daughter. What would you say regarding the safe use of tampons?

Hepatitis

Hepatitis is an inflammatory process in the liver that can be caused by several viruses. Types A, B, C (once called non-A and non-B), D, and E have been recognized. Hepatitis can also be caused indirectly from abuse of alcohol and other drugs. General symptoms of hepatitis include fever, nausea, loss of appetite, abdominal pain, fatigue, and jaundice (yellowing of the skin and eyes).[1]

Type A hepatitis is often associated with consuming fecal-contaminated food, such as raw shellfish, or water. Poor sanitation, particularly in the handling of food and diaper-changing activities, has produced outbreaks in child care centers. Experts estimate that up to two hundred thousand people per year experience this infection. This number far exceeds the reported 26,000 to 27,000 cases per year, suggesting that a very large reservoir exists among children, who are routinely asymptomatic prior to 6 years of age. Therefore, it is currently recommended that children living in states with high levels of reported hepatitis A be vaccinated, as well as children with weakened immune systems, and those who will travel outside the United States.

Type B hepatitis (HBV) is spread in various ways, including sexual contact, intravenous drug use, tattooing, body piercing, and even sharing electric razors. On the basis of these modes of transmission, college students should be aware of the potential risk that they too carry for HBV infection. Beyond the risk factors just identified, medical and dental procedures are also a potential means of transmitting the virus, including patient to practitioner, and practitioner to patient transmission. Chronic HBV infection has been associated with liver cirrhosis and is the principal cause of liver cancer. An effective immunization for hepatitis B is now available.

Although it is given during childhood, it should be seriously considered for older unvaccinated people and college students. In 2002 the American Academy of Pediatrics recommended that all newborns be immunized prior to leaving the hospital. A new vaccine against both hepatitis A and B is now available. Earlier concerns regarding hepatitis B vaccine and multiple sclerosis have been largely dismissed.

Hepatitis C is contracted in ways similar to hepatitis B (sexual contact, tainted blood, and shared needles). In the absence of immunization, the pool of infected people is in excess of four million and the death rate is expected to climb. Currently a dual-drug therapy for HCV involving multiple forms of interferon in combination with the drug ribavirin is the treatment of choice. It should also be noted that many infected persons remain asymptomatic for decades, and many persons infected with HCV recover from this liver-threatening infection. In a recent study a two-drug combination treatment resulted in a virus-free state for nearly 60% of a large group of infected persons treated for 1 year. In spite of encouraging news such as this, recovery from HCV infection seems less likely the case for infected African Americans, a phenomenon that cannot currently be explained.[34]

The newly identified type D (delta) hepatitis is very difficult to treat and is found almost exclusively in people already suffering from type B hepatitis, since the hepatitis D virus requires the presence of the hepatitis B virus in order to gain full pathogenicity. This virus, like type B hepatitis and HIV, makes unprotected sexual contact, including anal and oral sex, very risky. Hepatitis E, associated with water contamination, is rarely seen in this country other than in people returning from hepatitis E virus-endemic areas of the world.

Sudden Acute Respiratory Syndrome (SARS)

In February 2003, the world became aware of a previously unknown respiratory disease, initially thought to be a form of pneumonia. This disease, characterized by high fever (100.4+°F), chills, headaches, and, a few days later, a dry cough, was, in fact, a new viral disease, Sudden Acute Respiratory Syndrome (SARS). First reported in Hanoi, then in Singapore, mainland China, and other Asian countries, the disease quickly presented in Europe and North America. In actuality, the disease had first appeared in a rural area of China, during the fall of 2002, but the Chinese government had apparently chosen not to disseminate this information.

With the rapid spread of SARS, the World Health Organization and CDC issued travel advisories against unnecessary travel to several areas and cities of Asia, as well as to Toronto, Canada. At the same time, scientists isolated the virus responsible for the respiratory disease

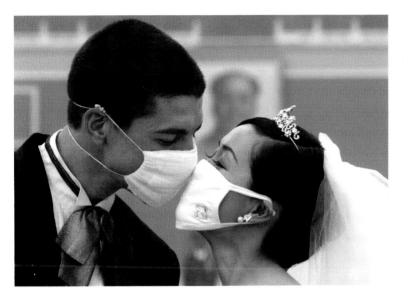

Attempts to prevent contracting SARS were widespread in China during 2003, as seen in this wedding photograph from Beijing.

and identified it as a member of the coronavirus family—a viral family with links to upper respiratory infection (colds). This particular virus, however, apparently entered the human germ pool in conjunction with the eating of civet cats—a delicacy in China—again demonstrating that many infectious conditions in humans have their origins in other animals— **zoonosis.**

With news of the SARS outbreak, the international scientific community began a cooperative effort to understand the disease's human-to-human transmission. It was quickly determined that the virus was transmitted by respiratory droplets. It was further determined that the frail, the elderly, and the young were at greatest risk, as well as persons in direct contact with symptomatic persons (family members and hospital staff). Soon thereafter, a diagnostic test was developed and treatment protocols became more focused and effective. These developments, in combination with concerted public health measures regarding the recognition of symptoms and curtailment of transmission opportunities, led to a rapid decline of reported new cases. On June 5, 2003, the World Health Organization declared that SARS had peaked and was subsiding in all infected areas.[35] By the WHO-defined end of the pandemic, August 15, 2003, 33 people in the United States had been infected and no one died, while worldwide 8,422 had been infected and 916 had died.[36] Clearly, in terms of a potentially pandemic disease, the global village had been condensed in size by international travel and commerce.

Monkeypox

During the summer of 2003, yet another example of a zoonosis, monkeypox, occurred in this country. Specifically, in three Midwest states a viral infection similar to smallpox and characterized by fever, rash, chills, and aches was diagnosed in 49 persons, with probable cases in 91 additional persons in other states. The common thread in all cases proved to be the purchase of pet prairie dogs from a variety of retailers. These retailers had, however, received their "dogs" from a single supplier in Illinois—"Phil's Pocket Pets."

Since the monkeypox virus is endogenous to Africa, and these prairie dogs came from the United States, what had served as the reservoir for the virus? The answer was eventually determined to be the large Gambian Rat (apparently another "pocket pet") imported from Ghana in Africa. Apparently physical contact, in some fashion, had occurred between the two different types of animals, thus providing a mode of transmission. Fortunately, no deaths were reported among the persons contracting the disease.

AIDS

AIDS (acquired immunodeficiency syndrome) has become the most devastating infectious disease in recent history and it is virtually certain to be the most devastating disease in history unless a cure is forthcoming. Setting aside for the present the international scope of the HIV/AIDS epidemic, statistics for the United States alone

---

Key Terms

zoonosis the transmission of diseases from animals to humans.

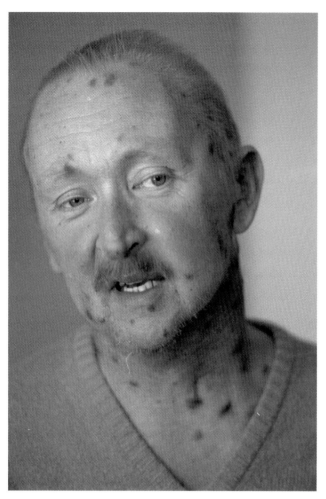

Kaposi's sarcoma, a rare skin cancer, is frequently seen in persons with AIDS.

gradually due to the effectiveness of newer medications, the financial burden that AIDS places on the health care system makes the disease demanding for all Americans.

Cause of AIDS

AIDS is the disease caused by HIV, a virus that attacks the helper T cells of the immune system (see pages 433–435). When HIV attacks helper T cells, people lose the ability to fight off a variety of infections that would normally be easily controlled. Because these infections develop while people are vulnerable, they are collectively called *opportunistic infections*. HIV-infected (HIV+) patients become increasingly vulnerable to infection by bacteria, protozoa, fungi, and several viruses. A variety of malignancies (see Chapter 11) also develop during this period of immune-system vulnerability.

HIV+ with AIDS was originally diagnosed based on the presence of specific conditions. Among these were *Pneumocystis carinii* pneumonia and Kaposi's sarcoma, a rare but deadly form of skin cancer. Gradually, experts recognized that additional conditions were associated with advancing deterioration of the immune system and thus added them to the list of AIDS conditions. This list now includes almost thirty definitive conditions, with more conditions being added as they become apparent. Among the conditions found on the current version of the list are toxoplasmosis within the brain, cytomegalovirus retinitis with loss of vision, lymphoma involving the brain, recurrent salmonella blood infections, and a wasting syndrome that includes invasive cervical cancer in women, recurrent pneumonia, and recurrent tuberculosis. Today, however, experts tend to assign the label of HIV+ with AIDS to HIV-infected people when their level of helper T cells drops below 250 cells per cubic millimeter of blood, regardless of whether specific conditions are present.

Spread of HIV

HIV cannot be contracted easily in comparison to other infectious conditions such as colds, flu, and some childhood infections that can spread quickly within a classroom or office complex. The chances of contracting HIV through casual contact with HIV-infected people at work, school, or home are extremely low or nonexistent. HIV is known to be spread only by direct sexual contact involving the exchange of bodily fluids (including blood, semen, and vaginal secretions), the sharing of hypodermic needles, transfusion of infected blood or blood products, and perinatal transmission (from an infected mother to a fetus or newborn baby). For HIV to be transmitted, it must enter the bloodstream of the noninfected person, such as through needles or tears in body tissues lining the rectum, mouth, or reproductive system. Current research also indicates that HIV is not transmitted by sweat, saliva, tears, or urine, although the virus may be found in very low concentrations in these fluids. The virus cannot enter the

paint a distressing picture. On the basis of data reported through December 2001, a total of 816,149 Americans have been diagnosed with AIDS, and 467,910 have died from its effects (or 57.3% of all cases).[38] Table 13.5 on page 440 shows the distribution of the disease on the basis of gender, age, and race/ethnicity through December 2001. When these are joined with data for persons with HIV (but not yet diagnosed as having AIDS), the scope of the disease is seen even more fully. Table 13.6 on page 450 presents HIV data through December 2001. Note that these data are limited to selected reporting areas and thus are not quite national in scope.

In addition to the human tragedy suggested by these statistics, the financial cost of treating the HIV/AIDS epidemic is sizable. Today it is estimated that annual medical care costs (including medications) for an infected individual is approximately $20,000, and that over $13 billion is expended annually by the public and third-party funding sources. Although these costs appear to be falling

Table 13.5 AIDS Cases by Sex, Age at Diagnosis, and Race/Ethnicity, Reported Through December 2001, United States

Male Age at Diagnosis (years)	White, Not Hispanic		Black, Not Hispanic		Hispanic		Asian/Pacific Islander		American Indian/ Alaska Native		Total[1]	
	No.	(%)	No.	(%)	No.	(%)	No.	(%)	No.	(%)	No.	(%)
Under 5	535	(0)	2,165	(1)	783	(1)	17	(0)	12	(1)	3,515	(1)
5–12	346	(0)	498	(0)	284	(0)	10	(0)	6	(0)	1,146	(0)
13–19	916	(0)	1,020	(0)	570	(0)	26	(0)	23	(1)	2,555	(0)
20–24	7,938	(3)	7,590	(3)	4,520	(4)	181	(3)	84	(4)	20,337	(3)
25–29	38,967	(12)	26,595	(12)	17,138	(14)	675	(13)	351	(17)	83,794	(12)
30–34	71,345	(23)	46,088	(20)	28,377	(23)	1,161	(22)	536	(26)	147,600	(22)
35–39	71,995	(23)	51,302	(22)	27,047	(22)	1,169	(22)	473	(23)	152,124	(23)
40–44	52,653	(17)	41,395	(18)	19,215	(16)	927	(17)	303	(15)	114,585	(17)
45–49	32,116	(10)	24,839	(11)	10,937	(9)	558	(10)	134	(7)	68,635	(10)
50–54	17,498	(6)	12,959	(6)	5,861	(5)	301	(6)	63	(3)	36,718	(5)
55–59	9,337	(3)	6,987	(3)	3,242	(3)	177	(3)	37	(2)	19,801	(3)
60–64	5,139	(2)	3,819	(2)	1,769	(1)	76	(1)	18	(1)	10,829	(2)
65 or older	4,249	(1)	3,242	(1)	1,455	(1)	76	(1)	17	(1)	9,048	(1)
Male Subtotal	**313,034**	**(100)**	**228,499**	**(100)**	**121,198**	**(100)**	**5,354**	**(100)**	**2,057**	**(100)**	**670,687**	**(100)**
Female **Age at Diagnosis (years)**												
Under 5	502	(2)	2,153	(3)	770	(3)	17	(2)	13	(3)	3,460	(2)
5–12	196	(1)	521	(1)	223	(1)	10	(1)	0	(0)	953	(1)
13–19	295	(1)	1,250	(1)	316	(1)	8	(1)	4	(1)	1,873	(1)
20–24	1,774	(6)	4,844	(6)	1,625	(6)	46	(6)	36	(8)	8,328	(6)
25–29	4,831	(16)	11,876	(14)	4,364	(15)	116	(14)	69	(14)	21,266	(15)
30–34	6,818	(22)	18,055	(21)	6,418	(22)	146	(18)	105	(22)	31,564	(22)
35–39	6,244	(20)	18,351	(22)	5,878	(21)	142	(18)	95	(20)	30,733	(21)
40–44	4,199	(14)	13,221	(16)	3,950	(14)	121	(15)	61	(13)	21,560	(15)
45–49	2,307	(7)	6,922	(8)	2,249	(8)	74	(9)	48	(10)	11,607	(8)
50–54	1,309	(4)	3,447	(4)	1,245	(4)	37	(5)	22	(5)	6,062	(4)
55–59	816	(3)	1,865	(2)	750	(3)	29	(4)	18	(4)	3,479	(2)
60–64	519	(2)	1,103	(1)	411	(1)	29	(4)	5	(1)	2,069	(1)
65 or older	1,044	(3)	1,073	(1)	355	(1)	28	(3)	4	(1)	2,507	(2)
Female Subtotal	**30,854**	**(100)**	**84,681**	**(100)**	**28,554**	**(100)**	**803**	**(100)**	**480**	**(100)**	**145,461**	**(100)**
Total[2]	**343,889**		**313,180**		**149,752**		**6,157**		**2,537**		**816,149**	

[1]Includes 545 males and 89 females whose race/ethnicity is unknown.
[2]Includes 1 person whose sex is unknown.

Source: HIV/AIDS Surveillance Report 2001.

Note: *HIV/AIDS Surveillance Report, Centers for Disease,* Centers for Disease Control and Prevention. 13(2): 1–47(inclusive), 2001.

body through the gastrointestinal system because digestive enzymes destroy the virus. An exception to this generalization, however, might exist, as studies conducted in Africa indicate that transmission can occur in conjunction with breast-feeding infants.[39] A second exception involves the transmission of HIV between infected persons and their uninfected sexual partners during episodes of unprotected oral sex when the uninfected persons have evident gingivitis and bleeding gums.[40]

Women are at much greater risk than men of contracting HIV through heterosexual activity because of the higher concentration of lymphocytes in semen (± 10 million lymphocytes/tsp.) than in vaginal secretions (± 1,200 thousand lymphocytes/tsp).[41] This susceptibility is seen in part by the increasing percentage of women with AIDS who were infected through heterosexual contact—from 8% in 1981, to 19% in 1993, and 36% in 2001.[38] Women under age 25 contract the virus

Table 13.6 HIV Infection Cases[1] by Sex, Age at Diagnosis, and Race/Ethnicity, Reported Through December 2001, from Areas with Confidential HIV Infection Reporting[2]

Male Age at Diagnosis (years)	White, Not Hispanic No.	(%)	Black, Not Hispanic No.	(%)	Hispanic No.	(%)	Asian/Pacific Islander No.	(%)	American Indian/ Alaska Native No.	(%)	Total[3] No.	(%)
Under 5	214	(0)	906	(2)	299	(2)	5	(1)	2	(0)	1,429	(1)
5–12	123	(0)	244	(0)	127	(1)	5	(1)	1	(0)	504	(0)
13–19	872	(2)	1,654	(3)	249	(2)	8	(1)	20	(3)	2,825	(2)
20–24	5,725	(11)	6,271	(11)	1,403	(10)	74	(12)	119	(17)	13,720	(11)
25–29	10,326	(20)	8,729	(16)	2,507	(18)	141	(22)	165	(24)	22,147	(18)
30–34	11,490	(23)	10,637	(19)	2,999	(21)	160	(25)	155	(22)	25,752	(21)
35–39	9,582	(19)	10,249	(19)	2,775	(20)	99	(16)	118	(17)	23,121	(19)
40–44	5,907	(12)	7,485	(14)	1,790	(13)	65	(10)	61	(9)	15,526	(13)
45–49	3,258	(6)	4,479	(8)	1,039	(7)	41	(6)	34	(5)	8,968	(7)
50–54	1,693	(3)	2,288	(4)	488	(3)	20	(3)	13	(2)	4,573	(4)
55–59	757	(1)	1,104	(2)	241	(2)	8	(1)	8	(1)	2,150	(2)
60–64	382	(1)	543	(1)	133	(1)	4	(1)	3	(0)	1,081	(1)
65 or older	335	(1)	523	(1)	124	(1)	6	(1)	2	(0)	1,005	(1)
Male Subtotal	**50,664**	**(100)**	**55,112**	**(100)**	**14,174**	**(100)**	**636**	**(100)**	**701**	**(100)**	**122,801**	**(100)**

Female Age at Diagnosis (years)	White, Not Hispanic No.	(%)	Black, Not Hispanic No.	(%)	Hispanic No.	(%)	Asian/Pacific Islander No.	(%)	American Indian/ Alaska Native No.	(%)	Total[3] No.	(%)
Under 5	214	(2)	1,039	(3)	307	(6)	8	(4)	8	(3)	1,583	(3)
5–12	61	(1)	242	(1)	97	(2)	2	(1)	2	(1)	407	(1)
13–19	739	(7)	2,716	(8)	256	(5)	9	(4)	23	(9)	3,762	(7)
20–24	1,776	(16)	5,036	(15)	657	(12)	47	(22)	47	(18)	7,628	(15)
25–29	2,117	(19)	5,885	(17)	919	(17)	51	(24)	46	(18)	9,096	(18)
30–34	2,111	(19)	6,183	(18)	1,032	(19)	37	(17)	44	(17)	9,498	(19)
35–39	1,719	(16)	5,203	(15)	837	(15)	24	(11)	47	(18)	7,896	(15)
40–44	1,041	(9)	3,556	(10)	588	(11)	19	(9)	30	(11)	5,280	(10)
45–49	604	(6)	2,014	(6)	367	(7)	6	(3)	13	(5)	3,038	(6)
50–54	290	(3)	984	(3)	207	(4)	4	(2)	0	(0)	1,497	(3)
55–59	140	(1)	480	(1)	107	(2)	2	(1)	0	(0)	744	(1)
60–64	63	(1)	271	(1)	47	(1)	1	(0)	1	(0)	384	(1)
65 or older	101	(1)	258	(1)	34	(1)	6	(3)	0	(0)	403	(1)
Female Subtotal	**10,976**	**(100)**	**33,867**	**(100)**	**5,455**	**(100)**	**216**	**(100)**	**261**	**(100)**	**51,216**	**(100)**
Total[4]	**61,641**		**88,981**		**19,629**		**852**		**962**		**174,026**	

[1]Includes only persons reported with HIV infection who have not developed AIDS.
[2]See table 3 for areas with confidential HIV infection reporting.
[3]Includes 1,514 males and 441 females whose race/ethnicity is unknown.
[4]Includes 9 persons whose sex is unknown.
Source: HIV/AIDS Surveillance Report 2001

principally through heterosexual contact. Figure 13-4 on page 451 shows the estimated number of new cases of HIV worldwide.

Signs and Symptoms of HIV Infection

Most people infected with HIV initially feel well and have no symptoms (that is, they are asymptomatic). Experts generally consider the *incubation stage* for HIV infection to be 6 months to 10 or more years, with the average approximately 6 years. Despite the long period between infection and the first clinical observation of damage to the immune system, antibodies to HIV may appear within several weeks to three months of contracting the virus. Of course, relatively few people are tested for HIV infection at any time during the incubation period. Thus infected people could remain

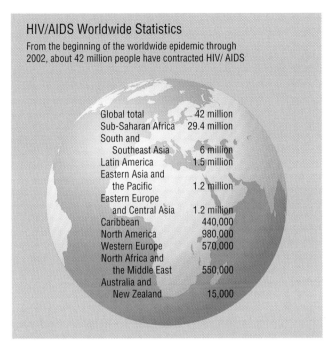

HIV/AIDS Worldwide Statistics

From the beginning of the worldwide epidemic through 2002, about 42 million people have contracted HIV/AIDS

Global total	42 million
Sub-Saharan Africa	29.4 million
South and Southeast Asia	6 million
Latin America	1.5 million
Eastern Asia and the Pacific	1.2 million
Eastern Europe and Central Asia	1.2 million
Caribbean	440,000
North America	980,000
Western Europe	570,000
North Africa and the Middle East	550,000
Australia and New Zealand	15,000

Figure 13-4 For every person counted in these statistics, there is a face and a story. What are you doing to protect yourself from HIV (AIDS)?

Source: UNAIDS and World Health Organization.

asymptomatic (currently described as HIV+ without symptoms) and be carriers of HIV for years before they experience signs of illness sufficient to warrant a physical examination.

Without symptoms of immune-system deterioration or AIDS-testing results, sexually active people need to redefine the meaning of monogamy. Couples must now account for the sexual partners they have both had over the past 10 years. Unfortunately, people do

this so infrequently that some observers are labeling today's young adults "a generation in jeopardy."

Most people infected with HIV, in the absence of early screening and prophylactic drug treatment, eventually develop signs and symptoms of a more advanced stage of the disease. These *prodromal stage* signs and symptoms include tiredness, fever, loss of appetite and weight, diarrhea, night sweats, and swollen glands (usually in the neck, armpits, and groin). At this point, they are said to be HIV+ with symptoms. (See Table 13.7.)

Given sufficient time, perhaps as long as 15 years, most infected people without prophylactic drug treatment will move beyond HIV with symptoms into the *acute stage.* At this point, the label HIV+ with AIDS is applied, either on the basis of clinically defined conditions or more likely on the basis of a helper T cell count below 250 per cubic millimeter of blood. A normal helper T cell range is 800 to 1,000. The efficacy of treatment is based in part on improvements in the T cell count over time.

A small percentage of infected people can suppress the infection and have survived for over two decades without developing AIDS, but experts do not fully understand this ability (possibly attributing it to a suppressor compound formed by specific immune system cells).

Diagnosis of HIV Infection

HIV infection is diagnosed through a clinical examination, laboratory tests for accompanying infections, and an initial screening test. Should the initial screening test produce a negative result, persons at risk for infection should be rescreened in 3 to 6 months. For persons reluctant to present themselves for screening in a clinical setting, home screening tests are also available. Regardless, once initial screening has been undertaken, to eliminate the small chance of a false positive having occurred, more sensitive

Table 13.7 The Spectrum of HIV Infection

	HIV+ without symptoms (asymptomatic)	HIV+ with symptoms	HIV+ with AIDS
External signs	No symptoms Looks well	Fever Night sweats Swollen lymph glands Weight loss Diarrhea Minor infections Fatigue	Kaposi's sarcoma *Pneumocystis carinii* pneumonia and/or other predetermined illnesses Neurological disorders One or more of an additional 30+ diagnosable conditions or a helper T cell count falls below 250 per cubic milliliter
Incubation	Invasion of virus to 10 years	Several months to 10 or more years	Several months to 10–12 or more years
Internal level of infection	Antibodies are produced Immune system remains intact Positive antibody test	Antibodies are produced Immune system weakened Positive antibody test	Immune system deficient Positive antibody test
Infectious?	Yes	Yes	Yes

tests can be administered, including the enzyme-linked immunosorbent assay (ELISA) and Western blot test. Although expensive and not completely reliable, even more recently developed tests are now available. One of these tests identifies the existence of viral mutations known to be drug resistant,[42] while another helps determine whether a particular drug will function in suppressing the contracted viral strain. This information helps physicians structure treatment protocols.

Treatment of HIV and AIDS

There is no cure for HIV infection and the resultant AIDS. It is critically important, however, that treatment begin upon diagnosis. Current treatment uses a combination of drugs drawn principally from two distinct groups: the *reverse-transcriptase inhibitors* and the *protease inhibitors.*

The reverse-transcriptase inhibitors block the action of reverse transcriptase, an enzyme the virus requires to replicate itself within the host's infected T helper cells. Currently a combination of two of the many available reverse-transcriptase inhibitors is used to formulate a portion of the drug "cocktail" employed in treating HIV infection.

Introduction of the protease inhibitors, in combination with the reverse-transcriptase inhibitors, has revolutionized the treatment of HIV infection. These drugs inhibit the ability of the virus to undertake the replication process. In most treatment protocols, one protease inhibitor is combined with two reverse-transcriptase inhibitors to complete the drug cocktail.

More recently, new combination protease inhibitor-based products have reached the market. These products that combine two or more protease inhibitors are intended to reduce the number of pills taken daily by HIV+ persons. Prior to the development of these products, a regimen of taking twenty or more pills needed to be followed each day. This demanding regimen leads to a high degree of *noncompliance,* or failure to follow directions, sometimes resulting in the cessation of medication use.

Protease inhibitors have revolutionized AIDS care, reducing HIV to undetectable levels in thousands of people. The number of deaths from AIDS has decreased dramatically, from 49,985 in 1995 to 14,499 in 2000.[38] However, people should not consider this improvement to mean that the emergency is over. In fact, when the drug cocktail therapy described above is discontinued, viral loads frequently move back toward pretreatment levels. This suggests the existence of well-protected sequestered (hidden) viruses within other tissues of the body.

In addition to reverse-transcriptase inhibitors and protease inhibitors, three recently introduced types of medications, including two entry inhibitors, two co-receptor inhibitors, and two fusion inhibitors, have been developed to further enhance the battle against HIV/AIDS.[43] Now, newer and even more potent "cocktails" are developed by combining both older and new medication. The treatment is deemed highly active antiretroviral therapy, or *HAART.* HAART has proven highly effective in extending the life of many persons with HIV/AIDS by significantly reducing the level of HIV (viral load) in the body. Decision as to what a given patient's HAART will consist of is determined by factors such as the viral load data and the presence of preexisting conditions.

In the final analysis, however, as effective as HAART is in improving the length and quality of life for persons with HIV/AIDS, mortality concerns remain, and life expectancy is compromised. The inability of persons with AIDS to move into and through the *decline stage* and on to the *recovery stage* reflects the relationship between the disease and the immune system itself. Although drug cocktails stabilize the downward movement of the helper T cell count for an extended period, the viral load moves rapidly upward when drugs are discontinued. Additionally, drug therapy is demanding on the overall body, opportunistic infections continue to develop, and preexisting conditions may often worsen, such as incipient cardiovascular disease.[44]

In addition to the antiviral drugs, physicians also have a variety of medications to treat the symptoms associated with various infections and malignancies that make up AIDS. These drugs, of course, cannot reverse HIV status or cure AIDS.

Researchers continue to search for vaccines to prevent HIV infection. One large-scale clinical trial involving a vaccine is now completed. The vaccine, AIDSVAX, that employed two genetically altered AIDS virus types (North American and European strains), did not, however, result in the anticipated level of protection. It did, however, provide a slightly higher level of protection for Blacks and Asian than for whites.[45] The FDA has advised the manufacturer that they will certify the vaccine for sale, if the level of protection can reach 30%.

The reality of HIV/AIDS in Africa and Asia is only now being recognized worldwide. With an estimated 29.4 million infected persons in Sub-Saharan Africa and an additional 6.0 million infected persons in Southeast Asia, the need for a vaccine specific to the viral strains of these areas is growing rapidly.[46] In late 2000, a radically new and relatively inexpensive vaccine using segments of HIV DNA attached to salmonella bacteria underwent its initial human trials in Uganda. Should this innovative approach prove safe and effective, then progress can be made in quelling the potential catastrophe that is taking form on these two continents. Conversely, in the absence of a vaccine (and the inability to effectively treat those currently infected), it is projected that African life expectancy will drop to 29 years and that more than 29 million orphans will need care. Similar consequences would be expected in areas of Asia.

Table 13.8 Selected Sexually Transmitted Diseases by Number of Cases, Sex, Age, Race, and Ethnicity. 2001 (and 1998)

Disease	Male	Females	15–19	20–24	25–29	White	Black	Hispanic	Asian Pacific Islander	American Indian Alaska Native
Chlamydia	141,138	547,247	254,176	252,425	93,776	206,348	319,667	136,617	13,590	13,165
Gonorrhea	117,541	184,217	101,065	116,226	56,084	58,323	271,871	26,190	2,935	2,439
Primary and Secondary Syphilis	4,132	1,968	387	836	876	1,387	3,813	754	55	90
		15–25	**26–39**	**40–64**						
Hepatitis B	5,929	3,887	1,757	4,357	3,117	3,958	855	850	683	80 (1998)
Hepatitis C	2,171	1,272	166	1,101	1,619	1,921	468	392	33	46 (1998)

Note: Similar data on AIDS appears in Table 13.5 page 449.

Sources: 2001 data: STD Surveillance 2001. National Center for HIV, STD, and TB Prevention Centers for Disease Control and Prevention, 2001. **http://www.cdc/gov.std/stats/TOC2001.htm** 1998 data: Table 13-8. *Understanding Your Health*, 7th ed. McGraw-Hill, 2002.

Developing a safe, effective, and affordable vaccine (as has been done for other infectious diseases) remains difficult because of the unique ability of HIV to alter its outer coat and quickly incorporate its genetic material into the host's helper T cells' genetic material, thus preventing the immune system from developing immune recognition.

Prevention of HIV Infection

Can HIV infection be prevented? The answer is a definite yes. HIV infection rates on college campuses are considered low (approximately 0.2%), but students can be at risk. Every person can take several steps to reduce the risk of contracting and transmitting HIV. All of these steps require understanding one's behavior and the methods by which HIV can be transmitted. Some appropriate steps for college-aged people are abstinence, safer sex, sobriety, and communication with potential sexual partners. To ensure the greatest protection from HIV, one should abstain from sexual activity. Other than this, the Changing for the Better box on page 456 lists recommendations for safer sex, sobriety, and the exchange of honest, accurate information about sexual histories.

In spite of the existence of these recommendations, it is increasingly apparent that it is difficult (or nearly impossible) for people to remember and then apply these guidelines. Accordingly, CDC is beginning a gradual "reversal-of-course" away from an emphasis on prevention, toward a more medical model based on testing, contact identification, and individual counsel. Initial testing, the beginning point of this model, will initially occur in homeless shelters, drug treatment centers, jails, and in conjunction with prenatal care. Is it possible that HIV screening will, at some point, become a component of the health record required as a part of college admission?

 TALKING POINTS In a job interview with a representative from a large pharmaceutical company, you are asked about your feelings regarding the affordability of HIV/AIDS medications in third world countries. What would your response be?

Sexually Transmitted Diseases

Sexually transmitted diseases (STDs) were once called venereal diseases (for Venus, the Roman goddess of love). Today the term *venereal disease* has been superseded by the broader terms *sexually transmitted disease* or *sexually transmitted infections*. Table 13.8 shows *the CDC* statistics on three of the reportable STDs by age, gender, and ethnicity. Experts currently emphasize the successful prevention and treatment of STDs rather than the ethics of sexuality. Thus one should consider the following points: (1) By age 25 years approximately one-third of all adults will have contracted a sexually transmitted disease—most often chlamydia, herpes simplex, or human papillomavirus infection; (2) a person can have more than one STD at a

> **Key Terms**
>
> **sexually transmitted diseases (STDs)** infectious diseases that are spread primarily through intimate sexual contact.

Table 13.9 Summary of Common Sexually Transmitted Diseases*

STD	Pathogen Name/Type	Symptoms
Chlamydia	*Chlamydia trachomatis* bacterium	Most women report no overt signs or symptoms. In men, gonorrhea-like signs and symptoms, including painful urination and a whitish pus discharge from the penis
Human papillomavirus (HPV, genital warts)	Human papillomavirus	Genital warts (condylomata acuminata), pinkish-white lesions in raised clusters on the penis, scrotum, labia, cervix, or around the anus.
Gonorrhea	*Neisseria gonorrhoea* bacterium	In men, a milky-white discharge from the penis, painful urination; women tend to be asymptomatic but can report frequent, painful urination, with a slimy yellow-green discharge from the vagina or urethra.
Herpes	Herpes simplex 1 virus (HSV-1) produces labial herpes; herpes simplex 2 virus (HSV-2) produces genital herpes	HSV-1 produces common fever blisters or cold sores around the lips and oral cavity; HSV-2 produces similar blisterlike lesions in the genital area, swollen lymph glands, muscular aches and pains, and fever.
Syphilis	*Treponema pallidum* bacterium	Primary stage marked by appearance of small, painless red pustule on skin or mucous membrane anywhere on body 10 to 90 days after exposure; forms a painless but highly infectious ulcer called a *chancre;* heals spontaneously in 4 to 8 weeks. If not treated, progresses to secondary, latent, and late stages.
Pubic lice	Pubic louse (insect)	Intense itching in the genital region.

Source: Centers for Disease Control and Prevention. Sexually transmitted disease treatment guidelines 2002. *MMWR* 51: (No. RR-6) [inclusive page numbers], 2002.

time; (3) the symptoms of STDs can vary over time and from person to person; (4) the body develops little immunity for STDs; and (5) STDs can predispose people to additional health problems, including infertility, birth defects in their children, cancer, and long-term disability. In addition, the risk of HIV infection is higher when sexual partners are also infected with STDs. Several of the most common STDs are summarized in Table 13.9 above.

This section focuses on the STDs most frequently diagnosed among college students (chlamydia, gonorrhea, human papillomavirus infection, herpes simplex, syphilis, and pubic lice). Complete the Personal Assessment on page 469

Table 13.9 *Continued*

Modes of Transmission	Treatment	Consequences if Not Treated
Sexual intercourse; can be transmitted to newborn during vaginal birth	Azithromycin: 1 g orally in a single dose Doxycycline: 100 mg orally twice a day for 7 days Erythromycin and ofloxacin are alternative medications.	In men, damage to prostate gland, seminal vesicles, and Cowper's glands; sterility; joint problems; heart complications. In women, PID; infection of uterine wall (endometrium), fallopian tubes, and surrounding structures; sterility and peritonitis.
Sexual activity	*Patient-Applied:* Podofilox solution or gel: applied by swab or finger twice a day for 3 days Imiquimod 5% cream: applied by finger 3 times a week for 16 weeks *Provider-Administered:* Cryotherapy: with liquid nitrogen or cryoprobe Podophyllin resin: small amount applied directly to each wart within a relatively small area TCA or BCA: applied in liquid form, repeated weekly if necessary Surgical removal: scissors, shave excision, curettage, or electrosurgery	In women, precancerous changes in the cervix; can become large enough to block the birth canal. In both sexes can become large enough to block the anus.
Sexual activity; oral sex can produce a gonorrheal infection of the throat; can be transmitted to the rectal areas of both sexes; can be transmitted to a newborn during birth	Cefixine: 400 mg orally (single dose) or Ceftriaxone: 125 mg IM (single dose) or Ciprofloxacin: 500 mg orally (single dose) or Ofloxacin: 400 mg orally (single dose) + azithromycin or doxycycline	Nausea, vomiting, fever, tachycardia (rapid heart beat), infection of upper or lower genital tract; can spread to tissues surrounding liver, peritoneum, heart, joints, or other structures.
Direct contact with a person who has an active infection; shared drinking glasses or utensils; intimate sexual contact; condoms may provide insufficient protection	*Initial Infection* (episodic and suppressive therapy protocols required later): Acyclovir: 400 mg orally 3/day (7–10 days) Acyclovir: 200 mg orally 5/day (7–10 days) Famciclovir: 250 mg orally 3/day (7–10 days) Valacyclovir: 1 g orally 2/day (7–10 days)	Recurrent infections are shorter and less severe than the initial episode.
Sexual intercourse	*Primary and Secondary:* Benzathine penicillin G: 2.4 million units IM (single dose) *Latent (early):* Benzathine penicillin G: 2.4 million units IM (single dose) *Latent (late):* Benzathine penicillin G: 7.2 million units (3 doses of 2.4 million once/week)	Secondary stage: general malaise, loss of appetite, fever, headache, hair loss, bone and joint pain, rash, sores in mouth and throat. Late (tertiary) stage: soft, rubbery tumors anywhere on the body that ulcerate and heal with scarring; damage to CNS and heart; disability; premature death.
Sexual contact; contact with contaminated bedsheets and clothes	Permethrin: 1% cream (applied for 10 minutes/washed off) Lindane: 1% shampoo (applied for 4 minutes/washed off) or Pyrethrins with piperonyl butoxide: (applied for 10 minutes/washed off) Bedding/clothing: wash (machine)/dry (hot cycle); no body contact for 72 hours	Lice rarely carry disease, but the itching they cause can be embarrassing and uncomfortable.

to determine your risk of contracting an STD. See the Changing for the Better box on page 456 for safer sex practices.

Chlamydia (Nonspecific Urethritis)

Chlamydia is thought to be the most prevalent STD in the United States today. Chlamydia infections occur an

Key Terms

chlamydia the most prevalent sexually transmitted disease; caused by a nongonococcal bacterium.

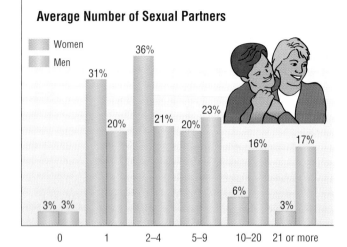

Average Number of Sexual Partners

Women
Men

Figure 13-5 Average number of sexual partners men and women have had since age 18. The fewer the number of partners you've had, the lower your risk of contracting HIV or an STD.

Source: RT Michael, JH Gagnon, EO Laumann, G Kolata: *Sex in America: a definitive study.*

estimated five times more frequently than gonorrhea and up to ten times more frequently than syphilis. Because of its high prevalence in sexually active adolescents, they should be screened for chlamydia twice a year, even in the absence of symptoms. Because chlamydia frequently accompanies gonorrheal infections, a dual therapy is often appropriate when gonorrhea is found. Sexually active people in the 20- to 24-year age range should also be considered for routine screening, particularly if they have a history of multiple sex partners and have not practiced a form of barrier contraception (see Figure 13-5 above).[47]

Chlamydia trachomatis is the bacterial agent that causes the chlamydia infection. Chlamydia is the most common cause of nonspecific urethritis (NSU). NSU describes infections of the **urethra** and surrounding tissues that are not caused by the bacterium responsible for gonorrhea. About 80% of men with chlamydia display gonorrhea-like signs and symptoms, including painful urination and a whitish pus discharge from the penis. As in gonorrheal infections and many other STDs, most women report no overt signs or symptoms. A few women might exhibit a mild urethral discharge, painful urination, and swelling of vulval tissues. The recommended treatment for chlamydia is either a single dose of azithromycin (1 g) or doxycycline (100 mg) given orally twice a day for 7 days. The infected person should carefully comply with instructions to abstain from sexual intercourse.[47]

Key Terms

urethra (yoo **ree** thra) the passageway through which urine leaves the urinary bladder.

Both sexual partners should receive treatment to avoid the ping-pong effect—the back-and-forth reinfection that occurs among couples when only one partner receives treatment. Furthermore, as with other STDs, having chlamydia once does not effectively confer immunity.

Unresolved chlamydia can lead to the same negative health consequences that result from untreated gonorrheal infections. In men the pathogens can invade and damage the deeper reproductive structures (the prostate gland, seminal vesicles, and Cowper's glands). Sterility can result. The pathogens can spread further and produce joint problems (arthritis) and heart complications (damaged heart valves, blood vessels, and heart muscle tissue).

In women the pathogens enter the body through the urethra or the cervical area. If the invasion is not properly treated, it can reach the deeper pelvic structures, producing a syndrome called **pelvic inflammatory disease (PID).** The infection may attack the inner uterine wall (endometrium), the fallopian tubes, and any surrounding structures to produce this painful syndrome. A variety of further complications can result, including sterility, ectopic pregnancies, and **peritonitis.** Infected women can transmit a chlamydia infection to the eyes and lungs of newborns during a vaginal birth. Detecting chlamydia and other NSUs early is of paramount concern for both men and women.

Human Papillomavirus

The appearance of another STD, **human papillomavirus (HPV),** is unwanted news. Because HPV infections are generally asymptomatic, the exact extent of the disease is unknown. A study of a group of sexually active college women found HPV infection in approximately 20% of the women. HPV-related changes to the cells of the cervix are found in nearly 5% of the Pap smears taken from women under age 30. Researchers currently believe that risk factors for HPV infection in women include: (1) sexual activity before age 20, (2) intercourse with three or more partners before age 35, and (3) intercourse with a partner who has three or more partners. The extent of HPV infection in men is even less clearly known, but it is probably widespread.

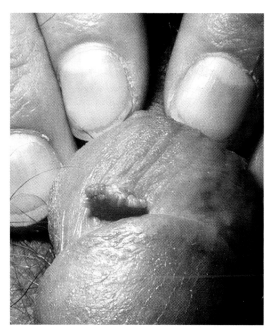

Figure 13-6 A human papillomavirus infection (genital warts).

HPV infection is alarming because some of the more than fifty forms of the virus are strongly associated with precancerous changes to cells lining the cervix, thus the importance of new viral pap smears (see Chapter 11). Additionally, visible genital warts (cauliflower-like, raised, pinkish-white lesions) are associated with viral forms 6 or 11, while viral forms 16, 18, 31, 33, and 35 foster changes in other areas[47] (Figure 13-6). Found most commonly on the penis, scrotum, labia, cervix, and around the anus, these lesions represent the most common symptomatic viral STD in this country. Although most genital wart colonies are small, they may become very large and block the anus or birth canal during pregnancy.

Treatment for HPV, including genital warts, may include patient-applied gels or creams or physician-administered cryotherapy, topical medication, or surgery

Key Terms

pelvic inflammatory disease (PID) an acute or chronic infection of the peritoneum or lining of the abdominopelvic cavity and fallopian tubes; associated with a variety of symptoms or none at all and a potential cause of sterility.

peritonitis (pare it ton **eye** tis) inflammation of the peritoneum, or lining of the abdominopelvic cavity.

human papillomavirus (HPV) sexually transmitted viruses, some of which are capable of causing precancerous changes in the cervix; causative agent for genital warts.

(see Table 13.9 on pages 454–455). Regardless of treatment, however, the viral colonies will probably return. One should use condoms to attempt to prevent transmission of HPV.

Gonorrhea

Another extremely common (600,000 cases/year estimated and 360,000 cases/year reported) STD, gonorrhea, is caused by a bacterium *(N. gonorrhoea)*. The incidence of gonorrhea rose 18% between 1997 and 2001,[48] perhaps, in part, because of decreasing fear of HIV/AIDS brought about by the effectiveness of the protease inhibitors being widely reported at that time. In men this bacterial agent can produce a milky-white discharge from the penis, accompanied by painful urination. About 80% of men who contract gonorrhea report varying degrees of these symptoms. This figure is approximately reversed for women: Only about 20% of women are symptomatic and thus report varying degrees of frequent, painful urination, with a slimy yellow-green discharge from the vagina or urethra. Oral sex with an infected partner can produce a gonorrheal infection of the throat (pharyngeal gonorrhea). Gonorrhea can also be transmitted to the rectal areas of both men and women.

An interesting finding relative to gonorrhea in adolescents appeared in the 28 April 2000 issue of the *Morbidity and Mortality Weekly Report*.[49] In that issue, it was reported that the incidence of gonorrhea within the adolescent population correlated closely with the consumption of beer, suggesting that alcohol consumption fosters a higher level of high-risk sexual behavior, including earlier onset of sexual activity, an increased number of partners, and less selectivity in choosing those partners. With heavy consumption of beer on many college campuses, this finding does not bode well for the highly asymptomatic female population.

Physicians diagnose gonorrhea by culturing the bacteria. Because of the paired occurrence of chlamydia and gonorrhea, dual therapy with doxycycline or azithromycin in combination with ofloxacin (see Table 13.9) is used in susceptible populations, particularly adolescent women. Outside of these groups, recommended treatment for uncomplicated cases involves the use of one of several antimicrobial drugs. Although prevalent in other areas of the world, drug-resistant strains are not extensive in the United States.[47] This said, however, it should be noted that a clear increase in drug-resistant strains has been reported along the West Coast, in various Pacific areas, such as Hawaii, other Pacific Islands, and Asia. Infected persons who might have contracted the disease while in these areas should report this information to their physicians.

Testing for gonorrhea is included as a part of prenatal care so that infections in mothers can be treated before they give birth. If the birth canal is infected, newborns can easily contract the infection in the mucous membranes of the eye.

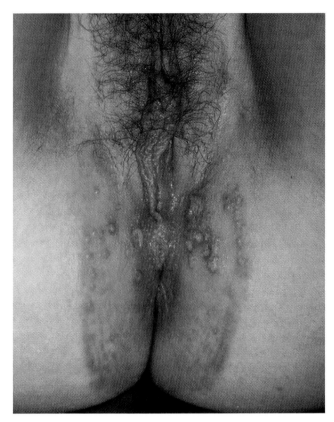

Figure 13-7 A severe herpes infection.

Herpes Simplex

Public health officials think that the sexually transmitted genital herpes virus infection rivals chlamydia as the most prevalent STD. To date about 45 million Americans have been diagnosed, although the asymptomatic (thus undiagnosed) population could increase this figure substantially. Herpes is really a family of more than fifty viruses, some of which produce recognized diseases in humans (chicken pox, **shingles,** mononucleosis, and others). One subgroup, called herpes simplex 1 virus (HSV-1), produces an infection called labial herpes (oral or lip herpes). Labial herpes produces common fever blisters or cold sores around the lips and oral cavity. Herpes simplex 2 virus (HSV-2) is a different strain that produces similar clumps of blisterlike lesions in the genital region (Figure 13-7). Laypeople call this second type of herpes the STD type, but both types produce identical clinical pictures. About 5 to 30% of cases are caused by HSV-1.[48] Oral-genital sexual practices most likely account for this crossover infection.

Herpes appears as a single sore or as a small cluster of blisterlike sores. These sores burn, itch, and (for some) become very painful. The infected person might also report swollen lymph glands, muscular aches and pains, and fever. Some patients feel weak and sleepy when they have blisters. The lesions may last from a few days to a few weeks. Viral shedding lasts a week on average; then the blisters begin scabbing, and new skin is formed. Even when the patient has become asymptomatic, viral transmission is still possible.

Herpes is an interesting virus for several reasons. It can lie dormant for long periods. For reasons not well understood but perhaps related to stress, diet, or overall health, the viral particles can be stimulated to travel along the nerve pathways to the skin and then create an active infection. Thus herpes can be considered a recurrent infection. Fortunately for most people, recurrent infections are less severe than the initial episode and do not last as long. Recommended treatment for an initial outbreak of herpes calls for the use of one of three medications: acyclovir, famciclovir, or valacyclovir. These medications are taken orally, multiple times each day, for seven to ten days (see Table 13.9). Because herpes may occur at intervals following initial treatment, two choices exist. One is to treat each recurrence as it arises (episodic recurrent treatment), and the second is to attempt to suppress recurrence through continuous use of medication (daily suppressive therapy) (see Table 13.9). The treatment choices described above appear to be equally effective for HSV-1 and HSV-2.[47] Additionally, physicians may recommend other medications for relief of various symptoms. Genital herpes is almost always diagnosed through a clinical examination.

At this time a much anticipated Phase III trial is under way in which a large number of women, known to be free of both HSV-1 and HSV-2, are testing a new vaccine manufactured by GlaxoSmith Kline Biologicals. Earlier, but in much smaller trials, it was found that the vaccine was effective in providing protection for about 70% of the female subjects, but far less so for males.[50] The current trial is being conducted in order to confirm these initial findings.

Currently, the best method of preventing herpes infection is to avoid all direct contact with a person who has an active infection. Do not kiss someone with a fever blister—or let them kiss you (or your children) if they have an active lesion. Do not share drinking glasses or eating utensils. Check your partner's genitals. Do not have intimate sexual contact with someone who displays the blisterlike clusters or rash. Condoms are only marginally helpful and cannot protect against lesions on the female vulva or the lower abdominal area of men. Be careful not to infect yourself by touching a blister and then touching any other part of your body. The Changing

for the Better box below gives helpful advice about talking with your partner if you have genital herpes.

Newborn babies are especially susceptible to the virus if they come into contact with an active lesion during birth. Newborns have not developed the defense capabilities to resist the invasion. They can quickly develop a systemic (general) infection (neonatal herpes) that is often fatal or local infections that produce permanent brain damage or blindness. Fortunately, most of these problems can be prevented through proper prenatal care. A cesarean delivery can be performed if viral particles might be present at birth, although this is done less often today than in the past.

Syphilis

Like gonorrhea, syphilis is caused by a bacterium (*Treponema pallidum*) and is transmitted almost exclusively by sexual intercourse. The incidence of syphilis, a

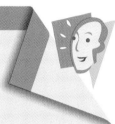

Changing for the Better

Talking with Your Partner about Herpes

My girlfriend told me she has herpes and said she's "taking care of everything." What can I do to get things out in the open?

Although herpes rarely has serious consequences, the lesions are infectious and tend to reappear. It is important to talk openly with your partner about this sexually transmitted disease. Here are some tips to make things easier:

- *Educate yourself.*
  Be aware that herpes is rarely dangerous. Learn when the disease is most contagious (during the eruption and blister stage), and realize that herpes can be spread even during the non-eruption, non-blister periods—traditionally defined as safe periods.
- *Choose the right time to talk.*
  Discuss herpes with your partner only after you have gotten to know each other.
- *Listen to your partner.*
  Be prepared to answer any questions that he or she may have.
- *Together, put things in perspective.*
  Keep a positive outlook.
  Remember that you are not alone.
  Be aware that using a condom and abstaining from coitus during the most infectious period can prevent transmission of the disease.
  Although there is no known cure, research continues on an antiviral drug.
  Join a local support group together.

InfoLinks

www.herpeszone.com/MainMenu.htm

Syphilis

Syphilis is a serious disease that, left untreated, can cause death. The chance of contracting syphilis during a single sexual encounter with an infected partner is now about 30%. Syphilis takes a well-established course after it is contracted.

Infection

The syphilis bacterium, *Treponema pallidum,* is a spirochete. It is transmitted from an infected person to a new host through intimate contact. Moist, warm tissue, such as that lining the reproductive, urinary, and digestive tracts, offers an ideal environment for the agent.

Incubation

Syphilis incubates without symptoms for 10 to 90 days, followed by the characteristic primary stage of the disease.

Primary Stage

The primary stage of syphilis lasts 1 to 5 weeks. A small, raised, painless sore called a *chancre* forms at this time. This highly infectious lesion is not easily identified in 90% of women and 50% of men; thus these people generally do not seek treatment. The chancre heals in 4 to 8 weeks.

Secondary Stage

The extremely contagious secondary stage of the disease occurs 6 to 12 weeks after initial infection. The infectious agents are now systemic, so symptoms may include a generalized body rash, a sore throat, or a patchy loss of hair. A blood test (VDRL) will be positive, and treatment can be effectively administered. If untreated, the second stage subsides within 2 to 6 weeks. A pregnant woman can easily transmit syphilis to her fetus during this stage. Congenital syphilis often results in stillbirth or an infant born with a variety of life-threatening complications. Early treatment of infected pregnant women can prevent congenital syphilis.

Latent Stage

After the secondary stage subsides, an extended period of noninfectiousness occurs. The infectious agents remain dormant within the body cells, and the infected person displays few clinical signs during this state.

Late Stage

Syphilis can recur for a third time 15 to 25 years after initial contact. In late-stage syphilis, tissue damage is profound and irreversible. The person suffers damage to the cardiovascular system, central nervous system, eyes, and skin, and death from the effects of the disease is likely.

Treatment

Depending on the stage, syphilis is treated with varying doses of Benzathine penicillin G. See Table 13.9 for protocol specifics.

CDC-reportable disease, is far lower than that of gonorrhea. In 1950 a record 217,558 cases of syphilis were reported in this country. The number of cases then fell steadily to fewer than 80,000 cases in 1980. From 1980 through 1990 the incidence climbed, reaching nearly 140,000 cases in 1990. Another decline then began, and in 1993 the number of cases dropped to 101,259. In 2000 the CDC reported that syphilis had fallen to the lowest level (5,972) in 42 years.

In spite of this downward trend, an increasing number of today's cases have been associated with HIV infections, largely among gay men in several larger cities. Syphilis cases among women continue to drop. See the Star box above for more information on this disease. Observers have noted an alarming increase in infant syphilis in children born to mothers who use drugs and support their habit through sexual activity.

Pubic Lice

Three types of lice infect humans: The head louse, the body louse, and the pubic louse all feed on the blood of the host. Except for the relatively uncommon body louse, these tiny insects do not carry diseases. They are, however, very annoying.

Pubic lice, also called crabs, attach themselves to the base of the pubic hairs, where they live and lay their eggs (nits). These eggs move into a larval stage after one week; after two more weeks, they develop into mature adult crab lice.

People usually notice they have a pubic lice infestation when they suffer intense itching in the genital region. Prescription and OTC creams, lotions, and shampoos are usually effective in killing both the lice and their eggs, although some reports suggest that lice are becoming resistant to OTC treatments.

Lice are not transmitted exclusively through sexual contact, but also by contact with bedsheets and clothes that may be contaminated. If you develop a pubic lice infestation, you must thoroughly treat yourself, your clothes, your sheets, and your furniture.

Vaginal Infections

Two common pathogens produce uncomfortable vaginal infections in women. The first is the yeast or fungus pathogen *Candida (Monilia) albicans,* which produces the yeast infection often called *thrush*. These organisms, commonly found in the vagina, seem to multiply rapidly when some unusual stressor (pregnancy, use of birth control pills or antibiotics, diabetes) affects a woman's body. This infection, now called vulvovaginal candidiasis (VVC),[47] is signaled by a white or cream-colored vaginal discharge that resembles cottage cheese. Vaginal itching and vulvar swelling are also commonly reported. Current treatment is based on the use of one of several prescription and OTC azole drugs.

Recently introduced nonprescription azole-based products offer effective home treatment. One should first consult with a physician before using these new products for the first time. (Men rarely report this monilial infection, although some may report mildly painful urination or a barely noticeable discharge at the urethral opening or beneath the foreskin of the penis.)

The protozoan *Trichomonas vaginalis* also produces a vaginal infection. This parasite can be transmitted through sexual intercourse or by contact with contaminated (often damp) objects, such as towels, clothing, or toilet seats, that may contain some vaginal discharge. In women, this infection, called *trichomoniasis*, or "trich," produces a foamy, yellow-green, foul-smelling discharge that may be accompanied by itching, swelling, and painful urination. Although topically applied treatments with limited effectiveness for trichomoniasis are available, only one highly effective oral medication is currently on the market.[47] Men infrequently contract trichomoniasis but may harbor the organisms without realizing it. They also should be treated to minimize reinfection of partners.[47]

The vagina is warm, dark, and moist, an ideal breeding environment for a variety of organisms. Unfortunately, some highly promoted commercial products seem to increase the incidence of vaginal infections. Among these are tight panty hose (without cotton panels), which tend to increase the vaginal temperature, and commercial vaginal douches, which can alter the acidic level of the vagina. Both of these products might promote infections. Women are advised to wipe from front to back after every bowel movement to reduce the opportunity for direct transmission of pathogenic agents from the rectum to the vagina. Avoiding public bathrooms when possible is also a good practice. Of course, if you notice any unusual discharge from the vagina, you should report this to your physician.

Cystitis and Urethritis

Cystitis, an infection of the urinary bladder, and urethritis, an infection of the urethra, occasionally can be caused by a sexually transmitted organism. Such infections can also be caused by the organisms that cause vaginitis and organisms found in the intestinal tract. A culture is required to identify the specific pathogen associated with a particular case of cystitis or urethritis. The symptoms are pain when urinating, the need to urinate frequently, a dull aching pain above the pubic bone, and the passing of blood-streaked urine.

Physicians can easily treat cystitis and urethritis with antibiotics when the specific organism has been identified. A newly introduced drug, Monurol, which requires only a single dose, has proved effective. Few complications result from infections that are treated promptly. If cystitis or urethritis is left untreated, the infectious agent could move upward in the urinary system and infect the ureters and kidneys. These upper-urinary-tract infections are more serious and require more extensive evaluation and aggressive treatment. Therefore one should obtain medical care immediately upon noticing symptoms.

A recent study involving urinary tract infections in mice, whose urinary tract infections are virtually identical to those in humans, demonstrated that the bacteria involved often avoid complete antibiotic elimination. This occurs when the bacteria clump into pods that are then covered by a "bio-film" produced by the organisms.[51] The film retards further antibody effectiveness, allowing the infection to be re-established when antibiotics have been cleared from the body.

Preventing cystitis and urethritis depends to some degree on the source of the infectious agent. One can generally reduce the incidence of infection by urinating completely (to fully empty the urinary bladder) and by drinking ample fluids to flush the urinary tract. Drinking cranberry juice has been found to reduce urinary tract infections.

TALKING POINTS Honesty regarding past sexual experiences is a critical issue in a decision to introduce sexual intimacy into a new relationship. What questions would you feel comfortable being asked by another person, and what questions would you be prepared to ask that person?

Nosocomial Infections

Where would you have to have been to have contracted a *nosocomial infection?* The answer is a hospital, a clinic, or a nursing home, or the office of a health care provider. Nosocomial infections are infections spread in conjunction with the delivery of health care services—most often from providers to patients or from patients to other patients. Persons who are hospitalized are particularly vulnerable to the development of a potentially fatal nosocomial infection.

It is estimated that each year approximately 2.2 million persons develop an infection directly linked to the health care system. Contact with infectious agents occurs in a variety of ways, including the failure of personnel to wash or glove their hands properly prior to conducting examinations, the use of contaminated medical equipment such as endoscopes and catheters, failure to maintain sterile operating areas during surgery, receiving intravenous medications contaminated during their manufacture, contact with visitors who are infectious, and, of course, sharing a semiprivate room with an infectious roommate.

Two factors make today's nosocomial infections particularly serious. The first, of course, is that these infections strike people who by virtue of being institutionalized are less than healthy. Second is the fact that the organisms most frequently associated with these infections are among the most pathogenic with which we have contact, staphylococcus aureus and enterococcus faecium, both of which are (or nearly are) resistant to vancomycin, our most biologically potent antibiotic.

Today, disease control officials debate the generally stated mortality (100,000 deaths/year) attributed to nosocomial infections. Some experts suggest that a relatively large percentage of the hospital and nursing home infections are in patients who are already terminal or so frail that infection was only an exacerbating factor in their demise. Accordingly, they believe that these deaths should not be included in the mortality statistics associated with nosocomial infections.

Because of the potential seriousness of nosocomial infections, persons entering the health care arena should discuss infection control with their physician, including the proper procedures for self-care, the possible need for greater isolation while an in-patient, and the desirability of restricting visitation.

Taking Charge of Your Health

- Since microorganisms develop resistance to antibiotics, continue taking all such medications until gone, even when the symptoms of the infection have subsided.
- Check your current immunization status to make sure you are protected against preventable infectious diseases.
- If you are parent, take your children to receive their recommended immunizations as necessary (see page 436).

- Because of the possibility of contracting HIV/AIDS and sexually transmitted diseases, incorporate disease prevention into all your sexual activities.
- Use the Personal Assessment on page 469 to determine your risk of contracting a sexually transmitted disease.
- If you have ever engaged in high-risk sexual behavior, get tested for HIV.

Summary

- We have made progress in reducing the incidence of some forms of infectious disease, but other infectious conditions are becoming more common.
- A variety of pathogenic agents are responsible for infectious conditions.
- A chain of infection with six potential links characterizes every infectious condition.
- Most infectious conditions progress through five distinct stages.
- One can acquire immunity for some diseases through both natural and artificial means. Children should be immunized according to a schedule.

- The immune system's response to infection relies on cellular and humoral elements.
- The common cold and influenza produce many similar symptoms but differ in their infectious agents, incubation period, prevention, and treatment.
- Tuberculosis and pneumonia are potentially fatal infections of the respiratory system.
- Mononucleosis and chronic fatigue syndrome are infections that produce chronic tiredness.
- Bacterial meningitis, a potentially fatal infection of the linings that cover the brain, is of increasing concern on college campuses.

- Lyme disease is a bacterial infection contracted through outdoor activities.
- Hantavirus pulmonary syndrome is caused by a virus carried by deer mice; human-to-human transmission has also been reported.
- Newly arrived in this country, the West Nile virus is a vector-borne infection that is now widely distributed in the United States.
- Toxic shock syndrome is a bacterial infection generally arising from the improper use of tampons.
- Hepatitis B (serum hepatitis) is a bloodborne infectious condition that produces serious liver damage. Other varieties are hepatitis A, C, D, and E.
- SARS, a potentially fatal respiratory infection, has reached North America from Asia.
- Monkeypox reflects the ability of infectious agents to move from animals to humans.
- HIV/AIDS is a widespread, incurable viral disease transmitted through sexual activity, through intravenous drug use, in infected blood products, or across the placenta during pregnancy.

- The definitive diagnosis of AIDS can be based on the presence of specific conditions or a reduced number of helper T cells.
- HIV and AIDS are currently best treated with a drug cocktail, using protease inhibitors and reverse-transcriptase inhibitors, in addition to three new categories of antiviral medications; an effective vaccine for prevention has not been developed. Concerns are rising regarding the unchecked spread of HIV/AIDS in areas of Africa and Asia.
- There are a variety of sexually transmitted conditions, many of which do not produce symptoms in most infected women and many infected men.
- Safer sex practices can reduce the risk of contracting STDs.
- Nosocomial infections are infections that develop in conjunction with the delivery of health care services, most often in hospitals and nursing homes.

Review Questions

1. What are the agents responsible for the most familiar infectious conditions?
2. Describe the six links in the chain of infection.
3. What are the five stages that characterize the progression of infectious conditions?
4. What are the two principal cellular/chemical components of the immune system, and how do they cooperate to protect the body from infectious agents, foreign protein, and abnormal cells?
5. How are the common cold and influenza similar? How do they differ in their causative agents, incubation period, prevention, and treatment?
6. What symptoms make mononucleosis and chronic fatigue syndrome similar? What aspects of each are different?
7. Why is bacterial meningitis of greater concern on the college campus than elsewhere?
8. Why is outdoor activity a risk factor for contracting Lyme disease?
9. During what type of activities would persons most likely expose themselves to a hantavirus infection? What is the reservoir for the hantavirus?
10. What role do birds play in the transmission of the West Nile virus? What insect is the vector?
11. What group of persons seems most susceptible to the development of toxic shock syndrome?

In what way is the infection most directly linked to the menstrual cycle?
12. How is hepatitis B transmitted, and which occupational group is at greatest risk of contracting this infection? How do forms A, C, D, and E compare with hepatitis B?
13. What is SARS? Where was its site of origin, and how did it most likely reach North America?
14. What "pocket pets" carried the monkeypox virus to humans, and how were these animals infected?
15. How is HIV transmitted? How are HIV/AIDS currently treated, and how effective is the treatment? In what areas of the world does the HIV/AIDS epidemic seem virtually unchecked? In terms of STD prevention, how can sexual practices be made safer?
16. What specific infectious diseases could be classified as STDs?
17. Why are women more often asymptomatic for STDs than men?
18. To what extent and in what manner can STD transmission be prevented?
19. What is a nosocomial infection, and in what settings are nosocomial infections most likely to develop?

References

1. Hamann B. *Disease identification, prevention, and control,* 2nd ed. McGraw-Hill, 2001.

2. Salidin KS. *Anatomy and physiology: unity of form and function,* 2nd ed. McGraw-Hill, 2001.

3. Parkham P. *The immune system.* Garland Publishing, 2000.

4. Vander A, Sherman J, and Luciano D. *Human physiology: the mechanisms of body function.* McGraw-Hill, 2004.

5. Korbling M, Estrov Z, Champlin R. Adult stem cells and tissue repair. *Bone Marrow Transplant* 32 Suppl 1: S23–24, 2003.

6. Burt RK, Traynor AE. SLE—hematopoietic stem cell transplantation for systemic lupus erythematosus. *Arthritis Res Ther* 5(5):207–209, 2003.

7. Ooi J, et al. Unrelated cord blood transplantation for adult patients with de novo acute myeloid leukemia. *Blood* August 21, 2003 (Epub).

8. Latkovic MS. The morality of human embryonic stem cell research and President Bush's decision: how should Catholics think about such things? *Linacre Q* 69(4):289–315, 2002.

9. Gershon D. Complex political, ethical and legal issues surround research on human embryonic stem cells. *Nature* 422(6934):928–929, 2003.

10. Straetemans M, et al. Review of randomized controlled trials on pneumococcal vaccination for prevention of otitis media. *Pediatr Infect Dis J* 22(6): 515–524, 2003.

11. DeStefano F, et al. Childhood vaccinations, vaccination timing, and risk of type 1 diabetes mellitus. *Pediatrics* 108(6):E112, 2001.

12. Destefano F, et al. Childhood vaccinations and risk of asthma. *Pediatr Infect Dis J* 21(6):498–504, 2002.

13. DeStefano F, Thompson WW. MMR vaccination and autism: is there a link? *Expert Opin Drug Saf* 1(2):115–120, 2002.

14. Immunization safety review: vaccinations and sudden unexpected death in infancy. *News.* The National Academies, 2003 **http://www.nap.edu**

15. McQuillan GM, et al. Serologic immunity to diphtheria and tetanus in the United States. *Ann Intern Med* 136(9):660–666, 2002.

16. Fendrick AM, et al. The economic burden of non-influenza-related viral respiratory tract infection in the United States. *Arch Intern Med* 163(4): 487–494, 2003.

17. Ball TM, et al. Influence of attendance at day care on the common cold from birth through 13 years of age. *Arch Pediatr Adolesc Med* 156(2):121–126, 2002.

18. Matthews CE, et al. Moderate to vigorous physical activity and risk of upper-respiratory tract infection. *Med Sci Sports Exer* 34(8):1242–1248, 2002.

19. Prevention and control of influenza, recommendations of the Advisory Committee on Immunization Practices (ACIP). *MMWR* 52,RR-08, 2003.

20. Division of Tuberculosis Elimination—2001 Surveillance Report. National Center for HIV, SID, and TB Prevention. CDC, 2003. **http://www.cdc.gov/nchstp,tb/surv/surv2001/content/Tl.htm**

21. Geng E, et al. Changes in the transmission of tuberculosis in New York City from 1900 to 1999. *N Engl J Med* 346(19):1453–1458, 2002.

22. Ewer K, et al. Comparison of T-cell based assay with tuberculin skin test for diagnosis of Mycobacterium tuberculosis infection in a school tuberculosis outbreak. *Lancet* 361(9364):1168–1173, 2003.

23. Oosterheert JJ, et al. Severe community-acquired pneumonia: what's in a name? *Curr Opin Infect Dis* 16(2):153–159, 2003.

24. Sisk JE, et al. Cost-effectiveness of vaccination against invasive pneumococcal disease among people 50 through 64 years of age: role of comorbid conditions and race. *Ann Intern Med* 1389(12):960–968, 2003.

25. Godshall SE, Kirchner JT. Infectious mononucleosis. Complexities of a common syndrome. *Postgrad Med* 107(7):183–184, 2000.

26. National Institute of Allergy and Infectious Disease (NIAID). *Chronic fatigue syndrome-etiological theories.* NIAID, 2000. **http://www.niaid.nih.gov/publications/cfs/etie.htm**

27. Bruce MG, et al. Risk factors for meningococcal disease in college students. *JAMA* 286(6):688–693, 2001.

28. *Meningococcaly disease.* Division of Bacterial and Mycotic Diseases. Centers for Communicable Disease and Prevention, 2003.

29. Nowakowski J, et al. Long-term follow-up with culture-confirmed Lyme disease. *Am J Med* 115(2):91–96, 2003.

30. Allan BF, Keesing F, Ostfeld RS. Effect of forest fragmentation on Lyme disease risk. *Conservation Biology* 17(1):267–272, 2003.

31. Toxic shock syndrome. *Topics in infectious diseases newsletter.* January 2002. **http://wordnet.com/au/Products/topics_in_infectious_diseases_Jan02.htm**

32. Armstrong GL, Bell BP. Hepatitis A virus infections in the United States: model-based estimates and implications for childhood immunizations. *Pediatrics* 109(5):839–845, 2002.

33. Dudclos P. Safety of immuni(s)ation and adverse events following vaccination against hepatitis B. *Expert Opin Drug Saf* 2(3):225–231, 2003.

34. Thomas DL, et al. The natural history of hepatitis C virus infection: host, viral, and environmental factors. *JAMA* 284(4):450–456, 2000.

35. *WHO: SARS outbreak "over the peak" around the world, including China.* Intelihealth: *Health News* (The Associated Press), June 5, 2003.

36. Summary table of SARS cases by country, 1 November 2002–7 August 2003. World Health Organization, August 15, 2003. **http://www.who.int/entity/crs/ sars/country/en/country2003_08_15.pdf**

37. *U.S. expands monkeypox probe to 15 states.* Intelihealth: *Health News* (The Associated Press), June 11, 2003.

38. *HIV/AIDS Surveillance Report, Centers for Disease,* Centers for Disease Control and Prevention. 13(2): 1–47(inclusive), 2001.

39. Ogundele MO, Coulter JB. HIV transmission through breastfeeding: Problems and prevention. *Ann Trop Paediatr* 23(2):91–106, 2003.

40. Edwards S, Crane C. Oral sex and the transmission of viral STIs. *JAMA* 74(1):6–10, 1998.

41. Cox FD. *The aids booklet,* 6th ed. McGraw-Hill, 2000.

42. Hirsch MS, et al. Antiretroviral drug resistance testing in adult HIV-1 infection: recommendations of an International AIDS society—USA Panel. *JAMA* 283(18):2417–2426, 2000.

43. Gulick RM (Presentor). *Current status of new antiretroviral drugs in development.* Topics in HIV Medicine. International AIDS Society-USA. Washington, DC, May 2002.

44. Hui D. HIV protease inhibitors and atherosclerosis. *J Clin Invest* 111(3):317–318, 2003.

45. HIV gp120 vaccine—VaxGen: AIDSVAX, AIDSVAX B/B, AIDSVAX B/E, HIV gp120 vaccine—Genentech, HIV gp120 vaccine AIDSVAX—VaxGen, HIV vaccine AIDSVAX-VaxGen. *Drug R.D.* 4(4):249–243, 2003.

46. Global estimates of the HIV/AIDS epidemic, as of end 2002. December 2002. **http://www.avert.org/ worldstats.htm**

47. Centers for Disease Control and Prevention. Sexually transmitted diseases treatment guidelines 2002. *MMWR* 51:(No. RR-6) [inclusive page numbers], 2002.

48. STD Surveillance 2001. National Center for HIV, STD, and TB Prevention. Centers for Disease Control and Prevention, 2001. **http://www.cdc.gov/ std/stats/TOC2001.htm**

49. Alcohol policy and sexually transmitted disease rates—United States 1981–1995. *MMWR* 49(16): 346–349, 2000.

50. Stanberry LR, et al. Glycoprotein-d-adjuvant vaccine to prevent genital herpes. *N Engl J Med* 347(21): 1652–1661, 2003.

51. Anderson GG, et al. Intracellular bacterial biofilm-like pods in urinary tract infections. *Science* 301(5629): 105–107, 2003.

As We Go to Press

It is very likely that human history is replete with examples where political or religiously influenced decisions have impacted on status of human infectious diseases. This contention being assumed, then an ongoing example is at hand. Today Nigeria, a country in which polio was eradicated, has recently experienced cases of polio; with additional infections currently reported in eight neighboring countries that were, until recently, polio free.

The western Africa reemergence of polio can be traced to a northern area of Nigeria in which local Islamic clergy began circulating the contention that the polio immunization program sponsored and implemented by the national government was using contaminated vaccines for the purpose of creating infertility in women. Growing resistance to the program ensued, and by August 2003, the program was terminated in this region's capital, Abuja. Intervention by the national government, the World Health Organization, and world Islamic leaders, has, to this date, proven ineffective in rebuilding trust in the polio immunization program, as cases of polio increased in number.

Within a few months of the discontinuation of the Nigerian program, new cases of polio infection were reported from the neighboring countries of the Ivory Coast, Ghana, Burkina Faso, Chad, Cameroon, and the Central African Republic. In response, a variety of world organizations, including Rotary International, UNICEF, and the CDC, announced plans to assist these countries in becoming polio-free again.

Prior to the spread of the infection to the eight countries named above, only India, Pakistan, Afghanistan, Egypt, Niger, and Nigeria were reporting new cases of polio.

the changing picture of infectious disease

Just a generation ago, many scientists believed we were wiping out infectious disease. Armed with improved sanitation, better hygiene practices, antibiotics, and pesticides, humankind had malaria, cholera, and tuberculosis (TB) on the run and smallpox and polio well on the way to extinction. In fact, infectious diseases were in decline until 1980, but as we enter the next century, the tide is turning. Ebola, HIV, Marburg virus, Lassa fever, Legionnaires' disease, hantavirus, and hepatitis C are but a few of the more than thirty new pathogens researchers have identified in the last few decades.

Previously unknown microbes have been evolving for thousands of years in animals and insects. They become threatening to humans only when conditions are right for transmission of the diseases from animals, including insects, to us, through a process called zoonosis.

Recent Global Epidemics

The Ebola virus struck in the African countries of Zaire and Sudan in 1976, and again in Sudan in 1979. In 1995 Ebola revisited Zaire, but in Gabon in 1996 it was recognized and stopped before it could take hold. In October 2000, Ebola reappeared in Uganda after not being reported in Africa for several years. The source of Ebola in nature is unclear. Monkeys do become infected but die quickly, as do humans. To be an effective reservoir or source of disease, an animal must be able to tolerate the disease organism and therefore remain active and alive for a longer time in which the virus can be spread. For example, monkeys may be the source of human immunodeficiency virus (HIV) because they harbor a similar virus, simian immunodeficiency virus

(SIV), but don't become sick. Of course, HIV/AIDS is a dangerous virus, but Ebola is more infective and runs a shorter disease course. As one author put it, "Ebola does in ten days what it takes AIDS ten years to accomplish."[1] This is terrible for the nine out of ten people infected with Ebola who die in a matter of days, but ironically by making its victims so sick so quickly, Ebola limits its own spread. Being deathly ill limits the social interactions of carriers.

Many other diseases also pose threats.[2] After a heat wave in 1988, mosquitos carrying dengue (pronounced "ding-ee") spread through Mexico. In 1991 an epidemic of cholera in South America killed 5,000 of the 500,000 people infected. A record year for infectious disease occurred in 1993, possibly set into effect by weather patterns associated with El Niño, which warmed the waters in the tropical Pacific. A year later, epidemic bubonic plague swept through India. In the summer of 1996, a dengue outbreak began in Latin America. By the time it ended, 140,000 people from Argentina to Texas had been infected, and 4,000 of those infected had died.[1]

Occurrence of New Infectious Diseases in the United States and Elsewhere

As the 1996 dengue outbreak illustrates, infectious disease is not just a problem for developing countries. In 1989 an airborne strain of Ebola, which fortunately was not dangerous to humans, was brought to Virginia in Philippine crab-eating monkeys that were to be distributed to research labs across the United States.

Hantavirus became an American problem in 1993. Following an extremely rainy year that was good for vegetation,

the rodent population exploded in the Four Corners area of New Mexico, Arizona, Colorado, and Utah. The rodent population spread hantavirus to sixteen states. This virus killed half of the ninety-four people it infected.[3] More recently, the first case of hantavirus transmission between humans occurred in Argentina. Apparently eighteen people, including five physicians, contracted the disease after having contact with sick patients.

The 1994 earthquake in Southern California provided more evidence to support the theory that new infectious diseases can spread to humans during environmental disturbances. The earthquake exposed a soil fungus that infected 200 people and killed 3.

Today zoonosis-related infections seem even more common as the American public becomes increasingly familiar with conditions such as Lyme disease, West Nile virus infections, SARS (sudden acute respiratory syndrome), and Monkeypox—all described in this chapter. Even more recently, potential zoonotic infectious agents have been identified, such as bacterial pathogens in fish raised through aquaculture (rainbow trout in Italy),[4] Avian (bird) influenza in China,[5] and flying squirrel-associated typhus in this country.[6] Of course, the relationship of these latter infections to the greater American public remains to be seen.

Leading the Fight for Public Health

The United States leads the international health community with its premier monitoring and response services provided by the Centers for Disease Control and Prevention (CDC).[7] Of course, international cooperation is vital, but we have seen why disease vigilance is in our own interest as well. To move from the reactive system now in place to a predictive one, some specific goals must be met.

A global network of epidemiological field stations should be established to detect and characterize outbreaks early, both here and abroad. Insect carriers of disease need to be managed in a variety of ways, including but not solely relying on pesticides. Further, insecticides and pesticides must be developed that are both effective and environmentally safe. Safe food and water must be made available to everyone, and new antibiotics and vaccines need to be developed. These goals are hard to achieve, particularly in the face of episodes of armed conflict within and between countries, growing religious intolerance that becomes transformed into national disputes, and a global economy that continues to separate the affluent developed countries from those far less developed and affluent.

Having entered a new millennium, Americans may encounter the threat of emerging diseases associated with biological weapons and regional armed conflict. This threat looms even larger when one realizes that some countries view these disease organisms as agents of war and are capable of using them as such. With about a dozen countries in possession or pursuit of biological weapons arsenals, the understanding of deadly pathogens becomes a matter of national security as well as global health. Interestingly in this regard, the principal reason that the United States military personnel gave in 2000 for not reenlisting in the armed forces was their fear of receiving the required anthrax vaccine developed for use by American forces in order to protect personnel from anthrax-based biological warfare.

For Discussion . . .

In your view, what is the most important step we can take to fight infectious disease? Do you think the United States does more than its share in monitoring these diseases? What kinds of precautions might prevent zoonosis infections from taking hold in this country? Do you know anyone who works in the public health field? If so, what does he or she do?

1. Monastersky R. Health in the hot zone. *Science News* 1996; 149(14):218–219.
2. Gubler DJ. Resurgent vector-borne diseases as a global health problem. *Emerg Infect Dis* 1998; 4(3):442–450.
3. Anon. Climate creates a hot zone. *Environment* 1996; 37(10):27.
4. Ghittino C, et al. Emerging pathologies in aquaculture: effects on production and food safety. *Vet Res Commun.* 2003 Sep; 27 Suppl 1:471–479.
5. Sims LD, et al. Avian influenza in Hong Kong 1997–2002. *Avain Dis.* 2003; 47(3 Suppl):832–838.
6. Reynolds MG, et al. Flying squirrel-associated typhus, United States. *Emerg Infect Dis.* 2003 Oct; 9(10):1341–1343.
7. Preventing emerging infectious diseases: a strategy for the 21st century: overview of the updated plan. *MMWR* (suppl) 1998; 47(15):1–14.

InfoLinks

www.who.int
www.cdc.gov/ncidod

personal assessment

what is your risk of Contracting a sexually transmitted disease?

A variety of factors interact to determine your risk of contracting a sexually transmitted disease (STD). This inventory is intended to provide you with an estimate of your level of risk.

Circle the number of each row that best characterizes you. Enter that number on the line at the end of the row (points). After assigning yourself a number in each row, total the number appearing in the points column. Your total points will allow you to interpret your risk for contracting an STD.

Age

						Points
1	3	4	5	3	2	_____
0–9	10–14	15–19	20–29	30–34	35+	

Sexual Practices

0	1	2	4	6	8	_____
Never engage in sex	One sex partner	More than one sex partner but never more than one at a time	Two to five sex partners	Five to ten sex partners	Ten or more sex partners	

Sexual Attitudes

0	1	8	1	7	8	_____
Will not engage in nonmarital sex	Premarital sex is okay if it is with future spouse	Any kind of premarital sex is okay	Extramarital sex is not for me	Extramarital sex is okay	Believe in complete sexual freedom	

Attitudes toward Contraception

1	1	6	5	4	8	_____
Would use condom to prevent pregnancy	Would use condom to prevent STDs	Would never use a condom	Would use the birth control pill	Would use other contraceptive measure	Would not use anything	

Attitudes toward STD

3	3	4	6	6	6	_____
Am not sexually active so I do not worry	Would be able to talk about STD with my partner	Would check out an infection to be sure	Would be afraid to check out an infection	Can't even talk about an infection	STDs are no problem–easily cured	

YOUR TOTAL POINTS _____

Interpretation

5–8	Your risk is well below average
9–13	Your risk is below average
14–17	Your risk is at or near average
18–21	Your risk is moderately high
22+	Your risk is high

To Carry This Further . . .

Having taken this Personal Assessment, were you surprised at your level of risk? What is the primary reason for this level? How concerned are you and your classmates and friends about contracting an STD?

sexuality and reproduction

Sexuality is an important part of our being. It colors the way we interact with the world around us and affects our goals, relationships, and roles in society.

1. **Physical Dimension**

   Sexuality is closely related to the physical dimension of health. For example, our bodies mature at puberty, we respond to sexual arousal, we make choices about contraception and pregnancy, and we adjust our sexual behavior as we age. Sexual experiences and relationships can be very complex and demanding because they are fueled by energy and time. They are enhanced when the body is well maintained, rested, and relatively free from illness.

2. **Emotional Dimension**

   One of the most stressful aspects of life is sexual intimacy. Feelings about your own sexual behavior can range from exhilaration to ambivalence to depression. Being comfortable with your sexuality comes from being guided by your core values, knowing how to express your sexual feelings openly, being able to set limits when appropriate, and understanding how to communicate effectively with your partner.

3. **Social Dimension**

   Because sexuality often involves interaction with others, the development of social skills in this area is imperative. For many, dating is an excellent arena in which to establish specific social skills. As a relationship becomes more serious, communication skills will grow. These skills are important factors in the process of mate selection and marriage for those who choose this path.

4. **Intellectual Dimension**

   As a relationship matures, opportunities abound for contemplation, analysis, and reflection. You may have to sort through your feelings, examine your values, and use lessons from past experiences as you take part in this process of introspection. You will also draw on your intellectual resources as you learn about reproductive anatomy, fertility, sexual response, contraception, and birth.

5. **Spiritual Dimension**

   As an intimate relationship progresses, you may have to explore your feelings about your sense of morality, the appropriateness of premarital sex, or the value of fidelity in a marriage or other long-term committed relationship. Dating, courtship, and particularly marriage offer opportunities to enhance your spirituality by extending sympathy, support, and love to another person. Some people even find the sexual act itself to be a way of expressing their spirituality.

6. **Occupational Dimension**

   Decisions about reproduction can have a significant effect on your occupational dimension of health. Women who are pregnant may have to work even when they are not feeling well. Then they must decide how much time to take off work after the child is born. They and their partners must also make difficult choices about long-term child care arrangements. The decisions they make will affect their occupational satisfaction and sense of fulfillment.

chapter fourteen

exploring the origins of sexuality

Chapter Objectives

Upon completing this chapter,
you should be able to:

- describe the genetic basis and the gonadal basis of sexuality.

- describe the psychosexual bases of sexuality, including gender identity, gender preference, gender adoption, and initial adult gender identification.

- define androgyny and discuss its role in our society.

- examine your attitudes toward masculine and feminine roles in our society.

- explain the structure and function of the male reproductive and female reproductive systems.

- discuss the issues related to male and female circumcision.

- trace the stages of the menstrual cycle.

- identify techniques for reducing menstrual pain.

- analyze the risks and benefits of hormone replacement therapy for reducing the symptoms of menopause.

- differentiate among the terms *reproductive sexuality, genital sexuality,* and *expressionistic sexuality.*

Online Learning Center Resources

www.mhhe.com/payne8e

Log on to our Online Learning Center (OLC) for access to these additional resources:

- Chapter key terms and definitions
- Learning objectives
- Student interactive question-and-answer sites
- Self-scoring chapter quiz
- Online assessments
- Key term flash cards

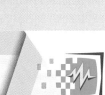

Talking It Over

"I Need Answers about Sex . . ."

OK, admit it. You don't know everything about sex. Why should you? If you're like most college students, your parents probably had a difficult time telling you about the "birds and the bees." Sure, they tried to tell you about what makes a baby, but they probably shied away from talking about topics like sexual expression, oral sex, sexual performance, sexual orientation, and masturbation. It's no wonder that you still have questions about sex. Fortunately, you can get many answers online.

CommunicationLinks

www.intelihealth.com
www.goaskalice.columbia.edu
www.webmd.com

Eye on the Media

Responsible Sexual Behavior by 2010

Be on the lookout for media reports that feature progress on the nation's health objectives for the year 2010. The government's *Healthy People 2010* report, a comprehensive, public health planning document for the United States, lists 467 health objectives in 28 focus areas. Especially significant for young adults (and their parents) will be reports that indicate progress made toward national goals in the area of "responsible sexual behavior." Responsible sexual behavior is one of the ten leading health indicators that are thought to be able to provide a snapshot of the health of the Nation.[1]

Success in the area of responsible sexual behavior will be largely determined by progress made in two key objectives:

Objective 25-11: *Increase the proportion of adolescents who abstain from sexual intercourse or use condoms if currently sexually active.*

Objective 13-6a: *Increase the proportion of sexually active persons who use condoms.*

These two key objectives were thought to be particularly important because of their overall ability to influence trends in sexual behavior, unintended pregnancies, sexually transmitted diseases, and HIV/AIDS.

For the first objective, *Healthy People 2010* established 95% as the target

Early in this new millennium, we have reached a better understanding of both the biological and psychosocial factors that contribute to the complex expression of our sexuality. As a society, we are now inclined to view human behavior in terms of a complex script written on the basis of both biology and conditioning.

Reflecting this understanding is the way in which we use the words *male* or *female* to refer to the biological roots of our sexuality and the words *man* or *woman* to refer to the psychosocial roots of our sexuality. In this chapter, we explore human sexuality as it relates to the dynamic interplay of the biological and psychosocial bases that form our masculinity or femininity.

Biological Bases of Human Sexuality

Within a few seconds after the birth of a baby, someone (a doctor, nurse, or parent) emphatically labels the child: "It's a boy," or "It's a girl." For the parents and society as a whole, the child's biological sexuality is being displayed and identified. Another female or male enters the world.

Genetic Basis

At the moment of conception, a Y-bearing or an X-bearing sperm cell joins with the X-bearing ovum to establish the true basis of biological sexuality.[1] A fertilized ovum with sex chromosomes XX is biologically female, whereas a fertilized ovum bearing the XY sex chromosome is biologically male. Genetics forms the most basic level of an individual's biological sexuality.

Gonadal Basis

The gonadal basis for biological sexuality refers to the growing embryo's development of *gonads.*[2] Male embryos develop testes about the seventh week after conception, and female embryos develop ovaries about the twelfth week after conception.

Structural Development

The development of male or female reproductive structures is initially determined by the presence or absence of hormones produced by the developing testes—androgens and müllerian inhibiting substance (MIS). With these hormones present, the male embryo starts to develop male reproductive structures (penis, scrotum, vas deferens, seminal vesicles, prostate gland, and Cowper's glands).

Because the female embryo is not exposed to these male hormones, it develops the characteristic female reproductive structures: the uterus, fallopian tubes, vagina, labia, and clitoris.

Biological Sexuality and the Childhood Years

The growth and development of the child in terms of reproductive organs and physiological processes have traditionally been thought to be "latent" during the childhood years. However, a gradual degree of growth occurs in both girls and boys. The reproductive organs, however, will undergo faster growth at the onset of puberty and will achieve their adult size and capabilities shortly thereafter.

Puberty

The entry into puberty is a gradual maturing process for young girls and boys. For young girls, the onset of menstruation, called *menarche,* occurs at about age 12 or 13 but may come somewhat earlier or later.[3] Early menstrual cycles tend to be anovulatory (ovulation does not occur). Menarche is usually preceded by a growth spurt that includes the budding of breasts and the growth of pubic and underarm hair.[4]

Young males follow a similar pattern of maturation, including a growth spurt followed by a gradual sexual maturity. However, this process takes place about two years later than in young females. Genital enlargement, underarm and pubic hair growth, and a lowering of the voice commonly occur. The male's first ejaculation is generally experienced by the age of 14, most commonly through **nocturnal emission** or masturbation. For many young boys, fully mature sperm do not develop until about age 15.

Reproductive capability only gradually declines over the course of the adult years. In the woman, however, the onset of **menopause** signals a more direct turning off of the reproductive system than is the case for the male adult. By the early to mid-fifties, virtually all women have entered a postmenopausal period, but for men, relatively high-level **spermatogenesis** may continue for a decade or two.[4]

The story of sexual maturation and reproductive maturity cannot, however, be solely focused on the changes that take place in the body. Now we will discuss the psychosocial processes that accompany the biological changes.

 TALKING POINTS Your twelve-year-old son comes to you and says that all of his male friends are starting to grow facial hair. He is worried that his own beard will never begin. What could you say to him that could ease his fears?

Psychosocial Bases of Human Sexuality

If you visualized growth and development of sexuality as a ladder (Figure 14-1), one vertical rail of the ladder would represent our biological sexuality. Arising at various points along this rail would be rungs representing the sequential unfolding of the genetic, gonadal, and structural components. These biological bases of our sexuality can be considered the "hard-wired" parts of our sexuality. They are rooted in the linkages of our parents' genetic backgrounds. These are the parts of our sexuality over which we have little control.

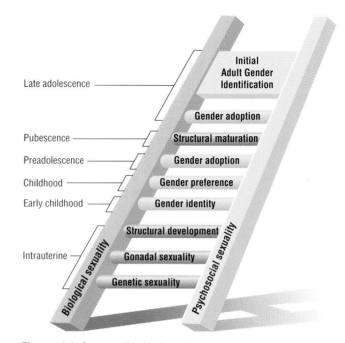

Figure 14-1 Our sexuality develops through biological and psychosocial stages.

Because humans, more so than any other life form, can rise above a life centered on reproduction, we have a second dimension or rail to our sexuality—our **psychosocial sexuality.** The reason we possess the ability to be more than reproductive beings is a question for the theologian or philosopher. We are considerably more complex than the hard-wired functions determined by biology. The process that transforms a male into a man and a female into a woman begins at birth and continues to influence us throughout the course of our lives.

It is during this transformation into a man or woman that we humans have some ability to influence our gender development. Here is where we occasionally are able to make decisions that influence both the way we view our-

Key Terms

nocturnal emission ejaculation that occurs during sleep; "wet dream."

menopause decline and eventual cessation of hormone production by the female reproductive system.

spermatogenesis (sper mat oh **jen** uh sis) process of sperm production.

psychosocial sexuality masculine and feminine aspects of sexuality.

selves as men or women and the way we are viewed as men or women by others. This is the part of our sexuality that is not completely hard-wired by our genetic background.

Gender Identity

Although expectant parents may prefer to have a child of one **gender** over the other, they frequently must wait until the birth of the baby to have their question answered. External genitals "cast the die," and femininity or masculinity begins to receive its traditional reinforcement by the parents and society in general. By the eighteenth month, typical children have both the language and the insight to correctly identify their gender. They have established a **gender identity.**[5] The first rung rising from the psychosocial rail of the ladder has been climbed.

Gender Preference

During the preschool years, children receive the second component of the scripting required for the full development of psychosocial sexuality—the preference for the gender to which they have been assigned. The process whereby **gender preference** is transmitted to the child is more than likely a less subtle form of the practices observed during the gender identity period (the first 18 months). Many parents begin to control the child's exposure to experiences traditionally reserved for children of the opposite gender. This is particularly true for boys; parents will often stop play activities they perceive as being too feminine.

Attitudes toward gender roles have become more flexible in recent years. Many parents now allow their children to pursue the activities they enjoy, regardless of whether the activities were once considered strictly masculine, such as playing baseball or building a model airplane, or feminine, such as growing flowers or cooking.

Parents should not become alarmed if their children or teenagers experiment with their gender identity through their appearance or activities. Such experimentation is natural and a part of finding the gender identity that best fits them. Such children often become very secure in their gender identity as adults.

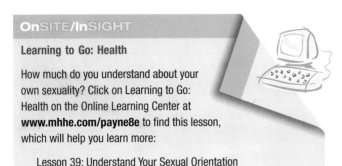

OnSITE/InSIGHT

Learning to Go: Health

How much do you understand about your own sexuality? Click on Learning to Go: Health on the Online Learning Center at **www.mhhe.com/payne8e** to find this lesson, which will help you learn more:

Lesson 39: Understand Your Sexual Orientation

With the recent acceleration in the importance of competitive sports for women, many of the skills and experiences once reserved for boys are now being fostered in young girls. What effect, if any, this movement will have on the speed at which gender preference is reached will be a topic for further research.

Gender Adoption

The process of reaching an initial adult gender identification requires a considerable period of time. The specific knowledge, attitudes, and behavior characteristic of adults must be observed, analyzed, and practiced. The process of acquiring and personalizing these "insights" about how men and women think, feel, and act is reflected by the term **gender adoption,** the first and third rungs below the initial adult gender identification rail of the ladder in Figure 14-1.

In addition to the construction of a personalized version of an adult sexual identity, it is important that the child and particularly the adolescent construct a gender schema for a member of the opposite gender. Clearly, the world of adulthood, with its involvement with intimacy, parenting, and employment, will require that men know women and women know men. Gender adoption provides an opportunity to begin constructing this equally valuable "picture" of what the other gender is like.

Initial Adult Gender Identification

By the time young people have climbed all of the rungs of the sexuality ladder, they have arrived at the chronological point in the life cycle when they need to construct an initial adult **gender identification.** You might notice that this label seems remarkably similar to the terminology used to describe one of the developmental tasks being used in this textbook. In fact, the task of forming an initial adult identity is closely related to developing an initial

---

Key Terms

gender general term reflecting a biological basis of sexuality; the male gender or the female gender.

gender identity recognition of one's gender.

gender preference emotional and intellectual acceptance of one's own gender.

gender adoption the long process of learning the behavior that is traditional for one's gender.

gender identification achievement of a personally satisfying interpretation of one's masculinity or femininity.

Just as women have broken into traditionally male careers, many men have taken on jobs and tasks that were once considered women's exclusive domain.

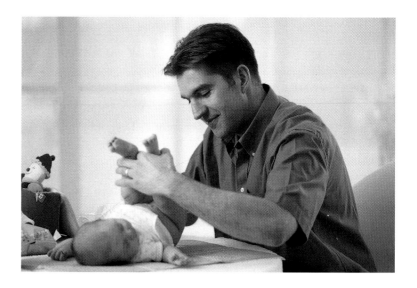

adult image of oneself as a man or a woman. Although most of us currently support the concept of "person" in many gender-neutral contexts (for some very valid reasons), we still must identify ourselves as either a man or a woman.

Androgyny: Sharing the Pluses

Our society has increasingly accepted an image of a person who possesses both masculine and feminine qualities. This accepted image has taken years to develop because our society traditionally has reinforced rigid masculine roles for men and rigid feminine roles for women.

In the past, from the time a child was born, we assigned and reinforced only those roles and traits that were thought to be directly related to his or her biological gender. Boys were not allowed to cry, play with dolls, or help in the kitchen. Girls were not encouraged to become involved in sports; they were told to learn to sew, cook, and baby-sit. Men were encouraged to be strong, expressive, dominant, aggressive, and career oriented, whereas women were encouraged to be weak, shy, submissive, passive, and home oriented.

These traditional biases have resulted in some interesting phenomena related to career opportunities. Women were denied jobs requiring above-average physical strength, admittance into professional schools requiring high intellectual capacities, such as law, medicine, and business, and entry into most levels of military participation. Likewise, men were not encouraged to enter traditionally feminine careers, such as nursing, clerical work, and elementary school teaching.

For a variety of reasons, the traditional picture has changed. **Androgyny,** or the blending of both feminine and masculine qualities, is more clearly evident in our society now than ever before. Today it is quite common to

see men involved in raising children (including changing diapers) and doing routine housework. On the other hand, it is also quite common to see women entering the workplace in jobs traditionally managed by men and participating in sports traditionally played by men. Men are not scoffed at when they are seen crying after a touching movie. Women are not laughed at when they choose to assert themselves. The disposal of many sexual stereotypes has probably benefited our society immensely by relieving people of the pressure to be 100 percent "womanly" or 100 percent "macho."

Research data suggest that androgynous people are more flexible and independent, have greater self-esteem, have more positive attitudes toward sexuality, and show more social skills and motivation to achieve.[5] Complete the Personal Assessment on page 493 to explore your own attitudes about sexuality and sex roles.

 TALKING POINTS How could you demonstrate to your grandmother that the blending of gender roles is a positive development?

Reproductive Systems

The most familiar aspects of biological sexuality are the structures that compose the reproductive systems. Each structure contributes in unique ways to the reproductive process. Thus with these structures, males have the ability

---

Key Terms

androgyny (an **droj** en ee) the blending of both masculine and feminine qualities.

Male Circumcision: No Longer an Automatic Choice

Should newborn boys still be routinely circumcised? Researchers no longer think so. For example, a committee of the Canadian Paediatric Society recently studied the issue and concluded that newborns should not be routinely circumcised. The study compared the costs and complications of the procedure itself, the incidence of urinary tract infections, sexually transmitted diseases, and cancer of the penis in both circumcised and uncircumcised males, and of cervical cancer in their partners. The committee concluded that routine circumcision cannot be justified.[1] This recommendation echoes that of the American Academy of Pediatrics and the Canadian Paediatric Society.

Another study reported that the rate of penile cancer in fact is lower in circumcised men, but that this difference alone is not sufficient to justify routine circumcision. Other researchers are more vehement, calling circumcision the mutilation of healthy organs. If parents do decide on circumcision, it should be performed only by a trained surgeon in a medical institution, as 85% of complications and nearly all disastrous circumcisions are performed by traditional, but medically untrained, circumcisers.[2] In addition, the surgeon should have adequate training in pain relief for this treatment, in view of the overwhelming evidence that newborn circumcision is painful.[3] The parents, in consultation with their physician, should make the final decision.

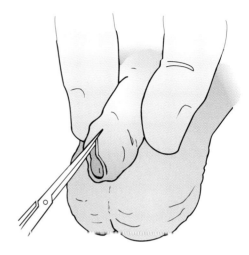

[1] Anonymous. Neonatal circumcision revisited. Fetus and Newborn Committee, Canadian Paediatric Society (review) *Can Med Assoc J* 1996 March 15; 154(6): 769–780.
[2] Azdemir E. Significantly increased complication risks with mass circumcisions. *Br J Urol* 1997; 80(1): 136–139.
[3] Howard CR, el al. Neonatal circumcision and pain relief: current training practices. *Pediatrics* 1998; 101 (3, part 1 of 2): 423–428.

to impregnate. Females have the ability to become pregnant, give birth, and nourish infants through breastfeeding. In addition, many of these structures are associated with nonreproductive sexual behavior.

Male Reproductive System

The male reproductive system consists of external structures of genitals (the penis and scrotum) and internal structures (the testes, various passageways or ducts, seminal vesicles, the prostate gland, and the Cowper's glands) (Figure 14-2A).

Male newborn babies are routinely circumcised by all Muslims and Jews. Millions of infants are circumcised in the United States and Canada annually. However, this routine practice has become a controversial subject.[6] Many researchers argue that male circumcision should no longer be an automatic choice, but rather that parents should consider the pros and cons. See the Star box above for a look at this debate.

The Testes

The testes (also called gonads or testicles) are two egg-shaped bodies that lie within a saclike structure called the scrotum. During most of fetal development, the testes lie within the abdominal cavity. They descend into the scrotum during the last two months of fetal life.

The testes are housed in the scrotum because a temperature lower than the body core temperature is required for adequate sperm development. The walls of the scrotum are composed of contractile tissue and can draw the testes closer to the body during cold temperatures (and sexual arousal) and relax during warm temperatures. Scrotal contraction and relaxation allow a constant, productive temperature to be maintained in the testes (Figure 14-2B).

A cross-sectional view of a single testis reveals an intricate network of structures called *seminiferous tubules*. Within these 300 or so seminiferous tubules, the process of sperm production (spermatogenesis) takes place. Sperm cell development starts at about age 11 in boys and is influenced by the release of the hormone **ICSH (interstitial cell-stimulating hormone)** from the pituitary gland. ICSH does primarily what its name suggests: It stimulates specific cells (called *interstitial cells*)

Key Terms

ICSH (interstitial cell-stimulating hormone) (in ter stish ul) a gonadotropic hormone of the male required for the production of testosterone.

Figure 14-2 The male reproductive system.
A, Side view, **B,** Front view.

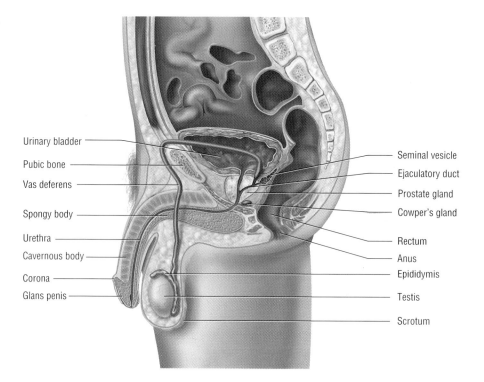

Urinary bladder
Pubic bone
Vas deferens
Spongy body
Urethra
Cavernous body
Corona
Glans penis

Seminal vesicle
Ejaculatory duct
Prostate gland
Cowper's gland
Rectum
Anus
Epididymis
Testis
Scrotum

A

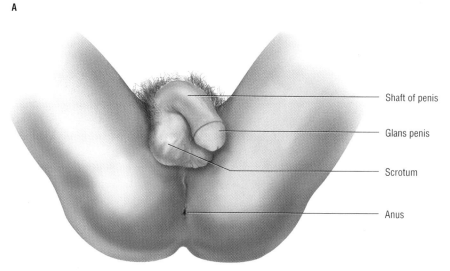

Shaft of penis
Glans penis
Scrotum
Anus

B

within the testes to begin producing the male sex hormone *testosterone*. Testosterone in turn is primarily responsible for the gradual development of the male secondary sex characteristics at the onset of puberty. By the time a boy is approximately fifteen years old, sufficient levels of testosterone exist so that the testes become capable of full spermatogenesis.

Before the age of about 15 most of the sperm cells produced in the testes are incapable of fertilization. The production of fully mature sperm *(spermatozoa)* is triggered by another hormone secreted by the brain's pitu-

itary gland— **FSH (follicle-stimulating hormone).** FSH influences the seminiferous tubules to begin producing spermatozoa capable of fertilization.

> **Key Terms**
>
> **FSH (follicle-stimulating hormone)** a gonadotropic hormone required for the initial development of ova (in the female) and sperm (in the male).

Ducts

Spermatogenesis takes place around the clock, with hundreds of millions of sperm cells produced daily. The sperm cells do not stay in the seminiferous tubules but rather are transferred through a system of ducts that lead into the epididymis. The epididymis is a tubular coil that attaches to the back side of each testicle. These collecting structures house the maturing sperm cells for 2 to 3 weeks. During this period the sperm finally become capable of motion, but they remain inactive until they mix with the secretions from the accessory glands (the seminal vesicles, prostate gland, and Cowper's glands).

Each epididymis leads into an 18-inch passageway known as the *vas deferens*. Sperm, moved along by the action of hairlike projections called *cilia*, can also remain in the vas deferens for an extended time without losing their ability to fertilize an egg.

Seminal Vesicles

The two vasa deferens extend into the abdominal cavity, where each meets with a *seminal vesicle*—the first of the three accessory structures or glands. Each seminal vesicle contributes a clear, alkaline fluid that nourishes the sperm cells with fructose and permits the sperm cells to be suspended in a movable medium. The fusion of a vas deferens with the seminal vesicle results in the formation of a passageway called the ejaculatory duct. Each ejaculatory duct is only about one inch long and empties into the final passageway for the sperm—the urethra.

Prostate Gland

This juncture takes place in an area surrounded by the second accessory gland—the *prostate gland*. The prostate gland secretes a milky fluid containing a variety of substances, including proteins, cholesterol, citric acid, calcium, buffering salts, and various enzymes. The prostate secretions further nourish the sperm cells and also raise the pH level, making the mixture quite alkaline. The alkalinity permits the sperm to have greater longevity as they are transported during ejaculation through the urethra, out of the penis, and into the highly acidic vagina.

Cowper's Glands

The third accessory gland, the Cowper's glands, serves primarily to lubricate the urethra with a clear, viscous mucus. These paired glands empty their small amounts of preejaculatory fluid during the arousal stage of the sexual response cycle. Alkaline in nature, this fluid also neutralizes the acidic level of the urethra. Viable sperm cells can be suspended in this fluid and can enter the female reproductive tract before full ejaculation by the male.[7] This may account for many of the failures of the "withdrawal" method of contraception.

The sperm cells, when combined with secretions from the seminal vesicles and the prostate gland, form a sticky substance called **semen.**[8] Interestingly, the microscopic sperm actually makes up less than 5% of the seminal fluid discharged at ejaculation. Contrary to popular belief, the paired seminal vesicles contribute about 60% of the semen volume, and the prostate gland adds about 30%.[1] Thus the fear of some men that a **vasectomy** will destroy their ability to ejaculate is completely unfounded (see Chapter 16).

During *emission* (the gathering of semen in the upper part of the urethra), a sphincter muscle at the base of the bladder contracts and inhibits semen from being pushed into the bladder and urine from being deposited into the urethra.[9] Thus semen and urine rarely intermingle, even though they leave the body through the same passageway.

Penis

Ejaculation takes place when the semen is forced out of the penis through the urethral opening. The involuntary, rhythmic muscle contractions that control ejaculation result in a series of pleasurable sensations known as *orgasm.*

The urethra lies on the underside of the penis and extends through the three cylindrical chambers of erectile tissue (two *cavernous bodies* and one *spongy body*). Each of these three chambers provides the vascular space required for sufficient erection of the penis. When a male becomes sexually aroused, the areas become congested with blood (*vasocongestion*). After ejaculation or when a male is no longer sexually stimulated, these

Key Terms
semen a secretion containing sperm and nutrients discharged from the urethra at ejaculation.
vasectomy a surgical procedure in which the vasa deferens are cut to prevent the passage of sperm from the testicles; the most common form of male sterilization.

DHEA (dehydroepiandrosterone) is a steroid hormone produced mainly by the adrenal glands. This hormone is the most abundant hormone in the human body. DHEA is converted by the body into other hormones, especially estrogen and testosterone. This hormone peaks in the bloodstream by age 25 and then gradually declines until about age 70, when levels of DHEA may be more than 80% lower than they once were.[1]

Recently, researchers have speculated that DHEA may be helpful in treating a variety of ailments. In fact, advocates of DHEA believe that this powerful hormone can reverse the aging process and bring back sexual vigor. Some claim that DHEA can fight off aging by boosting your sex drive, helping you lose weight, improving your immune system, warding off cancer and depression, and improving your mood, energy, and memory. DHEA might also be useful in combating chronic fatigue syndrome. However, large experimental trials of DHEA's impact have not been undertaken, so many health professionals remain cautious about the benefits (and risks) of taking DHEA.

It is plausible that DHEA may be useful only in those persons whose adrenal glands are not functioning properly and, thus, have low levels of natural DHEA.[2] Disorders in which low levels of DHEA are likely include Alzheimer's disease, certain cancers, diabetes, multiple sclerosis, lupus, and other immune function disorders. While DHEA supplementation might help persons with these and other diseases or conditions, this has not been clearly proven. Some physicians are big supporters of DHEA, while some remain skeptical.

Before you purchase DHEA supplements at your local health food store, speak with your physician about his or her understanding of DHEA's risks and benefits. Since it is clear that DHEA triggers additional hormone production in the body, you will want to avoid DHEA if you have a hormone-related cancer, such as breast, cervical, uterine, ovarian, or prostate cancer. If you are pregnant or breastfeeding, you should not take this supplement. Finally, be prepared for some of the same body changes that take place when people take steroids, including facial hair growth and a lowering of the voice in women and breast enlargement in men who take high doses.[1]

[1] Content article: DHEA www.my.webmd.com/content/article3187.13598, accessed 4 October 2000.
[2] Hamilton J. Hormone DHEA helps some women feel better, enjoy sex. http://my.webmd.com/content/article/1728.50092, accessed 4 October 2000.

chambers release the blood into the general circulation and the penis returns to a **flaccid** state.

The *shaft* of the penis is covered by a thin layer of skin that is an extension of the skin that covers the scrotum. This loose layer of skin is sensitive to sexual stimulation and extends over the head of the penis, except in males who have been circumcised. The *glans* (or head) of the penis is the most sexually sensitive (to tactile stimulation) part of the male body. Nerve receptor sites are especially prominent along the *corona* (the ridge of the glans) and the *frenulum* (the thin tissue at the base of the glans).

Later in life, men begin to experience some changes in their reproductive system. The level of androgens, or male hormones, decreases with age, and the size of the prostate gland often increases. A deficiency of androgens has been found to cause health concerns in older men, including a lack of strength and energy, changes in mood, lower interest in sex, decreased bone density, and a decrease in muscle mass.[10]

As a result, researchers are studying the benefits and risks of androgen replacement therapy in older men, similar to the hormone replacement therapy given to women. The benefits are an increase in bone and muscle mass, improved muscular and cardiovascular function, improved sexual function, and an overall better sense of well-being. The possible risks include an increased incidence of prostate disease, cardiovascular disease, and liver disease.[10,6] Androgen replacement therapy is available through prescription injections, transdermal patches, oral pills, and most recently through a gel applied daily to the upper arm, shoulders, or abdomen.[11]

Another steroid hormone, DHEA, is believed by some to reverse the aging process and revitalize sexual function (see the adjacent Considering Complementary Care box).

Female Reproductive System

The external structures (genitals) of the female reproductive system consist of the mons pubis, labia majora, labia minora, clitoris, and vestibule (Figure 14-3). Collectively these structures form the *vulva* or vulval area.

Mons Pubis

The mons pubis is the fatty covering over the pubic bone. The mons pubis (or mons veneris, "mound of Venus") is covered by pubic hair and is quite sensitive to sexual stimulation.

Labia Majora and Labia Minora

The *labia majora* are large longitudinal skin folds that cover the entrance to the vagina, whereas the *labia minora* are the smaller longitudinal skin folds that lie within the labia majora. These hairless skin folds of the labia minora join at the top to form the *prepuce*. The prepuce covers the glans of the *clitoris*, which is the most sexually sensitive part of the female body.

Key Terms

flaccid (fla sid) nonerect; the state of erectile tissue when vasocongestion is not occurring.

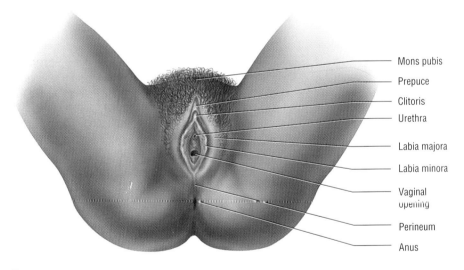

Figure 14-3
The female reproductive system.
A, Side view, **B,** Front view.

Fallopian (uterine) tube

Uterus

Urinary bladder

Pubic bone

Mons pubis

Urethra

Clitoris

Prepuce

Labia minora

Labia majora

Fimbriae

Ovary

Cervix

Cervical os (opening)

Rectum

Anus

Vagina

Bartholin's gland

Vaginal opening

A

Mons pubis

Prepuce

Clitoris

Urethra

Labia majora

Labia minora

Vaginal opening

Perineum

Anus

B

Clitoris

In terms of its tactile sensitivity, the clitoris is the most sensitive part of the female genitals. It contains a glans and a shaft, although the shaft is below the skin surface. It is composed of erectile tissue that can become engorged with blood. It is covered by skin folds (the clitoral prepuce) and can collect **smegma** beneath these tissue folds.[5]

Key Terms

smegma cellular discharge that can accumulate beneath the clitoral hood or the foreskin of an uncircumcised penis.

Female Circumcision

Although commonly referred to as female circumcision, the practice of surgically altering a young girl's vulva is more appropriately called female genital cutting (FGC) or female genital mutilation (FGM). This procedure is practiced in twenty-eight African countries, several countries in the Middle East, and among some Muslims in Indonesia and Malaysia.[1] Typically, the procedure takes one of three forms: the removal of the clitoral hood (circumcision), the removal of the clitoris and perhaps the labia minora (clitoridectomy), and the drastic removal of the clitoris, inner lips, and part of the outer lips (infibulation).

For people from Western cultures, these practices may seem barbaric. Often performed by native women with crude instruments in unsanitary conditions, FGC takes place without the use of anesthetics. Female infants or young girls are subjected to this ritualistic cutting. Obvious dangers include severe bleeding, infection, and the formation of scar tissue.[2]

Infibulation is sometimes extended to incorporate the sewing together the remaining parts of the labia majora. This is thought to ensure virginity in a woman, but poses major risks when a newlywed husband tries to force his penis through the sewn area. Sometimes a midwife must first cut through the scar tissue to open the entrance to the vagina. Years after FGC, women face the possibility of serious complications with childbirth.

It is estimated that FGC and FGM have taken place on 100 million women worldwide.[1] At face value, these procedures may seem gruesome to us in the West, yet we must pause to consider imposing our values on other cultures . . . cultures that readily accept these acts as important to the foundations of their belief systems.[2] To many of us, these procedures represent a sexist devaluation of women. Yet this is normative behavior for groups of people who believe in carrying traditional values for their society. FGC and FGM pose real ethical dilemmas for those of us in Western cultures. What are your thoughts on this?

[1] Hyde JS, DeLamater JD. *Understanding human sexuality,* 8th ed. McGraw-Hill, 2003.
[2] Masters WH, Johnson VE, Kolodny RC. *Human sexuality,* 5th ed. Addison Wesley, 1997.

Vestibule

The *vestibule* is the region enclosed by the labia minora. Evident here are the urethral opening and the entrance to the vagina (vaginal orifice). Also located at the vaginal opening are the *Bartholin's glands,* which secrete a minute amount of lubricating fluid during sexual excitement.

The hymen is a thin layer of tissue that stretches across the opening of the vagina. Once thought to be the only indication of virginity, the intact hymen rarely covers the vaginal opening entirely. Openings in the hymen are necessary for the discharge of menstrual fluid and vaginal secretions. Many hymens are stretched or torn to full opening by adolescent physical activity or by the insertion of tampons. In women whose hymens are not fully ruptured, the first act of sexual intercourse will generally accomplish this. Pain may accompany first intercourse in females with relatively intact hymens.

The internal reproductive structures of the female include the vagina, uterus, fallopian tubes, and ovaries.

Vagina

The *vagina* is the structure that forms a canal from the orifice, through the vestibule, to the uterine cervix. Normally the walls of the vagina are collapsed, except during sexual stimulation, when the vaginal walls widen and elongate to accommodate the erect penis. Only the outer third of the vagina is especially sensitive to sexual stimulation. In this location, vaginal tissues swell considerably to form the **orgasmic platform.**[12] This platform constricts the vaginal opening and in effect "grips" the penis (or other inserted object)—regardless of its size. Thus the belief that a woman receives considerably more sexual pleasure from men with large penises is not supported from an anatomical standpoint.

Uterus

The *uterus* (or *womb*) is approximately the size and shape of a small pear. This highly muscular organ is capable of undergoing a wide range of physical changes, as evidenced by its enlargement during pregnancy, its contraction during menstruation and labor, and its movement during the orgasmic phase of the female sexual response cycle. The primary function of the uterus is to provide a suitable environment for the possible implantation of a fertilized ovum, or egg. This implantation, should it occur, will take place in the innermost lining of the uterus—the *endometrium.* In the mature female, the endometrium undergoes cyclic changes as it prepares a new lining on a near-monthly basis.

The lower third of the uterus is called the *cervix.* The cervix extends slightly into the vagina. Sperm can enter the uterus through the cervical opening, or *cervical os.* Mucous glands in the cervix secrete a fluid that is thin and watery near the time of ovulation. Mucus of this consistency

> ### Key Terms
>
> **orgasmic platform** expanded outer third of the vagina, which grips the penis during sexual intercourse.

apparently facilitates sperm passage into the uterus and deeper structures. However, cervical mucus is much thicker during portions of the menstrual cycle when pregnancy is improbable, and during pregnancy, to protect against bacterial agents and other substances that are especially dangerous to the developing fetus.

The upper two-thirds of the uterus is called the *corpus* or *body*. This is where the fertilized ovum generally implants into the uterus.

Fallopian Tubes

The upper portion of the uterus opens into *two fallopian tubes,* sometimes called oviducts or uterine tubes, each about four inches long. The fallopian tubes are each directed toward an ovary. They serve as a passageway for the ovum in its weeklong voyage toward the uterus. In most cases, conception takes place in the upper third of the fallopian tubes.

Ovaries

The ovaries are analogous to the testes in the male. Their function is to produce the ovum, or egg. Usually, one ovary produces and releases just one egg each month. Approximately the size and shape of an unshelled almond, an ovary produces viable ova in the process known as *oogenesis.*

The ovaries also produce the female sex hormones through the efforts of specific structures within the ovaries. These hormones play multiple roles in the development of female secondary sex characteristics, but their primary function is to prepare the endometrium of the uterus for possible implantation of a fertilized ovum. In the average healthy female, this preparation takes place about thirteen times a year for a period of about 35 years. At menopause, the ovaries shrink considerably and stop nearly all hormonal production.

Menstrual Cycle

Each month or so, the inner wall of the uterus prepares for a possible pregnancy. When a pregnancy does not occur (as is the case throughout most months of a woman's fertile years), this lining must be released and a new one prepared. The breakdown of this endometrial wall and the resultant discharge of blood and endometrial tissue is known as *menstruation* (or *menses*) (Figure 14-4). The cyclic timing of this is controlled by a woman's hormones.

Girls generally have their first menstrual cycle, the onset of which is called *menarche,* around age 12 or 13. However, menarche ranges widely, from about age 9 to 17 years.[4] After a girl first menstruates, her cycles may be anovulatory for a year or longer before a viable ovum is released during her cycle. She will then continue this cyclic activity until age 45 to 55.

This text refers to a menstrual cycle that lasts 28 days. Be assured that few women display absolutely perfect

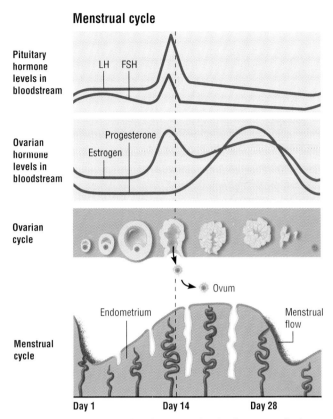

Menstrual cycle

Figure 14-4 The menstrual cycle involves the development and release of an ovum, supported by hormones from the pituitary, and the buildup of the endometrium, supported by hormones from the ovary, for the purpose of establishing a pregnancy.

Endometriosis

Endometriosis is a condition in which endometrial tissue that normally lines the uterus is found growing within the pelvic cavity. Because the tissue remains sensitive to circulating hormones, it is the source of pain and discomfort during the latter half of the menstrual cycle. Endometriosis is most commonly found in younger women and is sometimes related to infertility in women with severe cases.

In addition to painful cramping before and during menstruation, the symptoms of endometriosis include low back pain, pain during intercourse, painful bowel movements, heavy menstrual flow, and difficulty becoming pregnant. Many women with endometriosis, however, experience no symptoms.*

Treatment of endometriosis largely depends on its extent. Drugs to suppress ovulation, including birth control pills, may be helpful in mild cases. For more severe cases, surgical removal of the tissue or a hysterectomy may be necessary. For some women, endometriosis is suppressed during pregnancy and does not return after pregnancy.

*Content article. *Your guide to endometriosis.* WebMD. **www.my.webMD. com/CONTENT/ARTICLE/46/2953_501htm.** accessed July 10, 2003.

28-day cycles. Most women fluctuate by a few days to a week or more around this 28-day pattern.

Your knowledge about the menstrual cycle is critical for your understanding of pregnancy, contraception, menopause, and issues related to the overall health and comfort of women (see the Star box on page 483 for a discussion of endometriosis). Although seemingly complicated, each segment of the cycle can be studied separately for better understanding.

The menstrual cycle can be thought of as occurring in three segments or phases: the menstrual phase (lasting about one week), the preovulation (also lasting about one week), and the postovulation phase (lasting about two weeks). Day 1 of this cycle starts with the first day of bleeding, or menstrual flow.

Menstrual Phase

The *menstrual phase* signals the woman that a pregnancy has not taken place and that her uterine lining is being sloughed off. During a 5- to 7-day period, a woman will discharge about one-fourth to one-half cup of blood and tissue. (Only about one ounce of the menstrual flow is actual blood.) The menstrual flow is heaviest during the first days of this phase. Because the muscular uterus must contract to accomplish this tissue removal, some women have uncomfortable cramping during menstruation. Most women, however, report more pain and discomfort during the few days before the first day of menstrual flow. (See the discussion of menstrual pain on page 485.)

Today's methods of absorbing menstrual flow include the use of internal tampons and external pads. Caution must be exercised by the user of tampons to prevent the possibility of toxic shock syndrome (TSS) (see Chapter 13). Because menstrual flow is a positive sign of good health, women are encouraged to be normally active during menstruation.

Preovulation Phase

The *preovulation phase* of the menstrual cycle starts about the time menstruation stops. Lasting about one week, this phase is first influenced by the release of follicle-stimulating hormone (FSH) from the pituitary gland. FSH circulates in the bloodstream and directs the ovaries to start the process of maturing approximately twenty primary ovarian *follicles*. Thousands of primary egg follicles are present in each ovary at birth. These follicles resemble shells that house immature ova. As these follicles ripen under FSH influence, they release the hormone *estrogen*. Estrogen's primary function is to direct the endometrium to start the development of a thick, highly vascular wall. As FSH secretions are reduced, the pituitary gland prepares for the surge of the **luteinizing hormone (LH)** required to accomplish ovulation.[13]

In the days immediately before ovulation, one of the primary follicles (called the *graafian follicle*) matures fully.

The other primary follicles degenerate and are absorbed by the body. The graafian follicle moves toward the surface of the ovary. When LH is released in massive quantities on about day 14, the graafian follicle bursts to release the fully mature ovum. The release of the ovum is called **ovulation.** Regardless of the overall length of a woman's cycle, ovulation occurs 14 days before her first day of menstrual flow.

The ovum is quickly captured by the fingerlike projections (*fimbriae*) of the fallopian tubes. In the upper third of the fallopian tubes, the ovum is capable of being fertilized in a 24- to 36-hour period. If the ovum is not fertilized by a sperm cell, it will begin to degenerate and eventually be absorbed by the body.

Postovulation Phase

After ovulation, the *postovulation phase* of the menstrual cycle starts when the remnants of the graafian follicle restructure themselves into a **corpus luteum.** The corpus luteum remains inside the ovary, secreting estrogen and a fourth hormone called *progesterone*. Progesterone, which literally means "for pregnancy," continues to direct the endometrial buildup. If pregnancy occurs, the corpus luteum monitors progesterone and estrogen levels throughout the pregnancy. If pregnancy does not occur, high levels of progesterone signal the pituitary to stop the release of LH and the corpus luteum starts to disintegrate on about day 24. When estrogen and progesterone levels diminish significantly by day 28, the endometrium is discharged from the uterus and out the vagina. The postovulation phase ends, and the cycle is complete.

Related Conditions

Premenstrual Syndrome (PMS)

PMS is characterized by psychological symptoms, such as depression, lethargy, irritability, and aggressiveness, or somatic symptoms, such as headache, backache, asthma, acne, and epilepsy, that recur in the same phase of each menstrual cycle, followed by a symptom-free phase in

---

Key Terms

luteinizing hormone (LH) (**loo** ten eye zing) a gonadotropic hormone of the female required for fullest development and release of ova; ovulating hormone.

ovulation the release of a mature egg from the ovary.

corpus luteum (kore pus **loo** tee um) cellular remnant of the graafian follicle after the release of an ovum.

Dealing with Menstrual Pain

I am a 24-year-old woman who has a great amount of menstrual pain. What can I do to lessen this pain?

The medical term is *dysmenorrhea,* but most women know it as menstrual cramps, and most women suffer from it at one time or another. Fortunately, the medical profession seems to be paying more attention to this problem, and various treatments are being studied. Currently, the most popular treatments still seem to be exercise and prostaglandin inhibitors.

The periodic cramps can occur before and during the menstrual phase, when the uterus must contract to remove the uterine lining. These contractions are produced by prostaglandin hormones normally found in the body. The problem occurs when the body produces an excess of one of the prostaglandin hormones, and the result is excessive cramping and pain. Thus prostaglandin-inhibiting medications can be used to reduce the body's production of prostaglandins and thereby reduce the intensity of cramping. Antiprostaglandin medications include ibuprofen, aspirin, and some prescription medications.

Before beginning treatment, however, the first step is to see a physician to rule out other causes of the dysmenorrhea. If other underlying causes are eliminated, consider the following treatment suggestions:

- Consume a well-balanced diet, with limited salt and sugar intake. Reduce spicy foods, and drink six to eight glasses of water per day.
- Consider taking aspirin, ibuprofen, other over-the-counter medications, or prescription medications, with your physician's guidance. Do not take aspirin if you are allergic to aspirin or have anemia, ulcers, or intestinal bleeding.
- Try taking a warm bath or placing a hot water bottle on your abdomen.

Try the following exercise routine that targets menstrual cramping.

- Lie face up with the legs and knees bent; perform abdominal breathing about 10 times. Feel the abdomen slowly inflate and then slowly fall.
- Stand and hold the back of a chair; lift one heel off the floor, then the other. Repeat 20 times.
- Lie on your back; lift and bring your knees to your chin; repeat 10 times.

Other treatments currently being explored include herbal remedies, acupuncture, transcutaneous electrical nerve stimulation, and microwave diathermy.

---

each cycle. Some of the more frequently reported symptoms of PMS include tension, tender breasts, fainting, fatigue, abdominal cramps, and weight gain.

The cause of PMS appears to be hormonal. Perhaps a woman's body is insensitive to a normal level of progesterone, or her ovaries fail to produce a normal amount of progesterone. These reasons seem plausible because PMS-type symptoms do not occur during pregnancy, during which natural progesterone levels are very high, and because women with PMS seem to feel much better after receiving high doses of natural progesterone in suppository form. When using oral contraceptives that supply synthetic progesterone at normal levels, many women report relief from some symptoms of PMS. However, the effectiveness of a common form of treatment, progesterone suppositories, is now being questioned (see the Changing for the Better box above).

Until the effectiveness of progesterone has been fully researched, the medical community is unlikely to treat PMS through any approach other than a relatively conservative treatment of symptoms with the use of analgesic drugs (including prostaglandin inhibitors), diuretic drugs, dietary modifications (including restriction of caffeine and salt), vitamin B_6 therapy, exercise, and stress-reduction exercises. The exact nature of PMS has been further complicated by the classification of severe PMS as a mental disturbance by some segments of the American Psychiatric Association.

Fibrocystic Breast Condition

In some women, particularly those who have never been pregnant, stimulation of the breast tissues by estrogen and progesterone during the menstrual cycle results in an unusually high degree of secretory activity by the cells lining the ducts. The fluid released by the secretory lining finds its way into the fibrous connective tissue areas in the lower half of the breast, where in pocketlike cysts the fluid presses against neighboring tissues. Excessive secretory activity produces in many women a fibrocystic breast condition characterized by swollen, firm, or hardened tender breast tissue before menstruation.

Recently, researchers have begun to describe the importance of a healthy diet in preventing fibrocystic breast condition, in particular a low-fat diet. Because physicians cannot be certain whether fibroadenomas (benign breast cysts) will ever develop into a full-blown malignancy of the breast, some researchers still prefer to refer to this condition as precancerous, and use such terms as *proliferative breast disease.* Women with more extensive fibrocystic conditions can be treated with drugs that have a "calming" effect on progesterone production. Occasional draining of cysts can bring relief.

Alternatives to Hormone Replacement Therapy

You will remember from Chapter 10 that recent studies now question the benefits of hormone replacement therapy (HRT) for postmenopausal women. For the past few decades, it was thought that HRT not only helped women find relief from the uncomfortable symptoms of menopause (hot flashes, night sweats, vaginal dryness, mood swings, and insomnia) but that HRT also helped protect women from osteoporosis, and most importantly, cardiovascular disease.

However, in the largest study of its kind to examine the impact of HRT (specifically the most popular estrogen-progestin combination) on women's health, the National Heart, Lung, and Blood Institute found that HRT actually *increased* the incidence of breast cancer, heart attacks, blood clots, and strokes. Although the increase was not large (for example, women taking hormones were less than a tenth of 1% more likely to have a heart attack), it was enough to have this aspect of the Women's Health Initiative stopped in 2002, 3 years before completion of the study.[1] More recently, additional analysis of the data found that the estrogen-progestin pills can cause an aggressive form of breast cancer to develop.[2] Furthermore, the combination pills can encourage the breast tissue to become more dense, thus making it more difficult for physicians to detect tumors when they develop.[2]

It appears that taking an estrogen-only pill does not have the impact on the development of breast cancer as much as the combined estrogen-progestin regimen. A 2003 study of 975 postmenopausal women taking various combinations of hormone replacement therapy indicated that women taking estrogen alone had no appreciable increase in breast cancer, even if they had been using estrogen for many years.[3] However, the estrogen-only approach is recommended for women who have had hysterectomies, since estrogen taken by itself seems to play a role in causing uterine cancer.

Since the 2002 report[1], many women have stopped taking the combined estrogen-progesterone pills for menopausal symptoms. For women who still want this form of HRT, physicians generally recommend they take the lowest dosage for the least amount of time. Thus, women might think in terms of taking HRT for 2 to 5 years, not for a lifetime.

Another consequence of the recent concern is the increased interest in alternative approaches to HRT. For concerns about osteoporosis, there are alternative prescription drugs that can be helpful including alendronate (Fosamax) or raloxifens (Evista). A diet that adds calcium-rich foods (dairy products, leafy green vegetables, and sardines) in combination with Vitamin D promotes bone density. Weight-bearing exercise, such as walking and weight lifting, encourages bone growth as well.

Hot flashes and night sweats result from changing estrogen levels and are, perhaps, the most challenging acute symptoms to control. However, reducing the intake of spicy foods, caffeine, and alcohol may help. Vitamin E and soy products help some women, and the use of certain herbs (especially black cohosh) is being studied. For some women, the use of a prescription antidepressant (such as Prozac or Paxil) may reduce hot flashes.

Vaginal dryness can be helped by the use of over-the-counter lubricants and moisturizers, vaginal estrogen creams, and regular sexual activity. Insomnia can be countered with the use of good sleeping patterns (consistent bedtime hour, a small glass of warm milk, reduced caffeine, alcohol, and food intake before bed). Cardiovascular concerns at menopause can be reduced by a healthy lifestyle that includes not smoking, consuming healthy foods, monitoring blood cholesterol levels, and getting regular exercise.

Interestingly, physical activity cuts across most of the issues related to menopause. Physical activity has been demonstrated to help sleep patterns, provide emotional balance, encourage mental acuity, and bolster cardiovascular functioning. Physical activity also makes many people feel better about their bodies and, thus, become potentially more interested in sexual activity that can help maintain vaginal lubrication.

[1] Writing Group for the Women's Health Initiative Investigators. Risks and benefits of estrogen plus progestin in healthy postmenopausal women: principal results from the Women's Health Initiative Randomized Controlled Trial. *Journal of the American Medical Association,* Vol 288: No 3 (July 17, 2002), 321–333.

[2] Chlebowski RT, et al. Influence of estrogen plus progestin on breast cancer and mammography in healthy postmenopausal women: the Women's Health Initiative Randomized Trial. *Journal of the American Medical Association,* Vol 289: No 24 (June 25, 2003), 3243–3253.

[3] Li CI, et al. Relationship between long durations and different regimens of hormone therapy and risk of breast cancer. *Journal of the American Medical Association,* Vol 289: No 24 (June 25, 2003), 3254–3263.

Amenorrhea

Amenorrhea is a condition characterized by the absence of menstruation. The lack of menstruation, if not caused by aging or pregnancy, is categorized as either primary or secondary amenorrhea.[9] *Primary amenorrhea* occurs when girls have passed the age of 16 and have never menstruated. Perhaps these girls have not yet reached a critical body weight (with the increased ratio of body fat) to trigger the menstrual cycle to begin. Additionally, some girls may have inherited a familial tendency to mature later than most of their peers. At an appropriate time for their bodies, these girls will start to menstruate. However, in cases where the primary amenorrhea is determined to be caused by hormonal deficiencies or abnormal body structure, hormone therapy can be quite useful.

> ### Key Terms
>
> **amenorrhea** the absence of menstruation.

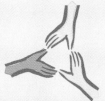
Secondary amenorrhea occurs when a previously menstruating woman ceases to menstruate. Likely reasons for secondary amenorrhea include pregnancy, breastfeeding, or the use of hormonal contraceptives. Less common reasons could be linked to unresolved stress, a reduction in body fat, hormonal irregularities, or serious athletic training. Other causes could be anorexia (see Chapter 6) or the female athlete syndrome (see Chapter 4). If a woman has not menstruated in 6 months and is not pregnant, not breastfeeding, and not using hormonal contraceptives, she should consult with her physician or medical care professional.[9]

Menopause

For the vast majority of women in their late forties through their mid-fifties, a gradual decline in reproductive system function, called *menopause*, occurs. Menopause is a normal physiological process, not a disease process. It can, however, become a health concern for some middle-aged women who have unpleasant side effects resulting from this natural ending of ovum production and menstruation.

As ovarian function and hormone production diminish, the hypothalamus, ovaries, uterus, and other estrogen-sensitive tissues must adjust. The extent of menopause as a health problem is determined by the degree to which **hot flashes,** night sweats, insomnia, vaginal wall dryness, depression and melancholy, breast changes, and the uncertainty of fertility are seen as problems.

Many of today's midlife women are likely to find menopause to be a relatively positive experience. The end of fertility, combined with children leaving home, makes the middle years a period of personal rediscovery for many women (see the Learning from Our Diversity box).

For women who are troubled by the changes brought about by menopause, physicians may prescribe **hormone replacement therapy (HRT).** This can relieve many

Key Terms

hot flashes unpleasant, temporary feelings of warmth experienced by women during and after menopause, caused by blood vessel dilation.

hormone replacement therapy (HRT) medically administered hormones to replace hormones lost as the result of menopause.

symptoms and offer benefits to help reduce the incidence of osteoporosis (see Chapters 4 and 5). However, HRT has recently been found to increase the risk of breast cancer and cardiovascular problems.[14,15] These concerns have caused many women to reconsider their use of HRT. The Star box on page 486 takes a closer look at HRT.

Additional Aspects of Human Sexuality

Earlier in this chapter, we identified the biological and psychosocial bases of our sexuality. In this section we explore three additional aspects of our sexuality—reproductive, genital, and expressionistic—around which many of our important decisions in life are made.* With these new perspectives in mind, you will be better able to see the complexity associated with our development as productive and satisfied beings.

Reproductive Sexuality

Of these three aspects of sexuality, *reproductive sexuality* reflects the most basic level of sexuality over which the adult must exercise discretion and display insight. Simply stated, reproductive sexuality is related to your knowledge of, desire for, and ability to participate in the act of *procreation.* Pregnancy, delivery, natural childbirth, breastfeeding, fertility control, and pregnancy termination are terms related to this dimension of sexuality. Demographic data indicate that most (but not all) of you will choose to be active in this dimension of your sexuality by becoming parents.

Genital Sexuality

Genital sexuality refers to the nonreproductive use of the reproductive organs. In comparison with the concept of reproductive sexuality, genital sexuality implies recreation and communication rather than procreation. The behaviors and meanings associated with the terms *orgasm, having sex, making love, oral-genital sex,* and *sexual responsiveness* are genital in their orientation.

In the most positive sense, sexual experiences that are genitally oriented should be sensual, erotic, and stimulating and should give the individual a sense of release. Genital sexuality reflects our gift to ourselves and to our partners as well. However, many forms of genital sexuality may not be condoned by certain groups of people or religions.

For some, genital sexuality can be a volatile experience. Far too frequently a genitally centered sexual experience results in an unanticipated and unwanted pregnancy.

---

*We cite no specific source for the terms *reproductive sexuality, genital sexuality,* and *expressionistic sexuality.* They are labels we and our colleagues use in instructional units associated with human sexuality.

In such circumstances the couple, or more often the female acting alone, is forced to make decisions that could significantly affect the future. An unexpected pregnancy, even for a relatively mature college person, may result in a series of compromises. In addition, the close association between genital sexuality and sexually transmitted diseases (including HIV infection) makes some sexual activities potentially dangerous.

For some people, genital sexuality becomes the mode of communication with which they feel most comfortable. In such cases, partners may know each other only in a very limited way. Growth in sexual technique may readily occur within the context of a genitally centered relationship, but

Discovering Your Spirituality

Sexuality as a Means of Spiritual Discovery

Few would argue that many of our expressions of sexuality are truly wonderful. For example, the enjoyment we can receive from a warm caress or an intimate kiss can be stimulating beyond imagination. The fact that our biological anatomy can function in ways that make us feel pleasure can be viewed as one of life's most rewarding gifts.

However, expressions of sexuality can extend beyond merely "feeling good." One's sexuality is an experience that encompasses the whole individual. It is much more than a biological act, a means of procreation, or an orgasmic release. While sexuality is all of these things, it also is a means of conveying intimacy to another person. Ultimately, sexuality is a form of intimate communication between two people. Through sexual expressions, one can convey feelings of love, devotion, caring, individuality, and openness. Of course, these feelings can also be communicated in nonsexual ways, but the depth of feelings that comes with sexual intimacy is especially powerful, and it is perhaps driven and enhanced by strong biological forces.

When sexuality is considered from this broader perspective, it can be viewed as a journey into personal understanding. This can evolve into a lifelong spiritual journey that constantly challenges one's values and stances on a variety of sexuality issues. In this spiritual journey, the brain, the body's most powerful sex organ, will play key roles. The brain will help one analyze feelings, moral and religious issues, relationship possibilities, and value stances. The brain will also serve to help one learn about sexual communication, sexual technique, and sexual pleasure.

As you read the sexuality material in this unit, you will see that sexuality encompasses the whole person, in a variety of ways and in a variety of circumstances. Sexual expression is much more than just "doing it." For those who think otherwise, remember that "People who are only interested in sex are probably not very interesting people." Look for the ways in which your sexuality is connected to other aspects of your life.

a fully developed relationship will not be formed. Genitally based relationships are rarely elevated to a much higher level.

Expressionistic Sexuality

Expressionistic sexuality represents the most broadly based dimension of yourself as a man or woman (see the Discovering Your Spirituality box on page 488). As the name implies, this is your expression of your current gender schema.

Cognitively, *affectively*, and behaviorally, you are playing out your initial adult gender identification. The way you dress, the occupation you pursue, and the leisure activities you develop are all aspects of this dimension of your sexuality.

Expressionistic sexuality encompasses the reproductive and genital dimensions of your sexuality, but it is more. It is the sexuality that will serve you most fully for the rest of your life. Most adults probably are conventional in their patterns of expressionistic sexuality, yet many people also express a variety of additional patterns (see Chapter 15).

Taking Charge of Your Health

- Take the Personal Assessment on page 493 to determine how traditional or nontraditional your attitudes are toward sexuality.
- If you wish to become more flexible and expand your social skills, identify ways in which you can increase your androgynous behavior. For example, learn to cook, expand your assertiveness skills, do volunteer work with children, join a club sports team, or learn how to invest in the stock market.
- Most college sexuality textbooks encourage readers to become familiar with their external reproductive "body parts." If you believe that this is important, study the illustrations in this chapter, locate

a handheld mirror, disrobe yourself, and identify these structures as best you can.
- If you are a woman who has a significant amount of menstrual pain, try some of the treatment suggestions in this chapter.
- If you are a man who is essentially "clueless" about the menstrual cycle and would like to understand it much better, study the information in this chapter. If you have a very close female friend and you wish to validate some of this information, ask her (diplomatically, of course) if you could get her "impressions" of this natural phenomenon.

Summary

- The biological basis of human sexuality includes genetic, gonadal, and structural components.
- The structural basis of sexuality begins as the male and female reproductive structures develop in the growing embryo and fetus. Structural sexuality changes as one moves through adolescence and later life.
- The psychosocial basis of human sexuality includes gender identity, gender preference, gender adoption, and initial adult gender identification.
- Androgyny is the blending of feminine and masculine qualities.
- The male and female reproductive structures are external and internal. The complex functioning of these structures is controlled by hormones.
- The menstrual cycle's primary functions are to produce ova and to develop a supportive environment for the fetus in the uterus.

- Endometriosis is a condition in which endometrial tissue that normally lines the uterus grows within the pelvic cavity, causing pain before and during menstruation and can lead to infertility.
- Fibrocystic breast condition is characterized by swollen, firm, or hardened tender breast tissue before menstruation.
- Hormone replacement therapy has benefits in treating the symptoms of menopause and of PMS but may carry risks for some women.
- Reproductive sexuality refers to aspects of sexuality related to procreation.
- Genital sexuality refers to the nonreproductive use of the reproductive organs.
- Expressionistic sexuality is the cognitive, affective, and behavioral expression of your gender.

Review Questions

1. Describe the following foundations of our biological sexuality: the genetic basis, the gonadal basis, and structural development.

2. Define and explain the following terms: gender identity, gender preference, gender adoption, and initial adult gender identification.

3. Define androgyny and explain its advantages.
4. Identify the major components of the male reproductive system. Trace the passageway for sperm.
5. Identify the major components of the female reproductive system. Trace the passageway for ova.
6. Identify and describe the four main hormones that control the menstrual cycle.
7. What are some of the nonpharmacologic techniques for reducing the symptoms of PMS?

8. What are the symptoms of fibrocystic breast condition and endometriosis?
9. Describe the difference between primary and secondary amenorrhea.
10. Name two circumstances in which hormone replacement therapy might be prescribed for women.
11. What is expressionistic sexuality?
12. What is genital sexuality?
13. What is reproductive sexuality?

References

1. Thibodeau GA, Patton KT. *Anatomy and physiology,* 5th ed. Mosby, 2003.
2. Sherwood L. *Human physiology: from cells to systems,* 5th ed. Brooks/Cole, 2004.
3. Hyde JS, DeLamater JD. *Understanding human sexuality,* 8th ed. McGraw-Hill, 2003.
4. Allgeier ER, Allgeier AR. *Sexual interactions,* 5th ed. Houghton Mifflin, 2000.
5. Crooks R, Baur K. *Our sexuality,* 8th ed. Wadsworth, 2001.
6. LeVay S, Valente, SM. *Human sexuality.* Sinauer Associates, Inc., 2003.
7. Kelly GF. *Sexuality today: the human perspective,* 7th ed. McGraw-Hill, 2004.
8. Masters WH, Johnson VE, Kolodny RC. *Human sexuality,* 5th ed. Addison Wesley, 1997.
9. Strong B, DeVault C, Sayad BW, Yarber WL. *Human sexuality: diversity in contemporary America,* 4th ed. McGraw-Hill, 2001.
10. Barclay L. *Unisex hormones?* WebMd Medical News Archive, (May 4, 2001) **www.webmd.com/content/article/32/1728_79051. htm,** accessed July 10, 2003.
11. Manos A. *FDA approves gel to treat low testosterone levels,* WebMd Medical News Archive, (March 2, 2000) **www.my.webmd.com/content/article/22/1728_55404.htm,** accessed July 10, 2003.
12. Greenberg JS, Bruess CE, Haffner DW. *Exploring the dimensions of human sexuality: 2002 update.* Jones and Bartlett, 2002.
13. Hatcher RA, et al. *Contraceptive technology,* 17th ed. Ardent Media, 1998.
14. Writing Group for the Women's Health Initiative Investigators. Risks and benefits of estrogen plus progestin in healthy postmenopausal women: principal results from the Women's Health Initiative Randomized Controlled Trial. *Journal of the American Medical Association,* Vol 288: No 3 (July 17, 2002), 321–333.
15. Hormone therapy is no heart helper. *Harvard Heart Letter,* Vol 13: No 2 (October 2002), 2–4.

As We Go to Press

Questions concerning "when life begins" have been debated for many years. This chapter has provided much technical information concerning the biological underpinnings of human life. *As we go to press,* President Bush just signed the April 2004 federal law called the Unborn Victims of Violence Act or UVVA. This law provides penalties for anyone convicted of harming a fetus while committing certain federal crimes, such as participating in a terrorist attack or a drug-related shooting.

The significance of this bill cannot be underestimated. In effect, the UVVA recognizes that a fertilized egg, embryo, or fetus has separate legal status from the pregnant woman. Opponents of this bill claim that its ultimate intention is to undermine the 1973 Supreme Court *Roe v. Wade* decision and elevate the legal status of a fetus to give it separate legal rights as a person. This recognition could eventually pave the way for a reversal of *Roe v. Wade.*

Proponents of the bill believe that an assault on a pregnant woman harms two victims and should result in two offenses against the perpetrator. It will be interesting to see how frequently federal prosecutors will attempt to enforce this law and whether its application will ever form the basis of an attempt to overthrow *Roe v. Wade.* What's your prediction about the impact of this new federal law?

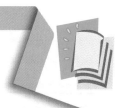

focus on

shifts in male sexuality

When Senator Bob Dole appeared on "Larry King Live" in late 1999 to discuss his prostate cancer operation, a groundbreaking conversation took place. The story goes that, during a commercial break, King asked his friend privately how he was dealing with one of the operation's grimmest side effects: impotence. Dole cheerfully replied there was a new drug, Viagra, that miraculously had cured the problem. When the talk-show host asked Dole if he would discuss it on the air, Dole said: Why not?[1]

A revolution was about to occur in our attitudes toward male sexual dysfunction and performance. Viagra flew through the paces of pop-culture acceptance. Leno and Letterman got a season of jokes off the subject. The media churned out stories about the drug. According to *The New York Times,* "There was Frank Bernardo, 70, who left his wife, declaring, 'It's time for me to be a stud again'; there was also Gen. Sani Abacha of Nigeria, who died in the midst of a Viagra-fueled encounter with two women in his magisterial bed."[1]

Most of the joking ended, however, after Viagra's sales surpassed $1 billion in the first year, and its maker, Pfizer, became the world's second-largest drug company. Although the drug's use has leveled off, almost 200,000 prescriptions are filled each week and 17 million Americans have tried the drug. The drug has been embraced at all social levels; Kmart and Wal-Mart have waged price wars selling the drug, and 4% of the total population of Palm Beach County have prescriptions.[1]

Already on its way to becoming one of the highest-selling new medications in history, Viagra has burst out of its original intended audience. Despite official pronouncements that it's meant only for men with erectile dysfunction, Viagra has

achieved a sort of cult status. Clubgoers use it as a recreational drug. Taking a couple of different rave drugs, for instance, Ecstasy or Special K, can kill the sex drive, and Viagra reportedly solves the problem.

Viagra also is popular in the gay subculture. "You have to realize that a lot of men come out of the closet when they are 30 or even 40, and then go nuts," says Eston Dunn, the health education coordinator for the Gay and Lesbian Community Center in Fort Lauderdale, Florida. "If you're heterosexual, you discover your sexuality at 15, and then you go nuts. That's why a lot of older gay men behave like 15-year-olds. In many ways, they really are 15, and a lot of them turn to Viagra to keep up with their own newfound enthusiasm." In the gay party scene, Dunn says, "you used to hear that cocaine lines were put out with straws. Now it's Viagra, like jelly beans in little candy dishes."[1]

Even nonimpotent heterosexual men are occasionally using the blue pill to make a good impression. Besides the stated effect of increasing blood flow to the penis and making it easier for a man to get and maintain an erection, Viagra also blocks the enzyme that deflates erections immediately after an orgasm, so users say the drug can lengthen intercourse and a man can have multiple orgasms. While Pfizer does not promote this cavalier use of the drug, the company has changed its ads from picturing 60-year-old guys to men who appear to be in their late 30s.

Viagra opened the door and legitimized the idea of enhancement drugs. In the summer of 2000, the media focused on another male sexual aid, AndroGel, a testosterone-replacement gel, which got American men thinking about their "T" levels. Patients taking testosterone supplements were said to be enjoying improved

libido and mood, bigger muscles, and stronger bones. Could testosterone gel be the next Viagra?

Some 55,000 prescriptions for AndroGel had been filled through November 2000, making it the most popular form of therapy for new testosterone-replacement patients.[2] The typical user is a man with low testosterone (hypogonadism). All men naturally experience a 1% annual decline in the hormone starting in their mid-30s so most users are in their 50s or older. Some 100,000 American males also have abnormally low testosterone levels.

The new development pioneered by Unimed, the Illinois-based distributor of AndroGel, is the convenient delivery system of the drug. Rather than receiving the hormone through a bulky scrotal patch or painful injections, the user can rub a clear, odorless gel on his abdomen or shoulder. Unlike Viagra (but like anabolic steroids or morphine), AndroGel is a controlled substance, so a physician will want to do blood tests to make sure the potential user is hypogonadal and then more blood tests to show he is free of preexisting conditions that might be exacerbated by the hormone. Finally, he would need to exhibit symptoms such as low sex drive or osteoporosis. Unlike Viagra, AndroGel isn't something you can just use for special occasions; you have to apply it every day to enjoy its benefits.

At least a dozen other drugs to treat male or female sexual performance problems are being developed by other companies. Not only will they be designed to improve the lives of those suffering from sexual disorders just now showing up in medical journals, but these drugs are expected to have an "enhancing" effect on normally functioning people.

Why now? Is science suddenly at a stage where researchers can find drugs for erectile dysfunction or other sexual performance enhancement? Medical experts say the emergence of a new class of drugs can have more to do with social changes than scientific discoveries. The emergence of a market for erectile dysfunction drugs is a classic example of how nonscientific forces can join to give new drugs an opportunity. For a long time the only treatments for sexual problems were for men, and they were primitive. Other than aphrodisiacs, there was only one solution for men with impotence: the penile implant, developed by urologists in 1973. Pfizer's great psychological breakthrough was in developing a treatment that didn't make the average person cringe in horror. In the short time since Viagra reached the market, the medical condition now known as erectile dysfunction has gone from a seldom-mentioned cause of embarrassment and misery to a billion-dollar industry.

The timing was right for Viagra in part because aging baby boomers are increasingly encountering the problem of erectile dysfunction, according to David F. Saks, the chief investment officer for Gruntal & Company's MedScience Fund. "There's a market out there," he says, that Viagra has not even begun to saturate. "The second, the third, the fourth drug will also have a market," he predicts.[3]

In addition, Pfizer paved the way for other drugs by running a sophisticated marketing campaign to make the erection problem a legitimate medical concern. "Part of that is giving them language that is not emotionally charged," says David

Brinkley, the worldwide team leader for Viagra at Pfizer. Pfizer insisted on calling the problem "erectile dysfunction" rather than "impotence." "'Erectile dysfunction' helps people feel more comfortable emotionally with it," says Mr. Brinkley. "It medicalizes the problem. It's not their fault anymore."[3]

What's next on the horizon? The pressure is on to improve something that was once an enjoyable side effect of procreation. Scientists, pharmaceutical companies, and physicians are racing to discover new and better drugs. Some are hormone treatments to restore desire and others are drugs to intensify the sensation of arousal. Researchers at the University of Edinburgh released a study in September 2000 saying that a hormonal male contraceptive has met with some success, raising the prospect that one day men will have access to a birth control method similar to the pill millions of women take. A testosterone "patch" is under development. And new Viagra-like medicines are currently in clinical trials, many also for women. Medical experts predict that female sexual dysfunction will soon cycle through the same paces as erectile dysfunction, leaving the term "frigidity" in the same wake as "impotence."

The real rush, though, is to create a drug to increase blood flow to the genitals that works simply—a pill or, even better, a quick-acting cream that is stabilized at room temperature so women can carry it in a purse like lipstick or men can toss it into a shaving kit.[1] The competition is intense, with blood flow drugs 1 to 5 years from market.

There are concerns that Viagra-type drugs will be misused like Prozac, as a Band-Aid approach to therapy, and that we may be treating the symptoms, not the problem. But as consumer demand for choice allows market forces to take more and more control of the health care industry, patients are redefining the purpose of "medicine." Rather than just being prevention oriented, we now want to enhance the average. The culture shift is perhaps that many average people have accepted the view that sex is an important part of good health, something to be enjoyed well into old age.

For Discussion . . .
How might sexual enhancement drugs cause us to rethink sex? Is the availability of Viagra over the Internet too much of a temptation for abuse of the drug? What do you think about the trend toward enhancement in sexual performance. Can this trend be compared to the personal enhancements that have come from the fields of cosmetic surgery (i.e., liposuction) or sports medicine (i.e., ergogenic aids)?

References
1. Hitt, J. The second sexual revolution. Magazine Desk, *The New York Times,* 20 February 2000.
2. Thornton, J. Testosterone supplements: not just for old guys anymore? *Men's Journal,* December 2000, pp. 81–84.
3. Kolata, G. Impotence is given another name, and a drug market grows. Health & Fitness, *The New York Times,* 18 April 2000.

personal assessment

sexual attitudes: a matter of feelings

Respond to each of the following statements by selecting a numbered response (1–5) that most accurately reflects your feelings. Circle the number of your selection. At the end of the questionnaire, total these numbers for use in interpreting your responses.

1 Agree strongly
2 Agree moderately
3 Uncertain
4 Disagree moderately
5 Disagree strongly

Men and women have greater differences than they have similarities. 1 2 3 4 5

Homosexuality and bisexuality are immoral and unnatural. 1 2 3 4 5

Our society is too sexually oriented. 1 2 3 4 5

Pornography encourages sexual promiscuity. 1 2 3 4 5

Children know far too much about sex. 1 2 3 4 5

Education about sexuality is solely the responsibility of the family. 1 2 3 4 5

Dating begins far too early in our society. 1 2 3 4 5

Sexual intimacy before marriage leads to emotional stress and damage to one's reputation. 1 2 3 4 5

Sexual availability is far too frequently the reason that people marry. 1 2 3 4 5

Reproduction is the most important reason for sexual intimacy during marriage. 1 2 3 4 5

Modern families are too small. 1 2 3 4 5

Family planning clinics should not receive public funds. 1 2 3 4 5

Contraception is the woman's responsibility. 1 2 3 4 5

Abortion is the murder of an innocent child. 1 2 3 4 5

Marriage has been weakened by the changing role of women in society. 1 2 3 4 5

Divorce is an unacceptable means of resolving marital difficulties. 1 2 3 4 5

Extramarital sexual intimacy will destroy a marriage. 1 2 3 4 5

Sexual abuse of a child does not generally occur unless the child encourages the adult. 1 2 3 4 5

Provocative behavior by the woman is a factor in almost every case of rape. 1 2 3 4 5

Reproduction is not a right but a privilege. 1 2 3 4 5

YOUR TOTAL POINTS_____

Interpretation

20–34 points   A very traditional attitude toward sexuality
35–54 points   A moderately traditional attitude toward sexuality
55–65 points   A rather ambivalent attitude toward sexuality
66–85 points   A moderately nontraditional attitude toward sexuality
86–100 points A very nontraditional attitude toward sexuality

To Carry This Further . . .

Were you surprised at your results? Compare your results with those of a roommate or close friend. How do you think your parents would score on this assessment?

chapter fifteen

Understanding sexual behavior and relationships

Online Learning Center Resources

www.mhhe.com/payne8e

Log on to our Online Learning Center (OLC) for access to these additional resources:

- Chapter key terms and definitions
- Learning objectives
- Student interactive question-and-answer sites

- Self-scoring chapter quiz
- Online assessments
- Key term flash cards

Talking It Over

Communicating Your Sexual Needs to Your Partner

For sexually active couples, communicating about sexual needs can be challenging. Start by being a good listener and supporting your partner's efforts at communication. Follow these guidelines:

- Ask nonthreatening, open-ended questions.
- Make your requests as specific as possible.
- Try not to be critical of your partner's shortcomings.

- Use sentences that start with "I" instead of "you."
- Choose a time to discuss your wishes and concerns that is separate from your sexual activities.

CommunicationLinks

www.goaskalice.columbia.edu
www.drdrew.com

Eye on the Media

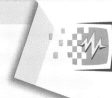

Advertising to Gays

An evolving form of advertising is currently being seen in the United States and abroad. This approach depicts gays and lesbians in positive ways (i.e., successful, attractive, happy); a far cry from historic, stereotypical views. What do these ads look like? Some ads might reflect couples whose relationship is one of sexual ambiguity. In many cases, the print ad or television commercial is so subtle that the sexual orientation implication is hidden.[1] Recently, however, especially on certain cable TV stations and in targeted print ads, the message is much more focused and direct.

To find out more about the blending of gay advertising into mainsteam media advertising, search the Web using "gay advertising" as key words. One site you will likely find is the website for The Commercial Closet

As we begin a new century and a new millennium, we have reached a greater understanding of the psychosocial factors that contribute to the complex expression of our sexuality. In this chapter, we explore human sexuality as it relates to the dynamic interplay of the psychosocial bases of sexual behavior and relationships. We begin by examining the human sexual response pattern.

The Human Sexual Response Pattern

Although history has many written and visual accounts of the human's ability to be sexually aroused, it was not until the pioneering work of Masters and Johnson[1] that the events associated with arousal were clinically documented. These researchers posed the following five questions, which gave direction to a series of studies involving the scientific evaluation of human sexual response.

Do the Sexual Responses of Men and Women Have a Predictable Pattern?

The answer to the first question posed by the researchers was an emphatic *yes.* A predictable sexual response pattern was identified;[1] it consists of an initial **excitement stage,** a **plateau stage,** an **orgasmic stage,** and a **resolution stage.** Each stage involves predictable changes in the structural characteristics and physiological function of reproductive and nonreproductive organs in both the male and female. These changes are shown in Figure 15-1.

Is the Sexual Response Pattern Stimuli-Specific?

The research of Masters and Johnson[1] clearly established a *no* answer to the second question concerning stimuli speci-ficity. Their findings demonstrated that several senses can supply the stimuli necessary for initiating the sexual response pattern. Although touching activities might initiate arousal in most people and maximize it for the vast majority of people, in both men and women, sight, smell, sound, and *vicariously formed stimuli* can also stimulate the same sexual arousal patterns.

What Differences Occur in the Sexual Response Pattern?

Differences Between Men and Women

In response to the third question, several differences are observable when comparing the sexual response patterns of men and women:

- With the exception of some late adolescent males, the vast majority of men are not multiorgasmic. The **refractory phase** of the resolution stage prevents

---

Key Terms

excitement stage initial arousal stage of the sexual response pattern.

plateau stage second stage of the sexual response pattern; a leveling off of arousal immediately before orgasm.

orgasmic stage third stage of the sexual response pattern; the stage during which neuromuscular tension is released.

resolution stage fourth stage of the sexual response pattern; the return of the body to a preexcitement state.

refractory phase that portion of the male's resolution stage during which sexual arousal cannot occur.

most men from experiencing more than one orgasm in a short time, even though sufficient stimulation is available.

- Women possess a **multiorgasmic capacity.** Masters and Johnson found that as many as 10% to 30% of all female adults routinely experience multiple orgasms.

- Although they possess multiorgasmic potential, some 10% of all women are *anorgasmic*— that is, they never experience an orgasm.[1] For many of these women, orgasms can be experienced when masturbation, rather than **coitus,** provides the stimulation.

- When measured during coitus, men reach orgasm far more quickly than do women. However, when masturbation is the source of stimulation, women reach orgasm as quickly as men.

More important than any of the differences pointed out is the finding that the sexual response patterns of men and women are far more alike than they are different. Not only do men and women experience the four basic stages of the response pattern, but they also have similar responses in specific areas, including the **erection** and *tumescence* of sexual structures; the appearance of a **sex flush;** the increase in cardiac output, blood pressure, and respiratory rate; and the occurrence of *rhythmic pelvic thrusting.*[1]

Differences Among Subjects Within a Same-Gender Group

When a group of subjects of the same gender was studied in an attempt to answer questions about similarities and differences in the sexual response pattern, Masters and Johnson noted considerable variation. Even when variables such as age, race, education, and general health were held constant, the extent and duration of virtually every stage of the response pattern varied.

Differences Within the Same Individual

For a given person the nature of the sexual response pattern does not remain constant, even when observed over a relatively short period. A variety of internal and external factors can alter this pattern. The aging process, changes in general health status, levels of stress, altered environmental settings, use of alcohol and other drugs, and behavioral changes in a sexual partner can cause one's own sexual response pattern to change from one sexual experience to another. Sexual performance difficulties and therapies are discussed in the Star box on page 500. For a discussion of aphrodisiacs, see the Considering Complementary Care box on page 501.

What Are the Basic Physiological Mechanisms Underlying the Sexual Response Pattern?

The basic mechanisms in the fourth question posed by Masters and Johnson are now well recognized. One factor, *vasocongestion,* or the retention of blood or fluid within a particular tissue, is critically important in the development of physiological changes that promote the sexual response pattern.[1] The presence of erectile tissue underlies the changes that can be noted in the penis, breasts, and scrotum of the male and the clitoris, breasts, and labia minora of the female.

A second mechanism now recognized as necessary for the development of the sexual response pattern is that of *myotonia,* or the buildup of neuromuscular tension within a variety of body structures.[2] At the end of the plateau stage of the response pattern, a sudden release of the accumulated neuromuscular tension gives rise to the rhythmic muscular contractions and pleasurable muscular spasms that constitute orgasm, as well as ejaculation in the male.[3]

What Role Is Played by Specific Organs and Organ Systems Within the Sexual Response Pattern?

The fifth question posed by Masters and Johnson, which concerns the role played by specific organs and organ systems during each stage of the response pattern, can be readily answered by referring to the material presented in Figure 15-1. As you study this figure, remember that direct stimulation of the penis and either direct or indirect stimulation of the clitoris are the principal avenues toward orgasm. Also, intercourse represents only one activity that can lead to orgasmic pleasure.[4]

Key Terms

multiorgasmic capacity potential to have several orgasms within a single period of sexual arousal.

coitus (**co** ih tus) penile-vaginal intercourse.

erection the engorgement of erectile tissue with blood; characteristic of the penis, clitoris, nipples, labia minora, and scrotum.

sex flush the reddish skin response that results from increasing sexual arousal.

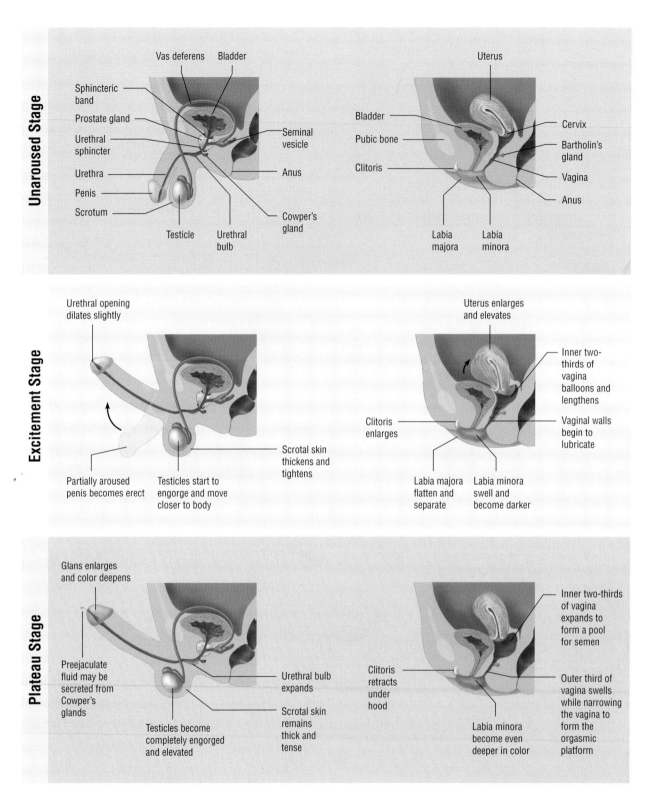

Figure 15-1 The sexual response pattern in men and women.

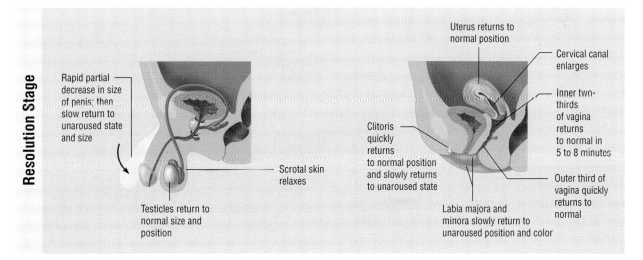

Orgasmic Stage

SENSATION OF ORGASM

Contractions occur in upper part of vas deferens

Prostatic portion of urethra fills with semen

Sphincteric band contracts

Urethral sphincter contracts

Seminal vesicle contracts

Urethral bulb expands further

Prostate gland contracts

Uterine contractions occur

Clitoris remains under hood

Contractions occur in anal sphincter

Contractions in outer third of the vagina occur rhythmically 3 to 15 times; the first of these contractions are spaced at 0.8-second intervals; later contractions are weaker and occur more slowly

EJACULATION

Semen is expelled; the first 2 or 3 contractions are strong and spaced 0.8 seconds apart

Sphincteric band remains contracted

Semen is released as urethral sphincter relaxes

Urethral bulb contracts

Pelvic floor muscles contract

BREAST CHANGES

① Unaroused stage

② Excitement stage
Breast size increases; nipples become erect; veins become more visible

③ Plateau and orgasmic stages
Breast size increases more; areola increases in size (making nipples appear less erect); skin color may become flushed from vasocongestion

Resolution Stage

Rapid partial decrease in size of penis; then slow return to unaroused state and size

Scrotal skin relaxes

Testicles return to normal size and position

Uterus returns to normal position

Cervical canal enlarges

Inner two-thirds of vagina returns to normal in 5 to 8 minutes

Clitoris quickly returns to normal position and slowly returns to unaroused state

Outer third of vagina quickly returns to normal

Labia majora and minora slowly return to unaroused position and color

Figure 15-1 *Continued*

Sexual Performance Difficulties and Therapies

For all of the predictability of the human sexual response pattern, many people find that at some point in their lives, they are no longer capable of responding sexually. The inability of a person to perform adequately is identified as a sexual difficulty or dysfunction. Sexual difficulties can have a negative influence on a person's sense of sexual satisfaction and on a partner's satisfaction. Fortunately, most sexual difficulties can be resolved through strategies that use individual, couple, or group counseling. Most sexual performance difficulties stem from psychogenic factors.

Difficulty	Possible Causes	Therapeutic Approaches
Women *Orgasmic Difficulties* Inability to have orgasm	Lack of knowledge about female responsiveness; inadequate sexual arousal; interpersonal problems with partner; anxiety, fear, guilt, anger, poor self-concept	Counseling to improve a couple's communication; educating a woman and her partner about female responsiveness; teaching a woman how to experience orgasm through masturbation
Vaginismus Painful, involuntary contractions of the vaginal muscles	Previous traumatic experiences with intercourse (rape, incest, uncaring partners); fear of pregnancy; religious prohibitions; anxiety about vaginal penetration of any kind (including tampons)	Counseling to alleviate psychogenic causes; gradual dilation of the vagina with woman's fingers or dilators; systematic desensitization exercises; relaxation training
Dyspareunia Painful intercourse	Insufficient sexual arousal; communication problems with partner; infections, inflammation; structural abnormalities; insufficient lubrication	Individual and couple counseling with a focus on relaxation and communication; medical strategies to reduce infections and structural abnormalities; additional lubrication
Men *Erectile Dysfunction* Inability to achieve an erection (impotence)	Chronic diseases (including diabetes, vascular problems, and chemical dependencies); trauma; numerous psychogenic factors (including anxiety, guilt, fear, poor self-concept)	Medical intervention (including possible vascular surgery, drugs, or the use of penile implants); couple counseling using sensate focusing, pleasuring, and relaxation strategies
Rapid Ejaculation Ejaculating too quickly after penile penetration; premature ejaculation	Predominantly psychogenic in origin; a man's need to prove his sexual prowess; anxiety associated with previous sexual experiences	Counseling to free the man from the anxiety associated with rapid ejaculation; altering coital position, masturbation before intimacy, use of the squeeze technique as orgasm approaches
Dyspareunia Painful intercourse	Primarily physical in origin; inability of the penile foreskin to retract fully; urogenital tract infections; scar tissue in seminal passageways; insufficient lubrication	Medical care to reduce infection or repair damaged or abnormal tissue; additional lubrication

Sexual Orientation

Sexual orientation refers to the direction in which people focus their sexual interests. People can be attracted to opposite-gender partners, same-gender partners, or partners of both genders.

Heterosexuality

Heterosexuality (or heterosexual orientation) refers to an attraction to opposite-gender partners. (*Heteros* is a Greek word that means "the other.") A heterosexual person is sometimes called *straight.* Throughout the world, this is the most common sexual orientation. For reasons related to species survival, heterosexuality has its most basic roots in the biological dimension of human sexuality. Beyond its biological roots, heterosexuality has significant cultural and religious support in virtually every country in the world. Worldwide, laws related to marriage, living arrangements, health benefits, child rearing, financial matters, sexual behavior, and inheritance generally support relationships that are heterosexual in nature. However, this may soon be changing (see the Focus On article on page 517).

Homosexuality

Homosexuality (or homosexual orientation) refers to an attraction to same-gender partners. The term *homosexuality* comes from the Greek word *homos,* meaning "same." The term *gay* can refer to males or females, while the word *lesbian* is used only in reference to females.[5]

The distinctions among the categories of sexual orientation are much less clear than their definitions might suggest. Most people probably fall somewhere along a continuum between exclusive heterosexuality and exclusive homosexuality. Kinsey in 1948 presented just such a continuum.[6]

Students often wonder "what makes a person gay?" This question has no simple answer. (College sexuality textbooks devote entire chapters to this topic.) Some research has pointed to differences in the sizes of certain brain structures as a possible biological or anatomical basis for homosexuality.[7] Other research proposes possible genetic, environmental, hormonal, or other foundations.

However, for sexual orientation in general, no single theory has emerged that fully explains this complex developmental process. The consensus of scientific opinion is that people do not choose their sexual orientation. Thus, being straight or being gay is something that "just happens." Most gays and lesbians report that no specific event "triggered" them into being gay. Many also indicate that they knew that their orientations were different from those of other children as far back as their prepuberty years.

Given the many challenges of being gay in a straight world, it would seem logical that gays and lesbians do not make conscious efforts to become gay. It is also highly unlikely that heterosexual persons actually choose to be straight. Sexual orientation is something that just unfolds. See the Discovering Your Spirituality box (page 502) for insight into some of the issues that gays and lesbians need to face.

Although operational definitions of sexual orientation may vary from researcher to researcher, Kinsey estimated that about 2% of American females and 4% of American males were exclusively homosexual.[6,8] More recent estimates place the overall combined figure at about 10% of the population. Clearly the expression of same-gender attraction is not uncommon.

TALKING POINTS How would you react if a close family member told you that he or she was gay? Could you be supportive or at least communicate your feelings without anger or criticism?

If you are openly gay, when you finally told your family and friends about your sexual orientation, a lot of things changed. But one thing probably stayed the same—you still feel like an outsider. Most of the couples holding hands on campus are young men and women. TV sitcoms are centered on heterosexual couples. They may include a gay character, but usually in a minor role. Popular magazines—through their ads, their features, their entire focus—are telling you how to be attractive to the opposite sex.

Being openly gay has probably made you wonder about some of the mixed messages you receive. The person who says it's OK that you're gay also seems to feel sorry for you—because you can't have a "normal" life and enjoy some of the things she does. Your mother makes remarks that suggest she still has hopes that someday you'll marry her best friend's son.

Feeling good about being gay in a straight world doesn't come easily. You've got to work at it. Start by finding support among your gay friends. Knowing that you're not alone is important—especially right after coming out. Realizing that other good, whole people are

gay helps to reinforce your self-esteem. Joining a campus gay organization is good for ongoing support, but don't limit yourself to that group. To grow as an individual, you also need to interact with and be part of heterosexual society.

Focus on what you value about yourself. Are you creative? Someone who gets things accomplished? A dependable friend? Think about the contributions you make—to your family, school, friends, church, and community. Remind yourself that you're a worthy person.

What do your friends appreciate about you? Do they value your advice? Like your sense of humor? Admire your courage? Think you're a strong leader?

Reinforcing the fact that you're a whole, worthy person is up to you. Listen to the "tapes" that are constantly playing in your head—both positive and negative. Edit out the negative thoughts, and turn up the volume on the positive ones. Take charge of what you think about yourself, rather than accepting what others think you are or should be.

Bisexuality

People who have the ability to be attracted to either gender are referred to as *bisexuals.* Bisexuals may fall into one of three groups: those who are (1) genuinely attracted to both genders, (2) gay but also feel the need to behave heterosexually, or (3) aroused physically by the same gender but attracted emotionally to the opposite gender. Some people participate in a bisexual lifestyle for extended periods, whereas others move quickly to a more exclusive orientation. The size of the bisexual population is not accurately known.[9] See the Learning from Our Diversity box (page 511) that describes some of the challenges for bisexual men and women.

Gender Identity Issues

Gender identity refers to the recognition of oneself as a male or female. As noted in Chapter 14, this recognition initially takes place within about eighteen months after birth. Most people then move through their lives, adopting many or all of the traditional gender roles for their biological sex. Most feel reasonably comfortable with who they are as a man or woman.

However, this typical pattern does not occur for everyone. Some individuals are not comfortable with their biological sex. They struggle with the issue of transsexualism. Other individuals are comfortable with their

gender identity, but find sexual pleasure from dressing in clothes that are more culturally "appropriate" for the opposite gender. These persons engage in transvestism.

Transsexualism

Transsexualism is an uncommon sexual variation in which a person rejects his or her biological sexuality. The male transsexual believes that he truly is a "woman trapped in a man's body." He desires to be the woman that he knows he is. Likewise, the female transsexual believes that she is a male existing in a woman's body. She desires to be the man that she knows she is. (It must be noted that sex therapists and psychiatrists do not view transsexuals as homosexual in their sexual orientation.)

For transsexuals, the periods of gender preference and gender adoption (see Chapter 14) are perplexing as they attempt, often with little success, to resolve the conflict between what their mind tells them is true and what their body displays. Adolescent and young adult transsexuals may cross-dress, undertake gay or lesbian relationships (which they view as heterosexual relationships), and

---

Key Terms

transsexualism a sexual variation in which a person rejects his or her biological sexuality.

experiment with hormone replacement therapy. Sometimes, transsexuals actively pursue a sex reassignment operation. Thousands of these surgeries have been performed at some of the leading medical centers in the United States. For more detailed information about transsexualism, including theories about the origins of transsexualism, you could consult a textbook used in college human sexuality courses or search the Internet for pertinent websites.

Transvestism

Public figures such as Dennis Rodman, Harvey Fierstein, and RuPaul have turned a spotlight on cross-dressing, or transvestism. The term **transvestism** is typically used to describe a heterosexual male who, from time to time, dresses as a woman. (Some gay men and women enjoy cross-dressing on occasion.) The practice of transvestism can range from simple sexual gratification from the wearing of feminine clothing, to the expression of the feminine side of the individual's personality. Although many transvestites wish to express the feminine aspects of their personality, most are satisfied with their gender role and their biological gender. Many are married and may or may not have shared this aspect of their personality with their partner.

One large study found that typical cross-dressers are virtually indistinguishable from non-cross-dressing men in their personality traits, sexuality, and measures of psychological wellness.[10]

Years ago, psychologists attempted to cure cross-dressers, but today most have recognized that cross-dressing is lifelong and that they can obtain better results by teaching the cross-dresser to accept his feminine side.

It is rare for a female to be a transvestite, perhaps because the norms for women's clothing are far less restrictive than those for men.[11] For example, while it might be quite normal to see your grandmother wearing a flannel shirt and bluejeans around the house, it would be surprising for you to see your grandfather watching NFL football wearing a frilly negligee.

Patterns of Sexual Behavior

Although sex researchers may see sexual behavior in terms of the human sexual response pattern just described, most people are more interested in the observable dimensions of sexual behavior.

Celibacy

Celibacy can be defined as the self-imposed avoidance of sexual intimacy. Celibacy is synonymous with sexual abstinence. People could choose not to have a sexually intimate relationship for many reasons. For some, celibacy is part of a religious doctrine. Others might be afraid of contracting a sexually transmitted disease. For most, however, celibacy is preferred simply because it seems appropriate for them. Celibate people can certainly have deep, intimate relationships with other people—just not sexual relationships. Celibacy may be short term or last a lifetime, and no identified physical or psychological complications appear to result from a celibate lifestyle.

 TALKING POINTS You have decided to remain celibate until you are ready to make a lifetime commitment to someone. How would you explain this to the person you are now dating?

Masturbation

Throughout recorded history, **masturbation** has been a primary method of achieving sexual pleasure. Through masturbation, people can explore their sexual response patterns. Traditionally, some societies and religious groups have condemned this behavior based on the belief that intercourse is the only "right" sexual behavior. With sufficient lubrication, masturbation cannot do physical harm. Today masturbation is considered by most sex therapists and researchers to be a normal source of self-pleasure.

Fantasy and Erotic Dreams

The brain is the most sensual organ in the body. In fact, many sexuality experts classify **sexual fantasies** and

---

Key Terms

transvestism atypical behavior in which a person derives sexual pleasure from dressing in the clothes of the opposite gender.

masturbation self-stimulation of the genitals.

sexual fantasies fantasies with sexual themes; sexual daydreams or imaginary events.

erotic dreams as forms of sexual behavior. Particularly for people whose verbal ability is highly developed, the ability to create imaginary scenes enriches other forms of sexual behavior.

Sexual fantasies are generally found in association with some second type of sexual behavior. When occurring before intercourse or masturbation, fantasies prepare a person for the behavior that will follow. As an example, fantasies experienced while reading a book may focus your attention on sexual activity that will occur later in the day.

When fantasies occur with another form of sexual behavior, the second behavior may be greatly enhanced by the supportive fantasy. Both women and men fantasize during foreplay and intercourse. Masturbation and fantasizing are inseparable activities.

Erotic dreams occur during sleep in both men and women. The association between these dreams and ejaculation resulting in a nocturnal emission (wet dream) is readily recognized in men. In women, erotic dreams can lead not only to vaginal lubrication but to orgasm as well.

Shared Touching

Virtually the entire body can be an erogenous zone when sensual contact between partners is involved. A soft, light touch, a slight application of pressure, the brushing back of a partner's hair, and gentle massage are all forms of communication that heighten sexual arousal.

Genital Contact

Two important purposes can be identified for the practice of stimulating a partner's genitals. The first is the tactile component of **foreplay.** Genital contact, in the form of holding, rubbing, stroking, or caressing, heightens arousal to a level that allows for progression into intercourse.

The second role of genital contact is that of *mutual masturbation to orgasm.* Stimulation of the genitals so that both partners have orgasm is a form of sexual behavior practiced by many people, as well as by couples during the late stage of a pregnancy. For couples not desiring pregnancy, the risk of conception is virtually eliminated when this becomes the form of sexual intimacy practiced.

As is the case in other aspects of intimacy, genital stimulation is best enhanced when partners can talk about their needs, expectations, and reservations. Practice and communication can shape this form of contact into a pleasure-giving approach to sexual intimacy.

Oral-Genital Stimulation

Oral-genital stimulation brings together two of the body's most erogenous areas: the genitalia and the mouth. Couples who engage in oral sex consistently report that this form of intimacy is highly satisfactory. Some people have experimented with oral sex and found it unacceptable, and some have never experienced this form of sexual intimacy. Some couples prefer not to participate in oral sex because they consider it immoral (according to religious doctrine), illegal (which it is in some states), or unhygienic (because of a partner's unclean genitals). Some couples may refrain because of the mistaken belief that oral sex is only for gays and lesbians. Regardless of the reason, a person who does not consider oral sex to be pleasurable should not be coerced into this behavior.

Because oral-genital stimulation can involve an exchange of body fluids, the risk of disease transmission is real. Small tears of mouth or genital tissue may allow transmission of disease-causing pathogens. Only couples who are absolutely certain that they are free from all sexually transmitted diseases (including HIV infection) can practice unprotected oral sex. Couples in doubt should refrain from oral-genital sex or carefully use a condom (on the male) or a latex square to cover the female's vulval area. Increasingly, latex squares (dental dams) can be obtained from drug stores or pharmacies. (Dentists may also provide you with dental dams, or you can make your own latex square by cutting a condom into an appropriate shape.)

Three basic forms of oral-genital stimulation are practiced by both heterosexual and homosexual couples.[12] **Fellatio,** in which the penis is kissed, licked, or sucked by the partner, is the most common of the three. **Cunnilingus,** in which the vulva of the female is kissed, licked, or penetrated by the partner's tongue, is only slightly less frequently practiced.

Mutual oral-genital stimulation, the third form of oral-genital stimulation, combines both fellatio and cunnilingus. When practiced by a heterosexual couple, the female partner performs fellatio on her partner while her male partner performs cunnilingus on her. Gay couples can practice mutual fellatio or cunnilingus.

Key Terms

erotic dreams dreams whose contents elicit a sexual response.

foreplay activities, often involving touching and caressing, that prepare individuals for sexual intercourse.

fellatio (feh **lay** she oh) oral stimulation of the penis.

cunnilingus (cun uh **ling** gus) oral stimulation of the vulva or clitoris.

Intercourse

Sexual intercourse (coitus) refers to the act of inserting the penis into the vagina. Intercourse is the sexual behavior that is most directly associated with **procreation.** For some, intercourse is the only natural and appropriate form of sexual intimacy.

The incidence and frequency of sexual intercourse is a much-studied topic. Information concerning the percentages of people who have engaged in intercourse is readily available in textbooks used in sexuality courses. Data concerning sexual intercourse among college students may be changing somewhat because of concerns about HIV infection and other STDs, but a reasonable estimate of the percentage of college students who have engaged in sexual intercourse is 60 to 75%.

These percentages reflect two important concepts about the sexual activity of college students. The first is that most college students are having intercourse. The second concept is that a large percentage (25% to 40%) of students are choosing to refrain from intercourse. Indeed, the belief that "everyone is doing it" may be a bit shortsighted. From a public health standpoint, we believe it is important to provide accurate health information to protect those who choose to have intercourse and to actively support a person's right to choose not to have intercourse.

Sexually active couples need to share their expectations concerning techniques and the desired frequency of intercourse.[13] Even the "performance" factors, such as depth of penetration, nature of body movements, tempo of activity, and timing of orgasm are increasingly important to many couples. Issues concerning sexually transmitted diseases (including HIV infection) are also critically important for couples who are contemplating intercourse. These factors also need to be explored through open communication.

A variety of books (including textbooks) provide written and visually explicit information on intercourse positions. Four basic positions for intercourse—*man above, woman above, side by side,* and *rear entry*—each offer relative advantages and disadvantages.

Anal Sexual Activity

Some couples practice **anal intercourse,** in which the penis is inserted into the rectum of a partner. Anal intercourse can be performed by both heterosexual couples and gay men. According to a year 2000 report in the journal *Archives of Sexual Behavior,* about 20 to 25% of college students have experienced anal intercourse.[14] The anal sphincter muscles contract tightly and tend to resist entry. Thus, couples who engage in anal intercourse must do so slowly, gently, and with adequate amounts of water-based lubricants. Because of the danger of tearing tissues in the rectal area, HIV transmission risk is increased if the inserting male is infected.[3] Unless it is absolutely certain that both partners are uninfected, the inserting male should always wear a condom. Even with a condom, disease transmission is possible, since during anal intercourse, condoms are more likely to tear than during penis-vaginal intercourse. Couples practicing anal sex must not follow anal insertion with insertion into the mouth or vagina because of the likelihood of transmitting infectious agents.

For many people, anal intercourse is not only unpleasant, but simply unnatural for humans. For others, the anal area is just another part of the human body that is especially sensitive to stimulation, and they enjoy the pleasurable sensations that come from intercourse or the insertion of a well-lubricated finger or sex toy. Some people enjoy kissing ("rimming") or touching in the anal area, but this should occur only when the anal area has been fully cleansed or covered with a sheet of protective plastic wrap. As with all sexual behavior, couples need to communicate clearly their feelings about any activity. If one partner is uncomfortable about an activity and wants to stop, his or her feelings must be supported by the other person. A desire for a particular sexual activity must not turn into sexual coercion or a sexual assault.

Until recently, thirteen states had laws on the books that banned **sodomy** (another term for anal sex as well as certain other sexual practices). However, a U.S. Supreme Court ruling *(Lawrence and Garner v Texas)* in June 2003 invalidated a Texas law that banned private consensual sex (in this case, sodomy) between adults of the same sex. Legal experts expected this Texas ruling to eventually invalidate the laws of the twelve other states that banned sodomy in one form or another.[15]

Secondary Virginity

Some individuals who have previously engaged in sexual intercourse have chosen to refrain from further sexual intercourse. They are said to be practicing **secondary virginity.** The practice of secondary virginity reflects a conscious choice for persons to wait until a time when they feel it's all right to resume intercourse.

Key Terms

procreation reproduction.

anal intercourse a sexual act in which the erect penis is inserted into the rectum of a partner.

sodomy generally refers to anal or oral sex; a legal term whose definition varies from state to state.

secondary virginity the discontinuation of sexual intercourse after initial exploration.

The decision to be a secondary virgin can be made for a number of reasons. Some prefer to return to abstinence for moral or religious reasons, while others wish to wait until there is more commitment in the relationship. Some come to the realization that they are not yet physically or emotionally ready for intercourse. Others do not want to risk pregnancy or the possibility of contracting a sexually transmitted disease. Some do not have the time or energy needed to become involved in a sexual relationship.

Those who choose secondary virginity are quick to point out its advantages. They no longer worry about certain risks, such as pregnancy or developing an STD. They no longer have to worry about the expense of contraception or the side effects from certain forms of birth control. Some feel great relief knowing that they are successfully following their own moral compass or religious beliefs. By pursuing secondary virginity, they can focus a great deal more time and energy on other important aspects of their relationship.

Sexuality and Aging

Students are often curious about how aging affects sexuality. This is understandable because we live in a society that idolizes youth and demands performance. Many younger people become anxious about growing older because of what they think will happen to their ability to express their sexuality. Interestingly, young adults are willing to accept other physical changes of aging (such as the slowing down of basal metabolism, reduced lung capacity, and even wrinkles) but not those changes related to sexuality.

Research shows that, although sexual activity does decline with age, the capacity to enjoy sex is not altered, and a significant proportion of older adults remain sexually active.[16]

As with other aspects of aging, certain anatomical and physiological changes will be evident, but these changes do not necessarily reduce the ability to enjoy sexual activity.[17] Most experts in sexuality report that many older people remain interested in sexual activity. Furthermore, those who are exposed to regular sexual activity throughout a lifetime report being most satisfied with their sex lives as older adults.[12]

As people age, the likelihood of alterations in the male and female sexual response cycles increases. In the postmenopausal woman, vaginal lubrication commonly begins more slowly, and the amount of lubrication usually diminishes. However, clitoral sensitivity and nipple erection remain the same as in earlier years. The female capacity for multiple orgasms remains the same, although the number of contractions that occur at orgasm typically is reduced.

In the older man, physical changes are also evident. This is thought to be caused by the decrease in the production of testosterone between the ages of 20 and 60 years. After age 60 or so, testosterone levels remain relatively steady. Thus many men, despite a decrease in sperm production, remain fertile into their eighties.[12] Older men typically take longer to achieve an erection (however, they are able to maintain their erection longer before ejaculation), have fewer muscular contractions at orgasm, and ejaculate less forcefully than they once did. The volume of seminal fluid ejaculated is typically less than in earlier years, and its consistency is somewhat thinner. The resolution phase is usually longer in older men. In spite of these gradual changes, some elderly men engage in sexual intercourse with the same frequency as do much younger men.

A significant proportion of older adults in nursing homes continue to be sexually active. Unfortunately, they face barriers such as a lack of privacy, chronic illness, lack of a willing partner, unsupportive attitudes of physicians and staff, feelings of unattractiveness, and a lack of knowledge about their own sexuality.[16]

Health care workers can help to remove these barriers by improving privacy, educating staff, arranging conjugal or home visits, encouraging several forms of sexual expression, and counseling interested patients.

Bonds Between People

As people develop their relationships, they often form bonds that start with friendship and dating activities and then move toward intimacy and love. Let's explore these stepping stones.

Friendship

One of the exciting aspects of college life is that you will probably meet many new people, some of whom will become your best friends. Because of your common experi-

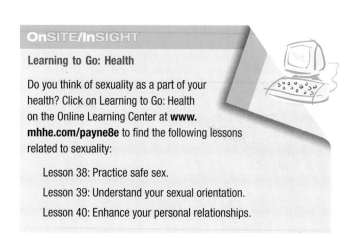

OnSITE/InSIGHT

Learning to Go: Health

Do you think of sexuality as a part of your health? Click on Learning to Go: Health on the Online Learning Center at **www.mhhe.com/payne8e** to find the following lessons related to sexuality:

Lesson 38: Practice safe sex.

Lesson 39: Understand your sexual orientation.

Lesson 40: Enhance your personal relationships.

Resolving Conflict Through Better Communication

Every relationship presents challenges to the individuals involved. Therapists would argue that couples who can learn to resolve conflict effectively have the best chance of maintaining long-term relationships. The hallmark of effective conflict resolution is that each person ends up feeling respected by his or her partner. Not surprisingly, this process is built on effective communication.

Here are some successful ways to communicate better to manage conflict:

- Show mutual respect. Remain calm.
- Identify and resolve the real issue.
- Be a good listener.
- Seek areas of agreement.
- Do not interrupt.
- Mutually participate in decision making.
- Be cooperative and specific.
- Focus on the present and future—not the past.
- Don't try to assign blame.
- Say what you are thinking and feeling.
- When talking, use sentences that begin with "I."
- Avoid using sentences that start with "You" or "Why."
- Set a time limit for discussing problems.
- Accept responsibility.
- Do something fun together.

ences, it is likely that you will keep in contact with a few of these friends for a lifetime. Close attachments to other people can have an important influence on all of the dimensions of your health.

What is it that draws friends together? With the exception of physical intimacy, many of the same growth experiences seen in dating and mate selection are also seen in the development of friendships. Think about how you and your best friend developed the relationship you now have. You probably became friends when you shared similar interests and experiences. Your friendship progressed (and even faltered at times) through personal gains or losses. In all likelihood, you cared about each other and learned to share your deepest beliefs and feelings. You cemented your bond by turning your beliefs into behaviors. You resolved conflicts (see Star box above).

Throughout the development of a deep friendship, the qualities of trust, tolerance, empathy, and support must be demonstrated. Otherwise the friendship can fall apart. You will soon note that the qualities seen in a friendship are very similar to the qualities noted in the upcoming description of companionate love (page 508). In both cases, people develop deep attachments through extensive familiarity and understanding.

Dating

A half-century ago, the events involved in a dating relationship were somewhat predictable. People met each other through their daily activities or groups of friends, and a formal request for a date was made. Ninety-nine times out of a hundred, the requestor was male and the invitee was female. After a period of formal and informal dates, the two made a commitment to steady dating or decided to "date around." If the relationship progressed, further commitments were made (for example, letter jackets, class rings, or other jewelry items were exchanged). After months or years of a committed relationship, the couple decided to get married. The man invariably asked for the woman's "hand" (after first receiving permission from her parents), and plans for a wedding ceremony were made.

Does this form of dating and mate selection exist as we move into the new millennium? For some couples, yes. The traditional way of dating and selecting a life partner works well for them. However, many young and midlife adults prefer a more flexible, less predictable format for dating and finding a person they might choose to marry. For example, more than ever, women are playing a more assertive role when it comes to initiating and establishing the ground rules for a relationship.

Interestingly, a large number of our students do not even like to use the word *dating* because it connotes a formalized pattern of behavior followed by their parents and grandparents. Many college students today seem to prefer "hanging out" with a group of 5 to 10 friends, instead of pairing off with a partner and doing only "couple activities."

When students do start to pair off and become exclusive in their dating, they tend to pursue a pattern called **serial monogamy.** In serial monogamy, a person dates one person exclusively until the relationship ends. Then another partner is found, and that couple dates exclusively for a period of time until that relationship eventually ends. In this pattern of dating, individuals do not date multiple people simultaneously. They go through mutually exclusive relationships, one after the other.

Students can fool themselves into believing that their dating patterns reflect **mutual monogamy.** Some couples

Key Terms

serial monogamy a pattern of dating in which a person is involved in a series of exclusive relationships, one after the other.

mutual monogamy a pattern of dating in which a person is involved exclusively with one partner.

believe that going out with another person as long as six months or a year reflects mutual monogamy. (Technically, for the six months or the year of going out, it can be called mutual monogamy.) When that relationship ends and a new one begins, however, the persons involved must understand that their dating pattern is developing into a serial pattern.

One critical health issue involved with serial monogamy is the increased possibility of exposure to infectious diseases, including all of the sexually transmitted diseases and HIV. While less risky than having indiscriminate sexual activities with multiple partners at the same time, serial monogamy still exposes a person to a new partner who may or may not be harboring a disease pathogen. Individuals who have a series of intimate relationships with multiple persons need to be especially vigilant in their safer sex practices. They need to understand clearly that their new partner could be exposing them to a rich pool of infectious diseases.

Intimacy

When most people hear the word **intimacy,** they immediately think about physical, sexual intimacy. However, sexuality experts and family therapists prefer to view intimacy more broadly, as any close, mutual, verbal or nonverbal behavior within a relationship. In this sense, intimate behavior can range from sharing deep feelings and experiences with a partner to sharing profound physical pleasures with a partner.

Intimacy is present in both love and friendship. You have likely shared intimate feelings with your closest friends, as well as with those you love. Intimacy helps us feel connected to others and allows us to feel the full measure of our own self-worth.

 TALKING POINTS Your teenage son equates intimacy with sex. How would you explain the emotional intimacy involved in marriage?

Love

Love may be one of the most elusive yet widely recognized concepts that describe some level of emotional attachment to another. Various forms of love include friendship and erotic, devotional, parental, and altruistic love. Other behavioral scientists[12] have focused primarily on two types of love most closely associated with dating and mate selection: *passionate love* and *companionate love.*

Passionate love, also described as romantic love or **infatuation,** is a state of extreme absorption in another. It is characterized by intense feelings of tenderness, elation, anxiety, sexual desire, and ecstasy. Often appearing early in a relationship, passionate love typically does not

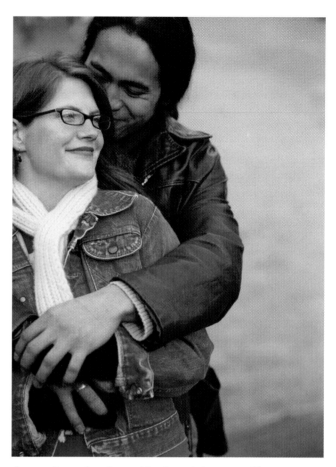

Companionate love is capable of sustaining mutual long-term growth.

last very long. Passionate love is driven by the excitement of being closely involved with a person whose character is not fully known.

If a relationship progresses, passionate love is gradually replaced by companionate love. This type of love is a less intense emotion than passionate love. It is characterized by friendly affection and a deep attachment that is based on extensive familiarity with the loved one.[12] This love is enduring and capable of sustaining long-term mutual growth. Central to companionate love are feelings of empathy for, support of, and toler-

Key Terms

intimacy any close, mutual, verbal or nonverbal behavior within a relationship.

infatuation an often shallow, intense attraction to another person.

ance of the partner. Complete the Personal Assessment on page 519 to determine whether you and your partner are truly compatible.

Relationships and Lifestyles

A variety of formal and informal relationships and lifestyles exist in our society. Here are a few of the most common ones.

Marriage

Just as there is no single best way for two people to move through dating and mate selection, marriage is an equally variable undertaking. In marriage, two people join their lives in a way that affirms each as an individual and both as a legal pair. They are able to resolve issues constructively (see the Changing for the Better box). However, for a large percentage of couples, the demands of marriage are too rigorous, confining, and demanding. They will find resolution for their dissatisfaction through divorce or extramarital affairs. For most, though, marriage will be an experience that alternates periods of happiness, productivity, and admiration with periods of frustration, unhappiness, and disillusionment with the partner. Each marriage is unique. Each marriage provides an opportunity for the partners to share a lifetime of experiences.[17]

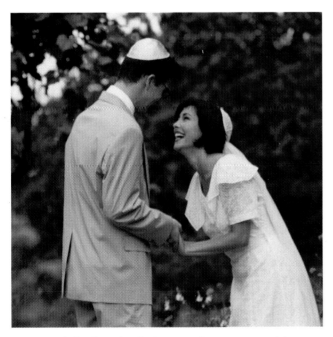

Recent statistics show that both men and women are waiting longer to get married.

Changing for the Better

Improving Marriage

Between working and taking classes, my wife and I both have heavy schedules. One thing that is not getting much attention is our relationship. What can we do to make our marriage better?

Few marital relationships are perfect. All marriages face occasional periods of strain or turmoil. Even marriages that do not exhibit major signs of distress can be improved, mostly through better communication. Marriage experts suggest that implementing some of these patterns can strengthen marriages:

- Problems that exist within the marriage should be brought into the open so that both partners become aware of the difficulties.
- Partners should balance the needs and expectations of each partner. They should make decisions jointly. Partners should support each other as much as they can. When one partner cannot actively support the other's goals, he or she should at least provide moral support and encouragement.
- Partners should establish realistic expectations. Partners should negotiate areas of disagreement. They should work together to determine how they will share resources.
- Participating in marriage counseling and marriage encounter groups can be helpful.

A sense of permanence helps sustain a marriage over the course of time. If the partners are convinced that their relationship can withstand difficult times, then they are more likely to take the time to make needed changes. Couples can develop a sense of permanence by implementing some of the patterns described above.

InfoLinks

www.competentcouples.com

As we move through the early years of this new century, we see certain trends in marriage. The most obvious of these is the age at first marriage. Today men are waiting longer than ever to marry. Now the average age at first marriage for men is 27 years.[18] In addition, these new husbands are better educated than in the past and are more likely to be established in their careers. Women are also waiting longer to get married and tend to be more educated and career oriented. Recent statistics indicate that the average age at first marriage for women is 25 years.[18]

Marriage still appeals to most adults. Currently, 76% of adults aged 18 and older are married, widowed, or divorced.[19] Thus about one-quarter of today's adults have not married. Within the last decade, the percentage of adults who have decided not to marry has nearly doubled.

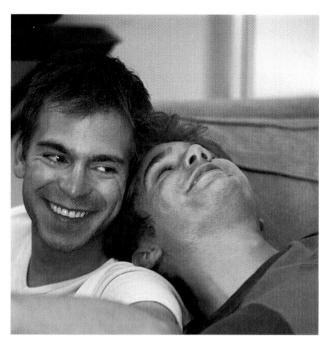

Legalization of same-sex marriage would grant gay couples a wide range of legal and economic rights.

Gay and Lesbian Partnerships

To believe that adult partnerships are reserved only for heterosexual couples is to avoid reality. In the United States and in many parts of the world, gays and lesbians are forming partnerships that, in many ways, mimic those of heterosexuals. It no longer is unusual to see same-sex men and women openly living together in one household. Gay and lesbian couples buy houses together and share property rights. As businesses restructure their employee benefits packages, gays and lesbians are covering their partners on health care plans and making them beneficiaries on their insurance policies and retirement plans.

A search of the literature will indicate that gay and lesbian partnerships have many of the same characteristics and problems of heterosexual couples.[3] Like straight couples, they struggle with interpersonal issues related to their relationship and their lifestyle. They work to decide how best to juggle their financial resources, their leisure time, and their friends and extended families. If they live together in an apartment or house, they must decide how to divide the household tasks.

If children are present in the household, they must be cared for and nurtured. These children could have come from an adoption, a previous heterosexual relationship, or, in the case of a lesbian couple, from artificial insemination. Research indicates that children raised in lesbian or gay families overwhelmingly grow up with a heterosexual orientation, and are like other children from heterosexual families in terms of their adjustment, mental health, social skills, and peer acceptance.[3]

One area in which gays and lesbians differ from heterosexual couples is in their ability to obtain a legal marriage. This inequity has been the focus of a national debate over same-sex marriage. For an extended discussion about same-sex marriage, turn to the Focus On article on page 517.

Forms of Marriage

To describe the nature of marital relationships, we use the classic categories of marital relationships proposed by Cuber and Harroff.[20] These marriage types should not be viewed as either good or bad. Rather, you should recognize one simple reality: These marriages are routinely found and apparently meet the needs of the individuals involved. Some of the types of marriages began in their current form. Others, however, evolved into their present form, having once been a very different type of marital relationship.

Conflict-Habituated Marriage

"We fought on our first date, our honeymoon was a disaster, and we've disagreed on everything of importance ever since." This frank description of a marital relationship characterized by confrontation, disagreement, and perhaps physical abuse reflects a *conflict-habituated marriage.* The central theme of this type of marital relationship is conflict, and its continuous presence suggests that the partners are making no attempt at resolution. Couples in long-term conflict-habituated marriages simply agree to disagree.

Devitalized Marriage

In the same way a dying person is said to possess failing signs, a *devitalized marriage* has lost its signs of life. Unlike the conflict-habituated marriage, which since its beginning was chronically impaired, the devitalized marriage was once a more active and satisfying marital relationship. However, the couple has lost its desire to keep the marriage dynamic.

The future of a devitalized marriage is difficult to predict. Some marriages of this type can be revitalized. Effective marriage counseling, a new job, or moving to a new community can rekindle a relationship. Other devitalized marriages are able to remain intact because one or both partners find vitality through an extramarital relationship. Some devitalized marriages persist at low levels of involvement and commitment with little hope for improvement. We would not be surprised if, for those of you who have witnessed the dissolution of your own or your parents' marriage, devitalization was an important factor in its ending.

Passive-Congenial Marriage

Passive means a low level of commitment or involvement, and the word *congenial* suggests warmth and friendliness. When these two words are combined as they are in

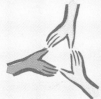
passive-congenial marriage, they describe perfectly the type of marital relationship sought by some couples.

For some of today's young professionals, the passive-congenial marriage offers a safe harbor from the rigors encountered in the competitive world of corporate business. Children may not be valued "commodities" in the passive-congenial marriage. The added financial and personal stressors related to child rearing could compromise an established lifestyle. You may be able to construct an image of a passive-congenial couple if you can picture two people meeting after work for a quiet dinner at a small restaurant, talking in muffled tones about their corporate battles, and planning their winter cruise.

Maintaining a passive-congenial marriage requires less time and energy than other forms of marriage. For two people who feel certain that their major contributions to society will be made through their efforts in the workplace, this marriage may be ideal. Certainly you may know many couples who are choosing this increasingly popular form of marriage.

Total Marriage

In the *total marriage,* little remains of the unique identities the two people had before their marriage took place. For reasons that are probably lost to the subconscious mind, two

people possessing individual personalities use marriage to fuse their identities into one identity—the total pair.

The total marriage requires that the individual partners set aside all aspirations for individual growth and development. Decisions are not made with "me" or even "you" as the center of attention. Rather, energies are directed toward what is best for "us." Life outside of the marital relationship and partner's presence does not exist, at least figuratively speaking. Eventually outsiders, when speaking about these individuals, can no longer truly speak about the man or the woman but are limited to speaking about the couple.

Vital Marriage

The *vital marriage* is intended to serve as an arena for the growth of both the individuals and the pair. The partners focus on "my growth," "your growth," and "our growth." In a vital marriage, personal goals may at times be subordinated for the good of the partner or the paired relationship. Yet both the partners (and the children) know that those once-subordinated goals will assume top priority when this becomes possible and desirable. The relationship has equality of opportunity.

In describing the vital marriage, we must point out that this type of marital relationship is not perfect, nor is

I have been with my boyfriend for nearly a year. We rarely argue, but we also rarely discuss our feelings, hopes, or dreams at any meaningful level. This is becoming a problem for me. What can I do to help improve our communication?

Developing a healthy intimate relationship is tough work, and it's okay to seek help and advice. Besides books and counselors, look around for the couples you know who seem to be happy with each other, who have the kind of relationship you want.

You probably learned your current communication skills as a child in your family. In functional families, the children learn to have conversations, express their feelings, solve problems, and ask for what they want.

Unfortunately, not all families have these skills, so if you would like to strengthen your relationship, or better prepare yourself for a relationship, consider the following communication tips:

- Admit to your partner that solving a problem is difficult, and if you are scared, say so.
- Understand that disagreement is healthy, and arguing between any two human beings in a relationship is inevitable. The *way* you disagree can be healthy or destructive.
- Listen to your partner's expression of feelings, not only about the current issue, but also about your partner's background. For example, your partner may be upset about an issue such as overspend-

ing, but also carry an undercurrent of fear that developed in a childhood of financial uncertainty.

- Do not interrupt or apologize too quickly. This can be a way of cutting off your partner. Do not assume that you know what your partner is thinking or feeling. Even if you are right, let your partner share his or her thoughts and feelings.
- Do not call your partner names or make broad, negative statements, even if you are very angry. Avoid broad indictments, such as "you always . . ." or "you are so . . ."
- Accept your partner's feelings and ideas. This does not necessarily mean you agree with them.
- Attempt to understand your partner's thoughts and feelings before you insist on being understood.
- If a discussion brings up intense feelings, and you have trouble sitting down and facing your partner, consider continuing the discussion during a brisk walk together.
- Sometimes you may be ready for a discussion, but your partner is not. But if your partner is never ready, you may have to reconsider his or her level of commitment.

InfoLinks

www.couples-place.com

---

it appropriate for all couples. In today's complex society, the vital marriage may be especially difficult to maintain (see the Changing for the Better box above).

Divorce

Marriages, like many other kinds of interpersonal relationships, can end. Today, marriages—relationships begun with the intent of permanence "until death do us part"—end through divorce nearly as frequently as not.

Why should approximately half of marital relationships end? Unfortunately, marriage experts cannot provide one clear answer to this question. Rather, they suggest that divorce is a reflection of unfulfilled expectations for marriage on the part of one or both partners, including the following:

- The belief that marriage will ease your need to deal with your own faults and that your failures can be shared by your partner
- The belief that marriage will change faults that you know exist in your partner
- The belief that the high level of romance of your dating and courtship period will be continued through marriage

- The belief that marriage can provide you with an arena for the development of your personal power, and that once married, you will not need to compromise with your partner
- The belief that your marital partner will be successful in meeting all of your needs

If these expectations seem to be ones you anticipate through marriage, then you may find that disappointments will abound. To varying degrees, marriage is a partnership that requires much cooperation and compromise. Marriage can be complicated. Because of the high expectations that many people hold for marriage, the termination of marriage can be an emotionally difficult process to undertake (see the Changing for the Better box on page 513).

The American attitude toward divorce swung like a pendulum during the last century. Divorce has gone from being an embarrassing, painful ordeal, to a common, relatively simple legal procedure. More recently, some observers have begun to question the wisdom of no-fault divorce.

Our society is concerned about the well-being of children whose parents divorce. Different factors, however, influence the extent to which divorce affects children. Included among these factors are the gender and age of the children, custody arrangements, financial support, and the remarriage of one or both parents. Many children must adjust to accept their new status as a member of a blended family.

Singlehood

For many people, being single is a lifestyle that affords the potential for pursuing intimacy, if desired, and provides an uncluttered path for independence and self-directedness. Other people, however, are single because of divorce, separation, death, or the absence of an opportunity to establish a partnership. The U.S. Bureau of the Census indicates that 42% of women and 38% of men over the age of 18 are currently single.[19]

Single people can have many different living arrangements. Some single people live alone and choose not to share a household. Other arrangements for singles include cohabitation, periodic cohabitation, singlehood during the week and cohabitation on the weekends or during vacations, or the platonic sharing of a household with others. For young adults, large percentages of single men and women live with their parents.

Like living arrangements, the sexual intimacy patterns of singles are individually tailored. Some singles practice celibacy, others pursue intimate relationships in a **monogamous** pattern, and others have multiple partners. As in all interpersonal relationships, including marriage, the levels of commitment are as variable as the people involved.

Cohabitation

Cohabitation, or the sharing of living quarters by unmarried people, represents yet another alternative to marriage. According to the U.S. Bureau of the Census, the number of unmarried, opposite-gender couples living together tripled between 1980 and 2000, from 1.6 million couples to over 4.8 million couples.[19] The number of reported same gender couples totaled nearly 600,000 in the year 2000.

Although cohabitation may seem to imply a vision of sexual intimacy between male and female roommates, several forms of shared living arrangements can be viewed as cohabitation. For some couples, cohabitation is only a part-time arrangement for weekends, during summer vacation, or on a variable schedule. In addition, **platonic** cohabitation can exist when a couple shares living quarters

Key Terms

monogamous (mo **nog** a mus) paired relationship with one partner.

cohabitation sharing of a residence by unrelated, unmarried people; living together.

platonic close association between two people that does not include a sexual relationship.

but does so without establishing an intimate relationship. Close friends, people of retirement age, and gay couples might all be included in a group called cohabitants.

How well do cohabitation arrangements fare against marriage partnerships in terms of long-term stability? A recent 2002 report prepared by the CDC's National Center for Health Statistics[21] indicated that unmarried cohabitations are generally less stable than marriages. The probability of a first marriage ending in separation or divorce within 5 years was found to be 20%, but the probability of a premarital cohabitation breaking up within 5 years was 49%. After 10 years, the probability of a first marriage ending was 33%, compared to 62% for cohabitations.

Single Parenthood

Unmarried young women continue to become pregnant and then become single parents in this country. There is also a significantly different form of single parenthood: the planned entry into single parenthood by older, better educated people, the vast majority of whom are women.

In contrast to the teenaged girl who becomes a single parent through an unwed pregnancy, the more mature woman who desires single parenting has usually planned carefully for the experience. She has explored several important concerns, including questions regarding how she will become pregnant (with or without the knowledge of a male partner or through artificial insemination), the need for a father figure for the child, the effect of single parenting on her social life, and, of course, its effect on her career development. When these questions have been resolved, no legal barriers stand in the way of her becoming a single parent.

A very large number of women and a growing number of men are actively participating in single parenthood as a result of a divorce settlement or separation agreement involving sole or joint custody of children. Increasing numbers of single persons are now adopting children. In the year 2000, single women headed up 7.6 million households with children under the age of 18. In contrast, single men headed up 1.8 million households in the year 2000 with children under age 18.[19]

Communication in Relationships

You may have noticed that one of the recurring messages in this chapter is the importance of effective communication between partners in a relationship. At the beginning of the chapter, you read about communicating sexual needs to a partner in the Talking It Over box on page 495. You saw the Star box (page 507) on resolving conflict through better communication. You also probably noticed the Changing for the Better boxes that discussed how to improve marriage (page 509), communication as the key to relationships (page 512), and how to cope with a breakup (page 513). Each of these behavior change boxes emphasized the value of effective communication. Furthermore, the chapter sections on friendship, dating, intimacy, love, and marriage become meaningless unless you realize that true satisfaction in these areas is grounded in effective communication.

When you think about it, effective communication is the basis for *all healthy relationships*. For this reason, we encourage all readers to take advantage of available opportunities to learn effective communication skills. You might find these opportunities in college courses that you select. Most speech and communication departments have courses in personal communication skills. Look for pertinent courses in psychology and counseling psychology departments. Most colleges and universities also offer one or more human sexuality courses in their psychology, sociology, or health science departments. The counseling center on your campus may offer programs that can improve your communication skills. Finally, your campus library or bookstore will have popular books that may be very useful.

 Taking Charge of Your Health

- Take the Personal Assessment on page 519 to learn how compatible you and your partner are.
- If being around someone whose sexual orientation is different from yours makes you feel uncomfortable, focus on getting to know that person better as an individual.
- If you are in an unhealthy relationship, take the first step toward getting out of it through professional counseling or group support.

- If you are in a sexual relationship, communicate your sexual needs to your partner clearly. Encourage him or her to do the same so that you can have a satisfying sex life.
- Consider whether your lifetime plan will include singlehood, marriage, cohabitation, single parenthood, or a gay partnership. Evaluate your current plan in relation to that plan.

Summary

- Men and women share the four stages of sexual response: excitement, plateau, orgasm, and resolution.
- Several senses can supply the stimuli necessary for initiating the sexual response pattern.
- Some differences have been shown in the sexual response patterns of men and women.
- Direct stimulation of the penis and direct or indirect stimulation of the clitoris are the principle avenues toward orgasm.
- The three sexual orientations are heterosexuality, homosexuality, and bisexuality.
- Celibacy is the self-imposed avoidance of sexual intimacy.
- Most sex therapists and researchers consider masturbation to be a normal source of self-pleasure.
- Shared touching, genital contact, oral-genital stimulation, and intercourse are common forms of sexual intimacy.
- Physiological changes may alter the way in which some older people perform sexually.
- The dating process has become more flexible and less formal and predictable during recent decades. Many young adults practice serial monogamy.

- Passionate love is gradually replaced by companionate love, which is characterized by deep affection and attachment.
- Communication skills are important in starting and maintaining a relationship.
- Intimacy is any close, mutual, verbal or nonverbal behavior within a relationship.
- Forms of marriage include conflict-habituated marriage, devitalized marriage, passive-congenial marriage, total marriage, and vital marriage.
- Although the legality of gay and lesbian marriages continues to be debated, committed relationships between members of the same sex often mimic the dynamics of heterosexual marriages.
- Although most people marry at some time in their lives, other relationships and lifestyles exist, including singlehood, cohabitation, and single parenthood.
- Many people enter marriage with unrealistic expectations, including the idea that they will no longer have to deal with their own faults.
- Most relationships can be improved through better communication.

Review Questions

1. What similarities and differences exist between the sexual response patterns of males and females? Do both women and men experience vasocongestion and myotonia?
2. Explain the differences between heterosexuality, homosexuality, and bisexuality. How common is each of these sexual orientations in our society?
3. Explain the difference between a person who is a transsexual and a person who is a transvestite.
4. Define celibacy, masturbation, sexual fantasies, erotic dreams, shared touching, genital contact, oral-genital stimulation, and sexual intercourse.
5. What precautions must be considered if a couple decides to engage in anal sexual activity?
6. Approximately what percentage of today's college students report having had sexual intercourse?

7. Identify the physiological changes that occur in men and women as they get older.
8. In what ways has advertising to gays become mainstream?
9. Identify and describe the five forms of marriage presented in this chapter.
10. What is meant by serial monogamy? What is meant by secondary virginity?
11. What are some differences between passionate love and companionate love?
12. In what ways do gay and lesbian partnerships differ from heterosexual partnerships?
13. Discuss current trends in the areas of singlehood, cohabitation, and single parenthood.
14. Describe the current status of the controversy over same-sex marriages?

References

1. Masters WH, Johnson VE. *Human sexual response.* Lippincott, Williams and Wilkins, 1966.
2. Strong B, DeVault C, Sayad BW, Yarber, WL. *Human sexuality: diversity in contemporary America,* 4th ed. McGraw-Hill, 2001.
3. Hyde JS, DeLamater JD. *Understanding human sexuality,* 8th ed. McGraw-Hill, 2003.
4. Bruess CE, Haffner DW, Greenberg JS. *Exploring the dimensions of human sexuality, 2002 update.* Jones and Bartlett, 2002.

5. Kelly GF. *Sexuality today: the human perspective,* 7th ed. McGraw-Hill, 2004.

6. Kinsey AC, Pomeroy WB, Martin CE. *Sexual behavior in the human male,* reprint edition. Indiana University Press, 1998.

7. Allen LS, Gorski RA. Sexual orientation and the size of the anterior commissure in the human brain. *Pract Nat Acad Sci USA* 89(15):7199–7202, 1992.

8. Kinsey AC, et al. *Sexual behavior in the human female,* reprint edition. Indiana University Press, 1998.

9. Masters WH, Johnson VE, Kolodny RC. *Human sexuality,* 5th ed. Addison-Wesley, 1997.

10. Brown GR, et al. Personality characteristics and sexual functioning of 188 crossdressing men. *J Nervous Mental Dis* 184(5):265–273, 1996.

11. Allgeier ER, Allgeier AR. *Sexual interactions,* 5th ed. Houghton Mifflin, 2000.

12. Crooks RL, Baur K. *Our sexuality,* 8th ed. Wadsworth, 2001.

13. LeVay S, Valente SM. *Human sexuality.* Sinauer Associates, 2002.

14. Baldwin JI, Baldwin JD. Heterosexual anal intercourse: an understudied, high-risk sexual behavior. *Archives of Sexual Behavior* 29(4), 357–373, 2000.

15. *Supreme Court strikes down Texas sodomy law,* **www.us.cnn.com/2003/LAW/06/26/scotus.sodomy/index/html,** 27 June 2003, accessed 22 July 2003.

16. Richardson JP, Lazur A. Sexuality in the nursing home patient (review). *Am Family Phys* 51(1): 121–124, 1995.

17. McAnulty RD, Burnette MM. *Exploring human sexuality: making healthy decisions,* Pearson, Allyn and Bacon, 2002.

18. Fields J, Casper LM. America's families and living arrangements: March 2000. *Current Population Reports* (U.S. Census Bureau), P20-537, p.9, 2001.

19. U.S. Bureau of the Census. *Statistical abstract of the United States: 2002,* ed. 122, U.S. Government Printing Office, 2002.

20. Cuber J, Harroff P. *Sex and the significant Americans.* Penguin Books, 1965.

21. Bramlett MD, Mosher WD. *Cohabitation, marriage, divorce, and remarriage in the United States.* U.S. Centers for Disease Control and Prevention, National Center for Health Statistics, Vital Health Statistics, 23(22), 2002.

As We Go to Press

As we go to press in the Spring of 2004, the marketing and sales of three oral prescription drugs to treat impotence is reaching a fever pitch. The oldest drug Viagra (Pfizer Pharmaceuticals) came on the market in 1998 and now has sales of over $1 billion annually. A second drug Levitra (GlaxoSmithKline) was approved by the Food and Drug Administration in early 2003. The newest drug Cialis (Eli Lilly & Co.) came to the market in early 2004, and was first nationally advertised during the January 2004 Super Bowl football game.

All three drugs act on an enzyme that helps relax small muscles in the penis and increase the flow of blood into the erectile chambers. Sexual stimulation is required for each of the drugs to work. The difference in the drugs is how long the drug works and how quickly it produces the erection. Reportedly, Viagra produces effects that last for about 4 hours, Levitra works for about 5 hours, and Cialis works for up to 36 hours. Viagra can work in as quickly as 30 minutes, Levitra in about 15 minutes, and Cialis around 30 minutes or more.

In the near future, be on the lookout for the development of prescription drugs that can enhance sexual performance in women. Pharmaceutical companies stand to reap tremendous sales with effective drugs in this area.

gay and lesbian unions: how close is our society to same-sex marriages?

What is the definition of a marriage? Must the marriage partners be only a man and a woman? Would allowing same-sex marriages weaken our society? Or would it make for a stronger society that is capable of recognizing commitments that legally bond men with men and women with women? These questions are being debated now on a scale that could not have been predicted even 5 years ago.

Same-sex marriages would grant gay couples an array of legal and economic benefits, including joint parental custody, insurance and health benefits, joint tax returns, alimony and child support, inheritance of property, hospital visitation rights, family leave, and a spouse's Social Security and retirement benefits.

Same-sex unions have been debated for many years. Some U.S. clergy were presiding over gay "marriages" in the 1980s, and hundreds of companies, businesses, associations and universities now offer benefits to same-sex partners of employees. Gay publications debated the subject in the 1950s. In his book *Same-Sex Unions in Premodern Europe,* the late John Boswell, a Yale University historian, suggested that ancient marriage ceremonies provide evidence that Greeks and medieval Christians celebrated same-sex relationships.[1]

The year 2000 became a defining year in the debate over same-sex marriages. In April 2000, the Vermont legislature passed the nation's first "civil union" law, which granted legal status to gay and lesbian couples. The law was signed into effect on July 1, 2000. By October 2000, the Health Department in Vermont had registered over 800 civil unions, with three-quarters of the couples coming from out-of-state.[2] This trend has continued since the law has been in effect. By the summer of 2003, 85% of Vermont's civil unions were granted to out-of-state couples.[3]

The law permits same-sex couples to obtain civil union licenses from the town clerk, similar to the way opposite-sex couples obtain marriage licenses. A judge, justice of the peace, or clergy member certifies the civil unions. Divorces between civil union partners are called "dissolutions" and are handled in family court, similar to opposite-sex divorces.[4]

Vermont's law confers on same-sex couples all the benefits that the state presently allows heterosexual married couples. However, Vermont's law does not affect federal programs, such as Social Security. Additionally, civil unions that take place in Vermont are not generally recognized by other states. In fact thirty-seven states and the federal government have passed laws that deny the recognition of gay and lesbian marriages. These laws are called Defense of Marriage Acts (DOMAs) and define marriage as the union of one man with one woman.[5]

By the summer of 2003, legal issues concerning same-sex marriage were making weekly headlines, not just in America, but in countries the world over. After the Canadian provinces of British Columbia and Ontario passed laws permitting same-sex marriage in June, the Canadian federal government put forth national legislation that was expected to make same-sex marriages available in all of Canada sometime in 2004.[6] If this were to happen, Canada would be following the path set by Germany (in 2001),[7] Holland (in 2001), and Belgium (in January 2003).[8]

In the United States, a State Supreme Court ruling in Massachusetts was expected in late summer 2003 in a case *(Goodridge v Department of Public Health)* in which seven gay and lesbian couples sued to have Massachusetts expand the definition of marriage to include same-sex couples. Another same-sex marriage suit was pending in New Jersey. While efforts to promote same-sex marriages in Hawaii and Alaska were unsuccessful, the California legislature was in the process of broadening the definition of domestic partnerships to include committed gay and lesbian couples. Such legislation, if passed, would grant to same-sex couples about one-third of the "rights, privileges, and obligations that the state automatically grants to married couples."[8]

Opponents of same-sex marriage were concerned that a June 2003 U.S. Supreme Court ruling *(Lawrence and Garner v Texas)* which struck down a Texas sodomy law banning private consensual sex between same-sex adults would open the door, eventually, for gay and lesbian marriages. The ruling effectively overturned similar sodomy laws that were still on the books in twelve other states.[9] At the time of this writing, efforts were underway among some members of the U.S. Congress to draft a constitutional amendment banning gay marriage. While President Bush was somewhat reluctant to support such an amendment, he did "support the notion that marriage is between a man and a woman."[10]

The July 2003 release of a Vatican document calling for Catholic politicians worldwide to oppose same-sex unions and marriages further added to the explosive nature of this debate. Political observers believe that this issue will be highly prominent in the 2004 political elections in the United States, perhaps on a par with issues involving the economy, foreign policy, and military capability. Indeed, politicians can expect to be asked where they stand on the issue of same-sex marriages.

Activists on both sides of this issue believe that this may be the greatest gay rights debate in history. Where do you stand on this issue? Should gay partners be granted the same legal right to marriage as heterosexual couples, or do you believe that legal marriage should be limited to its traditional definition of a union between a man and a woman?

References:

1. Boswell J. *Same-sex unions in pre-modern Europe,* reprint ed. Vintage Books, 1994.
2. *Civil unions are legal in Vermont.* **www.gaycivilunions.com**, accessed 2 December 2000.
3. Grossman J. *Will other states recognize Vermont's civil unions?* **www.cnn.com/2003/law/05/20/findlaw.analysis.grossman.civilunions.txt/**, 20 May 2003, accessed 22 July 2003.
4. *The Vermont Guide to Civil Unions.* **www.sec.state.vt.us/pubs/civilunions.html**, accessed 2 December 2000.
5. *FRC ready to respond to historic 'gay marriage' decision in Massachusetts,* media advisory, Family Research Council, **www.frc.org.org/?I=PR03G03**, 10 July 2003, accessed 22 July 2003.
6. Schneider B. *Canada acts on same-sex marriages,* **www.cnn.com/2003/allpolitics/06/20/ip.pol.opinion.canada.marriages/index.html**, 20 June 2003, accessed 22 July 2003.
7. *German gay marriage law backed,* **www.cnn.com/2002/world/europe/07/17/germany.marriage/index.html**, 17 July 2002, accessed 22 July 2003.
8. *Overview: same-sex marriages,* **www.religioustolerance.com/hom_marr.htm**, accessed 22 July 2003.
9. *Supreme Court strikes down Texas sodomy law,* **www.cnn.com/2003/law/06/26/scotus.sodomy/index.html**, 27 June 2003, accessed 22 July 2003.
10. *Bush uncertain about gay marriage ban,* **www.cnn.com/2003/allpolitics/07/02/bush.gay/index.html**, 2 July 2003, accessed 22 July 2003.

personal assessment

how compatible are you?

This quiz will help test how compatible you and your partner's personalities are. You should each rate the truth of these twenty statements based on the following scale. Circle the number that reflects your feelings. Total your scores and check the interpretation following the quiz.

1 Never true
2 Sometimes true
3 Frequently true
4 Always true

We can communicate our innermost thoughts effectively.	1	2	3	4
We trust each other.	1	2	3	4
We agree on whose needs come first.	1	2	3	4
We have realistic expectations of each other and of ourselves.	1	2	3	4
Individual growth is important within our relationship.	1	2	3	4
We will go on as a couple even if our partner doesn't change.	1	2	3	4
Our personal problems are discussed with each other first.	1	2	3	4
We both do our best to compromise.	1	2	3	4
We usually fight fairly.	1	2	3	4
We try not to be rigid or unyielding.	1	2	3	4
We keep any needs to be "perfect" in proper perspective.	1	2	3	4
We can balance the desires to be sociable and the need to be alone.	1	2	3	4
We both make friends and keep them.	1	2	3	4
Neither of us stays down or up for long periods.	1	2	3	4
We can tolerate the other's mood without being affected by it.	1	2	3	4
We can deal with disappointment and disillusionment.	1	2	3	4
Both of us can tolerate failure.	1	2	3	4
We can both express anger appropriately.	1	2	3	4
We are both assertive when necessary.	1	2	3	4
We agree on how our personal surroundings are kept.	1	2	3	4

YOUR TOTAL POINTS _____

Interpretation

20–35 points   You and your partner seem quite incompatible. Professional help may open your lines of communication.

36–55 points   You probably need more awareness and compromise.

56–70 points   You are highly compatible. However, be aware of the areas where you can improve.

71–80 points   Your relationship is very fulfilling.

To Carry This Further . . .

Ask your partner to take this test too. You may have a one-sided view of a "perfect" relationship. Even if you scored high on this assessment, be aware of areas where you can still improve.

chapter sixteen

managing your fertility

Chapter Objectives

Upon completing this chapter, you should be able to:

▌ explain the difference between the terms *birth control* and *contraception.*

▌ define the *theoretical effectiveness* and the *use effectiveness* of contraceptive methods and why they differ.

▌ discuss the advantages and disadvantages of each form of birth control.

▌ describe the four methods of periodic abstinence.

▌ explain how a woman can determine the days in which she is most fertile.

▌ identify the many ways in which contraceptive hormones can be delivered to females.

▌ differentiate between the combined oral contraceptive pill and the minipill.

▌ identify the circumstances under which emergency contraception might be used.

▌ identify and explain the procedures that produce male and female sterilization.

▌ understand which abortion procedures are used in each trimester of pregnancy.

Online Learning Center Resources

www.mhhe.com/payne8e

Log on to our Online Learning Center (OLC) for access to these additional resources:

- Chapter key terms and definitions
- Learning objectives
- Student interactive question-and-answer sites
- Self-scoring chapter quiz
- Online assessments
- Key term flash cards

Talking It Over

Choosing a Childless Lifestyle

There are many reasons a couple may choose not to have children. Here are some of the advantages and disadvantages:

Pros:

- more time for travel or work
- spontaneity remains possible
- uninterrupted privacy and intimacy
- easier to leave a bad relationship
- no contribution to overpopulation
- no worries of raising a child in a dangerous world
- less financial burden

Cons:

- possible regret over decision in the future
- feelings of selfishness and guilt

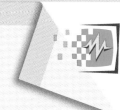

- no child/parent intimacy
- aloneness in old age
- no heirs
- no grandchildren for you or your parents
- loss of friends your own age who are parents

Can you think of other reasons for choosing to remain childless?

CommunicationLinks

www.now2000.com/cbc
www.avsc.org
www.nokidding.bc.ca

Eye on the Media

Information Online—Birth Control and Sexuality

The Internet offers a number of resources for locating information about contraception, birth control, and related topics. Planned Parenthood Federation of America provides one of the most comprehensive sites at **www.plannedparenthood.org.** Here you can find a wide selection of pamphlets, books, newsletters, and videotapes, as well as links to other websites.

If you're looking for birth control information, click on Planned Parenthood's "Frequently Asked Questions," "Fact Sheets,"

"Sexual Health Glossary," and "Links." Some of the frequently asked questions are:

- Am I pregnant?
- What can I do if I am pregnant?
- Do I have a sexually transmitted disease?
- What are the laws in my state about teens' access to abortion services and birth control?
- How can I get access to birth control?

Of course, answers follow each of these questions. Planned Parenthood believes that when people are empowered with knowledge, they are better able to make sound decisions about their health and sexuality.

The "Fact Sheets" option at Planned Parenthood's website provides various reports on specific topics, such as abortion, birth control, family planning, sexually transmitted diseases, and teen pregnancy and abortion. The "Sexual Health Glossary" is a listing of hundreds of terms related to sexuality. The "Links" option lists twenty-four topical categories, each one displaying links to related websites.

Three additional online sites offer reliable information about sexuality and reproductive choices. The first is the Alan Guttmacher Institute website at **www.agi-usa.org.** This institute is dedicated to protecting the reproductive choices of women and men throughout the world. It fulfills its mission by disseminating information and the results of scientific research on the subject. The Guttmacher Institute's menu of options includes abortion, law and public policy, pregnancy and birth, prevention and contraception, sexual behavior, and sexually transmitted diseases and youth.

The American Social Health Association's website is **www.ashastd.org.** This organization is dedicated to stopping the spread of sexually transmitted diseases. ASHA operates a network of national hotlines that answers over 2 million calls each year. The website's menu offers selections on sexually transmitted diseases, frequently asked questions, a sexual health glossary, and support groups.

The Sex Information and Education Council of the United States is a nonprofit organization dedicated to developing, collecting, and disseminating information about sexuality. SIECUS has its website at **www.siecus.org.** This organization promotes comprehensive sexuality education and advocates the right of individuals to make responsible sexual choices. SIECUS publishes and distributes thousands of pamphlets, booklets, and bibliographies each year to professionals and the general public.

If you wish to search for information about certain sexuality topics from a pro-life perspective, you might wish to examine the website for The Ultimate Pro-life Resource List at **www.prolifeinfo.org.** This site is supported by the non-profit Women and Children First organization. The Ultimate Pro-life Resource List provides links to information related to abortion alternatives, Roe *v.* Wade, euthanasia and assisted suicide, pregnancy help, pro-life news, and pro-life organizations.

How you decide to control your fertility will have an important effect on your future. Your understanding of information and issues related to fertility control will help you make responsible decisions in this complex area.

In the beginning of this chapter, we discuss the difference between birth control and contraception and introduce the concept of contraceptive effectiveness rates. We also take a look at why people use birth control. Then we discuss in detail the many birth control methods available today.

Birth Control versus Contraception

Any discussion about the control of your **fertility** should start with an explanation of the subtle differences between the terms **birth control** and **contraception.** These terms reflect different perspectives about fertility control. *Birth control* is an umbrella term that refers to all of the procedures you might use to prevent the birth of a child. Birth control includes all available contraceptive measures, as well as sterilization, use of the intrauterine device (IUD), and abortion procedures.

Contraception is a much more specific term for any procedure used to prevent the fertilization of an ovum.

Contraceptive measures vary widely in the mechanisms they use to accomplish this task. They also vary considerably in their method of use and their rate of success in preventing conception. A few examples of contraceptive methods are the use of condoms, oral contraceptives, spermicides, and diaphragms.

Beyond the methods mentioned, certain forms of sexual behavior not involving intercourse could be considered forms of contraception. For example, mutual masturbation by couples virtually eliminates the possibility of pregnancy. This practice, as well as additional forms of sexual expression other than intercourse (such as kissing, touching, and massage), has been given the generic

---

> **Key Terms**
>
> **fertility** the ability to reproduce.
>
> **birth control** all of the methods and procedures that can prevent the birth of a child.
>
> **contraception** any method or procedure that prevents fertilization.

There's More to Sex Than You Thought . . .

Are you ready for sex? If you're not sure, take time to think it over. If you start having sex before you're ready, you might feel guilty. You might feel bad because you realize this step isn't right for you now. Or your religious upbringing may make you feel as though you're doing something wrong. You also may not be ready for the emotional aspects of a sexual relationship. Most important, you will probably have difficulty handling the complexities of an unplanned pregnancy or a sexually transmitted disease.

If you do feel ready for sex, you still have a choice. Sex may be OK for you now. It may be personally fulfilling, something that enhances your self-esteem. Alternatively, you can choose to abstain from sex until later—another way of enhancing your self-esteem. You'll feel empowered by making the decision for yourself, rather than doing what is expected. Being strong enough to say "no" can also make you feel good about yourself. For some, making this decison may reflect a renewed commitment to spiritual or religious concerns.

If you're married, sex is a good way of connecting as a couple. It's something that the two of you alone share. It's a time to give special attention to each other—taking a break from the kids, your jobs, and your other responsibilities. It's a way of saying: "This relationship is important—it's something I value."

Going through a pregnancy together is another opportunity for closeness. From the moment you know that you're going to be parents, you're connected in a new way. Your focus becomes the expected child. You'll watch the fetus grow on ultrasound, go to parenting and Lamaze classes together, visit the doctor together, mark the various milestones, and share new emotions. When your child is born, you'll be connected as never before.

Whether you're thinking about starting to have sex, making the decision to wait, or examining the sexual life you have now, you can't ignore the possibilities and the consequences. Is the time right for you? Are you doing this for yourself or for someone else? What do you think you will gain from waiting? Do you expect your future partner to also have made the decision to wait? What do you expect to get from a sexual relationship—pleasure, intimacy, love? What do you expect to give? Do you want an emotional commitment? Do you view sex and love as inseparable? Do you understand how sex can enhance your spirituality? Taking time to consider these questions can make you feel good about yourself—no matter what you decide.

term **outercourse.** Outercourse protects against unplanned pregnancy and may also significantly reduce the transmission of sexually transmitted diseases, including HIV infection (see the Discovering Your Spirituality box above).

Reasons for Choosing to Use Birth Control

People use birth control for many reasons. Many career-minded individuals carefully plan the timing and spacing of children to best provide for their children's financial support without sacrificing their job status. Others choose methods of birth control to ensure that they will never have children. Some use birth control methods to permit safe participation in a wide variety of sexual behaviors. Fear of contracting a sexually transmitted disease prompts some people to use particular forms of birth control (see the Changing for the Better box on page 524).

Financial and legal considerations can be significant factors in the choice of certain birth control methods. Many people must of necessity take the cost of a method into account when selecting appropriate birth control. The cost of sterilization and abortion can prohibit some low-income people from choosing these alternatives, especially because federal funds do not support such procedures. A number of states have established statutes and policies that make contraceptive information and medical services relatively difficult to obtain.

Another important consideration in the use of birth control methods is the availability of professional services. An example of the effect of this factor may be the selection of birth control methods by college students. Some colleges and universities provide contraceptive services through their student health centers. Students enrolled in these schools have easy access to low-cost, comprehensive contraceptive services. Students enrolled in colleges that do not provide such complete services may find that access to accurate information and clinical services is difficult to obtain and that private professional services are expensive.

For many people, religious doctrine will be a factor in their selection of a birth control method. One example is the opposition of the Roman Catholic Church and other religious groups to the use of contraception other than natural family planning.

Key Terms

outercourse sexual activity that does not involve intercourse.

I have a new girlfriend and I think we are moving closer and closer to having sex. I know we should talk about birth control and disease prevention, but I don't know how to start. What should I do?

If you believe there is even a chance you will engage in any kind of sex, or if you think your partner may pursue sex with you, you should be prepared and discuss the possibility before being swept along by the heat of an encounter. In addition, you and your partner will feel more comfortable about your relationship and your sexual activity if you first discuss your feelings about contraception, disease prevention, and pregnancy. Consider the following topics:

- First, the fact that you are discussing contraception together does not necessarily mean that you will engage in sex. In addition, you can discuss abstinence as a very effective form of contraception.
- Discussing contraception and disease prevention with your partner is not rude. It is simply common sense.
- Talking about contraception is a way of sharing responsibility and intimacy. It can bring you closer.
- Which type(s) of contraception will you use? See the section below, Selecting Your Contraceptive Method, for help in making your choices.
- If you feel unsure about how to broach the subject or are undecided about any of the issues, consider discussing the subject with a

counselor or physician before you talk with your partner.

- Sort out your own feelings and understand all the alternatives, including their advantages and disadvantages, before you open the discussion.
- Pick the right occasion. Don't wait until you have begun sexual activity.
- Both partners have dignity and worth, and should be treated with dignity. If you and your boyfriend or girlfriend are discussing contraception and you have different views, you each have the right to your opinions. If necessary, you can agree to disagree.
- Listen carefully and ask questions. Speak honestly about your own feelings and beliefs.
- Who will pay for the contraceptive method? Will both partners share the cost?
- What will both of you do if the female partner becomes pregnant?

Have you discussed these issues in the past before initiating sex with a partner? Do you plan to discuss these issues in the future?

InfoLinks

www.arhp.org/success

Theoretical Effectiveness versus Use Effectiveness

People considering the use of a contraceptive method need to understand the difference between the two effectiveness rates given for each form of contraception. *Theoretical effectiveness* is a measure of a contraceptive method's ability to prevent a pregnancy when the method is used precisely as directed during every act of intercourse. *Use effectiveness,* however, refers to the effectiveness of a method in preventing conception when used by the general public. Use effectiveness rates take into account factors that lower effectiveness below that based on "perfect" use. Failure to follow proper instructions, illness of the user, forgetfulness, physician (or pharmacist) error, and a subconscious desire to experience risk or even pregnancy are a few of the factors that can lower the effectiveness of even the most theoretically effective contraceptive technique.

Effectiveness rates are often expressed as the percentage of women users of childbearing age who do not become pregnant while using the method for one year. For some methods the theoretical-effectiveness and use-

effectiveness rates are vastly different; the theoretical rate is always higher than the use rate. Table 16.1 presents data concerning effectiveness rates, advantages, and disadvantages of many birth control methods.

Selecting Your Contraceptive Method

In this section, we discuss some of the many factors that should be important to you as you consider selecting a contraceptive method. Completing the Personal Assessment on page 549 will help you make this decision.

Those who wish to exercise a large measure of control over their fertility can consider the following:

- It should be safe.
- It should be effective.
- It should be reliable.
- It should be reversible.
- It should be affordable.
- It should be easy to use.
- It should not interfere with sexual expression.

Table 16.1 Effectiveness Rates of Birth Control for 100 Women during 1 Year of Use

| Method | Estimated Effectiveness | | Advantages | Disadvantages |
	Theoretical	Use		
No method (chance)	15%	15%	Inexpensive	Totally ineffective
Withdrawal	96%	81%	No supplies or advance preparation needed; no side effects; men share responsibility for family planning	Interferes with coitus; very difficult to use effectively; women must trust men to withdraw as orgasm approaches
Periodic abstinence Calendar Basal body temperature Cervical mucus method Symptothermal	91%–99%	75%	No supplies needed; no side effects; men share responsibility for family planning; women learn about their bodies	Difficult to use, especially if menstrual cycles are irregular, as is common in young women; abstinence may be necessary for long periods; lengthy instruction and ongoing counseling may be needed
Cervical cap (no prior births)	91%	80%	No health risks; helps protect against some STDs and cervical cancer	Limited availability in some areas
Spermicide (gel, foam, suppository, film)	94%	74%	No health risks; helps protect against some STDs; can be used with condoms to increase effectiveness considerably	Must be inserted 5 to 30 minutes before coitus; effective for only 30 to 60 minutes; some concern about nonoxynol-9
Diaphragm with spermicide	94%	80%	No health risks; helps protect against some STDs and cervical cancer	Must be inserted with jelly or foam before every act of coitus and left in place for at least 6 hours after coitus; must be fitted by health care personnel; some women may find it awkward or embarrassing to use; some concern about nonoxynol-9
Male condom Male condom with spermicide	97% 99%	86% 95%	Easy to use; inexpensive and easy to obtain; no health risks; very effective protection against some STDs; men share responsibility for family planning	Must be put on just before coitus; some men and women complain of decreased sensation; some concern about nonoxynol-9
Female condom	95%	79%	Relatively easy to use; no prescription required; polyurethane is stronger than latex;	Contraceptive effectiveness and STD protection not as high as with male condom; couples may

continued

TALKING POINTS The method of birth control your partner prefers doesn't allow for spontaneous sex. How would you explain that this decreases your enjoyment?

Current Birth Control Methods

Abstinence

Abstinence as a form of birth control has gained attention recently on college campuses. This method is as close to 100 percent effective as possible. There have been isolated reports in medical literature of pregnancy without sexual intercourse, usually involving ejaculation by the male near the woman's vagina. Avoiding this situation should raise the effectiveness of abstinence to 100 percent.

Abstinence as a form of birth control has additional advantages in that it gives nearly 100 percent protection from sexually transmitted diseases, it is free, and it does not require a visit to a physician.

You can contract sexually transmitted diseases by other intercourse practices. A very common method is through oral sex with someone who has a cut, a fever blister, or a cold sore. Any sexual contact with an infected person makes transmission of STDs possible.

Withdrawal

Withdrawal, or **coitus interruptus,** is the contraceptive practice in which the erect penis is removed from the vagina just before ejaculation of semen. Theoretically this procedure prevents sperm from entering the deeper structures of

Key Terms

coitus interruptus (withdrawal) (**co** ih tus in ter rup tus) a contraceptive practice in which the erect penis is removed from the vagina before ejaculation.

Table 16.1 Effectiveness Rates of Birth Control for 100 Women during 1 Year of Use *continued*

Method	Estimated Effectiveness		Advantages	Disadvantages
	Theoretical	Use		
			provides some STD protection; silicone-based lubrication provided; useful when male will not use a condom	be unfamiliar with a device that extends outside the vagina; more expensive than male condoms
IUD ParaGard Progestasert Mirena	99%+ 98% 99%+	99% 98% n/a	Easy to use; highly effective in preventing pregnancy; does not interfere with coitus; repeated action not needed	May increase risk of pelvic inflammatory disease (PID) and infertility in women with more than one sexual partner; not usually recommended for women who have never had a child; must be inserted by health care personnel; may cause heavy bleeding and pain in some women
Combined pill (estrogen-progestin) Minipill (progestin only)	99%+ 99%+	95% 95%	Easy to use; highly effective in preventing pregnancy; does not interfere with coitus; regulates menstrual cycle; reduces heavy bleeding and menstrual pain; helps protect against ovarian and endometrial cancer	Must be taken every day; requires medical examination and prescription; minor side effects such as nausea or menstrual spotting; possibility of cardiovascular problems in a small percentage of users
Contraceptive ring (estrogen + progestin)	99%+	n/a	Easy to use after learning how to insert; remains in place 3 weeks	Like other hormonal methods, does not protect against STDs; requires physician prescription; possibility of cardiovascular problems in a small percentage of users
Contraceptive patch (estrogen + progestin)	99%+	n/a	Easy to apply; must change weekly for 3 weeks	No STD protection; requires physician prescription; possibility of cardiovascular problems in a small percentage of users
Depo-Provera	99%+	99%+	Easy to use; highly effective for 3-month period; continued use prevents menstruation	Requires supervision by a physician; administered by injection; some women experience irregular menstrual spotting in early months of use
Tubal ligation	99%+	99%+	Permanent; removes fear of pregnancy	Surgery-related risks; generally considered irreversible
Vasectomy	99%+	99%+	Permanent; removes fear of pregnancy	Generally considered irreversible

the female reproductive system. The use effectiveness of this method, however, reflects how unsuccessful the method is in practice (see Table 16.1).

Strong evidence suggests that the clear preejaculate fluid that helps neutralize and lubricate the male urethra can contain *viable* (capable of fertilization) sperm.[1] This sperm can be deposited near the cervical opening before withdrawal, which explains the relatively low effectiveness of this method. Furthermore, withdrawal does not protect users from the transmission of sexually transmitted diseases (STDs). It should never be considered a reliable contraceptive approach.

Periodic Abstinence

Four approaches are included in the birth control strategy called **periodic abstinence:** (1) the calendar method, (2) the basal body temperature (BBT) method, (3) the Billings cervical mucus method, and (4) the symptother-

mal method.[2] All four methods attempt to determine the time a woman ovulates. Figure 16-1 shows a day-to-day fertility calendar used to calculate fertile periods. Most research indicates that an ovum is viable for only about twenty-four to thirty-six hours after its release from the ovary. (After they are inside the female reproductive tract, some sperm can survive up to a week.) When a woman can accurately determine when she ovulates, she must refrain from intercourse long enough for the ovum to begin

> **Key Terms**
>
> **periodic abstinence** birth control methods that rely on a couple's avoidance of intercourse during the ovulatory phase of a woman's menstrual cycle; also called fertility awareness or natural family planning.

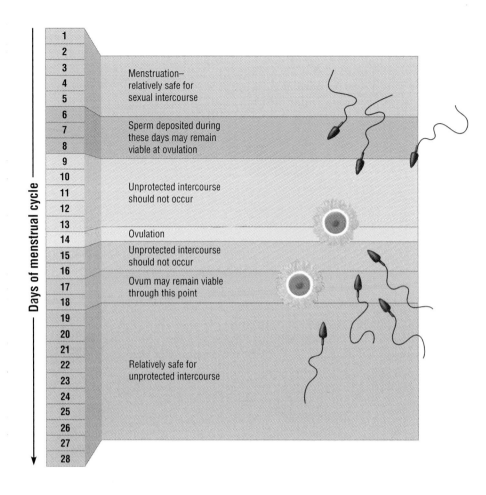

Figure 16-1 Periodic abstinence (fertility awareness or natural family planning) can combine use of the calendar, basal body temperature measurements, and Billings mucus techniques to identify the fertile period. Remember that most women's cycles are not consistently perfect 28-day cycles like those shown in most illustrations.

Days of menstrual cycle

1
2
3 — Menstruation–relatively safe for sexual intercourse
4
5
6
7 — Sperm deposited during these days may remain viable at ovulation
8
9
10 — Unprotected intercourse should not occur
11
12
13
14 — Ovulation
15 — Unprotected intercourse should not occur
16
17 — Ovum may remain viable through this point
18
19
20
21
22 — Relatively safe for unprotected intercourse
23
24
25
26
27
28

to disintegrate. Fertility awareness, rhythm, natural birth control, and natural family planning are other terms for periodic abstinence. Remember that periodic abstinence methods *do not* provide protection against the spread of STDs, including HIV infection.

Periodic abstinence is the only contraceptive method endorsed by the Roman Catholic Church. For some people who have deep concerns for the spiritual dimension of their health, selecting a method other than periodic abstinence may entail a serious compromise of beliefs.

The **calendar method** requires close examination of a woman's menstrual cycle for at least eight cycles. Records are kept of the length (in days) of each cycle. A *cycle* is defined as the number of days from the first day of bleeding of one cycle to the first day of bleeding of the next cycle.

To determine the days she should abstain from intercourse, a woman should subtract eighteen from her shortest cycle; this is the first day she should abstain from intercourse. Then she should subtract eleven from her longest cycle; this is the last day she must abstain from intercourse (see the Changing for the Better box on page 528).[3]

The *basal body temperature method* requires a woman (for about three or four successive months) to take her body temperature every morning before she rises from

bed. A finely calibrated thermometer, available in many drugstores, is used for this purpose. The theory behind this method is that there is a distinct correlation between body temperature and the process of ovulation. Just before ovulation, the body temperature supposedly dips and then rises about one degree Fahrenheit for the rest of the cycle. The woman is instructed to refrain from intercourse during the interval when the temperature change takes place.

Drawbacks of this procedure include the need for consistent, accurate temperature readings and the realization that all women's bodies are different. Some women may not fit the temperature pattern projection because of biochemical differences in their bodies. In addition, body temperature can fluctuate. Temperature kits cost about $5 to $8 in drugstores.

Key Terms

calendar method a form of periodic abstinence in which the variable lengths of a woman's menstrual cycle are used to calculate her fertile period.

The *Billings cervical mucus method* is another periodic abstinence technique. Generally used with other periodic abstinence techniques, this method requires a woman to evaluate the daily mucous discharge from her cervix. Users of this method become familiar with the changes in both appearance (from clear to cloudy) and consistency (from watery to thick) of their cervical mucus throughout their cycles. Women are taught that the unsafe days are when the mucus becomes clear and is the consistency of raw egg whites. Such a technique of ovulation determination must be learned from a physician or family planning professional.

Considering Complementary Care

Herbal Answers for Fertility Questions

Practitioners of most forms of alternative medicine and complementary care claim that they have solutions for individuals and couples having fertility problems. An examination of one form of complementary care, Chinese herbal medicine, supports this contention. Hundreds of Internet websites provide information about herbs' ability to bolster health and treat illness.

One commercial website, Baby Zone (**www.babyzone.com**), is fairly typical of the type of information one can quickly find. Baby Zone has a link called "Fertility and herbs" that identifies fifty-eight herbs touted to be helpful for nine male fertility problems and eighteen female fertility problems. Among the male problems are hormonal imbalance, low sperm count, low sperm motility, and impotence. Some of the female fertility problems are hormonal imbalance, anovulation (lack of ovulation), luteal phase defect, and endometriosis. There is even a category called "general fertility promoters" that describes various herbs that function broadly to improve fertility.

The list of fifty-eight herbs includes such unusual plants as astragalas, blue cohosh, chaste tree, dong quai, false unicorn, motherwort, rehmannia, and wild yam root. Other plants are much more common: alfalfa, cinnamon, dandelion, ginger, parsley, sage, rosemary, and wheat. This Internet source identifies typical doses and common forms for each of the herbs. Herbs are available in a variety of forms that could include whole herbs, teas, capsules, tablets, and extracts.

Perhaps one of the most important aspects of this website is the disclaimer that all users should read and take seriously before they decide to use any herb product. The first part of this disclaimer tells consumers that they must not consult the information unless they agree "not to hold Baby Zone or its associates liable for any errors or omissions." Additionally, the disclaimer reminds readers that the extent of the herbs' actions will never be completely known, that further research is recommended for herbal products, that users should consult with an experienced health care professional before starting herbal supplementation, that ill people need medical consultation, that pregnant and nursing women should never use supplements without medical supervision, that all herbs can contain some toxins, allergens, and carcinogenic agents, and that toxicity varies with individual users.

Reading the extensive disclaimer can make a potential user wary of the possible dangers of herbal supplementation without medical recommendation. However, complementary medicine, by definition, should "complement" traditional medicine. When viewed in this light, the use of the Internet for herbal answers to fertility questions becomes another information source that *may be helpful.* As with every consumer activity, "let the buyer beware."

The *symptothermal method* of periodic abstinence combines the use of the BBT method and the cervical mucus method.[3] Thus, some family planning professionals consider the symptothermal method a combination of all of the periodic abstinence approaches.

Those who wish to practice one of these periodic abstinence methods should consult a professional to learn how to chart their menstrual cycle and detect the physical signs that help predict the "unsafe" days. Besides the lack of protection against STDs, the periodic abstinence methods have the following potential problems:

- Partner may be uncooperative.
- Couple may take risks during "unsafe" days.
- Record-keeping may be poor.
- Illness and lack of sleep can affect body temperature.
- Vaginal infections and douches change mucus.
- Method cannot be used if the woman has irregular periods or temperature patterns.

Vaginal Spermicides

Spermicides are agents that are capable of killing sperm. When used alone, they offer a moderately effective form of contraception for the woman who is sexually active on an infrequent basis. Modern spermicides are generally safe (but see precaution below), reversible forms of contraception that can be obtained without a physician's prescription in most drugstores and supermarkets. Spermicides are relatively inexpensive. Applicator kits cost about $8 and refills cost around $4 to $8 (see Figure 16-2).

Spermicides, which are available in foam, cream, jelly, film, or suppository form, are made of water-soluble bases with a spermicidal agent in the base. Spermicides

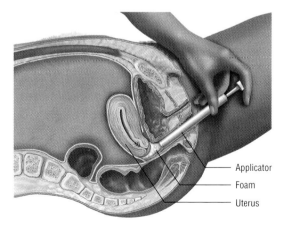

        —— Applicator
        —— Foam
        —— Uterus

Figure 16-2 Spermicidal foams and suppositories are placed deep into the vagina in the region of the cervix no longer than 30 minutes before intercourse.

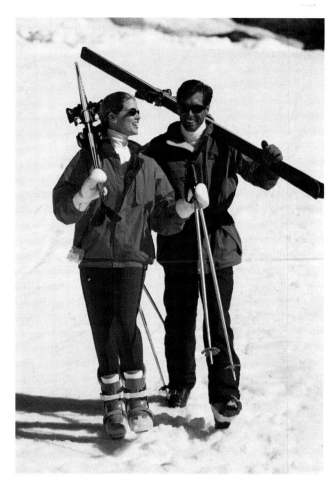

Choosing not to have children gives couples more time and money to pursue other interests.

are commonly used with other contraceptives, such as diaphragms, cervical caps, and condoms.

Spermicides are not specific to sperm cells; they also attack other cells. Until recently, nonoxynol-9, the most commonly used spermicidal agent, was thought to protect women from developing **pelvic inflammatory disease (PID).** Health professionals believed that nonoxynol-9 provided this protection by attacking and killing pathogens which caused various STDs.

However, the latest research indicates that nonoxynol-9 is not very effective in killing other pathogens. Nonoxynol-9 may actually *increase* the likelihood of disease transmission,

Key Terms

spermicides chemicals capable of killing sperm.

pelvic inflammatory disease (PID) a generalized infection of the pelvic cavity that results from the spread of an infection through a woman's reproductive structures.

Vaginal Contraceptive Film

A unique spermicide delivery system developed in England is vaginal contraceptive film (VCF). Vaginal contraceptive film is a sheet containing nonoxynol-9 that is inserted over the cervical opening. Shortly after insertion of the VCF, it dissolves into a gel-like material that clings to the cervical opening. The VCF can be inserted up to an hour before intercourse. Over the course of several hours, the material will be washed from the vagina in the normal vaginal secretions.

This spermicide is a nonprescription form of contraception that is as effective as other spermicidal foams and jellies. Users should be aware that the nonoxynol-9 spermicide may not be as effective against STDs as was formerly thought. A box of twelve sheets costs about $12.

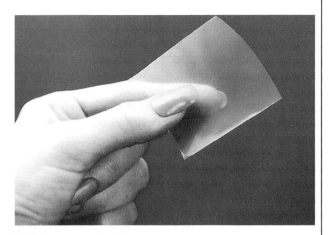

Vaginal contraceptive film.

including HIV transmission, because it can cause skin irritations and abrasions in a small percentage of users.[4] These irritated areas and abrasions can provide the avenue for passage into the bloodstream.

For this reason, couples should not depend on vaginal spermicides to stop the spread of infections from person to person. Condoms, when used consistently and correctly, provide much better disease protection and contraceptive effect than spermicides used alone. The latest research also indicates that condoms coated with nonoxynol-9 do not have enough of the spermicide to serve as a back-up contraceptive if the condom breaks.[5] Thus, some health centers and family planning agencies have stopped distributing condoms with nonoxynol-9 in the lubricant. If you and/or your partner have concerns about your use of spermicides, you should seek advice from your physician or health center.

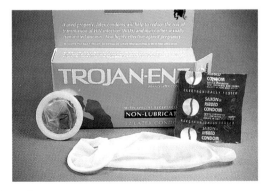

Male condoms.

Condoms

Colored or natural, smooth or textured, straight or shaped, plain or reservoir-tipped, dry or lubricated—the latex condom is approaching an art form. Nevertheless, the familiar **condom** remains a safe, effective, reversible contraceptive device. All condoms manufactured in the United States must be approved by the FDA.[6]

For couples who are highly motivated in their desire to prevent a pregnancy, the effectiveness of a condom can approach that of an oral contraceptive. A condom can be nearly 100% effective when used with contraceptive foam. For couples who are less motivated, the condom can be considerably less effective. Condoms cost from 25¢ up to $2.50.

The condom offers a measure of protection against sexually transmitted diseases. For both the man and the woman, chlamydial infections, gonorrhea, HIV infection, and other STDs are less likely to be acquired when the condom is used correctly (see the Changing for the Better box on page 532). Some lubricated condoms also contain a spermicide. However, recent research indicates that the use of the spermicide nonoxynol-9 may irritate tissues in some users and actually increase the likelihood of disease transmission. Also, the small amount of spermicide present in the condom's lubricant is not enough to consis-

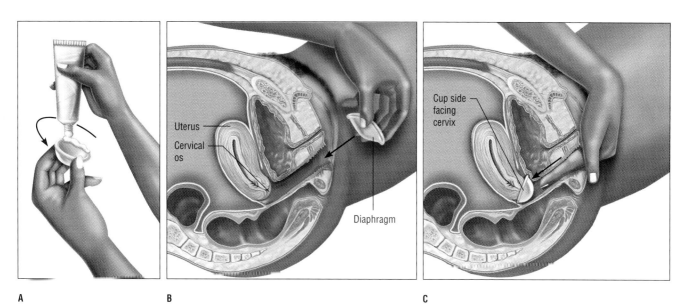

A   B   C

Figure 16-3 **A,** Spermicidal cream or jelly is placed into the diaphragm. **B,** The diaphragm is folded length-wise and inserted into the vagina. **C,** The diaphragm is then placed against the cervix so that the cup portion with the spermicide is facing the cervix. The outline of the cervix should be felt through the central part of the diaphragm.

tently prevent conception if the condom should break. Current recommendations are to use dry condoms or lubricated condoms without spermicide. Also, any additional lubricants used should be water-based lubricants.

The FDA has approved two types of non-latex condoms. The polyurethane male condom and the polyurethane female condom are available as one-time-use condoms (see the Star box on page 533).[3] These condoms are good alternatives for people who have an allergic sensitivity to latex, estimated to be up to 7% of the population.[7] Also, they are thinner and stronger than latex condoms and can be used with oil-based lubricants. Currently, these condoms are believed to provide protection against STDs that is close to that of latex condoms. The contraceptive effectiveness of the polyurethane condoms remains somewhat less than that of the male latex condom.[8,9]

Diaphragm

The **diaphragm** is a soft rubber cup with a springlike metal rim that rests in the top of the vagina. The diaphragm covers the cervical opening (Figure 16-3). During intercourse the diaphragm stays in place quite well and cannot usually be felt by either partner.

The diaphragm is always used with a spermicidal cream or jelly placed inside the cup and around the rim. When used properly with a spermicide, the diaphragm is a relatively effective contraceptive, and when combined with the man's use of a condom, its effectiveness is even greater.

Diaphragms must always be fitted and prescribed by a physician.[10] The cost of obtaining a diaphragm and keeping a supply of spermicide may be higher than that of other methods. Typically, it costs $13 to $25 for a diaphragm and

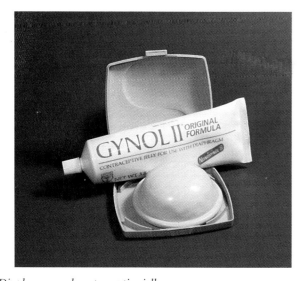

Diaphragm and contraceptive jelly.

Maximizing the Effectiveness of Condoms

I have used condoms a few times, but I was always in a hurry and never read the small print instructions. My current partner asked me if "I knew what I was doing" the last time we had intercourse. What do I need to know to use condoms more effectively?

These simple directions for using condoms correctly, in combination with your motivation and commitment to regular use, should provide you with reasonable protection:

- Keep a supply of condoms at hand. Condoms should be stored in a cool, dry place so that they are readily available at the time of intercourse. Condoms that are stored in wallets or automobile glove compartments may not be in satisfactory condition when they are used. Temperature extremes are to be avoided. Check the condom package for the expiration date.
- Do not test a condom by inflating or stretching it. Handle it gently and keep it away from sharp fingernails.
- For maximum effectiveness, put the condom on before genital contact. Either the man or the woman can put the condom in place. Early application is particularly important in the prevention of STDs. Early application also lessens the possibility of the release of preejaculate fluid into the vagina.
- Unroll the condom on the erect penis. For those using a condom without a reservoir tip, a 1/2-inch space should be left to catch the ejaculate. To leave this space, pinch the tip of the condom as you roll it on the erect penis. Do not leave any air in the tip of the condom.
- Lubricate the condom if this has not already been done by the manufacturer. When doing this, be certain to use a water-soluble lubricant and not a petroleum-based product such as petroleum jelly. Petroleum can deteriorate the latex material. Other oil-based lubricants, such as mineral oil, baby oil, vegetable oil, shortening, and certain hand lotions, can quickly damage a latex condom. Use water-based lubricants only!
- After ejaculation, be certain that the condom does not become dislodged from the penis. Hold the rim of the condom firmly

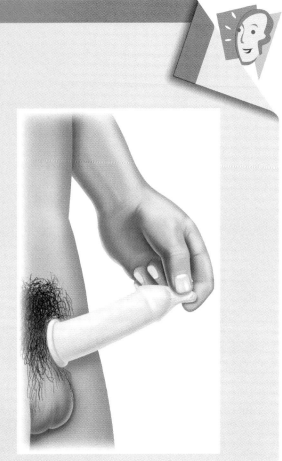

Directions: Pinch the end of the condom to leave 1/2 inch of space at the tip.

against the base of the penis during withdrawal. Do not allow the penis to become flaccid (soft) while still in the vagina.
- Inspect the condom for tears before throwing it away. If the condom is damaged in some way, immediately insert a spermicidal agent into the vagina or consider using emergency contraception (see page 538).

$4 to $8 for the spermicidal cream or jelly. An examination may cost between $50 and $125, but it will be less at family planning clinics. Also, a high level of motivation to follow the instructions *exactly* is important.

Diaphragms and other vaginal barrier methods (such as the cervical cap) do not provide reliable protection against STDs and HIV infection. Recent concerns about the spermicide nonoxynol-9 should prompt users to ask their physicians to recommend which spermicidal cream or jelly to use with diaphragms. If you are concerned about possible HIV infection, either avoid sexual activity or use a latex condom.

Cervical Cap

The **cervical cap** is a small, thimble-shaped device that fits over the entire cervix. The cap is held in place by suction rather than by pushing against anatomical structures

---

Key Terms

cervical cap a small, thimble-shaped contraceptive device designed to fit over the cervix.

The Female Condom

The Reality female condom is a soft, loose-fitting polyurethane sheath containing two polyurethane rings. Reality is inserted like a tampon and lines the inner contours of the vagina. The larger ring remains outside the vagina, and the external portion of the condom provides some protection to the labia and the base of the penis. Reality is coated on the inside with a silicone-based lubricant. Additional lubricant is provided for the outside of the sheath. This lubricant does not contain a spermicide. Female and male condoms should not be used at the same time since they might adhere to each other and cause slippage or displacement. The contraceptive effectiveness of the female condom is not as high as that of the male condom. However, as people become more familiar with using the female condom, its effectiveness may increase. Each female condom costs about $2.50.

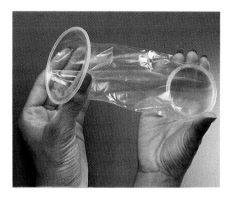

Female condom.

(Figure 16-4). As with the diaphragm, the cervical cap is coated with spermicide and prevents the sperm from reaching the egg. The cap carries no major health risks and is nearly equal to the diaphragm in effectiveness, although it can be slightly less effective for women who have already had a child.

The cervical cap comes in just four sizes and, thus, may be difficult to fit for some women.[8] A physician must prescribe the cervical cap and show the woman how to use it. With new concerns about the use of the spermicide nonoxynol-9, women are advised to ask their physicians which contraceptive or cream or jelly they should use with their cervical cap. The cost of a cervical cap is similar to that of a diaphragm.

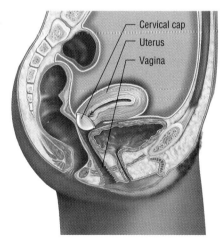

- Cervical cap
- Uterus
- Vagina

Figure 16-4 After the spermicidal cream or jelly is placed in the cervical cap, the cap is inserted into the vagina and placed against the cervix.

Contraceptive Sponge

The **contraceptive sponge** is a small, pillow-shaped polyurethane device containing nonoxynol-9 spermicide. The sponge is dampened with tap water and inserted deep into the vagina to cover the cervical opening. This device provides contraceptive protection for up to 24 hours, regardless of the number of times intercourse occurs. After the last act of intercourse, the device must be left in place for at least 6 hours. Once removed, the sponge must be discarded. The sponge must not be left in place for longer than 24 or 30 hours because of the risk of toxic shock syndrome. Used alone, the sponge does not provide reliable protection against STDs and HIV infection. Consult your physician if you are concerned about the use of nonoxynol-9 spermicide. In women who have not given birth to children, the contraceptive effectiveness of the sponge is similar to that of the diaphragm.

Prior to its removal from the market in 1995, when the manufacturer refused to upgrade its physical plant to meet new government safety regulations, the Today Sponge was the most popular female over-the-counter contraceptive. However, a different company, Allendale

> **Key Terms**
>
> **contraceptive sponge** a small, pillow-shaped contraceptive device that contains a spermicide; placed deep in the vagina to cover the cervical opening.

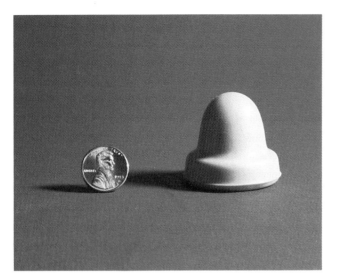

Cervical cap.

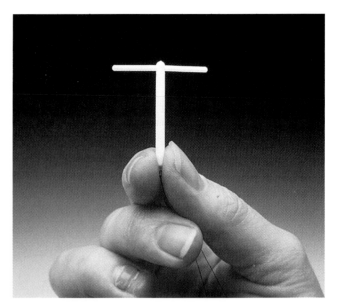

Progestasert IUD.

Pharmaceuticals, purchased the rights to the product and, at the time of this writing, is in the final stages of receiving FDA approval to return the Today Sponge to the U.S. market by early 2004.[11] The sponge is currently available in Canada. For the latest information on this product, see the Allendale website at *www.todayssponge.com*.

Intrauterine Device (IUD)

The **intrauterine device(IUD)** is the most popular reversible contraceptive method in the world, although the number of users in the United States is relatively small. The IUD is a safe, highly effective method of birth control. Experts still do not understand exactly how the IUD prevents pregnancy, but research suggests that IUDs may prevent conception or may prevent a fertilized ovum from implanting in the uterus. IUDs that contain synthetic hormones may cause the cervical mucus to thicken, thus reducing sperm movement into the uterus. Hormonal IUDs could also cause the uterine lining to become thinner and not permit a fertilized ovum to implant.[12]

Two types of IUDs are available in the United States: T-shaped IUDs containing progestin (Progestasert and Mirena) and a T-shaped IUD wrapped with copper wire (ParaGard). The two hormone-producing IUDs substantially reduce menstrual blood loss, but the Copper IUD may increase blood flow at menstruation. About 20% of women who use the Mirena IUD will stop having their periods.[13]

The Progestasert provides highly effective contraceptive protection for 1 year, the Mirena for 5 years, and the ParaGard for up to 10 years. Only a skilled physician can prescribe and insert an IUD. As with many other forms of contraception, IUDs do not offer protection against STDs, including the AIDS virus.[14]

The IUD is inserted into the uterus by a trained clinician. Along with a physical examination, the physician will ask several questions about the woman's lifestyle, and she should be honest about her sex life, because the IUD is not for all women. Women who have multiple partners or woman who do not practice safe sex might be advised not to use the IUD. The IUD can be an acceptable form of contraception, especially for women who are in their middle to late reproductive years, unable to take birth control pills, in a stable, monogamous relationship, and not at risk for STDs.

Two uncommon but potentially serious side effects of IUD use are uterine perforation (in which the IUD imbeds itself into the uterine wall) and pelvic inflammatory disease (PID, a life-threatening infection of the abdominal cavity). However, in women in monogamous relationships, the risk of PID is low.[15]

As Table 16.1 indicates, IUDs are very effective birth control devices, surpassed in effectiveness only by abstinence, sterilization, and hormonal (pill, injection, ring, patch) contraceptives. The choice of over one hundred million women worldwide, IUDs are used by fewer than 1%

> ### Key Terms
>
> **intrauterine device (IUD)** a small, plastic, medicated or unmedicated contraceptive device that prevents pregnancy when inserted in the uterus.

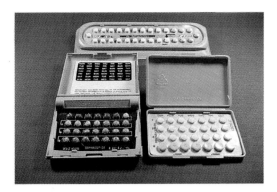

Oral contraceptives.

OnSITE/InSIGHT

Learning to Go: Health

Do you have questions about fertility? Click on Learning to Go: Health on the Online Learning Center at **www.mhhe.com/ payne8e** to explore these lessons on the topic:

Lesson 41: Choose a contraceptive that fits your lifestyle.

Lesson 42: Deal with an unintended pregnancy.

of women at risk of pregnancy in the United States.[3] The cost for an IUD ranges from $175 to $400, which includes an exam, insertion, and a follow-up visit.[12]

Oral Contraceptives

Developed in the 1950s, the **oral contraceptive pill** provides the highest effectiveness rate of any single reversible contraceptive method used today. "The pill" is the method of choice for over seventeen million users in the United States.[16]

Use of the pill requires a physician's examination and prescription. Because oral contraceptives are available in a wide range of formulas, follow-up examinations are important to ensure that a woman is receiving an effective dosage with as few side effects as possible. Matching the right prescription with the woman may require a few consultations.

All oral contraceptives contain synthetic (laboratory-made) hormones. The typical *combined pill* uses both synthetic estrogen and synthetic progesterone in each of twenty-one pills. With *triphasic pills,* the level of estrogen remains constant, but the level of progestin varies every 7 days. In 2003 the FDA approved the newest oral contraceptive (Seasonale) that contains active hormones for 84 days (12 weeks) followed by 1 week of pills containing inactive ingredients.[17] Women using this contraceptive pill would expect to have only four menstrual periods each year. This pill could become a highly popular choice for women. As with many forms of contraception, *oral contraceptives do not protect against the transmission of STDs, including HIV infection.* Also, the use of antibiotics may lower the pill's contraceptive effectiveness.

Oral contraceptives function in several ways. The estrogen in the pill tends to reduce ova development. The progesterone in the pill helps reduce the likelihood of ovulation (by lowering the release of luteinizing hormone). progesterone in the pill also causes the uterine wall to adequately and helps thicken cervical mucus, difficult for sperm to enter the uterus.

The physical changes produced by the oral contraceptive provide some beneficial side effects in women. Because the synthetic hormones are taken for 21 days and then are followed by **placebo pills** or no pills for 7 days, the menstrual cycle becomes regulated. Even women who have irregular cycles immediately become "regular." Because the uterine lining is not developed to the extent seen in a non-pill-taking woman, the uterus is not forced to contract with the same amount of vigor. Thus menstrual cramping is reduced, and the resultant menstrual flow is diminished. Research indicates that oral contraceptive use may provide protection against anemia, PID, noncancerous breast tumors, recurrent ovarian cysts, ectopic pregnancy, endometrial cancer, osteoporosis (thinning of the bones), and cancer of the ovaries.[3]

The negative side effects of the oral contraceptive pill can be divided into two general categories: (1) unpleasant and (2) potentially dangerous. The unpleasant side effects generally subside within two or three months for most women. A number of women report some or many of the following symptoms:

- Tenderness in breast tissue
- Nausea
- Mild headaches
- Slight, irregular spotting
- Weight gain

Key Terms

oral contraceptive pill a pill taken orally, composed of synthetic female hormones that prevent ovulation or implantation; "the pill."

placebo pills (pla **see** bo) pills that contain no active ingredients.

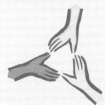

Learning from Our Diversity

The Male Contraceptive Pill

Having males be responsible for the medical control of fertility would be a big shift in the sexuality responsibility roles for men and women. Forty-five years after the breakthrough of the female contraceptive pill, researchers are gaining confidence that a version of a male contraceptive pill will be commercially available in the not-too-distant future, perhaps between 5 and 10 years.*

For decades, difficulties have surrounded the development of a male contraceptive pill. Although many people believe that the primary reason for the slow development was the fact that the researchers were male, the most plausible explanations deal with male physiology. The typical male ejaculate contains between 300 and 500 million sperm cells. A contraceptive method that is over 99% effective would still leave thousands and thousands of sperm cells available. In contrast, female contraceptives must block the viability of only one egg each cycle, arguably an easier task.

The drug being tested that blocks sperm development is actually a female hormone. While it is effective at blocking sperm production, it also reduces the amount of testosterone that the male produces. Without adequate levels of testosterone, the male sex drive diminishes considerably. For this reason, researchers are testing the effects of

replacement androgen, often in the form of an injection or an implant. It is also possible that a slow release patch, similar to the nicotine replacement patch, could be used in the future.

Critics claim that a safe, effective, and inexpensive form of male contraception already exists in the form of a vasectomy. They argue, why not use an approach that already has shown its effectiveness for years? Besides, are women going to trust a man who claims he is using an oral contraceptive pill? Would the pill also have to make a man's eyeballs turn blue as proof that he was using an effective method? When would a woman know that a man is being truthful? Unfortunately, the track record for honesty among couples in sexual relationships isn't particularly good.

Within the next decade, the obstacles that prevent a safe and effective male contraceptive pill from being manufactured may be overcome. But questions will still remain, especially for women, since after all is said and done, they will always be the ones who must bear the brunt (as well as the joy) of pregnancy, labor, and childbirth.

*Health news: Will men use a contraceptive pill? Will women trust them? InteliHealth Online, August 29, 2000, **www.intelihealth.com/enews?296075.**

- Fluctuations in sex drive
- Mild depression
- More frequent vaginal infections

 TALKING POINTS You've tried two different types of oral contraceptives and had unpleasant side effects with both. Your doctor says you should consider another birth control method, but you disagree. How could you talk with her about this in a matter-of-fact way?

The potentially dangerous side effects of the oral contraceptive pill are most often seen in the cardiovascular system. Blood clots, strokes, hypertension, and heart attack seem to be associated with the estrogen component of the combined pill. However, when compared with nonusers, the risk of dying from cardiovascular complications is only slightly increased among healthy young oral contraceptive users. Additionally, the present consensus is that oral contraceptive users place themselves at slightly increased risk of breast cancer and cervical cancer. This is especially true for women who used the higher-dosage oral contraceptives in the 1970s and also had a family history of breast cancer. However, it must be emphasized that this risk is quite small for users of today's lower-dose pills. Most health professionals agree that the risks related to

pregnancy and childbirth are much greater than those associated with oral contraceptive use. Certainly, a woman who is contemplating the use of the pill must discuss all of the risks and benefits with her physician. For a discussion on the male oral contraceptive, see the Learning from Our Diversity box above.

There are some **contraindications** for the use of oral contraceptives. If you have a history of blood clots, migraine headaches, liver disease, a heart condition, high blood pressure, obesity, diabetes, epilepsy, or anemia, or if you are too young to have started consistent menstrual cycles, the pill probably should not be your contraceptive choice. Providing a physician with a complete and accurate health history is important before a woman starts to take the pill.

Two additional contraindications are receiving considerable attention by the medical community. Cigarette smoking and advancing age are highly associated with a increased risk of potentially serious side effects. Incr

Key Terms

contraindications factors that make the us inappropriate or dangerous for a particr

ing numbers of physicians are not prescribing oral contraceptives for their patients who smoke. The risk of cardiovascular-related deaths is greatly enhanced in women over age 35. The risk is even higher in female smokers over 35. The data are quite convincing.[3]

For the vast majority of women, however, the pill, when properly prescribed, is safe and effective. Careful scrutiny of one's health history and careful follow-up examinations when a problem is suspected are essential elements that can provide a margin of safety. Monthly pill packs cost between $15 and $35 at drugstores and less at clinics. An exam may cost $35 to $125.[18]

Minipills

Some women prefer not to use the combined oral contraceptive pill. Thus to avoid some of the potentially serious side effects of the combined pill, some physicians are prescribing **minipills.** These oral contraceptives contain no estrogen—only low-dose progesterone.[19] The minipill seems to work by thickening cervical mucus, preventing ovulation, and perhaps preventing implantation of a fertilized ovum. The effectiveness of a minipill is slightly lower than that of the combined pill. *Breakthrough bleeding* and **ectopic pregnancy** are more common in minipill users than in combined-pill users. The cost of minipills is similar to that of combined pills.

Injectable Contraceptives

Depo-Provera is a highly effective (99%+) injectable progestin contraceptive that provides protection for 3 months. This hormone shot works by thickening the cervical mucus to keep the sperm from joining the egg, preventing the release of the egg, and preventing a fertilized egg from implanting in the uterus.

The most common side effects of Depo-Provera are irregular bleeding and spotting followed by *amenorrhea* (the absence of periods).[3] In particular, new users of

Depo-Provera report occasional breakthrough bleeding as the most common unpleasant side effect.[3] When the woman's body adjusts to the presence of this drug, breakthrough bleeding diminishes, and the most common side effect is amenorrhea. This is understandable, because the drug inhibits ovulation. Many women consider amenorrhea to be a desirable effect of Depo-Provera use. Women who stop using Depo-Provera may experience infertility for a period of up to one year.[3] The cost of Depo-Provera ranges from $30 to $75 per injection.[3]

In the year 2000, the Pharmacia Corporation received FDA approval to produce a monthly injectable contraceptive called Lunelle. Lunelle combined the hormones estrogen and progestin in its once-a-month shot. However, this product is no longer on the market since, in October 2002, Pharmacia stopped production and distribution of Lunelle.

Subdermal Implants

This form of contraception used six soft plastic rods filled with synthetic progesterone. Using a local anesthetic, a physician implanted these rods just beneath the skin of the woman's upper or lower arm. The rods released low levels of the hormone for 5 years. In 2002 Wyeth Pharmaceuticals stopped the production and distribution of subdermal implants.

Key Terms

minipills low-dose progesterone (progestin) oral contraceptives.

ectopic pregnancy a pregnancy in which the fertilized ovum implants at a site other than the uterus, typically in the fallopian tubes.

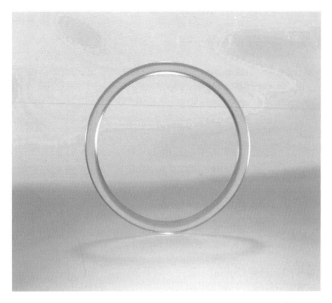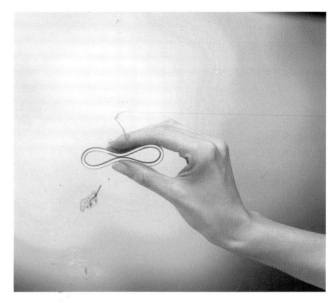

The NuvaRing contraceptive ring is a flexible ring about 2¹/₈ inches in diameter. When inserted into the vagina, it delivers a low dose of hormones similar to those found in oral contraceptives.

The Contraceptive Ring

One of the newest contraceptives on the market is the vaginal **contraceptive ring** (NuvaRing). Available by prescription in 2001, NuvaRing is a thin polymer ring (2⅛ inches in diameter and ⅛ inch thick) that contains synthetic estrogen and progestin. Users insert this device deep into the vagina where it remains for 3 weeks. At the end of the third week, the device is removed for a week and the woman has her period. The NuvaRing provides effective contraception (98–99% effective when used properly) for the entire 4-week time frame.[20]

The ring functions in a manner similar to the oral contraceptive pill: it reduces the chances of ovulation and thickens cervical mucus. Women who use the ring cannot at the same time use cervical caps or diaphragms as a backup method. The contraceptive ring does not protect against sexually transmitted diseases, including the virus that causes HIV/AIDS. The costs of the contraceptive ring are about $30–$35 per month for the device and $35–$125 for the exam.[18]

The Contraceptive Patch

In 2002 the Ortho Evra **contraceptive patch** became available to women. This patch contains continuous levels of estrogen and progestin delivered from a 1¾-inch square patch that is applied weekly to one of four areas on the woman's body: the buttocks, abdomen, upper chest (front and back, excluding the breasts), or upper outer arm.[21] The patch remains attached even while a woman bathes, swims, or exercises. After three weeks of patches, the woman uses no patch for the fourth week, during which time the woman has her period. The patch functions in a manner similar to the oral contraceptive pill. Like all hormonal measures of contraception, the patch does not protect against sexually transmitted diseases, including the virus that causes HIV/AIDS.

Emergency Contraception

Emergency contraception is designed to prevent pregnancy after unprotected vaginal intercourse such as when a condom breaks, when a couple uses no method of

---

Key Terms

contraceptive ring thin, polymer contraceptive device containing estrogen and progestin; placed deep within the vagina for a 3-week period.

contraceptive patch contraceptive skin patch containing estrogen and progestin; replaced each week for a 3-week period.

emergency contraception contraceptive measures used to prevent pregnancy within 72 hours after unprotected intercourse; also called post-coital or "morning after" contraception.

contraception, or when someone forces another to have intercourse. This method is also called post-coital or "morning after" contraception. Emergency contraception is available in two forms: emergency hormonal contraception and the insertion of an IUD. Both forms of contraception can be prescribed (or carried out) by a physician.

As of September 2003, five states (Alaska, California, Hawaii, New Mexico, and Washington) had enacted laws that permit a pharmacist to provide emergency contraception to customers in the absence of a prescription by a physician. However, the pharmacist is required to act within a collaborative agreement with a physician. This agreement clearly identifies the circumstances under which the pharmacist can dispense the emergency contraception.[22]

Emergency hormonal contraception involves the use of two doses of certain oral contraceptives.[3] The most commonly used oral contraceptives are the combined pills, which contain both synthetic estrogen and progesterone. The first dose of pills is taken within 72 hours of unprotected intercourse. A second dose is taken 12 hours later. If minipills (progesterone-only) are used for emergency contraception, the first dose must be taken within 48 to 72 hours after unprotected intercourse.

The insertion of an IUD is a less commonly used, but highly effective, form of emergency contraception. To function as a contraceptive, however, the Copper T 380-A IUD must be inserted within 5 days after unprotected intercourse.

Sterilization

All of the contraceptive mechanisms or methods already discussed have one quality in common: they are reversible. Although microsurgical techniques are providing medical breakthroughs, **sterilization** should still be considered an irreversible procedure.[23] When you decide to use sterilization, you no longer control your own fertility because you will no longer be able to produce offspring.

Therefore, couples considering sterilization procedures usually must undergo extensive discussions with a physician or family planning counselor to identify their true feelings about this finality. People must be aware of the possible changes in self-concept they might have after sterilization. If you are a man who equates fertility with masculinity, you may have trouble accepting your new status as a sterile man. If you are a woman who equates motherhood with femininity, you might have adjustment problems after sterilization. Some people later regret not being able to have children. Sterilization does not protect one against STDs, including HIV infection.

The male sterilization procedure is called a *vasectomy*. Accomplished with a local anesthetic in a physician's office, this 20- to 30-minute procedure consists of the surgical removal of a section of each vas deferens. After a small incision is made through the scrotum, the vas deferens is located and a small section removed. The remaining ends are either tied or *cauterized* (Figure 16-5A).

Immediately after a vasectomy, sperm may still be present in the vas deferens. A backup contraceptive is recommended until a physician microscopically examines a semen specimen. This examination usually occurs about six weeks after the surgery. After a vasectomy, men can still produce male sex hormones, get erections, have orgasms, and ejaculate. (Recall that sperm account for only a small portion of the semen.) Some men even report increased interest in sexual activity because their chances of impregnating a woman have been virtually eliminated.

What happens to the process of spermatogenesis within each testicle? Sperm cells are still being produced, but they are destroyed by specialized white blood cells called phagocytic leukocytes.

The future may hold a reversible form of vasectomy, as researchers experiment with injecting a plug-forming material into the vas deferens, with the intention that the plug could be removed at a later date if desired. The cost of a vasectomy ranges from $240 to $520.[18]

The most common method of female sterilization is called *tubal ligation*. During this procedure, the fallopian tubes are cut and the ends tied back. Some physicians cauterize the tube ends to ensure complete sealing (Figure 16-5B). The fallopian tubes are usually reached through the abdominal wall. In a minilaparotomy, a small incision is made through the abdominal wall just below the navel. The resultant scar is small and is the basis for the term *band-aid surgery*.

Female sterilization requires about twenty to thirty minutes, with the patient under a local or general anesthetic. The use of a laparoscope has made female sterilization much simpler than in the past. The laparoscope is a small tube equipped with mirrors and lights. Inserted through a single incision, the laparoscope locates the fallopian tubes before they are cut, tied, or cauterized. When a laparoscope is used through an abdominal incision, the procedure is called a *laparoscopy*.

Women who are sterilized still produce female hormones, ovulate, and menstruate. However, the ovum cannot move down the fallopian tube. Within a day of its release, the ovum will start to disintegrate and be absorbed by the body. Freed of the possibility of becoming pregnant, many sterilized women report an increase in sex drive and activity.

> ### Key Terms
>
> **sterilization** generally permanent birth control techniques that surgically disrupt the normal passage of ova or sperm.

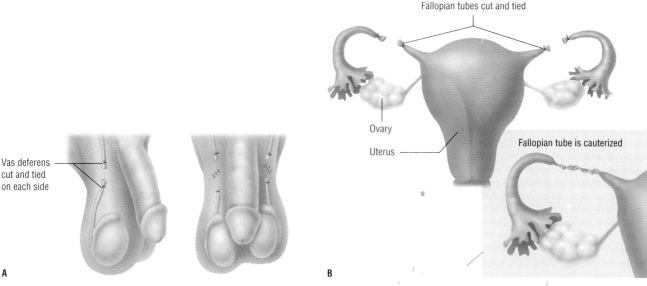

Figure 16-5 The most frequently used forms of male and female sterilization. **A,** Vasectomy. **B,** Tubal ligation.

Female sterilization is very effective, with failure rates of only 1 to 2 per 1,000 procedures. The complications tend to be few and minor, and there appear to be no serious long-term side effects. Tubal ligation costs range from $1,000 to $2,500.[18]

Two other procedures produce sterilization in women. *Ovariectomy* (the surgical removal of the ovaries) and *hysterectomy* (the surgical removal of the uterus) accomplish sterilization. However, these procedures are used to remove diseased (cancerous, cystic, or hemorrhaging) organs and are not primarily considered sterilization techniques.

 TALKING POINTS You and your husband have children. And you'd like to stop taking the pill for health reasons. Your husband says you're pressuring him to have a vasectomy. How can you keep the dialogue going in a cooperative way?

Abortion

Regardless of the circumstances under which pregnancy occurs, women may now choose to terminate their pregnancies. No longer must women who do not want to be pregnant seek potentially dangerous, illegal abortions. On the basis of current technology and legality, women need never experience childbirth. The decision will be theirs to make.

Abortion is a highly controversial, personal decision—one that needs serious consideration by each woman. On the basis of the landmark 1973 U.S. Supreme Court case *Roe v. Wade,* the United States joined many of the world's most populated countries in legalizing abortion within the following guidelines:

1. For the first 3 months of pregnancy (first trimester), the decision to abort lies with the woman and her doctor. Most abortions are performed in the first trimester.
2. For the next 3 months of pregnancy (second trimester), state law may regulate the abortion procedure in ways that are reasonably related to maternal health.
3. For the last weeks of pregnancy (third trimester) when the fetus is judged capable of surviving if born, any state may regulate or even prohibit abortion except where abortion is necessary to preserve the life or health of the mother. If a pregnancy is terminated during the third trimester, a living fetus would be considered a live birth and would not be allowed to die.

Each year, approximately 1.3 million women make the decision to terminate a pregnancy in the United States.[16] Thousands of additional women probably consider abortion but elect to continue their pregnancies.

Key Terms

abortion induced premature termination of a pregnancy.

First-Trimester Abortion Procedures

Menstrual Extraction Also referred to as *menstrual regulation, menstrual induction,* and *preemptive abortion,* menstrual extraction is a process carried out between the fourth and sixth week after the last menstrual period (or in the days immediately after the first missed menstrual period). It is generally performed in a physician's office under a local anesthetic or *paracervical* anesthetic. A small plastic *cannula* is inserted through the undilated cervical canal into the cavity of the uterus. When the cannula is in position, a small amount of suction is applied by a hand-held syringe. By rotating and moving the cannula across the uterine wall, the physician can withdraw the endometrial tissue.

Vacuum Aspiration Induced abortions undertaken during the sixth through ninth weeks of pregnancy are generally performed through *vacuum aspiration* of the uterine contents. Vacuum aspiration is the most commonly performed abortion procedure. This procedure is similar to menstrual extraction. Unlike menstrual extraction, however, vacuum aspiration may require **dilation** of the cervical canal and the use of a local anesthetic. In this more advanced stage of pregnancy, a larger cannula must be inserted into the uterine cavity. This process can be performed by using metal dilators of increasingly larger sizes to open the canal. After aspiration by an electric vacuum pump, the uterine wall may also be scraped to confirm complete removal of the uterine contents.

Dilation and Curettage (D & C) When a pregnancy is to be terminated during the ninth through fourteenth weeks, vacuum aspiration gives way to a somewhat similar procedure labeled **dilation and curettage,** or more familiarly, **D & C.** D & C usually requires a general anesthetic, not a local anesthetic.[3]

Like vacuum aspiration, the D & C involves the gradual enlargement of the cervical canal through the insertion of increasingly larger metal dilators. When the cervix has been dilated to a size sufficient to allow for the passage of a *curette,* the removal of the endometrial tissue can begin. The curette is a metal instrument resembling a spoon, with a cup-shaped cutting surface on its end. As the curette is drawn across the uterine wall, the soft endometrial tissue and fetal parts are scraped from the wall of the uterus. (The D & C is also used in the medical management of certain health conditions of the uterine wall, such as irregular bleeding or the buildup of endometrial tissue.)

As in the case of menstrual extraction, both vacuum aspiration and D & C are very safe procedures for the woman. The need to dilate the cervix more fully in a D & C increases the risk of cervical trauma and the possibility of perforation, but these risks are reported to be low. Bleeding, cramping, spotting, and infections present minimal controllable risks when procedures are performed by experienced clinicians.

Medical Abortion Mifepristone (RU-486) and methotrexate are drugs that can be used to induce a **medical abortion** during the first trimester of pregnancy. RU-486 was developed in France in the 1980s and has been widely used in Europe. Finally, after years of testing in the United States, the FDA gave approval to the so-called "abortion pill." The pill is being marketed under the name Mifeprex and is available only through physicians. The cost of using mifepristone is about the same as the cost of first-term, surgical procedures, or about $350–$575.[18]

Under the FDA's regimen, women must use mifepristone within 49 days of their last menstrual period. Mifepristone blocks the action of progesterone and causes the lining of the uterus to break down. Women take three pills at the first doctor visit and then return 48 hours later to take a second drug, misoprostol, which causes menstruation to occur, usually within about 5 hours.

A third visit to a physician is necessary to ensure that the woman is recovering well from medical abortion. Physicians will want to make certain that there is no infection or excessive bleeding and that the uterus is fully emptied. Over a decade of research studies have indicated that the use of mifepristone is around 95% effective, when used during the first 7 weeks of pregnancy.[24,25]

Methotrexate is a drug used since the 1950s for cancer treatment. Physicians have found that it is effective in inducing an early-term medical abortion. Thus physicians can use this drug in an off-label manner, with no specific protocols established.[3] Typically, a woman receives an injection of methotrexate and, during an office visit 3 to 7 days later, receives prostaglandin, usually through vaginal suppositories. The fetal contents are expelled, generally within 12 hours. With the recent FDA approval of mifepristone (RU-486), it is likely that the use of methotrexate will

---

> **Key Terms**
>
> **dilation** gradual expansion of an opening or passageway, such as the cervix.
>
> **dilation and curettage (D & C)** (kyoo re **taage**) a surgical procedure in which the cervical canal is dilated to allow the uterine wall to be scraped.
>
> **medical abortion** an abortion caused by the use of prescribed drugs.

decline. If these and other new drugs continue to gain favor with women and their physicians, it is likely that more women will use physicians' offices, rather than abortion clinics, for abortion services.

Second-Trimester Abortion Procedures

When a woman's pregnancy continues beyond the fourteenth week of gestation, termination becomes a more difficult matter. The procedures at this stage become more complicated and take longer to be completed, and complications become more common.

Dilation and Evacuation Vacuum aspiration and D & C can be combined in a procedure called *dilation and evacuation (D & E)* (Figure 16-6). D & E is a primary procedure for abortions between 13 and 15 weeks.[3]

Hypertonic Saline Procedure From the sixteenth week of gestation to the end of the second trimester, intrauterine injection of a strong salt solution into the amniotic sac is the procedure most frequently used. The administration of intrauterine **hypertonic saline solution** requires a skilled operator so that the needle used to introduce the salt solution enters the amniotic sac. When the needle is in place, some amniotic fluid is withdrawn, allowing the saline solution to be injected.

Some physicians support the saline procedure by dilating the cervix with *laminaria* or another dilatory product and administering the hormone oxytocin to stimulate uterine contractions. The onset of uterine contractions will expel the dehydrated uterine contents within 24 to 36 hours.

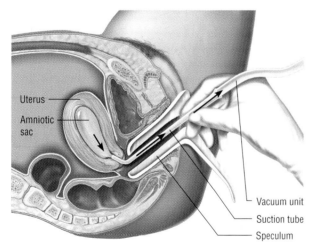

Uterus
Amniotic sac

Vacuum unit
Suction tube
Speculum

Figure 16-6 During dilation and evacuation, the cervix is dilated and the contents of the uterus are aspirated (removed by suction). This procedure is used to perform abortions up to 16 weeks' gestation.

Prostaglandin Procedure The use of prostaglandin is the third type of abortion procedure employed during the second trimester. Prostaglandins are hormonelike chemicals that have a variety of useful effects on human tissue. Produced naturally within the body, these substances influence the contractions of smooth muscle. Because the uterine wall is composed entirely of smooth muscle, it is particularly sensitive to the presence of prostaglandins. When prostaglandin is administered in sufficient quantity (through either a uterine intramuscular injection or a vaginal suppository), uterine contractions become strong enough to expel the fetal contents.

Third-Trimester Abortion Procedures

If an abortion is required in the latter weeks of the gestational period, a surgical procedure in which the fetus will be removed or a procedure in which the entire uterus is removed (hysterectomy) can be undertaken. As you can imagine, these procedures are more complicated and involve longer hospitalization, major abdominal surgery, and an extended period of recovery.

In the late 1990s, the United States House of Representatives and the U.S. Senate voted to ban a rarely used third-trimester abortion procedure referred to as intact D and E (dilation and extraction). Lawmakers believed that this procedure, also called *partial-birth abortion,* was too gruesome to be permitted. President Clinton vetoed this ban, and because the Senate failed to override his veto, the ban on partial-birth abortion did not become federal law.

At the state level, however, many individual state governments had already passed laws banning partial-birth abortions. On June 30, 2000, the Supreme Court invalidated a Nebraska law that prohibited this procedure. This ruling called into question the constitutionality of other existing states' laws concerning this third-trimester procedure.

At the time of this writing (in September 2003), thirty-one states had enacted laws related to partial birth abortion. However, in nineteen of these states, court orders had specifically blocked the enforcement of the laws. Partial birth ban laws in nine states (Indiana, Mississippi, Montana, North Dakota, Oklahoma, South Carolina, South Dakota, and Tennessee) had not yet been challenged in the courts. Only four states (Georgia, Kansas, New Mexico and Utah) had partial birth ban statutes that were considered clearly enforceable.[26]

> **Key Terms**
>
> **hypertonic saline solution** a salt solution with a concentration higher than that found in human fluids.

A Final Word

In the heat of passion, people often fail to think rationally about the potential outcomes of unprotected sex. Therefore, the time to prepare for the romantic moment is *before* you are in a position where you don't want to think about the possibility of an unintended result. If you choose to be sexually active, find a form of protection that works well for you and use it consistently. If you choose not to be sexually active, realize that this is a viable choice that can be 100% effective.

Taking Charge of Your Health

- Use the Personal Assessment on page 549 to help you determine which birth control method is best for you.
- If you have a partner, discuss your personal preferences with him or her.
- Talk to your doctor about the health aspects of different types of birth control boforo malcing your dcci3ion.

- Find out as much as you can about the newest types of contraception (Seasonale, NuvaRing, Mirena, and Evra).
- Think about your likelihood of becoming pregnant or contracting an STD, and discuss with your partner how you might handle these possibilities if they should occur.

Summary

- *Birth control* refers to all of the procedures that can prevent the birth of a child.
- *Contraception* refers to any procedure that prevents fertilization.
- Each birth control method has both a theoretical effectiveness rate and a use effectiveness rate. For some contraceptive approaches, these rates are similar (such as hormonal methods), and for others the rates are very different (such as condoms, diaphragms, and periodic abstinence).
- Many factors should be considered when deciding which contraceptive is best for you.
- Recent research indicates that the spermicide nonoxynol-9 may increase the spread of STDs among some users.
- Stcrilization (vaseʟtoy aʈd lubal ligation) is usually considered an irreversible procedure.
- The birth control pill is safe and effective for the vast majority of women, but it does not protect against sexually transmitted diseases.

- Among the newest contraceptives are "the ring" and "the patch."
- Female condoms are currently available in drugstores without a prescription.
- Two types of IUDs are available: a hormone-containing IUD and a copper-wrapped IUD.
- Emergency contraception is safe and effective in preventing pregnancy when used within 3 days of unprotected intercourse.
- The FDA has approved the drug mifepristone (RU-486) to induce a medical abortion during the first trimester of pregnancy.
- Currently, abortion remains a woman's choice under the guidelines of the 1973 *Roe v. Wade* decision and various state restrictions.
- Abortion procedures vary according to the stage of the pregnancy.

Review Questions

1. Explain the difference between the terms *birth control* and *contraception*. Give examples of each.
2. Explain the difference between theoretical and use effectiveness rates. Which is always higher?
3. Identify some of the factors that should be given careful consideration when selecting a contraceptive method. Explain each factor.

4. What is periodic abstinence? Identify and describe each of the four approaches to this birth control strategy.
5. Describe how vaginal spermicides work and how effective they are as a contraceptive.
6. What are the current concerns over the use of the spermicide nonoxynol-9?

7. What are the differences between the diaphragm and the cervical cap?
8. What are the two types of IUDs that are available in the United States?
9. How do minipills differ from the combined oral contraceptive?
10. What is emergency contraception? For what circumstances might this be used?
11. In what form is Depo-Provera delivered to a woman?
12. How does the contraceptive ring (NuvaRing) differ from the contraceptive patch (Evra)?
13. Describe the various sterilization procedures.
14. Identify and describe the different abortion procedures that are used during each trimester of pregnancy.
15. In which trimester of pregnancy are most abortions performed?
16. What is a medical abortion?

References

1. McAnulty RD, Burnette MM. *Exploring human sexuality: making healthy decisions.* Allyn and Bacon, 2001.
2. Strong B, DeVault C, Sayad BW, Yarber WL. *Human sexuality: diversity in contemporary America,* 4th ed. McGraw-Hill, 2001.
3. Hatcher RA, et al. *Contraceptive technology,* 17th ed. Ardent Media, 1998.
4. WebMD Medical News. *Warning for spermicide nonoxynol-9* (January 17, 2003), **www.my.webmd. com/content/article/59/66773.htm**, accessed September 15, 2003.
5. Davis JL. *Spermicide promotes HIV,* WebMD Medical News (September 26, 2002), **www.webmd. com/content/article/50/40570.htm**, accessed September 15, 2003.
6. Allgeier ER, Allgeier AR. *Sexual interactions,* 5th ed. Houghton Mifflin, 2000.
7. DeNoon D. *Best condoms still latex,* WebMD Health (March 21, 2003), **www.my.webmd.com/content/article/62/71710.htm**, accessed September 11, 2003.
8. Planned Parenthood Federation of America. *Your contraceptive choices,* **www.plannedparenthood.org**, accessed September 10, 2003.
9. Steiner MJ, et al. Contraceptive effectiveness of a polyurethane condom and a latex condom: a randomized controlled trial. *Obstetrics and Gynecology* 101(3):539–547, 2003.
10. Greenberg JS, Bruess CE, Haffner DW. *Exploring the dimensions of human sexuality.* Jones and Bartlett, 2000.
11. Allendale Pharmaceuticals, telephone interview, September 11, 2003.
12. Planned Parenthood Federation of America. *Your contraceptive choices: IUD,* **www.plannedparenthood.org/bc/cchoices3.html#IUD**, accessed September 12, 2003.
13. Berlex Laboratories Website. *Changes in menstruation,* **www.mirena-us.com**, accessed September 15, 2003.
14. Crooks R, Baur K. *Our sexuality,* 8th ed. Wadsworth, 2001.
15. Adlind V. Modern intrauterine devices. *Bailliers Clin Obstet Gynaecol* 10(1):55-57, 1996.
16. U.S. Bureau of the Census. *Statistical abstract of the United States: 2002,* 122nd ed. U.S. Government Printing Office.
17. U.S. Food and Drug Administration. *FDA approves Seasonale oral contraceptive,* FDA Talk Paper (September 5, 2003), **www.fda.gov/bbs/topics/ANSWERS/2003/ANS01251.html**, accessed September 8, 2003.
18. Planned Parenthood Federation of America. *Birth control,* **www.plannedparenthood.org/bc/**, accessed September 10, 2003.
19. Hyde JS, DeLameter JD. *Understanding human sexuality,* 8th ed. McGraw-Hill, 2003.
20. Columbia University Health Education Program. *The NuvaRing—another birth control option,* **www.goaskalice.columbia.edu,** (November 11, 2002), accessed September 10, 2003.
21. Ortho-McNeil Pharmaceutical. *The first birth control patch receives FDA approval* (press release November 20, 2001), **www.ortho-mcneil.com/news/archive/pr/news_evra.htm**, accessed November 27, 2001.
22. The Alan Guttmacher Institute. *State policies in brief: Access to emergency contraception* (September 1, 2003),www.agi-usa.org/pubs/spib_EC.pdf, accessed September 7, 2003.
23. Kelly GF. *Sexuality today: the human perspective,* 7th ed. McGraw-Hill, 2004.
24. *FDA approves 'abortion pill.'* (September 28, 2000), **www.cnn.com/health/women/09/28/abortion.pill**, accessed October 15, 2000.
25. Creinin MD, et al. Mifepristone and misoprostol and methotrexate/misoprostol in clinical practice for abortion. *American Journal of Obstetrics and Gynecology* 188(3): 664–669, 2003.
26. The Alan Guttmacher Institute. *State policies in brief: Bans on 'partial-birth' abortion* (September 1, 2003), **www.agi-usa.org/pubs/spib_BPBA.pdf**, accessed September 7, 2003.

The political circumstances surrounding so-called "partial-birth abortion" procedures have changed very much since the manuscript for this edition (see pages 542–543) was finished. The U.S. Congress passed the "Partial-Birth Abortion Ban Act" and in November 2003 President George W. Bush signed the bill into law. Shortly thereafter, a number of organizations (including the American Civil Liberties Union, the National Abortion Federation, and the Planned Parenthood Federation of America) went to court and won temporary restraining orders to effectively block the immediate implementation of the new law.

As we go to press in April 2004, three trials (in California, New York and Nebraska) are under way that challenge the wording and constitutionality of the new law. Critics of the law claim that the wording is vague and fails to protect women's health and reproductive choices. Proponents of the law contend that the procedure is not medically necessary to protect a woman's health and that it causes undue, inhumane pain to the fetus.

By the time you read this, verdicts in these suits will likely have been rendered. Do you know the current status of this law?

Childless by Choice: new options for women and Couples

Any aspect of reproduction is bound to be emotionally charged. Choosing not to reproduce is a subject that is rarely discussed openly.[1] Although there have been childless (some prefer the term *child-free*) women and couples throughout history, ours is one of the first generations of women who can bypass motherhood by their own will.[1] Safe, reliable contraception and paid employment have broadened possibilities for women, allowing them to choose motherhood without being absorbed by it or to reject motherhood for themselves and not be stigmatized by that choice.[2]

Making the Choice

Sterilization of males and females is the leading form of birth control. Forty-six percent of women ages 40 to 44 have been sterilized.[2] However, this procedure is more rare among younger women and those with no children. Many of these women rely on the second leading method of birth control, the oral contraceptive pill.[2]

Forty-two percent of all women of childbearing age have not yet given birth. Some will become mothers, and others will not.[3] For some this is a conscious choice. Others have children without thinking, or under pressure, while the rest postpone having children until it is biologically too late. One-third of women who decide to remain childless do so before they marry.[4] Their future spouses rarely disagree with their choice, probably because these women have been leaning away from motherhood all along and tend to select men who agree with their choice or with whom childbearing would not be probable or possible. Marrying men who already have children or are unwilling or

physically unable to have them removes some of the burden of choice from the woman.[1] Nine out of ten childless couples actively decide to remain so, whereas only two-thirds of parents make a deliberate decision to have children; the remaining one-third do so by default or accident.[4]

The rate of voluntary childlessness in this country is highest among Asian Americans and whites (7.7%) and American Indians (6%). African Americans have a 3% rate of voluntary childlessness, and the rate for Hispanic Americans is 1.6%.[4] Voluntary childlessness occurs among all socioeconomic groups rather than being the prerogative of privileged women, as once believed.[3]

The vast majority of women do become mothers by the age of 45. Since society views parenthood as natural, people rarely ask them why they had children. However, the opposite question is frequently asked of the minority of women who aren't mothers.

Why Women Choose Not to Be Mothers

One author sums up the complexity of the choice to remain childless in the following way: "A variety of factors make women psychologically receptive to considering the childless alternative, and then a combination of what happens to them and how they choose to live causes them ultimately to embrace it." It is a combination of history, personality, and circumstance that leads some women to choose the unconventional life of a nonmother.

Characteristics of Childless Women and Couples

As a group, women who remain childless are typically firstborn or only children, untraditional, better educated, more

cosmopolitan, less religious, and more likely to have a profession than mothers. They also tend to gravitate toward independent professions in which they can have more control of their working hours and conditions.[1] Nonmothers have the most education and best paid jobs of all American women.[3]

The wife in a childless marriage almost always works and frequently earns more money than her husband. Husbands in these unions tend to share more of the household responsibilities than men do when children are present.[1] These unconventional men and women have unconventional marriages as well. These couples may be older when they marry, and many have been married before. Differences in age, ethnicity, and social class between the partners are common.

Contrary to popular belief, nonmothers are not cold or selfish. They can be deeply committed, nurturing, and generous, but on their own terms. Many prefer not to give up control of their lives to the unpredictability of child rearing. They also recognize that they can't put their own goals aside for a prolonged period of time without fostering resentment and anger. Nonmothers are so completely committed to whatever they undertake that they know they couldn't live up to their own standards of parenting and don't want to impose similar unrealistic expectations on a child.[1] For these women, the satisfaction of child rearing would not offset the costs.

The Role of Fathers

A woman without children has traditionally been called "barren," which implies an emptiness and causes others to question her femininity. No comparable term exists for a man without children, and no questions of his masculinity are raised.[1] Thus childlessness highlights different issues for both sexes, as does parenting. More men than women reject parenthood after having children, which is evidenced by the soaring birthrate for single mothers.[3] Some women decide not to bring children into the world with partners who are less than totally committed to raising them.[4]

This concern is often valid. Parenthood more commonly and more drastically alters a woman's life than a man's.[1] American fathers spend an average of 38 seconds a day with their babies, 26 minutes a day with preschoolers, and 16 minutes a day with school-aged children. Although many fathers do take an active role in caring for their children, half of all fathers have never changed a diaper and three-quarters take no responsibility for child care. The remainder of the responsibility for parenting usually falls to the mothers, and this extra burden can be emotionally draining.[4]

Pros and Cons of a Childless Lifestyle

The Talking It Over box on page 521 presents an abbreviated list of the pros and cons of choosing not to have children. These reasons are examples, and there are many more on each side of the issue, many of which are uniquely personal. Also bear in mind that the same reasons that motivate some people to become parents cause others to avoid parenthood.[3]

The advantages of the childless lifestyle are supported by a recent study that found that couples were happiest before their first baby arrived.[5] Their marital happiness then suffered a long drop as their children grew, reaching its lowest point during a child's teen years. The couples did not approach their pre-baby levels of satisfaction until their last child was on his or her own. Childless couples were found to be as happy as couples are before babies arrive, and, without the long cycle of child rearing, their happiness tended to stay at this high level over time.

Some people have babies for the wrong reasons, such as to try to fix something in their lives. This is an impossibly large burden for a child. A baby can't revitalize an unhappy marriage, improve poor self-esteem, or lessen feelings of depression, frustration, or disappointment with work, friends, or family. Ultimately the desire to raise a child, not anxiety over your own past, present, or future, is the only good and fair reason to give birth. It is typical to approach this decision with avoidance, uncertainty, mixed emotions, and conflicting desires. People who choose to remain childless may rethink their decision and reevaluate the pros and cons many times in their lives.[1]

Society's View

Although it is more acceptable now, voluntary childlessness is still viewed negatively in American society. Motherhood automatically brings status, structure, and a sense of purpose, whereas women who are childless by choice are often unfairly judged to be self-indulgent and immature. Instead of accepting childlessness as a personal choice, many people perceive it as a threat to society as a whole. The notion of remaining childless makes many people uneasy. Those who choose to remain childless often hear such prying questions and statements as:

- "Don't you think you're being selfish?"
- "You will be lonely when you're old."
- "You will change your mind after you have kids."
- "Do you dislike children?"
- "Don't you have any maternal instinct?"
- "Is it a physical problem?"

Parents of a childless couple may fear that the decision their child has made reflects poorly on their own parenting skills.[1] At family gatherings, childlessness is often spoken of in hushed tones, as if the woman or couple has a disease. With pity in their voices, family members may whisper, "She doesn't [they don't] have any children."[1] They may add the word *yet* and tell stories of women in their 40s who have given birth, as if there is still hope for a cure.

One of the most significant factors in determining how many children a couple has, if any, may be religion and how strictly the couple practices it. Muslims, for example, have a higher fertility rate than non-Muslims, and Catholics have a higher fertility rate than Protestants or Jews.[2]

Living with the Decision

Historically, women were rewarded for producing male heirs to carry on the family name and daughters to take care of their parents in old age.[2] In today's society, a woman's earning ability, rather than her fertility, provides her security.[3]

The 22% of women born between 1956 and 1972 who will not bear children are in their own ways confronting what it has always meant to be born female.[2,6] While there have been notable childless women in history, their attitudes toward childlessness are unknown. Their personal stories, along with other feminine wisdom about whether or not to bear children, have been distorted, lost, or ignored.[3] This silence makes the decision even more difficult.

Women who end up rejecting motherhood for themselves are usually not rejecting the institution of motherhood itself. On the contrary, they value it as something that requires special qualities and skills, rather than something just anyone can do. Those who choose not to take that course are different but not in any way defective as women.

For childless couples, friends replace the family as lifelines. Like-minded friends foster self-acceptance, while friends with children provide special bonding and involvement for the childless couple as special "aunts" and "uncles" or "adopted" neighbors to their children.[1]

Whether you decide to have children or not, the issue will probably never be completely resolved for you or anyone else. Nobody has it all. No one lives a life without limitations, and no one makes choices without loss. As long as you make a genuine, conscious choice for your own reasons, your choice will most likely be right for you.

For Discussion . . .

If you don't have children, do you plan to become a parent one day? Why or why not? How do you view childless couples? Is there a person with no children of his or her own who was special to you during your childhood?

References

1. Safer J. *Beyond motherhood.* Pocket Books, 1996.
2. Bartlett J. *Will you be a mother? Women who choose to say no.* New York University Press, 1995.
3. Lisle L. *Without child: challenging the stigma of childlessness.* Ballantine Books, 1996.
4. Lang SS. *Women without children: the reasons, the rewards, the regrets.* Pharos Books, 1996.
5. Elias M. Couples in pre-kid, no-kid marriages happiest. *USA Today* 1997 March 12:1D.
6. Thomas IM. Childless by choice. *Hispanic* 1995; 8(4)50–52.

personal assessment

which birth control method is best for you?

To assess which birth control method would be best for you, answer the following questions, and check the interpretation below.

Do I: Yes   No

1. Need a contraceptive right away?   ____   ____
2. Want a contraceptive that can be
   used completely independent of   ____   ____
   sexual relations?
3. Need a contraceptive only once in a   ____   ____
   great while?
4. Want something with no harmful   ____   ____
   side effects?
5. Want to avoid going to the doctor?   ____   ____
6. Want something that will help protect   ____   ____
   against sexually transmitted diseases?
7. Have to be concerned about affordability?   ____   ____
8. Need to be virtually certain that   ____   ____
   pregnancy will not result?
9. Want to avoid pregnancy now but want   ____   ____
   to have a child sometime in the future?
10. Have any medical condition or   ____   ____
    lifestyle that may rule out some form
    of contraception?

Interpretation

If you have checked *Yes* to number:

1. Condoms and spermicides may be easily purchased without prescription in any pharmacy.
2. Sterilization, oral contraceptives, hormone rings, patches, or injections, cervical caps, and periodic abstinence techniques do not require that anything be done just before sexual relations.
3. Diaphragms, condoms, or spermicides can be used by people who have coitus only once in a while. Periodic abstinence techniques may also be appropriate but require a high degree of skill and motivation.

4. IUD use should be carefully discussed with your physician. Sometimes the use of oral contraceptives or hormone products results in some minor discomfort and may have harmful side effects.
5. Condoms and spermicides do not require a prescription from a physician.
6. Condoms help protect against sexually transmitted diseases. Nonoxynol-9 may increase STD transmission in some users. No method (except abstinence) can guarantee complete protection.
7. Be a wise consumer: check prices, ask pharmacists and physicians. The cost of sterilization is high, but there is no additional expense for a lifetime.
8. Sterilization provides near certainty. Oral contraceptives, hormone injections, or a diaphragm-condom-spermicide combination also give a high measure of reliable contraceptive protection. Periodic abstinence, withdrawal, and douche methods should be avoided. Outercourse may be a good alternative.
9. Although it is sometimes possible to reverse sterilization, it requires surgery and is more complex than simply stopping use of any of the other methods.
10. Smokers and people with a history of blood clots should probably not use oral contraceptives or other hormone approaches. Some people have allergic reactions to a specific spermicide or latex material. Some women cannot be fitted with a diaphragm or cervical cap. The woman and her health care provider will then need to select another suitable means of contraception.

To Carry This Further . . .

There may be more than one method of birth control suitable for you. Always consider whether a method you select can also help you avoid an STD. Study the methods suggested above, and consult Table 16.1 to determine what method may be most appropriate.

chapter seventeen

becoming a parent

Online Learning Center Resources

www.mhhe.com/payne8e

Log on to our Online Learning Center (OLC) for access to these additional resources:

- Chapter key terms and definitions
- Learning objectives
- Student interactive question-and-answer sites

- Self-scoring chapter quiz
- Online assessments
- Key term flash cards

Talking It Over

Discussing Adoption Options

Approximately two million couples consider adopting a child each year in the United States. Only about 20,000 healthy children are available for adoption, and traditional adoption methods can take a long time. However, older children, children with disabilities, and children already in foster care are available immediately. Increasingly, couples are seeking children to adopt from foreign countries. In 1998, a total of 15,774 children from abroad were adopted by Americans.

Prospective parents need to prepare for adoption by considering the impact the child will have on the existing family, as well as the family's ability to provide for the adopted child's emotional and physical needs. It is also helpful if the adoptive parents can acquire information about the child's family medical history, prenatal care, and pre-adoption life.

CommunicationLinks

www.adoption.org
www.adopt.org
www.calib.com/naic

Eye on the Media

Grandparents' Visitation Rights

According to the American Association of Retired Persons (AARP), 6.3 percent of children under the age of 18 live in homes that are headed by grandparents. This amounts to 4.5 million children under age 18. Of these 4.5 million children, about one-third have no parent present in the grandparent-headed household. Clearly, some grandparents are playing larger roles than are the parents in the lives of many of their grandchildren. Some grandparents are gaining custody of their grandchildren, and others are adopting their grandchildren. The AARP website **(www.aarp.org)** offers information (and website links) for grandparents who are raising children.[1]

Some grandparents who want to play a larger role in the lives of their grandchildren find it difficult to spend time with them, usually because the child's parents (or parent) do

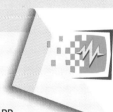

Eye on the Media *continued*

not want their children to be with their grandparents. Parental objections to grandparent visitation vary widely and can range from a parent's belief that the child does not have enough spare time (due to school and extracurricular activities) to maintaining the position that the grandparents are unfit to visit alone with the child. The parents may feel that it is not in the best interests of the child to be with the grandparents.

Issues of custody and visitation are frequently resolved in the courts. During the summer of the year 2000, a major United States Supreme Court decision held that grandparents *do not necessarily* have the right to visit their grandchildren, if the parent objects to the visit. In the *Troxel v. Granville* case, the Supreme Court ruling invalidated a Washington state law that allowed *any person* the right to seek time with a child if the judge believed it to be in the best interests of the child. The Troxels had sought to spend more time with their granddaughters, after the girls' father (who was the Troxels' son) died. The mother objected to the amount of time sought by the Troxels. Ultimately, the Supreme Court supported the mother.[2] The Court, however, did not rule that all nonparent visitation laws are unconstitutional, and many states' laws concerning visitation are likely to remain in place.

This Court decision was significant because it upheld the view that biological connections to grandchildren are not necessarily the sole criterion for visitation rights, even if the biological grandparents are determined to be generous, kind people. In this decision, the parents' wishes superseded those of the grandparents. It will be interesting to see if other state laws concerning grandparents' visitation will be challenged in the future. At stake may be the home lives of many children and, ultimately perhaps, the definition of what constitutes a family in the United States.

[1] AARP. *For grandparents.* **www.aarp.org/grandparents/,** accessed September 24, 2003.
[2] Lithwick D. *Children's time: the real issue in grandparents' rights case.* CNN.com, **www.CNN.com/2000/LAW/06/COLUMNS/FL.LITHWICK.TROXEL,06.23,** 23 June 2000, accessed 1 November 2000.

Although birth control is especially important for many young couples, most couples eventually want to have children and raise a family. In the past, couples had their children very quickly after either high school or college. Now the trend seems to be to wait longer before having children. Most likely, educational, economic, contraceptive, and occupational factors have laid the groundwork for this trend. To the relief of many people, medical research indicates that women over the age of 30 or 35 are quite capable of having healthy babies.

Parenting Issues for Couples

Before deciding to have children, couples should frankly discuss the effects that pregnancy and a newborn child will have on their lives (see the Discovering Your Spirituality box on page 553). In addition, anyone who is sexually active should consider these same issues, because very few contraceptive methods are 100% effective all the time, and pregnancy can result from nearly any act of intercourse. For those students contemplating single parenthood, we ask that you consider these issues as they relate to your particular situation and to excuse our consistent use of plural pronouns. In any event, couples should discuss some or all of the following basic considerations:

- What effect will pregnancy have on us individually and collectively?
- Why do we want to have a child?
- What effect will a child have on the images we have constructed for ourselves as adults?

- Can we afford to have a child and provide for its needs?
- How will the responsibilities related to raising a child be divided?
- How will a child affect our professional careers?
- Are we ready now to accept the extended responsibilities that can come with a new child?
- How will we rear our child in terms of religious training, discipline, and participation in activities?
- Are we ready to part with much of the freedom associated with late adolescence and the early young adult years?
- How will we handle the possibility of being awakened by 6 o'clock or earlier each morning for the next few years?
- What plans have we made in the event that our baby (or fetus) has a serious birth defect?
- Are we capable of handling the additional responsibilities associated with having a disabled child?
- Are we comfortable with the thought of bringing another child into an already overcrowded, violent, bigoted, and polluted world?

If these questions seem strikingly negative in tone, there is indeed a reason for this. We believe that all too frequently the "nuts and bolts" issues related to childbearing and parenting are ignored or at least are placed on the back burner (see the Learning from Our Diversity box on page 555). Although it is important for future parents to consider how cute and cuddly a new baby will be, how holidays will be enhanced with a new child, and how pleased the grandparents will be, we consider these issues

Parenthood Expands Personal Growth

Becoming a parent is almost always an exciting experience. Through 9 months of pregnancy, anticipation of the baby increases on a daily basis. What sex will the baby be? How much hair will he or she have? How large will the baby be? Will the baby be a healthy child? Will the labor and delivery go smoothly? How will the household be changed as a result of the baby? How will the parents interact with each other after the baby enters the picture?

All of these parental thoughts are centered on the baby and its presence. This is natural. Carrying a pregnancy to term and adjusting to the new baby are exciting, challenging, and exhausting experiences for the parents. There are times when new parents wonder how they ever got themselves into this situation. But there are many more times when parents are likely to be immensely thankful and proud to be parents of a newborn child.

Sometimes as we watch the growth and development of a newborn baby, we fail to think about the opportunities parenthood provides for the parents themselves to grow and develop. Parenthood presents an extra dimension to the lives of most parents. Although one can see this extra dimension in a number of ways, perhaps the most noticeable change is in the depth and quality of human relationships.

Perhaps most easily seen is the connection between mother and child. Living together, sharing nutrients (ideally only good ones), and protecting each other for 9 months forges a spiritual bond between mother and child that remains for a lifetime. They experience labor and delivery in a way unique to themselves. Although fathers may be able to sense how strong this bond is, they never can fully understand or feel how close this mother-child connection is and how strong it tends to remain. *Parenthood is a life-altering experience for a woman.*

After becoming parents, fathers also tend to forge close, intimate bonds with their children, but these bonds are more likely related to the interactions they experience with the children as they grow and develop. Sometimes to their surprise, fathers find out that they have marvelous capabilities to adjust to the new demands a baby presents. Many fathers develop unexpected talents at nurturing their children. Perhaps because of this, more and more fathers are choosing to stay at home and raise their children, while their spouse works to support the family financially. This arrangement was virtually unheard of just three decades ago. *Indeed, parenthood is also a life-altering experience for a man.*

Parenthood encourages men and women to expand their focus from themselves (and their careers, their interests, their friends) to a broader spectrum of other people. This spectrum will certainly include the child, but also health care providers, teachers, school officials, their child's friends, the friends' parents and perhaps religious leaders, law enforcement personnel, and sports coaches. Parents will be required to expand their communication skills, their patience, and their insights as they try to raise their children the best way they can. Through this struggle comes added personal growth for the parents.

A final area in which parenthood offers a new dimension for the parents concerns the intimate bond between the parents themselves. Although it doesn't always happen (and the divorce statistics tell a compelling story), the process of conceiving a child, birthing a child, and raising a child to adulthood can make two people grow together in a way unmatched by any other experience. Older adult couples will often say that their most significant shared experience was raising their children. Many agree that it was through this experience that they gained a depth of understanding about each other that enriched their lives and established their most intimate connection. *In this sense, parenthood is a spiritual, life-altering experience for the parents.*

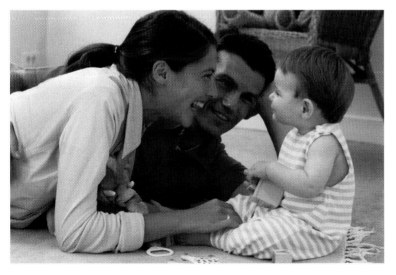

For many young couples, the rewards of raising a family outweigh the stress that inevitably accompanies parenthood.

secondary to the serious realities of having a child enter your lives. Complete the Personal Assessment on page 577 to explore your feelings about parenting.

TALKING POINTS If you think you would like to have children some day, would you feel comfortable discussing these issues with your partner? How would you start the conversation?

Human Cloning: An Ethical Dilemma

Today's most controversial issue related to parenting is reproduction through **human cloning.** With the 1997 breakthrough cloning of the Scottish sheep Dolly, the possibility of human cloning emerged within the scientific community. To clone a human, the procedure would involve the following steps:[1]

- Doctors would surgically retrieve an egg from the female donor.
- The nucleus of this egg would be removed.
- A cell is taken from a cloning subject (a male or female).
- Through an electrical jolt, the cloning subject's cell is fused with the **enucleated egg.** This creates a clonal zygote. Shortly after, this clonal zygote divides over and over and develops into a clonal embryo.
- The clonal embryo is implanted in the womb of a surrogate mother.
- After nine months, a genetically matched reproduction of the cloning subject is born.

Although this step-by-step process may seem simple, it has never been accomplished with human subjects. In fact, it took scientists 277 attempts to produce Dolly, the cloned sheep.[1] The technical expertise to clone humans has not been fully developed, although some scientists believe it could be on the near horizon, if public policy would fully support this area of research.

However, public policy currently does not support human cloning. Several countries and a few states have passed laws banning human cloning.[1] The U.S. Food and Drug Administration (FDA) has warned researchers that any attempts at human cloning must first get FDA approval, which the FDA claims will not be forthcoming. Both the American Society for Reproductive Medicine and the National Academy of Sciences have voiced their opposition to human cloning.[2] Many public opinion polls have indicated that Americans are overwhelmingly against the use of cloning to produce babies.[3]

However, the potential use of a particular type of cloning has received much more popular public support in America. This is the use of cloning to reproduce body parts, tissues, and specific organs for use in medical trans-

plant procedures. A baby is never reproduced in this cloning procedure.[2] In organ and tissue cloning, sometimes called **therapeutic cloning,** the clonal embryo is not implanted into a surrogate mother, but allowed to grow (divide) into a number of premature cells called **stem cells.** These stem cells have the potential to grow into any kind of body cell.

Theoretically, scientists could develop techniques that would cause these stem cells to grow into tissues or organs that would match the tissues or organs in the person who donated the genetic material. Because of this genetic match, these cloned organs would not be rejected after the transplant surgery. In essence, this technology permits a person's own body to be a human repair kit. Some predict that, in the not too distant future, scientists will be able to grow replacement organs like hearts, livers, and skin and replacement neurons for persons who suffer from Parkinson's or Alzheimer's disease.

On the other side of the fence are those who wonder if cloning represents "science gone mad." Some believe that any kind of cloning is unethical because it interferes with nature. Altering a woman's eggs, reprogramming cells, and tampering with embryos is something that is *simply wrong.* Regardless of the position you take on this issue, you can expect to see more scientific advances regarding cloning, especially therapeutic cloning.

Becoming a Parent Through a Stepfamily

Some people will become parents through a marriage in which one or both adult partners bring children from a previous relationship.[4] This newly constituted household is called a *stepfamily.*

Although some people call this a blended family, the Stepfamily Association of America believes the preferred term is a stepfamily. Children in stepfamilies do not lose their individual identities and instantly "blend" into a new family while losing attachments to the parent who is not a part of the new marriage. Things are rarely that smooth. If both parents remarry, a child may become a member of

Key Terms	
human cloning	the replication of a human being.
enucleated egg	an ovum with the nucleus removed.
therapeutic cloning	the use of certain human replication techniques to reproduce body tissues and organs.
stem cells	premature cells that have the potential to turn into any kind of body cell.

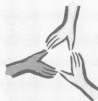

Learning from Our Diversity

Pregnancy and Parenting After Forty

Women who become pregnant in their forties are not a new phenomenon. Many young people and baby boomers today were delivered by mothers who were 40 or more years old. What is new is women becoming pregnant for the first time at an age when many women begin menopause.

The reasons for the delay are several. Some couples may have tried to conceive for years and only succeeded when in their forties. Other women and couples delayed pregnancy in order to build their careers, travel, or become more financially secure. In addition, fertility technology, such as in vitro fertilization, microsurgery, and the use of donor eggs or sperm, have finally given many couples the baby they long wanted.

The trend of later childbearing began in the late 1970s, when better-educated baby-boom women began entering the workforce. For women 40 to 44, the rate of first babies increased from 0.3 to 1.4 per 1,000, still a small percentage but a significant jump.[1]

The common belief that men can father babies well into middle age is supported not only by anecdotal evidence (such as Tony Randall, Larry King, and Michael Douglas), but also recent research that shows that sperm function in older men does not differ significantly from that of younger men.[2]

Women traditionally were discouraged from becoming pregnant for the first time in their forties because of the health risks to the mother and the risk of birth defects for the baby. It is true that women 40 and older suffer more complications during childbirth, and the risk of having a baby with Down syndrome or another genetic abnormality increases as a mother ages.[1]

The chances of having a cesarean delivery are about 40% higher than in a younger woman.[3] The number of women over 40 with gestational diabetes and high blood pressure is higher, and many have more difficulty with labor and deliver babies that are underweight or premature. In addition, the risk of fetal death is higher in women over 35 years old.[4]

Women who want to have a baby should use this information to prevent the problems, however, rather than let it discourage them from having a baby at all, researchers say.

Women who want to start families in their forties should consider the following points:

- Infertility can become a problem with age, but fertility drugs such as Clomid or treatments such as in vitro fertilization can help.
- The rate of miscarriage is higher among older women, so immediate prenatal care is vital.
- Early genetic testing can ease the fears about birth defects. Tests can reveal the presence of Down syndrome, Tay-Sachs disease, cystic fibrosis, and sickle-cell anemia.
- Cesarean sections are more common in older mothers.

On the plus side, another study recently reported that women who are able to give birth after age 40 (not including those who become pregnant through the use of fertility treatments) may be "slow to age" and live longer.[1] This can be good news to older moms who wonder whether they will have the energy to chase a toddler.

[1] Blackburn B. Moms starting families in 40s test odds. *USA Today* 1997; Sept 24:14A.
[2] Haidl G, Jung A, Schill WB. Aging and sperm function. *Hum Reprod* 1996; 11(3):558–560.
[3] Later age pregnancy. Preparing for the happy, healthy event of after 40. *Health Oasis,* Mayo Clinic, 1998. **www.mayohealth.org/mayo/9708/htm/aged_p.htm**
[4] Fretts RC et al. Increased maternal age and risk of fetal death. *N Engl J Med* 1995; 333(15):953–957.

---

two stepfamilies and, perhaps, face even more obstacles concerning family loyalty. It is natural for children to wonder where they fit in or where they belong. Calling a newly constituted family a blended family may set up too many unrealistic expectations for children and adults and make adjustments more difficult. For example, children may balk when told that they are to consider their new family to be the family that deserves all their attention and loyalty.[4]

It is beyond the scope of this chapter to outline the challenges (and joys) that come with becoming a parent through a stepfamily arrangement. The Stepfamily Association of America, a nonprofit support group for persons involved in stepfamily relationships, indicates that for stepfamilies to be successful, parents should:

- Nurture and enrich the couple relationship.
- Reveal and understand emotions.
- Have realistic expectations.
- Develop new roles.
- Seek support and see the positive.

Throughout the merging of families into stepfamilies, clear communication, honest feelings, and a positive attitude about one's new role can help the process run more smoothly. It is quite possible that new family relationships can be wonderful experiences for all involved.

Parenting Across Cultures

In their recent text *Transcultural Health Care,* Purnell and Paulanka describe the various ways ethnic groups in America tend to view babies and young children.[5] In the Amish culture, children are seen as gifts from God. They

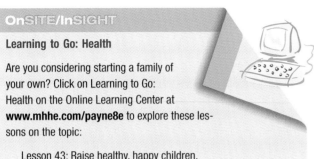

are very welcomed into families. Amish families have an average of seven children per family and, unlike in other ethnic groups in America, this fertility pattern has not changed for the past century. Large families prize children because they are not only gifts from God, but they are also valuable resources on low tech, labor-intensive family farms.

Children are considered a blessing to Jewish families. Children are to be afforded an education that prepares them for progress in society as well as increased understanding of their Jewish heritage. To that end, many Jewish children attend public school but also attend Hebrew school a couple of afternoons each week during the school year. Jewish children play important roles in most of the holiday celebrations and religious services. Parents are expected to treat their children fairly and to be flexible, caring, and attentive to discipline.[5]

Although there is much change taking place as Chinese increase their assimilation into the United States, many Chinese American families still hold on to Chinese traditions. Children are highly valued, but the number of children in a family tends to be small, perhaps because of China's one-child rule. Independence is usually not fostered, and parents make many decisions for the children even into young adulthood. Teens are expected to work hard in school, score well on exams, and help with chores around the home.[5]

In discussing Arab Americans' views of children, Purnell and Paulanka write that high fertility rates tend to be favored because of the belief that "God decides family size" and because families follow Islamic dictates regarding birth control, treatment of infertility, and abortion. Procreation is considered the primary reason for a marriage, since it enhances family strength. As with a number of cultures around the world, pregnancy tends to occur early in the marriage, and the preference for boys over girls is a reality. The sex of a child can be a great concern for the pregnant woman, and observers will often note the way in which the mother "carries" her baby during the pregnancy (girls are thought to be carried high and boys to be carried low).[5]

Pregnancy: An Extension of the Partnership

Pregnancy is a condition that requires a series of complex yet coordinated changes to occur in the female body. This chapter follows pregnancy from its beginning, at fertilization, to its conclusion, with labor and childbirth. Fathers-to-be share many of the joys and worries of pregnancy and childbirth. For a look at the concerns that expectant fathers may feel, see the Changing for the Better box on page 557.

Physiological Obstacles and Aids to Fertilization

Many sexually active young people believe that they will become pregnant (or impregnate someone) only when they want to, despite their haphazard contraceptive practices. Because of this mistaken belief, many young people do not consistently use contraceptives. Young adults must remember that, to ensure the survival of our species, our bodies were designed to promote pregnancy. It is estimated that about 85 percent of sexually active women of childbearing age will become pregnant within one year if they do not use some form of contraception.[6]

With regard to pregnancy, each act of intercourse can be considered a game of physiological odds. Obstacles exist that may reduce a couple's chance of pregnancy, including the following.

Obstacles to Fertilization

1. *The acidic level of the vagina is destructive to sperm.* The low pH of the vagina will kill sperm that fail to enter the uterus quickly.
2. *The cervical mucus is thick during most of the menstrual cycle.* Sperm movement into the uterus is more difficult, except during the few days surrounding ovulation.
3. *The sperm must locate the cervical opening.* The cervical opening is small and may not be located by most sperm.
4. *Half of the sperm travel through the wrong fallopian tube.* Most commonly, only one ovum is released at ovulation. The two ovaries generally "take turns" each month. The sperm have no way of "knowing" which tube they should enter. Thus it is probable that half will travel through the wrong tube.
5. *The distance sperm must travel is relatively long compared with the tiny size of the sperm cells.* Microscopic sperm must travel about seven or eight inches after they are inside the female.
6. *The sperm's travel is relatively "upstream."* The anatomical positioning of the female reproductive structures necessitates an "uphill" movement by the sperm.

7. *The contoured folds of the tubal walls trap many sperm.* These folds make it difficult for sperm to locate the egg. Many sperm are trapped in this maze.

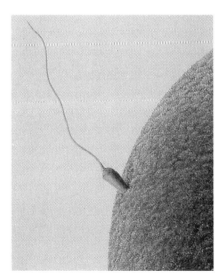

The surface of an ovum is penetrated by sperm at fertilization.

There are also a variety of aids that tend to help sperm and egg cells join. Some of these are listed next.

Aids to Fertilization

1. *An astounding number of sperm are deposited during ejaculation.* Each ejaculation contains about a teaspoon of semen.[7] Within this quantity are between 200 and 500 million sperm cells. Even with large numbers of sperm killed in the vagina, millions are able to move to the deeper structures.

2. *Sperm are deposited near the cervical opening.* Ejaculation into the vagina by the penis places the sperm near the cervical opening.

3. *The male accessory glands help make the semen nonacidic.* The seminal vesicles, prostate gland, and Cowper's glands secrete fluids that provide an alkaline environment for the sperm. This environment helps sperm be better protected in the vagina until they can move into the deeper, more alkaline uterus and fallopian tubes.

4. *Uterine contractions aid sperm movement.* The rhythmic muscular contractions of the uterus tend to cause the sperm to move in the direction of the fallopian tubes.

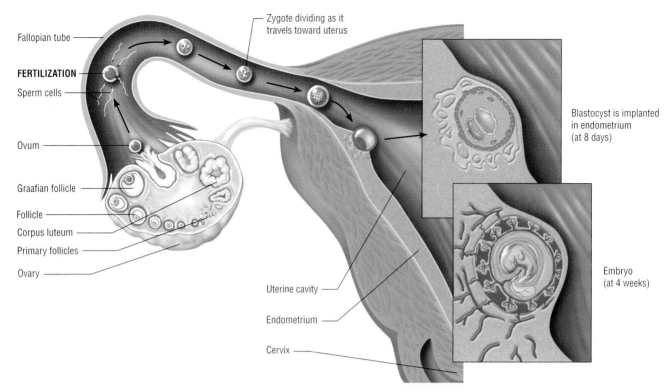

Figure 17-1 After its release from the follicle, the ovum begins its week-long journey down the fallopian tube. Fertilization generally occurs in the outermost third of the tube. Now fertilized, the ovum progresses toward the uterus, where it embeds itself in the endometrium. A pregnancy is established.

5. *Sperm cells move rather quickly.* Despite their tiny size, sperm cells can move about one inch per hour. Powered by sugar solutions from the male accessory glands and the whiplike movements of their tails, sperm can reach the distant third of the fallopian tubes in less than eight hours as they swim in the direction of the descending ovum.

6. *After they are inside the fallopian tubes, sperm can live for days.* Some sperm may be viable for up to a week after reaching the comfortable, nonacidic environment of the fallopian tubes. Most sperm, however, will survive an average of forty-eight to seventy-two hours. Thus they can "wait in the wings" for the moment an ovum is released from the ovary (Figure 17-1).

7. *The cervical mucus is thin and watery at the time of ovulation.* This mucus allows for better passage of sperm through the cervical opening when the ovum is most capable of being fertilized.

Signs of Pregnancy

Aside from pregnancy tests done in a professional laboratory, a woman can sometimes recognize early signs and symptoms. The signs of pregnancy have been divided into three categories.

Presumptive Signs of Pregnancy

Missed period after unprotected intercourse the previous month

Nausea on awakening (morning sickness)

Increase in size and tenderness of breasts

Darkening of the areolar tissue surrounding the nipples

Probable Signs of Pregnancy

Increase in the frequency of urination (the growing uterus presses against the bladder)

Increase in the size of the abdomen

Cervix becomes softer by the sixth week (detected by a pelvic examination by a clinician)

Positive pregnancy test (see the Star box on page 559)

Positive Signs of Pregnancy

Determination of a fetal heartbeat

Feeling of the fetus moving (quickening)

Observation of the fetus by ultrasound or optical viewers

Home Pregnancy Tests

Think you might be pregnant? A home pregnancy test is simple to do and can give you an accurate answer in 2 to 5 minutes.

Improved technology has made the urine home pregnancy test about as accurate as blood tests—99% under perfect conditions—although in actual use it may be less than that.*

Using a woman's urine, a home pregnancy test detects the presence of human chorionic gonadotropin (hCG), a hormone produced only during pregnancy. The tests contain monoclonal antibodies, which are molecules coated with a substance that bonds to the pregnancy hormone. If the hormone is present, a colored stripe, dot, or other symbol appears in the test windows. The tests also contain "control" windows to indicate whether the device has functioned properly.

Although the makers of today's tests say their products can detect hCG as soon as the very day a missed period was supposed to begin, they also advise taking the test again a few days later to confirm the result. If the result is positive, see a doctor as soon as possible.

*Williams RD. Healthy pregnancy, healthy baby. *FDA Consumer,* March–April 1999; 33(2):18–22.

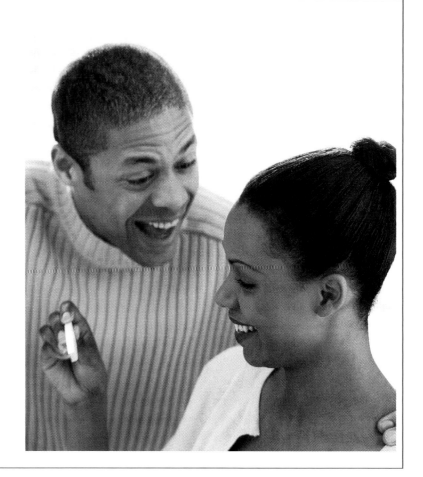

Agents That Can Damage a Fetus

A large number of agents that come into contact with a pregnant woman can affect fetal development. Many of these (rubella and herpes viruses, tobacco smoke, alcohol, and virtually all other drugs) are discussed in other chapters of this text. The best advice for a pregnant woman is to maintain close contact with her obstetrician during pregnancy and to consider carefully the ingestion of any over-the-counter (OTC) drug (including aspirin, caffeine, and antacids) that could harm the fetus.

Women should also avoid exposure to radiation during pregnancy. Such exposure, most commonly through excessive x-rays or radiation fallout from nuclear testing, can irreversibly damage fetal genetic structures. In addition, pregnant women should avoid Accutane, a drug prescribed for the treatment of cystic acne that can severely damage the fetus.

Intrauterine Development

Intrauterine development takes place over the course of three **trimesters.** Most pregnancies last from 38 to 42 weeks. For purposes of illustration, we will consider each

trimester to be 13 weeks. The growth and development during these trimesters occurs in a typical pattern for most pregnancies. (To read about emotional changes during pregnancy, see the Changing for the Better box on page 562.)

First Trimester

The first 13-week trimester starts at conception, when the egg and sperm unite to form a structure called the **zygote.** The zygote, or fertilized egg, undergoes a series of cellular changes as it grows and makes its week-long journey down the fallopian tube to the uterus. About the tenth day after conception, the zygote, now called a **blastocyst,** imbeds itself into the endometrial lining of the uterus.

> ### Key Terms
>
> **trimester** a 3-month period; human pregnancies encompass three trimesters.
>
> **zygote** a fertilized ovum.
>
> **blastocyst** early stage of the developing life form that imbeds into the endometrial lining of the uterus.

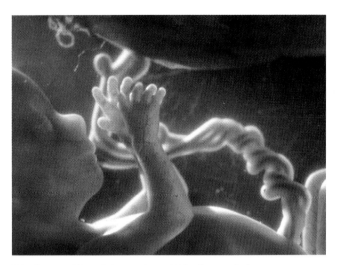

The fetus at 16 weeks' gestation within the amniotic sac.

From the end of 2 weeks after conception until the end of the eighth week, the growing structure is called an **embryo.** After 8 weeks and until the birth, it is called a **fetus.**

The first trimester is characterized by rapid cellular growth. By the end of the first trimester, the fetus weighs only about 1 oz., yet most body organs are formed and the fetus can move.[8] It is currently thought that about half of all pregnancies end in **spontaneous abortion** during the early weeks of the first trimester, usually before the woman realizes she is pregnant. These miscarriages usually result from a genetic defect or a serious developmental problem.

Second Trimester

The second trimester is characterized by continued growth and maturation. During this time, the organs continue to grow and physicians can hear the fetal heartbeat with a stethoscope. The bone structures are fully evident during the second trimester. The fetus starts to look more and more like an infant.

Additionally, the mother's breast weight increases by about 30 percent because of the deposition of 2 to 4 pounds of fat. This fat serves as a reserve energy source for the mother should she decide to nurse her baby. For this reason, good maternal nutrition is essential during the second trimester.

Third Trimester

The third trimester is another critical time for the developing fetus. At the beginning of this trimester, the fetus generally weighs 2 to 3 pounds. Over the final 13 weeks of gestation, the fetus will double in length and multiply its weight by up to five times.

This is also the time when the fetus absorbs considerable amounts of the minerals iron and calcium from the mother. For this reason, the mother must maintain sound eating patterns and avoid her body's depletion of mineral stores, perhaps by taking a vitamin and mineral supplement containing iron, which would reduce her risk of developing anemia during the final trimester.[8]

Childbirth: The Labor of Delivery

Childbirth, or *parturition,* is one of the true peak life experiences for both men and women. Most of the time, childbirth is a wonderfully exciting venture into the unknown. For the parents, this intriguing experience can provide a stage for personal growth, maturity, and insight into a dynamic, complex world.

During the last few weeks of the third trimester, most fetuses will move deeper into the pelvic cavity in a process called *lightening.* During this movement, the fetus' body will rotate and the head will begin to engage more deeply into the mother's pelvic girdle. Many women will report that their babies have "dropped."

Another indication that parturition may be relatively near is the increased reporting of *Braxton Hicks contractions.*[9] These uterine contractions, which are of mild intensity and often occur at irregular intervals, may be felt throughout a pregnancy. During the last few weeks of pregnancy (*gestation*), these mild contractions can occur more frequently and cause a woman to feel as if she is going into labor **(false labor).**

Labor begins when uterine contractions become more intense and occur at regular intervals. The birth of a child can be divided into three stages: (1) effacement and dilation of the cervix, (2) delivery of the fetus, and (3) expulsion of the placenta (Figure 17-2). For a woman having her first child, the birth process lasts an average of

---

Key Terms

embryo developmental stage from the end of the second week after conception until the end of the eighth week.

fetus developmental stage from the beginning of the ninth week after conception until birth.

spontaneous abortion any cessation of pregnancy resulting from natural causes; also called a miscarriage.

false labor conditions that resemble the start of true labor; may include irregular uterine contractions, pressure, and discomfort in the lower abdomen.

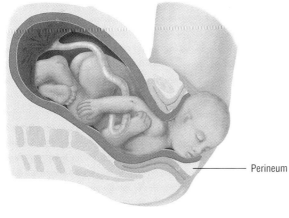

A First Stage

Placenta

Umbilical cord

Uterus

Cervical opening

Birth canal

Uterine contractions thin the cervix and enlarge the cervical opening.

Figure 17-2 Labor, or childbirth, is a three-stage process. During effacement and dilation, the first stage (**A**), the cervical canal is gradually opened by contractions of the uterine wall. The second stage (**B**), delivery of the fetus, encompasses the actual delivery of the fetus from the uterus and through the birth canal. The delivery of the placenta, the third stage (**C**), empties the uterus, thus completing the process of childbirth.

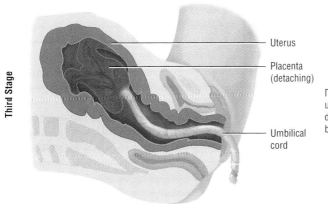

B Second Stage

Uterine contractions are aided by mother's voluntary contractions of abdominal muscles.

Fetus moves through dilated cervical opening and birth canal.

Perineum

C Third Stage

Uterus

Placenta (detaching)

Placenta detaches from uterine wall and is delivered through the birth canal.

Umbilical cord

twelve to sixteen hours. The average length of labor for subsequent births is much shorter—from four to ten hours on the average. Labor is very unpredictable: Labors that last from 1 to 24 hours occur daily at most hospitals. (See the Considering Complementary Care box on page 563 for a discussion of midwifery.)

Stage One: Effacement and Dilation of the Cervix

In the first stage of labor the uterine contractions attempt to thin (*efface*) the normally thick cervical walls and to enlarge (*dilate*) the cervical opening.[10] These contractions are directed by the release of prostaglandins and the hormone oxytocin into the circulating bloodstream. In women delivering their first babies, effacement will occur before dilation. In subsequent deliveries, effacement and dilation usually occur at the same time.

The first stage of labor is often the longest. The cervical opening must thin and dilate to a diameter of ten centimeters before the first stage of labor is considered complete.[11] Often this stage begins with the dislodging of the cervical mucous plug. The subsequent *bloody show* (mucous plug and a small amount of blood) at the vaginal opening may indicate that effacement and dilation have begun. Another indication of labor's onset may be the bursting or tearing of the fetal amniotic sac. "Breaking the bag of waters" refers to this phenomenon, which happens in various measures in expectant women.

The pain of the uterine contractions becomes more intense as the woman moves through this first stage of labor. As the cervical opening effaces and dilates from 0 to 3 centimeters, many women report feeling happy, exhilarated, and confident. In the early phase of the first stage of labor, the contractions are relatively short (lasting from 15 to 60 seconds) and the intervals between contractions range from 20 minutes to 5 minutes as labor progresses. However, these rest intervals will become shorter and the contractions more forceful when the woman's uterus contracts to dilate 4 to 7 centimeters.

In this second phase of the first stage of labor, the contractions usually last about one minute each and the rest intervals drop from about five minutes to one minute over a period of five to nine hours.

The third phase of the first stage of labor is called *transition*. During transition, the uterus contracts to dilate the cervical opening to the full 10 centimeters required for safe passage of the fetus out of the uterus and into the

For the past century, most of the women in the United States who went into labor followed a fairly standard procedure. This included a trip to the hospital and a lengthy wait in a labor room. The actual birth then took place in a delivery room, which was a surgical room equipped to handle most medical emergencies. Doctors and nurses were always close by to watch the expectant mother and to track the high-tech monitors.

This scenario is rapidly changing with the increased use of midwives, many of whom help deliver babies within hospital settings, at free-standing birthing centers, or in the homes of the pregnant women. Two types of nurse-midwives are certified by the American College of Nurse-Midwives (ACNM). A Certified Nurse-Midwife (CNM) is trained and certified in the two disciplines of nursing and midwifery, while the Certified Midwife (CM) has training and certification in midwifery. All Certified Nurse-Midwives have baccalaureate degrees and over 70% also have master's or doctoral degrees.[1]

Both CNMs and CMs operate within a framework of a health care system that provides for consultation, collaborative management, or referral to additional medical care according to the health needs and condition of the pregnant woman. If the woman needs specialized help during the pregnancy or emergency care during labor, certified midwives do not hesitate to access the traditional medical system. Since 99% of midwife deliveries take place within hospitals, this care is usually easily attainable. Presently, less than 1 percent of midwife-assisted births occur at free-standing birthing centers or in private homes.[2]

For many years, the traditional medical establishment discounted the use of midwives, believing that midwives were incapable of providing professional prenatal care and birthing assistance to women. However, this position has softened considerably. Indeed, most pregnancies and births follow a natural, standard pattern in which trained midwives can function in a very cost-effective, low-tech, patient-friendly manner.

Today, over 9% of all births in the United States are attended by midwives. In the year 2000, certified midwives attended 297,902 births.[2] With certified midwifery training programs in place at some of the most prestigious universities in the country (for example, Vanderbilt University, Baylor College of Medicine, the University of Michigan, and Yale University), this trend will likely continue.

[1] American College of Nurse-Midwives. *Basic facts about nurse-midwives,* **www.midwife.org**, (12 December 2002), accessed 1 October 2003.
[2] Martin JA et al. Births: final data for 2000. *National Vital Statistics Reports* 50:5 (12 February 2002), pp. 1–102.

vagina (birth canal).[12] This period of labor is often the most painful part of the entire birth process. Fortunately, it is also the shortest phase of most labors. Lasting between 15 and 30 minutes, transition contractions often last 60 to 90 seconds each. The rest intervals between contractions are short and vary from 30 to 60 seconds.

An examination of the cervix by a nurse or physician will reveal whether full dilation of 10 centimeters has occurred. Until the full 10-centimeter dilation, women are cautioned not to "push" the fetus during the contractions. Special breathing and concentration techniques help many women cope with the first stage of labor.

Stage Two: Delivery of the Fetus

When the mother's cervix is fully dilated, she enters the second stage of labor, the delivery of the fetus through the birth canal. Now the mother is encouraged to help push the baby out (with her abdominal muscles) during each contraction. In this second stage the uterine contractions are less forceful than during the transition phase of the first stage and may last 60 seconds each, with a 1- to 3-minute rest interval.

This second stage may last up to two hours in first births.[7] For subsequent births, this stage will usually be much shorter. When the baby's head is first seen at the vaginal opening, *crowning* is said to have taken place. Generally the back of the baby's head appears first. (Infants whose feet or buttocks are presented first are said to be delivered in a *breech position.*) After the head is delivered, the baby's body rotates upward to let the shoulders come through. The rest of the body follows quite quickly. The second stage of labor ends when the fetus is fully expelled from the vagina. In the past, deliveries were often performed with an *episiotomy,* a surgical incision of the **perineum** intended to prevent lacerations (tearing) when the baby was delivered.

Immediately after the birth, and again 5 minutes later, the newborn's physical health frequently is evaluated by obstetrical assistants using the Apgar score system. The baby will be judged (rated either 0, 1, or 2) on five criteria including appearance (color), pulse, response to foot

Key Terms

perineum in the female, the region between the vulva and the anus.

stimulation, muscle tone, and respiration. After 5 minutes, 98% of infants score 7 or above. An Apgar score of less than 5 after 5 minutes indicates the possibility of a serious defect.

Newly delivered babies often look "unusual." Their heads are often cone-shaped as a result of the compression of cranial bones that occurs during the delivery through the birth canal. Within a few days after birth, the newborn's head will assume a much more normal shape. Most babies (of all races) appear bluish at first until they begin regular breathing. All babies are covered with a coating of *vernix,* a white, cheeselike substance that protects the skin.

Stage Three: Delivery of the Placenta

Usually within 30 minutes after the fetus is delivered, the uterus will again initiate a series of contractions to expel the placenta (or *afterbirth*). The placenta is examined by the attending physician to ensure that it was completely expelled. Torn remnants of the placenta could lead to dangerous hemorrhaging by the mother. Often the physician manually examines the uterus after the placenta has been delivered.

After the placenta has been delivered, the uterus continues with mild contractions to help control bleeding and start the gradual reduction of the uterus to its normal, nonpregnant size. This final aspect of the birth process is called **postpartum.** External abdominal massage of the lower abdomen seems to help the uterus contract, as does an infant's nursing at the mother's breast. For suggestions for successfully breastfeeding your baby, see the Changing for the Better box above.

Cesarean Deliveries

A **cesarean delivery** (cesarean birth, C-section) is a procedure in which the fetus is surgically removed from the mother's uterus through the abdominal wall. This type of delivery, which is completed in up to an hour, can be performed with the mother having a regional or a general anesthetic.

Key Terms

postpartum the period after the birth of a baby during which the uterus returns to its prepregnancy size.

cesarean delivery (si **zare** ee an) surgical removal of a fetus through the abdominal wall.

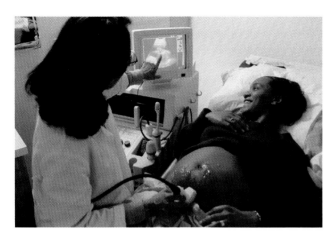

Ultrasound scans are used to check the growing fetus for possible abnormalities, as well as size, development, position, and many other factors.

In 2002, the percentage of deliveries by cesarean section reached an all-time high of 26.1%.[13] The increasing use of cesarean deliveries is questioned by some medical experts, although others point to the need for this kind of delivery when one or more of the following factors are present:

- The fetus is improperly positioned.
- The mother's pelvis is too small.
- The fetus is especially large.
- The fetus shows signs of distress.
- The umbilical cord is compressed.
- The placenta is being delivered before the fetus.
- The mother's health is at risk.

Although a cesarean delivery is considered major surgery, most mothers cope well with the delivery and post-surgical and postpartum discomfort. The hospital stay is usually a few days longer than for a vaginal delivery. The mother can still nurse her child and may still be able to have vaginal deliveries with later children. More and more hospitals are allowing the father to be in the operating room during cesarean deliveries. Fortunately, research indicates that early **bonding** between child, mother, and father can still occur with cesarean deliveries. Cesarean deliveries are much more expensive than vaginal deliveries.

Complications in Pregnancy and Childbirth

Most women progress through pregnancy and delivery without complications, but once in a great while something goes wrong. Complications are usually the result of genetics, an environmental factor (such as the use of drugs or alcohol by the mother), or some combination of these (see the Star box on page 566). Pregnant women should remember that the following complications are unusual if they are consuming a healthy diet, avoiding agents that can damage a fetus, such as alcohol and drugs, and following their doctor's recommendations (see the Changing for the Better box on page 567).

- *Ectopic pregnancy:* This is a pregnancy in which the embryo implants outside the uterus, most often in a fallopian tube. It can be serious and even life threatening, especially if not discovered early, but treatment can remove most of the risk for the mother while preserving future fertility.

- *Miscarriage:* Early miscarriage is very common, occurring in as many as half of all conceptions, often passing unnoticed by the woman. It is usually related to a chromosomal abnormality or other problem in the fetus. Late miscarriage, on the other hand, is usually related to the mother's condition, her exposure to drugs or other toxins, or problems of the placenta.

- *Gestational diabetes:* This is a temporary condition in which the mother's body does not produce enough insulin to handle the increased blood sugar of pregnancy. Symptoms include unusual thirst, frequent urination, and fatigue. If treated, it is not a threat to the mother or baby.

- *Hyperemesis gravidarum:* This term literally means "excessive vomiting during pregnancy." This is a very unusual condition that is more serious than typical morning sickness. If untreated, it can result in malnutrition, dehydration, or damage to the fetus. It can be treated, however, with measures ranging from rest and antacids to hospitalization if necessary.

- *Preeclampsia (pregnancy-induced hypertension; toxemia):* This is a condition in which the woman's blood pressure becomes elevated during pregnancy; it occurs in one of every ten to twenty pregnancies, and if untreated, preeclampsia can be serious and even life threatening. Fortunately, physicians almost invariably identify the disease if the mother is receiving regular prenatal care, and a poor outcome is rare. Treatment depends on the severity of the disease and can include

Testing for Birth Defects

Many women undergo tests during pregnancy to check for birth defects, genetic disorders, and other problems.* A few of the most common tests are ultrasound scans, the alpha-fetoprotein (AFP) test, amniocentesis, and chorionic villi sampling (CVS). Each of these can be helpful in diagnosing problems, but the tests are not necessary for every pregnancy. Check with your doctor about what tests, if any, are appropriate for you.

Ultrasound—Ultrasound technology uses high-frequency sound waves to form pictures of the fetus on a computer screen. The test can verify a due date, determine causes of bleeding, check the overall health, development, sex, and position of the baby, measure the amniotic fluid, and check the condition of the placenta. There are no known risks from the tests, and many women have one or two ultrasounds in routine pregnancies. However, there is little scientific evidence that normal pregnancies benefit from ultrasound tests.

Alpha-fetoprotein Screening (AFP)—A simple blood test that poses no risk to the fetus, AFP screening measures the levels of alpha-fetoprotein in the mother's blood. Abnormal levels can indicate a brain or spinal cord defect, the presence of twins, a miscalculated due date, or an increased risk of Down syndrome. Because AFP levels can be elevated for a number of reasons, a positive test is usually repeated or followed up by other tests before a diagnosis is made. Very few women with elevated AFP levels are found later to have babies with birth defects.

Amniocentesis—This test examines the cells shed by the fetus into the surrounding amniotic fluid. Performed about 16 weeks into pregnancy, the test involves inserting a long, thin needle through the mother's abdomen to extract fluid from the womb. The cells must be cultured in a laboratory and it may take up to a month for test results to be ready. The test is a reliable indicator of chromosomal abnormalities such as Down syndrome or genetic disorders such as Tay-Sachs disease, Hunter's syndrome, and others. While usually safe, amniocentesis can trigger cramping, leakage of amniotic fluid, and vaginal bleeding, and it may increase the risk of miscarriage by about 0.5 to 1 percent. The test is only done on women at increased risk of having babies with genetic disorders or to assess the maturity of the baby's lungs in the last trimester.

Chorionic Villi Sampling (CVS)—Performed between 10 and 12 weeks of pregnancy, CVS can detect the same genetic abnormalities as amniocentesis. It involves inserting a catheter or needle into the womb and extracting some of the chorionic villi (cells from the tissue that will become the placenta). The chorionic villi contain the same chromosomes as the fetus. The test is relatively safe, but it has a greater risk of miscarriage than amniocentesis. While there has been some concern that the test itself may be associated with limb deformities, many geneticists believe that CVS performed between 10 and 12 weeks of pregnancy does not increase that risk.

* Williams RD. Healthy pregnancy, healthy baby. *FDA Consumer*, March–April 1999; 33(2):18–22.

---

an immediate induction of labor or hospitalization of the mother until the fetus is sufficiently developed to survive outside the uterus.

- *Eclampsia:* The final stage of preeclampsia, this disease is very unusual when the mother is receiving regular prenatal care. Symptoms include convulsions and coma. Treatment includes preventing convulsions and inducing labor or performing a cesarean delivery as soon as possible.

- *Intrauterine growth retardation (IUGR):* This term is used to describe insufficient growth of the fetus, which can occur because of genetic factors, maternal disease, or fetal malnutrition. With regular prenatal care, this disease can be identified and reversed.

- *Premature rupture of the membranes (PROM):* Rupture of the chorionic membranes, often called "breaking of the water," can occur prematurely. Infection is a risk because the protective membrane has been broken. Doctors typically try to delay delivery as long as possible up to about thirty-seven weeks.

- *Premature labor:* Labor that begins after the fetus is considered viable and before term, at about thirty-

seven weeks, is called *premature labor*. It carries a variety of risks, but in many cases premature labor can be halted, and the mother can carry the baby to term. Quick medical attention is paramount.

- *Fetal distress:* This term describes a category of fetal problems, in particular a lack of oxygen caused by any of a variety of factors. The treatment usually is immediate delivery, by cesarean if necessary.

TALKING POINTS Are there people in your life that you can comfortably ask, "What was it like to go through labor and delivery?" Will you feel open enough to express any personal concerns you might have about your own fears of this process?

Preconceptional Counseling

Prenatal diagnosis and counseling is one of the most beneficial advances in medical technology. Genetic counselors can provide timely, accurate, and complete information to patients, while maintaining the attitude that the patient's values should guide the decisions.

My husband and I are thinking about starting a family in the near future. What can we do to ensure the healthiest baby possible?

Having a healthy pregnancy and delivering a healthy child actually should start before conception. In their book *The Twelve-Month Pregnancy,* Barry Herman, MD, and Susan Perry, PhD, emphasize the importance of the preconception weeks in getting your baby off to a good start.[1] They encourage expectant moms to adopt a healthy lifestyle while they are trying to become pregnant. They advise women to stop smoking, stop drinking alcoholic beverages, eat well, get physical exercise, avoid or treat infections, avoid unnecessary exposure to toxic chemicals, and ask a physician before consuming any drug (prescription or over-the-counter).

It is well established that tremendous embryonic and fetal growth and development take place during the first weeks after conception. Women often do not know that they are pregnant until after they miss a menstrual period. If they wait to alter their lifestyle until after they are certain of the pregnancy, they could inadvertently be putting the child's health at risk. So, it's best to plan ahead . . . prior to conception.

Once the pregnancy is established, it is important to follow some additional guidelines:[2]

- Arrange for prenatal care.
- Consume a well-balanced diet.
- Take a vitamin supplement that contains folic acid.
- Exercise according to your physician's recommendation.
- Avoid and treat infections.
- Avoid alcohol, tobacco, and other drugs.
- Limit your caffeine intake.
- Stay away from x-rays, hot tubs, and saunas.
- Stay away from toxic chemicals.

An expectant dad can also participate in this healthy approach by matching the woman's lifestyle changes. This provides sound emotional support for the pregnancy and, as an added bonus, improves the health status of the dad.

[1] Herman B, Perry SK. *The Twelve-month pregnancy: what you need to know before you conceive to ensure a healthy beginning for you and your baby,* 2nd ed. Lowel House, 1997.
[2] Williams RD. Healthy pregnancy, healthy baby. *FDA Consumer,* March–April 1999; 33(2):18–22.

You should seek genetic counseling *before* attempting to conceive a child if you or your partner fall into any of the following categories:[14]

- History of multiple spontaneous abortions
- Consanguinity (partners are related by blood)
- Birth defect, possible genetic condition, neuromuscular or neurologic condition, or abnormalities of physical sexual development in the patient or families
- Ethnic background with increased risk of recessive genetic disease
- Maternal age of 35 or more years at delivery
- Paternal age of 55 or more years
- Positive maternal test for Down syndrome or trisomy 18
- Positive maternal test for an open neural tube defect
- Carrying a gene for a recessive disease that is more common in some ethnic populations
- Exposure to a known or suspected **teratogenic agent** (capable of causing birth abnormality)

The genetic counselor might use a variety of methods for gathering information about the couple, including DNA testing, other medical tests, medical records, family histories, and autopsy reports. When couples receive genetic counseling before conception and learn that they have a high risk of conceiving a child with birth defects, they then

Key Terms

teratogenic agent any substance that is capable of causing birth defects.

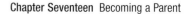

have a variety of options still open to them, such as artificial insemination by a donor, ovum donation, and adoption.

In addition, some couples can also reduce the risk of birth defects by changing their behavior or diet. For example, taking folic acid supplements has been shown to reduce the risk of neural tube defects. Abstaining from alcohol during pregnancy eliminates the risk of fetal alcohol syndrome. Stopping smoking reduces the risk of fetal intrauterine growth retardation, placental abruption (premature detachment of the placenta from the uterine wall), and fetal death. Women with the disease phenylketonuria who eliminate phenylalanine from their diet before pregnancy drastically reduce the risk of mental retardation in their children.[14]

If you have already become pregnant, you still should work with your physician to identify risk factors in your first prenatal visit, to allow time for tests to be conducted and medical records to be reviewed. Tests commonly performed for those at risk are chorionic villi sampling (CVS) and amniocentesis.

In the second trimester, tests commonly performed include targeted ultrasound and screening for Down syndrome, trisomy 18, and open neural tube defects. Couples who learn of an increased risk through a second-trimester test tend to be significantly more anxious than those who learned of the risk earlier in the pregnancy. In general, couples should attempt to receive genetic counseling and testing while they still have the legal option to terminate the pregnancy.

 TALKING POINTS You have a concern that makes you want to get preconceptual counseling, but your partner balks at this. How can you get a dialogue going so that you can change his or her mind about this?

Infertility

Most traditional-age college students are interested in preventing pregnancy. However, increasing numbers of other people are trying to do just the opposite: They are trying to become pregnant. It is estimated that about one in six couples has a problem with *infertility*. These couples wish to become pregnant but are unsuccessful.

Causes of Infertility

What causes infertility? About 40% of infertility problems are attributed to male factors and about 40% are explained by female factors. Approximately 10% of the problems stem from a combination of female and male factors, while the remaining 10% come from unknown origins.[15]

Problems of infertility that may come from males include low sperm count, inability of the sperm to move properly, or structural abnormalities of the sperm. Female factors related to infertility center on lack of ovulation and obstructions in the fallopian tubes.

Enhancing Fertility

A number of approaches can be used to increase sperm counts. Among the simple approaches are the application of periodic cold packs on the scrotum and the replacement of tight underwear with boxer shorts. When a structural problem reduces sperm production, surgery can be helpful. Most experts (reproductive endocrinologists) suggest that couples have intercourse at least a couple of times in the week preceding ovulation. Frequent intercourse tends to lower sperm counts, so couples should not have sex more than every 36 hours.[16]

Artificial Insemination

Men can also collect (through masturbation) and save samples of their sperm to use in a procedure called *artificial insemination by partner*. Near the time of ovulation, the collected samples of sperm are deposited near the woman's cervical opening. In a related procedure called *artificial insemination by donor*, the sperm of a donor are used. Donor semen is screened for the presence of pathogens, including the AIDS virus.

Surgical Remedies

Causes of infertility in women center mostly on obstructions in the reproductive tract and the inability to ovulate. The obstructions frequently result from tissue damage (scarring) caused by infections. Chlamydial and gonorrheal infections often produce fertility problems. In certain women the use of IUDs has produced infections and PID; both of these increase the chances of infertility. Other possible causes of structural abnormalities include scar tissue from previous surgery, fibroid tumors, polyps, and endometriosis. A variety of microsurgical techniques may correct some of these complications.

One of the most recent innovative procedures involves the use of **transcervical balloon tuboplasty.** In this procedure a series of balloon-tipped catheters are inserted through the uterus into the blocked fallopian tubes. After they are inflated, these balloon catheters help open the scarred passageways.

⌐ **Key Terms** ⌐

transcervical balloon tuboplasty the use of inflatable balloon catheters to open blocked fallopian tubes; a procedure used for some women with fertility problems.

When a woman has ovulation difficulties, pinpointing the specific cause can be very difficult. Increasing age produces hormone fluctuations associated with lack of ovulation. Being significantly overweight or underweight also has a serious effect on fertility. However, in women of normal weight who are not approaching menopause, it appears that ovulation difficulties are caused by failure of synchronization between the hormones governing the menstrual cycle. Fertility drugs can help alter the menstrual cycle to produce ovulation. Clomiphene citrate (Clomid), in oral pill form, or injections of a mixture of luteinizing hormone (LH) and follicle-stimulating hormone (FSH) taken from the urine of menopausal women (Pergonal) are the most common fertility drugs available. Both are capable of producing multiple ova at ovulation (see Focus On article on pages 573–575).

Assisted Reproductive Technology (ART)

For couples who are unable to conceive after drug therapy, surgery, and artificial insemination, the use of one of four assisted reproductive technologies (ART) can be helpful. One option is *in vitro fertilization and embryo transfer (IVF-ET)*. This method is sometimes referred to as the "test tube" procedure. Costing around $10,000 per attempt, IVF-ET consists of surgically retrieving fertilizable ova from the woman and combining them in a glass dish with sperm. After several days, the fertilized ova are transferred into the uterus. IVF-ET accounts for 98% of all ART procedures.[17]

A second test tube procedure is called *gamete intrafallopian transfer (GIFT)*. Similar to IVF-ET, this procedure deposits a mixture of retrieved eggs and sperm directly into the fallopian tubes.

Fertilized ova (zygotes) can also be transferred from a laboratory dish into the fallopian tubes in a procedure called *zygote intrafallopian transfer (ZIFT)*. One advantage of this procedure is that the clinicians are certain that ova have been fertilized before the transfer to the fallopian tubes. GIFT and ZIFT combined account for fewer than 2% of ART procedures.[17]

The fourth (and newest) procedure is *intracytoplasmic sperm injection (ICSI)*. This is a laboratory procedure in which a single sperm cell is injected into a woman's retrieved egg. The fertilized egg is then transplanted into the woman's uterus. The cost and technical expertise involved in ICSI make it a seldom-used procedure for infertile couples.

Surrogate Parenting

Surrogate parenting is another option that has been explored, although the legal and ethical issues surrounding this method of conception have not been fully resolved. Surrogate parenting can take several forms. Typically, an infertile couple will make a contract with a woman (the surrogate parent), who will then be artificially inseminated with semen from the expectant father. In some instances the surrogate will receive an embryo from the donor parents. The surrogate carries the fetus to term and returns the newborn to the parents. In some cases, women have served as surrogates for their close relatives. Because of the concerns about true "ownership" of the baby, surrogate parenting may not be a particularly viable or legal option for many couples.

Options for Infertile Couples

The process of coping with infertility problems can be an emotionally stressful experience for a couple. Hours of waiting in physicians' offices, undergoing many examinations, scheduling intercourse, producing sperm samples, and undergoing surgical or drug treatments place multiple burdens on a couple. Knowing that other couples are able to conceive so effortlessly adds to the mental strain. Fortunately, support groups have been established to assist couples with infertility problems. Some of these groups are listed in the Star box on page 570.

What can you do to reduce the chances of developing infertility problems? Avoiding sexually transmitted diseases is one crucial factor. Barrier methods of contraception (condom, diaphragm) with a spermicide reportedly cut the risk of developing infertility in half. The risk from multiple partners should encourage responsible sexual activity. Men and women should avoid working around hazardous chemicals or using psychoactive drugs. Being overweight or underweight, smoking, and heavy alcohol consumption are risk factors that reduce one's fertility.[18] Maintaining overall good health and having regular medical (and, for women, gynecological) checkups are good ideas. Because infertility is directly linked with advancing age, couples may not want to indefinitely delay having children.

Adoption

For couples who have determined that biological childbirth is impossible, adoption offers an alternative.[19] Adopted children currently represent about 2% of all children in the United States (see the Talking It Over box on page 551).

As the supply of adoptable infants has decreased, young women considering putting their babies up for adoption have gained new leverage. Couples determined to adopt a healthy infant have increasingly turned to independent adoptions arranged by a lawyer, or they may negotiate directly with the birth mother. Independent adoptions now surpass those arranged by social service agencies.

Foster Parenting

The number of children in foster care who are waiting to be reunited with their biological parents or awaiting adoption has risen steadily since the mid-1980s. Experts attribute the rise to family problems caused by parental drug abuse, unemployment, alcoholism, and other difficulties. Currently about one-half million children a year spend time in foster homes.

Like adoption, foster parenting has presented a variety of ethical and legal issues, especially the debate between "the best interests of the child" and parental rights.

TALKING POINTS You have tried for a couple of years to get pregnant, and now you are ready to consider some of the newest options to increase the chances of conception. Your partner seems unwilling to spend much money for these high-tech procedures. You are ready to spend some of your retirement savings in this effort. How can you and your partner best come to an agreement on this issue?

Taking Charge of Your Health

- Use the Personal Assessment on page 577 to help you think about your feelings about parenting.
- Talk to your partner (or roommate) about any ethical concerns that you think might be involved in human cloning.
- With the accuracy that exists with home pregnancy tests, do you envision yourself ever using one?

- If you are pregnant or think you might be pregnant, challenge yourself to avoid any agents that might damage your fetus.
- If you plan to become a parent one day, choose lifestyle behaviors that will enhance (not reduce) your fertility.

Summary

- Couples have many important issues to discuss before deciding to have children.
- Having children through human cloning raises many ethical issues.
- Parents in stepfamilies face challenges as children merge into different living arrangements.
- Several physiological factors can be either aids or obstacles to fertilization.
- Women can often recognize the presumptive and probable signs of pregnancy; a physician can determine positive signs of pregnancy.
- Expectant fathers can experience many of the same symptoms and emotions as expectant mothers.
- Pregnant women, and women attempting to become pregnant, should avoid agents that can damage the fetus, including all drugs (prescription, over-the-counter, and illicit), tobacco smoke, and alcohol.
- The 9 months of pregnancy can be divided into three trimesters. The fetal growth and development during each trimester is unique.
- Childbirth takes place in three distinct stages: effacement and dilation of the cervix, delivery of the fetus, and delivery of the placenta.
- Complications during pregnancy and delivery are varied and can be caused by genetics, environmental factors, or a combination of these.
- Regular prenatal care is vital and can help prevent or reverse complications of pregnancy.
- Preconceptual counseling can provide much information to prospective parents.
- For couples with fertility problems, numerous strategies can be used to help conception take place.

Review Questions

1. What important issues should couples discuss before they decide to have children?
2. What is the difference between human cloning and therapeutic cloning?
3. How would you define the term *stepfamily*?
4. What are some obstacles and aids to fertilization presented in this chapter? Can you think of others?
5. What are the presumptive, probable, and positive signs of pregnancy?
6. Briefly describe the changes in intrauterine development during each trimester.
7. Identify and describe the events that occur during each of the three stages of childbirth. Approximately how long is each stage?
8. Who should seek genetic counseling? How can the counselor assess the couple's risk of having a child with birth defects?
9. What is meant by the term *preconceptional counseling*?
10. List and describe several complications that can occur during pregnancy and delivery.
11. What can be done to reduce chances of infertility?
12. Explain the IVF-ET, GIFT, ZIFT, and ICSI procedures.
13. What options do couples have when they cannot conceive a child?

References

1. Bonsor K. *How human cloning will work,* **www.science.howstuffworks.com/human-cloning.htm,** accessed 24 September 2003.
2. DeNoon D. *Cloning FAQs and fiction,* **www.my.webmd.com/content/article/57/66221.htm,** (6 January 2003), accessed 24 September 2003.
3. Warner J. *Most Americans against human cloning,* **www.my.webmd.com/content/article/59/66746.htm,** (16 January 2003), accessed 24 September 2003.
4. Stepfamily Association of America. *Stepfamily fact sheet,* **www.stepfamilies.org,** accessed 23 September 2003.
5. Purnell LD, Paulanka BJ. *Transcultural health care: a culturally competent approach,* 2nd ed. F.A. Davis, 2003.
6. Hatcher RA et al. *Contraceptive technology,* 17th ed. Irvington, 1998.
7. Hyde JS, DeLameter JD. *Understanding human sexuality,* 8th ed. McGraw-Hill, 2003.
8. Wardlaw GM, Hampl JS, Disilvestro RA. *Perspectives in nutrition,* 6th ed. McGraw-Hill, 2003.
9. Allgeier EA, Allgeier AR. *Sexual interactions,* 5th ed. Houghton Mifflin, 2000.
10. LeVay S, Valente SM. *Human sexuality.* Sinauer Associates, Inc, 2003.

11. Kelly GF. *Sexuality today: the human perspective,* updated 7th ed. McGraw-Hill, 2004.

12. Strong B, DeVault C, Sayad BW, Yarber WL. *Human sexuality: diversity in contemporary America,* 4th ed. McGraw-Hill, 2001.

13. National Center for Health Statistics. U.S. birth rate reaches record low: births to teens continue 12-year decline; cesarean deliveries reach an all-time high, *NCHS Press Release* (25 June 2003), **www.cdc.gov/nchs/releases/03news/lowbirth.htm,** accessed 1 October 2003.

14. Kuller JA, Chescheir NC, Cefalo RC. *Prenatal diagnosis and reproductive genetics.* Mosby-Year Book, 1996.

15. McAnulty RD, Burnette MM. *Exploring human sexuality: making healthy decisions,* 2nd ed. Pearson Allyn & Bacon, 2003.

16. WebMd. *Health guide A–Z: infertility—home treatment,* **www.my.webmd.com/content/healthwise/130/32439,** accessed 2 October 2003.

17. WebMd. *A couple's guide: trying to conceive,* **www.my.webmd.com/content/article/73/87996,** accessed 3 October 2003.

18. RESOLVE. *Preserving your fertility: risk factors,* **www.resolve.org/,** accessed 8 October 2003.

19. Adoption. **www.adoption.org,** accessed 7 October 2003.

As We Go to Press

As we go to press, the Food and Drug Administration (FDA) is informing the public about the potentially dangerous use of ultrasound technology to produce "keepsake videos" for parents-to-be. Ultrasound imaging is a common diagnostic medical procedure that uses high-frequency sound waves to record moving images (sonograms) of organs, tissues, or blood flow inside the body. Physicians use ultrasound to check the size, location, number and age of fetuses, fetal movements, birth defects, numbers of fingers and toes, breathing and heartbeat. This information can be very important for legitimate medical reasons.

However, a growing number of expectant parents seem to be more interested in using ultrasound to determine the baby's sex, facial features and hair. Across the country, the FDA reports that parents are obtaining these keepsake videos in strip malls and shopping center stores with names such as Fetal Fotos, Peek-a-Boo, Baby Insight, and Womb with a View. In laboratory studies, ultrasound produces mechanical vibrations in tissues and elevates tissue temperature. While there is no solid evidence that ultrasound can harm a fetus, the consensus of professional opinion is that the casual use of ultrasound should be avoided.

The FDA has jurisdiction over ultrasound technology. Making keepsake videos represents an unapproved use of a medical device. Additionally, the use of this equipment requires a physician's prescription. Few keepsake facilities are requiring doctors' prescriptions. *As we go to press,* the FDA is starting to take action against these businesses. (See **www.fda.gov** for the latest information.)

supertwins: the boom in multiple births

During World War II their parents gave them patriotic names, such as Franklin, Delano, and Roosevelt, or Franklin D. (for Roosevelt) and Winnie C. (a girl named for Winston Churchill).[1] You may know them as Rachel, Richard, Rebecca, and Ryan or Courtney, Brittany, and Tiffany. They're supertwins—multiple-birth siblings such as triplets, quadruplets, quintuplets, and even sextuplets and more. From 1989 to 1993, an average of 1,057 sets of triplets, 241 sets of quads, and 32 sets of quints were born each year in the United States.[1] More recently, the McCaugheys of Iowa gave birth to septuplets on November 19, 1997. All of their septuplets are home and doing well. Nkem Chukwu and her husband Lyke Louis Udobi of Texas were not as lucky with their octuplets. One of the eight died shortly after delivery in 1998.

Such multiple births are controversial for several reasons, including the increased risk they bring to the mother and the fetuses.

The Good, the Bad, and the Unusual

A special type of bonding occurs among multiple-birth siblings that ranges from reading one another's moods to saving another's life, as in the case of twin girls Brielle and Kyrie.[1,2] Kyrie, at 2 pounds 3 ounces, was doing well, but Brielle, the smaller twin, at 2 pounds, had had trouble breathing, an irregular heart rate, and a low blood oxygen level since birth. Then Brielle's condition suddenly became critical. The hospital staff tried every medical procedure they thought might help, to no avail. As a last resort, they put the girls in the same incubator, as some European hospitals do. Amazingly, Brielle's condition immediately improved

and within minutes her blood oxygen level was the best it had been since birth. Studies have confirmed that double bedding of multiple-birth babies reduces the length of their hospital stay.[2]

On the darker side, sometimes multiple births, or the prospect of them, are exploited by parents. The Dionne quintuplets, now over 60 years old, were the middle 5 of 13 children. When their father sold the rights to exhibit his daughters, the Ontario government made them wards of the state. But the government ended up exploiting them in a bizarre glass playground "Quintland" display, which attracted 10,000 visitors a month. When they were returned to their parents, they were made to feel guilty for their unusual birth and the ensuing familial discord.[3] The surviving quints have written a book about their experiences and have helped teach the world that multiples are not something to be exploited.

Recently, in England, a woman abused fertility drugs by taking them even though she was already fertile and ignoring her physician's instructions while on the drugs. She became pregnant with eight fetuses. She refused to undergo multifetal pregnancy reduction, which would have given the remaining fetuses a better chance of survival, because she had sold her story to a tabloid and would get more money for each baby born. All eight fetuses died at 19 weeks' gestation.[4]

Fertility Drugs and Techniques

Since the birth of the first "test tube baby" (conceived by in vitro fertilization) in 1978, the number of assisted pregnancies and multiple births has escalated. The use of fertility drugs and techniques that

stimulate ovulation sometimes causes the release of multiple eggs per cycle.[1,5]

The infertility rate among married couples is 8.5%. While this rate has remained relatively constant in recent years, the number of couples seeking help for infertility has tripled.[6] Less than half of the couples who receive fertility treatment ever give birth, but one-fourth of those who *do* achieve a pregnancy give birth to more than one child.[1,6] This happens for a number of reasons. First, some fertility drugs are so strong that they cause multiple eggs to be released during one cycle. Second, some treatments are developed too quickly and are administered under too little supervision.[7] And third, fertility services are so competitive and lucrative ($67,000 to $114,000 per delivery[3]) that many clinics go to great lengths to increase the likelihood of pregnancy, such as implanting up to eight embryos in a woman's uterus. In the United Kingdom, a doctor can lose his or her license for implanting more than three embryos, but no such laws have been passed in the United States.[8] Usually, few or no embryos develop; if too many develop, however, multifetal pregnancy reduction is often suggested.[7] This abortion procedure is usually performed by injecting potassium chloride into the most accessible embryos to increase the odds of survival for the others.[9]

The whole process of fertility treatment has been described as an emotional roller coaster.[1] The parents often want children desperately but can't conceive naturally. The drugs and hormones women are given to promote pregnancy can cause great emotional distress. If a couple does achieve a pregnancy, exhilaration can turn to fear when they find out how many embryos are developing.

Will they be able to care for that many children? What if some or all of the babies are sick, or die? Should some be aborted to give the others a better chance? Many fertility clinics do an unsatisfactory job of counseling couples about the likelihood of success and the risks associated with the procedures, so couples often must answer these tough questions without all the information they need.[7]

Medical Complications

After conception, the fertility specialist's job is finished. Everything that goes on during the course of pregnancy and delivery is in the hands of another physician, usually an obstetrician with a specialty in high-risk pregnancy. These physicians must discuss with the parents any risks and concerns that were not addressed earlier.[7]

Each additional fetus shaves roughly 3.5 weeks off the normal 40-week gestation period.[9] Prematurity brings with it a host of problems. The babies are about a third of the weight or less of single babies and much more likely to be ill. The death rate before or soon after birth is 19 times higher for triplets than single babies.[1] From birth to 28 days, the death rate for multiples is still 7 times higher than for singles.[7] Surviving babies suffer higher rates of cerebral palsy and other neurological problems.[10]

Of course, multiple babies have longer hospital stays and are more likely to require intensive care during their stay than single babies. Although the issue of "drive-through" deliveries, in which mother and baby are released within 24 hours, has become a controversial topic lately, the average stay for a single baby is 4.6 days, compared with 8.2 days for twins and 34 days for triplets.[1,6] During their stays, 15% of single infants need intensive care, while 50% of twins and 75% of triplets, quads, and quints require this level of care.[6] Research has shown that most of the heavy use of medical resources in multiple births is due to lower gestational age and lower birth weight.[11]

Multiple births also increase the mother's need for care. The risks of cesarean delivery, anemia, hypertension,

postpartum hemorrhage, and kidney failure are all greater in mothers of supertwins.[1,6] And this specialized care is extremely expensive: The estimated cost of a single birth is $9,850, compared with $37,950 for twins and $109,764 for triplets.[6] Hospital costs for quints can easily exceed half a million dollars.[1] If an insurance company covers this cost, we all pay in the form of increased premiums and deductibles. If they do not pay, it can spell financial ruin for the family. And these medical and financial complications all occur even before the newborns come home.

Public and Private Life

Parents of supertwins say the stress kicks in after about six months. Until then, they're busy just trying to meet their constant needs, which during the first 3 months involves feeding each of three to six babies seven to eight times per day.[1] Because of the stress of the babies' medical problems, financial strain, and pure exhaustion, child abuse is 2.5 to 9 times more likely in families with twins, compared with singles, and parents of supertwins are more likely to divorce.[1,7]

However, some people take it all in stride. One father of quintuplets regards the parenting of his five 3½ and one 7-month-old babies as character building. He's manufactured his own stairstep stroller, and he and his wife handle the 20 minutes of buckling, toy stowing, negotiating with the kids, and answering the questions of strangers whenever they go somewhere, with smiles on their faces.[1]

Some strangers beam at the sight of this unusual family, while others grimace and turn away. When people lightly tell their mother, "I'm glad it's you and not me," she answers in all seriousness, "Me too." The father sums up their situation this way: "Sure, it's a lifestyle change, but you take one day at a time, people help, and things work out."[1]

Family, friends, strangers, and even local and national companies do help out. Discounts on diapers and baby food, two years' worth of free formula, a night's stay

at a local motel, discounts on vans, and money to start college funds are examples of public generosity to the families of quads and quints. But along with public generosity comes public nosiness. One family answered a knock on the door from a senior citizens' tour bus group that wanted the parents to wake up the kids for a picture. More commonly, strangers think they can touch the children or ask personal questions of the parents, such as "Are they natural?" and "So, have you had your tubes tied?" and so on.[1]

Two nonprofit support groups help families cope with the unique stressors that multiple-birth families face. The Triplet Connection, based in California, and Mothers of Supertwins (MOST), based in New York, were both founded in the 1980s by triplet moms to provide reliable, accessible information to the families of supertwins.[1] With the sincere help of most people and organizations like these, parents can increase the odds that the more will truly be the merrier.

For Discussion . . .

Do you know any sets of twins or supertwins? How are their lives and those of their parents different from other families? What would you do if you or your partner was pregnant with supertwins? Do you think society has an obligation to help support supertwin families?

References

1. Jackson DD. People say, you poor thing and I'm thinking I have four healthy kids. *Smithsonian* 1996; 27(6):30–39.
2. Sheehan N. A sister's helping hand. *Reader's Digest* 1996; 148(889): 155–156.
3. Came B. A family tragedy. *Maclean's* 1994; 107:40–43.
4. Luscombe B. Eight at once is too many. *Time* 1996; 148(18):103.
5. Anonymous. Where are they now? *Time* 1996; 148(7):18.
6. Anonymous. The high cost of having some babies gets higher by the numbers. *Science News* 1994; 146(6):95.

7. Anonymous. And baby makes three or more: the ethics of fertility treatment are mainly a private matter. *The Economist* 1996; 340(7979):16.

8. Seligmann J. Fewer bundles of pain. Fertility doctors introduce reforms to reduce premature and multiple births. *Newsweek* 1996; 127(10):63.

9. Cowley G, Springen K. More is not merrier: when fertility drugs work too well. *Newsweek* 1996; 128(9):49.

10. Doyle P. The outcome of multiple pregnancy. *Hum Reprod* (11 Suppl) 1996; 4:110–117.

11. Ettner SL, Christiansen CL, Callahan TL, Hall JE. How low birth weight and gestational age contribute to increased inpatient costs for multiple births. *Inquiry* 1997–1998; 34(4): 325–339.

InfoLinks

www.mostonline.org
www.nomotc.org

personal assessment

how do you feel about parenting?

Respond to each of the following items based on your own
opinions about parenting. Circle the letters that best match
your response.

SA **Strongly agree**
A   **Agree**
U   **Undecided**
D   **Disagree**
SD **Strongly disagree**

1. One cannot parent successfully without, at the same time, being a generally successful adult member of the community.	SA	A	U	D	SD
2. It is inappropriate to view parenting as a method of achieving immortality.	SA	A	U	D	SD
3. Parenting requires that one be willing to make major personal sacrifices for the benefit of the child.	SA	A	U	D	SD
4. Parenting adds a large measure of vitality to an adult's life.	SA	A	U	D	SD
5. Parenting demands greater creativity than any other adult pursuit.	SA	A	U	D	SD
6. A person who cannot comfortably make decisions for others should not consider parenting.	SA	A	U	D	SD
7. A family cannot exist in the absence of children.	SA	A	U	D	SD

To Carry This Further . . .

After completing this personal assessment, join three of your
classmates in comparing and discussing your responses. What
suggestions were made to help increase your awareness of all that
parenting involves?

Consumer and safety issues

Part Six includes chapters on consumer health and safety. The decisions you make in each of these areas can have a profound effect on your well-being in each dimension of your health.

1. **Physical Dimension**
   The physical dimension of health is directly influenced by consumer decisions, such as the physician you choose. And, of course, it is crucial to learn how to protect yourself from physical harm caused by intentional or unintentional injury.

2. **Emotional Dimension**
   The effect of an overcrowded, highly industrialized society on your emotional health is often evident. Yet an even more powerful influence is the potential for violence or unintentional injury. Many people who are rape survivors or victims of other crimes feel fearful or angry for years afterward. Those who have behaved violently themselves may find that the knowledge of their actions erodes their emotional health.

3. **Social Dimension**
   Good health care consumers are made, not born. The decisions you make about your health are shaped by many people. Your doctor, for example, may give you information about behavior change, or your insurance agent may offer you several managed care options from which to choose. Effective interaction with these professionals and many other people can help you meet your health care needs.

4. **Intellectual Dimension**
   Understanding violence-related issues and consumer options requires critical thinking skills. Isolating causes of safety-related

problems and devising workable solutions are complex tasks. In addition, you must be able to analyze a number of variables to make difficult decisions about your health.

5. **Spiritual Dimension**
   Nurturing our spirituality and caring for the well-being of others are inextricably intertwined. As we search for solutions to complex social and health-related issues, we must often make difficult decisions: For example, will we someday deny health insurance coverage to persons based on the existence of high-risk health behaviors such as tobacco use and a sedentary lifestyle? Or, might we someday legally define smoking by parents as a form of child abuse? To build a better world for future generations may be the most serious challenge to our spiritual commitment to serve others.

6. **Occupational Dimension**
   Your occupational health can be enhanced by making sound decisions about your health care and personal safety. For example, choosing a health care provider who emphasizes prevention and positive behavior change will promote your overall well-being and minimize the number of days you are unable to work because of illness. In addition, avoiding intentional and unintentional injuries will allow you to perform at your peak.

chapter eighteen

becoming an informed health care consumer

Talking It Over

Health Care: Where Do You Stand?

Health care is more than a political "hot potato." It's a high-priority issue that affects everyone, even if you're young and healthy. You probably realize that the U.S. health care system isn't perfect. What can you, as a college student, do?

- Keep yourself informed by reading and talking about health care issues.
- Write e-mails about your health care concerns to your legislators.

- Consider where candidates stand on health care issues when you vote.
- Join an advocacy group that is working to improve health care.

CommunicationLinks
www.health.gov/healthypeople
www.capweb.net

Eye on the Media

The Internet—Your New Health Superstore

In 2000, an estimated 33 million Americans explored the Internet in search of information, products, and services related to their health. A majority, an estimated 53%, will search for information about specific conditions, such as cancer or hypertension. Smaller but still impressive percentages of people will look for information about dieting and nutrition, fitness, women's health, and pharmaceuticals. In fact, the health books, supplements, medications, and devices found through these visits generated sales of about $1.7 billion in 2003.

The biggest challenge for you as a health consumer is determining the credibility of the information you find on the Internet. How can you know that this information (and accompanying products or services) is trustworthy and that the persons responsible for

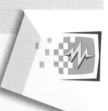

Eye on the Media *continued*

the information, products, or services are motivated by concern for your health and well-being rather than just by profit? Recognized authorities offer these guidelines to help you:

- Who does the website belong to? Is it sponsored by an institution of higher education, a professional society, a government or not-for-profit agency, or a recognized pharmaceutical company? If not, who is responsible for the information? Remember, virtually anyone can develop a web page and begin disseminating information.
- Is the information carefully referenced, showing sources such as government reports, professional journal articles, or respected reference publications? Are the references clearly documented and cur-

rent? Is the web page updated regularly? Does the information appear to agree with the titles of its own references?

- Does the content of the information seem to have a critical or negative bias toward a particular profession, institution, or treatment method? Is the information more discrediting of others than supportive of itself?
- Are "significant breakthroughs" promised in a way that suggests that only this source has the "ultimate answer" to certain problems? Does this answer involve throwing out your prescriptions, going against your physician's orders, or considering suicide as a way of escaping the pain and difficulties associated with your illness?

If you are skeptical about the credibility of any health care information you find online,

submit the information to a respected health care professional or organization for assessment. If you and your physician find suspicious information or fraudulent health claims, report this to the Federal Trade Commission. Today, most health care practitioners feel comfortable with well-informed patients. Many will welcome the chance to learn about your sources of information and share with you any concerns they might have about them.

Once you feel secure about distinguishing reliable and valid information from questionable or fraudulent information, you will be able to make better judgments and choices. Together, you and your health care provider can use that information in the management of your health care and in planning your approach to a healthier lifestyle.

Health care providers often evaluate you by criteria from their area of expertise. The nutritionist knows you by the food you eat. The physical fitness professional knows you by your body type and activity level. In the eyes of the expert in health consumerism, you are the product of the health information you believe, the health-influencing services you use, and the products you consume. When you make your decisions about health information, services, and products after careful study and consideration, your health will probably be improved. However, when your decisions lack insight, your health, as well as your pocketbook, may suffer.

Health Information

The Informed Consumer

What aspects of health do people seem most interested in having information about? To which products and services do they most want access? In a 2001 poll conducted for the Kaiser Family Foundation to determine the health interests of American youth (15 to 24 years of age), the following areas were found: diseases (50%), sexual health (44%), weight loss/gain (25%), drugs and alcohol (23%), depression/mental illness (23%), violence (23%), smoking (19%), eating disorders (15%), acne/skin care (15%), local clinics (15%), and sexual assault (10%).[1] In light of the breadth of these interest areas and the complexity associated with each, it is very likely that most people turn to a variety of sources for the information and access that they seek. Some sources will be

easily accessed, while others will be more difficult to find but perhaps contain more valid information. In the section that follows you will be introduced to several sources of health-related information. Complete the Personal Assessment on page 615 to rate your own skills as a consumer of health-related information, products, and services.

Sources of Information

Your sources of information on health topics are as diverse as the number of people you know, the number of publications you read, and the number of experts you see or hear. No single agency or profession regulates the quantity or quality of the health-related information you receive. Readers will quickly recognize that all are familiar sources and that some provide more accurate and honest information than others.

Family and Friends

The accuracy of information you get from a friend or family member may be questionable. Too often the information your family and friends offer is based on "common knowledge" that is wrong. In addition, family members or friends may provide information they believe is in your best interest rather than facts that may have a more negative effect on you.

Unfortunately, some family members and friends today also might give biased health information because they are participating in a pyramid-type sales organization that sells health products. Some people might urge you to use a particular line of food supplements or vitamins or even ask you to join their sales team.

Advertisements and Commercials

Many people spend much of every day watching television, listening to the radio, and reading newspapers or magazines. Because many advertisements are health oriented, these are significant sources of information. The primary purpose of advertising, however, is to sell products or services. One newer example of this intertwining of health information with marketing is the "infomercial," in which a compensated studio audience watches a skillfully produced program that trumpets the benefits of a particular product or service. In spite of the convincing nature of these infomercials, however, the validity of their information is often questionable. This was the case in 2000 when the FTC ordered the producers of The Enforma System for weight loss—*Fat Trapper* and *Exercise in a Bottle*—to repay customers $10 million for having used spurious information in selling their product.

In contrast to advertisements and commercials, the mass media routinely offer public service messages that give valuable health-related information.

Labels and Directions

Federal law requires that many consumer product labels, including all medications and many kinds of food (see Chapter 5), contain specific information. For example, when a pharmacist dispenses a prescription medication, he or she must give a detailed information sheet describing the medication.

Many health care providers and agencies give consumers informative information about their health problems or printed directions for preparing for screening procedures. Generally, information from these sources is accurate and current and is given with the health of the consumer foremost in mind.

Folklore

Because it is passed down from generation to generation, folklore about health is the primary source of health-related information for some people.

The accuracy of health-related information obtained from family members, neighbors, and coworkers is difficult to evaluate. As a general rule, however, one should exercise caution relying on its scientific soundness. A blanket dismissal is not warranted, however, because folk wisdom is occasionally supported by scientific evidence. In addition, the emotional support provided by the suppliers of this information could be the best medicine some people could receive. In fact, for some ethnic groups, indigenous health care is central to overall health care. For example, within the Chinese American community, practitioners of traditional healing arts represent primary health care. Even though

many Americans would consider this form of care "folk medicine," it is highly valued and trusted by those who find it familiar. Additionally, what would be considered folklore represents important sources of dependable and valid health information to members of this ethnic group.

Testimonials

People strongly want to share information that has benefited them. Others may base their decisions on such testimonials. However, the exaggerated testimonials that accompany the sales pitches of the medical quack or the "satisfied" customers appearing in advertisements and on commercials and infomercials should never be interpreted as valid endorsements.

Mass Media

Health programming on cable television stations, stories in lifestyle sections of newspapers, health care correspondents appearing on national network news shows, and the growing number of health-oriented magazines are sources of health information in the mass media.

Specific reliance on the mass media sources can be seen in a survey conducted for the National Council on Aging, when it was reported that for persons between the ages of 46 and 64, television was the most widely turned to source of health-related information (36%), while magazines (34%), newspapers (17%), the Internet (8%), and radio (2%) followed behind.[2]

Health-related information in the mass media is generally accurate, but it is sometimes presented so quickly or superficially that its usefulness is limited. The consumer who wants more complete coverage of a health topic might acquire it by subscribing to a cable channel devoted partly or entirely to health-related programming, such as *The Learning Channel.*

Practitioners

The health care consumer also receives much information from individual health practitioners and their professional associations. In fact, today's health care practitioner so clearly emphasizes patient education that finding one who does not offer some information to a patient would be difficult. Education improves patient **compliance** with health care directives, which is important to the practitioner and the consumer.

Another important development in the trend toward patient education is the evolution of the hospital as an

compliance willingness to follow the directions provided by another person.

educational institution. Because the American Medical Association advocates patient education activities in hospitals, wellness centers, and other health facilities, it now refuses to endorse health products with its logo, which would create a conflict of interest.

Online Computer Services

The development of computer technology in the last decade has opened new sources of health information. Today, more than 100 million Americans (out of 270 million) have access to online services. However, the extent to which the Internet is used to access health-related information seems uncertain. A recent study found that only about 20% of American adults sought health-related information on the Internet during 2002,[3] while two earlier studies suggested much higher percentages (75%–80% and 40%). Regardless of the extent of its use, the Internet offers expansive collections of information, including text and video, to people interested in health.

To make certain that this increasingly important source of health information provides the most reliable information possible, twenty of the most frequently visited health-related sites joined forces in creating a code of ethics to ensure that information (and products sold via the sites) was valid and reliable. This voluntary code of ethics was implemented in November 2000. The Star box on page 584 lists several of the more popular websites for health-related information.

How should health-related information gleaned from the Internet be used, particularly when communicating with health care providers? Howard LeWine, MD, offers the following suggestions[4]:

- Inform your health care provider that you are accessing the Internet for information related to your particular area of concern. Know the name of the site you're using; your provider might already be familiar with the site, or wish to access it in preparation for your discussion.

- Do not bombard your provider with questions whenever you come across information that might be related to your health concern. Keep notes and discuss all of your findings at one time.

- Be prepared to *discuss* your information with your provider; don't use Web information to second-guess his or her position. Bear in mind that health concerns are too complex to generalize from the kind of one-size-fits-all information provided by even the most reliable websites, and must be evaluated on a case-by-case basis by a physician who has actually examined you.

- Always recognize that health-related information involves knowledge from many disciplines and uses highly technical language; media-based sources may grossly oversimplify in an effort to be accessible to lay persons.

 TALKING POINTS A family member considers herself good at diagnosing health problems. Since she hasn't been wrong in years, she no longer relies on physicians. What questions could you ask her to point out the dangers associated with her approach?

Health Reference Publications

A substantial portion of all households own or subscribe to a health reference publication, such as the *Encyclopedia of Complementary Health Practices,*[5] the *Physicians' Desk Reference* (PDR),[6] or a newsletter such as *The Harvard Medical School Health Letter* or *The Johns Hopkins Medical Letter: Health After 50.* Some consumers also use personal computer programs and videocassettes or CDs featuring health-related information.

Reference Libraries

Public and university libraries continue to be popular sources of health-related information. One can consult with reference librarians and check out audiovisual collections and printed materials. More and more of these holdings can be accessed through the home computer.

Consumer Advocacy Groups

A variety of nonprofit consumer advocacy groups patrol the health care marketplace (see the Star box on page 585). These groups produce and distribute information designed to help the consumer recognize questionable services and products. Large, well-organized groups, such as The National Consumers' League and Consumers Union, and smaller groups at the state and local levels champion the right of the consumer to receive valid and reliable information about health care products and services.

Voluntary Health Agencies

Volunteerism and the traditional approach to health care and health promotion are virtually inseparable. Few countries besides the United States can boast so many national voluntary organizations, with state and local affiliates, dedicated to improving health through research, service, and public education. The American Cancer Society, the American Red Cross, and the American Heart Association all are voluntary (not-for-profit) health agencies. Consumers can, in fact, expect to find a voluntary health agency for virtually every health problem. College students should also note that volunteerism on their part, perhaps with a health agency like the Red Cross or the AHA, is both a personally satisfying experience and an activity viewed favorably by potential employers.

Government Agencies

Government agencies are also effective sources of information to the public. Through meetings and the release of

Internet Sites for Health Information

The following are some of the most visited health information–related Internet sites, both governmental and nongovernmental.

AMA Health Insight www.ama-assn.org

This site provides easily understood information and allows users to search online for physicians, hospitals, and sources of health information.

America's Doctor www.americasdoctor.com

This site provides the opportunity to have real-time chat room conversations with physicians, as well as providing bulletin boards and shopping sites.

Centers for Disease Control and Prevention www.cdc.gov

This site is the federal government's primary site for disease-related statistics, including a link to the Morbidity and Mortality Weekly Report (MMWR).

Health Central www.healthanswers.com

This site contains general health information as well as reports by the media physician Dean Edell.

Healthfinder www.healthfinder.gov

This site is the government's directory of authoritative health information sites, providing links to each.

InteliHealth www.intelihealth.com

Sponsored by Aetna U.S. Healthcare, this site features Harvard Medical School's Consumer Health Information.

Mayo Clinic Health Oasis www.mayohealth.org

This site is one of the oldest and most used, featuring information from the internationally respected Mayo Clinic.

MedScape www.medscape.com

Organized by medical specialties, this site is geared to both physicians and the general public.

National Institutes of Health www.nih.gov/health

This site links the public to the various governmental health institutes and to the National Library of Medicine's Medline Plus.

WebMD www.webmed.com

This site has informational sections geared to health care professionals and sites intended for the general public.

information to the media, agencies such as the Food and Drug Administration, Federal Trade Commission, United States Postal Service, and Environmental Protection Agency publicize health issues. Government agencies also control the quality of information sent out to the buying public, particularly through labeling, advertising, and the distribution of information through the mail. The various divisions of the National Institutes of Health regularly release research findings and recommendations to clinical practices, which in turn reach the consumer through clinical practitioners.

Despite their best intentions, federal health agencies are often less effective than the public deserves. A variety of factors, including inadequate staff, poor administration, lobbying by special interest groups, and political pressures prevent these federal agencies from enforcing consumer-protection legislation. As a result, the public is left with a sense of false confidence in the consumer protection provided by the federal government.

State governments also distribute health-related information to the public. State agencies are primary sources of information, particularly in the areas of public health and environmental protection. For an example of health care activism at work, see the Learning from Our Diversity box on page 585.

Qualified Health Educators

Health educators work in a variety of settings and offer their services to diverse groups. Community health educators work with virtually all of the agencies mentioned in this section; patient educators function in primary care settings; and school health educators are found at all educational levels. Health educators are increasingly being employed in a wide range of wellness-based programs in community, hospital, corporate, and school settings.

Health Care Providers

The sources of health information just discussed can greatly help us make decisions as informed consumers. The choices we make about physicians, health services, and medical payment plans will reflect our commitment to remaining healthy and our trust in specific people who are trained in keeping us healthy. Refer to the Changing for the Better boxes on pages 587 and 588 for tips on choosing a physician and a hospital.

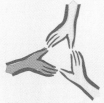

Learning from Our Diversity

Americans with Disabilities Act—New Places to Go

Although federal laws designed to end discrimination on the basis of gender and race were enacted in the United States decades ago, a law designed to address discrimination on the basis of physical and mental disabilities was not enacted until 1990. This law, the *Americans with Disabilities Act (1990),* has done a great deal to level the playing field for the disabled, both on the college campus and in the larger community. On campuses today, it's common to see students whose obvious disabilities would have prevented them from attending college before this law was enacted. Students with cerebral palsy, spina bifida, spinal cord injuries, sensory impairments, and orthopedic disabilities share living quarters, lecture hall seats, and recreational facilities with their nondisabled classmates.

Equally important are those students whose disabilities are largely unobservable. Students with learning disabilities, mental disabilities,

and subtle but disabling chronic health conditions such as Crohn's disease, lupus, and fibromyalgia may pass unnoticed. Yet their lives are equally challenged.

The Americans with Disabilities Act does not suggest that preferential treatment be given to students with disabilities, nor does it allow students to be unaccountable for their behavior. Instead, it seeks to create an environment—on the college campus and beyond—where people, regardless of disability, can learn new things, form meaningful relationships, and develop independence.

This law has the power to remove the physical and emotional barriers that can hinder a person with a disability from succeeding. For the first time, it allows students with disabilities to go where everyone else can—and beyond.

Consumer Protection Agencies and Organizations

Federal Agencies

Office of Consumer Affairs, Food and Drug Administration

U.S. Department of Health and Human Services
5600 Fishers Lane
Rockville, MD 20857
(301) 827-5006
www.fda.gov/oca/aboutoca.htm

Federal Trade Commission
Consumer Inquiries
Public Reference Branch
6th Street and Pennsylvania Avenue
Washington, DC 20580
(202) 326-2222
www.ftc.gov

Fraud Division
Chief Postal Inspector
U.S. Postal Inspection Service
475 L'Enfant Plaza
Washington, DC 20260-2166
(202) 268-4299
www.usps.gov

Consumer Information Center
Pueblo, CO 81009
(719) 948-3334
www.pueblo.gsa.gov

U.S. Consumer Product Safety Commission Hotline
(800) 638-CPSC

Consumer Organizations

Consumers Union of the U.S., Inc.
101 Truman Avenue
Yonkers, NY 10703
(914) 378-2000
www.consumerreports.org

Professional Organizations

American Medical Association
515 N. State Street
Chicago, IL 60610
(312) 464-5000
www.ama-assn.org

American Hospital Association
1 N. Franklin Street
Chicago, IL 60606
(312) 422-3000
www.aha.org

American Pharmaceutical Association
2215 Constitution Avenue, NW
Washington, DC 20037
(202) 628-4410
www.aphanet.org

Communication Between Patients and Their Health Care Providers

In the complex world of modern health care, it is of critical importance that patients communicate important information to their health care providers, and, in turn, that they understanding as fully as possible the information that they receive from their providers. Below are 10 valuable suggestions from the Joint Commission on Accreditation of Healthcare Organizations and the U.S. Government's Agency for Healthcare Research and Quality.

- Take part in every decision about your health care.
- If you are not prepared to ask questions on your own behalf, ask a family member or friend to fill this role for you.
- Tell your physician and pharmacist about every drug you are taking, including prescription drugs, OTC drugs, vitamins, supplements, and herbal products—bring them with you.
- Make certain that you get the results of every test, and understand what they mean.
- If you do not hear about test results, never assume that everything is all right. Call your doctor's office and ask.
- Whenever possible, choose a hospital where many patients receive the same procedure that you are to receive. Ask your physician or the hospital for the actual numbers.
- Ask hospital personnel if they have washed their hands before they begin touching you.
- If you are having surgery, make sure that your, your physician, and your surgeon all agree on what will be done during the operation.
- Insist that your surgeon write his or her initials or words such as "yes" or "this side" on the part of the body to be operated on. Put "no" on the opposite body part.
- When you are discharged, ask your doctor to explain your treatment plan, including changes in medications, restrictions on activity, and additional therapies you will need.

In many situations involving medical care, carefully communicated comments and questions between providers and patients can be the basis of the successful resolution of a health problem, versus unnecessary delay, pain, discomfort, or even death.

Source: Ellis L. *How you can help guard against errors.* June 28, 2002.
http://www.intelihealth.com

Why We Consult Health Care Providers

Most of us seek care and advice from medical and health practitioners when we have a specific problem. A bad cold, a broken arm, or a newly discovered lump can motivate us to consult a health care professional. Yet *diagnosis* and *treatment* are only two reasons that we might require the services of health care providers.

We also might encounter health practitioners when we undergo *screening.* Screening most often involves a cursory (or noninvasive) collection of information that can quickly be compared to established standards, themselves often based on gender, age, race, or the presence of preexisting conditions. Your earliest experience with screening may have been in elementary school, where physicians, nurses, audiologists, and dentists sometimes examine all children for normal growth and development patterns. As an adult, your screening is more likely to be done on an individual basis by a physician's staff as a routine portion of every office visit when they collect baseline information such as height, weight, and blood pressure measurements. You may also encounter community-based screening when you stop at your local shopping mall's health fair and have your blood pressure taken or cholesterol checked. In both settings, the extent to which your data becomes incorporated into a larger data pool determines whether this screening is community-based or simply personally informing. Although screening should be considered much less precise than actual diagnosis, screening serves to identify people who should seek further medical examination.

Consultation is a fourth reason that knowledgeable consumers seek health care providers. A consultation is the

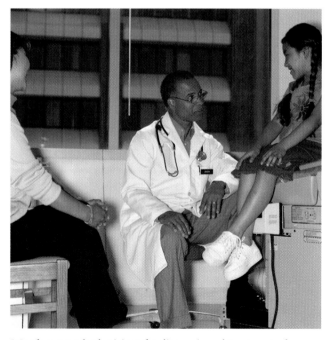

We often consult physicians for diagnosis and treatment of common ailments.

use of two or more professionals to deliberate a person's specific health problem or condition. Consultations are especially helpful when **primary care health providers,** such as family practice physicians, gynecologists, pediatricians, internists, and general practice dentists, require the opinion of specialists. Using additional practitioners as consultants can also help reassure patients who may have doubts about their own condition or about the abilities of their physician.

Prevention is a fifth reason we might seek a health care provider. With the current emphasis on trying to stop problems before they begin, using health care providers for prevention is becoming more common. People want information about how to prevent needless risks and promote their health, and they seek such advice from physicians, nurses, dentists, exercise physiologists, patient educators, and other health promotion specialists.

When prevention becomes a routine component of your personal health care, you will annually receive, in addition to the baseline measurements of height, weight,

and blood pressure, more in-depth assessments such as a blood chemistry assessment, lipid profile, and cardiogram. Women will also likely receive a ViraPap test, breast examination, mammography, and pelvic examination, while men will likely receive a Prostate Specific Antibody (PSA) test, digital prostate examination, and testicular examination.

Physicians and Their Training

In every city and many smaller communities, the local telephone directory lists physicians in a variety of medical

---

Key Terms

primary care health providers health care providers who generally see patients on a routine basis, particularly for preventive health care.

specialties. These health care providers hold the academic degree of Doctor of Medicine (MD) or Doctor of Osteopathy (DO).

At one time, **allopathy** and **osteopathy** were clearly different health care professions in terms of their healing philosophies and modes of practice. Today, however, MDs and DOs receive similar educations and engage in very similar forms of practice. Both can function as primary care physicians or as board-certified specialists. Their differences are in the osteopathic physician's greater tendency to use manipulation in treating health problems. In addition, DOs often perceive themselves as being more holistically oriented than MDs.

Medical and osteopathic physicians undergo a long training process. They usually take 4 years of initial undergraduate preparation with a heavy emphasis on the sciences—biology, chemistry, mathematics, anatomy, and physiology. Most undergraduate schools have preprofessional courses of study for students interested in medical or osteopathic schools.

After they are accepted into professional schools, students generally spend 4 or more years in intensive training that includes advanced study in the preclinical medical sciences and clinical practice. When they complete this phase of training, the students are awarded the MD or DO degree and then take the state medical license examination. Most newly licensed physicians complete a residency at a hospital. Residency programs vary in length from 3 to 4 years. When they conclude their residency programs, including board-related examinations, physicians are granted board-certified status. Interestingly, since the late 1990s, applications for medical schools have been in a state of decline, and that, in turn, influences residency programs.[7] The Star box on page 590 describes several of

the more familiar specialties. In addition to state and specialty board certification, comprehensive national certification of physicians is a frequently discussed possibility. At this time, no nationally required and all-encompassing certification of physician competency is required. It should be noted, however, that with the advent of the Internet, something approaching this type of information is available through websites such as *HealthGrade*, described in the Changing for the Better box entitled Choosing a Physician on page 587.

Complementary, Alternative, and Integrative Care Practitioners

In addition to medical and osteopathic physicians, several other forms of health care offer alternatives within the large health care market. Included within this group of complementary or alternative forms of practice are chiropractic, acupuncture, homeopathy, naturopathy, herbalism, reflexology, and ayurveda.[8] Also, see the Considering

---

Key Terms

allopathy (ah **lop** ah thee) a system of medical practice in which specific remedies (often pharmaceutical agents) are used to produce effects different from those produced by a disease or injury.

osteopathy (os tee **op** ah thee) a system of medical practice in which allopathic principles are combined with specific attention to postural mechanics of the body.

Complementary Care box on page 591 for a discussion on therapeutic touch. Although the traditional medical community has long scoffed at these fields of practice as ineffective and unscientific, many people use these forms of health care and believe strongly that they are as effective as (or more effective than) allopathic and osteopathic medicine. As a result of this belief, today many physicians are better informed about complementary care methods and more comfortable discussing them with patients. Following are brief descriptions of some of the more popular of these complementary care fields and the practitioners that function within them. Readers are also reminded of the Considering Complementary Care box on page 13 of Chapter 1, which discusses the controversial nature of various fields of complementary or alternative care.

Chiropractic

Historically (and, to varying degrees, today) the underlying premise of chiropractic is that misalignment or subluxation of the spinal (vertebral) column is the primary cause of illness, and, thus, its realignment is the appropriate treatment for illness. Accordingly, chiropractic medical practice is primarily limited to vertebral adjustments, where manual manipulation of the spine its used to correct misalignments. Recent studies have shown that **chiropractic** treatment of some types of low-back pain can be more effective than conventional care. With about 50,000 practitioners in the United States, chiropractic is the third-largest health profession, used by 15 to 20 million people. Some chiropractors use only spinal manipulation, while others use additional medical technologies, including dietary supplementation and various noninvasive technologies similar to those used by physical therapists and athletic trainers, including massage.

In spite of the fact that chiropractors undergo nearly the same number of years of training as do primary care physicians and take courses closely aligned with those taken by physicians, current laws restrict the scope of chiropractic practice to those techniques initially consistent with the original theoretical basis of their discipline, "one cause—one cure of all illnesses and diseases." Unless carefully controlled research, as specified by the National Center for Complementary and Alternative Medicine,[9] finds spinal subluxation/manipulation to be a salient cause/cure of illness (which seems unlikely), chiropractic medicine is likely to remain a user-friendly, highly popular but highly limited approach to health care. There is, however, a current trend of including chiropractic physicians within allopathic medical groups, principally to treat those conditions clearly associated with postural injuries or conditions. If chiropractic physicians can accept this slightly subordinate role for the foreseeable future, while seeing their discipline evolve in the direction of osteopathic medicine (even transforming their schools into schools of osteopathic medicine), then chiropractic may move out of complementary/alternative/integrative medicine into the mainstream.

Acupuncture

Acupuncture is, for Americans, the most familiar component of the 3,000-year-old Chinese medical system. This system is based on balancing the active and passive forces with the patient's body to strengthen the qi ("chee"), or life force. The system also employs herbs, food, massage, and exercise.

Acupuncturists place hair-thin needles at certain points in the body to stimulate the patient's qi. These points are said to correspond to different organs and bodily functions and, when stimulated, help the body's own defenses fight illness. More specifically, the scientific communities suggest that acupuncture speeds up the electrical conductivity within the central and peripheral nervous systems, enhances the production of biological opiates, and alters the production of specific neurotransmitters within various areas of the nervous system.[10]

Of all the Chinese therapies, acupuncture is the most widely accepted in the West. Researchers have produced persuasive evidence of acupuncture's effectiveness as an anesthetic and as an antidote to chronic pain, migraines, dysmenorrhea, and osteoarthritis.[11] In addition, some

> **Key Terms**
>
> **chiropractic** manipulation of the vertebral column to relieve misalignments and cure illness.
>
> **acupuncture** insertion of fine needles into the body to alter electroenergy fields and cure disease.

Medical Specialties

The American Board of Medical Specialties is a nonprofit organization that represents a variety of medical specialty boards.* Each board is composed of expert physicians already qualified in a particular field.

These specialty boards evaluate physicians who wish to practice in a specific area of medicine. Some of the more common specialty areas consumers might encounter are:

Specialty	Scope of Practice
Allergy and immunology	Treatment of immune system–related disorders
Anesthesiology	Use of drugs to sedate or anesthetize
Cardiovascular surgery	Various forms of heart surgery
Colon and rectal surgery	Perform surgery on the lower portions of the gastrointestinal tract
Dermatology	Skin diseases and disorders
Emergency medicine	Care of accident victims
Family practice	Broad-based family medical care
Geriatrics	Diseases and disorders of older adults
Gynecology	Female reproductive health care
Internal medicine	Nonsurgical treatment of internal organ systems
Medical genetics	Consulting, screening, counseling, and research on inherited genetic abnormalities
Nephrology	Kidney diseases and disorders
Neurology	Diseases and disorders of the nervous system
Nuclear medicine	Utilize non-x-ray forms of radiation to diagnose and treat an array of health conditions
Obstetrics	Prenatal care and child delivery
Oncology	Treatment of unusual growths and tumors
Ophthalmology	Disorders of the eye
Orthopedic surgery	Surgery for structural disorders of the bones and joints
Otolaryngology	Ear, nose, and throat problems
Pathology	Diagnosis of disease through the examination of body tissues
Pediatrics	Childhood health concerns
Physical medicine and rehabilitation	Formulate and administer a range of therapies, including physical and occupational therapies, to aid patients in their recovery from illnesses and injuries
Plastic surgery	Perform cosmetic and reconstructive surgery on an array of body areas
Psychiatry and neurology	Mental and emotional diseases or disorders
Radiology	Use of radiation to diagnose and treat diseases and injuries
Thoracic surgery	Operate upon structures within the chest cavity
Urology	Treatment of urinary tract diseases and male reproductive dysfunctions

*Governed by these medical boards are 85 practice specialties.

Therapeutic Touch (Biofield Therapy)

The biofield (or energy field) is believed by therapeutic touch practitioners to dwell within and immediately surround the body. For thousands of years, practitioners of biofield therapy, as exemplified by therapeutic touch, have attempted to identify irregularities or contractions in this electrical field and through appropriate touching (or near-touching of the body), restore its appropriate configuration. Once the biofield is aligned appropriately, the negative forces that have been disruptive to the physical and emotional balance required for healthful living are released. A second perception of biofield therapies is that through manipulation of the biofield a pathway or entry point is established that allows other health modalities, such as medications, to influence the restoration of the holistic balance needed for good health.

Practitioners of biofield therapies, including healing touch, therapeutic touch, and SHEN (Specific Human Emotional Nexus) therapy, describe their practice as noninvasive, deeply relaxing, gentle, and both safe and effective. Treatment sessions are usually conducted in a quiet and relaxed location, with the patient fully clothed and lying on a softly padded table or in bed. Sessions generally last from several minutes to an hour, often including a period of dialogue between the patient and the practitioner, and may be delivered for several days or for only a day or two.

Sessions may be delivered within a hospital (prior to or following surgery) or in the home following discharge from the hospital. Therapeutic touch is generally an adjunct therapy to more conventional therapies, given in conjunction with cancer treatment or during post-surgical recovery or as part of the treatment to alleviate the anxiety associated with traumatic injury recovery.

Nurses are the most likely practitioners of therapeutic touch and related therapies in the hospital setting. In fact, it is in nursing journals that the most literature related to the practice is found. When therapeutic touch is used in a wellness-oriented manner, it is most often delivered by a certified practitioner. This is often a nurse practicing in a fee-for-service manner, a chiropractor, a naturopathic physician, or a psychologist.

The scientific literature regarding the effectiveness of therapeutic touch is very difficult to interpret. This is largely because of the difficulty of establishing double-blind experiments to study a therapeutic approach (that is, experiments in which neither practitioner nor patient knows whether the actual therapy versus a sham therapy is being delivered). A second difficulty is the problem of quantifying the outcome of the therapy. At this point it appears that therapeutic touch is somewhat effective in reducing anxiety, enhancing mood, improving sleep, and producing a higher level of relaxation among patients experiencing various emotionally traumatic medical treatments, such as breast cancer surgery. Its efficacy in enhancing holistic health and a sense of wellness is based largely on self-reported improvement and various inventories designed to assess feeling states.

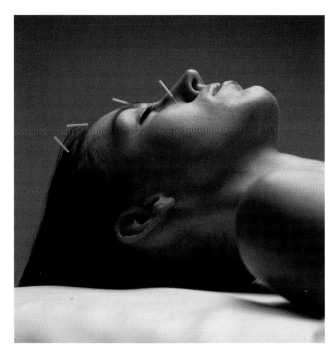

Acupuncture has received increasing acceptance within the Western medical community.

have suggested that acupuncture can help patients overcome addictions to alcohol, drugs, and tobacco.

Reflexology

Reflexology uses principles similar to those of acupuncture but focuses on treating certain disorders through massage of the soles of the feet. To date, however, there is relatively little data regarding its effectiveness, when evaluated under carefully controlled conditions. However, among reflexology studies available through the National Library of Medicine (Pubmed), three reflect the uncertainty of its role in integrative medical care. A study conducted in Israel found that active reflexology therapy versus a sham (calf area massage) was beneficial in alleviating motor, sensory, and urinary difficulties in persons with multiple sclerosis.[12]

> **Key Terms**
>
> **reflexology** massage applied to specific areas of the feet to treat illness and disease in other areas of the body.

A British study in which reflexology was used as a portion of palliative (enhanced comfort) care produced higher and more consistent reports of comfort than among patients who did not receive the reflexology component in their care.[13] In contrast, a Danish study in which middle ear infections in children were treated exclusively with reflexology versus antibiotics found reflexology to be ineffective as a treatment modality.[14] The National Center for Complementary and Alternative Medicine has yet to fund carefully controlled research into the effectiveness of reflexology.

Homeopathy

Widely accepted in Europe, **homeopathy** is the leading alternative therapy in France. Homeopathy uses infinitesimal doses of herbs, minerals, or even poisons to stimulate the body's curative powers. The theory on which homeopathy is based, the *law of similars,* contends that if large doses of a substance can cause a problem, tiny doses can trigger healing. A few small studies showed homeopathy to be at least somewhat effective in treating hay fever, diarrhea, and flu symptoms, but members of the scientific community call the studies flawed or preliminary and suggest that the placebo effect was occurring. Much more informative, however, are reports from three meta-analysis studies, funded by the National Center for Complementary and Alternative Medicine, involving the reassessment of 240 individual studies, in which it was concluded that major methodology weaknesses existed in most studies of homeopathy studies conducted to date. It was further concluded that on the basis of these studies there was no strong evidence in favor of homeopathy over conventional treatment methods. The Center recommended that larger, more carefully controlled studies be conducted.[15]

An interesting new dimension to the marketing of homeopathy as an effective alternative to conventional medical care relates to the contention of some homeopathy physicians that the "molecular essence" of their homeopathic medicines can be sent via the Internet, thus allowing treatment to occur through cyberspace.[16]

Naturopathy

The core of naturopathic medicine is what Hippocrates called *medicatrix naturae,* or the healing power of nature. Proponents of **naturopathy** believe that when the mind and the body are in balance and receiving proper care, with a healthy diet, adequate rest, and minimal stress, the body's own vital forces are sufficient to fight off disease. Getting rid of an ailment is only the first step toward correcting the underlying imbalance that allowed the ailment to take hold, naturists believe. Correcting the imbalance might be as simple as rectifying a shortage of a particular nutrient, or as complex as reducing overlong work hours, strengthening a weakened immune system, and identifying an inability to digest certain foods.

Naturopathy was popular in the nineteenth century and began a comeback in the 1970s in the Pacific Northwest, spurred by the back-to-nature themes of the counterculture. In some states, naturopaths are licensed, and health insurance plans must cover treatment they provide.

Herbalism

Herbalism may be the world's oldest and most widely used healing form. Herbalists make herbal brews for treating a variety of ills, such as depression, anxiety, and hypertension. In some cases, scientific research supports the herbalists' beliefs. For example, studies have found St. John's wort to be more effective than a placebo and one of the older tricyclic antidepressants in alleviating mild depression, and that garlic reduces cholesterol and blood pressure, while black cohosh (a member of the buttercup family) and soy can relieve hot flashes and other menopause symptoms.

However, the potential side effects of many dietary supplements have raised questions about the dangers associated with particular herbs, especially of products containing ephedra, a stimulant used to enhance athletic performance or stimulate weight loss.[17] The Food and Drug Administration began to consider taking increased control over the testing and safety of all dietary supplements following the ephedra-related death of Baltimore Orioles pitcher Steve Belcher in February 2003; more than 150 deaths have been linked to the supplement.[18] In December 2003, after extensive studies, the FDA officially banned the sale and use of ephedra, to be implemented in April 2004.[19] However, it is important to recognize that most supplements are not studied in this manner, and that virtually no regulation of the supplements industry currently exists.

Ayurveda

Even older than Chinese medicine, India's **ayurveda** takes a preventive approach and focuses on the whole person.

Key Terms

homeopathy (hoe mee **op** ah thee) the use of minute doses of herbs, minerals, or other substances to stimulate healing.

naturopathy (na chur **op** ah thee) a system of treatment that avoids drugs and surgery and emphasizes the use of natural agents to correct underlying imbalances.

herbalism an ancient form of healing in which herbal preparations are used to treat illness and disease.

ayurveda (ai yur **vey** da) traditional Indian medicine based on herbal remedies.

Choosing the Best Complementary Medical Practitioner for You

I'm interested in exploring complementary approaches to medicine, but I feel uncertain about how to proceed. What steps should I take?

Perhaps you are one of the millions of people who feel that their doctors don't encourage them to ask questions, don't seek their opinion about their medical condition, or don't take a thorough medical history. Perhaps you want advice on improving your health rather than just a quick diagnosis and prescription.

For whatever reasons, millions of Americans are turning to complementary medical practitioners, such as doctors of naturopathy, Chinese medicine, or ayurveda. Unfortunately, the patient looking for these alternatives faces other problems: practitioners' training may be weak, they might not be licensed or covered by insurance, they are hard to find, and they usually are not permitted to prescribe drugs unless they also happen to be medical doctors. This means that you must do some legwork to find a good provider who can meet your needs.

Consider the following tips for finding the practitioner who is right for you.

- *Don't forget the family physician.* Family-practice medicine is enjoying a surge in the United States, and many of these doctors tend to think holistically.
- *Find a physician who believes in complementary therapies.* Your doctor's attitude toward the treatment can be just as important as your own.
- *Give the treatment time.* Complementary therapies encourage the body to do its own healing. This often takes time. Seek a physician who is confident in your self-healing ability, so you won't become discouraged if it takes some time.

- *Request natural healing.* Natural healing tends to change the internal conditions so that pathogens are less likely to gain a foothold; conventional medicine seeks to destroy the pathogen. Natural healing searches for the causes of symptoms, while conventional medicine treats symptoms.
- *Know your disease.* Find books that describe your conditions and offer complementary as well as conventional treatments. This way you can discuss your treatment with your physician and create an effective treatment plan.
- *Treat yourself.* Don't overuse your health care provider, whether conventional or complementary. For many conditions, you can be your own best doctor; of course, persistent or severe symptoms should send you to the physician.
- *Learn whether the treatment is covered by insurance.* Coverage of complementary treatment differs sharply by state. Some insurance groups are beginning to pay for more complementary medicine, and HMOs are hiring some complementary specialists.
- *Talk to professional associations.* Most of the more established complementary fields have associations that can give you a list of providers. Use it as a start.
- *Interview the practitioner.* Before making an appointment, talk with the physician over the telephone. Then, in the practitioner's office, take notes, even use a tape recorder, to make certain you understand. Watch for a physician who is a good listener, a good communicator, and open-minded.

InfoLinks

http://nccam.nih.gov

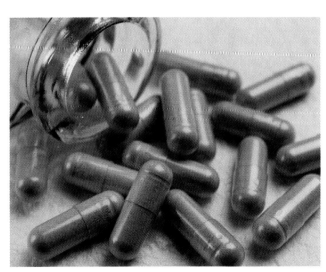

Herbal supplements such as ginseng may be beneficial to some, but consumers should be informed about potential side effects as these products are not required to carry warning labels.

This system employs diet, tailored to the patient's constitutional type, or dosha; herbs; yoga and breathing exercises; meditation; massages; and purges, enemas, and aromatherapy. Practitioners of ayurveda report success in treating rheumatoid arthritis, headaches, and chronic sinusitis.

If you would like to consult a practitioner in one of the alternative disciplines but you don't know where to start, see the Changing for the Better box above for some tips on choosing a provider in alternative medicine.

At the urging of many people in both the medical and complementary health care fields, the National Institutes of Health requested federal funding to establish a scientific center for the study of alternative medical care. Today the National Center for Complementary and Alternative Medicine assembles information about alternative approaches to medical care and provides a framework for well-controlled research into the effectiveness of each approach. Double-blind studies, so called because neither the participants nor the researchers know which treatment each participant is receiving, are being conducted. The first substantial recommendation regarding an alternative form of care, acupuncture, was released in 1998.

It will be interesting to note whether all the branches of complementary medical care will want their theories of treatment and prevention tested under the rigorous criteria used by the National Center for Complementary and Alternative Medicine and to see how they respond if the results are not favorable.

Restricted-Practice Health Care Providers

We receive much of our health care from medical physicians. However, most of us also use the services of various health care specialists who also have advanced graduate-level training. Among these professionals are dentists, psychologists, podiatrists, and optometrists.

Dentists (Doctor of Dental Surgery, DDS) deal with a wide range of diseases and impairments of the teeth and oral cavity. Dentists undergo undergraduate predental programs that emphasize the sciences, followed by 4 additional years of study in dental school and, with increasing frequency, an internship program. State licensure examinations are required. As with physicians, dentists can also specialize by completing a postdoctoral master's degree in fields such as oral surgery, **orthodontics,** and **prosthodontics.** Dentists are also permitted to prescribe therapy programs (such as the treatment of temporo-mandibular joint [TMJ] dysfunction) and drugs that pertain to their practices (primarily analgesics and antibiotics).

As discussed in Chapter 2, *psychologists* provide services to help patients understand behavior patterns or perceptions. More than forty states have certification or licensing laws that prohibit unqualified people from using the term *psychologist.* The consumer should examine a psychologist's credentials. Legitimate psychologists have received advanced graduate training (often leading to a PhD or EdD degree) in clinical, counseling, industrial, or educational psychology. Furthermore, these practitioners will have passed state certification examinations and, in many states, will have met further requirements that allow them to offer health services to the public. Psychologists may have special interests and credentials from professional societies in individual, group, family, or marriage counseling. Some are certified as sex therapists.

Unlike psychiatrists, who are medical physicians, psychologists cannot prescribe or dispense drugs. They may refer to or work collaboratively with medical physicians about clients who might benefit from drug therapy.

Podiatrists are highly trained clinicians who practice podiatric medicine, or care of the feet (and ankles). Although not MDs or DOs, doctors of podiatric medicine (DPM) treat a wide variety of conditions related to the feet, including corns, bunions, warts, bone spurs, ham-

mertoes, fractures, diabetes-related conditions, athletic injuries, and structural abnormalities. Podiatrists perform surgery, prescribe medications, and apply orthotics (supports or braces), splints, and corrective shoes for structural abnormalities of the feet.

Doctors of podiatric medicine follow an educational path similar to that taken by MDs and DOs, consisting of a 4-year undergraduate preprofessional curriculum, 4 additional years of study in a podiatric medical school, and an optional residency of 1 or 2 years. Board-certified areas of specialization include surgery, orthopedics, and podiatric sports medicine. Hospital affiliation generally requires board certification in a specialized area.

Optometrists are eye specialists who primarily treat vision problems associated with **refractory errors.** They examine the eyes and prescribe glasses or contact lenses to correct visual disorders. Additionally, optometrists prescribe prescription medications, such as antibiotic drops for application in the eye. Optometrists sometimes attempt to correct certain ocular muscle imbalances with specific exercise regimens. Optometrists must complete undergraduate training and additional years of coursework at one of sixteen accredited colleges of optometry in the United States or two Canadian colleges before taking a state licensing examination.

Opticians are technicians who manufacture and fit eyeglasses or contact lenses. Although they are rarely licensed by a state agency, they perform the important function of grinding lenses to the precise prescription designated by an optometrist or ophthalmologist (physicians who have specialized in vision care). To save money and time, many consumers take an optometrist's or ophthalmologist's prescription for glasses or contact lenses to optician-staffed retail stores that deal exclusively with eyewear products.

Nurse Professionals

Nurses constitute a large group of health professionals who practice in a variety of settings. Their responsibilities usually depend on their academic preparation. Registered

---

| Key Terms |

orthodontics a dental specialty that focuses on the proper alignment of the teeth.

prosthodontics a dental specialty that focuses on the construction and fitting of artificial appliances to replace missing teeth.

refractory errors abnormal patterns of light wave transmission through the structures of the eye.

nurses (RNs) are academically prepared at two levels: (1) the technical nurse, and (2) the professional nurse. The technical nurse is educated in a 2-year associate degree program. The professional nurse receives 4 years of education and earns a bachelor's degree. Both technical and professional nurses must successfully complete state licensing examinations before they can practice as RNs.

In light of the important role that nurse professionals play in today's health care system, it is worrisome that a significant shortage of nurses exists. On the basis of enrollment data for nursing programs in this country, and the number of nurses who have apparently left the workforce for various reasons, the current shortage of registered nurses is estimated to be 110,000. Projecting through 2008, it is estimated that the shortage will have increased to 450,000.[20] Compounding the shortage of nurses is an equally acute shortage of nursing faculty to staff the nursing education programs that currently exist. As can be imagined, the demand for nurses has increased salaries, generated competition between health care institutions to recruit nurses, and increased the nurse-to-patient ratio to dangerously high levels in many areas of the country. In this final regard, it is estimated that as many as 20,000 unnecessary deaths that occur annually in American hospitals and nursing facilities can be attributed to the shortage—about one-fifth of all deaths attributed to medical errors.[21]

Many professional nurses continue their education and earn master's and doctoral degrees in nursing or other health-related fields. Some professional nurses specialize in a clinical area (such as pediatrics, gerontology, public health, or school health) and become certified as *advanced practice nurses* (APNs). Currently four APN fields, including nurse midwives, nurse anesthetists, nurse practitioners, and nurse case managers, can be found in larger communities. Working in close association with physicians, APNs perform an array of diagnositic, treatment, and administrative activities once limited to physicians. The ability of these highly trained nurses to function at this level gives communities additional primary care providers and frees physicians to deal with more complex cases. With the expansion of managed care, the role of APNs is growing. This increases access to medical care and allows physicians to use their time more cost effectively.

Licensed practical nurses (LPNs) are trained in hospital-based programs that last 12 to 18 months. Because of their brief training, LPNs' scope of practice is limited. Most LPN training programs are gradually being phased out.

Allied Health Care Professionals

Our primary health care providers are supported by a large group of allied health care professionals, who are often responsible for highly technical services and procedures. These professionals include respiratory and inhalation therapists, radiographic technologists, nuclear medicine technologists, pathology technicians, general medical technologists, operating room technicians, emergency medical technicians, physical therapists, occupational therapists, cardiac rehabilitation therapists, dental technicians, physician assistants, and dental hygienists. Depending on the particular field, the training for these specialty support areas can take from 1 to 5 years of postsecondary school study. Programs include hospital-based training leading to a diploma through associate, bachelor's, and master's degrees. Most allied health care professionals must also pass state or national licensing examinations.

Self-Care/Home Care

The emergence of the **self-care movement** suggests that many people are becoming more responsible for maintaining their health. They are developing the expertise to prevent or manage many types of illness, injuries, and conditions. They are learning to assess their health status and treat, monitor, and rehabilitate themselves in a manner that was once thought possible only through a physician or some other health care specialist.

The benefits of this movement are that self-care can (1) reduce health care costs, (2) provide effective care for particular conditions, (3) free physicians and other health care specialists to spend time with other patients, and (4) increase interest in health-related activities.

Self-care is an appropriate alternative to professional care in three areas. First, self-care may be appropriate for certain acute conditions that have familiar symptoms and are limited in their duration and seriousness. Common colds and flu, many home injuries, sore throats, and nonallergic insect bites are often easily managed with self-care. That said, there are some symptoms that might seem somewhat familiar that should not be responded to through self-care, but rather by seeing a physician promptly. These include feeling of pressure or squeezing in the chest, a sudden severe headache, markedly blurred vision, difficulty talking or walking, dizziness and confusion, blood in urine or stool, unrelieved depression, and a cough with a yellow-green discharge.[22] Self-care might be useful at some point, but not until the symptoms have been evaluated by a physician.

Key Terms

self-care movement the trend toward individuals' taking increased responsibility for prevention or management of certain health conditions.

Good Health—What's It Worth, Now and Later?

The average life expectancy for women in the United States today is 80 years. For men, it's 76 years. That's a dramatic change from just a few generations ago. Thanks to tremendous advances in medical science and technology, many people are enjoying healthy, happy, and spiritually fulfilling lives well into their final years.

But this longevity comes with a price tag. It means that making healthful choices every day—including eating a balanced diet, getting exercise and adequate rest, and making opportunities for emotional and spiritual expression—takes on new importance. If you're going to live 10 "extra" years, what do you want to do with that time? Probably many of the things you're doing now, plus some different ones. Are you going to be able to meet the challenge—healthwise?

Taking charge of your health right now, when you're young and healthy, can be one of the most empowering things you do. By consciously choosing a healthy lifestyle—limiting your intake of alcohol, avoiding drugs and cigarette smoking, and limiting your sexual partners—you are building the foundation for good health in your later years.

If you should ever have a serious health problem, you'll be better equipped to handle it if you're used to taking care of yourself. You'll feel comfortable being involved in your treatment decisions and doing whatever you can to control the quality of your life. You'll see your health crisis as a challenge you need to deal with, instead of viewing yourself as a helpless victim.

Taking charge of your own health—by being an informed health care consumer, by choosing a healthy lifestyle, and by fostering a positive attitude—brings a sense of peace. It's knowing that you're doing everything you can to take care of yourself. It's enhancing the quality of your life today and preparing for an active and rewarding tomorrow.

A second area in which self-care might be appropriate is therapy. For example, many people administer injections for diabetes mellitus, allergies, and migraine headaches and continue physical therapy programs in their homes. Asthma and hypertension are also conditions that can be managed or monitored with self-care.

A third area in which self-care has appropriate application is health promotion. Weight loss programs, physical conditioning activities, smoking cessation, and stress-reduction programs are particularly well suited to self-care (see the Discovering Your Spirituality box above).

As the U.S. population ages, it is becoming increasingly common for family members to provide home care to older relatives. As the number of frail older people increases, home care can significantly reduce the need for institutional care. Home care also can be delivered by home health care specialists. In fact, this form of care is proving so cost-effective that some insurance programs, including *Medicare* and *Medicaid,* cover portions of the cost of home health care for older adults (see the Star boxes on Medicare and Medicaid on pages 601 and 602).

With the rapid development of the home health care industry during the 1980s and 1990s, concerns mounted about the lack of regulation over aspects of the industry, particularly the background and training of personnel, and existence of fraud in the billing of services to Medicare and Medicaid. Although personnel issues remain to some degree, the financial aspects of professional home care have been addressed at the federal level. In 1999 the Healthcare Integrity and Protection Data Bank was established to better supervise the billing by home health care providers for services covered under Medicare and Medicaid.[23]

A decision to provide family-based home care, particularly for older adults, is often made for admirable and understandable reasons, including love for the relative who needs care and the high cost of professional home care and institutional care. For the millions of families who have made this decision, providing home health care can be highly rewarding. It also can be very demanding, however, because of the needs and limitations of the person who requires care and the compromises the caregivers must make. Particularly when a spouse or family decides to provide care without the assistance of professional caregivers, they can jeopardize their own health long before the recovery or death of the person for whom they are caring. Even when their physical stamina seems unaffected, factors such as fatigue, emotional strain, postponement of personal and family goals, loss of social contact, and even physical abuse of caregivers by those receiving care can be substantial.

Health Care Facilities

Most of us have a general idea of what a hospital is. However, all hospitals are not alike. They usually fall into one of three categories—private, public, or voluntary. *Private hospitals* (or proprietary hospitals) function as profit-making hospitals. They are not supported by tax monies and usually accept only clients who can pay all their expenses. Although there are some exceptions, these hospitals are generally smaller than tax-supported voluntary hospitals. Commonly owned by a group of business investors, a large hospital corporation, or a group of physicians, these hospitals sometimes limit their services to a few specific types of illnesses.

Public hospitals are supported primarily by tax dollars. They can be operated by government agencies at the state level (such as state mental hospitals) or at the federal level (such as the Veterans Administration Hospitals and various military service hospitals such as Walter Reed Army Hospital). Large county or city hospitals are frequently public hospitals. These hospitals routinely serve indigent segments of the population. They also function as *teaching hospitals.*

The most commonly recognized type of hospital is the *voluntary hospital.* Voluntary hospitals are maintained as nonprofit public institutions. Often supported by religious orders, fraternal groups, or charitable organizations, these hospitals usually offer a wider range of comprehensive services than do private hospitals or clinics. Voluntary hospitals are supported by patient fees (covered by health insurance), Medicare reimbursement, and Medicaid and public assistance reimbursement.

In the last decade, hospitals, particularly private and voluntary hospitals, have expanded their scope of services. Today hospitals often operate *wellness centers,* stress centers, cardiac rehabilitation centers, chemical dependence programs, health education centers, and satellite centers for well-baby care and care for the homeless. During the 1990s two trends were observed in terms of hospital organization and ownership. These included the acquisition of small hospitals (such as county hospitals and smaller community hospitals) by larger regional hospitals and the reorganization of voluntary hospitals as for-profit hospitals. Both trends reflected the rapid movement of medical care in the direction of *managed care,* the term referring to the more profit-focused, cost-efficient, and third-party-controlled care reflective of the application of corporate strategies to the delivery of health care services. Whether these trends will be as obvious in the current decade is uncertain, as the federal government looks more critically at managed care and the dissatisfaction of the public and the medical community with its restrictive approach to delivering health care services.

Other health care facilities include clinics (both private and tax-supported), nursing homes (most of which are private enterprises), and rehabilitation centers. Rehabilitation centers are often supported by charitable organizations devoted to the care of chronically ill or handicapped people, orthopedically injured people, or burn victims.

In recent years, many private, 24-hour drop-in medical emergency and surgical centers have appeared. These clinics have their own professional staffs of physicians, nurses, and allied health professionals. They compete directly with larger hospital-based facilities. Some clinics specialize in women's health needs, including gynecological care, prenatal care, and childbirth services.

Patients' Institutional Rights

Regardless of the type of institution in which you are a patient, you have a variety of rights. These are intended to protect you from unnecessary harm and financial loss. The hospital too can expect your cooperation as a patient.

As a patient, you can expect all of the following from the institution:

- To be treated with respect and dignity
- To be afforded privacy and confidentiality consistent with federal and state laws, institutional policies, and the requirements of your insurance carrier
- To be provided services on request, as long as they are reasonable and consistent with appropriate care
- To be fully informed of the identity of the physicians and staff providing care
- To be kept fully updated about your condition, including its management and your prognosis for recovery
- To be informed of any experimental or other research/educational projects that may be utilized in your treatment and to refuse such treatment
- To have the opportunity to specify advance directives (a living will, a life-prolonging statement, or the appointment of a health care representative) in order to facilitate health care decisions
- To receive an explanation of your bill for services regardless of the source of payment
- To present a complaint and receive a response about any aspect of your care or treatment and to have your complaint taken seriously
- To be involved in ethical considerations that arise during the course of your care

The institution can expect you, as a patient:

- To keep all appointments
- To provide all background information pertinent to your condition
- To treat hospital personnel with respect
- To ask questions and seek clarification about matters that affect you
- To follow the treatment prescribed by your physician
- To be considerate and respectful of other patients and to ensure that your visitors are considerate and respectful as well

- To satisfy your financial obligation to health care providers through the provision of insurance information and by arranging credit where applicable

As a patient, you may at any time:

- Refuse treatment
- Seek a second opinion
- Discharge yourself from the institution

Health Care Costs and Reimbursement

There are many avenues for receiving health care. However, being able to pay for quality health care is one of the greatest concerns of the American public. According to the latest available statistics (2002), 41.2 million Americans are without health insurance. This figure is down from 42.5 million in 1999. When the lack of health insurance is viewed from the perspective of income groups, 14.5% earning less than $25,000 lack health insurance, 13.5% that earn between $25,000 and $49,999 lack coverage, while only 6.6% earning between $50,000 and $75,000 or more are without health insurance. Race and ethnicity also influence the availability of health insurance. Viewed from this perspective, 33.2% of Hispanics, 19.0% of Blacks, and 18.2% of Asians, while only 10.0% of non-Hispanic whites lack health insurance coverage.[24] Regardless of category, persons in this country who lack health insurance are truly living "dangerously." Furthermore, Americans are less optimistic today about their ability to maintain adequate health insurance coverage, find reasonably priced health care, and afford long-term homebound or nursing home care than ever before. Unfortunately, the word *crisis* is appropriate to use when talking about our ability to afford high-quality health care today.

Cost is a basic concern about health care. It is estimated that in 2000 Americans spent $1.295 trillion on health care, and by 2007 this expenditure will increase to $2.13 trillion. Stated another way, in 2000 Americans incurred an average of $4,547 per person in health care–related costs. This amount is expected to increase to $7,100 per person by the year 2007. No developed country spends a greater percentage (14.2% in 2000) of its gross domestic product on health care than does America.[25] In 2000 the U.S. Government spent more than $1,424 billion on health care for its citizens; that figure is expected to top $1,907 billion in 2005.[25] Table 18.1 breaks down annual health care expenditures in the United States.[26]

As a result of factors such as the high cost of modern medical technology, an emphasis on long life at any cost, the growing number of older people with chronic conditions that require expensive long-term care, and the AIDS epidemic, controlling the cost of medical care is one of the most complex problems facing the nation. Nevertheless,

Table 18.1 Per Capita Health Care Expenditures (in Dollars)

Category	Out of Pocket	Third-Party Payments (Insurance & Government)
Personal Health Care		
1970	116	181
1980	256	667
1990	555	1,809
2000	726	3,220
Hospital Care		
1970	12	119
1980	23	414
1990	40	947
2000	34	1,434
Physicians' Services		
1970	27	37
1980	62	130
1990	124	439
2000	106	782
Other Professional Services		
1970	4	3
1980	14	13
1990	53	81
2000	108	165
Drugs/Medical Nondurables		
1970	37	5
1980	75	17
1990	156	75
2000	216	222
Dental Services		
1970	20	2
1980	38	19
1990	59	62
2000	96	117
Vision Services		
1970	8	1
1980	16	4
1990	40	14
2000	56	27
Nursing Home Care		
1970	11	9
1980	31	44
1990	84	111
2000	107	232

Note: The sum of individual categories may not equal the amount shown under *Personal Health Care* due to the exclusion of some categories.

Source: Health Care Financing Administration. *National health care expenditures projections tables—1972–2007,* Tables 2a, 2b, 3b, 4b, 5b, 6b, 8b, 8d, 9b, 10b. November 2000. **www.hcfa.gov/stats/NHE-proj/tables/default.htm**

more than forty different plans have been advanced since 1990 to respond to this problem. These range from only modest changes in the current system, to tax-credit strategies and mandatory employment-based insurance, to a federally controlled national health plan. Today government officials seem to be particularly interested in lowering the cost of prescription drugs for older Americans. Two principal plans are under discussion. One plan assigns prescription drug coverage to Medicare, while the other involves a greater role for third party payers (insurance companies), in combination with prescription drug discount plans offered by pharmaceutical companies. In December 2003, President Bush signed the Medicare Prescription Drug Improvement and Modernization Act. Hailed as an answer to rising drug costs for seniors, the act was widely criticized as still being too costly for many seniors (see the Star box on page 601).

Health Insurance

Health insurance is a financial agreement between an insurance company and an individual or group for the payment of health care costs. After paying a premium to an insurance company, the policyholder is covered for specific benefits. Each policy is different in its coverage of illnesses and injuries. Merely having an insurance policy does not mean that all health care expenses will be covered. Most health insurance policies require various forms of payments by the policyholder, which includes deductible amounts, fixed indemnity benefits, coinsurance, and exclusions. In 2000 Americans spent $372.8 billion on private health insurance, and they are expected to spend $643.4 billion by 2007.[27]

A *deductible* amount is an established amount that the insuree must pay before the insurer reimburses for services. For example, a person or family may have to pay the first $200 of the year's medical expenses before insurance begins providing any coverage.

A policy with *fixed indemnity* benefits will pay only a specified amount for a particular procedure or service. If the policy pays only $1,000 for an appendectomy and the actual cost of the appendectomy was $1,500, then the policy owner will owe the health care provider $500. A policy with full-service benefits, which pays the entire cost of a particular procedure or service, may be worth the extra cost.

Policies that have *coinsurance* features require that the policy owner and the insurance company share the costs of certain covered services, usually on a percentage basis. One standard coinsurance plan requires that the policyholder pay 20% of the costs above a deductible amount, and the company pays the remaining 80%.

An *exclusion* is a service or expense that is not covered by the policy. Elective or cosmetic surgery procedures, unusual treatment protocols, prescription drugs, and certain kinds of consultations are common exclusions. Illness and injuries that already exist at the time of purchase (preex-isting conditions) are often excluded. In addition, injuries incurred during high-risk activities (ice hockey, hang gliding, mountain climbing, intramural sports) might not be covered by a policy.

Health insurance can be obtained through individual policies or group plans. Group health insurance plans usually offer the widest range of coverage at the lowest price and are often purchased cooperatively by companies and their employees. In 2003 companies with health insurance benefits spent on average $6,656.00 for each employee's family health insurance plan—a 28% increase over 2000 costs.[28] Fortunately, no employee is refused entry into a group insurance program. However, when employees leave the company, their previous group coverage can follow them for a prescribed period of time only, usually 18 to 24 months. Today, as many large American companies continue to lay off employees, the eventual loss of health insurance becomes a serious personal and family crisis.

Individual policies can be purchased by one person (or a family) from an insurance company. These policies are often much more expensive than group plans and may provide much less coverage. Still, people who do not have access to a group plan should attempt to secure individual policies, because the financial burdens resulting from a severe accident or illness that is not covered by some form of health insurance can be devastating. Many colleges and universities offer annually renewable health insurance policies that students can purchase. The Changing for the Better box on page 600 gives the consumer some questions to consider before purchasing a health insurance policy.

Health Maintenance Organizations

Health maintenance organizations (HMOs) are health care delivery plans under which health care providers agree to meet the covered medical needs of subscribers for a prepaid amount of money. For a fixed monthly fee, enrollees are given comprehensive health care with an emphasis on preventive health care. Enrollees receive their care from physicians, specialists, allied health professionals, and educators who are hired (group model) or contractually retained (network model) by the HMO.

Managed care, and HMOs in particular, was a reaction to the sharply climbing costs of health care in the 1980s. Businesses, which paid a large portion of health care costs through employee-benefit plans, complained that no one in the health care loop had an incentive to control costs. Employers complained that consumers paid only a deductible and a small copayment, giving them little cause to question prices; doctors faced little financial oversight; and insurance companies merely rubber-stamped the bills.

When HMOs presented an alternative, employers began offering their workers incentives to select HMOs over traditional fee-for-service coverage and thus attempted to rein in the runaway costs of health care. HMOs now cover nearly 70 million Americans. Increases in membership continued until 2000, when many HMOs that participated in Medicare supplement plans discontinued participation and, thus, discontinued service to their previously enrolled older adult members. The escalating cost of prescription medications was the principal factor in this decision. In all HMOs the annual cost of membership continues to rise, particularly for persons enrolled in the for-profit HMOs. This increase reflects the rising cost of services that must be provided to members.

HMOs are usually the least expensive but most restrictive type of managed care. The premiums are 8% to 10% lower than traditional plans, they charge no deductibles or coinsurance payments, and copayments are $5 to $10 per visit. However, you are limited to using the doctors and hospitals in the HMO's network, and you must get approval for treatments and referrals.

In theory, HMOs were to be the ideal blend of medical care and health promotion. Today, however, many observers are concerned that too many HMOs are being too tightly controlled by a profit motive in which physicians are being paid large bonuses to *not* refer patients to specialists or are prevented by "gag rules" from discussing certain treatment options with patients because of their costs to the HMOs.

Concerns, in addition to the "gag rules" mentioned above, have also arisen over the years. Among these have been concerns related to the right of members to sue their HMOs for medical negligence, the provision of better ob-gyn coverage, and the development of a more efficient mechanism to appeal denial of services. The latter is among the most distressing aspects of HMO membership to most members.

In spite of the problems just mentioned, HMOs remain, in theory, more cost-efficient than the traditional

Medicare

Since it was established in 1965, *Medicare* has been a key provider of health coverage for the nation's elderly. Medicare is a federally funded health insurance program for persons 65 years of age and older, as well as for persons of any age who have particular disabilities or permanent kidney failure. Funding for Medicare comes primarily from federal payroll taxes and is administered by the Health Care Financing Administration, within the Department of Health and Human Services.

In its current configuration Medicare is divided into two portions. Part A (the hospital insurance portion) helps pay for care while in hospitals, as well as for care in skilled nursing facilities and hospice care, and for some home health care. Persons become eligible for Part A coverage upon turning 65 years of age, on the basis of having paid Medicare taxes while working.

Part B is an optional portion of Medicare that can be chosen at the time of becoming eligible for Part A, or at selected times following initial eligibility. Unlike Part A, there is a monthly charge for Part B coverage. Currently that charge is $54.00 per month, but is subject to annual adjustment. Part B helps pay for doctors' services, outpatient hospital care, and some other medical services not covered under Part A, including physical and occupational therapy, medical devices, and some home health care. Routine dental and vision care are not covered.

Because of the universal nature of Medicare Part A and the affordable monthly charge for Part B, group health insurance plans to which many retirees belong will require that Medicare be the "first payer" for services, thus allowing the group plan to be responsible for only that portion of health-related charges not covered by Medicare.

The Medicare Prescription Drug Improvement and Modernization Act of 2003 provides new prescription coverage options for Medicare recipients. It provides prescription coverage through third-party providers for a premium of about $35 per month. After meeting an annual deductible of $250, Medicare would cover 75% of the costs of prescription drugs, up to $2,250 per year; there is then a gap in coverage until out-of-pocket expenses reach $3,500 in a single year, at which point Medicare would again kick in and cover 90% of further costs.

Source: *Medicare & you: the knowledge to make good decisions.* U.S. Department of Health and Human Services, Health Care Financing Administration. Publication No. HCFA-02179. May 2002; Rosenbaum, David E. Bush Signs Law to Cover Drugs for the Elderly. *The New York Times,* December 9, 2003.

---

fee-for-service healthcare model. Cost containment is achieved, in part, because most of the medical services within a group model HMO are centralized, there is little duplication of facilities, equipment, or support staff. Central filing of records gives all the HMO physicians access to a single file for each client. This saves time, administrative costs, and the overlapping of care. Many HMOs also routinely use health-promotion activities.[29]

Other new approaches to reducing health costs are independent practice associations (IPAs) and preferred provider organizations (PPOs). An IPA is a modified form of an HMO that uses a group of doctors who offer prepaid services out of their own offices and not in a central HMO facility. IPAs are viewed as "HMOs without walls." A PPO is a group of private practitioners who sell their services at reduced rates to insurance companies. When a policyholder chooses a physician who is in that company's PPO network, the insurance company pays the entire physician's fee. When a policyholder selects a non-PPO physician, the insurance company pays only a portion of that physician's fee. Today, more than 80% of Americans with health benefits are enrolled in a managed care plan (HMO, IPA, or PPO).[28] In some areas of the country, such as California, Oregon, and Washington, over 90% of persons with benefits are in managed care plans. For a discussion on Medicare and Medicaid, see the Star boxes on pages 601 and 602.

Extended Care Insurance

With the aging of the population and the greater likelihood that nursing home care will be required (at nearly $57,000 per year in 2002), insurers have developed extended care policies.[29, 30] When purchased at an early age (by mid-50s), these policies are much more affordable than if purchased when a spouse or family member will soon require institutional care. However, not all older adults will need extensive nursing home care, so an extended care policy could be an unnecessary expenditure.

Access to Health Care

With 41.2 million Americans lacking any health insurance and with nearly a quarter of those with insurance being underinsured, Americans are finding it increasingly difficult to access their country's highly sophisticated health care system. The unemployed poor, working poor, and minorities have the most difficulty accessing health care. African Americans, Hispanic Americans, and Native Americans have the worst health status of all Americans, yet they receive the fewest health care services. Even for older Americans with Medicare, gaping holes exist in the types of care covered (for example, glasses and hearing aids are not covered) and the prices of prescription medications far exceed the coverage provided. Thus, as America

Medicaid

Unlike Medicare (see Star box on page 601), a program that is almost exclusively for persons 65 years of age or older, *Medicaid* is a program designed to assist in meeting the health care needs of qualified persons regardless of age. Also, unlike Medicare, which is a federal program entirely funded through Medicare tax withholdings (Part A) and user-paid elected enrollment fees (Part B), Medicaid is a federal- and state-funded program administered by each of the individual states.

Qualification for receiving Medicaid assistance can be perplexing. Federal Medicaid law sets mandatory eligibility standards, while optional eligibility standards allow each state to tailor many aspects of the program to fit its unique needs. Central to the majority of federally mandated eligibility standards is the current Federal Poverty Level (FPL), as well as standards related to the Aid to Families with Dependent Children (AFDC) program and the Temporary Assistance to Needy Families (TANF) program. Optional eligibility standards allow states to define some aspects of eligibility for pregnant women, disabled children, certain working disabled persons, and those designated as Medically Needy.

Federally mandated Medicaid services are wide ranging, and include hospital services, physician services, laboratory/X-ray procedures, immunizations, family planning services, home health care services, transportation for medical care services, and nursing home services. This final service is of critical importance to older adults in that it pays for the majority of nursing home care required by this age group. Optional services, which are under state control, include prescription drugs, rehabilitation and physical therapy services, prosthetic devices, vision services, hearing services, and dental services, to include a few.

Source: *Opportunities to use Medicaid in support of access of health services: basic description of the Medicaid program.* Department of Health and Human Services, Health Care Financing Administration (HCFA). December 2000. **http://www.hrsa.gov/ medicaidprimer/medicare_program.htm**

---

enters the twenty-first century, its people are expressing growing concern about the extent to which their health care needs will be met. As political opposition remains strongly against a national health care system, the United States joins South Africa to make them the only two major industrialized nations lacking a comprehensive and unified approach to meeting the health care needs of their populations.

Health-Related Products

As you might imagine, prescription and over-the-counter (OTC) drugs constitute an important part of any discussion of health-related products.

Prescription Drugs

Caution: Federal law prohibits dispensing without prescription. This FDA warning appears on the labels of approximately three-fourths of all medications. Prescription drugs must be ordered for patients by a licensed practitioner. Because these compounds are legally controlled and may require special skills in their administration, the public's access to these drugs is limited.

Although the *Physicians' Desk Reference* lists more than 2,500 compounds that can be prescribed by a physician, only 200 drugs make up the bulk of the nearly 3,010 million new prescriptions and refills dispensed by 43,600 pharmacies in 2001.[31] Total retail prescription sales of $145 billion for 2000 represents a 15% increase over the previous year's sales. This upward trend reflects in large part the greater variety of prescription medications being prescribed each year by physicians. It is projected that by the year 2012 approximately $446 billion will be spent on prescription medications.[26] The rapid expansion of online pharmacies now occurring is unlikely to influence the number of prescriptions filled, though their presence will likely affect the sales of "brick and mortar" drugstore chains.

Research and Development of New Drugs

As consumers of prescription drugs, you may be curious about the process by which drugs gain FDA approval. The rigor of this process may be the reason that only about one hundred new drugs are approved annually.

The nation's pharmaceutical companies constantly explore the molecular structure of various chemical compounds in an attempt to discover important new compounds with desired types and levels of biological activity. Once these new compounds are identified, companies begin extensive in-house research with computer simulations and animal testing to determine whether clinical trials with humans are warranted. Of the 125,000 or more compounds under study each year, only a few thousand receive such extensive preclinical evaluation. Even fewer of these are then taken to the FDA to begin the evaluation process necessary to gain approval for further research with humans. When the FDA approves a drug for clinical trials, a pharmaceutical company can obtain a patent, which prevents the drug from being manufactured by other companies for the next 17 years.

The $500+ million price tag for bringing a new drug into the marketplace reflects this slow, careful process. If the 7 years of work needed to bring a new drug into the marketplace go well, a pharmaceutical company enjoys the remaining 10 years of legally protected retail sales. Today new "fast-track" approval procedures at the FDA are progressively reducing the development period, particularly for desperately needed breakthrough drugs like those used to treat AIDS. Concern was expressed in 2000 that this "rush to approval" forced the FDA to utilize the services of independent evaluators, many of whom had ties to the pharmaceutical industry that would have influenced their assessments of a drug's readiness for marketing. Additional areas of concern related to the research and development of prescription medications include the extent to which the pharmaceutical industry will continue to voluntarily use children (and pregnant women) in reassessment of drug dosages initially determined for adults; and the decrease in the FDA's approval of new drugs from 24 in 2001 to 17 in 2002 and *new drug investigation* requests submitted to the FDA from 60 in 1995 to 23 in 2002.

Generic versus Brand-Name Drugs

When a new drug comes into the marketplace, it carries three names: its **chemical name,** its **generic name,** and its **brand name.** While the 17 year patent is in effect, no other drug with the same chemical formulation can be sold. When the patent expires, other companies can manufacture a drug of equivalent chemical composition and market it under the brand name drug's original generic name. Because extensive research and development are unnecessary at this point, producing generic drugs is far less costly than developing the original brand name drug. Nearly all states allow pharmacists to substitute generic drugs for brand name drugs, as long as the prescribing physician approves. In 2002 the list of approved generic drugs was increased by 80 additional inclusions. For those interested in viewing all of the current approved generics, the FDA updates each month its Generic Drug Approvals list.[32]

 TALKING POINTS Your mother insists on using the brand-name drug that she has used for years to control her arthritis pain, even though her doctor has prescribed a generic version that has recently become available. What might you say to help her consider the less expensive option?

In recent years the pharmaceutical industry has actively attempted to extend the patent protection on several of the most profitable drugs on the market because their period of protected sales is expiring. In some cases the manufacturers have appealed directly to Congress for waivers to the current patent law, contending that they need the additional time to recoup research and development costs. Other manufacturers have quietly "layered" additional patents onto their products to prevent manufacturers of generic versions from using the same shape or color used in brand name versions, even though the chemical formulations are no longer protected. In another approach, manufacturers of highly profitable brand name drugs have offered to pay manufacturers of generic drugs to not make generic versions of their products once the patent protection has expired.

Today a variety of reference books are available to inform consumers about the availability of generic drugs and the prescription drugs that they can legally be substituted for. *Mosby's Drug Consult* series is a widely used reference focusing on both brand name drugs and generic equivalents. Updated annually, this publication is currently available in the 2004 edition.[33]

Over-the-Counter Drugs

When people are asked when they last took some form of medication, for many the answer might be, "I took aspirin (or a cold pill, or a laxative) this morning." In making this decision, people engaged in self-diagnosis, determined a course for their own treatment, self-administered their treatment, and freed a physician to serve people whose illnesses are more serious than theirs. None of this would have been possible without readily available, inexpensive, and effective OTC drugs (see the Star box on page 604).

While 2,500 prescription drugs are available, there are perhaps as many as 300,000 different OTC products, routinely classified into twenty-six different families (see the Star box on page 604). Like prescription drugs, nonprescription drugs are regulated by the FDA. However, for OTC drugs, the marketplace is a more powerful determinant of success.

The regulation of OTC drugs is based on a provision in a 1972 amendment to the 1938 Food, Drug, and Cosmetic

> **Key Terms**
>
> **chemical name** name used to describe the molecular structure of a drug.
>
> **generic name** common or nonproprietary name of a drug.
>
> **brand name** specific patented name assigned to a drug by its manufacturer.

The Attraction of Canadian Prescription Drugs

On a weekday morning automobiles pull into the parking lot of an Indianapolis shopping mall, car doors open, and within a few minutes fifty or more people are waiting. In a few minutes they are joined by a comfortable new motor coach. The bus fills quickly and soon departs for a 5-hour drive to Windsor, Canada, via Detroit. Yet another "drug run" is under way to the closest point in Canada in order that Hoosier senior citizens can purchase American-made prescription medication in a foreign country more cheaply than at home. A comparison of prices gives credence to the sensibility of making this exhausting daylong trip. For example, a 90-pill supply of the prescription drug Zocor, used to lower blood cholesterol, will cost more than $350 from an American pharmacy; in Canada, a patient can purchase the same amount of the same medication for $140.

Why are drugs manufactured in this country, that are in compliance with the rigorous safety and effectiveness standards of both Canada and the United States, priced more cheaply in Canada than in the United States? The answer to that question reflects the buying power of Canada's provincial health care programs that have forced American manufacturers to set lower Canadian wholesale prices in order to compete in their group-sales driven marketplace. A far less "structured" health care marketplace in this country, in combination with a "supportive" FDA and FTC, has allowed the American pharmaceutical industry to charge wholesale prices considerably higher than those charged to our "neighbor to the north." Thus, a disproportionate portion of the profit made by the American pharmaceutical industry comes from the pockets of its own citizens; while those in a foreign country enjoy the benefits of our technology. Understandably, a similar trip northward is planned for the next week.

Source: What's the difference? *USA Today,* July 25, 2003, p. 5A.

Act. As a result of that action, OTC drugs were placed in three categories (I, II, and III) based on the safety and effectiveness of their active ingredient(s). Today, only category I OTC drugs that are safe, effective, and truthfully labeled are to be sold. The FDA's drug-classification process also allows some OTC drugs to be made stronger and some prescription drugs to become nonprescription drugs by reducing their strength through reformulation. Whether the reformulation of a prescription drug into an OTC formulation is always to the consumer's advantage is questionable. For example, in 2003 Prilosec, a drug for reducing esophageal reflux disease, became available over the counter. Although

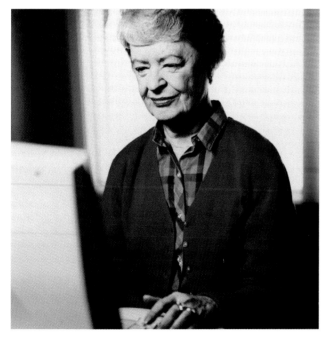

Using the Internet to comparison shop is one way of becoming a wise consumer of health care products and services, such as insurance policies and medications.

Categories of Over-the-Counter (OTC) Products

- Antacids
- Antimicrobials
- Sedatives and sleep aids
- Analgesics
- Cold remedies and antitussives
- Antihistamines and allergy products
- Mouthwashes
- Topical analgesics
- Antirheumatics
- Hematinics
- Vitamins and minerals
- Antiperspirants
- Laxatives
- Dentrifices and dental products
- Sunburn treatments and preventives
- Contraceptive and vaginal products
- Stimulants
- Hemorrhoidals
- Antidiarrheals
- Dandruff and athlete's foot preparations

Dietary Supplements and the Self-Care Movement

Currently, more than 60 million Americans are using an array of vitamins, minerals, herbal products, hormones, amino acids, and glandular extracts in their quest for improved health. People turn to dietary supplements rather than the dietary recommendation discussed in Chapter 5 for many reasons, including concern over their own morbidity and mortality, dissatisfaction with today's impersonal health care system, distrust in the safety of the food supply, and people's increasing inability to control other aspects of life. As a result, we are now spending more than $12 million annually on dietary supplements— many of which appear unnecessary and some of which may be unsafe and ineffective. Recall that dietary supplement makers are not required to submit evidence of safety or effectiveness to the Food and Drug Administration, as is the case with prescription medications and, to a lesser degree, the OTC products.

In spite of the lack of available data on safety and effectiveness, the traditional medical community is showing increasing interest in the potential benefits of dietary supplements. A growing number of teaching hospitals are establishing departments of complementary medicine, and medical students are learning about the documented role (to the extent that it is known) that these supplements can play in promoting health. Additionally, major international pharmaceutical companies are beginning to market dietary supplements. The reputation and resources of these companies are likely to generate more carefully controlled research into the safety and efficacy of these products. However, the extent to which the National Center for Complementary and Alternative Medicine (within the National Institutes of Health) will undertake carefully controlled studies of dietary supplements remains uncertain. Until studies have been completed, the public should be aware that only three supplements have received approval from the FDA to include specific health claims on their labels. These include folic acid and its ability to facilitate neural tube closure, calcium and its contribution to the prevention of osteoporosis, and a highly qualified claim for omega-3 fatty acids in the reduction of cardiovascular disease.

Prilosec as an OTC drug is less expensive than it was as a prescription product, it is now no longer covered by health insurance. The loss of insurance coverage (usually 80% of the price once deductibles are met) makes the medication as expensive, if not more expensive, than it was initially, at least for patients who have prescription coverage. Of course, by being an OTC, a doctor appointment and resultant prescription are not required, but even this savings will soon be offset by the lack of insurance coverage if the medication is used over a long period of time.

Like the proposed label shown in Figure 18-1, current labels for OTC products reflect FDA requirements. The labels must clearly state the type and quantity of active ingredients, alcohol content, side effects, instructions for appropriate use, warning against inappropriate use, and risks of using the product with other drugs (polydrug use). Unsubstantiated claims must be carefully avoided in advertisements of these products.

Advance Medical Directives

Have you talked to your family about what kind of care you would want to receive in the event of a severe injury or illness? Would you feel prepared to make decisions regarding medical care, extreme lifesaving measures, or organ donation for other members of your family?

Many people do not wish to think about what would happen if they were rendered completely incapacitated and unable to speak for themselves. But determining in advance the kind of treatment you wish to receive in the event of a terminal illness or severe injury can lift a terrible burden off of your family and loved ones, who might be hard pressed to make those decisions for you. For this reason, many people are using legal documents called advance medical directives to articulate their wishes regarding lifesaving measures, organ donation, and the decision whether treatment is burdensome or beneficial with hopes for recovery. The advance directive is not called upon until two physicians have determined that the patient's condition is terminal, irreversible, and incurable, and the individual is unable to communicate his or her wishes or considered no longer capable of decision making.

One of the most common of these medical directives is the living will, a document that confirms a person's desires to die peacefully and with a measure of dignity should a time arrive when there is little hope for recovery from a terminal illness or severe injury. Living will statutes exist in all fifty states and in the District of Columbia. An estimated 25% of U.S. adults have signed living wills.[34]

A second important document that can assist terminally ill or incapacitated patients is the **medical power of attorney** for health care document. This legal document

Figure 18-1 The FDA will soon require over-the-counter drugs to carry standardized labels, such as the one at right.

Drug Facts

Active Ingredient (in each tablet) **Purpose**
Chlorpheniramine maleate 2 mg   Antihistamine

Uses temporarily relieves these symptoms due to hay fever or other upper respiratory allergies:

■ sneezing ■ runny nose ■ itchy, watery eyes ■ itchy throat

Warnings
Ask a doctor before use if you have
■ glaucoma ■ a breathing problem such as emphysema or chronic bronchitis
■ trouble urinating due to an enlarged prostate gland

Ask a doctor or pharmacist before use if you are taking tranquilizers or sedatives

When using this product
■ you may get drowsy ■ avoid alcoholic drinks
■ alcohol, sedatives, and tranquilizers may increase drowsiness
■ be careful when driving a motor vehicle or operating machinery
■ excitability may occur, especially in children

If pregnant or breast-feeding, ask a health professional before use.
Keep out of reach of children. In case of overdose, get medical help or contact a Poison Control Center right away.

Directions

adults and children 12 years and over	take 2 tablets every 4 to 6 hours; not more than 12 tablets in 24 hours
children 6 years to under 12 years	take 1 tablet every 4 to 6 hours; not more than 6 tablets in 24 hours
children under 6 years	ask a doctor

Other information
■ store at 20-25° C (68-77° F) ■ protect from excessive moisture

Inactive ingredients D&C yellow no. 10, lactose, magnesium stearate, microcrystalline cellulose, pregelatinized starch

---

authorizes another person to make specific health care decisions about treatment and care under specified circumstances, most commonly when patients are in long-term vegetative states and cannot communicate their medical wishes. This document helps inform hospitals and physicians which person will help make the critical medical decisions. Usually this person is a loving relative. It is recommended that people complete both a living will and a medical power of attorney for health care documentation.

You might also consider organ donation. On any given day, more than eighty thousand Americans are on waiting lists for organ transplants.[35] For some, the decision to donate body tissue and organs after death is rewarding and comforting. To become an organ donor, you must fill out an organ donor card indicating your wishes to become an organ donor and specifying what organs and tissues you would want to donate in the event of your death. In many states, you can put this information on your driver's license. However, it is also crucial that you discuss your wishes with family members so that they understand them and are able to inform medical professionals of your wishes if you should die suddenly.

 TALKING POINTS Have you discussed the importance of a living will with your parents or grandparents? How might you approach the subject?

Health Care Quackery and Consumer Fraud

A person who earns money by marketing inaccurate health information, unreliable health care, or ineffective health products is called a fraud, quack, or charlatan.

Prepaying a Funeral

The disposition of human remains is a complicated reality in today's world. Factors ranging from public health laws to the emotional needs of survivors dictate that we plan ahead, if time permits. Accordingly, a growing percentage (currently estimated to be 30%) of Americans are preplanning and prepaying for their funerals. Federal Trade Commission laws and some state regulations give structure to the process, but it behooves individual consumers to work carefully with a reputable funeral home.

Although the cost of funerals can vary widely depending on the areas of the country and the personal desires of individuals, the average American funeral, less cemetery plot, grave opening/closing and marker, is approximately $6,000. Among the specific components of this cost are professional services charges ($1,213), embalming ($420), other preparations of body (cosmetics, hair) ($150), visitation and viewing ($275), funeral service at funeral home ($350), transfer of remains to funeral home (usually from a hospital or nursing home)($154), hearse for local use ($185), other vehicles (flower car/family car) ($85),

acknowledgement cards ($18), casket ($2,330, and vault ($950)). Cremation of the body, rather than burial or entombment, will lower this cost to some degree.

Today many people wish to pay funeral expenses before their death, thus freeing grieving family members from the task of "guessing" what final arrangements were desired. In order to make certain that this process can be carried out in standardized manner, that is both professional and fair, the Federal Trade Commission has established the following rules to regulate preplanned and prepaid funerals. According to these rules:

- Funeral directors must provide a list of itemized prices in person and, if you ask, over the phone.
- You have the right to choose the goods and services you want (with some exceptions). The funeral home cannot require you to buy a package of preselected goods and services.
- If a state law requires you to buy a particular item, the funeral provider must disclose it on the price list, with reference to the specific law.

- The funeral provider may not refuse, or charge a fee, to handle a casket you bought elsewhere.
- If you want to buy a casket, the funeral home must provide you with descriptions of the selections and prices before showing you the caskets.
- A funeral provider that offers cremation must make alternative containers available.

Once preplanning is completed and a contract signed, the consumer can prepay for the service or purchase an insurance policy that will cover the funeral costs when death occurs. After prepaying, the purchaser should be certain that the money is deposited by the funeral provider into a funeral trust account at an insured (FDIC) lending institution. A copy of all relevant information and documents should be given to responsible family members for safekeeping, rather than being left in a safe deposit box. Additionally funeral related instruction should not be written into a will, but, rather, discussed with family members at a time well before death seems likely.

Consumer fraud flourished with the old-fashioned medicine shows of the late 1880s. Unfortunately, consumer fraud still flourishes. You need look no further than large city newspapers to see questionable advertisements for disease cures and weight loss products. Quacks have found in health and illness the perfect avenues to make maximum gain with minimum effort.

When people are in poor health, they may be afraid of becoming disabled or dying. So powerful are their desires to live and avoid suffering that people are vulnerable to promises of health improvement or a cure. Even though many people have great faith in their physicians, they also want access to experimental treatments or products touted as being superior to currently available therapies. When tempted by the promise of help, people sometimes abandon traditional medical care. Of course, quacks recognize this vulnerability and present a variety of "reasons" to seek their help (see the Changing for the Better box on page 608). Gullibility, blind faith, impatience, superstition, ignorance, or hostility toward professional expertise eventually carry the day. In spite of

the best efforts of agencies at all levels, no branch of government can protect consumers from their own errors of judgment that so easily play into the hands of quacks and charlatans.

Regardless of the motivation that leads people into consumer fraud, the outcome is frequently the same. First, the consumer loses money. The services or products are grossly overpriced, and the consumers have little recourse to help them recover their money. Second, the consumers often feel disappointed, guilty, and angered by their own carelessness as consumers. Far too frequently, consumer fraud may lead to unnecessary suffering.

Key Terms

consumer fraud marketing of unreliable and ineffective services, products, or information under the guise of curing disease or improving health; quackery.

Planning an Organ Donation

I've thought about organ donation for a long time, and now I am ready to document my wishes. What steps do I need to take to do this?

Donating organs is one of the most compassionate, responsible acts a person can perform. Only a few simple steps are required:

1. You must complete a uniform donor card. Obtain a card from a physician, a local hospital, or the nearest regional transplant or organ bank.
2. Print or type your name on the card.
3. Indicate which organs your wish to donate. You may also indicate your desire to donate all organs and tissues.

4. Sign your name in the presence of two witnesses, preferably your next of kin.
5. Fill in any additional information (such as date of birth, city and state in which the card is completed, and date the card is signed).
6. Tell others about your decision to donate. Some donor cards have detachable portions to give to your family.
7. Always carry your card with you.
8. If you have any questions, you can call the United Network for Organ Sharing (UNOS) at 1-888-TXINFO1, or visit this organization's website at **www.unos.org.**

Uniform Donor Card

Of _____
(print or type name of donor)

In the hope that I may help others, I hereby make this anatomical gift, if medically acceptable, to take effect upon my death. The words and marks below indicate my wishes.
I give: ☐ any needed organs or parts
☐ only the following organs or parts

_____
specify the organ(s), tissue(s), or part(s)

for the purposes of transplantation, therapy, medical research or education:
☐ my body for anatomical study if needed.
Limitations or special wishes, if any:_____

National Kidney Foundation
Please detach and give this portion of the card to your family.

This is to inform you that, should the occasion ever arise, I would like to be an organ and tissue donor. Please see that my wishes are carried out by informing the attending medical personnel that I have indicated my wishes to become a donor. Thank you.

_____
Signature   *Date*
For further information write or call:
National Kidney Foundation
30 East 33rd Street, New York, NY 10016
(800)-622-9010

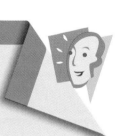

Recognizing Quackery

I don't want to get taken in by health care quackery. What should I be on the lookout for?

"Duck" when you encounter these!

- Makes promises of quick, dramatic, simple, painless, or drugless treatment or cures
- Uses anecdotes, case histories, or testimonials to support claims
- Displays credentials or uses titles that might be confused with those of the scientific or medical community, such as Stan Smith, Ph.D. (in results)
- Claims a product or service provides treatment or cure for multiple or all illnesses and conditions
- States that this treatment or cure is either secret or not yet available in the United States

- States that medical doctors should not be trusted because they do more harm than good with their approaches to diagnosis and treatment
- Reports that most disease is due to a faulty diet and can be treated with nutritional supplements
- Promotes the use of hair analysis to diagnose illnesses or deficiencies
- Claims that "natural" products are superior to those sold in drugstores or dispensed by physicians
- Supports the "freedom of choice" concept that should allow you to try something even though it has not been proved safe and effective

Becoming a Skilled Health Care Consumer

After reading this discussion of health information, services, and products, you should be a wiser, more prepared consumer. However, information alone is not enough. Consider these six suggestions to help you become a more skilled, assertive consumer:

1. *Prepare yourself for consumerism.* In addition to this personal health course, your university may offer a course on consumerism. Libraries and bookstores offer trade books on a variety of consumer topics. Consumer protection agencies can guide you in some subjects. Government agencies also may help you in your choices.
2. *Comparison shop.* In our free-enterprise system, virtually every service or product can be duplicated on the open market. Very few items or services are one-of-a kind. Take the time to study your choices before you purchase a product or service.
3. *Insist on formal contracts and dated receipts.* Under the consumer laws in most states, you have a limited time in which to void a contract. Formal documentation of your actions as a consumer will give you the maximum protection available.
4. *Obtain written instructions and warranties.* Be certain of the appropriate use of any product you purchase. If you use a product inappropriately, you might void its warranty. Be familiar with what you can reasonably anticipate from the products and services you buy. In addition, be aware that a written warranty supersedes any verbal assurances a salesperson might make.
5. *Put your complaints in writing.* A carefully constructed record of your complaints is vital. Accurate records of the names and addresses of all companies and people with whom you have done business will enable you to document your actions as a consumer.
6. *Press for resolution of your complaints.* As a consumer, you are entitled to effective products and services. If your consumer complaints are not resolved, you have legal recourse through the courts. You should not hesitate to assert your rights, not only for your own sake, but for consumers who might later become victims.

Consumerism is an active relationship between you and a provider. If the provider is competent and honest and you are an informed and active consumer, both of you will profit from the relationship. However, if the provider is not competent or honest, you can protect yourself by employing the preceding six suggestions.

Taking Charge of Your Health

- Keep yourself well informed about current health issues and new developments in health care.
- Analyze the credibility of the health information you receive before putting it into practice.
- Select your health care providers by using a balanced set of criteria (see pages 587 and 588)
- Explore alternative forms of health care, and consider using them as a complement to traditional health care.

- In selecting a health care plan, compare various plans on the basis of several key factors, not simply cost (see page 600).
- Assemble a complete personal/family health history as soon as possible. Be sure to include information from older family members.
- Comply with all directions regarding the appropriate use of prescription and OTC medications.
- Write a living will and encourage family members to do the same.

Summary

- Sources of health information include family, friends, commercials, labels, the Internet, and information supplied by health professionals, as well as others.
- Physicians can be either Doctors of Medicine (MDs) or Doctors of Osteopathy (DOs). They receive similar training and engage in similar forms of practice.
- Although alternative health care providers, including chiropractors, naturopaths, herbalists, and acupuncturists, meet the health care needs of many people, systematic study of these forms of health care is only now under way.

- Restricted-practice health care providers play important roles in meeting the health and wellness needs of the public.
- Nursing at all levels is a critical health care profession. Advanced practice nurses represent the highest level of training within nursing.
- Self-care is often a viable approach to preventing illness and reducing the use of health care providers.
- Our growing inability to afford health care services has reached crisis proportions in the United States.
- More than 41 million Americans, not just the poor, have problems getting health care. Minorities

have the most limited access to health care services of all Americans.

- Health insurance is critical to our ability to afford modern health care services.
- HMOs provide an alternative way of receiving health care services, although the influence of the profit motive in their operation is a concern.
- Medicare and Medicaid are governmental plans for paying for health care services.
- The development of prescription medication is a long and expensive process for pharmaceutical manufacturers. The cost of prescription medica-

tion is the most rapidly increasing aspect of health care affordability.
- OTC products have a role to play in the treatment of illness, but their safe use is based on following label directions.
- Advance medical directives can help physicians and/or family members make appropriate medical decisions for you in the event that you are unable to make them for yourself.
- Critical health consumerism, including avoiding health quackery, requires careful selection of health-related information, products, and services.

Review Questions

1. Determine how you would test the accuracy of the health-related information you have received in your lifetime.
2. Identify and describe some sources of health-related information presented in this chapter. What factors should you consider when using these sources?
3. Describe the similarities between allopathic and osteopathic physicians. What is an alternative health care practitioner? Give examples of the types of alternative practitioners.
4. What are the theories underlying acupuncture and ayurveda?
5. Describe the services that are provided by the following limited health care providers: dentists, psychologists, podiatrists, optometrists, and opticians. Identify several allied health care professionals. What levels of training and expertise exist within nursing?
6. In what ways is the trend toward self-care evident? What are some reasons for the popularity of this movement?
7. How do private, public, and voluntary (proprietary) hospitals differ?
8. What is health insurance? Explain the following terms relating to health insurance: deductible amount, fixed

indemnity benefits, full-service benefits, coinsurance, exclusion, and preexisting condition.
9. What is a health maintenance organization? How do HMO plans reduce the costs of health care? What are IPAs and PPOs?
10. What do the chemical name, brand name, and generic name of a prescription drug represent? How long is the patent protection for a prescription medication?
11. What role do Medicare and Medicaid play in meeting the health care needs of the American public? Which portion of Medicare is universal? What elective options does Medicare offer?
12. What are the three criteria that must be met by an OTC drug? In comparison with prescription medication and OTC drugs, what regulatory control does the FDA have over dietary supplements?
13. What does an advance medical directive do? What is a living will? How does it differ from medical power of attorney?
14. What is health quackery? What federal agencies have some ability to limit its presence? What can a consumer do to avoid consumer fraud?

References

1. Rideout V. *Generation Rx.com.* International Communications Research, Kaiser Family Foundation. 2001. **http://www.kff.org/2001/200111211a/ GenerationRx.pdf**
2. The National Council on the Aging. Media sources of health info. As reported in *USA Today,* 26 October 1999, 9d.
3. Baker L, et al. Use of the Internet and e-mail for health care information: results from a national survey. *JAMA* 289(18):2400–2406. 2003.
4. LeWine H. Quick tips for using online health information with your physician. Harvard Special Commentary, October 9, 2002. **http://www. intelihealth.com**

5. Clark C, Gordon RJ, Harris B (editors). *Encyclopedia of complementary health practice.* Springer, 1999.

6. *Physicians desk reference pocket guide to prescription drugs.* Simon and Schuster, Inc., 2002.

7. Tieman J. Med school downer. Applications decline for third year in a row, experts cite anti–affirmative action initiatives. *Mod Health* 30(38):18–19, 2000.

8. Sierpina VS. *Integrative health care: complementary and alternative therapies for the whole person.* F.A. Davis, 2000.

9. National Center for Complementary and Alternative Medicine. National Institutes of Health. September 2003. **http://www.nccam.nih.gov**

10. *Acupuncture: Mechanism of action.* National Center for Complementary and Alternative Medicine. September 2003. **http://www.bccan.nih.gov/health/acupuncture/#nccam**

11. NIH panel issues consensus statement on acupuncture (press release), 5 November 1997. **http://www.gov/news/plr/nov97/od.or.htm**

12. Siev-Ner I, et al. Reflexology treatment relieves symptoms of multiple sclerosis: a randomized controlled study. *Mult Scler* 9(4):356–361. 2003.

13. Gambles M, Crooke M, Wilkinson S. Evaluation of a hospice based reflexology service: a qualitative audit of patient perceptions. *Eur J Oncol Nurs* 6(1):37–44, 2002.

14. Kholler M. Children with ear disorders who are treated by reflexologists or general practitioners. *Ugeskr Laeger* 165(19):1994–1999, 2003.

15. Questions and answers about homeopathy. National Center for Complementary and Alternative Medicine. 2003. **http://www.nih.gov/health/homeopathy/index.htm#a1**

16. Jaroll L. Homeopathic e-mail: can the "memory" of molecules be transmitted via the Internet? *Time,* 7 May 1999, 153(19).

17. Shekelle PG, et al. Efficacy and safety of ephedra and ephedrine for weight loss and athletic performance: a meta-analysis. *JAMA* 289(12):1537–1545. 2003.

18. Associated Press. U.S. Bans Ephedra, Drug linked to Deaths. December 30, 2003.

19. Fontanarosa PB, Rennie D, DeAngelis CD. The need for regulation of dietary supplements—lessons from ephedra. *JAMA* 289(12):1568–1570, 2003.

20. Norris S, Morgan R. Providers issue brief: nursing shortages: year end report—2002. *Issue Brief Policy Track Serv,* December 31, 2002, 1–14.

21. Aiken LH, et al. Hospital nurse staffing and patient mortality, nurse burnout, and job satisfaction. *JAMA* 288(16):1987–1993. 2002.

22. Eastman PD. Now, do-it-yourself care. *AARP Bulletin Online.* January 2002. **http://www.aarp.org.bulletin/yourhealth/articles/a2003-08-05-doityourself.html**

23. *Federal Register* 64(243):71041. Rules and Regulations. December 20, 1999.

24. *People without health insurance coverage for the entire year by race and ethnicity: 2002 and 2003.* U. S. Census Bureau, Current Population Survey 2002 and 2003 Annual Social and Economic Supplements. **http://www.census.gov/hhes/hlthins02/hi02t3.pdf**

25. Health Care Financing Administration. *National health care expenditures projections tables— 1972–2007,* Table 1. November 2000. **http://www.hcfa.gov/NHE-Proj/t01.htm**

26. *National health care expenditure amounts, and average annual percent change by type of expenditure (Table 2).* Centers for Medicare & Medicaid Services. Department of Health and Human Services. **http://www.cms.hhs.gov/statistics/nhe/projections-2002/t2.asp**

27. Health Care Financing Administration. *Personal health care expenditures, average percent change, percent distribution and per capita amounts, by source of funds for selected calendar years 1970–2007,* Table 2a. November 2000. **http://www.chfa.gov/stats/NHE-proj/t02b.htm**

28. *Employer health benefits: 2003 annual survey.* The Kaiser Family Foundation and Health Research and Educational Trust. 2003.

29. McKenzie JF, Pinger RR, Kotecki JE. *An introduction to community health,* 4th ed. Jones and Bartlett. 2002.

30. *Average annual cost of nursing home care.* The Metlife Assisted Living Market Telephone Survey 2002. **http://www.massmutual.com/mmfg/pdf/nursing_home_cost.pdf**

31. *Statistical abstract of the United States: 2002 (122nd ed).* U.S. Census Bureau. U.S. Department of Commerce. 2003 (Tables No 102 and 1001).

32. *Generic drug approvals.* FDA/Center for Drug Evaluation and Research. January 2003. **http://www.fda.gov/cder/ogd/approvals/default.htm**

33. *Drug consult 2004; the comprehensive reference for generic and brand name drugs,* Mosby's Drug Consult, 2004. Mosby. 2004.

34. Partnership for caring. Facts about advance directives. 10 October 2000. **www.partnershipforcaring.org**

35. United Organ Sharing Network. Accessed January 27, 2004. **http://www.unos.org/**

The inability to adequately communicate in one's own language is, by definition, illiteracy. For some this inability is so widespread that even the ability to read or write is absent. For others illiteracy exists only in terms of selected aspects of the language, such as the highly technical language of an academic discipline, or within the jargon of a group based on the uniqueness of experiences or interests. For the typical American, medical (health care) illiteracy is a likely reality.

In a recently released report of a study conducted by the Agency for Healthcare Research and Quality, it was disclosed that 90 million Americans have very little understanding of the instructions given to them by health care practitioners, often involving information critical to prevention or recovery from serious health problems. Underlying this medical illiteracy is a multitude of problems, not all of which are the "fault" of the laypersons. In no particular order, these include:

- the highly technical language of the medicine, with long complicated words and terms, many having suffixes derived from Latin.
- the age, illness/discomfort, or sensory impairment of persons receiving medically related instructions.
- the failure of practitioners to "quiz" their patients about "what is it that I just finished instructing you to do?"
- the lack of fluency in English of many patients and the inability of practitioners or their staff to speak languages other than English.
- the absence in the homes of most patients of an easy-to-read home health reference book that would make complicated instructions or the abbreviated information on prescription and OTC medication labels easier to understand.
- the complicated legal language associated with health consent forms that often obscure understanding by virtually all persons, except those with a medical/legal background.

In response to the literacy concerns identified by the report just released, the following recommendations were made by the agency responsible for the study:

. . . Government-sponsored research on methods for improving health care literacy.

. . . Health care professional schools should teach their students (future practitioners) how to better communicate with laypersons.

. . . Health care–related literacy should be required in elementary through college curricula.

. . . Health care third party payers (insurance companies, Medicare, Medicaid) should strongly encourage providers to increase their efforts in communicating effectively.

In the final analysis, the absence of literacy in the health care field is too dangerous and expensive to allow for continued stagnation. Health care is too important and expensive for the general public to remain complacent in understanding the care they need and are paying for.

using health information on the internet

So you want to find some information on health. Maybe you have a paper due in this class. Maybe you need more information on a condition that you or a loved one has. Or maybe you simply want to take advantage of the latest information on fitness and nutrition to make healthful decisions. No matter what information you're looking for, you can probably find it on the Internet. But be wary as you search—a great deal of misinformation is also available, and it may be hard for the average consumer to separate health fact from health fiction.

You can be relatively certain that government sites and links contain reliable information. In fact, the U.S. Department of Health and Human Services has established a site to provide consumer information. It can be accessed under Health/General Health or directly at **www.healthfinder.gov**. This site was launched in April 1997 to improve consumer access to federal health information online. As Healthfinder points out in its introductory paragraph, information alone can't take the place of health care you may need, but it can make you an informed partner in your own health care. This site leads you to selected online publications, databases, websites, support and self-help groups, government agencies, not-for-profit organizations, and universities that provide reliable health information to the public.

Unfortunately, the government does not have the resources to filter out all false and misleading health care information. Many people mistakenly believe that advertising claims must be true or advertisers would not be allowed to continue making them. Not enough time, money, and regulators are available to assess the validity of each and every health claim. However, health care professionals and consumer advocates can give us the tools we need to determine the reliability of health information for ourselves.

What Is Quackery and How Can You Spot It?

One prominent consumer advocate is Stephen Barrett, a retired physician and nationally renowned author. In 1969 he founded the Lehigh Valley Committee against Health Fraud, which more recently changed its name to Quackwatch. Investigation of questionable claims, answering of inquiries, distribution of reliable publications, reporting of illegal marketing, and improvement of the overall quality of health information on the Internet are all tasks that this group takes on.

Quackery is more difficult to spot than most people think. Whereas fraud is deliberate deception and more easily recognized and corrected, quackery involves the use of methods that are not scientifically valid. Information purveyed by quacks cannot be scientifically confirmed or denied, and this is where the problem arises. There is no way to separate the good from the bad or the harmful from the benign or helpful.

Anecdotes and Testimonials

Some alternative health care methods have been accepted by the scientific community, having met reliable criteria for safety and effectiveness. Other methods are in the experimental stages. These methods are unproven but are based on plausible, rational principles and are undergoing responsible testing. But many other alternative health remedies are groundless and completely lack scientific rationale. Instead of scientific tests, people who promote these methods rely on anecdotes and testimonials to "prove" the effectiveness of their products. Perhaps you have noticed that claims of effectiveness are not found on the products themselves, but rather in brochures placed in conspicuous locations very near the products. This use of testimonials is unique to the dietary supplement market and reflects the virtual absence of regulatory power held by the FDA and FTC. The FDA does allow a limited number of claims related to structural/functional benefits and a very small number of disease-related health claims.

Intelligent Consumer Behavior

Americans waste $50 million to $150 million per year on bogus mail-order health remedies. Many of these products are now available on the Internet. You can avoid wasting your money in this way by not buying any of these products without medical advice from your physician or other health care professional. And don't be fooled by money-back guarantees; they're usually as phony as the products that they back.

Be wary of characteristic quackery ploys. Purveyors of quackery may say that they care about you, but their care, even if it were sincere, cannot make useless medicine work. These products are commonly touted as having no side effects. If this is true, then the product is too weak to have any effect at all. Quacks will encourage you to jump on the bandwagon of their time-tested remedy, as if popularity and market longevity are surrogates for effectiveness. When they do claim that their products are backed by scientific studies, these studies turn out to be untraceable, misinterpreted, irrelevant, nonexistent, or based on poorly designed research.

The costs of buying into health care quackery are more than financial. The psychological effects of disillusionment and the physical harm caused by the method itself or by abandoning more effective care are much worse.

HONcode Principles

Any reputable health information site on the Internet subscribes to the HONcode Principles. These principles are put forth and monitored by the Geneva-based Health On the Net Foundation and have arisen from input from webmasters and medical professionals in several countries. According to these principles, any medical advice appearing at a site must meet the following requirements:

- It must be given by medically trained and qualified professionals unless a clear statement is made that the information comes from a non-medically qualified individual or organization.
- The information must be intended to support, not replace, the physician-patient relationship.
- Data relating to individual patients and visitors to a medical website are confidential.
- Site information must have clear references to source data and, where possible, specific links to that data.
- Claims related to the benefit or performance of a treatment, product, or

service must be supported by appropriate, balanced evidence.
- The webmaster's e-mail address should be clearly displayed throughout the website.
- Commercial and noncommercial support and funding for the site should be clearly revealed.
- There must be a clear differentiation between advertising at the site and the original material created by the institution operating the site.

Be skeptical about any health information you find on the Internet that does not meet these criteria. Ask your physician whether the information is accurate, or move on to a more reliable site.

Assessing Health Care Information

The Internet is a valuable health care tool. Reliable information is supplied by government health agencies, research universities, hospitals, disease foundations, and other experts. However, not all health sites are reputable. As the saying goes, you can't believe everything you read, even if it's on the Internet. Anyone can create an online resource that looks professional. Ordinary people who believe they've been helped by a product, companies trying to sell products and services, and even cheats and quacks are all out there spouting their information. To protect yourself, you must be an informed consumer of information. To evaluate the credibility

of an online source, ask yourself the following questions:

1. Who maintains the information?
2. Is it linked to other reputable sources of medical information?
3. When was it last updated?
4. Is it selling a product?

While the Internet cannot and should not replace visits with a physician, reliable information obtained on the Internet can make us more active partners in our own health care. It can give us information we can use to stay healthy and prevent disease. It can help us to ask our doctors the right questions and educate us so that we're not afraid to ask them. It can connect us to people who are experiencing the same things as we are. It can help us learn about our health, receive support from others, and make sound health care decisions based on fact—not fiction.

For Discussion . . .

Which health-related sites have you visited on the Internet? Did you find them informative? Reliable? Fun? What could be done to improve the status of health information on the Internet?

InfoLinks

www.hon.ch
www.nnlm.nlm.nih.gov/gmr/publish/ eval.html

personal assessment

are you a skilled health consumer?

Circle the selection that best describes your practice. Then total your points for an interpretation of your health consumer skills.

1   Never
2   Occasionally
3   Most of the time
4   All of the time

1. I read all warranties and then file them for safekeeping.
   1   2   3   4

2. I read labels for information pertaining to the nutritional quality of food.
   1   2   3   4

3. I practice comparative shopping and use unit pricing, when available.
   1   2   3   4

4. I read health-related advertisements in a critical and careful manner.
   1   2   3   4

5. I challenge all claims pertaining to secret cures or revolutionary new health devices.
   1   2   3   4

6. I engage in appropriate medical self-care screening procedures.
   1   2   3   4

7. I maintain a patient-provider relationship with a variety of health care providers.
   1   2   3   4

8. I inquire about the fees charged before using a health care provider's services.
   1   2   3   4

9. I maintain adequate health insurance coverage.
   1   2   3   4

10. I consult reputable medical self-care books before seeing a physician.
    1   2   3   4

11. I ask pertinent questions of health care providers when I am uncertain about the information I have received.
    1   2   3   4

12. I seek second opinions when the diagnosis of a condition or the recommended treatment seems questionable.
    1   2   3   4

13. I follow directions pertaining to the use of prescription drugs, including continuing their use for the entire period prescribed.
    1   2   3   4

14. I buy generic drugs when they are available.
    1   2   3   4

15. I follow directions pertaining to the use of OTC drugs.
    1   2   3   4

16. I maintain a well-supplied medicine cabinet.
    1   2   3   4

YOUR TOTAL POINTS _____

Interpretation

16–24 points   A very poorly skilled health consumer
25–40 points   An inadequately skilled health consumer
41–56 points   An adequately skilled health consumer
57–64 points   A highly skilled health consumer

To Carry This Further . . .

Could you ever have been the victim of consumer fraud? What will you need to do to be a skilled consumer?

chapter nineteen

protecting your safety

Chapter Objectives

After studying this chapter, you should be able to:

▌ define the terms *intentional* and *unintentional injuries* and give three examples of each.

▌ discuss the different types of domestic violence, including intimate partner violence, child maltreatment, and the maltreatment of elders.

▌ list some ways to reduce one's risk of becoming a victim of violent crime in your home, in your car, or on campus.

▌ explain the particular way guns contribute to violent crime statistics.

▌ name at least five groups who are targets of hate crimes.

▌ list five things you can do to avoid perpetrating a date rape if you are male.

▌ list five things you can do to reduce your risk of becoming a date rape victim if you are female.

▌ list ten things you can do to reduce your risk of becoming seriously injured in a motor vehicle crash.

▌ compare the risk of a fatal injury occurring while riding a motorcycle to the risk of a fatal injury while riding in a car and explain the difference.

▌ list ten things one can do to prevent injuries from occurring in the home.

▌ explain what identity theft is, and list several steps you can take to protect yourself from it.

Online Learning Center Resources

www.mhhe.com/payne8e

Log on to our Online Learning Center (OLC) for access to these additional resources:

- Chapter key terms and definitions
- Learning objectives
- Online assessments

- Key term flash cards
- Student interactive question-and answer sites
- Self-scoring chapter quiz

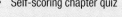

Talking It Over

Helping a Friend End Abuse

Although the boyfriend of one of your friends has been threatening her, she isn't taking the situation seriously. What should you say?

- Explain that domestic violence includes emotional, psychological, physical, and sexual abuse in which one person tries to control another.
- Encourage your friend to tell you how she feels about the situation. Getting her to admit that she is frightened is the first step toward recognizing that she needs help.

- Explain that your friend's safety is more important than "loyalty" to her boyfriend.
- Provide information on support that's available.

CommunicationLinks

www.feminista.com/vln4
www.ndvh.org

Eye on the Media

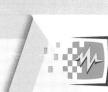

Images of Terrorism: The World Trade Center Disaster

Where were you on the morning of September 11, 2001? How did you hear the news about the terror attacks on New York and Washington? The entire nation stood stunned as TV cameras captured a passenger jet crashing into one of New York's twin towers, followed a few minutes later by a second plane that hit the second tower. Soon after, it was reported that a third plane had hit the Pentagon, and a fourth had crashed in a field in Pennsylvania.

Most of the day's horrors were captured by television cameras, as well as by a few film crews who happened to be filming in Manhattan that day. Americans watched in horror as networks played and replayed footage of each plane hitting the World Trade Center, and of the fires that ensued; they saw office workers running for their lives and witnessed fireman and other rescue workers going back into buildings that were clearly unsound to guide people out of the burning towers. And finally, they saw the two towers crumble to the ground.

Eye on the Media *continued*

For three full days the major TV networks suspended their regular programming to cover the disaster in depth. No commercials, no sit-coms, no soap operas, and no David Letterman or Jay Leno for days. When Letterman returned to the air, it wasn't to tell jokes but to have Dan Rather talk about the tragic events, and viewers saw the normally staunch newsman's eyes fill with tears. When *Saturday Night Live* featured New York Mayor Rudolph Giuliani, it was as a respected guest, not as a target for a spoof. By Saturday morning the cartoons were back—for the children. In fact, many networks geared toward children—most notably PBS—tailored their programming to offer them more comforting fare, and provided special public service announcements advising parents on how to help their children feel safe despite their own uncertainty.

In the weeks and months that followed, the media helped provide a sense of unity to a vast, grieving nation. But the constant coverage of the tragedy and its aftermath—including footage of the attacks, and of rescue workers searching the rubble of Ground Zero for the bodies of their fallen comrades—took a toll on many people watching. People lost sleep and felt depressed. Some worried about having to get on an airplane again. Young children had an especially difficult time—wondering why this happened and whether *they* would be victims of a terrorist attack. Some children touched buildings to make sure they were "safe" before going inside.

Today, Americans are acutely aware of the possibility of terror attacks on our soil. The international news media regularly report on anti-American sentiments in Middle Eastern countries. The Department of Homeland Security continually evaluates the national threat level, with a system ranging from Code Green (low) to Code Red (severe). When the national threat level was raised from Yellow (elevated) to Orange (heightened) in December of 2003, it was major news. Many media outlets—especially the 24-hour news channels—report on the nation's state of alert every day. Continual coverage of the War on Terror—first in Afghanistan and then in Iraq—only adds to Americans' concern for their safety and for that of American troops abroad.

Do you worry about another attack? How closely do you follow media coverage of national and international terror issues? Are you aware of the nation's state of alert on any given day? Do you watch the news differently from the way you watched it before September 11, 2001?

In recent years, several high-profile violent crimes have been the subject of intense media scrutiny and public outrage: the killings of Matthew Shepard and James Byrd, Jr., and the terrorist attack on the World Trade Center in New York City, for example, have received exhaustive media coverage. Heinous sexual assaults and murders of children—Megan Kanka, JonBenet Ramsey, and Girl X in Chicago—have also generated much attention and angered the public. The killing of students and a teacher at Columbine High School by two students shocked the nation and caused residents of Littleton, Colorado, to wonder sadly what had happened to their "safe" community.

Domestic violence directed at women and children is all too common, and many people fear becoming a random victim of a homicide, robbery, or carjacking. Law enforcement officials contend that gang activities and hard-core drug involvement are significant factors that have led to violent behavior in our society.

Although violence may seem to be focused in urban areas, no community is completely safe. Even people who live in small towns and rural areas now must lock their doors and remain vigilant about protecting their safety. Crime on college campuses, much of which is a direct result of alcohol use, remains a threat. For tips on avoiding becoming a victim of a violent crime, see the Changing for the Better box on page 619.

For some students the content in this chapter may be the most important information in this textbook. Becoming a victim of violent behavior or sustaining an unintentional injury can harm your health as much (or more than) any of your own unhealthy behavior. The goal of this chapter is to help you understand the scope of violence and unintentional injury in our society and learn what you can do to avoid becoming a victim. Complete the Personal Assessment on page 643 to see whether you are adequately protecting your own safety.

Reducing Risk Factors

Many factors influence your risk of suffering an injury or becoming a victim of crime. Some of these you cannot change. For example, the greatest percentage of violent crimes tend to be committed by, and suffered by, the young. This risk is multiplied for those who are young and African American, and for those who live in an area with gang activity.

However, you *can* affect many of the other risk factors for injury or crime, as you will learn throughout this chapter. For example, alcohol plays a major role in driving, motorcycle, and boating accidents. You can reduce your risk of accidents by avoiding alcohol and drugs while you enjoy these activities. Likewise, boxes throughout this chapter will show you how to avoid becoming a victim of date rape, how to avoid accidents in your car, and how to maintain a safe and comfortable home.

Intentional Injuries

Intentional injuries are injuries that are committed on purpose. With the exception of suicide (which is self-directed), intentional injuries reflect violence committed by one person acting against another person. Criminal acts that result in intentional injuries include homicide, robbery, rape, sexual assault, aggravated assault, and simple assault. These acts may be carried out in the context of interpersonal or domestic violence, gang violence, hate crimes, or terrorism. Each year in the United States, intentional violence results in nearly fifty thousand deaths and another 2 million nonfatal injuries.[1]

In 2001, more than twenty-four million crimes were committed against U.S. residents age 12 and older, according to data collected in the National Crime Victimization Survey. Of these, one in four (5.7 million) was a violent crime (rape, sexual assault, robbery, aggravated assault, or simple assault). The good news is that these fig-

ures continue the downward trend in criminal victimization that began in 1994. The 2001 rate is about half the 1994 rate.[2,3]

Homicide

Homicide, or murder, is the intentional killing of one person by another. Sadly, the United States leads the

---

Key Terms

intentional injuries injuries that are purposely committed by a person.

homicide the intentional killing of one person by another person.

---

industrialized world in homicide rates. The 2000 murder rate, however, was 5.5 per 100,000 inhabitants. Fortunately, this rate reflects an annual decline since 1991, when the homicide rate was 9.8 per 100,000 population.[4] In fact, this was the lowest rate since 1965.[4]

Criminal justice experts are trying to pinpoint why U.S. homicide rates are dropping. No single answer has emerged but speculation centers on better community policing efforts; the 1994 passage of the broad Federal Crime Bill; legislation, such as the Brady Law; and a variety of tough state laws, such as the "three strikes and you're out" provision, that mandate life sentences without parole for repeat violent offenders. If recent incarceration rates do not change, an estimated 1 in 20 people (5.1%) will serve time in a state or federal prison. The chances of going to prison are higher for men (9%) than for women (1.1%).[5]

One clear trend is the extent to which illegal drug activity is related to homicide. A variety of research studies from large cities indicate that 25% to 50% of all homicides are drug related.[6] Most of these murders are associated with drug trafficking, including disputed drug transactions. For the country taken as a whole, this figure is much lower. For 2000, only 4.4% of homicides were drug related.[7] However, statistics reveal that high percentages of both homicide assailants and victims have drugs in their system at the time of the homicide.[6]

Another clear trend is that handguns are the weapons of choice for homicides. It was the proliferation of handguns and their use in violent crimes that led to the passage of the so-called Brady Law.

Domestic Violence

Family life in the 1990s is a far cry from that portrayed in the popular 1950s and 1960s television shows like "The Donna Reed Show," "Father Knows Best," and "The Adventures of Ozzie and Harriet." The composition of families has changed considerably. In the 1950s a common family pattern included children being raised by both parents. Generally, the father was the income earner and the mother stayed at home and managed the growing family.

Today, family patterns are much more complex. Children are more frequently being raised in blended families or in families headed by single parents. In 2002 nearly 20 million children under 18 lived with one parent.[8] A much higher percentage of women are employed outside the home. Because of pressing family economic concerns, many children take care of themselves during after-school hours. Sociologists indicate that families, and the individuals in those families, are under more stress than ever. Nonetheless, reports of some types of family violence have decreased in recent years. Yet domestic violence remains a serious concern in our society.

Intimate Partner Violence

Intimate partner violence (IPV) refers to violence committed against a domestic partner. Most often the victims are women, and a significant percentage of these women are spouses or former spouses of the assailant. IPV can include murder, rape, sexual assault, robbery, aggravated assault, and simple assault. Violent acts that constitute abuse range from a slap on the face to murder.

A 2001 report released by the Bureau of Justice Statistics revealed encouraging findings. The report indicated that intimate nonlethal violence had declined 48% since 1993, from a rate of 5.8 nonfatal intimate victimizations per 1,000 persons to just 3 per 1,000 persons. The rate of decline was greater for female victims (49%) than for male victims (42%).[9] Two reasons have been proposed for this decline in intimate partner violence: better services for families at risk, and an improving economy during the period covered by the report.[10] Actually, rates of IPV began to edge upward in 2001, perhaps as a result of rising unemployment.

Murders by intimates in 2000, the most recent year for which statistics are available, reached the lowest levels since 1976. In 2000 1,687 murders were reported among intimate partners, whereas nearly three thousand such murders took place in 1976. As has been the case for many years, three of every four victims of intimate murder were females.[10]

The most vulnerable female victims are African American and Hispanic, live in large cities, are young and unmarried, and are from lower socioeconomic groups. However, these trends do not mean that only women from these classifications are vulnerable to violent behavior. Women across all economic, racial, and age categories are potential victims.

One of the real difficulties related to intimate violence is the vast underreporting of this crime to law enforcement authorities. The U.S. Department of Justice estimates that about half of the victims of intimate violence do not report the crime to police. Too many victims view their violent situations as private or personal matters and not actual crimes. Despite painful injuries, many victims view the offenses against them as minor. Even psychological abuse, the least frequently reported form of intimate violence, can lead not to feelings of loss of control and emotional dysfunction, but also to a wide array of physical health problems. Victims of psychological abuse are twice as likely as

---

Key Terms

intimate partner violence violent victimization committed by current or former spouses, boyfriends, or girlfriends.

others to report chronic pain, spastic colon, irritable bowel syndrome, infections, and migraine headaches.[11]

Of course, it is easy to criticize the victims of intimate violence for not reporting the crimes committed against them, but this may be unfair. Why do women stay in these relationships? Many women who are injured may fear being killed if they report the crime. Women may also fear for the safety of their children. Women who receive economic support may fear being left with no financial resources.

However, help is available for victims of intimate abuse. Most communities have family support or intimate violence hot lines that abused people can call for help. Communities are establishing shelters where abused women and their children can seek safety while their cases are being handled by the police or court officials. If you are being abused or know of someone who is the victim of intimate violence, do not hesitate to use the services of these local hot lines or shelters. Also, check the resources listed in the Health Reference Guide at the back of this text.

 TALKING POINTS A close friend confides that her boyfriend sometimes "gets rough" with her. She's afraid to talk to him about it because she thinks that will make things worse. What immediate steps would you tell her to take?

Child Maltreatment

Like many cases of intimate partner violence, **child maltreatment** tends to be a silent crime. It is estimated nearly one million children are victims of child abuse and neglect each year.[12] Some children are victims of repeated crimes, and since many victims do not report these crimes, the actual incidence of child abuse is difficult to determine.

Child maltreatment includes child abuse and child neglect. Children are abused in various ways. Physical abuse reflects physical injury, such as bruises, burns, abrasions, cuts, and fractures of the bones and skull. Sexual abuse includes acts that lead to sexual gratification of the abuser. Examples include fondling, touching, and various acts involved in rape, sodomy, and incest. Psychological abuse is another form of child abuse. Certainly, children are scarred by family members and others who routinely damage their psychological development. However, this form of abuse is especially difficult to identify and measure.

Child neglect is failure to provide a child with adequate clothing, food, shelter, and medical attention. The incidence of child neglect is approximately three times the incidence of physical abuse and about seven times the incidence of child sexual abuse. Child maltreatment deaths are more often associated with child neglect than with any type of abuse.[12] Educational neglect, such as failure to see that a child attends school regularly, is one of the most common types of child neglect. Each form of abuse can have devastating short- and long-term consequences for the child.

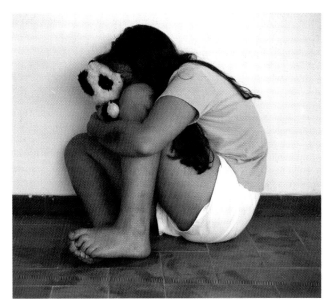

Child maltreatment can be psychologically as well as physically damaging.

Research studies in the various areas of child maltreatment reveal some interesting trends. Abused children are much more likely than are nonabused children to grow up to be child abusers themselves. It is also now understood that abused children are more likely to suffer from poor educational performance, increased health problems, and low levels of overall achievement. Abused children are significantly more likely than are nonabused children to become involved in adult crime and violent criminal behavior. Finally, neglected children's rates of arrest for violence were almost as high as those of physically abused children.[13]

It is beyond the scope of this book to discuss in detail how to reduce child abuse. However, the violence directed against children can likely be lessened through a combination of early identification measures and violence prevention programs. Teachers, friends, relatives, social workers, counselors, psychologists, police, and the court system must not hesitate to intervene early in cases of suspected child abuse. In fact, every adult is responsible for reporting suspected child abuse and neglect. To do so, persons should call their local police department or Child Protective Services (within the Department of Public Welfare) and request assistance in filing a report. So long as the report is filed in good conscience (without malice)

Key Terms

child maltreatment the act or failure to act by a parent or caretaker which results in abuse or neglect of a child or which places the child in imminent risk of serious harm.

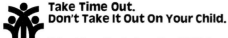

12 alternatives
to lashing out at your child.

**The next time everyday pressures
build up to the point where
you feel like lashing out—STOP!
And try any of these simple alternatives.**

You'll feel better . . . and so will your child.

1. Take a deep breath. And another. Then remember <u>you</u> are the adult . . .

2. Close your eyes and imagine you're hearing what your child is about to hear.

3. Press your lips together and count to 10. Or better yet, to 20.

4. Put your child in a time-out chair. (Remember the rule: one time-out minute for each year of age.)

5. Put yourself in a time-out chair. Think about why you are angry: is it your child, or is your child simply a convenient target for your anger?

6. Phone a friend.

7. If someone can watch the children, go outside and take a walk.

8. Take a hot bath or splash cold water on your face.

9. Hug a pillow.

10. Turn on some music. Maybe even sing along.

11. Pick up a pencil and write down as many helpful words as you can think of. Save the list.

12. Write for parenting information: Parenting, Box 2866, Chicago, IL 60690.

**Take Time Out.
Don't Take It Out On Your Child.**

® National Committee for Prevention of Child Abuse

CHILD ABUSE PREVENTION CAMPAIGN
MAGAZINE AD NO. CA-2835-90—7" x 10"
Volunteer Agency: Lintas: Cambell-Ewald. Campaign Director: Beth M. Pritchard, S.C. Johnson & Son, Inc.

Figure 19-1 Alternatives to hitting your child.

there will be no negative ramifications for the person filing. The later the intervention, the more likely that the abuse will have worsened. When an individual has abused once, he or she is likely to do it again.

Violence prevention programs can help parents and caregivers learn how to resolve conflicts, improve communication, cope with anger, improve parenting skills, and challenge the view of violence presented in movies and television. These programs may help to stop violence before it begins to damage the lives of young children. Figure 19-1 provides simple alternatives parents can choose to avoid hitting a child.

Maltreatment of Elders

Among the nation's 35 million adults 65 years of age and older, between one and two million have been injured, exploited, or otherwise mistreated.[14,15] Particularly vulnerable are women over the age of 75 years. Nearly half (47%) of the abusers are the children of the victims, and 85% are family members.[16]

Many older adults are hit, kicked, attacked with knives, or denied food and medical care; others are robbed of their Social Security checks and automobiles. These crimes probably reflect a combination of factors, particularly the stress of caring for failing older people by middle-aged children who also face the additional demands of dependent children and careers. In many cases, the middle-aged children were themselves abused, or there may be a chemical dependence problem. The alternative, institutionalization, is so expensive that it is often not an option for either the abused or the abuser.

Although protective services are available, abuse of older adults is frequently unseen and unreported. In many cases, the older adults themselves are afraid to report their children's behavior because of the fear of embarrassment that they were not good parents to their children. Regardless of the cause, however, abuse of older adults must be reported to the appropriate protective service so that intervention can occur.

Gangs and Youth Violence

In the last 30 years, gangs and gang activities have been increasingly responsible for escalating violence and criminal activity. Before that time, gangs used fists, tire irons, and occasionally, cheap handguns ("Saturday night specials") as tools of enforcement. Now, gang members do not hesitate to use more lethal semiautomatic weapons.

Sixty-six percent of gang members live in large cities (more than 25,000 population),[17] where many socially alienated, economically disadvantaged young people live. Convinced that society has no significant role for them, gang members can receive support from an association of peers that has well-defined lines of authority. Rituals and membership initiation rites are important in gang socialization. Gangs often control territories within a city. Frequently, gangs are involved in criminal activities, the most common of which are illicit drug trafficking and robberies. In the late 1990s, gang-related murders and drive-by shootings contributed to the high death rate among young people and especially inner-city youth. In 1999 the rate of gang-related murders of young persons reached, on average, 24 deaths every two days—the equivalent of a classroom of dead young persons (below the age of 20) every other day. Perhaps no single example of youth violence, with a measure of gang affiliation included, is more vivid than the April 20, 1999, shootings that occured at Columbine High School in Littleton, Colorado. On that day Eric Harris and Dylan Klebold, dressed in their gang-affiliated black trench coats, entered their high school and began a planned and systematic gun and bomb rampage that resulted in the deaths of fourteen students and one teacher. To this day, no one is certain why Harris and Dylan, and their

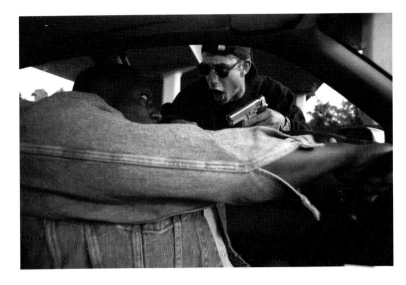

The prevalence of firearms in American society—especially among young men—is especially troubling. Guns are involved in more than half of all homicides and suicides, and are often used during violent crimes such as robberies and carjackings.

closest friends, felt such anger toward and sense of disenfranchisement from their classmates and community.

It is not only older male teenagers and young adults who are members of today's gangs. Law enforcement officials see younger people (ages 12, 13, and 14) joining gangs. Some gangs have recently included young women as members, and some cities report a growing number of all-female gangs. Some female gangs are reported to be every bit as ruthless as the male gangs. Only about 6% of gang members were female in 2000.[17]

Attempting to control gang and youth violence is particularly expensive for communities. When you consider that for every gang-related homicide, there are about one hundred nonfatal gang-related intentional injuries, it becomes obvious that gang violence is an expensive health care proposition. Furthermore, gang and youth violence takes an enormous financial and human toll on law enforcement, the judicial system, and corrections departments.

Fortunately, the recent decline in murders and other serious crimes also applies to gang-related crimes. Once again, some observers credit more aggressive police tactics for the decline. Some of the tactics being used to meet this problem are the aggressive "quality of life" policing in some cities and President Clinton's COPS program (Community Oriented Policing Services) to hire new police officers and put them on foot patrols, where they become acquainted with residents. Others believe that the drop in crime should be attributed to factors such as a stronger economy and the fading of the crack market. In Boston, a campaign aimed at youth gangs offered summer jobs to gang members, combined with threats of federal prison sentences for gun violence. In a 2-year period since that time, no youngsters under 17 have been shot and killed in Boston. Regardless, reducing gang and youth violence will be a continuing challenge for the nation in the 21st century.

Gun Violence

Guns are being used more widely than ever in our society and in other parts of the world. The fatality rate for gun injuries is 30% higher than the fatality rate for injuries of all causes (less than 1%).[18] More than 60% of the homicides and 55% of the suicides committed each year in the United States involve the use of guns. As previously mentioned, gun violence is a leading killer of teenagers and young men, especially African American men, and the use of semiautomatic assault weapons by individuals and gang members is common. Colleges and universities are not immune to gun violence. A recent study found that 4.3% of college students had a working firearm at college. Of these, nearly half stated that they had the gun for protection.[19] Accidental deaths of toddlers and young children from loaded handguns is another dimension of the violence attributable to guns in our society. In addition, guns are often used in **carjackings.**

The proliferation of firearm use has prompted serious discussions about the enactment of gun control laws. For years, gun control activists have been in direct battle with the National Rifle Association (NRA) and its congressional supporters. Gun control activists want fewer guns manufactured and greater controls over the sale and possession of handguns. Gun supporters believe that such

Key Terms

carjacking a crime that involves a thief's attempt to steal a car while the owner is behind the wheel; carjackings are usually random and unpredictable, and they frequently involve handguns.

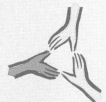

Learning from Our Diversity

Violence against the Disabled

No one is totally free from the risk of senseless violence—children, adults, or college students. No single group, however, is a more tragic target of violence than the disabled. Despite the protective efforts of laws such as the Fair Housing Amendments Act, the Americans with Disabilities Act, and the Rehabilitation Act, the disabled remain an easily victimized segment of the population.

Because of the high level of vulnerability that disabled persons face, national advocacy groups, such as All Walks Of Life, are working to assist the disabled, their caregivers, and the general population in reducing the risk of violence to this group. However, much can also be accomplished on an individual basis. If you are an able-bodied college student, you can probably implement the following suggestions on your campus:

- Encourage your disabled peers to remain vigilant by staying tuned in to their environment. Remind them that simply because they appear disabled does not guarantee that they will be protected from harm.
- Support your disabled friends in the challenges imposed by their limitations, particularly when they are in unfamiliar environments or experiencing unusual situations.
- Suggest that your peers with disabilities carry, or wear a personal alarm device. Such devices, also frequently carried by

able-bodied students, can be purchased in bookstores or sporting goods stores.
- Remind your disabled friends to inform others about their schedule plans, for example, when they will be away from school and when they are likely to return.
- Encourage people with disabilities to seek the assistance of an escort (security personnel) when leaving a campus building or a shopping mall to enter a large parking area.
- Be an advocate for your disabled friends. For example, if residence hall room doors do not have peepholes at wheelchair height, find out if the doors can be modified.

One additional approach remains controversial. That is the teaching of self-defense techniques to people with disabilities. Groups that advocate instruction to the disabled in the martial arts, such as judo, remind us that "doing nothing will produce nothing." Others contend that a limited ability to use a martial art leads to a false sense of confidence that encourages a disregard for other forms of protection. They further argue that if disabled persons try to counter aggression with ineffectively delivered martial arts techniques, they may anger their attacker and actually increase the aggression against themselves.

controls are not necessary and that people (the criminals) are responsible for gun deaths, not simply the guns. This debate will certainly continue.

Bias and Hate Crimes

One sad aspect of any society is how some segments of the majority treat certain people in the minority (see the Learning from Our Diversity box above). Nowhere is this more violently pronounced than in **bias and hate crimes.** These crimes are directed at individuals or groups of people solely because of a racial (61%), religious (14%), ethnic (11%), sexual orientation (13%), or other difference attributed to the victims. Victims of hate crimes are often verbally abused, their property is damaged or destroyed, and too frequently they are physically attacked. Two recent hate-motivated killings shocked the nation. One case involved the beating death of Matthew Shepard, a gay college student who was taken from a Wyoming bar, driven to a rural area, tied to a fence post, and savagely beaten to death. Aaron McKinney, one

Key Terms

bias and hate crimes criminal acts directed at a person or group solely because of a specific characteristic, such as race, religion, sexual orientation, ethnic background, or other difference.

Putting Fear in Perspective

Your neighbor, an elderly adult, stays locked in her house all day, afraid to open the door to anyone. Too many hours of watching local TV news, you think. But it's not just older people who are living in fear. Parents, women, gays, and minorities are all looking over their shoulders.

Some parents who walked to school when they were children wouldn't think of letting their kids do that. What about child molesters and kidnappers? A young woman at a party guards her drink all night—afraid that someone might put a drug in it. She's afraid of being raped. The gay person who goes to his old neighborhood to visit his grandmother feels uneasy. Is it his imagination, or are people looking at him in a threatening way? An African American man walking down the street hears a racial slur. Should he ignore it, or stop and say something?

All of these situations call for caution. If you're a parent, you need to be careful about your child's safety. But your child can walk to school—accompanied by you, another parent, or an older child. If you're a woman, you can keep an eye on your drink at a party without making that the focus of your attention. If you're a gay man who feels uncomfortable in an unfamiliar part of town, stay focused on where you're going. Walk quickly and confidently, without being intimidated. If you're a minority member who's being taunted, keep your dignity and remain calm.

Putting fear in perspective takes practice. First, stay reasonable. Recognize that acts of violence represent the extreme elements of society. There's a good reason you probably haven't met many (or any) murderers, robbers, or rapists. They make up a small segment of society. The people you usually encounter, who are basically good, represent the large majority. Second, be aware. Pay attention to what's going on around you. See things in a neutral way. If you do, you'll realize when an argument is about to turn into a fistfight or worse. Third, use common sense. Don't put yourself at risk, but don't stop living. You can't build your life around avoiding a potential act of violence. Fourth, trust your senses. If someone is walking too close to you and you feel uncomfortable, cross the street and go into a store. Last, practice what-if situations. For example, what would you do if you were in your car at a stoplight and someone held a gun up to your window? Considering your possible actions ahead of time, without dwelling on them, is one way of preparing yourself for real-life threats.

Living in fear is something that happens gradually—as fear takes control of a person's life. But that doesn't need to happen to you. You can take control of fear in a healthy, positive way—to build a life of rich experiences balanced by caution and good sense.

of the two men accused in the killings, based his defense on "gay panic," contending that he was traumatized by a homosexual advance as a young child. A second case that shocked the nation was that of James Byrd, Jr., a young African American man who was accosted by two white men as he walked along a rural roadway in Texas. After being beaten, spray-painted black, and chained to the rear of a pickup, Byrd was then dragged behind the truck for an extended distance. The trauma experienced by Byrd was so severe that he was decapitated and his torso dismembered.

Typically, the offenders in bias or hate crimes are fringe elements of a larger society who believe that the mere presence of someone with a racial, ethnic, or religious difference is inherently bad for the community, state, or country. Examples of groups commonly known to commit bias and hate crimes in the United States are skinheads, the Ku Klux Klan, and other white supremacist groups. Increasingly, state and federal laws have been enacted to make bias and hate crimes serious offenses.

With a small but growing presence of neo-Nazi groups in Europe and clear evidence that ethnic cleansing took place in Kosovo, Bosnia, Serbia, Croatia, Rwanda, Iraq, and the former Soviet Union, bias and hate crimes are a worldwide problem. The recent push on college campuses to promote multicultural education and the celebra-

tion of diversity may help today's generation of college graduates understand the importance of tolerance and inclusion and avoid bigotry and exclusion.

Stalking

In recent years the crime of **stalking** has received considerable attention. Stalking refers to an assailant's planned efforts to pursue an intended victim. Most stalkers are male. (One notable exception was the convicted female stalker of talk show host David Letterman.) Many of these stalkers are excessively possessive or jealous and pursue people with whom they formerly had a relationship. Some stalkers pursue people with whom they have had only an imaginary relationship.

Some stalkers have served time in prison and have waited for years to "get back" at their victims. In some

<hr>

Key Terms

stalking a crime involving an assailant's planned efforts to pursue an intended victim.

cases, stalkers go to great lengths to locate their intended victims and frequently know their daily whereabouts. Although not all stalkers plan to batter or kill their victims, their presence and potential for violence are enough to create an extremely frightening environment for the intended victim and family. See the Discovering Your Spirituality box on page 625 about putting your fear into perspective.

Fortunately, since 1990 virtually all states have enacted or tightened their laws related to stalking and have created stiff penalties for stalkers. In many areas the criminal justice system is proactive in letting possible victims of stalking know, for example, when a particular prison inmate is going to be released. In other areas, citizens are banding together to provide support and protection for people who may be victims of stalkers.

A recent report indicates that about 13% of college women are stalked in a given year.[20] If you think you are or someone you know is being stalked, contact the police (or a local crisis intervention hot line number) to report your case.

 TALKING POINTS You suspect that someone is stalking you, but your friends think you're being dramatic. How would you get objective advice on what to do?

Sexual Victimization

Ideally, sexual intimacy is a mutual, enjoyable form of communication between two people. Far too often, however, relationships are approached in an aggressive, hostile manner. These sexual aggressors always have a victim—someone who is physically or psychologically traumatized. *Sexual victimization* occurs in many forms and in a variety of settings. In this section we briefly look at sexual victimization as it occurs in rape and sexual assault, sexual abuse of children, sexual harassment, and the commercialization of sex.

Rape and Sexual Assault

As violence in our society increases, the incidence of *rape* and *sexual assault* correspondingly rises. The victims of these crimes fall into no single category. Survivors of rape and sexual assault include young and old, male and female. They can be mentally retarded people, prisoners, hospital patients, or college students. We are all potential victims, and self-protection is critical. Read the Star box above to learn about the myths surrounding rape.

Sometimes a personal assault begins as a physical assault that may turn into a rape. Rape is generally considered a crime of sexual aggression in which the victim is forced to have sexual intercourse. Current thought concerning rape characterizes this behavior as a violent act

Myths about Rape

Despite the fact that we are all potential victims, many of us do not fully understand how vulnerable we are. Many people hold several myths (false assumptions) about rape, including the following:

- *Women are raped by strangers.* In approximately half of all reported rapes, the victim has some prior acquaintance with the rapist. Increasingly, women are being raped by husbands, dating partners, and relatives.
- *Rapes almost always occur in dark alleys or deserted places.* The opposite is true. Most rapes occur in or very near the victim's residence.
- *Rapists are easily identified by their demeanor or psychological profile.* Most experts indicate that rapists do not differ significantly from nonrapists.
- *The incidence of rape is overreported.* Estimates are that only one in five rapes is reported.
- *Rape happens only to people in low socioeconomic classes.* Rape occurs in all socioeconomic classes. Each person, male or female, young or old, is a potential victim.
- *There is a standard way to escape from a potential rape situation.* Each rape situation is different. No one method to avoid rape can work in every potential rape situation. Because of this, we encourage personal health classes to invite speakers from a local rape prevention services bureau to discuss approaches to rape prevention.

that happens to be carried out through sexual contact. (See the Changing for the Better box on rape awareness on page 627.)

Psychiatrists and psychologists have long contended that the psychodynamic underlying the act of rape is that of a deviant urge to control and dominate others that is in no way related to the fulfillment of sexual desire. They support this contention by pointing out that rapists often experience impotence during the rape, that rapists are emotionally aroused by images of violent behavior directed toward women, and that rapists choose as victims those women that they perceive to be most vulnerable. These traits are viewed by mental health professionals as being largely unrelated to sexually based needs.

In stark contrast to the prevailing interpretation presented above, in a recent book by two evolutionary biologists, rape is conceptualized as an extreme expression of the evolutionary urge to reproduce common to all males.[21] According to the authors, their controversial theory in no way excuses rape, nor does it speak against the incarceration of rapists, but it rather suggests an alternative interpretation of rape's underlying causation that might eventually lead society to determine more effective ways to prevent the crime from occurring. Although thought provoking, this interpretation is unlikely to change many minds about the heinous nature of the act.

Acquaintance and Date Rape

Sexual victimization can occur in relationships. *Acquaintance rape* refers to forced sexual intercourse between individuals who know each other. *Date rape* is a form of acquaintance rape that involves forced sexual intercourse by a dating partner. Studies on a number of campuses suggest that about 20% of college women report having experienced date rape; a recent report from the Bureau of Justice Statistics puts the figure at about 3% per year. This figure includes completed and attempted rapes.[22] A higher percentage of women report being kissed and touched against their will. Alcohol is frequently a significant contributing factor in these rape situations. (See Chapter 8 concerning alcohol's role in campus crime.) Some men have reported being psychologically coerced into intercourse by their female dating partners. In many cases the aggressive partner will display certain behaviors that can serve as warning signs (see the Changing for the Better box on page 628).

In addition to alcohol as an adjunct to acquaintance rape or date rape, the use of additional drugs such as rohypnol (roofies), ketamine hydrochloride (Special K), and gamma-hydroxybutyrate (GHB) (see Chapter 7) are playing a greater role in date rapes reported on or near college campuses. Because of the inconspicuous nature of these drugs, they are easily incorporated into drinks without intended victims knowing it. The effects of these drugs are disinhibition, increasing confusion (including the inability to give sexual consent), relaxation of voluntary muscles, and eventual unconsciousness.[23] The amnestic effect of these drugs reduces the ability of victims to supply information important in the apprehension of date rapists.

Psychologists believe that aside from the physical harm of date rape, a greater amount of emotional damage may occur. Such damage stems from the concept of broken trust. Date rape survivors feel particularly violated because the perpetrator was not a stranger; it was someone they initially trusted, at least to some degree. Once that trust has been broken, developing new relationships with other people becomes much more difficult for the date rape survivor.

Nearly all survivors of date rape seem to suffer from *posttraumatic stress syndrome.* They can have anxiety, sleeplessness, eating disorders, and nightmares. Guilt concerning their own behavior, self-esteem, and judgment of other people can be overwhelming, and the individual may require professional counseling. Indeed, all students should be aware of the risk of date rape.

Sexual Abuse of Children

One of the most tragic forms of sexual victimization is the sexual abuse of children. Children are especially vulnerable to sexual abuse because of their dependent relationships with parents, relatives, and caregivers (such as babysitters, teachers, and neighbors). Often, children are unable to readily understand the difference between appropriate and inappropriate physical contact. Abuse may range from blatant physical manipulation, including fondling, to oral sex, sodomy, and intercourse.

I've heard that there are warning signs for date rape. What signs should I be alert for?

First, consider your partner's behaviors. Many, but not all, date rapists show one or more of the following behaviors: a disrespectful attitude toward you and others, lack of concern for your feelings, violence and hostility, obsessive jealousy, extreme competitiveness, a desire to dominate, and unnecessary physical roughness. Consider these behaviors as warning signs for possible problems in the future. Reevaluate your participation in the relationship.

Below are some specific ways both men and women can avoid a date rape situation.

Men

- *Know your sexual desires and limits.* Communicate them clearly. Be aware of social pressures. It's OK not to score.
- *Being turned down when you ask for sex is not a rejection of you personally.* Women who say no to sex are not rejecting the person; they are expressing their desire not to participate in a single act. Your desires may be beyond control, but your actions are within your control.
- *Accept the woman's decision.* "No" means "No." Don't read other meanings into the answer. Don't continue after you are told "No!"
- *Don't assume that just because a woman dresses in a sexy manner and flirts that she wants to have sexual intercourse.*

- *Don't assume that previous permission for sexual contact applies to the current situation.*
- *Avoid excessive use of alcohol and drugs.* Alcohol and other drugs interfere with clear thinking and effective communication.

Women

- *Know your sexual desires and limits.* Believe in your right to set those limits. If you are not sure, STOP and talk about it.
- *Communicate your limits clearly.* If someone starts to offend you, tell him so firmly and immediately. Polite approaches may be misunderstood or ignored. Say "No" when you mean "No."
- *Be assertive.* Often men interpret passivity as permission. Be direct and firm with someone who is sexually pressuring you.
- *Be aware that your nonverbal actions send a message.* If you dress in a sexy manner and flirt, some men may assume you want to have sex. This does not make your dress or behavior wrong, but it is important to be aware of a possible misunderstanding.
- *Pay attention to what is happening around you.* Watch the nonverbal clues. Do not put yourself into vulnerable situations.
- *Trust your intuitions.* If you feel you are being pressured into unwanted sex, you probably are.
- *Avoid excessive use of alcohol and drugs.* Alcohol and other drugs interfere with clear thinking and effective communication.

Because of the subordinate role of children in relationships involving adults, sexually abusive practices often go unreported. Sexual abuse can leave emotional scars that make it difficult to establish meaningful relationships later in life. For this reason, it is especially important for people to pay close attention to any information shared by children that could indicate a potentially abusive situation. Most states require that information concerning child abuse be reported to law enforcement officials.

Sexual Harassment

Sexual harassment consists of unwanted attention of a sexual nature that creates embarrassment or stress. Examples of sexual harassment include unwanted physical contact, excessive pressure for dates, sexually explicit humor, sexual innuendos or remarks, offers of job advancement based on sexual favors, and overt sexual assault. Unlike more overt forms of sexual victimization, sexual harassment may be applied in a subtle manner and can, in some cases, go unnoticed by coworkers and fellow students. Nevertheless, sexual harassment produces stress that cannot be resolved

until the harasser is identified and forced to stop. Both men and women can be victims of sexual harassment.

Sexual harassment can occur in many settings, including employment and academic settings. On the college campus, harassment may be primarily in terms of the offer of sex for grades. If this happens to you, think carefully about the situation and document the specific times, events, and places where the harassment took place. Consult your college's policy concerning harassment. Next, you should report these events to the appropriate administrative officer (perhaps the affirmative action officer, dean of academic affairs, or dean of students). You may also want to discuss the situation with a staff member of the university counseling center.

If harassment occurs in the work environment, the victim should document the occurrences and report them to the appropriate management or personnel official. Reporting procedures will vary from setting to setting. Sexual harassment is a form of illegal sex discrimination and violates Title VII of the Civil Rights Act of 1964.

In 1986 the United States Supreme Court ruled that the creation of a "hostile environment" in a work setting was sufficient evidence to support the claim of sexual harassment. This action served as an impetus for thousands of women to step forward with sexual harassment allegations. Additionally, some men are also filing sexual harassment lawsuits against female supervisors.

Not surprisingly, this rising number of complaints has served as a wake-up call for employers. From university settings to factory production lines to corporate board rooms, employers are scrambling to make certain that employees are fully aware of actions that could lead to a sexual harassment lawsuit. Sexual harassment workshops and educational seminars on harassment are now common and serve to educate both men and women about this complex problem.

Violence and the Commercialization of Sex

It is beyond the scope of this book to explore whether sexual violence can be related to society's exploitation or commercialization of sex. However, sexually related products and messages are intentionally placed before the public to try to sway consumer decisions. Do you believe that there could be a connection between commercial products, such as violent pornography in films and magazines, and violence against women? Does prostitution lead directly to violence? Do sexually explicit "900" phone numbers or pornography on the Internet cause an increase in violent acts? Can the sexual messages in beer commercials lead to acquaintance rape? What do you think?

Identity Theft

In today's cashless, wired society, we make several transactions each day in which personal information is transferred: we write checks, pay bills online, use credit and debit cards for purchases, and withdraw cash from ATMs; we might be asked to provide a social security number when we write a check, or give our phone number or address when we shop at a particular store. Each of these transactions provides an opportunity for thieves to obtain your personal information and use it fraudulently.

Identity theft has been on the rise since the early 1990s. Thieves have many ways of obtaining personal data, including stolen mail (or mail diverted with a "change of address" form); sorting through garbage for discarded bills or receipts that include account numbers; posing as a landlord or employer to obtain people's credit report; stealing records—either electronically (hacking) or physically removing them—from offices where the victim is a customer, patient, student, or employee. Thieves use falsely obtained names, addresses, and social security numbers to open credit card accounts and bank accounts, purchase cell phone services, and secure loans to buy automobiles and other big-ticket items. They might even avoid paying taxes by working under false social security

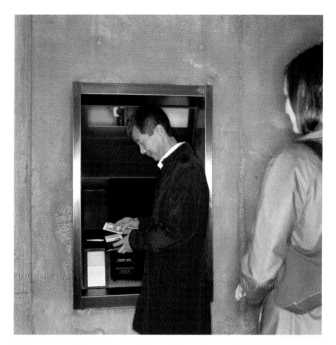

Being aware of your surroundings when using an ATM is important for personal safety.

numbers, or use your identity for other purposes—if they are arrested, for example. Identity thefts can drain a person's bank account and ruin their credit rating before a person knows they've become a victim. Often the crime is not discovered until a person wants to make a major purchase—like a house or a car—that requires a credit check.

There are several steps that you can take to avoid becoming a victim of identity theft. The most important step involves ordering copies of your credit reports each year to make sure that there are no fraudulent accounts in your name. Other steps are outlined in the Star box on page 630.

Campus Safety

Although many of the topics in this chapter are quite unsettling, students and faculty must continue to lead normal lives in the campus environment despite potential threats to our health. The first step in being able to function adequately is knowing about these potential threats. You have read about these threats in this section on intentional injuries; now you must think about how this information applies to your campus situation.

The campus environment is no longer immune to many of the social ills that plague our society. At one time the

> **Key Terms**
>
> **identity theft** a crime involving the fraudulent use of a person's name, social security number, credit line, or other personal financial or identifying information.

Reducing Your Risk for Identity Theft

The Federal Trade Commission outlines several steps to minimize your risk for identity theft:

- Order a copy of your credit report from each of the three major credit bureaus, and review it carefully to make sure it's accurate.
- Place passwords on your credit card, bank and phone accounts. Avoid obvious passwords such as birthdays, mother's maiden name, or social security numbers.
- Keep personal information in your home secure. Be vigilant about guarding your

mail and your trash; use a document shredder when discarding sensitive papers like credit card bills. Make sure your home computer has firewall protection.
- Ask about information security procedures in your workplace or at your school.
- Carefully read all your bills to make sure that you recognize all purchases and charges.
- Do not give out your personal information. Be especially wary of e-mail and phone solicitations requesting such information.

- Watch your wallet. Be wary of pickpockets, and carry only the identification and credit cards you need. Do not carry your social security card with you unless it is absolutely necessary.
- If you are a victim of identity theft, visit the FTC's website **(http://www.consumer. gov/idtheft/)** for valuable information on how to file a complaint and restore your credit.

Source: Federal Trade Commission. *ID Theft: When Bad Things Happen to Your Good Name.*

---

university campus was thought to be a safe haven from the real world. Now there is plenty of evidence to indicate that significant intentional and unintentional injuries can happen to anyone at any time on the college campus.

For this reason, you must make it a habit to think constructively about protecting your safety. In addition to the personal safety tips presented earlier in this section, remember to use the safety assistance resources available on your campus. One of these might be your use of university-approved escort services, especially in the evenings as you move from one campus location to another. Another re-

source is the campus security department (campus police). Typically, campus police have a 24-hour emergency phone number. If you think you need help, do not hesitate to call this number. Campus security departments frequently offer short seminars on safety topics to student organizations or residence hall groups. Your counseling center on campus might also offer programs on rape prevention and personal protection.

If you are motivated to make your campus environment safer, you might wish to contact an organization that specifically focus on campus crime. Safe Campuses

---

Considering Complementary Care

Safety and Health Care Decisions

In today's complex world of health care, four generalizations regarding the interfacing of traditional allopathic health care and complementary health care can be made. First, as adults age, they are increasingly likely to be under the care of several health care providers, in addition to their primary care physician. In fact, many middle-aged and older adults may be seeing three or more specialists, such as cardiologists, rheumatologists, and endocrinologists, in addition to their family physician or internist. As a result, these individuals may be taking multiple prescription medication simultaneously. Second, over 40% of adults report that they are using complementary care, including taking a vast array of dietary supplements. Third, less than 20% of adults mention the use of such complementary health care to their physicians, and an even smaller percentage of physicians question patients about their use of complementary health care. Fourth, despite its $50 million budget and newly designated independent status, the National Center for Alternative and Complementary Medicine has yet to carefully evaluate the effectiveness and safety of all the many

forms of health care and the vast array of dietary supplements available in the marketplace.

When these factors are combined, the potential for unanticipated and dangerous drug interactions exists. It is, therefore, imperative that patients proactively inform their physicians about the type and extent of complementary health care they are using. It is equally important that physicians ask their patients about any alternative forms of care being received and any dietary supplements being taken. When this information is not taken into consideration in the patient's plan of care, the complementary care itself may become a negative factor. Therefore, until a great deal more is understood about complementary medical care procedures and the nature of prescription medication–dietary supplement interactions, the use of complementary care should be limited to preventive and palliative measures. In addition, such care should be discontinued during periods of treatment with prescription medications and chemotherapeutic agents or prior to undergoing surgery.

Should I Have a Watch Dog?

Some people feel safer with an animal companion around. Others have had bad experiences with pets and find them a nuisance and expensive as well. Does keeping a dog increase one's personal safety? And if so, what kind of dog is best . . . a *watch* dog? . . . a *guard* dog?

The difference between watch dogs and guard dogs is that a watch dog will bark to alert owners of an approaching stranger, but will not usually attack. The sound of a barking dog may be enough to deter an intruder. A guard dog may also deter by barking, but is also "large enough to intimidate and, if necessary, attack an intruder."[1]

If your planning to obtain a watch dog, you should be aware that some breeds are better that others. According to PetPlace.com, the American Eskimo, Boston terrier, Chihuahua, French bulldog, Pekingese, and Irish setter are among those breeds that make good watch dogs.

However, there are several disadvantages to owning a dog. There are considerable veterinary expenses involved as well as the cost of dog food. Also, there is the question of what to do with your dog when you need to be away for a few days and cannot take the dog with you. Perhaps the biggest concern is safety. In 2001 an estimated 4.7 million bites occurred in the United States, and approximately, 799,700 of those required medical care.[2] Research has shown that the majority (80%) of bites incurred by those under 19 years of age were inflicted by a family

dog (30%) or a neighbor's dog (50%). Also, during 1997–1998, 75% of fatal dog bites were inflicted on family members or guests on the family's property.

Therefore, one should carefully consider the safety advantages and disadvantages of dog ownership. If you decide that owning a dog is right for you and your family, do some research and make sure that the dog you select is a safe one.

[1]PetPlace Staff. Top Watch Dogs: Breeds that protect the family. **www.PetPlace.com/**
[2]Centers for Disease Control and Prevention. Nonfatal dog bite-related injuries treated in hospital emergency departments—United States, 2001. Morbidity and Mortality Weekly Report 52(26):605–610. 2003. **www.cdc.gov/mmwr/preview/mmwrhtml/mm5226a1.htm**

Now is a nonprofit student group that tracks legislation, provides educational seminars, and monitors community incidents involving students. For information about Safe Campuses Now, including how to start a chapter on your campus, call (706) 354-1115. Visit the web page for Safe Campuses Now (www.uga.edu\safecampus). This organization is located at the University of Georgia. We encourage you to become active in making your campus a safer place to live.

Unintentional Injuries

Unintentional injuries are injuries that have occurred without anyone's intending that any harm be done. Common examples include injuries resulting from car crashes, falls, fires, drownings, firearm accidents, recreational accidents, and residential accidents. Each year, unintentional injuries account for nearly 100,000 deaths and 29 million visits to hospital emergency departments.[24]

Unintentional injuries are very expensive for our society, both from a financial standpoint and from a personal and family standpoint. Fortunately, to a large extent it is possible to avoid becoming a victim of an unintentional injury. By carefully considering the tips presented in the safety categories that follow, you will be protecting yourself from many preventable injuries.

Since this section of the chapter focuses on a selected number of safety categories, we encourage readers to consider some additional ones (see the Considering Complementary Care box on page 630). To review important points in the area of first aid skills, consult Appendix 1 in this text.

Finally, we encourage you to take a first aid course from the American Red Cross. American Red Cross first aid courses incorporate a significant amount of safety prevention information along with the teaching of specific first aid skills.

Residential Safety

Many serious accidents and personal assaults occur in dorm rooms, apartments, and houses. As a responsible adult, you should make every reasonable effort to prevent these tragedies from happening. One good idea is to discuss some of the following points with your family or roommates and see what cooperative strategies you can implement:

- Fireproof your residence. Are all electrical appliances and heating and cooling systems in safe working order? Are flammable materials safely stored?
- Prepare a fire escape plan. Install smoke or heat detectors.
- Do not give personal information over the phone to a stranger.
- Use initials for first names on mailboxes and in phone books.
- Install a peephole and deadbolt locks on doors.
- If possible, avoid living in first floor apartments. Change locks when moving to a new place.

Key Terms

unintentional injuries injuries that have occurred without anyone's intending that harm be done.

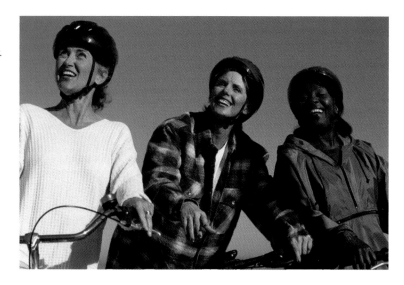

Wearing proper safety gear—including a helmet—is an essential safety measure when biking or skating. Obeying traffic laws and using proper hand signals are equally important.

- Put locks on all windows.
- Require repair people or delivery people to show valid identification.
- Do not use an elevator if it is occupied by someone who makes you feel uneasy.
- Be cautious around garages, laundry rooms, and driveways (especially at night). Use lighting for prevention of assault.

Some people report feeling safer at home with a dog. Statistics on whether dogs actually improve safety are hard to come by, but one should consider several factors before acquiring a dog for protection (see Star box on page 631).

Recreational Safety

The thrills we get from risk taking are an essential part of our recreational endeavors. But a significant number of injuries occur in recreational settings. For example, bicycle riding accounted for more than 412,000 emergency department visits in 2001.[25] Some injuries occur because we fail to consider important recreational safety information. Do some of the following recommendations apply to you?

- Seek appropriate instruction for your intended activity. Few skill activities are as easy as they look.
- Make certain that your equipment is in excellent working order.
- Involve yourself gradually in an activity before attempting more complicated, dangerous skills.
- Enroll in an American Red Cross first aid course to enable you to cope with unexpected injuries.
- Remember that alcohol use greatly increases the likelihood that people will get hurt.
- Protect your eyes from injury (see the Changing for the Better box on page 633).

- Learn to swim. Most drowning victims are people who never intended to be in the water.
- Obey the laws related to your recreational pursuits. Many laws are directly related to the safety of the participants.
- Be aware of weather conditions. Many outdoor activities turn to tragedy with sudden shifts in the weather. Always prepare yourself for the worst possible weather.

Bicycle Safety

With a little common sense and a few precautions, bicycling can be a very safe and enjoyable aerobic activity. Remember these key points:

- Wear a helmet. More than any other precaution, wearing a helmet is paramount and can save your life.
- When cycling at night or when visibility is poor, wear brightly colored reflective clothing.
- Use hand signals so drivers around you know what you plan to do.
- Obey traffic signals just like any other vehicle on the road. You have a right to bicycle on the road, but you also have the same responsibilities as other vehicles. Don't run stop signs or red lights!
- Brake carefully, and use both hand brakes at the same time. Using only the front brake can send you over the handlebars, and using only the back brake can cause a skid. On long downhills or in wet weather, gently tap the brakes to retain control. Be especially careful in wet weather, when wet brake pads are not very helpful.

Boating Safety

Most boating deaths result from drowning, when the victim was not wearing a personal flotation device (PFD). Of the 675 boaters who drowned in 1996, most could have been saved if they had been wearing a PFD, according to the U.S. Coast Guard. Eight out of ten victims in fatal boating accidents are not wearing life jackets.[26]

The other major cause of boating accidents and fatalities is "operator error," including (1) inattention, not looking in the direction in which one is moving, (2) carelessness, going out in bad weather or water conditions or while intoxicated, and (3) speeding. In particular, intoxication is a factor in more than half of all boating accidents. Too many casual boaters assume that rules of boating safety do not apply to them. Every boater should learn how to handle high winds, storms, whitecaps, rough waters, and heavy boat traffic. Most boat dealers can give you information about PFDs, "rules of the road," and Coast Guard safety regulations.

Even some experienced boaters tend to go too fast. Some modern watercraft tend to climb out of the water at higher speeds, and less hull in the water means less stability. With less stability, the boat tends to rock from side to side, and this rocking is a warning that you are about to lose control.

Firearm Safety

In 2000, the last year for which statistics are available, 14,037 Americans died as a result of homicides committed with a firearm, another 808 died from firearm-related accidents, and 214 died from discharged firearms where intent was not determined.[27] Most homicides are, in fact, committed using firearms, with handguns accounting for the vast majority of murders. (Shotguns and rifles tend to be more cumbersome than handguns and thus are not as frequently used in murders, accidents, or suicides.)

More than half of all murders result from quarrels and arguments between acquaintances or relatives. With many homeowners arming themselves with handguns for protection against intruders, it is not surprising that more than half of all gun accidents occur in the home. Children are frequently involved in gun accidents, often after they discover a gun they think is unloaded. On a positive note in this regard, youth gun deaths have declined significantly since the mid-1990s. In 1994, tragically, 5,833 children and adolescents died at the hands of firearms. This number declined to 3,593 youth gun-related deaths in 1997 and 3,180 in 1998.[28] Firearm deaths continued to decline in all age groups in 1999.[29]

Handgun owners are reminded to adhere to the following safety rules:

- Make certain that you follow the gun possession laws in your state. Special permits may be required to carry a handgun.
- Make certain that your gun is in good mechanical order.
- If you are a novice, enroll in a gun safety course.
- Consider every gun to be a loaded gun, even if someone tells you it is unloaded.
- Never point a gun at an unintended target.
- Keep your finger off the trigger until you are ready to shoot.
- When moving with a handgun, keep the barrel pointed down.
- Load and unload your gun carefully.
- Store your gun and ammunition safely in separate locked containers. Use a trigger lock on your gun when not in use.
- Take target practice only at approved ranges.

- Never play with guns at parties. Never handle a gun when intoxicated.
- Educate children about gun safety and the potential dangers of gun use. Children must never believe that a gun is a toy.

 TALKING POINTS You do not have a firearm in your home, but you're not sure whether your neighbors do, and your child enjoys playing at their house. How might you go about asking your neighbor if they have a gun in their home?

Motor Vehicle Safety

The greatest number of injury deaths in the United States occur on highways and streets. Young people (ages 16–24 years) are more likely to be involved in a fatal motor vehicle crash than persons of any other age (Figure 19-2). The most dangerous times to drive are 12 midnight to 3 A.M. on Saturdays and Sundays.[30] If the driver has been drinking and is driving a subcompact car or motorcycle, the likelihood of a fatal crash is even more pronounced.

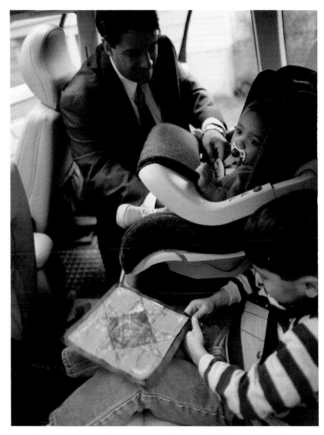

Consistent use of safety restraints during childhood can help make buckling up a life-long habit.

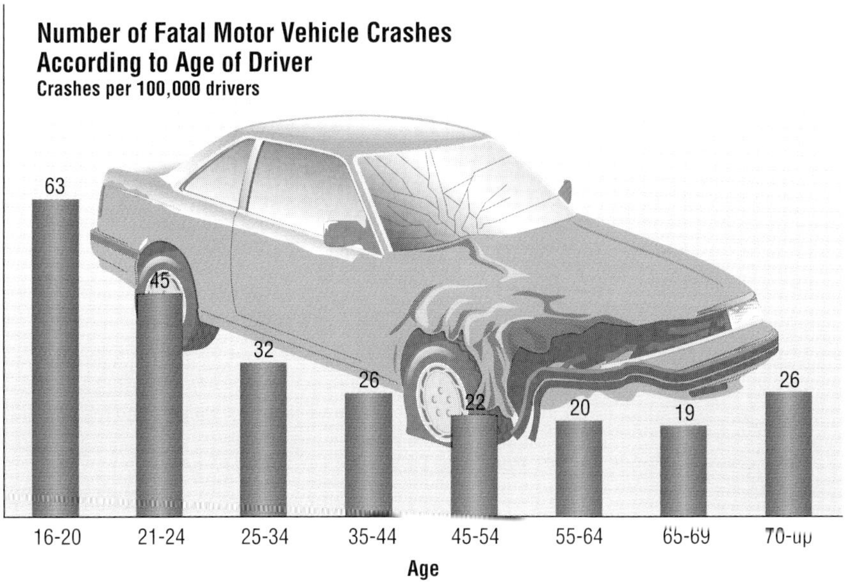

Number of Fatal Motor Vehicle Crashes According to Age of Driver
Crashes per 100,000 drivers

Age	Crashes
16-20	63
21-24	45
25-34	32
35-44	26
45-54	22
55-64	20
65-69	19
70-up	26

Figure 19-2 Driving is a dangerous activity for those under age 25. What could be done to reduce the number of driving fatalities among this age group?

Motor vehicle crashes also cause disabling injuries. With nearly two million such injuries each year, all college students should be concerned about avoiding motor vehicle crashes. With this thought in mind, we offer some important safety tips for motor vehicle operators:

- Make certain that you are familiar with the traffic laws in your state.

- Do not operate an automobile or motorcycle unless it is in good mechanical order. Regularly inspect your brakes, lights, and exhaust system.

- Do not exceed the speed limit. Observe all traffic signs.

- Always wear safety belts, even on short trips. Require your passengers to buckle up. Always keep small children in child restraints.

- Never drink and drive. Avoid horseplay inside a car.

- Be certain that you can hear the traffic outside your car. Keep the car's music system at a reasonable decibel level. (See the Star box below concerning cell phone use while driving.)

Cell Phone Safety While Driving

Cell phones that fit easily into a pocket or purse are being used in every place imaginable, including restaurants, theaters, subways, parks, golf courses, and, of course, in cars. And it's in cars that the use of cellular phones is most controversial. A variety of studies and reports indicate a four- to nine-fold increase in the potential for car crashes associated with the driver's use of a cell phone. In July 2001, the state of New York passed the country's first *statewide ban* on the use of hand-held cellular phones while driving. Violators of this ban are subject to a $100 fine for the first offense. Since then, at least 24 other states have passed laws regulating cell phone use while operating a motor vehicle.*

Research suggests the use of a cell phone decreases driver concentration and delays driver reaction time. The use of mounted, hands-free phones may improve safety, although the safety benefit has been controversial. Experts in traffic safety are careful to point out that there are too many other factors associated with driving to make it fair to blame behind-the-wheel phone use for all or most accidents. These complicating factors include adverse weather conditions, the structural integrity of the cars, the age and health of the drivers, radio, CD, or cigarette use, and interactions between drivers and passengers. The influence of other drivers on the road must also be considered.

If you must use your cell phone in a car, consider these common sense rules: Get off the main road to a safe parking area to make your call, especially if the call is an important one or one that might upset you. If you must talk while driving, opt for a hands-free phone. Dial when your car is stopped. Keep calls very brief. Don't try to dial or talk in heavy traffic. Keep your eyes on the road. (Or, let a passenger make the call!)

*Governor's Highway Safety Association. Cell Phone Restrictions—State and Local jurisdictions, 2003 **www.statehighwaysafety.org/html/stateinfo/ cellphone_laws**

Drowsy Driving

The Danger of Driving While Sleepy

Falling asleep at the wheel is something that no one thinks will happen to them, yet drowsy driving is estimated to cause up to 200,000 accidents per year on American roads.

Sleepiness is a significant cause of traffic fatalities. Up to 3% of all yearly vehicular deaths in the United States can be attributed to driving while drowsy, yet Americans remain uneducated about this problem. Sleepiness undermines a person's ability to make sound decisions and reduces attention span considerably. Any condition that impairs the judgment of drivers should be taken seriously. It has been estimated that 100 million Americans fail to get enough sleep and that up to 50% of all accident-related fatalities (not just driving fatalities) can be attributed to sleep deprivation.

Tips to Avoid Drowsy Driving

Because of the stealthy manner in which sleep can overtake you, it is important to evaluate your condition before getting behind the wheel and also while you are on the road. It is also important to prevent regular sleep deprivation. We must reduce the risk of falling asleep while driving by using common sense. The following suggestions should help reduce your chances of driving while drowsy:

- Get plenty of sleep. About 8 hours of sleep per night is desirable. If this is not practical, try to catch up on sleep when possible (take naps, sleep more on weekends, etc.).
- Take breaks while driving. Stop at least every 2 hours on long trips. If possible, avoid driving alone so the driving duties can be split. Don't eat heavy meals, and avoid too much caffeine.
- Stay alert. Talk, listen to the radio, sing, or do whatever you can to keep from drifting off. Don't let all of the passengers in the car sleep; having someone to converse with can help keep the driver alert.
- Don't get too comfortable. Getting too relaxed can promote dozing off. Avoid using cruise control. Reduce use of the heater, and keep the windows open when possible.
- Don't drink and drive. This is true anytime, but even a small amount of alcohol in the system can intensify the effects of fatigue on the body.
- Remember that some prescription and OTC medications can cause drowsiness and should not be used when driving. When beginning a medication, be certain to read labels, cautionary statements on packages, and information inserts regarding alertness.
- If you feel yourself drifting off or you think you may be in danger of falling asleep, stop driving. Dozing off for a few seconds (a phenomenon known as *microsleep*) is a significant warning sign of fatigue. Don't try to fight through fatigue while driving. Pull off the road at a safe place and take a nap if you need to.

- Give pedestrians the right-of-way.
- Drive defensively at all times. Do not challenge other drivers (see the Focus On article on pages 641–642). Refrain from drag racing.
- Look carefully before changing lanes.

- Be especially careful at intersections and railroad crossings.
- Carry a well-maintained first aid kit that includes flares or other signal devices.
- Drive even more carefully during bad weather.
- Do not drive when you have not had enough sleep (see the Star box on drowsy driving above).

In spite of the best efforts that people make to prevent motor vehicle crashes, when they occur there is, of course, not only damage to property but also the very real possibility of injury and even death. Also affected are family members and friends who pay an emotional price as they experience the loss of companionship when people for whom they care a great deal have been in serious motor vehicle crashes. The effects of motor vehicle-related injuries and injury deaths are also felt in the workplace where they result in economic losses of employers and employees alike.

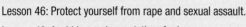

Learning to Go: Health

Are you proactive about your personal safety? Click on Learning to Go: Health on the Online Learning Center at **www.mhhe.com/payne8e** to check out the following lessons:

Lesson 46: Protect yourself from rape and sexual assault.

Lesson 48: Avoid becoming a victim of crime.

Lesson 50: Keep yourself safe at home.

Lesson 51: Play it safe when you're having fun.

Lesson 52: Drive safely and defensively.

Lesson 53: Shield yourself from road rage.

TALKING POINTS You're in a car with a friend when another driver starts tailgating you very closely. Your friend, who is driving, slows down to annoy the tailgater. How would you convince your friend that his action is dangerous?

Motorcycle Safety

Some emergency-room physicians call motorcycles "murder-cycles" because of their experience with motorcycle crash victims. The statistics support this grim view. With the death rate for motorcycles at 33.4 per 100,000 vehicle miles of travel compared to a death rate for cars of 1.3, motorcycles are 26 times more deadly.[30]

If you choose to ride a motorcycle, you can improve your chances of avoiding injury or death by following these suggestions:

- Most important of all, wear a helmet. A variety of studies have supported the effectiveness of helmets in preventing head injuries. Warriors and athletes have worn helmets for centuries to protect themselves from head injuries. Modern examples include construction workers, football players, race car drivers, and military aircraft pilots.

- Wear boots, gloves, and heavy clothing to protect your skin from serious injury when you slide on pavement in a crash.

- Get proper training, such as the Motorcycle Safety Foundation course offered in some states.

- Your risk increases in wet weather. Consider whether a ride in the rain is necessary.

- Do not ride after taking medication that can affect your alertness or performance.

- Never ride after drinking alcohol or taking drugs. About half of motorcyclists killed in accidents had alcohol in their blood.

- Ride defensively. Remember that many drivers do not see you or may not give you the right-of-way you deserve.

For all of the reasons discussed in conjunction with automobile accidents, motorcycle accidents can influence the well-being of a wide array of people. However, because of the very high probability of serious injury and death associated with these accidents, the distress suffered by family, friends, witnesses, and coworkers may be even more extensive.

Home Injury Prevention for Children and Elders

Approximately one person in ten is injured each year at home. Children and elders spend significantly more hours each day in a home setting than do young adults and adults. These groups are at greater risk of unintentional injury at home. (See the Changing for the Better box on page 637). Here are some important tips to remember. Can you think of others?

For Everyone

- Be certain that you have adequate insurance protection.

- Install smoke detectors appropriately.

- Keep stairways clear of toys and debris. Install railings.

- Maintain electrical and heating equipment.

- Make certain that family members know how to get emergency help.

For Children

- Know all the ways to prevent unintentional poisoning.

- Use toys that are appropriate for the age of the child.

- Never leave young children unattended, especially infants.

- Keep any hazardous items (guns, poisons, etc.) locked up.

- Keep small children away from kitchen stoves.

For Elders

- Protect elders from falls by removing damaged carpet, improving lighting near stairs, installing handrails, and repairing broken walks, steps, and porches.

- Be certain that elders have a good understanding of the medications they may be taking. Know the side effects.

- Encourage elders to seek assistance for home repairs.

- Make certain that all door locks, lights, and safety equipment are in good working order.

For young children who are mostly at home and elders whose dependence on homes is often an issue of restricted mobility and a sense of insecurity, homes should be dependably safe environments. Implementing the suggestions made in this section can help make a home safer.

Taking Charge of Your Health

- Use the Personal Assessment on page 643 to determine how well you manage your own safety.
- Assess your behaviors and those of your dating partners for signs of potential date rape by reviewing the Changing for the Better box on page 628.
- Check you residence for the safety strategies listed on page 637. Make the necessary changes to correct any deficiencies.
- Review the motor vehicle safety tips on page 634. If you need to make changes to your car or your driving, begin working on them at once.

- Check the recommendations for recreational safety on page 632 and put them into practice. Be assertive about using these measures when you are participating in activities with others.
- Find out about the security services available on your campus, and take advantage of them. Post the 24-hour-help phone number in your room and carry it with you.
- Minimize your risk for identity theft by taking the steps outlined in the Star box on page 630.

Summary

- Everyone is a potential victim of violent crime.
- Each year in the United States, intentional injuries cause nearly fifty thousand deaths and millions of additional nonfatal injuries.
- The national rate of serious crimes such as murder, rape, and robbery has been falling in recent years.
- Homicide is the leading cause of death for young male African Americans. Handguns are the weapon of choice for homicides.
- About half of all homes in the United States have a gun, for a total of about 230 million guns.
- In spite of changes in family structure, fatal and nonfatal, intimate partner violence has declined since 1993.
- Forms of child maltreatment include child abuse and child neglect. Child neglect is the most common form.
- Bicyclists and motorcyclists can best protect their safety by wearing helmets.
- Bias and hate crimes, as well as the crime of stalking, are increasingly recognized as serious, violent acts.
- Rape and sexual assault, acquaintance rape, date rape, and sexual harassment are forms of sexual victimization in which victims often are both physically and psychologically traumatized.
- The use of date rape drugs is a reality on today's college campuses.
- Unintentional injuries are injuries that occur without anyone intending that harm be done.
- The numbers of fatal and nonfatal unintentional injuries are exceedingly high.
- Recreational activities such as boating, bicycling, hunting, and simply being active at home place people at an increased level of risk.

Review Questions

1. Identify some of the categories of intentional injuries. How many people are affected each year by intentional injuries?
2. What are some of the most important facts concerning homicide in the United States? How are most homicides committed?
3. Identify changes in the traditional family structure in America. What factors contribute to domestic violence?
4. What reasons might explain why so many women do not report domestic violence?
5. Aside from the immediate consequences of child maltreatment what long-term problems do many abused and/or neglected children face?
6. List some examples of groups that are known to have committed bias or hate crimes.
7. Explain some of the myths associated with rape. How can date rape be prevented?
8. What are the date rape drugs now appearing on college campuses, and how are they employed by rapists?
9. Identify some examples of behaviors that could be considered sexual harassment. Why are employers especially concerned about educating their employees about sexual harassment?
10. Identify some common examples of unintentional injuries. Point out three safety tips appropriate for safe bicycling, boating, firearm use, and driving automobiles and motorcycles. How can you make your home a safer environment?
11. In what ways can individuals protect themselves from identity theft?

References

1. Center for Disease Control and Prevention, National Center for Injury Prevention and Control, WISQARS (Web-based Injury Surveillance Query and Reporting Systems), March 7, 2003, **www.cdc. gov/ncipc/wisqars/**
2. Bureau of Justice Statistics. *National Crime Victimization Survey: Criminal Victimization 2001, Changes 2000–01 with Trends 1993–2001.* U.S. Department of Justice, NCJ 194610, September 2002.
3. Bureau of Justice Statistics. U.S. Department of Justice, Office of Justice Programs, *National Crime Victimization Survey, Violent Crime Trends, 1973–2001,* **www.ojp.usdoj.gov/bjs/glance/tables/ viortrdtab.htm**
4. Bureau of Justice Statistics. *Homicide Trends in the U.S., Long-Term Trends,* U.S. Department of Justice, Office of Justice Programs, November 2002, **www.ojp.usdoj.gov/bjs/homicide/tables/ totalstab.htm**
5. Bureau of Justice Statistics. *Criminal offenders statistics: lifetime likelihood of going to state or federal prison,* U.S. Department of Justice, November 2000.

6. Bureau of Justice Statistics. U.S. Department of Justice, Office of Justice Programs, *Homicide Trends in the United States,* November 21, 2002.

7. Bureau of Justice Statistics. U.S. Department of Justice, Office of Justice Programs, *Drug Use and Crime,* January 2000, **www.ojp.usdoj.gov/bjs/dcf/duc.htm#to**

8. U.S. Census Bureau. *Children's Living Arrangements and Characteristics: March 2002.* Washington, D.C., 2003.

9. Bureau of Justice Statistics. U.S. Department of Justice, Office of Justice, *Crime Data Brief, Intimate Partner Violence, 1993–2001,* NCJ 197838, February 2003.

10. McKenzie JF, Pinger RR, Kotecki JF. *An Introduction to Community Health,* 4th ed. Jones & Bartlett, 2002.

11. Coker AI, et al. Physical health consequences of physical and psychological intimate partner violence. *Arch Fam Med* 9(5):451–457, 2000.

12. United States Department of Health and Human Services, Administration on Children, Youth and Families. *Child Maltreatment 2001.* Washington, D.C.: U.S. Government Printing Office, 2003, **http://www.acf.hhs.gov/programs/cb/publications/cm01/cm01.pdf**

13. National Institute of Justice. *The cycle of violence revisited.* Washington D.C.: U.S. Department of Justice, Office of Justice Programs, NIJ, Research in Progress Seminar Series, February, 1996.

14. U.S. Census Bureau. *The 65 years and over population: 2000, Census 2000 Brief.* U.S. Department of Commerce, Economics and Statistics Administration, 2001, **http://www.census.gov/prod/2001pubs/c2kbr01-10.pdf**

15. National Research Council. *Elder Mistreatment: Abuse, Neglect, and Exploitation in an Aging America.* Washington D.C.: The National Academies Press, 2003.

16. Office for Victims of Crime, Statistical Overviews. *Elder Abuse and Neglect.* Washington, D.C.: U.S. Department of Justice, Office of Justice Programs, 2001, **www.ojp.usdoj.gov/ovc/ncvrw/2001/stat_over_7.htm**

17. Office of Juvenile Justice and Delinquency Prevention. *OJJDP Fact Sheet: National youth gang survey trends from 1996 to 2000.* Washington, D.C., U.S. Department of Justice, Office of Justice Programs, 2002.

18. Centers for Disease Control and Prevention. *Surveillance for Fatal and Nonfatal Firearm-related Injuries—United States, 1993–1998.* Morbidity and Mortality Surveillance Summaries 50(ss02):1–32, 2001.

19. Miller M, Hemenway D, Wechsler H. Guns and Gun Threats at College. *J Am Coll Hlth* 51(2):57–65.

20. Bureau of Justice Statistics. *Special Report: Hate Crimes Reported in NIBRS, 1997–1999.* U.S. Department of Justice, Office of Justice Programs, NCJ 186765, Washington, D.C., 2001.

21. Thornhill R, Palmer CT, Wilson M. *A natural history of rape.* MIT Press, 2000.

22. National Institute of Justice. *The Sexual Victimization of College Women.* U.S. Department of Justice, Bureau of Justice Statistics, Washington, D.C., 2001.

23. Schwartz RH, Milteer R, LeBeau MA. Drug-facilitated sexual assault ('date rape'). *South Med* 93(6):558–561, 2000.

24. Federal Trade Commission. ID THEFT: When bad things happen to your good name. **www.consumer.gov/idtheft** 2002.

25. National Safety Council. *Injury Facts, 2003 Edition.* Itasca, IL, 2003.

26. U.S. Coast Guard. *Boating Safety.* **www.uscgboating.org/stats.htm 2003**.

27. Minimo AM, Smith BL. *Deaths: Preliminary data for 2000.* National Vital Statistics Reports 49(12):1–40.

28. *Deaths: final data for 1998.* National Center for Health Statistics. November 2000. **www.cdc.gov/nchs/data/nvsr/nvs48_11.pdf**

29. *Deaths: final data for 1999.* National Center for Health Statistics. September 2001. **www.cdc.gov/nchs/data/nvsr/nvsr49/nvsr49_08.pdf**

30. National Highway Traffic Safety Administration. *Traffic Safety Facts 2001.* Washington, D.C., U.S. Department of Transportation. DOT HS 809 484, 2002.

As We Go to Press

A recently released report by the AAA Foundation for Traffic Safety reveals that drivers whose ages are 65 years and older are 1.78 times more likely to die in car crashes than drivers ages 55 to 64. Cognitive skills and vision decline with age, the report noted. Drivers over 75 were more than 2.59 times more likely to die in car crashes, while those 85 and over were 3.72 times as likely to die when compared with drivers 55 to 64 years of age. Seniors are also more likely to be involved in left turn crashes as they age.

These statistics are important because the proportion of Americans who are seniors is growing. By 2030 one in five Americans will be 65 or older. Among the many resources available for seniors is the website: **www.seniordrivers.org**

The report noted that teenage drivers remain the age group at highest risk for injury or death in traffic crashes.

Source: **http://www.aaafoundation.org/multimedia/index.cfm?button-SeniorInjur.**

rage on the road: the danger of aggressive driving

The driver behind you is following so closely that you can't see his license plate in your rear view mirror. Or maybe the car in front of you is hogging the passing lane and won't even do the speed limit. Surprise! A driver in the next lane slips in front of you, without using a turn signal, into a space that is only a carlength because you slowed down so she wouldn't hit you. On another road, it's more of the same. Someone feels compelled to pull out in front of the last car in a line of traffic rather than wait a fraction of a second for the road to be clear. People run stop signs and stop lights that are long since yellow. At merges, drivers drag race until someone "chickens out" when the lane ends, rather than take turns. And there are those people who speed past the line of cars forming for an exit or lane closure and try to cut in at the front of the line. Add four-letter words, horn honking, and a couple of hand gestures and you have all of the elements of a daily commute. These rude and unthinking drivers set the stage for highway aggression and danger.

At this point, it is important to make a distinction between two concepts that are often used interchangeably—*aggressive driving* and *road rage*. Aggressive driving commonly involves dangerous and illegal acts, such as speeding, entering intersections on the caution light, and following another car too closely. Technically, this is not road rage. However, it may precipitate responses that lead to road rage. In actual road rage, drivers use their automobiles as weapons (or weapon platforms) with the intent of harming others, usually other drivers.

Motorists are aware of an increasing sense of danger on America's congested highways. An unthinking act or no provocation at all can result in a deadly face-off with a complete stranger. During the period 1990 through 1996, aggressive drivers have killed 218 people and injured another 12,610, at a frequency that increased by about 7% each year.[1] This is just the tip of the iceberg. For every incident serious enough to result in a police report or newspaper story, hundreds or thousands of other incidents take place that are never reported. The problem has become so severe that, according to a National Highway Safety Administration report, the public is more concerned about aggressive drivers than about drunk drivers.

During the average commute and on leisure excursions, millions of American drivers are conditioned to accept stupid, uncivilized driving. The hostile and aggressive behavior of the instigators and those who react to them reinforces the belief that belligerence works. Of course, belligerence does not work—it only causes anger to escalate, which can result in accidents, property damage, injury, and death. Various weapons are used when traffic altercations become violent. Conventional weapons, such as firearms, knives, clubs, and tire irons, were used in 44% of reported violent traffic altercations. The vehicle itself became the weapon in 23% of the cases, and in 12% of the incidents the car and a conventional weapon were both used. In several unusual cases, pepper spray, eggs, golf clubs, and even a crossbow were involved.[1]

Characteristics of Aggressive Drivers

Although there is no profile *per se* of the typical aggressive driver, most aggressive drivers are men between the ages of 18 and 26. Many of these men are poorly educated, and some have criminal records or histories of violence and substance abuse, but hundreds of others are successful men and women, of all ages, with no such history.[1]

Between the sexes, men are angered most by police presence and slow driving, whereas illegal behavior and traffic obstructions tend to frustrate women. When all factors are added in, though, men and women do not differ in total driving anger scores.[2] Increasingly, women are acting on their anger. Only 4% of recorded aggressive driving incidents involved women drivers,[2] but during the last 15 years the number of fatal accidents involving women drivers has increased dramatically while men's risks have dropped.[3] Most of the increase for women has occurred because more women are on the road at riskier times, but women are also increasingly displaying the more aggressive driving tactics common among men.

Individually, people generally think of themselves as better-than-average drivers. This holds true even among younger people, who consider themselves to be good drivers. But perceptions and reality are not always identical. While some people are aware of their aggressive tendencies on the road, other people see themselves as innocent and the issue of aggressive driving as everyone else's problem. The truth is, we're all human and can let our emotions run away from us. Many professionals suggest that you tape-record your vocalizations in the car to become aware of and change your own negative and intense driving behavior.[4]

Causes of Aggressive Driving

Violent traffic disputes result not from single incidents but from personal attitudes and accumulated stress in motorists' lives. Specifically, drug use, domestic arguments or violence, racism, the desire to evade or attack police, and the everyday stresses of home, work, and commuting can lead to aggressive driving.[1] For the general population, the anonymity and physical excitement of driving, combined with a feeling of control and power and the ability to drive away, sow the seeds of aggression.[5] Some people drive to "win" rather than to arrive safely at their destination. Adding to this climate are overpowered cars, driver's licenses that are easy to qualify for, and sporadically lax enforcement of traffic laws.

Unfortunately, and perhaps tellingly, the people who spend the most time on the road are the least effective at dealing with its stressors. Long-distance commuters have higher blood pressure, less tolerance for frustration, and more frequent negative moods than do short- or medium-distance commuters.[6] Carpooling, not only saves gas and miles on the car, but it also lessens the negative effects of commuting, especially over long distances, for everybody in the carpool.

Avoiding Aggressive Drivers

The best way to stay out of driving conflicts is not to be an aggressive driver yourself. You can do a number of things to reduce your stress and thus reduce the tendency toward aggression. First, allow plenty of time for your trip. We tend to overschedule our days and not allow enough time to get from one place to the next. Sure, under perfect conditions you could cover X number of miles in X amount of time, but weather, traffic, and road construction are facts of life. Not building extra travel time into our schedules causes us to run late when we encounter these variables and then get angry and possibly aggressive. Other ways to reduce stress are to listen to soothing music, improve the comfort of your vehicle, and probably most important,

understand that you can't control the traffic—only your reaction to it.[1]

If traffic really pushes your buttons, you may want to avoid peak commuting hours. If your company doesn't have a flextime policy, you can go in a little earlier and leave a little later. If you're still tempted to let another driver have it, imagine that you're being videotaped. How would you react if the world were watching? Or imagine that the driver in the other car is someone you love—a spouse, parent, grandparent, sibling, or friend. How would you treat them? Practice driving courtesy and keep the following points in mind:

- Do not make obscene gestures.
- Use your horn sparingly.
- Do not block the passing lane.
- Do not switch lanes without signaling.
- Do not block the right-hand turn lane.
- Do not take more than one parking space.
- If you are not disabled, do not park in a space reserved for disabled people.
- Do not allow your door to hit the car parked next to you.
- Do not tailgate.
- If you travel slowly, pull over and allow traffic to pass.
- Avoid unnecessary use of high-beam headlights.
- Do not let the car phone distract you.
- Do not stop in the road to talk to a pedestrian or another driver.
- Do not inflict loud music on neighboring cars.

Avoid engaging other drivers by following the limousine drivers' rule: Duty bound to protect their passengers, they do not make eye contact with other drivers.[7] If another driver is following you, don't drive home. Instead, drive to a public place, ideally a police station. This or using your cell phone to call for help is usually enough to scare off the offending driver.

Of course, it's hard not to respond when challenged. It may help to look at the other driver's mistakes and actions

objectively and not take them personally. Treat their poor behavior as their problem; don't make it yours. Remember how dangerous the situation can become.

It's not one driver's job to teach other drivers proper manners.[4] In all certainty, you won't be successful. Instead, try being extra nice to a fellow driver. Courtesy can be as contagious as aggression.

For Discussion . . .

What aspect of driving makes you the angriest? How do you handle the situation? Do you recognize any of your own bad driving habits in the list above? What can be done about the problem of aggressive driving?

References

1. AAA Foundation. *Road rage on the rise.* 1997. **www.webfirst.con/aaa**
2. Deffenbacher JL, Oetting ER, Lynch RS. Development of a driving anger scale. *Psychological Reports* 1994; 74(1):83–91.
3. Guerin B. What do people think about the risks of driving? Implications for traffic safety interventions. *J. App Soc Psychol* 1994; 24(11):994–1021.
4. James L, Hahl D. *Dr. Driving says.* 1999. **www.aloha.net/~dyc/surveys/tables.html**
5. Thurber S. Don't drive under the influence of emotion. *Safety and Health* 1994;150(1):66–68.
6. Spilner M. Destress your commute. *Prevention* 1995;47(3):60–62.
7. Cook WJ. Mad driver's disease: a survival guide for handling highway nuts, from a recovering lunatic. *U.S. News and World Report* 1996;121(19):74–76.

InfoLinks

www.drivers.com
www.safety.gmu.edu

personal assessment

how well do you protect your safety?

This quiz will help you measure how well you manage your personal safety. For each item below, circle the number that reflects the frequency with which you do the safety activity. Then, add up your individual scores and check the interpretation at the end.

3   I regularly do this
2   I sometimes do this
1   I rarely do this

1. I am aware of my surroundings and do not get lost.
    3   2   1
2. I avoid locations in which my personal safety would be compromised.
    3   2   1
3. I intentionally vary my daily routine (such as walking patterns to and from class, parking places, and jogging or biking routes) so that my whereabouts are not always predictable.
    3   2   1
4. I walk across campus at night with other people.
    3   2   1
5. I am careful about disclosing personal information (address, phone number, social security number, my daily schedule, etc.) to people I do not know.
    3   2   1
6. I carefully monitor my alcohol intake at parties.
    3   2   1
7. I watch carefully for dangerous weather conditions and know how to respond if necessary.
    3   2   1
8. I do not keep a loaded gun in my home.
    3   2   1
9. I know how I would handle myself if I were to be assaulted.
    3   2   1
10. I maintain adequate insurance for my health and my property.
    3   2   1
11. I keep emergency information numbers near my phone.
    3   2   1
12. I keep my first aid skills up-to-date.
    3   2   1
13. I use deadbolt locks on the doors of my home.
    3   2   1
14. I use the safety locks on the windows at home.
    3   2   1
15. I check the batteries used in my home smoke detector.
    3   2   1
16. I have installed a carbon monoxide detector in my home.
    3   2   1
17. I use adequate lighting in areas around my home and garage.
    3   2   1
18. I have the electrical, heating, and cooling equipment in my home inspected regularly for safety and efficiency.
    3   2   1
19. I use my car seat belt.
    3   2   1
20. I drive my car safely and defensively.
    3   2   1
21. I keep my car in good mechanical order.
    3   2   1
22. I keep my car doors locked.
    3   2   1
23. I have a plan of action if my car should break down while I am driving it.
    3   2   1
24. I use appropriate safety equipment, such as flotation devices, helmets, and elbow pads, in my recreational activities.
    3   2   1
25. I can swim well enough to save myself in most situations.
    3   2   1
26. I use suggestions for personal safety each day.
    3   2   1

TOTAL POINTS _____

Interpretation
Your total may mean that:

72–78 points	You appear to carefully protect your personal safety.
65–71 points	You adequately protect many aspects of your personal safety.
58–64 points	You should consider improving some of your safety-related behaviors.
Below 58 points	You must consider improving some of your safety-related behaviors.

To Carry This Further . . .
Although no one can be completely safe from personal injury or possible random violence, there are ways to minimize the risks to your safety. Scoring high on this assessment will not guarantee your safety, but your likelihood for injury should remain relatively low. Scoring low on this assessment should encourage you to consider ways to make your life safer. Refer to the text and this assessment to provide you with useful suggestions to enhance your personal safety. Which safety tips will you use today?

chapter twenty

the environment and your health

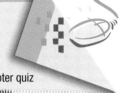

Talking It Over

Talking—and Acting—Like an Environmentalist

One of your classmates claims to be an avid environmentalist who loves hiking, camping, and other outdoor activities. He is involved with several organizations that lobby the government for environmental reform. So, when you see him drive a large, gas-guzzling SUV up to the recycling center, where he deposits neatly sorted paper, bottles, and cans for recycling, does this image strike you as contradictory? Do you think he recycles to ease a guilty conscience about driving an SUV? Would it matter more if you were standing in the middle of New York City (far from any dirt roads), or in Salt Lake City (surrounded by vast wildlands)? If his love of the great outdoors requires a larger vehicle (to haul camping gear, kayak, etc.), might he have made a more environmentally sound choice?

CommunicationLinks:

www.thedetroitproject.com
http://www.ecocenter.org/auto.shtml

Eye on the Media

Does Eco-Terrorism Really Work to Protect Our Environment?

On August 23, 2003, several automobile dealerships were attacked by arsonists who left graffiti claiming that they destroyed or damaged gas-guzzling SUVs to protect the environment. The unknown perpetrators claimed to be acting in accordance with the Earth Liberation Front, or ELF. According to their Internet website, ELF is an international underground organization that uses "direct action" (called eco-terrorism by others) in the form of economic sabotage to stop the destruction of the natural environment. Since 1997, the ELF in North America has caused over $100 million in damages to entities who profit from the destruction of life and the planet. ELF-linked arson fires have destroyed many buildings associated with urban sprawl and economic developments in previously natural habitats.

Many people are angered by the degradation of our shared natural environment, but is direct action/eco-terrorism ever justified in a democratic society? For some, the degradation or destruction of a local wetland, a forested mountaintop, or a local river or lake is a personal loss, like the death of an old friend. Others are depressed by news of species extinctions and the destruction of rain forests and coral reefs due to human exploitation of natural resources. Many people are frustrated by the perception that well-funded corporate interests have bought out our democratic political system so that they can exploit our shared natural lands. Some wonder, "If the system is unfair, why not take direct action to right these wrongs?"

Those who participate in eco-terrorism may feel at the time that they are "part of the solution," but are they really? To shift the course of the global human population toward a more ecologically sustainable path will require many changes, large and small, governmental and personal. Does eco-terrorism really change people's attitudes and behaviors toward protecting our environment? Will eco-terrorism stimulate governments toward more ecologically sound policies, or cause a societal backlash against all groups who work to protect the environment? Does direct action against environmental "bad guys" discourage their activities, or allow them to claim "victim" status that brings them assistance in proceeding with their destructive practices?

One likely motivation for ELF's acts of economic sabotage is to get environmental problems on the national agenda; to make people more aware and motivated to act in the political process. Certainly, this strategy worked well for the civil rights movement. The TV pictures of peaceful black demonstrators being viciously attacked by white police officers and their dogs caused our entire nation to wake up to the problem of institutional racism. To date, the main results from actions by ELF are short-lived news stories that show damage to expensive SUVs and burned-out buildings. These news stories never show pictures of environmental damage associated with the manufacture of the SUVs or economic development of natural habitats. All the public sees is waste of resources in the burned hulks of automobiles, the vandalism of extremists. This does not seem to be a particularly effective way to draw public attention to environmental problems. Even worse, some anti-environment commentators use widely televised actions of ELF to discredit the entire environmental movement. Using the media to get environmental issues on the national agenda is a good thing only if it advances positive changes that provide real environmental protection.

Environmental issues are important concerns for many college-age students as they perceive disturbing trends that may affect their future health and well-being. News programs regularly present the latest bad news about environmental problems such as over-population, pollution, global warming, damage to the ozone layer, loss of wilderness to economic exploitation, and endangered species. Movies such as *Water World, Blade Runner, Batman, The Matrix,* and *The Terminator* depict various fictional futures that are dismal environmental disasters. Some college students join environmental organizations that work to clean up litter, encourage recycling, regulate pollution emissions, control human population growth, and protect endangered species and natural areas. Others feel there is nothing they can do about such monumental environmental issues. They lose hope for a future where the world will be a good place to live and raise a family, and may become depressed and apathetic. The impact of environmental quality on your health is influenced by both the nature of your environment and your intellectual, emotional, social, and spiritual responses to that environment.

Your **environment** includes a range of conditions that can influence your health, such as the availability of resources (oxygen, water, food) and environmental characteristics, such as temperature, humidity, toxins, allergens, pathogens, noise, and radiation. Conditions in your environment operate across a wide range of spatial scales, from the air immediately surrounding your body to the global earth, air, and ocean system. Your physical health is influenced primarily by your *personal environment,* comprised of conditions immediately around your body, in the home, neighborhood, and workplace. However, this personal environment is influenced by conditions in the larger *community* and *regional environment,* including such conditions as air pollution and water pollution. These local and regional conditions are influenced by conditions of the *global environment,* such as climate and solar radiation.

Your health can be influenced by changes in environmental conditions at the home/workplace, community/region, or global levels. Excessive noise in the workplace or neighborhood can significantly impact your sense of well-being and your ability to work effectively. High ozone levels in the air of your community can limit your ability to enjoy outdoors activities and cause or exacerbate asthma. Environmental conditions in a particular community and region can enhance or limit opportunities for various types of employment, and so affect occupational health. Few people ever visit a tropical rain forest, wilderness area, or whale sanctuary, but many feel their

---

Key Terms

environment the physical conditions (temperature, humidity, light, presence of substances) and other living organisms that exist around your body.

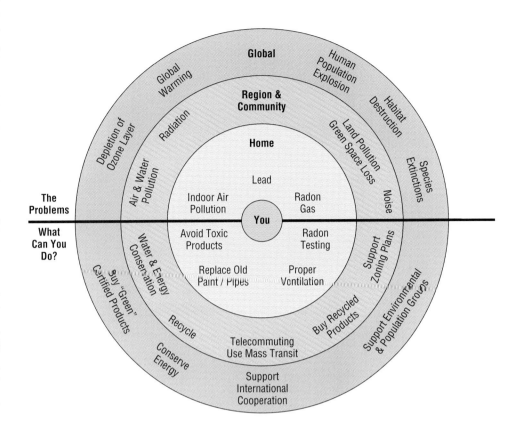

Figure 20-1 Spatial scales of environmental health risks and appropriate personal responses to environmental problems.

emotional and spiritual well-being is diminished when they hear these remote places are threatened or destroyed.

The goal of this chapter is to help you identify aspects of your environment that can significantly affect various dimensions of your health, and to suggest ways that you can exert some level of personal control over these environmental influences. The range of options for personal action to improve your environment include altering personal behaviors and buying habits, becoming involved in the political process surrounding governmental actions on environmental issues, and supporting various nongovernmental organizations that work to address major environmental problems. Different specific environmental conditions and personal responses will be important at the various spatial scales of your environment (home/workplace, community/region, and global). Figure 20-1 displays a range of environmental problems that exist at various spatial scales of your environment, and a range of personal responses that might be appropriate at each level.

The Personal Environment: Home, Neighborhood, Workplace

On average you spend about 90 percent of your time indoors,[1] in your home, workplace, local stores, and entertainment venues. The indoor air you breathe, the water you drink from the tap on your sink, and the radiation and noise in your immediate surroundings are environmental factors that have the most direct and obvious impact on your health. Some indoor environmental problems cause immediate and obvious health effects, such as headaches, dizziness, nausea, or allergic reactions. Other kinds of environmental problems act in subtle, cumulative ways over many years, causing major health problems such as cancer or neurological damage that may not become apparent until permanent damage is done.

Of all the different environmental influences that can affect your health, you have the greatest degree of control over factors in your personal environment. You are responsible for maintaining the appliances in your home so that they do not produce excessive air pollution. You have a great degree of control over the amount of ventilation you have in your home, allowing you to vent pollutants out from the indoor environment. You choose which products you will purchase and bring into your home, and can avoid products that may expose you to toxic chemicals. You can choose to not smoke tobacco, and to insist that others do not smoke in your home or workspace. In your personal environment, you can identify sources of health risk and have them removed from your home or notify those responsible for environmental safety at your workplace.

In this section you will learn to identify important environmental health risks in your personal environment,

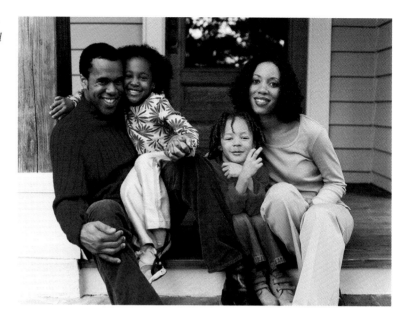

Protecting your family from environmental hazards begins at home. Have your home tested for radon gas, lead paint, asbestos, and other household pollutants, and take the necessary steps described in your text to reduce their impact on your family's health.

learn the effects of these environmental factors on your health, and see what you can do to minimize associated risks of health problems.

Indoor Air Quality

Indoor air quality within buildings can be influenced by a wide range of factors, including ventilation, humidity, gases given off by building construction materials, furniture and flooring materials, and combustion by-products from stoves and furnaces. When there is a problem with one or more of these factors, people in the affected building can experience a wide range of symptoms, from headaches and itchy eyes to unconsciousness and death. This section covers some of the most important health risks associated with indoor air quality.

Carbon Monoxide

Carbon monoxide is a highly toxic gas that is colorless, odorless, and tasteless, and so is not detectable by the un-aided senses. Average levels in homes without gas stoves vary from 0.5 to 5 parts per million (ppm). Levels near properly adjusted gas stoves are often 5 to 15 ppm, and those near poorly adjusted stoves may be 30 ppm or higher.[1] The various sources of indoor carbon monoxide also produce nitrogen oxides and small particulates that contribute to indoor air pollution.

Health effects of carbon monoxide vary from mild discomfort to death, due to interference with oxygen transport by the blood. At low concentrations (1 to 70 ppm), effects of carbon monoxide are barely noticeable by most people. Persons who suffer from heart disease may feel chest pain. At concentrations between 70 to 150 ppm, your vision and coordination may be impaired and you may suffer from headaches, dizziness, mental confusion, and/or nausea. Regular exposure to these levels in the home or workplace can cause flu-like symptoms that rapidly disappear after you leave the location where you are exposed.[1] At very high concentrations (> 150 ppm), carbon monoxide poisoning can render you unconscious and then kill you.[2] Nitrogen oxides produced along with

OnSITE/InSIGHT

Learning to Go: Health

Are you concerned with the world around you? Click on Learning to Go on the Online Learning Center at **www.mhhe.com/payne8e** to explore this topic in the following lessons:

Lesson 59: Foster a sustainable environment

Lesson 60: Pinpoint the health effects of pollution.

Key Terms

indoor air quality characteristics of air within homes, workplaces, and public buildings, including the presence and amount of oxygen, water vapor, and a wide range of substances that can have adverse effects on your health.

carbon monoxide a gaseous by-product of the incomplete combustion of natural gas, kerosene, heating oil, wood, coal, gasoline, and tobacco.

Religious Perspectives on Human-Environment Relationships

In an article written by Lynn White (published in *Science,* 1967), he states that the root of all the environmental problems today can be found in Judeo-Christian (including Islamic) scripture. According to scripture of these religious traditions, the purpose of all of creation was to meet the needs and uses of humankind. This established a dualism (human versus not human) that did not exist in earlier religions that perceived divinity in all of creation. White proposed that the Judeo-Christian dualism encourages exploitation and dominion over nature by humans, resulting in the many environmental problems facing us today.

Earth-based religions of many indigenous cultures of the world (pre-Christian Europe, Native American, African) believed that many or all aspects of the natural world were manifestations of one or more gods. Humans were perceived as being at the mercy of these powerful, sometimes petty and vindictive, natural forces, and often performed religious rituals to gain favors or atone for sins against Nature. Many of these cultures appear to have lived in ecological balance with their environment. Whether this balance was the consequence of their religious beliefs, their small populations, their limited technologies, or the combination of these factors is unknown.

Modern-day Earth-based religions include Paganism, Wicca, Druidism (a resurrection of pre-Roman European Celtic religious traditions), and Goddess religions. These modern versions of ancient traditions also worship the natural world as a manifestation of the energy of God or Creation. People who follow these religious traditions are often dedicated to protecting the environment.[1]

Traditional Hinduism also lacks the distinction between humankind as separate from the rest of Creation. Hindus believe that humans, gods, and Nature are all parts of a single organic whole. In Hindu tradition, God is present in all of Nature, and the natural forces that impact on daily life are manifestations of the Creator. Because divine forces sustain all life on Earth, Hindus believe they should live in harmony with Creation. Many religious rituals serve to appease Mother Earth and seek forgiveness for any violations of Nature. Any abuse of Nature is considered a sacrilegious act. These traditional beliefs encourage Hindus to live in balance with their environment. However, in their efforts to develop a modern economic system in India, many Hindus have abandoned these traditional beliefs. In recent decades India has suffered from the same environmental degradation as many other developed nations.[2]

In the Islamic tradition, humankind is considered the most favored of God's creation, and all the rest of Creation is deemed subservient to human needs and uses. However, Islamic tradition also holds that all living things in Nature are partners of humankind, deserving of respect and their own existence. Passages in the Qur'an (Koran) state that it is the duty of humankind to deal with the environment and other species in a loving, caring, and respectful manner. Islamic tradition also stipulates that humankind should be good stewards of natural resources and should not pollute clean waters with their wastes. Muslims are encouraged to put the common good ahead of personal benefit, and to be moderate in consumption, including the use of natural resources. Taken together, these passages from the Qur'an encourage Muslims to protect and manage their environment for the common good.[3]

While the Judeo-Christian and Islamic religious traditions have scriptural passages that could be seen as justifying environmentally destructive behavior, they also have distinctly environment-friendly teachings. In the Judeo-Christian tradition, God created the heavens and Earth, the land and waters, the plants and animals, and humankind. At the end of each day of Creation, the Bible states that God saw each of his creations was "good." Some theologians interpret these statements to mean that the Creator valued all aspects of Creation, not just humankind. In subsequent biblical passages, several references are made regarding human responsibility to be "good stewards" over the other parts of Creation. However, other passages in the Bible are less environmentally friendly, including statements that humankind should "go forth and multiply" and "subdue the Earth." These passages are often cited by those who seek a religious basis to justify unchecked human population growth and environmental destruction in pursuit of human goals.

The National Religious Partnership for the Environment is an umbrella organization for Christians and Jews who believe that protecting the environment is a mandate well-founded in their scriptural traditions.[4] This association of religious congregations works to increase awareness of the environmental message in the Bible and Torah. A main objective of this association is to enhance the activity of its members in the political process in support of environmental protection. For people who are committed to protecting the environment and dedicated to their Judeo-Christian religion, this organization offers a community of like-minded people working toward similar goals.

[1]Pagan and Earth-based Religions. **http://www.beliefnet.com/index/ index_10015.html**
[2]Adhopia A. Hinduism Promotes Environmental Protection. 2001. **http://www.indianest.com/analysis/018.htm**
[3]Alhilaly TH. Islam and Ecology. 1993. **http://www.ummah.com/islam/ taqwapalace/fitness/microcosmpage2.html**
[4]National Religious Partnership for the Environment. **http://www.nrpe.org**

carbon monoxide can cause irritation to the eyes, nose, and throat, and impair respiratory function. Small particulates produced by these same sources irritate and damage lung tissues.

You can minimize your exposure to carbon monoxide and risk of poisoning by keeping all appliances that burn gas or other fuels in proper working order (to ensure complete combustion) and ensuring proper ventilation.

You should have your gas-burning furnace and stove regularly inspected and repaired, as necessary. You should use the manufacturer-specified fuel in space heaters, and ensure proper ventilation of space heaters, woodstoves, charcoal and gas grills, and fireplaces, as directed by the manufacturer. You should avoid letting your car idle inside a garage, especially if it is attached to your home.[1] Never spend any long period of time close to the exhaust vent of a gas engine. Recent news reports have described several deaths of young people who were "body surfing" by holding on to the back of a power boat. They inhaled the exhaust from the engine, were rendered unconscious by carbon monoxide poisoning, and died before proper medical treatment could be obtained.

Installing a carbon monoxide detector will let you monitor levels of this gas in your home, and will sound an alarm if levels exceed safety standards. Every year, 300 people in the United States die from carbon monoxide poisoning.[3] In many cases, improperly maintained furnaces or incorrectly used space heaters vent carbon monoxide into the home. If this occurs while the occupants are sleeping, they may never wake up. A carbon monoxide alarm can prevent this tragedy from happening to you.

Volatile Organic Compounds

Volatile organic compounds (VOCs) are emitted from products such as paint, paint stripper, cleaning solvents, wood preservatives, aerosol sprays, cleaners, disinfectants, insect repellents and pesticides, air fresheners, stored fuels and automotive products, hobby supplies such as wood glue, and recently dry-cleaned clothing. Formaldehyde is a specific VOC that commonly enters the indoor environment due to emissions from pressed wood products (hardwood plywood wall paneling, particleboard, fiberboard) and furniture made with these pressed wood products. Urea-formaldehyde foam used for home insulation can emit this gas into the indoor environment.[4] Studies have found that levels of several VOCs average two to five times higher indoors than outdoors. During and for several hours immediately after certain activities, such as paint stripping, levels of VOCs may be 1,000 times background outdoor levels.[4]

The health effects of volatile organic compounds will vary, depending on which specific substance is involved. Immediate effects of many VOCs include irritation to the eyes, nose, and throat, headaches, loss of coordination,

Key Terms

volatile organic compounds a wide variety of chemicals that contain carbon and readily evaporate into the air.

and/or nausea. Longer term exposure to some VOCs can result in damage to the liver, kidney, and central nervous system. Some VOCs have been shown to cause cancer in animals, and some are suspected or known to cause cancer in humans.

There are several ways you can limit your exposure to toxic volatile organic compounds. First, you can minimize your use of products that contain these substances by choosing cleaning supplies, paints, and glues that do not contain VOCs. For example, you could use latex interior house paint rather than an oil-based paint. If you must use a product that contains VOCs, use it in accordance with manufacturer's directions and provide for plenty of ventilation to reduce levels indoors. If you want to strip the paint off that antique cabinet, do it in the backyard or garage (with the door open) instead of in the family room. Never mix household care products, as this may result in chemical reactions that emit toxic VOCs.[4] Also, you should buy only as much of the VOC-containing product as you will need for your current project and dispose of the unused portion in an appropriate manner as soon as possible. Many communities have regularly scheduled and advertised "Tox-Away Days." You can drop off these toxic household products at specified locations for proper disposal. Never simply pour these products down the sink or storm drain, since this will pollute local waterways and may be illegal.

Tobacco Smoke

Secondhand tobacco smoke is an indoor air pollutant widely recognized as a major health risk, especially for children. For example, this pollutant can increase the risk for acute asthma attacks that require hospital emergency care. There is some evidence that regular exposure to tobacco smoke increases the risk of developing asthma in the first place.[5] Exposure to tobacco smoke in the home is also associated with increased risk of Sudden Infant Death Syndrome (SIDS), childhood bronchitis, pneumonia and ear infections, cardiovascular disease, and cancer. The health effects of indoor tobacco smoke are covered in more detail in Chapter 9.

Asbestos

Asbestos is a building material that was widely used for insulation, floor tiles, and for its fire retardant and noise-dampening properties. Health effects of asbestos exposure include cancers of the lung and abdomen, and irreversible scarring of the lungs that can result in reduced respiratory function. These dire effects most commonly occur only after many years of exposure, usually in the workplace.[6] When the serious health risks associated with exposure to asbestos became known, governmental agencies banned several asbestos products, and manufacturers voluntarily limited other uses of asbestos. Today, asbestos is most commonly found in older buildings, including homes, schools, and factories. The greatest risk of exposure to asbestos occurs when insulation, floor tiles, and other asbestos-containing substances deteriorate with age, or are damaged during building renovation or repair. These activities release the microscopic asbestos fibers into the air, from which they are inhaled into the lungs. However, intact and undisturbed, asbestos-containing products are relatively safe.[6]

You can minimize your risk of exposure to inhaled asbestos fibers by leaving undamaged asbestos-containing materials alone, and by hiring qualified contractors to remove damaged asbestos. Before you remodel an old house, you should determine whether or not asbestos is present. If so, do not try to do the remodeling yourself. Never cut, rip, or use a sander on any material that contains asbestos. Some oven mitts, ironing board pads, and woodstove gaskets contain asbestos; you should follow manufacturer's recommendations for replacing and disposing of such materials as they become worn.[6]

Biological Pollutants

There are many sources of **biological air pollutants** within your personal environment. Disease-causing viruses and bacteria (common cold, flu, measles) are put into the air when infected people or animals sneeze or cough. Contaminated central air handling systems can be breeding grounds for mold, mildew, and bacteria and can then distribute these contaminants throughout the home. *Humidifier fever* is associated with exposure to toxins produced by microorganisms that can grow in ventilation systems.[7] *Legionnaire's disease* is a sometimes fatal pneumonia-like disease caused by bacteria that grow in moist indoor environments, such as air conditioning systems, cooling towers, showers, and whirlpool spas.[8] Some people have allergic reactions (itchy eyes, runny nose, sneezing, coughing, stuffy chest, shortness of breath, headache, and/or dizziness) to spores from mold that grows on moist surfaces inside buildings. Some research indicates that exposure to indoor mold can more than double your risk of developing adult onset asthma.[5] Pollen from plants around the home or workplace can cause allergic reactions (hay fever) in many people. Household pets, rats, mice, and cockroaches are sources of saliva, urine, feces, and skin dander that can also stimulate strong allergic reactions.[7]

You can minimize your exposure to biological indoor air pollutants by maintaining the relative humidity in your home within the range of 30% to 50%. This will minimize the growth of many microorganisms that can cause health problems. Control indoor air humidity by installing exhaust fans in bathrooms and kitchens (major sources of water vapor), venting places where water vapor accumulates (attics, basements, and crawl spaces), and using air conditioning or a dehumidifier. You should also eliminate standing water, rugs that have been damaged by leaks or floodwater, and any other wet surfaces.[7]

To minimize allergic reactions to biological indoor air pollutants, you should regularly clean and vacuum your home. While this will not completely eliminate dust mites, pollen, and animal dander, cleaning can substantially reduce the amounts of these allergens and the severity of allergy symptoms. Allergic individuals should leave the house while it is being vacuumed because this may temporarily increase airborne levels of mite allergens and other biological contaminants. You should also try to keep your house free of rodents and cockroaches as these pests are sources of potent allergens.[7]

Radon

Radon is an environmental health risk that seeps into buildings from the soil surrounding their foundation. It is invisible, odorless, and tasteless, and can be detected only by using radon detectors. Uranium, the source of radon, can be found in most parts of the world, and this element is present in rock and soil in parts of all fifty states of the United States. Once radon is produced by decay of uranium, this gas moves through the ground to the air above. Some radon gas may dissolve into groundwater. When radon undergoes radioactive decay, it emits radiation in the form of alpha particles and other by-products that are also radioactive. These radioactive by-products can attach to dust and other particles in the air and these particles can be inhaled.

It is estimated that indoor radon is at a level sufficient to increase risk of lung cancer in one of every fifteen homes in the United States.[9] The U.S. Surgeon General has warned that exposure to radon gas is the second leading cause of lung cancer in the United States. The National Academy of Sciences estimates that radon exposure causes about 15,000 lung cancer deaths in the United States every year.[10] This risk from radon is especially high for cigarette smokers. Lung damage is caused by radioactive particles formed as by-products from decay of radon

that are inhaled and trapped deep within the lungs. As the particles continue the radioactive decay process, they emit bursts of energy that damage adjacent lung tissue. There are no obvious short-term effects from this damage, but with long-term exposure this damage can cause lung cancer.[10] There is some evidence that consuming water that is contaminated by radon gas can increase the risk of stomach cancer. The National Academy of Sciences estimates consumption of radon in drinking water causes 19 stomach cancer deaths per year in the United States.[11]

The key to minimizing the health risk of radon exposure is to have your home tested. You can purchase an inexpensive "do-it-yourself" test kit in some hardware stores and other retail outlets. If you can't find a radon test kit locally, you can purchase one from the National Safety Council's Radon Hotline (800-767-7236). After the kit is exposed to the air in your home for a specified time period, it must be returned to a laboratory for analysis.

If unsafe levels of radon are detected in your home, you should work with a contractor who is certified to install a radon reduction system in your home. This will often involve installing a venting system just below the concrete slab of the house foundation. This venting system will intercept the radon gas before it enters your home and vent it outside the home where it can be dissipated by wind. You should also have cracks in the slab, basement walls, or foundation of the home repaired to reduce seepage of radon gas through these spaces. However, just sealing the cracks, without installing the belowground venting system, does not adequately reduce indoor radon levels. If you live in a region where high radon levels are common and you plan to build a new home, you should work with your contractor to install radon-resistant features during construction. The average cost to install radon-resistant features in an existing home is $800 to $2,500. The average cost to install radon-resistant features in a new home during construction is $350 to $500 (a 128% to 400% savings).[9] For a map of radon risk zones in the United States, see **http://www.epa.gov/iaq/radon/zonemap.html**.

Lead

Lead is a toxic metal that was widely used in house paint, as a gasoline additive, and in plumbing solder for metal

Key Terms

radon a naturally occurring radioactive gas that is emitted during the decay of uranium in soil, rock, and water.

pipes. As the health consequences of lead toxicity became better know, several of these uses of lead were banned, including lead-based house paint and leaded gasoline. However, lead is a very stable substance that remains in the environment today, long after its use was banned.

Lead exposure most commonly occurs in older homes, built before 1970. Many of these homes contain substantial amounts of lead-based paint, and older metal plumbing may contain lead solder. In late 1991, more than 10 years after lead-based paint was banned, the Secretary of the U.S. Department of Health and Human Services called lead, "the number one environmental threat to the health of children in the United States."[12] Exposure to lead from old paint occurs when the paint breaks down into paint flakes and dust, which are then inhaled or swallowed by children. Lead can also leach from solder in old plumbing and be ingested when people drink tap water.[12]

While lead additives in gasoline were banned by 1990, lead from automobile exhaust fumes was already deposited in soils and can still be found in high concentrations near major highways and city streets. Airborne dust from dirt tracked into the house on shoes can transfer this contaminant to the indoor environment.

Lead has serious health effects when ingested or inhaled, especially for children. Lead can affect virtually all organ systems of the body, but is particularly damaging to the nervous system, kidneys, and blood. *Acute lead toxicity* (blood lead level greater than 80 micrograms per deciliter) can lead to convulsions, coma, and death. However, blood lead levels as low as 10 micrograms per deciliter in children can delay physical and mental development, lower IQ, reduce attention span, and increase behavioral problems.[12]

You can minimize your exposure to lead by replacing deteriorated lead house paint and lead soldered plumbing, and by keeping your home clean of roadside dirt that

may be contaminated with residual lead from automobile exhaust. If the lead-based paint in your old house is in good condition, leave it alone; it does not pose a hazard *if it is intact.* However, if the old paint is flaking or producing paint dust, you should have it removed by a contractor that is certified for lead abatement. Do not try to remove lead-based paint yourself, as you may inhale large amounts of paint dust or volatilized lead.

If you are exposed to lead contamination, eating a balanced diet that is rich in calcium and iron can reduce the effects of lead toxicity.[12] If you live in an older house with metal plumbing, you should have the tap water tested for lead. Lead is not readily excreted by the body, and will tend to accumulate over time. There are chelating drug treatments that help the body to excrete lead and reduce toxicity effects, but they have adverse side effects and are generally used only to treat acute lead toxicity.[13]

Drinking Water

The safety of drinking water in your home is affected by environmental factors both in the home or neighborhood and in the larger community. The water supply for rural homes is often a well that draws from groundwater, and can be much affected by environmental conditions around the home and neighborhood. In urban areas a municipal water supply system draws from rivers or lakes and then treats the water to make it safe to drink. The community/regional environment plays the dominant role in determining the safety of water from municipal suppliers. However, municipal water can be contaminated by the personal environment as it passes through pipes in the home. Environmental health issues relating to drinking water as influenced by conditions in your home and neighborhood will be covered here. Issues related to municipal water supply are presented later in this chapter.

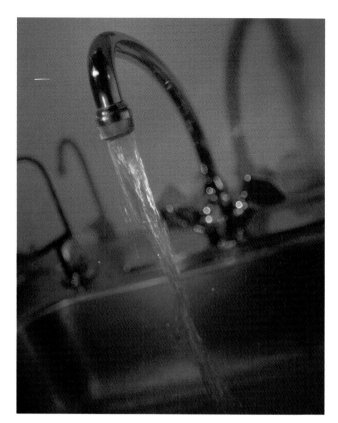

Tap water is a key source of pollutants in the home.

Approximately 23 million people in the United States obtain their drinking water from groundwater (i.e., from private wells), streams, or cisterns that collect rainwater.[14] These households are responsible for ensuring the safety of their own drinking water. Private drinking water supplies that rely on surface waters, or wells that tap shallow groundwater layers, are at risk of contamination by pathogens from home septic systems, contaminants from leaking underground fuel storage tanks, improper disposal of various household chemicals (cleaners, automotive fluids, and pesticides), and agricultural chemicals applied to surrounding farm fields.

Nitrate from agricultural fertilizer that leaches into shallow groundwater supplies poses a widespread health risk in rural areas. The U.S. Geological Survey estimates that 10% to 20% of groundwater sources of drinking water may have levels of nitrate contamination that pose risks to human health.[15] Excessive consumption of nitrate in contaminated drinking water can cause serious illness and death. Nitrate interferes with the oxygen-transport function of the blood (methemoglobinemia). This effect is most pronounced in children, resulting in "blue-baby" syndrome.[15,16] Nitrate can also cause reproductive problems and is linked to development of several types of cancer.[15]

Rural wells contaminated by nitrate may also have high levels of other agricultural chemicals. Some researchers have suggested that agricultural pesticides and herbicides can contribute to the development of testicular cancer and reduced sperm production in men, breast cancer in women, and nervous system disorders in children.[17]

Leaching of substances from pipes in the plumbing of older homes is another potential source of contamination to drinking water in the home.[18] Metallic pipes can release toxic metals such as lead and copper into the water. Polyvinyl chloride (PVC) pipes manufactured before 1977 may release toxic vinyl chloride into the water. Vinyl chloride is a known human carcinogen.

Leaching of toxic substances from pipes into the drinking water supply is most problematic in small diameter pipes (less than a 2-inch diameter), with high water temperatures, and when the water is stagnant in the pipes for long periods (more than 24 hours).[18] A relatively easy way to reduce contaminants from household plumbing in your drinking water is to regularly flush fresh water through the plumbing. Let the water run from the tap for a couple of minutes before taking water to drink, especially first thing in the morning and if you have been away from home for long time periods. In some cases it may be advisable to replace the old plumbing, but this can be very expensive.

Private water supplies should be tested annually for nitrate and **fecal coliform bacteria.** If you suspect there may be a problem with radon or pesticide contamination, you may need to test your water even more frequently.[14] Testing will generally require that you send samples of your water to a laboratory that tests water quality. You can get a listing of local certified laboratories from your local or state public health department. Some local health departments test private water for free. A private laboratory will charge $10 to $20 to perform a nitrate and bacteria test. Testing for pesticides or organic chemicals may cost from several hundred to several thousand dollars. Most laboratories mail back the sample results within a few days, or several weeks if the analyses are more complex. The results will indicate the concentrations of contaminants and indicate whether each contaminant exceeds a drinking water quality standard.

If your drinking water contains contaminants that exceed safety standards, you should retest the water supply immediately and contact your public health department for assistance. High bacteria concentrations can sometimes be easily controlled by disinfecting a well. Water filters may also remove some contaminants. However, other problems may require a new source of water, such as a deeper well. Alternatively, you may need to rely on bottled water until a new water source can be obtained.[14] You can obtain technical assistance with residential drinking water supply problems from the organization Farm*A*Syst/ Home*A*Syst (see the websites **http://www.uwex.edu/ farmasyst** or **http://www.uwex.edu/homeasyst**).

Noise

Noise can be defined as any undesirable sound. What constitutes "undesirable sound" will vary from one person to the next, but it often involves loud sounds that occur at irregular intervals and are not controllable by the listener.[19] In the personal environment of the home, neighborhood, and workplace, noise may include overly loud music, barking dogs, motorcycles and cars with broken or missing muffler systems, loud machinery, appliances and power tools, airplanes flying overhead, and train whistles.

The health effects of environmental noise depend on the intensity, frequency, and nature of the noise. Excessively loud noise can cause physical damage to sensory tissues in your ears, resulting in partial or total hearing loss that can be temporary or permanent. This physical damage will depend on both the intensity (as measured in decibels) and the duration of exposure to the loud noise. For example, sitting in front of the speaker column at a large rock concert, with noise levels at 120 decibels for over 2 hours, can result in immediate pain and long-term or permanent hearing loss. Ironically, the tissues that are damaged by excessively loud sounds are those responsible for hearing high frequency sounds associated with nor-

mal conversation, not the tissues that actually hear the damaging sound. Loud noise sources rob you of one of your most important senses, the ability to hear the unamplified human voice.

Even noise at lower levels can cause adverse health effects. The American Speech-Language-Hearing Association reports that low level noise can elevate blood pressure, reduce sleep, cause fatigue, and disturb digestion. These physical effects of low level noise can impact emotional, intellectual, social, and occupational health. Effects reported by the World Health Organization include increased frustration and anxiety, impaired ability to concentrate, reduced productivity and ability to learn, and increased absenteeism and accidents. These effects of noise can increase your feeling of stress and diminish your ability to tolerate minor irritations; you may exhibit anger and aggression that are out of proportion to the immediate source of your irritation.[19] This antisocial behavior may have negative consequences in your personal relationships and occupational health.

A common source of long-term exposure to loud sound that causes hearing loss in many young people is amplified music. Occasional loud rock music at 110 to 120 decibels may cause only temporary damage. However, daily exposure to such sound levels will cause permanent hearing loss. A number of aging rock stars have admitted to significant hearing loss that they attribute to standing in front of huge amplifiers night after night. Many rock musicians performing today stand behind the main speaker columns or wear ear protection. Jacking up the volume in your headphones, or the powerful amplifier in your car stereo, may be fun today, but is it worth a lifetime of incessant ringing in your ears and diminished hearing later in life? See Changing for the Better on page 656 for tips on reducing health risks associated with noise pollution.

The Community and Regional Environment

The community and regional environment is comprised of the outdoor air you breathe, local rivers and lakes that provide water and recreation opportunities, surrounding lands (urban, industrial, suburban, rural, agricultural, natural communities), and all the people and other

---

Key Terms

fecal coliform bacteria a category of bacteria that live within the intestines of warm-blooded animals; the presence of these bacteria is used as an indicator that water has been contaminated by feces.

Changing for the Better

Reducing Health Risks of Noise Pollution

What is all the fuss about a little noise? It's not like noise can hurt you, right?

In addition to limiting your exposure to loud music, there are a number of other actions you can take to reduce your personal contribution to noise pollution and to protect yourself against adverse health effects from noise, including:

1. Keep the sound-muffling components of your vehicle exhaust system in proper working order.
2. If your dog is outdoors barking, bring it inside. It is not fair to your neighbors to just let it bark. If the barking problem persists, consider various products and programs that train your dog to stop barking.
3. Avoid using power tools, lawn mowers, leaf blowers, and loud power boats, or playing loud music in the late evening or early morning.
4. If you work around loud machinery or power tools, or regularly shoot firearms, always use ear plugs or sound-absorbing earmuffs.
5. Furnish your home and work space with sound-absorbing materials, such as carpeting, heavy drapes, and cork wall and ceiling tiles.
6. Choose the location of your residence to minimize the number of potential sources of irritating noise. There is a reason why the rent or purchase price for a residence near a major highway or airport is usually cheaper than at a location with fewer sources of noise.

For more information about reducing noise pollution:
http://www.nonoise.org

species that live in these areas. A wide range of human activities can degrade this community environment in ways that affect personal health. Air, water, and land pollution include many substances that have significant negative effects on physical health. Loss of natural areas and other recreational and aesthetic "green space" to roads, cities, and industrial development can adversely affect your perceived quality of life, with negative effects on emotional and spiritual health. Degraded environmental conditions in many communities discourage new economic development and may limit occupational health.

While you can exert some influence on the environmental conditions in your community, the influence of any one individual is usually small. Your control over how the community environment affects your personal health is often limited to controlling your exposure to known health risks, such as contaminated water and land, or out-

door air pollution. You can also choose to reduce your own contributions to community/regional air, water, and land pollution through conservation of energy and water and recycling solid waste.

Because one person cannot have a significant impact on community environmental problems, many people join organizations that work to improve the environment and quality of life in their community. By working with others of like mind in the political process and in environmental organizations, you become "part of the solution" to major environmental problems that can affect your health and that of your family. For many people, getting involved in solving local environmental problems can provide significant benefits to emotional and spiritual health.

In this section you will learn about aspects of the community and regional environment that can affect your health, and what you can do to exert some level of personal control over these environmental influences.

Air Pollution

Air pollution includes substances that naturally occur in the air (pollen, microbes, dust, sea salt, volcanic ash) and substances produced by human activities (engine exhaust, ozone, various volatile organic compounds, and acid rain). In this section on community and regional environmental influences on health, we focus on those components of air pollution that are produced within a specific region and that have substantial health effects within that community or region.

The primary sources of human-caused air pollutants are various kinds of internal combustion engines associated with electric power plants, industry, and transportation (trucks, automobiles, and farm/construction equipment). Oil refineries and chemical production factories also contribute to air pollution in some communities. Electric power stations, industrial facilities, and chemical factories are classified as *point sources* that produce large amounts of pollution from a single location. Automobiles, trucks, heavy construction/farm equipment, gas stations, lawn mowers, and charcoal grills are *nonpoint sources* of air pollutants. Individually, nonpoint sources produce relatively small amounts of pollution, but when added together account for a large proportion of community air pollution.

Air pollutants that are directly produced by internal combustion engines include *carbon monoxide, nitrogen*

Key Terms

air pollution refers to a wide variety of substances found in the atmosphere that can have adverse effects on human health, crop productivity, and natural communities.

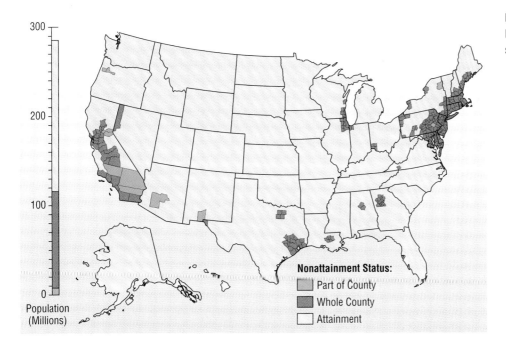

Figure 20-2 Counties classified by EPA as in "nonattainment" of ozone standards in the year 2003.

Nonattainment Status:
- Part of County
- Whole County
- Attainment

dioxide, sulfur dioxide, hydrocarbons and *particulate matter.* Carbon monoxide is a toxic gas that impairs respiration, as described under indoor air quality in the previous section. Nitrogen and sulfur oxides interact with water vapor in the air to form small particulates (diameter < 2.5 μm) that are inhaled into the deepest parts of the lungs. These substances can damage lung tissues, reduce lung capacity, cause coughing and chronic bronchitis, and make worse such ailments as hypersensitivity to allergens, asthma, emphysema, and heart disease. The U.S. Environmental Protection Agency estimates that over 70 million people in the United States live in counties where levels of small particulate air pollutants exceed human health standards for at least some part of the year.[23] It has been estimated that small particulate air pollution causes as many as 50,000 to 100,000 premature deaths in the United States per year.[21] In addition to these direct effects, nitrogen oxides may act as a fertilizer, stimulating pollen production in many plant species (such as ragweed) and worsen pollen-related allergic reactions in humans.[15]

Tropospheric ozone is another important regional air pollutant that is linked to chemicals in exhaust fumes from internal combustion engines. This substance is produced when hydrocarbons, nitrogen oxides, and other small particle matter chemically interact in the presence of sunlight. The result is a brownish haze over affected cities, often called *smog.*

Ozone levels are particularly high in locations with warm, sunny climates (Southern California) and where natural vegetation produces volatile organic compounds that contribute to the photochemical process that produces ozone (eastern U.S.). The U.S. Environmental Protection Agency estimates that over 110 million people in the United States live in counties where ozone levels exceed human health standards for at least some part of the year.[20] Most of these people live in Southern California and near the East Coast between Virginia and southern Maine (see Figure 20-2).

Inhalation of ozone can cause lung damage that reduces lung capacity. This is a particular health risk to individuals who suffer from asthma, emphysema, or heart disease. On days when ozone concentrations are highest, local hospital emergency room visits associated with respiratory distress increase from 10% to 20%.[22] There is also some evidence that childhood exposure to ozone can actually cause children to become asthmatic.[23]

Air toxics are a diverse collection of hazardous air pollutants produced mainly by electric power plants and

---

Key Terms

tropospheric ozone ozone is comprised of three oxygen atoms that are bound into a single molecule; tropospheric ozone refers to this substance as it occurs in the lower layer of the atmosphere, close to the ground.

air toxics a class of 188 toxic air pollutants identified by the U.S. Environmental Protection Agency as known or suspected causes of cancer or other serious health effects, such as reduced fertility, birth defects, or adverse environmental effects.

Smog over a major U.S. city.

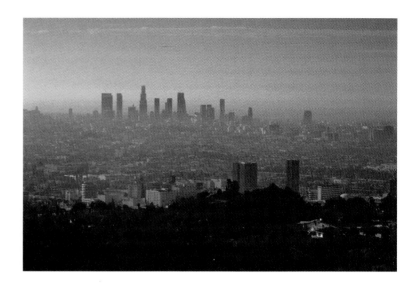

industrial sources that constitute a widespread environmental health risk in the United States. When lifetime cancer risks for all carcinogenic air toxics are combined, 200 million people in the U.S. live in counties where that risk exceeds 10 in one million, and 20 million people live in areas where the risk exceeds 100 in one million.[24] However, these risk estimates are based on a lifetime of exposure to toxic air pollutant levels as they were last inventoried in 1996. With continued progress on reducing toxic air pollution, risks associated with air toxics might be expected to decrease in the future. Since Congress passed the Clean Air Act in 1970, substantial progress has been made in reducing most human-caused air pollution in the U.S. However, further reduction of air pollution poses serious technological and/or economic challenges, and efforts to strengthen regulations often face tough political opposition. For more information about air toxics, go to the U.S. EPA website **http://www.epa.gov/ttn/atw.**

Unfortunately, the degree to which you can control your own exposure to regional air pollution and the associated health risks is limited. In many larger urban areas, where air pollution levels are highest, weather reports in newspapers and on television often include information about air pollution. This is because weather conditions have a strong influence on air pollution levels. Hot, dry weather promotes tropospheric ozone formation. When there is little wind, or when there is limited vertical mixing of the atmosphere, air pollutants are not dispersed and can accumulate to dangerous levels near the ground. If you live in a large city, you should pay attention to air pollution information. This information is often conveyed in color-coded alerts. A "yellow" air pollution alert means people who suffer from respiratory or cardiac diseases, or hypersensitivity to allergens, should stay indoors. An "orange" air pollution alert indicates that everyone should limit their outdoor activities to the minimum possible.

You can also help to lower air pollution levels by limiting contributions from your own automobile, lawn mower exhaust, and charcoal grill. You can carpool, use mass transit, or telecommute (work at home via a computer network) to reduce air pollution associated with automobile exhaust. You can fill your car gas tank, mow your lawn, and use your grill during the cooler evening hours to reduce your contribution to tropospheric ozone. You can conserve electricity to reduce emissions of air toxics, sulfur and nitrogen oxides, and particulates from electric power plants. In areas of the United States where air pollution is especially problematic, local laws may require that you do some of these things on days when conditions result in a "pollution emergency."

Water Pollution

Humankind has had a very schizophrenic relationship with our rivers and lakes. Water is an essential resource for all living things on our planet, including humans and the plants and animals we use for food. We also value our rivers and lakes for the recreational opportunities and aesthetic benefits they provide. Yet for decades, we used these water bodies as convenient dumps for our sewage and industrial wastes.

The problem of water pollution came to national attention on a day in 1968 when children playing with matches set on fire chemical pollutants that covered the Cuyahoga River in Ohio. The subsequent public outcry resulted in major national legislation, including the Clean Water Act of 1972 and the Safe Drinking Water Act of 1974. Since then, substantial progress has been made in reducing water pollution and insuring safe drinking water supplies.

The job of cleaning rivers and lakes in the U.S. is not complete, and people who come in close contact with contaminated waters or fish from these areas are still at risk for a variety of health problems. Water pollutants in surface waters come from obvious point sources (sewer overflows, confined livestock feedlot operations, sometimes called "factory farms") and from nonpoint sources such as water runoff from urban streets and agricultural areas that carries various chemicals and animal waste into local rivers. In some areas, water drainage from mines carries toxic metals into nearby streams. Toxic air pollutants can be deposited into water bodies in rainfall. Some of the most troublesome water pollutants in the U.S. today are described below.

Biological water pollutants from untreated sewage and drainage from leaking home septic systems include various species of disease-causing viruses, bacteria, and protozoa found in rivers and lakes. These organisms cause diseases that are at best uncomfortable (diarrhea) and at worst potentially lethal (dysentery, hepatitis, typhoid fever, and cholera). In the late 1800s, diseases associated with drinking water contaminated by biological pollution were the third leading cause of death in the United States.[25]

The largest sources of biological water pollutants in surface waters of the U.S. today are overflows from combined septic and storm sewers during heavy rainfall events, and animal wastes that are carried by runoff of rainfall from agricultural areas. While much has already been done to eliminate biological contamination from municipal sewer systems, billions of dollars are still required to dig up old combined sewer systems and replace them with separate systems for sewage and storm water runoff. As large animal "factory farms" have become more common in rural America, government agencies have established regulations for the proper handling of the huge amounts of animal sewage that are generated. Even so, violations of regulations and occasional accidents result in contamination of local surface waters with animal waste.

At present, your personal risk of exposure to biological water pollution in the United States is relatively small. Public health departments monitor local surface waters for the presence of fecal coliform bacteria in every county in the U.S. While they may or may not cause illness or disease, the presence of fecal coliform organisms is an indicator that water has been contaminated by sewage. All municipal drinking water systems, and many private households, in the U.S. treat their water to kill pathogenic organisms. By the end of the 20th century, deaths due to water pathogens in the drinking water supply were very rare in the United States.[25]

A wide variety of other **toxic pollutants** can be found in surface and groundwater sources of drinking water. These substances include naturally occurring toxic elements (such as arsenic and mercury) produced by breakdown of minerals in certain kinds of rock. Various human activities produce a wide range of toxic chemicals that find their way into surface waters of the U.S., including metals, solvents, plastics, and PCBs (polychlorinated biphenols). Some toxic substances have both natural and human-caused sources, including arsenic and mercury.

Agricultural pesticides can be significant toxic water pollutants in parts of the United States where large areas of land are used for crop production. These chemicals include insecticides, fungicides, and herbicides to kill organisms that consume or compete with crop plants. While these chemicals are applied to croplands, they are often carried into local streams and rivers by runoff of rainfall.

While the dumping of toxic substances into surface waters is now illegal, some of these toxins are very stable and can be found in large quantities in the sediments of rivers and lakes that were polluted before 1972. Cleaning up these toxic sediments can be very costly. A recent decision to dredge and dispose of PCB-contaminated sediments in the Hudson River near Albany, New York, will cost hundreds of millions of dollars.

Health effects of agricultural chemicals and other toxic substances depend on the specific chemical.[27] Taken as a group, these substances have been linked to adverse effects on the blood, liver, spleen, kidney, adrenal gland, thyroid gland, reproductive system (fertility), and cardiovascular system. Some are known or suspected human *carcinogens* (substances that cause cancer), *mutagens* (substances that cause cell mutations), or *teratogens* (substances that cause birth defects). Obvious health effects that occur immediately after exposure to high concentrations of these substances include nausea, fatigue, headache, skin and eye irritation, or tremors. The risks for these adverse immediate health effects are greatest for workers who come in direct contact with the concentrated chemicals. More insidious are health effects such as cancer and birth defects that develop slowly, imperceptibly, after long-term exposure to low concentrations of these chemicals in the environment.

Many toxic chemicals and pesticides also have adverse consequences for natural systems, causing declines and extinctions of species and degradation of biological communities and ecosystems. For example, DDT was a widely used insecticide that has been blamed for the near extinction of many large bird species, including eagles, hawks, falcons, condors, and pelicans. While this was not a direct impact on human physical health, many people felt that the decline of these and other wildlife species diminished their emotional and spiritual health.

> ### Key Terms
>
> **biological water pollutants** disease-causing organisms that are found in water.
>
> **toxic pollutants** substances known to cause cancer or other serious health effects.

The best way for you to minimize physical health risks posed by consuming biological or toxic contaminants is to be well informed. Read the annual water quality report from your municipal water supplier. If your water supplier fails to meet health standards, consider drinking bottled, boiled, or filtered water until the supplier fixes the problems.

The U.S. Environmental Protection Agency has set **maximum contaminant level (MCL)** standards for the amounts of the biological pollutants, pesticides, and toxic chemicals that are allowed in municipal drinking water supplies.[25] MCLs are set at levels that minimize human health risks, but also take into account the limits of available treatment technology and the costs of meeting the standards. Municipal water suppliers are required to report any violations of MCLs to state and federal environmental agencies.

Many municipal water suppliers will provide consumers with annual reports that list the amounts of biological contaminants, agricultural pesticides, and toxic substances that are detected in their water. If your supplier does not provide a report, you can access the supplier's annual report to the U.S. Environmental Protection Agency at **http://www.epa.gov/safewater/dwinfo.htm**. These reports list the mean and range (minimum and maximum) concentrations for all regulated contaminants for all samples analyzed in a year. Look at the maximum value to determine if your water system occasionally fails to adequately remove any regulated contaminants.

You can also be exposed to toxic substances by eating contaminated fish or wild game. Some toxic substances, such as mercury and PCBs, accumulate to high levels in the bodies of shellfish, fish, and waterfowl that consume contaminated water. This problem can occur even in remote, apparently pristine areas if there are natural sources of toxic substances such as mercury. People who regularly consume wild food animals from contaminated waters may be at high risk of adverse health effects.

To reduce health risks associated with consuming wild game, you should be aware of health advisories for consuming contaminated fish or game. These advisories are often stated in terms of limits on how much fish or meat should be consumed in a specified time period. Pregnant women should be especially careful of consuming shellfish, fish, or wild game; mercury and PCBs can cause birth defects in the fetus they carry. These health advisories are usually issued by the public health department or state agencies responsible for fish and game.

You can also be exposed to waterborne pollutants, with associated health risks, as a result of recreational activities, such as swimming, boating, and backpacking. You can limit your personal risk of exposure to health risks from contaminated water by being aware of "Don't swim" warnings for your local rivers and lakes, usually issued by

the public health department. If you are backpacking in an apparently pristine wilderness area, never assume that crystal clear water in the mountain stream is safe to drink. Backpackers should always filter, boil, or chemically treat drinking water to kill pathogens that may be present even in such remote water sources.

 TALKING POINTS How can you approach your political representatives about environmental policy? What are some effective ways of keeping health-related environmental issues on the national agenda?

Land Pollution

We do not consume land or soil into our bodies the way we do air and water, but pollution of land can still result in serious adverse health effects. Disposal of toxic wastes often involves burying them in the ground. When done with proper safeguards, this disposal method can isolate these dangerous materials so they can do no harm to humans or natural systems. If done improperly, these toxic pollutants leach into groundwater or are carried into surface waters by the runoff of rain, where they cause serious ecological problems and pose significant human health risks.

Occasionally, housing developments are built on top of old toxic waste disposal sites, and the residents are exposed to toxic substances by inhaling or swallowing contaminated dust and soil, drinking contaminated water, or through chemicals leaching into their basements. One of the worst cases of such a mistake was the infamous Love Canal incident in New York State during the 1970s.[26] Schools and housing developments were built near an abandoned waste disposal site, into which many different toxic chemicals and sewage had been deposited. Children swimming in contaminated water holes suffered from skin lesions. Families living in the houses had children born with birth defects. In the end, the state of New York bought the homes and moved the families to other locations. While toxic waste disposal is now strictly regulated, and old toxic waste dumps are being cleaned up under the EPA Superfund program, there remain thousands of sites like Love Canal around the United States. These toxic

---

Key Terms

maximum contaminant level (MCL) the highest concentration of a contaminant that is allowed in drinking water, as established and regulated by the U.S. Environmental Protection Agency.

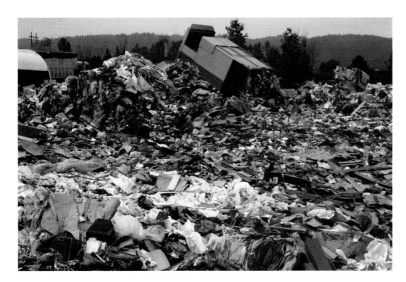

Finding someplace to put our garbage will continue to present a major environmental and health dilemma as we progress into the twenty-first century. Solid waste buried in landfills can pollute the surrounding air and water, creating health risks for people and wildlife that live in the surrounding areas.

waste sites are ticking time bombs waiting for ignorant or unscrupulous developers and unwary homebuyers.

Most land pollution today is associated with the disposal of **solid waste.** *Municipal solid waste* consists of everyday items such as product packaging, grass clippings, furniture, clothing, bottles, food scraps, newspapers, appliances, paint, and batteries. Other solid waste produced by business and industry includes waste tires, concrete, asphalt, bricks, lumber, and shingles from demolished buildings, and *sewage sludge* (solids remaining after wastewater treatment). In 1999 the U.S. population produced 230 million tons of solid waste, or about 4.6 pounds of waste per person per day (or 1,680 pounds per person per year).[27]

Municipal sanitation departments and private disposal companies are very efficient at removing these wastes from our homes and businesses and putting them someplace where we don't see them. These waste disposal locations include sanitary landfills (wastes are compacted and buried under soil), ocean dumping in garbage barges (with trash sometimes escaping to wash up on beaches), and incinerators (where solid wastes are burned).

While out-of-sight often means out-of-mind, these solid wastes do not "go away," but rather, they accumulate. Many municipal and regional sanitary landfills are reaching their capacity and must be closed. No one wants a new landfill located near their home, so it is politically and legally difficult to locate new landfills. Sometimes wealthy states pay to export their solid wastes to landfills in poorer states that have weaker environmental regulations. Sometimes, toxic wastes are shipped to poor underdeveloped countries with no environmental regulations. However, even these poorer countries are beginning to realize that accepting toxic wastes in return for money does not serve their long-term best interests and some have banned this practice.

As we run out of places to dump our solid waste, some have proposed that we burn it in large incinerators. However, many concerns have been raised about incinerators because they can release toxic substances into the atmosphere. Furthermore, the ash from these incinerators contains concentrated toxic chemicals in forms that can easily leach into ground and surface waters.

Most of the potential health effects of land pollution have already been described in this chapter under the topics of air and water pollution. Most human exposure to pollutants that are deposited on land occurs when those toxic substances end up in the air or water. You can limit your risk of these health effects by being aware of where solid wastes are disposed, both at the present time and in the past. You should be particularly aware of proximity to a local landfill or waste disposal site if your water source is a private well that draws from groundwater that might be contaminated. Municipal water systems are required to regularly monitor their water for pollutants. If your water comes from a private well, it is very much in your best interests to do likewise.

You can reduce your personal contribution to the solid waste problem of your community by following the Three R's: Reduce, Reuse, Recycle. You can reduce the amount of solid waste you produce by consuming less and

Key Terms

solid waste pollutants that are in solid form, including nonhazardous household trash, industrial wastes, mining wastes, and sewage sludge from wastewater treatment plants.

The High-Tech Revolution and E-Waste

The much heralded high-tech revolution has a hidden dark side, mountains of accumulating obsolete electronic equipment that contain large amounts of toxic substances. During the period from 1997 to 2007, it is estimated that over 500 million computers must be disposed of. These computers will contain 6.2 billion pounds of plastic, 1.6 billion pounds of lead, 3 million pounds of cadmium, 1.9 million pounds of chromium, and 632,000 pounds of mercury. Lead, cadmium, chromium, and mercury are highly toxic metals, and can cause a wide range of severe health effects if they end up in the air, drinking water, or food supply.[1,2]

Computers contain over 1,000 different substances, many of which are toxic. This makes recycling a complex, labor-intensive process that can cost more than the value of the recycled materials. Only 6% of obsolete computers disposed of after 1998 were recycled. The remainder was deposited in landfills across the country. It is estimated that 70% of heavy metals such as lead and mercury going into U.S. landfills today comes from electronic waste. Several states, including California and Massachusetts, have banned disposal of computer monitors in landfills to protect groundwater.[1]

While recycling of computers is seen as the ideal solution to the problem of waste disposal, it is estimated that 50% to 80% of computers "recycled" before the year 2002

were actually shipped to poor Asian countries. Workers in these countries disassemble computers to recover useful materials for very low wages and with minimal or no protection from the toxic materials to which they are exposed. These countries have weak or poorly enforced environmental regulations, so materials that cannot be recycled are dumped into rivers or burned in open air pits. These practices expose the recycling workers and surrounding local populations to toxic substances. In one city in China, river water had 190 times the pollution levels allowed under World Health Organization standards, and drinking water had to be transported from 18 miles away.[1]

The practice of shipping toxic computer waste to underdeveloped countries is now banned by an international treaty, but the United States is the only developed nation that has not ratified this treaty. The "free market" justification for the practice of shipping toxic computer waste to underdeveloped countries is that this provides jobs and helps poor people. The question is whether or not it is moral to give poor people the choice between poverty or poisons?[1]

Given that the use of computers and electronics will only increase in the future, many argue that we must develop environmentally responsible computer recycling systems. In 2002 Rep. Mike Thompson introduced The Computer Hazardous-Waste Infrastructure

Program (CHIP) Act that would require the Environmental Protection Agency to help set up computer recycling across the United States. The program would be funded by a fee of up to $10 on all retail sales of desktop and laptop PCs and computer monitors. Similar legislation is also appearing in many state legislatures. The electronics industry does not favor charging consumers a fee on new computers, but rather wants to charge consumers the fee when they return their old computers to the manufacturer. Some computer manufacturers are already initiating computer take-back programs. However, development of a comprehensive national strategy for responsibly addressing the computer waste problem continues as of this writing.

The other, and perhaps most important, approach to the computer waste problem is to develop electronic equipment that is less toxic and more easily recycled. This will require development of, and investment in, new technologies. In our free market system, this will happen only when the electronics manufacturers must share the cost of dealing with computer waste.

[1]Puckett J, et al. Exporting Harm:The High-Tech Trashing of Asia. The Basal Action Network and Silicon Valley Toxics Coalition, 2002.
[2]U.S. Environmental Protection Agency. WasteWise Update: Electronics Reuse and Recycling, 2003. **http://www.epa.gov/wastewise/pubs/wwupda14.pdf**

---

accepting less packaging materials on the products you buy. You can compost your yard waste for use as a mulch and fertilizer in flower beds, or use a lawn mower with a mulching blade to eliminate grass clippings and leaves in the autumn. Reusing items such as bottles, zipper-closure storage bags, cloth shopping bags, and cloth diapers reduces the amount of solid waste you throw away each week. Many items in typical household trash (newspapers and magazines, aluminum and steel cans, glass bottles, and many plastic containers) can be recycled and the materials used to make new products. Diverting these solid wastes away from the landfill toward reuse can greatly reduce the solid waste problem of your community. However, recycling will only work if you also buy products that are made from recycled materials, such as recycled paper and plastic "wood" products.

Loss of Green Space

Loss of **green space** represents another kind of land pollution that can affect your quality of life and health. In many parts of the United States, green space is being converted to housing developments, shopping malls, industrial

> ### Key Terms
>
> **green space** areas of land that are dominated by domesticated or natural vegetation, including rural farmland, city lawns and parks, and nature preserves.

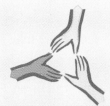

Learning from Our Diversity

Native Americans and the Environment

An essay by David Lewis, in *Native America in the Twentieth Century: An Encyclopedia,* published in 1994 by Garland Publishers of New York, describes the historical and modern environmental ethic of Native Americans. Many early environmentalists were inspired by their perceptions of the close relationship between Native Americans and their natural environment. Before contact with Euroamericans, Native American cultures perceived that their spiritual and physical universes were one. They felt connected with the animate and inanimate beings of their environment, and managed its bounty carefully so as not to upset the spirits who kept their world in balance and supplied all necessary resources. They acknowledged the power of the Earth and considered the hunter and hunted as equal partners in the larger scheme of things. They practiced rituals with the animals they killed, the agricultural fields they tended, and the resources they consumed to ensure a continued supply.

Romantic modern misconceptions that Native Americans "left no mark on the land" ignore much cultural and historical evidence that they used fire and water to transform their landscapes.* When necessary, Native Americans adjusted their environments to meet their cultural and material needs. However, Native Americans were careful students of their functional environments. They strived for maximum sustained yield, not maximum production. Their use of natural resources was based on reciprocity and balance.* This approach to stewardship of natural resources is certainly worthy of admiration, and a worthy goal for modern society.

Modern Native American communities are often far removed from their traditional land ethic, a fact that sometimes places them at odds with environmentalists. However, environmental problems on Native American lands must be placed in the perspective of the total destruction of their cultures and environment at the hands of Euroamericans. There are instances when control of natural resources on Indian reservations has been returned to Native Americans, with disastrous environmental consequences. However, these Native American communities have been forced to live on remote, marginal lands, with few

apparent natural resources, and lacking virtually all the native plants and animal species upon which their traditional practices depended. These communities suffer in the depths of poverty, and sometimes seek any economic development regardless of the environmental cost. In desperation, some accept toxic waste dumps onto their lands, and others strip the land of its forests to meet the immediate needs of their communities. Often, these environmentally destructive decisions are made by Euroamerican government agents on behalf of their Native American clients.

Another point of disagreement between Native Americans and modern environmentalists involves traditional hunting of species that are now considered threatened or endangered, such as the bald eagle, bowhead whale, and Florida panther. The rights of Native Americans to these traditional hunting practices, intimately connected with their religion and culture, is protected by the American Indian Religious Freedom Act of 1978. Environmentalists who oppose these hunts seem to pick and choose which Native American traditions to admire and which to condemn. They fail to recognize that the religious practice of the hunts is part of a larger tradition that motivated Native Americans to seek balance with their environment.

As Native American communities struggle to meet their most basic needs and maintain their cultural traditions in a hostile modern world, we should be careful about harshly judging their departures from traditional land ethics. There is a diversity of opinion within Native American communities, just as in other communities. Some people seek to be modern, while others yearn for the traditional values of an earlier day. Traditional land ethics are much more recent history for Native Americans than are similar, pre-Christian, Earth-centered religions of Euroamericans. Nonetheless, both communities struggle with the question of how best to manage our environment for present and future generations.

*Lewis DR. Essay on Native American Environmental Issues. In: *Native Americans and the Environment.* 2000. **http://www.cnie.org/nae/docs/intro.html**

---

sites, and highways. Hundreds of large, brightly lit signs along the highways pollute the visual environment. Wildlife species disappear from your community and surroundings as their habitats are destroyed.

While development of green space for human uses may provide job opportunities and be beneficial for your occupational health, it can also detract from recreational and aesthetic aspects of your community. If you find that you must travel farther and longer from home or work to find a safe and enjoyable location to jog or bicycle, you may exercise less often. Your sense of "quality of life" is diminished when you no longer see wild

animals in your backyard or you feel that your community is becoming ugly. Many people feel their emotional and spiritual health are diminished when formerly green space is converted to asphalt parking lots and commercial buildings.

Some communities have created land-use (zoning) plans that allow for economic development while protecting recreational and aesthetic values in their communities. These zoning plans can be controversial, as they try to balance the rights of private property owners with the welfare of the entire community. You can contribute toward protecting environmental quality in your community by supporting land-use planning and enforceable zone laws that protect green space while allowing for responsible economic development.

Radiation

Radiation is a general term that refers to various forms of energy that are emitted by atoms and molecules when they undergo change, including radio waves, infrared, visible light, ultraviolet, X-rays, and gamma rays. Each kind of radiation has different effects on biological materials and health. **Ionizing radiation** causes damage to biological structures such as DNA that can result in serious adverse health effects. Ionizing radiation is produced by nuclear reactions, and sources include medical X-rays, naturally occurring radioactive minerals such as uranium, various radioactive materials used by industry, nuclear reactors and their waste products, and nuclear bomb explosions. **Non-ionizing radiation** most commonly causes adverse health effects simply by heating tissues, resulting in burns. These effects are generally less severe than the effects from ionizing radiation. Sources of non-ionizing radiation include sunlight and electromagnetic fields generated by all electrical and electronic devices. (See Focus On article on page 676 for more on non-ionizing radiation).

The health effects of exposure to X-rays and gamma radiation depend on many factors, including the duration, type, and dose of radiation, and your individual sensitivity. Heavy exposure to these forms of radiation can occur if you are near a nuclear bomb blast or downwind of a major nuclear reactor accident. In such cases, exposure can cause *radiation sickness,* including intense fatigue, nausea, weight loss, hair loss, fever, bleeding from the mouth, and compromised immune system, usually resulting in death.

On April 26, 1986, a major nuclear reactor accident at the Chernobyl nuclear power plant in the Soviet Union exposed hundreds of thousands of people to nuclear radiation. Leading Soviet scientists estimate that 10,000 miners and soldiers who sealed the damaged nuclear reactor immediately after the accident died of radiation sickness. Over 200,000 people in the surrounding communities had to be relocated at a cost of $26 billion. Families exposed to the radioactive fallout from the explosion have had an increased occurrence of birth defects and cancer. A much less severe accident in 1979 at the Three Mile Island nuclear power plant in eastern Pennsylvania released radioactive gases into the atmosphere. Subsequent studies indicated that people who lived in the surrounding community at the time of the accident acquired higher rates of lung cancer and leukemia than the general population.

Exposure to lower levels of nuclear radiation can cause damage to eyes, skin, and reproductive organs, and may result in birth defects in children. Low-level exposure

to radioactive materials could occur if a truck or train transporting low-level wastes were involved in a wreck, or if a nuclear waste disposal site leaked and radioactive substances were dispersed at low concentrations in air or water. Since September 11, 2001, government officials have warned about the possibility of terrorists using *"dirty bombs,"* wherein conventional explosives are combined with radioactive materials. The resulting dispersion of bits of radioactive matter by the conventional bomb blast and wind would contaminate land well beyond the area affected by the blast.

In the coming years, huge amounts of radioactive waste must be safely collected and permanently stored where it cannot escape back into our environment. For decades, nuclear reactors that generate 20% of the U.S. electricity supply have been accumulating highly radioactive wastes on-site. During this time, the U.S. government has been working to develop appropriate technologies and find sites to store these wastes permanently. The most likely location is in underground salt caves below Yucca Mountain, Nevada. The geology of this location causes officials to believe that nuclear waste stored there would not be carried back to the surface by groundwater movement. Various technologies have been developed to contain nuclear wastes within large "casks" and/or embedded in concrete or glass-like substances to make the radioactive substances immobile. Nuclear wastes will be extremely toxic for thousands of years, and no one knows if our technologies will be able to contain them until they become harmless.

A major health concern raised about the U.S. nuclear waste disposal program is the need to transport large quantities of highly radioactive waste by truck or train across the highways and rails of the United States. If you live next to an interstate highway or a major railroad line, it is possible that containers of high-level radioactive waste will be passing through your community on a regular basis. Much research has been done to devise containers that can withstand the worst imaginable wreck. Many people do not want these wastes to be transported through their

---

Key Terms

ionizing radiation electromagnetic radiation that is capable of breaking chemical bonds, such as X-rays and gamma rays.

non-ionizing radiation electromagnetic radiation that cannot break chemical bonds, but may excite electrons (ultraviolet radiation) or heat biological materials (infrared, radio frequency, and microwave radiation).

community, but the current situation is not safe either. Hundreds of tons of high-level radioactive waste are dispersed across the country in shallow, water-filled temporary holding tanks adjacent to nuclear power plants. This problem will only get worse as older nuclear power plants are retired, and hundreds of tons of concrete and steel that are somewhat radioactive must be disposed of.

The Global Environment

The global environment is comprised of the atmosphere, oceans, continental land masses, and all the living organisms that exist on Earth. Interactions among these components of the global environment influence the characteristics of solar radiation at the ground level, climate (temperature, precipitation, seasonal variation), production of food plants and animals, availability of freshwater, energy requirements for heating and cooling of human habitations, the geographic distribution of diseases, the composition of natural communities (deserts, tundra, rain forest), and the survival and extinction of species.

Some of the characteristics of the global environment have obvious and direct effects on human physical health, such as the presence of disease-causing organisms or solar UV radiation that can increase the risk of skin cancer. Other effects of the global environment on personal health are less well documented, such as the adverse effects on emotional or spiritual health associated with the extinction of species or destruction of beautiful natural communities. Many scientists warn that the global environment is being degraded by the combined forces of ever more powerful technology being used by a rapidly increasing global human population. In this section we briefly describe major concerns regarding the global environment and how these might affect personal health. We end this section and the chapter with some thoughts about how you can take some degree of personal control over these global environmental problems and their influence on your health.

Human Population Explosion

Many scientists warn that the human population is increasing at a rate that cannot be sustained by the resources of the Earth. There are currently over 6 billion people in the global human population, and this is projected to increase to over 10 billion in the next 50 years. It took all of human history until 1830 for the global population to reach 1 billion people. It took only 25 years, between 1975 and 1999, to increase from 4 to 6 billion. Every year the world's population grows by about 78 million people, with 97% born into the poorest countries.[28]

To grasp the implications of this expansion of the human population, consider the vast problems we face with the current population, including depletion of natural resources (freshwater, food, and oil), air and water pollution, conflict and political upheaval, starvation, and destruction of natural communities. Now imagine trying to solve these problems in the 21st century with twice as many people trying to make a living and raise a family on the same Earth.

The effects of the human population explosion on personal health depend on who you are and where you live. Many of the poorer nations of Asia, Africa, and South America will not be able to feed their people; starvation and associated diseases will be major health problems for these populations. Growing populations in dry regions are exceeding their freshwater supply, and hundreds of millions of people must drink from contaminated water sources. Every year, 5 million children die from waterborne diarrhea diseases associated with unsanitary drinking water.[28] By 2025, 2.5 billion people may live in regions where available freshwater is insufficient to meet their needs.

In many extremely poor countries, hungry people will destroy most or all of the remaining natural communities (tropical rain forests, African savanna) in vain efforts to grow food on lands that are not suited for agriculture. Six hundred thousand square miles of forest were cut down worldwide in the 1990s to meet demand for wood products and to expand farm and grazing land. How much will remain in a world with 10 billion people? Overcultivation of farmlands to meet the demand for food has already degraded the fertility of a land area equivalent to that of the United States and Canada combined.[28] Hungry people who live on oceanic islands often destroy their coral reefs trying to make a living by using dynamite or cyanide to catch fish. In Africa hungry people hunt wild game for food, putting more and more species at risk of extinction.

Competition among nations for limited supplies of water and oil is often a root cause of political tensions, terrorism, and war. Political upheaval in the Middle East, recent terrorist attacks on U.S. targets, and the war in Iraq can be partially explained by competition for scarce resources (water, land, and oil). The genocide that killed hundreds of thousands in Rwanda in 1994–95 has been traced to inequitable distribution of land and associated hunger in some parts of that country.[29] Many fear that such social instability and strife will be the inevitable result of competition for scarce resources, associated with excessive human population growth and overconsumption of limited resources.

The solutions to the human population growth problem are simple in theory, but often complex in their implementation. Basic population ecology theory states that the rate of population growth can be reduced if: (1) women have fewer children over their lifetime, and

(2) if they delay the start of their reproduction. A somewhat counterintuitive pattern is that population growth rate slows when infant survival rate is increased by better health care. It has been documented in many countries that women choose to have fewer children if they are confident that the children they do have will survive. Where infant mortality is high, women will often choose to have more children than they want or can afford as a "bet hedge" to ensure that at least some will live to adulthood.

Simply providing education opportunities to girls can have major and long-lasting effects that act to reduce population growth. Girls who have the opportunity to go to school and become educated delay having their first child; educated women have half the pregnancies of their uneducated sisters.[28] Educated women are more likely to be able to find employment outside the home. This has two effects: working women are too busy to care for large numbers of children, and women with an independent income have greater status and influence in deciding how many children they will have. Of course, universal access to birth control information and affordable contraception are also needed to allow women to have only as many children as they desire.

While this combination of commonsense actions can drastically reduce future human population growth, these proactive initiatives are often held hostage to political and cultural controversies. The sad result is that human populations may ultimately be controlled by increased death rates associated with starvation, disease, and war, rather than reduced birth rates.

Global Climate Change

A wide range of human activities add **greenhouse gases** to the atmosphere that trap heat and cause a net gain of energy and increase in temperature in the Earth system. This increase in global temperature is called the "Greenhouse Effect" or "Global Warming." Human-caused sources of greenhouse gases include both industrial and agricultural activities, including the burning of fuels, conversion of natural communities (grasslands, forests, and wetlands) to human uses, and methane emissions from large herds of cattle, flooded rice fields, and leaks from natural gas pipelines.

There is clear evidence that the concentration of greenhouse gases in the atmosphere has increased substantially since the beginning of the Industrial Revolution in the late 1700s. The average concentration of carbon dioxide in the atmosphere has increased 31% during this time period. Atmospheric methane, tropospheric ozone, and nitrous oxide concentrations have increased by 151%, 35%, and 17%, respectively.[30] Most of the increase in atmospheric carbon dioxide is associated with burning of fossil fuels.[31]

There is growing evidence that increases in atmospheric greenhouse gases are associated with changes in global climate. Chemical analyses of gas bubbles in glacial ice core samples from the polar ice caps indicate that atmospheric carbon dioxide and methane concentrations have been closely related to changes in global temperature through several cycles of ice ages and warm periods during the past 420,000 years; when carbon dioxide and methane concentrations increased, so did atmospheric temperature.[32] Coincident with the current increase in atmospheric concentrations of greenhouse gases, average global surface temperature was higher during the decade of the 1990s than at any other time in the historical record of weather data.[30]

Many scientists around the world believe that the changes in global climate described above are the first evidence of global climate change related to human activities. However, there is still controversy regarding the relative contributions of humans versus natural processes, and whether or not this warming trend is a short-term phenomenon or the beginning of a long-term trend.

Because climate is such a fundamental characteristic of the environment, global warming is expected to have diverse and widespread effects, including melting of the polar ice caps, rising sea level, inundation of coastal areas (including major coastal cities), and increased frequency and severity of hurricanes and other destructive weather events. Effects of climate change on human health include increased heat stress in tropical and subtropical areas, loss of life in storms and floods, expansion of the range of disease-carrying insects (such as mosquitoes) from subtropical regions into temperate regions (such as the United States), increased abundance of waterborne pathogens, decreased air and water quality, and decreased food availability associated with severe weather and water shortages.

Ecological effects of global warming include increased frequency of wildfires and insect pest outbreaks that destroy forests, and widespread death of coral reefs associated with higher water temperature. Many scientists project large scale decline and extinction of species that cannot adapt to changes in climate and cannot migrate to more suitable areas because of barriers associated with

---

Key Terms

greenhouse gases a category of gases in the atmosphere that allow solar radiation to pass through the atmosphere to the Earth, but then trap the heat that is radiated from the Earth back toward space; greenhouse gases include water vapor, carbon dioxide, methane, nitrous oxide, and tropospheric ozone.

Organizations Related to Environmental and Population Control Concerns

Population Issues

The organizations listed below provide material and informational support to women and men worldwide who seek to protect their reproductive health and to control their family size.

United Nations Family Planning Organization: **http://www.unfpa.org**

International Planned Parenthood Federation: **http://www.ippf.org**

The Population Institute: Provides information on the social and environmental consequences of rapid population growth, and advocacy for governmental support of voluntary family planning programs. **http://www.populationinstitute.org**

Environmental Political Advocacy Groups

The private environmental organizations listed below use the political and legal system to promote responsible use of the Earth's ecosystems and resources, and to provide information to the public about a full range of environmental issues. Some also employ scientists, policy analysts, and lawyers in support of lobbying and litigation in support of environmental protection.

Sierra Club: **http://www.sierraclub.org**

Wilderness Society: **http://www.wilderness.org**

National Wildlife Federation: **http://www.nwf.org**

Natural Resources Defense Council: **http://www.nrdc.org**

Environmental Defense Fund: **http://www.environmentaldefense.org**

The League of Conservation Voters: A political action organization that provides information to voters on the voting records of politicians regarding environmental issues. This organization also campaigns to elect candidates who support environmentally responsible policies. **http://www.lcv.org**

Conservation of Natural Communities and Endangered Species

The Nature Conservancy: Uses private donations to purchase, protect, and manage important natural communities and habitats in the United States and throughout the world (116 million acres worldwide, as of 2003). **http://nature.org**

World Wildlife Fund: Privately funded organization that works to protect endangered species and threatened habitats around the world, and to reduce pollution and climate change. **http://www.panda.org**

Sources of Environmental Information

World Resources Institute: A privately funded "think tank" that compiles environmental and economic data from around the world and publishes environmental policy analyses to promote a worldwide transition to an ecologically sustainable, socially just society. **http://www.worldwatch.org**

U.S. Environmental Protection Agency: The agency within the U.S. federal government responsible for monitoring environmental quality and enforcing environmental laws and regulations. This agency provides a wide range of environmental information to the public. **http://www.epa.gov**

---

human roads, cities, and farms. These ecological changes could adversely impact emotional and spiritual health as cherished natural wonders are degraded or disappear entirely under the onslaught of climate changes.

The primary means proposed for reducing and reversing global warming associated with human activities is to reduce the burning of fossil fuels such as oil and coal and increase the proportion of our energy needs that are met by other technologies. Many suggest that a combination of energy conservation, increased efficiency of automobiles and electrical appliances, and a gradual shift to alternate power sources for cars (fuel cells and/or hydrogen) and electricity (photovoltaic cells, wind turbines, geothermal energy, nuclear power) can get this job done. These transitions will require major shifts in the national and global economies, continuing innovation and technology development, and many small changes in everyday life of humans on planet Earth.

Your ability as an individual to take personal responsibility for addressing the global warming problem is limited, but all good things must start with individuals willing to do the right thing. You can reduce your personal contribution to global warming by conserving electricity at home, driving the most fuel-efficient automobile that meets your needs, using mass transit where available, recycling/reusing, and purchasing appliances that are rated as highly efficient. As technologies improve, you may someday be able to contribute to the electricity needs of your home using photovoltaic roof coverings and solar or geothermal energy for heating and cooling. Using compact fluorescent lighting is more expensive initially than standard lighting, but less costly over the long run. Fluorescent lighting uses much less electricity and has a much longer life span than standard incandescent light bulbs. Government action will be required to support widespread conservation practices in industry and business. You could join and be active in environmental organizations that work to address global warming. When politicians see their constituents want to protect our common global environment, they may find the political will to do the right thing.

TALKING POINTS How can you encourage your children to develop sound habits regarding their environment and their personal health? What changes can you make in your own habits to serve as a better example for them?

Stratospheric Ozone Depletion

The *stratospheric ozone layer* is a concentration of ozone molecules located about 10 to 25 miles above the Earth's surface. This "ozone layer" contains about 90% of the planet's ozone. Stratospheric ozone is a naturally occurring gas formed by the interaction of atmospheric oxygen and components of solar radiation.

Unlike tropospheric (low-elevation) ozone, which has many adverse health and ecological effects, the stratospheric ozone layer has beneficial health effects by protecting living organisms on the Earth's surface from harmful solar ultraviolet (UV) radiation. For people, overexposure to UV rays can lead to skin cancer, cataracts (clouding of the lens of the eye), and weakened immune systems. Increased UV can also lead to reduced crop yield and disruptions in the ocean's food chain.

It has been well-documented that chemical reactions between stratospheric ozone and certain human-made air pollutants can significantly reduce the ozone layer, causing increased UV radiation at the Earth's surface. The chemicals that cause ozone depletion include chlorofluorocarbons or CFCs (used as coolants in many air conditioning and refrigeration systems, in insulating foams, and as solvents), halons (used in fire suppression systems), and methyl bromide (used in pesticides). When these substances are released to the atmosphere and rise to the stratosphere, they release either chlorine or bromine molecules. One chlorine molecule can destroy 100,000 ozone molecules, and these substances can remain in the atmosphere for years.[33]

The vast majority of this depletion of the ozone layer occurs in the atmosphere above the north and south polar regions. In one year, ozone levels above Antarctica decreased by 60%. While the polar "ozone holes" allow the greatest amount of UV radiation to reach the ground in these sparsely populated areas, the ozone layer has decreased by 5% to 10% above the United States. These decreases in the stratospheric ozone layer have been associated with as much as a 50% increase in UV radiation at the ground level in Antarctica.[33]

In response to the well-documented links between certain air pollutants and depletion of the ozone layer, and links between UV radiation and adverse health and ecological effects, the world community has worked to eliminate the use of ozone-depleting chemicals. For example, a complete ban on the production of halons and CFCs went

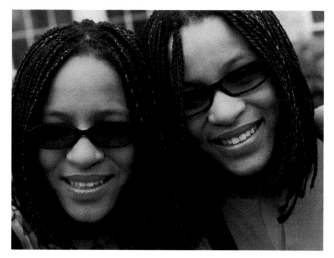

When you buy sunglasses, look for the UV-protection rating.

into effect in the mid-1990s. As the amounts of ozone-depleting chemicals in the atmosphere decrease, the ozone layer will recover to natural levels by the year 2050.[33]

To limit your risk of skin cancer and other UV-related health problems, you should limit your exposure to direct sunlight, and when you are outside you should wear sunscreen on exposed skin. You should also wear sunglasses that are rated as eliminating over 95% of UV radiation. When traveling to parts of North America, Europe, South Africa, South America, and Australia that are close to the polar ozone holes, you should be aware of UV index information presented by the popular media. During months when the polar ozone holes are larger, you may want to further restrict your exposure to direct sunlight.

TALKING POINTS Your sister is a sun worshipper who loves the look of a deep, dark tan. How might you persuade her to protect her skin from the rays of the sun?

Loss of Natural Habitats and Species Extinctions

On every continent, an exploding human population armed with even more powerful technology is altering or completely taking over the habitats of other species that share our planet. Sixteen to 23% of the total land surface of Earth has been converted entirely for human uses, including row crop fields, grazing lands, and urban/industrial areas. As much as 40% to 50% of the land surface has been transformed or degraded by human activities.[34]

The Earth has lost almost half (7.5 billion acres) of its original forest cover to human exploitation. Every year, another 40 million acres is cleared for farming or logged for timber. Only 20% of the original forest cover on Earth remains ecologically intact and able to support its full complement of species, mostly in the northern parts of Canada and Siberia. In the lower 48 states of the United States, only 1% of the original pristine forest present at the time of European settlement remains today, located in three scattered parks/wilderness areas.[35]

As much as 30% of the African continent is at risk for **desertification,** mainly due to overgrazing by livestock, excessive brush and tree cutting for fuel, and inappropriate agricultural practices.[36] This problem is most severe when expanding populations of poor people try to feed themselves using nonsustainable food production methods on dry lands. As these lands are degraded, the human populations shift to new dry land natural communities, and the expanding deserts can support neither humans nor wildlife populations.

The worldwide human population currently uses 50% of the Earth's freshwater runoff, 70% of which is used for agricultural irrigation. In some major river drainages, water diversion is so great that no water reaches the ocean (e.g., the Colorado River in the southwest U.S.). Dams for electric power generation, flood control, and irrigation have impacted all but 6% of rivers in the world.[35]

Human impact on the biosphere is not limited to the land. Sixty percent of the human population lives within 100 km of an ocean coast, and humans consume 25 to 35% of the energy flow in coastal ocean waters. As of 1995, 22% of all ocean fisheries for human consumption were overexploited (resulting in population crashes of the targeted fish species), and another 44% were being exploited at their maximum sustainable level. In addition, 27 million tons of nontargeted fish species are caught, killed, and dumped back into the ocean each year, constituting 33% of the total catch.[34] Overharvesting has put most of the world's whale species at risk of extinction. Recent plans by the U.S. Navy to deploy a powerful sonar system that will produce loud noises throughout the world's oceans may further jeopardize whales and other marine mammals.

Many coastal wetlands, mangrove forests, and coral reefs are destroyed or degraded by human activities. As much as 50% of worldwide mangrove forests have been transformed or destroyed.[34] In Indonesia, with the largest coral reef system in the world, 70% of the reefs have been severely degraded by dynamite fishing. Worldwide, 30% of all coral reefs have been destroyed by human activities, pollution, and coral bleaching that may be associated with global warming. Coastal water pollution has been linked to increased frequency of harmful algae blooms that cause extensive fish kills, massive "dead zones" where nothing else can live, and increased risk of shellfish poisoning for humans who eat seafood.[34]

The cumulative effects of all these human-caused changes to the Earth's land and oceans have increased the species extinction rate by 100 to 1,000 times over rates estimated for the period before human domination. Scientists estimate that 25% of bird species known to science have gone extinct in the last 2,000 years. Of those species currently alive and known to science, 11% of birds, 18% of mammals, 5% of fish, and 8% of plants are threatened with extinction. These numbers do not account for the thousands or millions of species not yet known to science that are likely going extinct as their habitats are destroyed. The primary causes of these extinctions are habitat loss due to human transformations of land and water and overharvesting of species by humans.[35]

The effects on personal health associated with worldwide loss of natural communities and species extinctions are highly variable from person to person. Pharmaceutical companies have found many substances produced by species in various natural communities to be useful sources of drugs to treat human illnesses. A well-known example is Taxol, a substance derived from an endangered tree species found in the old-growth forests of the U.S. Pacific Northwest that is a potent drug to fight breast cancer. As the richness of species on Earth is depleted by extinction, we lose a wealth of genetic material that could be of great importance to human health. The degradation and loss of natural ecosystems also undermines the systems that function to make Earth a livable planet, contributing to such problems as global climate change, freshwater shortages, and increased frequency of destructive flooding.

Some have proposed that human evolution predisposes us to desire green spaces and diverse biological systems; this is called the *Biophilia hypothesis*.[37] That is, we are most happy when we are surrounded by natural beauty. Many have written about the human psychological benefits from natural communities. John Muir, a famous early environmentalist in the United States, wrote:

> Climb the mountains and get their good tidings.
> Nature's peace will flow into you as sunshine flows into trees.
> The winds will blow their own freshness into you,
> and the storms their energy,
> while cares drop off like autumn leaves.

Wallace Stegner wrote a passage that appears in the Wilderness Act passed by the U.S. Congress in 1964 to

---

Key Terms

desertification a process that converts lands that historically supported grasslands, shrublands, or dry forest to nonproductive desert.

protect areas of intact ecosystems in the United States for the enjoyment of future generations:

> It was a lovely and terrible wilderness, such a wilderness as Christ and the prophets went out into; harshly and beautifully colored, broken and worn until its bones are exposed, its great sky without a smudge or a taint from Technocracy, and in hidden corners and pockets under its cliffs, the sudden poetry of springs. Save a piece of country like that intact, and it does not matter in the slightest that only a few people every year will go into it. That is precisely its value . . . We simply need that wild country available to us, even if we never do more than drive to its edge and look in. For it can be a means of reassuring ourselves of our sanity as creatures, a part of the geography of hope.

Both Muir and Stegner refer to the psychological benefits that humans derive simply from the knowledge that natural communities and wildlife species still exist, as they always have, somewhere on our planet. Now, try to imagine how you would feel about a world completely dominated and degraded by a massive human population; no great herds of caribou, zebra, and wildebeest moving like a tide across the landscape; no wolves, lions, tigers, or elephants to excite the imagination; no Monarch butterflies sipping nectar in your backyard on their migration from Maine to Mexico; no dolphins and orcas playing in the ocean waves; no humpback whales singing in the depths; no great, ancient trees stretching out of sight toward a clear blue sky; no expansive grasslands rippling in the breeze as far as the eye can see; the sky and waters tainted with pollution; the climate itself hostile to human civilization. The effects of such a dark and dismal world on the human psyche are unimaginable to me. The thought of forever losing the natural wonders of our planet could have profound adverse consequences for emotional, psychological, and spiritual well-being. For many, the thought of such a dark future can cause anger, frustration, depression, hopelessness, and despair.[38]

How can you or any one person exert any degree of personal control over such a great and complex threat to your physical, emotional, and spiritual health? Let's start with the little things: conserve energy, recycle and reuse what you can, limit your consumption of the world's resources to what you need, and join together with others of like mind to provide political and financial support to organizations that are working to solve these big problems (see the photo above and the listing in the Star box on page 667). If you want to make a bigger personal commitment to solving global environmental problems, you could limit your own family size to no more than two children. For a list of many more ways to reduce your personal impact on the Earth, go to the website **http://www.earthshare.org/get_involved/earth_saving_tips.html**, and take a look at the Changing for the Better box on page 671.

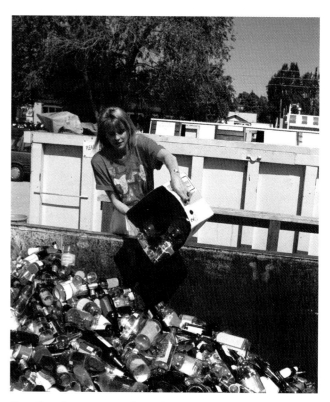

Recycling glass, paper, and metal can reduce land pollution and consumption of natural resources.

Another way you can reduce the negative environmental effects of your personal consumption of natural resources is to "buy green" when you can (see the Considering Complementary Care box on page 671). There are often multiple ways to meet human needs for food, clothing, and shelter, some of which are very destructive and degrade the natural heritage of the Earth. In recent years, environmental organizations have begun certification programs so that the consumer can identify which products are produced by "Earth-friendly" means (for more information, go to the website **http://www.newdream.org/buygreen/**). Examples of such products include sustainably harvested timber, shade-grown coffee, and organic food and cotton. Often these products are more expensive, as the means of their production lack the efficiency of mechanized, chemically dependent, environmentally destructive production systems. When you "buy green," you support Earth-friendly producers and may reduce the economic push to destroy more natural communities and species. Many "buy green" organizations also work to improve the economic conditions of small rural villages where the producers of their products live. These efforts at economic development are often associated with improved education opportunities that lead to reduced birth rates, slowing global human population growth that is the root cause for many environmental problems.

Considering Complementary Care

Is Organic Food Good for the Environment?

Certified "organic" food in the United States is produced under guidelines set out by the Organic Foods Production Act. The guidelines in this law stipulate materials and practices that enhance the balance of natural systems and that integrate parts of the farming system into an ecological whole.

The primary goal of organic agriculture is to optimize the health and productivity of interdependent communities of soil life, plants, animals, and people. Organic farmers that produce grain, fruits, and vegetables may not use synthetic pesticides or fertilizers. Meat producers must feed their livestock only organically produced feedstuffs. In addition, many organic meat producers forgo the use of growth hormones and antibiotics that stimulate livestock growth rates. While organic foods have not been shown to be any more nutritious than non organic food, organic foods have fewer chemical residues that may adversely impact human health.[1]

The description of organic food above suggests that organic farming practices are good for the environment. Organic farming puts far less pollution into local water and air, and fewer chemicals into the food supply. Local farmers can often make greater profits through direct sales of organic produce to local cooperatives or other consumer-supported agriculture organizations. This may help to preserve local green space against encroachment by suburban developers. Hence, organic farming can certainly be good for the local community environment.

Whether or not organic farming is good for the global environment is an open question. While organic farms produce less pollution, they also produce less food per acre. Lower production per acre, higher labor costs, and the small number of organic farmers often make organic foods an expensive luxury for the well-to-do. Many environmentalists call for a widespread shift from chemical-dependent agriculture to more ecologically sustainable organic farming. However, it is doubtful that organic farming on existing agricultural lands could feed the current human population of 6 billion people. A worldwide shift to organic farming would likely require an expansion of agricultural lands into national parks, nature preserves, and wilderness areas. This loss of natural habitats would result in massive species extinctions.[2] On the other hand, there is some uncertainty as to whether or not intensive, chemical-dependent agricultural systems will provide a sustainable food supply. Chemical fertilizers can replace lost nutrients, but can't repair compacted soil, nor replace eroded topsoil. Pesticides and herbicides can control pests and weeds now, but these species are already displaying signs of increased resistance that may prevent control in the future.

At the moment, your personal choices to buy organically grown, locally produced foods are probably most beneficial to your local environment, and may benefit your personal health. It is much less clear whether or not a widespread shift to organic farming would be beneficial to the larger global environment.

[1]Cable News Network Interactive. In-Depth: Organic Food. 1998. **http://www.cnn.com/HEALTH/indepth.food/organic/index.html**
[2]Center for Global Food Issues. Growing More Food per Acre Leaves More Land for Nature. 2002. **http://www.highyieldconservation.org**

Changing for the Better

Taking Personal Action with a Positive Attitude Can Make a Difference

All environmental problems and their associated health risks begin with personal choices regarding resource consumption, waste disposal, and electing leaders who set policies and regulations. When you make your choices, consider the environmental consequences and act in ways that promote a healthy environment for all people and other living things on Earth.

- Be aware of environmental hazards in the air, water, and materials in your personal environment and work to minimize or eliminate these hazards.
- Reduce your own consumption of natural resources, and dispose of wastes responsibly.
- Be aware of government policies regarding natural resource exploitation, pollution, and habitat destruction.
- Vote for leaders who are more concerned with the quality of the environment of all people and other species than they are for economic special interests.

- When that small voice inside you says, "Forget it, there is nothing I can do," don't listen! That voice is leading you toward a life of cynicism and despair. For your own psychological, emotional, and spiritual well-being, have faith that the actions of individuals can accumulate to bring about world change.*

The combined actions of 6 billion people making personal choices will determine the future of the Earth's environment, and so, the future of humankind on Earth. The solutions to the great environmental problems looming in the future begin with you, today. Your positive actions and faith in fellow humans to do the right thing will not only benefit the future, but also enhance your emotional well-being in the present.*

*Ellison K. A question of faith. *Frontiers in Ecology and the Environment* 1(1): 56, 2003.

Taking Charge of Your Health

- Protect yourself from ultraviolet light. Always wear sunscreen, and make sure your sunglasses filter out UV rays.
- Have your home tested for radon, and install a radon reduction system if necessary.
- Install a water filtration device to remove contaminants from your drinking water.
- Keep your car in proper running condition to reduce the amount of noise and air pollution it produces.

- Reduce your personal impact on the environment by reducing your consumption of energy and recycling and reusing what you can, and using Earth-friendly products in your home.
- Take personal action on environmental issues using the suggestions outlined in the Changing for the Better box on page 671.

Summary

- Your environment contains a wide range of substances, living organisms, and forms of energy that may substantially impact one or more dimensions of your personal health.
- Environmental influences on personal health operate over a wide range of spatial scales, from the personal spaces of your home and workplace, to the common spaces of your community and region, to the global environment that supports all life on Earth.
- The most direct environmental risks to your physical health are related to the presence of toxic substances or pathogenic organisms (pollutants) in the air and water of your personal and community environments.
- You can exert the greatest degree of control over your exposure to pollutants within the personal environment of your home and workplace. You can identify environmental health risks in your personal environment, and then eliminate or reduce these risks by changing your buying habits and eliminating pollutant sources.
- Air pollution in major urban areas can cause significant adverse health effects, especially for people who suffer from respiratory or cardiac disease.
- While you have no control over community air pollution, you can limit your exposure to these toxic substances by being aware of daily pollution levels and by restricting your outdoor activities when these levels are high.
- Much progress has been made in reducing community water pollution, but water in many rivers and lakes still contains chemicals and pathogens that can adversely affect your health.
- You should seek out information about any health advisories for wild foods you obtain from local rivers, and advisories regarding recreational use of those rivers.
- The U.S. Environmental Protection Agency monitors and regulates the quality of drinking water from

municipal water suppliers, but it is up to you to ensure the safety of your drinking water if it comes from a private well.
- Improper disposal of toxic solid wastes in landfills designed for household waste is a major source of regional surface and groundwater pollution.
- You should never dispose of toxic household products (batteries, automotive fluids, pesticides, oil-based paint products) by simply putting them in the household trash or pouring them down a drain. Take them to specially designated toxic disposal locations.
- Loss of green space in your community and regional environment, associated with urban sprawl and unregulated land development, can diminish your perceived quality of life, and reduce opportunities for exercise, which is important for maintaining good physical health.
- While you have limited personal control over the environment of your community and region, you can still work to enhance your environment by joining others of like mind in groups that advocate environmental protection through the democratic political process.
- A rapidly expanding global human population, armed with increasingly more powerful technologies, is now degrading the global environment that sustains all life on Earth.
- At the current rate of human population growth, most scientists of the world warn of increased starvation and disease, decreased standards of living, and increased conflict over progressively decreasing supplies of natural resources.
- Human population growth can be substantially slowed by simply providing girls and women opportunities to become educated and gainfully employed, and access to contraception.
- Pollutants produced by humans are responsible for changes in the atmosphere that are altering climate

patterns and allowing harmful solar radiation to reach the surface of the Earth.

- Changes in the global environment have potential to increase risks to human health, and to significantly harm many other species and natural communities.
- While individuals can do little to address global environmental problems, the solutions all start

with individual choices about family size, resource consumption, and political candidates. The best path to a livable future for humankind is to do your part and have faith that others will do theirs.

Review Questions

1. What is radon, and what are the health risks associated with it? What actions can you take to minimize the health risks of radon?

2. Identify the sources and the potential health effects of the following common indoor air pollutants: carbon monoxide, volatile organic compounds, and biological pollutants such as mold, mildew, pollen, and pet dander. Describe actions you could take to minimize health risks from these pollutants.

3. What health risks are associated with lead and asbestos? What actions can you take to minimize these risks?

4. Describe actions you should take to safeguard drinking from a well on your own property.

5. Define the concept of "noise" in a way that clarifies how a particular type of music could be noise to some, but not noise to others.

6. What are the physical and emotional health effects of noise? What actions could you take to minimize the health risks of noise?

7. Describe the distinction between a "point source" versus a "non-point source" of community/regional air or water pollution. Which type of pollution source do you think is most easily controlled? Explain your answer.

8. Tropospheric ozone and small particulate matter are community and regional air pollutants that have been linked to serious health risks. For each of these substances, describe the main human sources, the effect(s) on human physical health, and what actions you could take to minimize your own risk of adverse health effects from these air pollutants.

9. What are "air toxics" and where do you think you are most likely to be exposed to these substances? What do you think you could do to minimize your personal health risk from air toxics?

10. What is "biological water pollution" and what is the main source of this pollution in your community's rivers, streams, and/or lakes? What are the health risks associated with biological water pollution? What can you do to minimize the risk to your personal health from this type of pollution?

11. Who is responsible for ensuring the safety of your drinking water if the source is a municipal water company? What can you do to minimize any health risks associated with your drinking water in this circumstance?

12. What is the main health risk associated with land pollution from solid waste landfills? What can you do to minimize your personal contribution to this type of pollution?

13. What is "green space," and why is it important to your personal health? What personal actions could you take to protect green space in your community or region?

14. Which do you think is the best plan for dealing with radioactive wastes from U.S. nuclear reactors: storing it on the site of the reactor or shipping it across the country to the Yucca Mountain underground storage facility? Explain your answer in terms of the health risks posed by each option.

15. What policies should the U.S. foreign aid agencies implement in poor underdeveloped countries to help them reduce their population growth rate? Explain how these policies would work toward this goal.

16. Global warming and stratospheric ozone depletion are large-scale changes in the global environment with uncertain, but potentially significant, health consequences. For each of these global changes, describe the cause(s) of environmental change, the potential health effects, and what might be done to minimize these effects.

17. Loss of natural habitats and species extinctions are major ecological problems, but do these phenomena represent any risk to *your* personal health? Your answer should reflect your own perceptions, and should provide some explanation for your assessment.

18. A well-known environmentalist slogan is, "Think globally, but act locally." Based on what you've learned in this chapter, describe how you think this slogan applies to your personal actions in response to environmental health risks.

References

1. U.S. Environmental Protection Agency. Healthy Buildings, Healthy People: A Vision for the 21st Century. 2003. **http://www.epa.gov/iaq/hbhp/index.html**
2. Consumer Product Safety Commission. Carbon Monoxide Questions and Answers. CPSC Document #466. 2003. **http://www.cpsc.gov/cpscpub/pubs/466.html**
3. U.S. Environmental Protection Agency. The Senseless Killer. 2003. **http://www.epa.gov/iaq/pubs/senseles.html**
4. U.S. Environmental Protection Agency. The Inside Story: A Guide to Indoor Air Quality. 1995. **http://www.epa.gov/iaq/pubs/insidest.html**
5. Thorn J, et al. Adult-Onset Asthma Linked to Mold and Tobacco Smoke Exposure. *Allergy* 56: 287–292, 2001.
6. U.S. Environmental Protection Agency. Sources of Indoor Air Pollution: Asbestos. 2003. **http://www.epa.gov/iaq/asbestos.html**
7. U.S. Environmental Protection Agency. Sources of Indoor Air Pollution: Biological Pollutants. 2003. **http://www.epa.gov/iaq/biologic.html**
8. Centers for Disease Control. Legionellosis: Legionnaire's Disease (LD) and Pontiac Fever. 2001. **http://www.cdc.gov/ncidod/dbmd/diseaseinfo/legionellosis_g.htm**
9. National Safety Council. Radon. 2002. **http://www.nsc.org/ehc/radon.htm**
10. National Academy of Sciences. Biological Effects of Ionizing Radiation (BEIR) VI Report: "The Health Effects of Exposure to Indoor Radon." 1998. National Academy Press. **http://books.nap.edu/books/0309056454/html/**
11. National Academy of Sciences. Risk Assessment of Radon in Drinking Water. 1999. **http://www.nap.edu/books/0309062926/html/index.html**
12. U.S. Environmental Protection Agency. Sources of Indoors Air Pollution: Lead (Pb). 2003. **http://www.epa.gov/iaq/lead.html**
13. U.S. Department of Health and Human Services, Public Health Service, Agency for Toxic Substances and Disease Registry. Case Studies in Environmental Medicine: Lead Toxicity. 1995. **http://www.atsdr.cdc.gov/HEC/HSPH/caselead.html**
14. U.S. Environmental Protection Agency. Water on Tap: A Consumer's Guide to the Nation's Drinking Water. 2003. **http://www.epa.gov/safewater/wot/howsafe.html**
15. Townsend AR, et al. Human health effects of a changing global nitrogen cycle. *Frontiers in Ecology* 1: 240–246.
16. U.S. Environmental Protection Agency. Technical Factsheet on: Nitrate/Nitrite. 2002. **http://www.epa.gov/safewater/dwh/t-ioc/nitrates.html**
17. Gray LE, Ostby J. Effects of pesticides and toxic substances on behavioral and morphological reproductive development: endocrine versus no-endocrine mechanisms. *Toxicology and Industrial Health* 14: 159–184, 1998.
18. U.S. Environmental Protection Agency. Permeation and Leaching. 2003. **http://www.epa.gov/safewater/tcr/pdf/permleach.pdf**
19. Bell PA. Noise, pollution, and psychopathology. In: AMA Ghadirian and Lehmann HE (eds.). *Environment and Psychopathology.* Springer Publishing Co., New York, 1993.
20. U.S. Environmental Protection Agency. Draft Report on the Environment: Outdoor Air Quality. 2003. **http://www.epa.gov/indicators/roe/html/roeAirOut.htm**
21. Dockery DW and CA Pope III. Acute Respiratory Effects of Particulate Air Pollution. Annual Review Public Health 15: 107–132, 1994.
22. U.S. Environmental Protection Agency. Asthma Triggers—Related Topics—Ozone. 2003. **http://www.epa.gov/iaq/asthma/triggers/ozone.html**
23. McConnell R, Berhane K, Gilliland F, London S, Islam T, Gauderman WJ, Avol E, Margolis H, and Peters J. Asthma in exercising children exposed to ozone. The Lancet 359: 386–391, 2002.
24. U.S. Environmental Protection Agency. The National Air Toxics Assessment. 2002. **http://www.epa.gov/ttn/atw/nata**
25. U.S. Environmental Protection Agency. Drinking Water and Your Health, What You Need to Know, List of Drinking Water Contaminants & MCLs. 2003. **http://www.epa.gov/safewater/mcl.html#1**
26. Beck EC. The Love Canal Tragedy. 2002. **http://www.epa.gov/history/topics/lovecanal/01.htm**
27. U.S. Environmental Protection Agency. Municipal Solid Waste: Basic Facts. 2003. **http://www.epa.gov/epaoswer/non-hw/muncpl/facts.htm**
28. The Population Institute. **http://www.populationinstitute.org/**
29. Gasana J. Remember Rwanda? *World Watch* 15(5): 24–33, 2002.
30. Intergovernmental Panel on Climate Change. Climate Change 2001: Summary Report: Synthesis for Policy Makers. 2001. **http://www.ipcc.ch/pub/un/syreng/spm.pdf**
31. Bacastow R and Keeling DC. Atmospheric carbon dioxide and radiocarbon in the natural carbon cycle: II. Changes From AD 1700 to 2070 as Deduced From a Chemical Model. In: Woodwell GM and Pecan EV (eds.). *Carbon and the Biosphere.*

BHNL/CONF 720510, Springfield VA: National Technical Information Service, 1974.

32. Petit JR, et al. Climate and atmospheric history of the past 420,000 years from the Vostok ice core, Antarctica. *Nature* 399: 429–436, 1999.

33. U.S. Environmental Protection Agency. The Science of Ozone Depletion. 2003. **http://www.epa.gov/docs/ozone/science/index.html**

34. Vitousek P, et al. Human domination of Earth's ecosystems. *Science* 277: 494–499, 1997.

35. World Resources Institute. 2003. **http://www.wri.org**

36. United Nations. Food and Agriculture Organization. **http://www.fao.org/desertification/default.asp?lang=en**

37. Wilson E. *Biophilia: The Human Bond with Other Species.* Harvard University Press, Cambridge, MA, 1984.

38. Gardner GT and Stern PC. *Environmental Problems and Human Behavior.* Allyn & Bacon, a Simon & Schuster Co. Needham Heights, MA, 1996.

As We Go to Press

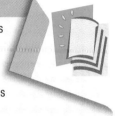

Recent research in the journal *Environmental Science and Technology* reports that Americans are exposed to more cancer-causing air pollutants than is indicated by standard air quality assessments. Most air pollution data for the U.S. is collected at centrally located outdoor monitoring sites. However, most people spend over 90% of their time indoors. For this recent study, the investigators rigged 71 study subjects with lapel-mounted air filters that absorbed volatile organic compounds (VOCs). For 14 VOCs that are designated as "hazardous," the personal lapel-mounted sensors contained concentrations that were 3 to 60 times higher than samples taken at outdoor air quality monitors. Several of these VOC's are documented carcinogens. Environmental concentrations of many hazardous VOCs have decreased in recent years due to regulations developed under the Clean Air Act. Nonetheless, the results of this study indicated that even non-smokers' personal exposure to airborne carcinogens is surprisingly high.

Fortunately, it is fairly easy to reduce your personal exposure to these hazardous substances. You should avoid cigarette smoke and air fresheners. You should hang recently dry-cleaned clothing in a well-ventilated area for a few hours. You should use cleaning agents and other household chemicals that contain VOCs only in well-ventilated spaces.

radiation from cell phones and electrical devices: environmental health hazard or not?

In 1992 a lawsuit filed in a Florida court alleged that radio frequency radiation (RFR) from cell phones caused the brain cancer and subsequent death of a woman. The concern and controversy about potential health effects of exposure to RFR has lasted long after this lawsuit was dismissed for lack of evidence. The potential problem with many cell phones is that the radio transmitter is placed next to the head, and millions of people are exposed to this radiation every day.

Scientific evidence for adverse health effects caused by RFR is limited. Some studies that exposed lab rats to constant, high levels of radio frequency radiation claim to have documented damage to DNA in brain cells that might later cause cancer. However, the amount of RFR to which these rats were exposed far exceeded the amount that a person would receive from normal use of a cell phone. Also, other animal studies found no cancer-related effects of exposure to RFR. Several large-scale epidemiological studies in a number of countries have compared the occurrence of various cancers of the brain and head between people who do and do not use cell phones. None of these studies found a link between exposure to cell phone RFR and cancer.

At the time of this writing, there is no scientifically credible evidence that using a cell phone poses a health risk beyond distracting you while driving. [1,2] However, cell phones have been in widespread use for only a relatively short period of time. There is no way to determine if long-term exposure to low levels of RFR from a cell phone placed close to the head has cumulative effects that might pose a health risk.

If you are concerned about potential long-term health effects of RFR, and must use a cell phone for long periods of time, you might use a head set so that the transmitter in the phone can be placed away from your body. The intensity of RFR decreased rapidly over even very short distances to levels so low that it is very unlikely to be a health risk.

For information about potential health effects of radio frequency radiation sources in the workplace, go to the following website of the U.S. Dept. of Labor, Occupational Safety and Health Administration: **http://www.osha-slc.gov/ SLTC/radiofrequencyradiation.**

Other kinds of non-ionizing radiation are a ubiquitous component of the environment of technologically advanced societies like that of the United States. Every electric wire and electronic device emits some form of non-ionizing radiation, including microwave, infrared, and ultraviolet radiation. Sources of non-ionizing radiation include microwave ovens, televisions, tanning lamps and black lights, home alarm systems, electric blankets, electric clothes dryers and ovens, and electricity transmission lines.

The health effects of various forms of non-ionizing radiation associated with modern electronic gadgets and electrical power lines are topics of some public controversy. A few studies have suggested that exposure to non-ionizing radiation or magnetic fields around electrical devices or power lines may slightly increase risk for some cancers. [3,4] For example, one of these studies estimated that up to 8% of childhood leukemia cases in the U.S. were associated with living in proximity to power lines. However, the vast majority of studies of health effects of non-ionizing radiation have failed to find any increased risk of adverse health effects associated with household electronics or living in close proximity to high voltage power lines [5,6] (for a comprehensive review of the scientific literature, go to the website of J.E. Moulder, professor of radiation oncology at the Medical College of Wisconsin, **http://www.mcw.edu/ gcrc/cop/powerlines-cancer-FAQ/ toc.html#C55**).

In a world where environmental health hazards are common, we must be careful to not blindly accept unsubstantiated claims regarding new hazards. However, we must also consider which is the lesser of two evils, to ban a product that is safe, or to allow a hazardous product on the market that causes damage to human health or natural systems. Sometimes governmental policies and regulations err on the side of caution, banning products even if there is only a hint of potential adverse effects. Sometimes dangerous products pass initial testing, only to cause devastating consequences when they are released into the environment. Just because a study fails to detect adverse effects of a new product does not mean that the product is safe. Finding the correct balance between caution and progress is difficult, both for governmental agencies and for individuals making choices in their own lives.

For Discussion . . .

How often do you use a cell phone? Do you worry about the effects of radio frequency radiation? What about other forms of non-ionizing radiation? Why or why not?

References

1. Foster KR. Are mobile phones safe? Institute of Electrical and Electronic Engineers (IEEE) Spectrum Online Volume 37, Number 8, 2000. http://www.spectrum.ieee.org/publicfeature/aug00/prad.html

2. U.S. Food and Drug Administration. *Cell Phone Facts: Consumer Information on Wireless Phones.* 2002.

3. Ahlbom A, Day N, et al. A pooled analysis of magnetic fields and childhood leukemia. *British Journal of Cancer* 83: 692–698, 2000.

4. UK Childhood Cancer Study Investigators. Childhood cancer and residential proximity to power lines. *Brit J Cancer* 83: 1573–1580, 2000.

5. Savitz DA and Loomis DP. Magnetic field exposure in relation to leukemia and brain cancer mortality among electric utility workers. *American Journal of Epidemiology* 141(2): 123–128, 1995.

6. Greenland S, Sheppard AR, et al. A pooled analysis of magnetic fields, wirecodes, and childhood leukemia. *Epidemiology* 11: 624–634, 2000.

personal assessment

are you an environmentalist?

When asked, many people will say that they are an "environmentalist," including political leaders who are widely criticized for decisions perceived by others to be environmentally destructive. So what is an "environmentalist"? One definition of environmentalism is that it is an ideology that values and reveres Nature, and works to protect and preserve natural systems for both ethical reasons and because humankind depends on these systems for life. However, beyond this general statement environmentalists encompass a wide diversity of beliefs and practices. For some, their environmental beliefs are a form of religion, others function mainly in the political process, and some operate like terrorist groups who use violence to fight human economic development on behalf of Earth.[1] The wide diversity of beliefs and practices encompassed under "environmentalism" creates a situation where almost anyone could claim to be an environmentalist. Perhaps more useful criteria for determining if you are an environmentalist would be: (1) your awareness of how various human activities create environmental health hazards or degrade natural systems; (2) your willingness to consider your own role in creating environmental problems; and (3) your willingness to act in ways that reduce your personal risk from environmental hazards and your contribution to the causes of these hazards. These three criteria define a hierarchy of commitment to environmental protection. First you have to know a problem exists. Then you have to recognize your own part in creating that problem. The last, and most difficult, step is that you must be willing to reduce or eliminate your contribution to environmental problems. Your answers to the following questions will help you think about where you really stand on protecting the environment for yourself, your community, and all the rest of life on Earth.

Awareness of Environmental Problems

1. Have you ever read the water quality assessment provided by the supplier of your drinking water?
2. If your drinking water is from a well, do you know about potential sources of contamination (landfills or other waste disposal sites, large agricultural areas, confined feedlot livestock operations) in your watershed?
3. If your drinking water supply is from a well, do you know if your water contains potentially harmful contaminants?
4. Do you know whether or not your community wastewater treatment system occasionally dumps raw sewage into the local river during high rainfall events?
5. If you use a gas furnace or kerosene space heater, do you know whether or not these appliances are functioning properly so as to maximize energy efficiency and minimize risks from indoor air pollution?
6. Have you ever made a note of air pollution alerts or information about high ultraviolet radiation published in a local newspaper or presented on a local TV news program?
7. Have you ever searched for information on air, water, and land pollution in your community?
8. When you eat fish, are you aware of health advisories regarding contaminants in fish (e.g., mercury, PCBs) and recommendations that you limit the amount of the fish you consume?
9. When you purchase products, do you look at packaging materials for warnings that the product contains toxic chemicals?
10. When you listen to loud music, do you think about potential long-term damage to your hearing and the nuisance noise you create for your neighbors?
11. Do you know if your community (city, county, state) has a land-use management (zoning) plan?
12. When you see new economic developments (malls, superstores, warehouses, suburban housing developments) being constructed, do you wonder if wildlife habitat is being destroyed?
13. Do you know the proposed human causes of global warming and the potential consequences of this change in climate?
14. Do you know the causes and potential health effects of depletion of the stratospheric ozone layer?
15. Do you know the link between the wood you buy at a store like Menard's, Lowe's, and Home Depot and species extinctions?

Willingness to Consider Your Personal Environmental Impact

16. When you think about having a family of your own, do you worry about contributing to a rapidly growing human population that is responsible for widespread environmental degradation?
17. When you think about purchasing a vehicle, do you consider fuel efficiency more important than "image" sold by advertisers?
18. When you consider purchasing any product, do you consider the resources used, and pollution created, to produce that product?
19. When you purchase an electric appliance or a gas-powered device, do you consider energy efficiency?
20. When planning to build a new home, do you consider how your choices regarding location and amount of land could contribute to loss of green space and natural habitat?
21. When you use or dispose of household, yard, and automotive chemicals and fluids, do you consider that you may be contributing to local water pollution?
22. When you hear about global warming, do you recognize that your own use of electricity and gas-powered vehicles contributes to this problem?

23. Did you know that if you vent your home or automotive air conditioning system coolant while performing do-it-yourself maintenance, you are contributing to the depletion of the stratospheric ozone layer?

24. When you purchase lumber, do you wonder if the wood you are buying was harvested using environmentally sound practices, or if critical wildlife habitats or wilderness was destroyed to produce the lumber?

25. Do you consider how your vote in public elections can affect government policies that impact the environment?

Willingness to Alter Your Lifestyle to Protect Yourself and the Environment

26. Would you limit the number of your own children to one or two so as to reduce your contribution to the problem of global human population explosion?

27. When you purchase a vehicle, is energy efficiency your main concern?

28. Would you use mass transit to travel from home to work, if it were available, to reduce your contribution to local air pollution and need for paving more land to expand highways?

29. When you buy a home, would you seek to minimize the distance from work and schools to reduce gas consumption, minimize air pollution, and reduce demand for construction of new roads?

30. When you buy a home, would you look for a smaller, energy-efficient home to minimize your contribution to natural resource exploitation and pollution associated with energy consumption?

31. When you buy lighting, do you buy energy-efficient lights (compact fluorescent and LED lightbulbs) that are initially more expensive, but more efficient and less expensive over the long term?

32. When furnishing your home, would you seek out water-efficient toilets, faucets, and shower heads that conserve freshwater and reduce demands on wastewater treatment systems?

33. Do you set the thermostat in your home to cooler temperatures in winter and warmer temperatures in summer to conserve energy?

34. Would you invest money and effort to better insulate your home so as to reduce energy needed for heating and cooling?

35. When buying food, would you be willing to pay more for organically grown foods that were produced without the use of pesticides and fertilizers that pollute the surrounding environment?

36. Would you buy locally grown foods to support farmers (and their green spaces) in your community and reduce energy spent on long-distance transport?

37. When purchasing wood products, would you buy more expensive wood that is certified to have been harvested using environmentally sound practices?

38. Would you be willing to have something less than the perfect lawn so that you avoid using fertilizers and pesticides that contaminate local waterways?

39. Would you limit your personal consumption of material goods to mainly those things you need, so as to reduce exploitation of natural resources?

40. When you dispose of household chemicals, automotive fluids, and spent batteries, do you make the extra effort to be sure they do not end up polluting the environment, like taking them to a Tox-Away Day location?

41. Do you make the effort to recycle paper, glass, plastic, and metals?

42. When you make purchases, do you look for products made from recycled materials (e.g., post-consumer recycled paper, "plastic wood," fleece clothing made from recycled plastic)?

43. Do you limit the noise that you produce (loud music, loud car or motorcycle engines, barking dogs) to reduce noise pollution in your neighborhood?

44. Do you contribute financial support to environmental groups that promote conservation and protection of natural resources through the legal and political systems?

45. When you consider candidates for public office, do you vote for the candidates who have strong records or position statements for environmental protection?

If the majority of your answers to questions 1 to 15 are "Yes," you are likely "environmentally aware." That is, you pay attention to news stories about environmental issues or have taken an environmental science course.

If most of your answers to questions 1 to 25 are "Yes," you are "environmentally conscious." That is, you are not only aware of the problems, but beginning to think about how these problems are related to your own lifestyle.

If the majority of your answers to questions 26 to 45 are "Yes," you are likely "environmentally active." That is, you are personally involved in efforts to address environmental problems through your own lifestyle choices and through the political process.

[1]Wikipedia (The Free Encyclopedia). **http://www.wikipedia.org/wiki/Environmentalism**

appendix 1

first aid

Accidents are the leading cause of death for people ages 1 to 37. Injuries sustained in accidents can often be tragic. They are grim reminders of our need to learn first aid skills and to practice preventive safety habits.

First aid knowledge and skills allow you to help people who are in need of immediate emergency care. They also can help you save yourself if you should become injured. We recommend that our students enroll in American Red Cross first aid and safety courses, which are available in local communities or through colleges or universities. In this appendix, we briefly present some information about common first aid emergencies. (Please note that our information is *not* a substitute for comprehensive American Red Cross first aid instruction.)

First Aid

- Keep a list of important phone numbers near your phone (your doctor, ambulance service, hospital, poison control center, police and fire departments).
- In case of serious injury or illness, call the appropriate emergency service immediately for help (if uncertain, call "911" or "0").

Common First Aid Emergencies

Specific Problem	What To Do
Asphyxiation Victim stops breathing and skin, lips, tongue, and fingernail beds turn bluish or gray.	Tip head back with one hand on forehead and other lifting the lower jaw near the chin. Look, listen, and feel for breathing. If not breathing, place your mouth over victim's mouth, pinch the nose, get a tight seal, and give 2 slow breaths. Do pulse check. If no pulse is detected, CPR must be administered (Note: Some states require CPR training for those who administer CPR). If there is a pulse but no breathing, give breaths once every 5 seconds for an adult, once every 3 seconds for a child, once every 3 seconds for infants (do not exaggerate head tilt for babies). Recheck pulse and breathing every minute.
Bleeding Victim bleeding severely can quickly go into shock and die within 1 or 2 minutes.	Use universal precautions. With the palm of your hand, apply firm, direct pressure to the wound with a clean dressing or pad. Elevate the body part if possible. Do not remove blood-soaked dressings; use additional layers, continue to apply pressure, and elevate the site.
Choking Accidental ingestion or inhalation of food or other objects causes suffocation that can quickly lead to death. There are over 3,000 deaths annually, mostly of infants, small children, and the elderly.	The procedure of giving abdominal thrusts is easy to learn; however, the correct technique must be learned from a qualified instructor. The procedure varies somewhat for infants, children, adults, pregnant women, and obese people.

continued

Specific Problem	What To Do
Hyperventilation A situation in which a person breathes too rapidly; often the result of fear or anxiety; may cause confusion, shortness of breath, dizziness, or fainting. Intentional hyperventilation before an underwater swim is especially dangerous, since it may cause a swimmer to pass out in the water and drown.	Have the person relax and rest for a few minutes. Provide reassurance and a calming influence. Having the victim take a few breaths in a paper bag (not plastic) may be helpful. Do not permit swimmers to practice hyperventilation before attempting to swim.
Bee Stings Not especially dangerous except for people who have developed an allergic hypersensitivity to a particular venom. Those who are not hypersensitive will experience swelling, redness, and pain. Hypersensitive people may develop extreme swelling, chest constriction, breathing difficulties, hives, and shock signs.	For nonsensitive people: Scrape stinger from skin and apply cold compresses or over-the-counter topical preparation for insect bites. For sensitive people: Get professional help immediately. Scrape the stinger from skin; position the person so that the stung body part is below the level of the heart; help administer prescribed medication (if available); apply cold compresses.
Poisoning Often poisoning can be prevented with adequate safety awareness. Children are frequent victims.	Call the poison control center immediately; follow the instructions provided. Keep syrup of ipecac on hand.
Shock A life-threatening depression of circulation, respiration, and temperature control; recognizable by a victim's cool, clammy, pale skin; weak and rapid pulse; shallow breathing; weakness; nausea; or unconsciousness.	Keep the victim calm; loosen tight clothing. Help the victim to a comfortable, reclining position with legs elevated 8–12 inches (if there are no head, neck, back, or internal injuries, in which case, do not move the person at all; if breathing is difficult, help the person to sit or semi-recline). Prevent loss of body heat; cover if necessary. Do not give food or fluids. Seek further emergency assistance.
Burns Burns can cause severe tissue damage and lead to serious infection and shock.	Minor burns: immerse in cold water 10–15 minutes; dry; apply antibiotic agent and loose sterile dressing; do not apply butter or grease to burns. Major burns: immerse in cold water; cover affected area with sterile or clean dressings; do not try to clean the burn area or break blisters. Seek medical attention. Chemical burns: flood the area with running water.
Broken Bones Fractures are a common result of car accidents, falls, and recreational accidents.	Do not move the victim unless absolutely necessary to prevent further injury. Immobilize the affected area. Give care for shock while waiting for further emergency assistance.

Epilepsy: Recognition and First Aid

Seizure Type	What It Looks Like	Often Mistaken For	What To Do	What Not To Do
Convulsive Generalized tonic-clonic (also called grand mal)	Sudden cry, fall, rigidity, followed by muscle jerks, frothy saliva on lips, shallow breathing or temporarily suspended breathing, bluish skin, possible loss of bladder or bowel control, usually last 2–5 minutes; normal breathing then starts again; there may be some confusion and/or fatigue, followed by return to full oonccioucnoss	Heart attack Stroke Unknown but life-threatening emergency	Protect from nearby hazards Loosen ties or shirts collars Place folded jacket under head Turn on side to keep airway clear; reassure when consciousness returns Look for medical identification *after* seizure subsides or protective steps have been taken If single seizure lasted less than 5 minutes, ask if hospital evaluation wanted If multiple seizures, or if one seizure lasts longer than 5 minutes, seek medical attention	Don't put any hard implement in the mouth Don't try to hold tongue; it can't be swallowed Don't try to give liquids during or just after seizure Don't use artificial respiration unless breathing is absent after muscle jerks subside, or unless water has been inhaled Don't restrain
Nonconvulsive	This category includes many different forms of seizures, ranging from temporary unawareness (petit mal) to brief, sudden, massive muscle jerks (myoclonic seizures)	Daydreaming, acting out, clumsiness, poor coordination, intoxication, random activity, mental illness, and many others	Usually no first aid necessary other than to provide reassurance and emotional support If behavior during seizure places person in potentially hazardous situation (e.g., traffic, machinery), gently guide person away from hazard Medical evaluation is recommended	Do not shout at, restrain, expect verbal instructions to be obeyed, or grab a person having a nonconvulsive seizure (unless danger threatens)

appendix 2

body systems

The Circulatory System

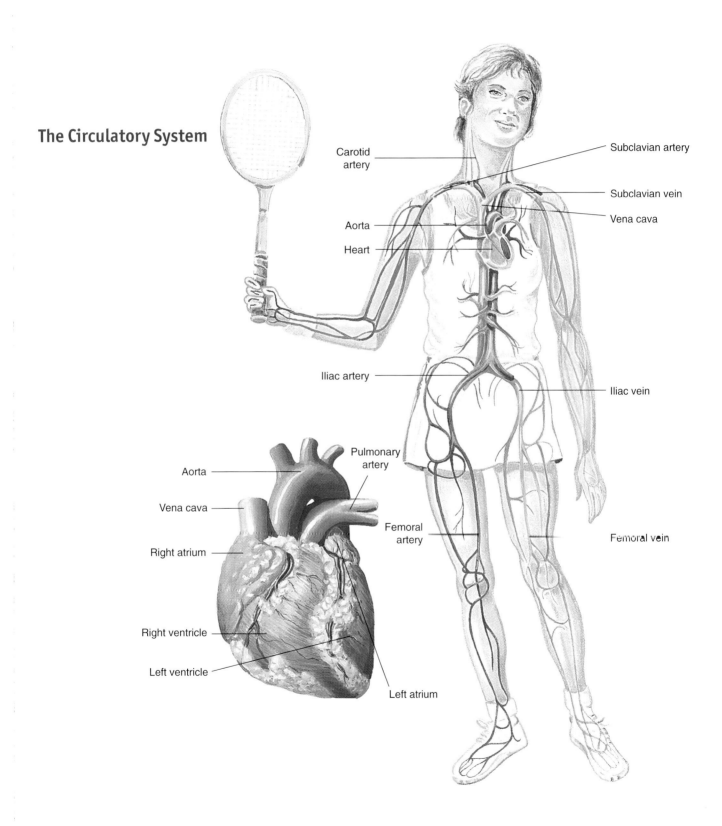

Carotid artery

Subclavian artery

Subclavian vein

Vena cava

Aorta

Heart

Iliac artery

Iliac vein

Aorta

Pulmonary artery

Vena cava

Right atrium

Femoral artery

Femoral vein

Right ventricle

Left ventricle

Left atrium

The Respiratory System

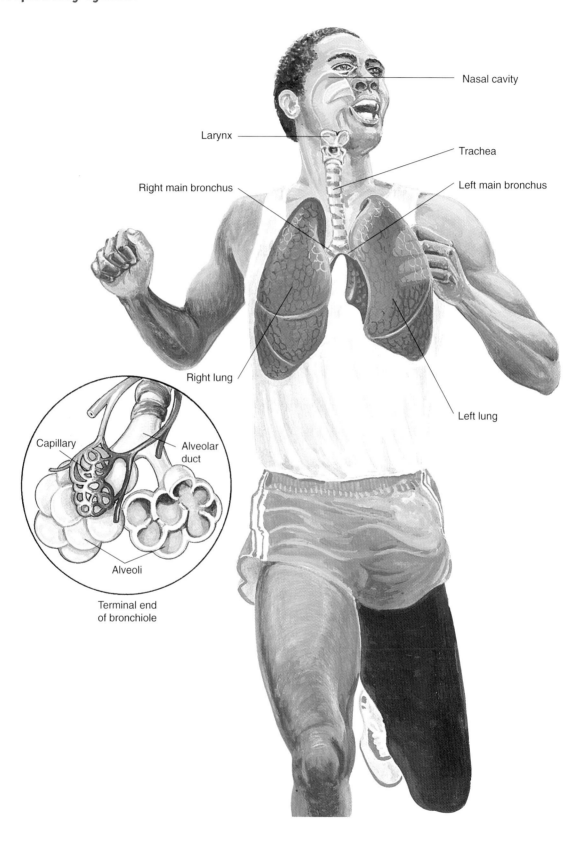

Nasal cavity

Larynx

Trachea

Right main bronchus

Left main bronchus

Right lung

Left lung

Capillary

Alveolar duct

Alveoli

Terminal end of bronchiole

The Muscular System

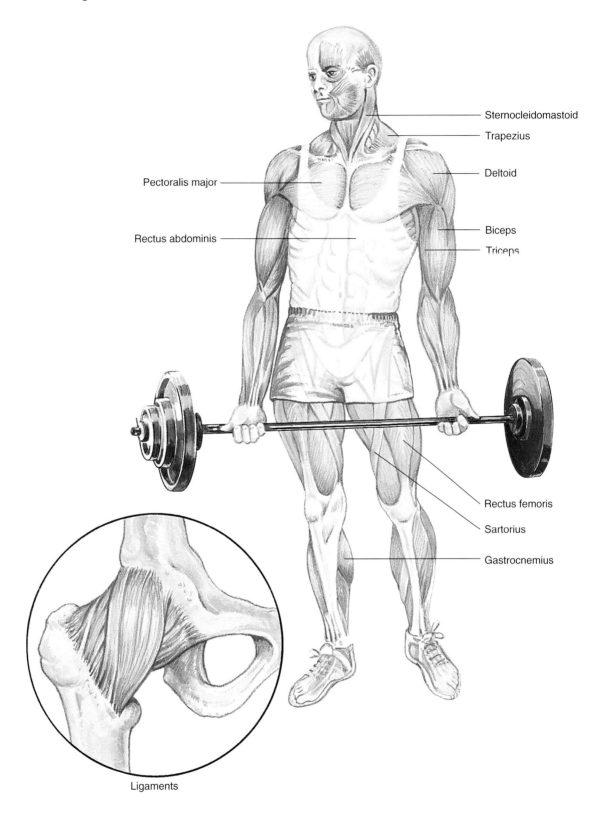

Sternocleidomastoid

Trapezius

Deltoid

Pectoralis major

Biceps

Triceps

Rectus abdominis

Rectus femoris

Sartorius

Gastrocnemius

Ligaments

The Skeletal System

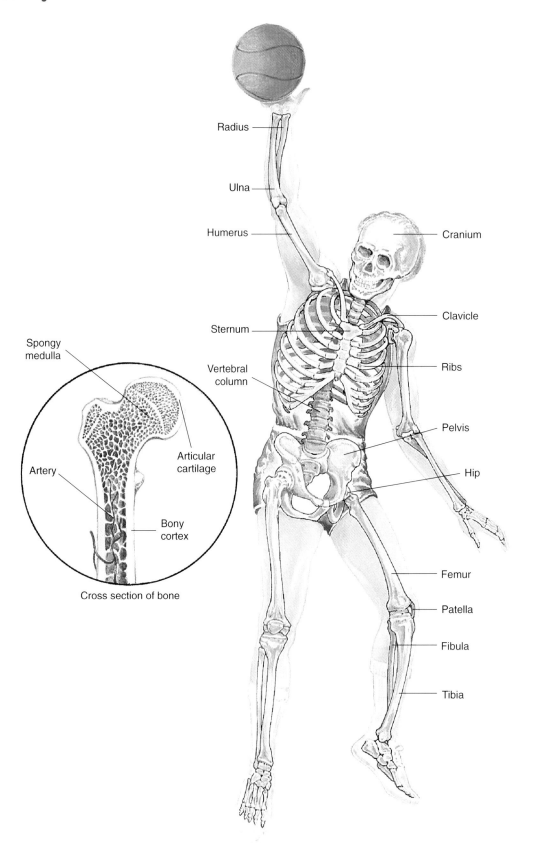

Radius

Ulna

Humerus

Sternum

Vertebral column

Spongy medulla

Artery

Articular cartilage

Bony cortex

Cross section of bone

Cranium

Clavicle

Ribs

Pelvis

Hip

Femur

Patella

Fibula

Tibia

The Nervous System

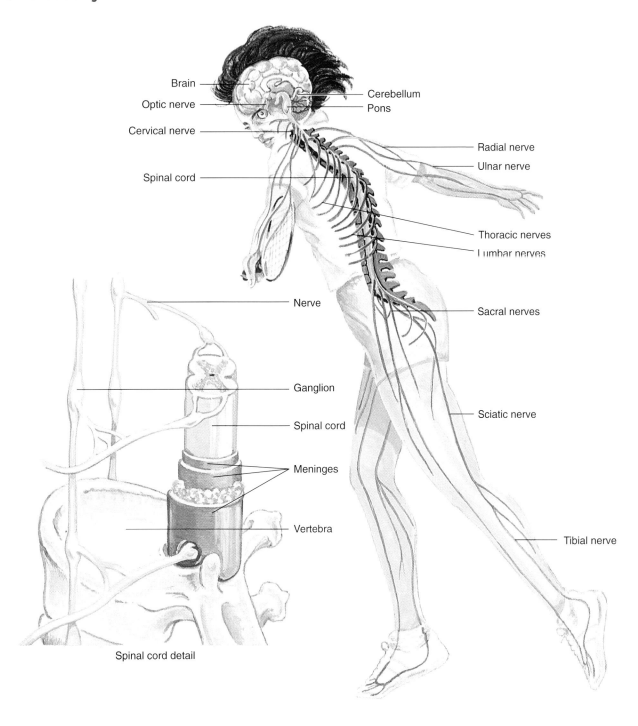

Brain

Optic nerve

Cervical nerve

Spinal cord

Cerebellum

Pons

Radial nerve

Ulnar nerve

Thoracic nerves

Lumbar nerves

Nerve

Sacral nerves

Ganglion

Spinal cord

Meninges

Sciatic nerve

Vertebra

Tibial nerve

Spinal cord detail

The Digestive System

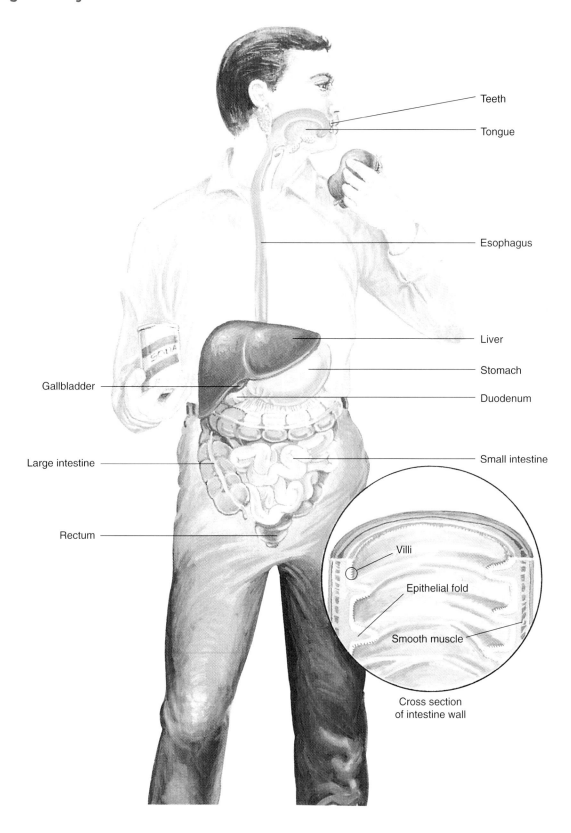

Teeth

Tongue

Esophagus

Liver

Stomach

Gallbladder

Duodenum

Large intestine

Small intestine

Rectum

Villi

Epithelial fold

Smooth muscle

Cross section
of intestine wall

The Urinary System

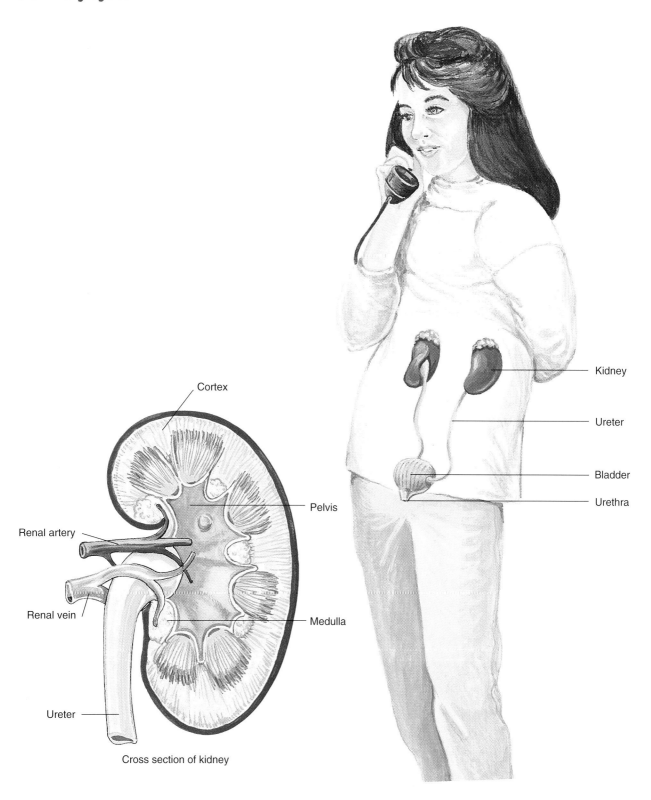

Cortex

Renal artery

Renal vein

Ureter

Cross section of kidney

Pelvis

Medulla

Kidney

Ureter

Bladder

Urethra

The Endocrine System

NOTE: Refer to Figures 14-2 and 14-3 for detailed anatomical illustrations of the reproductive systems.

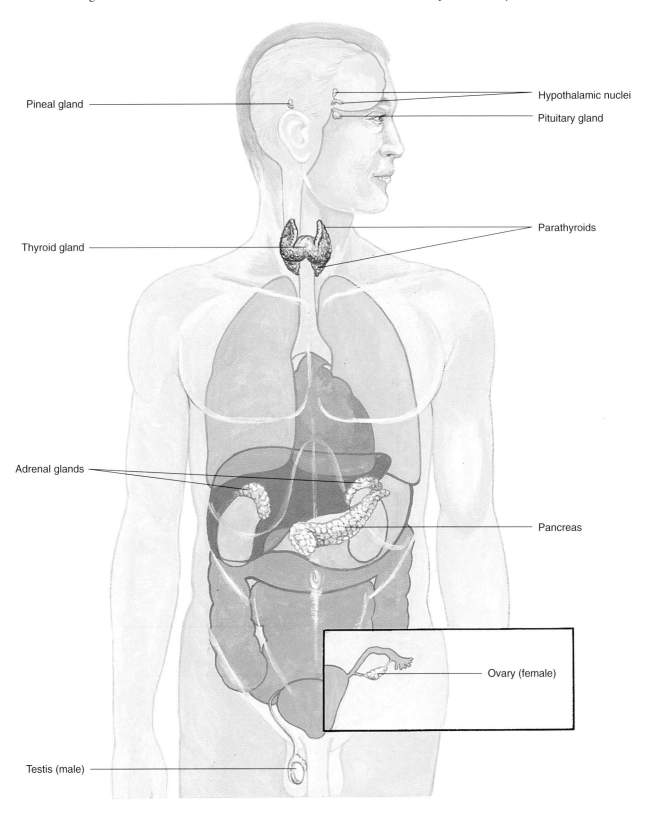

Pineal gland

Hypothalamic nuclei

Pituitary gland

Parathyroids

Thyroid gland

Adrenal glands

Pancreas

Ovary (female)

Testis (male)

appendix 3

Canadian health

by Professor Don Morrow, The University of Western Ontario

Composed of 10 provinces and 3 territories, Canada is a huge geographic land mass with a relatively small population—some 30 million people. The population is mainly concentrated along the lower one-third of the country. Historically, relationships with its southern neighbor, the United States, have been good, although Canadians perceive themselves as distinctly different from Americans. The most obvious distinction is the bilingual nature of the country, English and French, with a significant concentration of the French-speaking population located in the province of Quebec. Unlike the United States, Canada has not experienced a major civil war. Still, escalating tensions over the potential for Quebec's separation from Canada's confederation to become a sovereign state have given rise to a great deal of discussion, reflection, and concern about nationhood and our current political structure. Clearly, the prospect of Quebec and succession threatens the integrity of Canada as a nation and as a society.

One unifying element in Canadian society has been its comprehensive program of national health insurance, in which coverage is provided to all citizens directly through government, without the involvement of insurance companies. The major responsibility for health care rests with the provinces, while the federal government has served as policymaker, along with assuming some direct health-care responsibilities for special populations such as Native Canadians, the three territories, and the military. The umbrella for Canadian health is a national health insurance program. The envy of many developed countries, this program represents a cost of about 10% of the gross domestic product; however, the expenses of maintaining the program have exceeded anyone's forecast. For example, in 1993 the total cost of the health-care system was some $55 billion, almost double the amount of just seven years earlier. Clearly, changes in concept, structure, and funding are needed if government is to continue offering any health-care system. This section outlines the history, nature, and future directions of health and health care in Canada. Further readings are listed at the end.

Historical Background

The first universal hospital insurance program in Canada was implemented in the province of Saskatchewan shortly after the end of World War II; by 1960 the other nine provinces had established similar programs, with federal legislation enacted for a national program in 1971 (Frankel et al. 1996; Pederson et al. 1994). In the early 1980s this federal, political infrastructure became the Canadian Health Promotion Directorate. Without question, the landmark federal initiative was the publication and dissemination in 1974 of the document titled *A New Perspective on the Health of Canadians.* The impact of this document nationally and internationally cannot be overstated. It received worldwide attention for its recasting of the concept of health toward what is now called *health promotion.* Whereas health traditionally had been equated with the health-care system, the *Perspective's* thrust was toward the broad concept of a *health field* that included all matters affecting health. This *health field concept* embraced four avenues or elements:

- health care organization: the "system" of health care
- the environment
- lifestyle
- human biology

Such a concept was radical for the mid-1970s. It challenged the prevalent and ingrained equation that level of health equals quality of medicine. While applauding Canada's health care system as "second to none in the world," the *New Perspective* underlined "ominous" counterforces threatening the standard of living, public health protection and advances in medical science; such counterforces as environmental pollution, city living, abuse of alcohol, tobacco, and other drugs, eating patterns, and sedentary habits of indolence were identified for concern and action. In effect, the *Perspective* paper provided a whole new way of conceptualizing health as much broader than the traditional "medical model" of health and health care that had been so strongly focused on disease and illness.

The Health Field Concept

Careful to recognize that "the provision of personal health services to the general public is clearly a matter of provincial jurisdiction," the 1974 document highlighted the existence of national health problems that know no provincial boundaries and that arise from causes embedded in the social fabric of the nation as a whole (page 6). To convince health professionals and the public alike, the *New Perspective* showed that major causes of illness, defined as number of hospitalization days, were diseases of the cardiovascular system, followed by accidents and violence, then mental illness; in turn these were directly related to the interplay of the four elements identified as the health field concept. Thus, ill health was shown to be the direct result of self-imposed risks like drug abuse, poor diet, and insufficient exercise as well as of careless driving, promiscuity, and so forth. Also tied to the health field concept were environmental problems such as urbanization, working conditions, rapid social change, and economic deprivation. The paradox so clearly illuminated in the *New Perspective* was that of lip-service agreement on the importance of research and prevention in health improvement, juxtaposed against the continued tendency to increase disproportionately the amount of money spent on existing illnesses and their treatment. The health field concept was characterized as comprehensive, as allowing for a workable system of analysis, and as bringing focus to neglected areas. The document's authors believed this reconfigured understanding of health would greatly assist in identifying factors that contribute to sickness/death and in determining actions that could improve the quality of health. In this regard the *New Perspective* offered 74 suggestions or proposals to analyze health-care issues and to develop more effective health-care policy.

Not only was the *New Perspective* document symbolic of major health reform, but it was also the first federal government articulation of a comprehensive and inclusive view of health that went far beyond the World Health Organization definition, "Health is a state of complete physical, mental, and social well-being and not merely the absence of disease and infirmity," so entrenched in health-care systems worldwide. In reality, however, this 1974 perspective was ahead of its time; and it presented a viewpoint that challenged the status quo as represented by the Canadian medical establishment, the country's health-care institutions, and the collective consciousness of Canadians themselves. It was just too easy to cling to the old equation of level of health = quality of medicine/health care. Moreover, economic prosperity and growth masked the significance of such threats to health as environmental and lifestyle factors. Further, it was widely held that the *New Perspective* was too narrow, and that it intended to "blame the victim" for health problems. What was needed, critics said, was a more socially oriented view of health and health education, one that accounted more directly for environmental and social factors, to place health in context in Canadian society.

The Ottawa Charter

Major indicators of change were witnessed in the early 1980s. The city of Vancouver in British Columbia, Canada's westernmost province, hosted a "Shifting Medical Paradigm Conference" in 1980; formulated to usher in a shift from the medical, disease-prevention/treatment model, this conference represented more of a challenge to Western medical tradition, rather than offering any concrete concept of health promotion. Of somewhat greater impact was the Toronto-based 1984 conference, "Beyond Health Care," which stressed the need for transitions in public health policy to promote healthy cities and communities (Pederson et al. 1994). The most important piece of health legislation or reform was produced in 1986 when the *Ottawa Charter for Health Promotion* was created after a conference on health promotion hosted in Ottawa, the nation's capital. Spiraling health-care costs were the major force behind the reform initiatives that resulted in the *Charter;* however, individual and agency initiatives in the spirit of health reform complemented the federal document.

The *Charter* took bold and needed steps to move the concept of health away from the treatment of illnesses and the attendant technologies toward a concept and policy that truly focused on health. Instead of trying to change the definition of health—so sacred to many health professionals—the *Charter* used the concept of *health promotion,* or "the process of enabling people to increase control over, and to improve their health." Health in this sense was perceived as a resource for everyday life, not the goal or objective of living. This concept underscored the importance of quality of everyday life in the process of health in preference to the traditional statistical emphasis on longevity or illness. Health promotion was envisioned in this document as a process rather than as a set of risk factor outcomes or as the "social work of medicine" (Pederson et al. 1994). Health promotion was not merely presented as the responsibility of the health-care sector but as an arena of shared personal and social resources and decisions. The *Charter* identified the fundamental conditions and resources for health:

- peace
- shelter
- education
- food
- income
- stable economic system

- sustainable resources
- social justice
- equity

In short, this set of Maslow-like conditions reflected the multifaceted nature of the concept of health. Moreover, the *Charter* gained worldwide attention for its identification and explanation of strategies for change:

- Build healthy public policy.
- Create supportive environments.
- Strengthen community action.
- Develop personal skills.
- Reorient health services.

Set against the action orientations of *advocate, enable,* and *mediate,* the prerequisites for health and the strategies for change were aligned for a new conceptual and realistic vision of health and its promotion. Once again Canada played a leadership role in framing and operationalizing the concept of health promotion, just as it had in changing the medical perception of health care in 1974 via the *New Perspective* document.

A Framework for Health Promotion

The World Health Organization and Health and Welfare Canada were responsible for hosting the 1986 Ottawa conference and establishing an action-oriented *Charter* that challenged participating organizations, governments, and individuals to pursue a "health for all" goal for the year 2000 and beyond. In the same year, the federal Minister for Health and Welfare, Jake Epp, took the *Charter* out of the realm of abstract conceptualization by articulating and promoting a practical model to achieve the *Charter's* goal. It was called *A Framework for Health Promotion* and it is configured in the chart below.

Some explanation will be helpful. The *Framework* paper identified three major challenges that were not being addressed by current health policies and practices. First, disadvantaged groups had a significantly lower life expectancy, poorer health, and higher prevalence of disability than the average Canadian. Second, various forms of preventable diseases and injuries continued to undermine the health and quality of life of the citizenry. Third, the lack of support for chronically ill, disabled, or emotionally stressed people was pronounced and serious; improved coping mechanisms and support services were needed. Such challenges, the document stated, warranted mechanisms for relief. First, self-care, or the decisions and actions individuals take in the interests of their own health, was intrinsic to health promotion. Second, through mutual aid, people could help each other cope; and third, the creation of conditions and surroundings conducive to health was strongly recommended. These three strategies could be implemented in provinces, municipalities, and communities to enhance health.

The *Framework* received large-scale promotion and, like the 1974 federal document (*New Perspective*), it was criticized for being too vague in its strategies. Nonetheless, the *Framework* must be credited with targeting health promotion as the central focus of health reform and direction in Canada. Because health is constitutionally defined as a provincial concern, federal policy could serve only to stimulate, challenge, and frame new concepts and tactics for health. Together with the *Charter,* the *Framework* represented new commitments that both provoked and empowered changes in health in line with the World Health

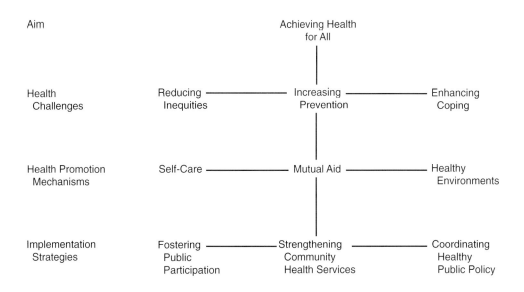

Organization's enabling definition of health promotion defined in the *Charter* just described. If health promotion was to involve social responsibility, then the federal initiatives in 1986 did establish a new framework for health promotion. The challenge of "health for all" seems ambitious and lofty; however, if health can be perceived as an attitude and a process more than an end in itself, then the goal of health for all seems more realistic. Cost containment may well be an engine that drives health-care reform in Canada, yet reform is absolutely necessary, as is the reduction of health expenditures everywhere.

Current Provincial Perspectives

The acid test of any policy initiative is, of course, its implementation. In 1988 the Canadian Public Health Association, inspired by the three key strategies presented in the *Framework* model, created the Strengthening Community Health Program with a view toward focusing and applying health promotion at the community level. This program had its roots in the Ottawa *Charter* and might best be examined by considering a cross-Canada description of health promotion during the late 1980s and early 1990s. Most of the material discussed in this section is synthesized from Pederson's comprehensive book, *Health Promotion in Canada* (1994). The intent here is to provide a brief overview of the provincial and community responses to federal policy and strategy.

On the west coast, the province of British Columbia has been successful in inducing some one hundred communities to join a vibrant "healthy community" movement inspired directly by the *Framework* document. Government initiatives in that province are directed toward recognizing, promoting, and linking community actions that reflect health promotion activities such as community health plans, conferences, surveys, and educational programs. By contrast, in neighboring Alberta, we see conflicting perspectives about health promotion that range from full commitment at one extreme to the notion that it represents an unaffordable luxury. Nevertheless, the provincial government in Alberta stresses changes related to promoting healthy lifestyles and addressing health determinants.

Saskatchewan, the first province to adopt a universal hospital insurance program, has a decades-old health action strategy of creating coalitions through which communities have been encouraged and supported in health promotion activities with dramatic success. In 1992, this province's government released a major health reform initiative, *A Saskatchewan Vision for Health,* which is based on two principles for action: the concept of wellness as the goal of health services, and community control of health service delivery. In the same year, the fourth prairie province, Manitoba, published its *Quality Health for Manitobans* paper to support health promotion for its 1 million inhabitants. Manitoba boasts seven strong healthy community projects based on a partners-for-health agreement between the government and the communities involved.

In central Canada, the most populous and arguably the most prosperous area of the country, responses to the *Charter* and the *Framework* are significantly different. The 10 million people in Ontario have seen lengthy policy statements on the province's *Nurturing Health* documents, but very little in the way of developments at the community or grassroots level of health reform. Instead the Ontario government seems intent on taking only the broad social view of health that is grounded in the determinants of health and the health-care system. Quebec's 7 million people (about 80% of whom are French speaking) and their governing bodies have given only token acknowledgment to federal initiatives in health promotion. The province has had very few "champions" of the concept of health promotion and very little political pressure for reform. As a unit, the Atlantic provinces are victims of inequity because they live in a distinctly poorer economic environment. Many of the communities in these four provinces are single-industry towns. As a result, change is slow and at best some of these provinces are just beginning to move toward the concept and practice of health promotion. Including the Yukon Territory, which is under direct federal health jurisdiction, it is evident that across Canada the contemporary trend is toward community or grassroots initiatives in health promotion. It will be helpful to examine the trends in health care as a means of viewing the community and provincial moves toward health reform in a larger context.

Health Practices and Health Status

As we have seen in our review of provincial programs, health-care structures are rooted in the individual social ideologies of each province. Less evident is the effect of these programs on the actual health practices or health status of the Canadian population. If over $55 billion is currently spent on health care in Canada, it is useful to ascertain where the money is being spent in relation to health concepts, practices, and reform policies. In a recent publication, *The Sociology of Health and Health Care,* the authors point out that health-care expenditures in Canada consume a greater proportion of our gross national product than is the case in most other industrialized nations. This information is critical in discussing and understanding Canadian health. Just over one-third of total provincial budgets are expended on health, and by far the majority (75%) of that money goes to institutional and physician services, that is, for health care itself, not for prevention or programs for change (Sutherland and Fulton, 1990). Canadian life expectancy in general has increased, but the reasons for the increase have less to do with improvements in health care and more to do with positive changes in standard of living related to living conditions, nutrition and nutritional practices, and decreases in the rate of infant mortality. Frankel and other authors are careful to point out that increased life expectancy carries greater risks for decreases in the quality of life; for example, life expectancy does not automatically imply disability-free life expectancy. If social class is isolated, no matter which measure of socioeconomic status is used, higher income earners and people working in more prestigious jobs experience lower mortality rates and longer life expectancy even when the latter is adjusted for quality measures. Overall, changes in longevity among the Canadian population do not necessarily mean proportional changes in health status. The converse of this statement is equally instructive; in countries like Hungary and Finland, where life expectancy has decreased in spite of costly health-care systems, suicide and lifestyle risk have actually increased (Sutherland and Fulton, 1990). Thus, it is important to interpret longevity data in context with other measures or indicators of health and health status.

In this decade, cardiovascular diseases and cancer remain the most significant causes of death for both sexes from the age of 25 years onward (*Action Statement*). Mortality rates continue to be considerably higher for males than for females throughout the life span. The irony here is that females in Canada report higher rates of illness and higher rates of use of health services than do males (Frankel et al. 1996). Whether the latter tendency represents a cultural and/or gender difference in the approach to health behavior, it is a significant sex difference worthy of greater exploration and analysis. From a Canadian and a global perspective, it is critical to recognize the epidemic proportions of depression, anxiety, stress, loneliness, and insecurity (Sutherland and Fulton, 1990), all of which contribute to a decline in the quality of life and lifestyle— more evidence to underline the importance of health promotion that is beyond mere physical health or well-being.

Health workers make up about 8% of the Canadian labor force. Of that percentage, about three-quarters work in the nation's approximately 1,200 hospitals. The Canadian health-care system constitutes the largest social service sector in the country, and it is the third largest employer in the nation (Frankel et al. 1996). Sutherland and others contend that since the 1970s, Canada has had "too many physicians." This is a debatable point when the stature of physicians is so elevated in our society and when hospitals themselves serve as such powerful symbols of wealth and power. What is remarkable and worthy of reconsideration is the rejection of "alternative" forms of health practitioners like naturopaths, homeopaths, and practitioners of Eastern forms of medicine (acupuncture, for example). Also, in spite of community-based health policy reforms, the whole notion of community health centers is slow to gain acceptance by traditional medical personnel, who perceive them as threatening to their power and independence. The concept of community health-care centers is based on a team or shared approach to health delivery, which challenges the current top-down approach. Community health centers support a variety of health-care personnel only some of whom are medical doctors, in order to serve health consumers. To date, only the province of Quebec has achieved significant inroads in establishing such centers (Frankel et al. 1996), solid evidence that health promotion may be more of a factor in that province than its perceived lack of compliance with either the *Charter* or the strategies of the *Framework* documents.

Action Statement for Health Promotion

Lifestyle, special environments, age, sex, wealth, power, institutional dominance, biological factors, and a wide variety of other variables interact in Canada, as they do elsewhere in the world, to characterize the status of health in any given time period or social grouping. And still the mirage of the importance of the health-care system continues to overwhelm health-care reform and to monopolize human and economic resources. To renew efforts toward greater health promotion, with optimal health as a goal, the Canadian Public Health Association in 1996 recommitted itself to the strategies of the *Charter* and the *Framework*. In July of 1996, the association published a working paper called *Action Statement for Health Promotion in Canada,* with the following introductory comment:

> This *Action Statement* is the product of a two-year consultation process involving more than 1000 people. Participants in the process were mainly health professionals and volunteers who work to promote health. Other participants came from areas such as social services, education, recreation, environment and law enforcement. These people share the values and ways of working that define health promotion, even though they may not call themselves health promoters. Together we represent a community of shared purpose.

The Canadian Public Health Association is a group within the Population Health Directorate of the federal ministry, Health Canada. The *Action Statement* is a policy developed for provinces and health-care workers to consider and implement in local areas. Notice that paid professionals in the health-care industry, such as physicians and hospital personnel, are conspicuous by their absence in this process of formulating an action statement. Instead it is a grassroots commitment based on shared values with respect to the goals of health promotion. The wisdom or necessity of not using health professionals/workers in strategic policy is not the issue here; instead it is important to examine the direction of this proposal and then to look at examples of what has been happening recently in health promotion in the country.

The *Action Statement,* significantly, represents a recommitment to the framework established in the 1986 *Charter* as a viable approach to health promotion; 10 years after the charter was published, the *Action Statement* refines the document's focus to the mid-1990s. Noting global trends with respect to the escalation of poverty levels, rapidly increasing unemployment, and economic decisions and practices that threaten the environment and consolidate wealth and power in private corporations with few legal responsibilities to the common good, the *Action Statement* recommends that priorities be set to affirm and share the vision and values of health promotion. The statement also calls for the creation of alliances across and between different community and health sectors; honing knowledge, skills, and the capacity to improve health; emphasizing political commitment and the development of healthy public policies; working to ensure that health system reform truly promotes health both inside and outside the health-care system. Of major importance in this statement is the recognition that improving health is a vital component of human development. Instead of reiterating ill-health data, the *Action Statement* succinctly summarized the implications of that data in sifting out the following critical health determinants:

- healthy childhood development
- adequate incomes
- small gaps between the rich and poor
- absence of discrimination based on gender, culture, race, and sexual orientation
- lifelong learning opportunities
- healthy lifestyles
- meaningful work opportunities with some control over decision making
- social relationships that respect diversity
- freedom from violence or its threat
- freedom from exposure to infectious disease
- protection of humans from environmental hazard
- protection of the environment from human hazards

The *Action Statement* takes a refreshing approach to health status data by interpreting what it means to work toward health as a process with direction instead of merely reporting the state of ill health. Further, the statement recognizes that health promotion has a firm values base. For example, of the six value statements given in the

document, one stresses the value that individual liberties must be respected with a priority given to the common good, and another stresses that individuals must be treated with dignity and respect. Although these might seem like obvious commonsense principles, explicitly recognizing and stating them provides some validation for perceiving health in its fullest sense: physical, emotional, mental, and spiritual.

Also important, relative to this *Action Statement,* is the learning gained from the 1986 commitment to health promotion. The document stresses that strategic principles must be understood in guiding the development and implementation of health promotion:

- Health promotion addresses health issues in social and environmental context.
- Health promotion supports a holistic approach to all aspects of healthy development.
- Health promotion requires a long-term perspective; time must be taken to create awareness and build understanding about health determinants.
- Health promotion supports a balance between centralized and decentralized decision making on policies affecting people.
- Health promotion is multisectional in that cooperation must be achieved between people and organizations to dovetail with program initiatives in the health sector.
- Health promotion draws on formal knowledge in the social, economic, political, medical, and environmental sciences and on personal experience.
- Health promotion emphasizes public accountability.

Apparently much has been learned about solidifying and implementing health promotion from a strategic perspective. In particular, it is recognized that, while change in health policy and behavior must come, it will come slowly; newer or "sexier" health initiatives are not the answer. Instead the *Action Statement* confirms health promotion from an empowerment perspective. Strategies require some concrete tactics for implementation, and the *Action Statement* supplies strong suggestions in that regard. Once again, the *Charter* is used as a springboard to reinvigorate specific thrusts in health promotion. With respect to advocating healthy public policy, the statement accurately highlights the shaping power of policies in determining how money, power, and material resources flow through institutions of health and thereby offer the determinants of health behavior and outcomes. During the past 10 years, the emphasis in policy making has been on support for creating and developing healthy lifestyles; more emphasis must now be placed on policies that create healthy living conditions and that give voice to society's least powerful groups. To that end, the *Action Statement* provides a comprehensive list of priorities and tactics for action in policy making.

Community Focus

Equally stressed in this 1996 document is the dominant and proven need to *strengthen communities* in the health promotion thrust. Because communities already share common space, identities, interests, and concerns through various agencies and activities, the *Action Statement* mentions several action priorities to provide community training opportunities, funding, support from/for community networks, and the development of evaluation methods for continued monitoring and improvement. The evidence is clear in Canada that changes in health promotion will not come from the institutionalized health-care sector. The provincial initiatives toward health promotion described earlier demonstrate that change in the area of health promotion works best at the community, grassroots level. Related to this fact is the third tactic identified in the *Action Statement:* the absolute necessity to *reform health systems.* The document narrows its focus to two specific objectives: to shift the emphasis from treating disease to improving health; and to increase the effectiveness and efficiency of the health-care system.

Both of these objectives form part of most provincial policy statements on health reform. Still, the reality of health system reform lags considerably behind the recognition that it is needed. Political debate and public attention tend to be focused on insured medical treatments and reducing the number of hospital beds; cuts in primary health care are widespread. For example, in Ontario, the *Toronto Daily Star* gave full-page coverage to the appointment of retired Queen's University former dean of medicine Duncan Sinclair to the chair of the province's Health Services Restructuring Committee (*TDS,* September 15, 1996). Sinclair's task, the article said, was to "shake up/down the Ontario hospital system" to rid the system of duplication and to "ensure there is a health care system for future generations." This is a prime example of praiseworthy reductions in cost but failure to address the broad determinants of health: closing hospitals is not the sole answer to health reform. Instead, according to the *Action Statement,* family- and community-based care must be improved with stronger health protection programs and access to client-centered primary health-care services. To achieve real benefits from and by health promotion, the knowledge base about health determinants and regional health profiles must be increased and stronger alliances or coalitions must be fostered among different organizations that share the common goal of health promotion, and can effect real change in the broad determinants of health. Ultimately, as the *Action Statement* points out, if efforts to develop health promotion efforts in Canada are to succeed, they must be allied to similar efforts throughout the global community.

Current Initiatives and Future Directions

In Canada's health promotion survey in 1990, in which some 13,000 people across the country were interviewed regarding health status, practices, and beliefs, self-reports were compiled to assess the status of health promotion in the population. The respondents reported very little change in health status. The rich and the well educated were more likely to report good to excellent health status than those with less wealth and education. The same survey showed findings about social relationships, environmental health practices, personal health practices, alcohol and other drug use, nutritional practices, heart disease prevention, leisure time physical activity, cancer prevention practices, injury control and safety, sexual health, and dental health. The conclusion, once again, is that health education is absolutely critical as a catalyst for improvement in health behaviors.

Similarly, in 1991 Angus published an extensive "Review of Significant Health Care Commissions and Task Forces in Canada Since 1983–84," sponsored by the Canadian Medical Association. His finding? At the root of all of these commissions and reforms is the desire to rebalance and redirect the system in three important ways: toward greater emphasis on disease prevention and health promotion; toward community-based health-care alternatives; and toward greater accountability of the health-care system. Clearly, Canada has committed itself to the whole concept and implementation of health promotion. Is it working? This question is difficult to answer, because generalizations are impossible. The following section examines specific pockets of information and examples in an effort to find out if and how health promotion is being implemented in Canada.

The Implementation of Health Promotion

A positive sign of knowledge-based, applied research is the work of the Canadian Fitness and Lifestyle Research Institute (CFLRI). This organization's mission is to "enhance the well being of Canadians through research and communication of information about physically active lifestyles to the public and private sectors." The Institute seeks to understand active living by addressing fitness issues from the complementary perspectives of the health professions, the social and psychological sciences, and the physiological and biological sciences. In 1994 the CFLRI published its findings on "Health Promotion at Work: Results of the 1992 National Workplace Survey." The Institute recognized that because some 13 million Canadians are employed, the workplace is a very important environment and avenue for health promotion. Some 45,000 Canadian companies claim to have health promotion programs in place to varying degrees. The most popular lifestyle or health promotion intervention on the part of employees is in the realm of smoking cessation. Some 3,500 companies with 20 or more employees responded to the survey and provided information about such health determinants as stress, harassment, discrimination, financial uncertainty, conflicts at work, fatigue, and levels of physical activity. The survey data show that workplace health promotion efforts are increasing and expanding. Only businesses in Quebec were more likely to claim that health is the sole responsibility of the employee. Workplaces must continue to be targeted for health promotion and reform. Philosophically, however, such efforts run counter to the value system in a capitalist society. Capitalism is based on the values of material gain and inequality, reflected in most workplaces by the very fact of work and its goals. Health promotion, in contrast, is rooted in equality of opportunity and benefits as well as in the quality of everyday life rather than material ends or goals. This contradiction in values is one that must be resolved to functionally support and implement health promotion initiatives.

ParticipACTION

If data don't convince people—and the history of health data and ill-health data confirm that most people are not scared easily by statistical trends—then there must be alternatives to persuasion. In Canada, one of the most successful campaigns focused on healthy behavior has been ParticipACTION, a non-government movement to promote healthy lifestyles. Established in the early 1970s, this not-for-profit organization was initially commissioned by the federal government to campaign for improved fitness and lifestyle improvement. ParticipACTION's objective was to market physical fitness as one would market toothpaste or any other product. The organization used two key marketing strategies: (1) to employ modern marketing methods in advertising; and (2) to finance itself from the private sector, not the public purse. To implement the first strategy, the organization developed a four-cornered approach to marketing fitness: educate, motivate, remind, and provide solutions about/for physical fitness. The group leans heavily on private corporations to achieve its goals and is distinguished by its clever use of advertising. In its 30-year history, ParticipACTION has had to compete with service agencies and charities like the United Way for advertising time and space. Annual reviews of its efforts show impressive cost-benefit ratios for its advertising. It is difficult to open any newspaper today and not find some small ad or teasing clip provided by this organization, which is highly effective in targeting the population at the grassroots level.

ParticipACTION also publishes *Active Living,* a national magazine that provides resource information to educators, health professionals, fitness leaders, and others in the broad spectrum of health interests in Canada. This publication and the efforts of ParticipACTION to involve itself in wider aspects of health and behavior change and information exchange are clear indicators of health promotion at work.

Food Guides and Eating Patterns

A growing body of evidence suggests that symptoms and causes of ill health are directly attributable to eating choices and patterns. Canada has long been famed for its *Food Guide to Healthy Eating,* a simple, one-sheet "recipe" for appropriate daily food selection from the four main food groups. Heavy marketing emphasis is placed on low-fat foods, reducing portion sizes, focusing on "grazing" foods, and becoming better consumers by paying attention to food labels. The Heart and Stroke Foundation of Canada, long committed to decreasing the incidence and prevalence of these disorders, actively promotes *heart-smart* foods, and has supported the publication of a heart-healthy cookbook.

Another excellent example of promoting health through healthier eating is a highly successful recipe book called *Looneyspoons: Low-Fat Food Made Fun,* written by two sisters in Ontario. Using the teasing style employed in ParticipACTION campaigns, the book taps into the day-to-day experiences and interests of ordinary people. Chapter titles include, "If You Bake It, They Will Come," and, "Meatless in Seattle." Straightforward low-fat tasty recipes are presented with lighthearted comments like, "Low-fat eating is for those who are thick and tired of dieting," and "Dieting is the penalty for exceeding the feed limit." Even the recipe titles have flair and appeal: "Pita-the-Great," "Scalloping Gourmet," "Mission Shrimpossible," and "Veal of Fortune" are a few examples. Such an innovative approach to healthy behavior through nutritious eating is a solid and useful response to serious problems like obesity and anorexia nervosa, which so negatively affect the health and health costs of Canadians.

Wellness

Newspapers in Canada carry stories regularly about communities hosting "health fairs," local gatherings at which the public has easy access to health-care personnel, resources, and information. Similarly, educational curricula reflect growing trends toward teaching and learning about health. For example, the *Food Guide to Healthy Eating* is known to most elementary school children across Canada. In secondary schools, such as those in Ontario, the most senior course in physical education contains an entire, comprehensive section on "wellness" and "psychological and social development" related to a framework of holistic health education. Several universities have implemented wellness or well-being research; teaching and study centers patterned themselves after the phenomenally successful National Wellness Center in Stevens Point, Wisconsin, but with greater emphasis on the research component and mandate in postsecondary education.

Promoting Men's Health

In Canada, as in the United States and other Western Hemisphere countries, women are far more likely to seek help in matters of health than men—despite the fact that men have distinct health problems and earlier incidences of disease and premature death than do women. Part of the reason for this gender-based difference in response to health initiatives and reform lies in social conditioning; traditionally, men have been expected to be stoic, invulnerable, almost bulletproof in their day-to-day lives. Until recently, boys have been brought up to be self-reliant, to suppress "soft" emotions, and to "prove" their toughness through sports, hazardous jobs, war, and high-risk behaviors like workaholism, social isolation, and avoidance of intimacy. There are no clear answers to the dramatic difference in men's and women's responses to health promotion, but new approaches must be identified as the role of men in Canadian society continues to change.

A Regional Example

If health promotion is grounded in community-based programs and reform, then we must have evaluations and information bases for those communities. A comprehensive study, "Community Health and Well Being in Southwestern Ontario," recently was compiled to provide epidemiological information on the determinants of health and health status of the region, a community of some 1.5 million people, or about 13 percent of the province's total population. Results of this study show that the region has significantly higher rates of mortality from heart attacks and other cardiovascular diseases and diabetes. Hospitalization rates are at least 10 percent higher for these same problems than in the rest of Ontario. The residents of this community smoke more, eat more fat, exercise less, and have more body fat than residents of Ontario as a whole—not surprising given the mortality and hospitalization findings presented above.

The area has a higher proportion of seniors and residents aged 15 and over with less than a grade 9 education than do other parts of the province.

Significantly, the study found that the only factor that predicts life expectancy of a community is its poverty rate (not the number of hospital beds available or other traditional data); the higher the poverty level, the higher the rate of premature mortality. These findings are important for many reasons. First, they dramatically illustrate once again that health status does not equal health care. Further, they show that social environment, physical environment, and biological endowment (how well one chooses his/her parents!) all are determinants of health as is the individual's responses to those factors. Lifestyle factors, the study's authors stress, are not the sole or even the primary cause of poor health; rather, they are symptoms of a variety of social, psychological, and economic factors, perhaps the most important of which is low income. In fact, low income may be such a key health variable that it "may set off a domino effect on other health hazards." Community-based studies like this appear to contribute significantly to ongoing efforts toward health promotion and corresponding evaluation in Canada.

Summary

Health promotion is a slow process, but the changes occurring in health delivery and health behavior toward enhancement of quality lifestyles are rapid. The ability to diagnose symptoms from such sources as the Internet and its resources are a boon, as well as a challenge to traditional health procedures and forms of care. Clearly, changes in health cannot be the responsibility of government: individuals in communities must assume increasing responsibility for promoting health as a process, not a static end or achievable goal. In reality, health, like most forms of human behavior, is an attitude, one that is based on personal, social, and cultural values and practices. Until Canada or any other nation recognizes that fact, the achievement of true health will remain an elusive goal.

Sources and Further Reading

Action Statement for Health Promotion in Canada, Ottawa: Canadian Public Health Association, July, 1996.

Active Learning, September 1992, Volume 1, Number 4.

Alder, R., Vingilis, E., Mai, V., editors. London, Ontario: Middlesex-London Health Unit and the Faculty of Medicine, The University of Western Ontario, 1996.

Craig, C. L., Beaulieu, A., Cameron, C. *Health Promotion at Work: Results of the 1992 National Workplace Survey*. Ottawa: Canadian Fitness and Lifestyle Research Institute, 1994.

Crichton, A., Hsu, D., Tsand, S. *Canada's Health Care System: Its Funding and Organization.* Ottawa: Canadian Hospital Association, 1990.

Epp, J. *Achieving Health for All: A Framework for Health Promotion.* Ottawa: Health and Welfare Canada, 1986.

Frankel, G., Speechley, M., Wade, T. J. *The Sociology of Health and Health Care: A Canadian Perspective.* Toronto: Copp Clark Ltd., 1996.

Lazear, D. *Seven Ways of Knowing.* Palatine, IL: Skylight Publishing, 1991.

Ottawa Charter for Health Promotion. Ottawa: World Health Organization and Health and Welfare Canada, 1986.

Pederson, A., O'Neill, M., Rootman, I. *Health Promotion in Canada: Provincial, National and International Perspectives.* Toronto: W. B. Saunders Canada, 1994.

Podleski, J., Podleski, G. *Looneytoons: Low-Fat Food Made Fun.* Ottawa: Granet Publishing Inc., 1996.

Stephens, T., Fowler, G. D., editors. *Canada's Health Promotion Survey 1990: Technical Report.* Ottawa: Ministry of Supply and Services Canada, 1993.

Sutherland, R. W., Fulton, M. J. *Health Care in Canada: A Description and Analysis of Canadian Health Services.* Ottawa: The Health Group, 1990.

appendix 4

Canada's food guide to healthy eating

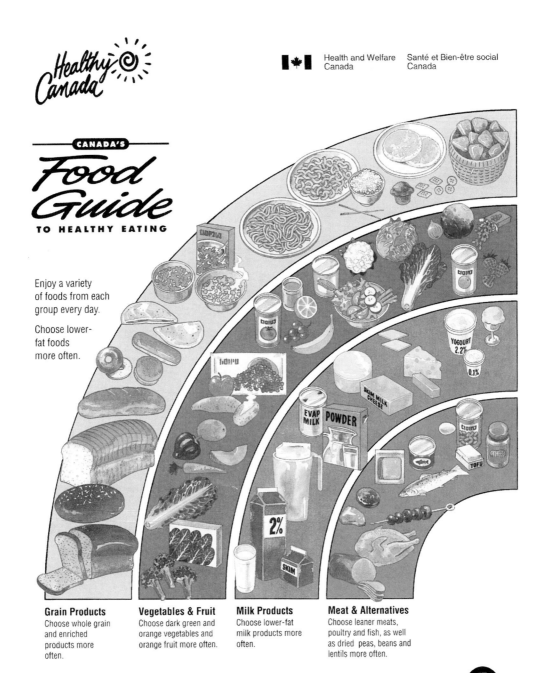

Healthy Canada

■♦■ Health and Welfare Canada   Santé et Bien-être social Canada

CANADA'S
Food Guide
TO HEALTHY EATING

Enjoy a variety of foods from each group every day.

Choose lower-fat foods more often.

Grain Products
Choose whole grain and enriched products more often.

Vegetables & Fruit
Choose dark green and orange vegetables and orange fruit more often.

Milk Products
Choose lower-fat milk products more often.

Meat & Alternatives
Choose leaner meats, poultry and fish, as well as dried peas, beans and lentils more often.

Canada

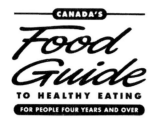

CANADA'S
Food Guide
TO HEALTHY EATING
FOR PEOPLE FOUR YEARS AND OVER

Different People Need Different Amounts of Food

The amount of food you need every day from the 4 food groups and other foods depends on your age, body size, activity level, whether you are male or female and if you are pregnant or breast-feeding. That's why the Food Guide gives a lower and higher number of servings for each food group. For example, young children can choose the lower number of servings, while male teenagers can go to the higher number. Most other people can choose servings somewhere in between.

Grain Products
5-12
SERVINGS PER DAY

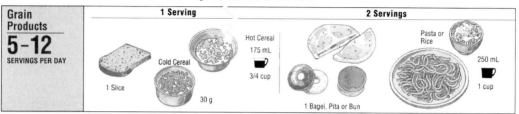

Vegetables & Fruit
5-10
SERVINGS PER DAY

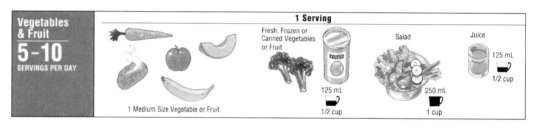

Milk Products
SERVINGS PER DAY
Children 4–9 years: 2–3
Youth 10–16 years: 3–4
Adults: 2–4
Pregnant & Breast-feeding
Women: 3–4

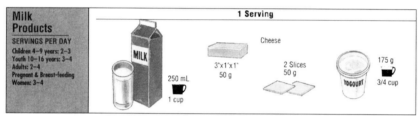

Other Foods

Taste and enjoyment can also come from other foods and beverages that are not part of the 4 food groups. Some of these foods are higher in fat or Calories, so use these foods in moderation.

Meat & Alternatives
2-3
SERVINGS PER DAY

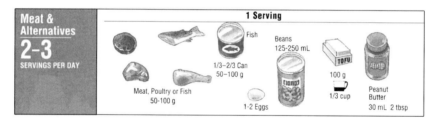

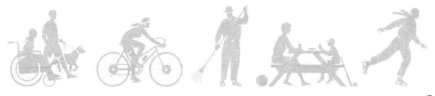

Enjoy eating well, being active and feeling good about yourself. That's VITALIT

© Minister of Supply and Services Canada 1992 Cat. No. H39-252/1992E No changes permitted. Reprint permission not required.
ISBN 0-662-19648-1

glossary

A

abortion induced premature termination of a pregnancy.

absorption the passage of nutrients or alcohol through the walls of the stomach or intestinal tract into the bloodstream.

abuse any use of a legal or illegal drug in a way that is detrimental to health or well-being.

acquired immunity (AI) the major component of the immune system; forms antibodies and specialized blood cells capable of destroying pathogens.

acupuncture the insertion of fine needles into the body to alter electroenergy fields and treat disease.

acute has a sudden onset and a prompt resolution.

acute alcohol intoxication a potentially fatal elevation of BAC, often resulting from heavy, rapid consumption of alcohol.

acute rhinitis the common cold; the sudden onset of nasal inflammation.

adaptive thermogenesis the physiological response of the body to adjust its metabolic rate to the presence of food.

addiction compulsive, uncontrollable dependence on a substance, habit, or practice to such a degree that cessation causes severe emotional or physiological reactions.

additive effect the combined (but not exaggerated) effect produced by the concurrent use of two or more drugs.

adipose tissue tissue made up of fibrous strands around which specialized cells designed to store liquefied fat are arranged.

aerobic energy production the body's primary means of energy production, used when the respiratory and circulatory systems can process and transport sufficient oxygen to muscle cells to convert fuel energy.

agent the causal pathogen of a particular disease.

agoraphobia a fear of being in situations from which there is no escape or where help would be unavailable should an emergency arise; often associated with panic disorder.

air pollution refers to a wide variety of substances found in the atmosphere that can have adverse effects on human health, crop productivity, and natural communities.

air toxics a class of 188 toxic air pollutants identified by the U.S. Environmental Protection Agency as known or suspected causes of cancer or other serious health effects, such as reduced fertility, birth defects, or adverse environmental effects.

alarm stage the first stage of the stress response involving physiological, involuntary changes which are controlled by the hormonal and nervous system; the fight or flight response is activated in this stage.

alcoholism a primary, chronic disease with genetic, psychosocial, and environmental factors influencing its development and manifestations.

allopathy (ah **lop** ah thee) a system of medical practice in which specific remedies (often pharmaceutical agents) are used to produce effects different from those produced by a disease or injury.

alveoli(al **vee** oh lie) thin, saclike terminal ends of the airways; the site at which gases are exchanged between the blood and inhaled air.

amenorrhea cessation or lack of menstrual periods.

amino acids the building blocks of protein; manufactured by the body or obtained from dietary sources.

anabolic steroids(ann uh **bol** ick) drugs that function like testosterone to produce increases in weight, strength, endurance, and aggressiveness.

anal intercourse a sexual act in which the erect penis is inserted into the rectum of a partner.

anaerobic energy production the body's alternative means of energy production, used when the available oxygen is insufficient for aerobic energy production. Anaerobic energy production is a much less efficient use of stored energy.

androgyny (an **droj** en ee) the blending of both masculine and feminine qualities.

angina pectoris (an **jie** nuh **peck** tor is) chest pain that results from impaired blood supply to the heart muscle.

anorexia nervosa an eating disorder in which the individual weighs less than 85% of their expected weight, and has an intense fear of gaining weight; in females, menstruation ceases for at least 3 consecutive months; people with anorexia perceive themselves as overweight, even though they are underweight.

antagonistic effect the effect produced when one drug reduces or offsets the effects of a second drug.

antibodies chemical compounds produced by the body's immune system to destroy antigens and their toxins.

artificially acquired immunity (AAI) a type of acquired immunity resulting from the body's response to pathogens introduced into the body through immunizations.

asbestos a term used to refer to a class of minerals that have a fibrous crystal structure.

asphyxiation death resulting from lack of oxygen to the brain.

atherosclerosis the buildup of plaque on the inner wall of arteries.

attention deficit hyperactivity disorder (ADHD) an above-normal rate of physical movement; often accompanied by an inability to concentrate on a specified task; also called *hyperactivity*.

autoimmune disorders disorders caused by the immune system's failure to recognize the body as "self"; thus the body mounts an attack against its own cells and tissues.

axon the portion of a neuron that conducts electrical impulses to the dendrites of adjacent neurons; neurons typically have one axon.

ayurveda (ai yur **vey** da) traditional Indian medicine based on herbal remedies.

B

balanced diet a diet featuring selections from each of the food groups in the Food Guide Pyramid.

ballistic stretching a "bouncing" form of stretching in which a muscle group is lengthened repetitively to produce multiple, quick, forceful stretches.

bariatrician a physician who specializes in the study and treatment of obesity.

basal metabolic rate (BMR) the amount of energy (expressed in calories) the body requires to maintain basic functions.

basic needs deficiency needs that are viewed as essential and fundamental, including physiological safety, belonging, and love and esteem needs.

behavior therapy a behavior modification therapy based upon the learning principles of reinforcement therapy, stimulus-response, and conditioning responses to change behavior.

benign noncancerous; tumors that do not spread.

beta blockers drugs that reduce the workload of the heart, which results in angina pectoris.

beta endorphins mood-enhancing, pain-reducing, opiatelike chemicals produced within the smoker's body in response to the presence of nicotine.

bias and hate crimes criminal acts directed at a person or group solely because of a specific characteristic, such as race, religion, ethnic background, sexual orientation, or other attribute.

binge drinking the consumption of five drinks or more on one drinking occasion.

binge eating disorder an eating disorder formerly referred to as compulsive eating disorder; binge eaters use food in the same way to cope as bulimics do, but do not engage in compensatory purging behavior.

biological air pollutants living organisms or substances produced by living organisms that cause disease or allergic reactions, including bacteria, molds, mildew, viruses, dust mites, plant pollen, and animal dander, urine, or feces.

biological water pollutants disease-causing organisms that are found in water.

biopsychological model a model that addresses how biological, psychological, and social factors interact and affect psychological health.

bipolar disorder a mood disorder characterized by alternating episodes of depression and mania.

birth control all of the methods and procedures that can prevent the birth of a child.

blackout a temporary state of amnesia experienced by an alcoholic; an inability to remember events that occur during a period of alcohol use.

blood alcohol concentration (BAC) the percentage of alcohol in a measured quantity of blood; BAC can be determined directly, through the analysis of a blood sample, or indirectly, through the analysis of exhaled air.

body image our subjective perception of how our body appears.

body mass index (BMI) a numerical expression of body weight based on height and weight; used to determine desirable body weight.

bolus theory a theory of nicotine addiction based on the body's response to the bolus (ball) of nicotine delivered to the brain with each inhalation of cigarette smoke.

bradycardia slowness of the heartbeat, as evidenced by a resting pulse rate of less than 60 beats per minute.

brand name the specific patented name assigned to a drug by its manufacturer.

bulimia nervosa an eating disorder in which individuals engage in episodes of binging, consuming unusually large amounts of food and feeling out of control, and engaging in some form of compensatory purging behavior to eliminate the food.

C

calcium channel blockers drugs that reduce the workload of the heart; used in the long-term management of angina pectoris.

calendar method a form of periodic abstinence in which the variable lengths of a woman's menstrual cycle are used to calculate her fertile period.

calipers a device used to measure the thickness of a skinfold from which percent body fat can be calculated.

calories units of heat (energy); specifically, one calorie (used here to mean *kilocalorie*) equals the heat required to raise one kilogram of water one degree Celsius.

carbohydrates chemical compounds composed of sugar units; the body's primary source of energy.

carbon monoxide a gaseous by-product of the incomplete combustion of natural gas, kerosene, heating oil, wood, coal, gasoline, and tobacco.

carcinogens environmental agents, including chemical compounds within cigarette smoke, that stimulate the development of cancerous changes within cells.

cardiac muscle specialized muscle tissue that forms the middle (muscular) layer of the heart wall.

cardiorespiratory endurance the ability of the heart, lungs, and blood vessels to process and transport oxygen required by muscle cells so that they can contract over a period of time. Cardiorespiratory endurance is produced by exercise that requires continuous, repetitive movements.

cardiovascular pertaining to the heart (cardio) and blood vessels (vascular).

carjacking a crime that involves a thief's attempt to steal a car while the owner is behind the wheel; carjackings are usually random and unpredictable, and they frequently involve handguns.

catabolizing the metabolic process of breaking down tissue for the purpose of converting it into energy.

CAT scan computerized axial tomography scan; an x-ray procedure designed to illustrate structures within the body that would not normally be seen through conventional x-ray procedures.

cellulite tissue comprised of fat cells intertwined around strands of fibrous connective tissue.

cerebrovascular occlusions (ser ee bro **vas** kyou lar) blockages to arteries supplying blood to the cerebral cortex of the brain; the most common type of stroke.

cervical cap a small, thimble-shaped contraceptive device designed to fit over the cervix.

chemical name the name used to describe the molecular structure of a drug.

chemoprevention cancer prevention using food, dietary supplements, or medications thought to bolster the immune system or reduce the damage caused by carcinogens.

child maltreatment the act or failure to act by a parent or caregiver which results in abuse or neglect of a child or which places the child in imminent risk of serious harm.

chiropractic manipulation of the vertebral column to relieve malalignment and cure illness.

chlamydia the most prevalent sexually transmitted disease; caused by a nongonococcal bacterium.

cholesterol a primary form of fat found in the blood; lipid material manufactured within the body, as well as derived from dietary sources.

chronic develops slowly and persists for an extended period of time.

chronic bronchitis persistent inflammation and infection of the smaller airways within the lungs.

chronic fatigue syndrome (CFS) an illness that causes severe exhaustion, fatigue, aches, and depression; mostly affects women in their thirties and forties.

chronic stress refers to remaining at a high level of physiological arousal for an extended period of time; it can also occur when an individual is not able to immediately react to a real or perceived threat.

cilia (**sill** ee uh) small, hairlike structures that extend from cells that line the air passages.

circadian rhythms the internal, biological clock that helps coordinate physiological processes to the 24-hour light/dark cycle.

clinical depression a psychological disorder in which individuals experience a lack of motivation, decreased energy level, fatigue, social withdrawal, sleep disturbance, disturbance in appetite, diminished sex drive, feelings of worthlessness, and despair.

club drug one of a variety of psychoactive drugs typically used at raves, bars, and dance clubs.

cognitive-behavioral therapy an action-oriented form of therapy that assumes that maladaptive, or faulty, thinking patterns cause maladaptive behavior and negative emotions; treatment focuses on changing an individual's thoughts or cognitive patterns in order to change his or her behavior and emotional state.

cohabitation sharing of a residence by two unrelated, unmarried people; living together.

coitus (**co** ih tus) penile-vaginal intercourse.

coitus interruptus (withdrawal) (**co** ih tus in ter **rup** tus) a contraceptive practice in which the erect penis is removed from the vagina before ejaculation.

cold turkey immediate, total discontinuation of use of a drug; associated withdrawal discomfort.

collateral circulation the ability of nearby blood vessels to enlarge and carry additional blood around a blocked blood vessel.

colonoscopy (co lun **os** ko py) examination of the entire length of the colon, using a flexible fiberoptic scope to inspect the structure's inner lining.

compliance willingness to follow the directions provided by another person.

condom a latex shield designed to cover the erect penis and retain semen upon ejaculation; "rubber."

congestive heart failure inability of the heart to pump out all the blood that returns to it; can lead to dangerous fluid accumulations in veins, lungs, and kidneys.

consumer fraud the marketing of unreliable and ineffective services, products, or information under the guise of curing disease or improving health; quackery.

contraception any method or procedure that prevents fertilization.

contraceptive patch contraceptive skin patch containing estrogen and progestin; replaced each week for a three-week period.

contraceptive ring thin, polymer contraceptive device containing estrogen and progestin; placed deep within the vagina for a three-week period.

contraindications factors that make the use of a drug inappropriate or dangerous for a particular person.

coronary arteries vessels that supply oxygenated blood to heart muscle tissues.

coronary artery bypass surgery a surgical procedure designed to improve blood flow to the heart by providing alternate routes for blood to take around points of blockage.

corpus luteum (kore pus **loo** tee um) the cellular remnant of the graafian follicle after the release of an ovum.

c-reactive protein a chemical compound found in the blood that is associated with inflammation; high levels are related to increased risk of coronary heart disease.

cross-tolerance transfer of tolerance from one drug to another within the same general category.

cruciferous vegetables (crew **sif** er us) vegetables that have flowers with four leaves in the pattern of a cross.

crystal methamphetamine a dangerous form of methamphetamine that quickly produces intense physical and psychological exhilaration when smoked.

cunnilingus (cun uh **ling** gus) oral stimulation of the vulva or clitoris.

cyanosis blue coloration of the lips, skin, and nail beds caused by inadequate oxygenation of the blood.

D

degenerative a slow but progressive deterioration of the body's structure or function.

dehydration abnormal depletion of fluids from the body; severe dehydration can be fatal.

dementia the loss of cognitive abilities, including memory and reason.

dendrite the portion of a neuron that receives electrical stimuli from adjacent neurons; neurons typically have several such branches or extensions.

dependence a general term that refers to the need to continue using a drug for psychological or physical reasons or both.

depressants a category of drugs that sedate the user by slowing central nervous system function; they produce tolerance and strong psychological and physical addiction in users.

desertification a process that converts lands that historically supported grasslands, shrub lands, or dry forest to nonproductive desert.

designated driver a person who abstains from or carefully limits alcohol consumption to be able to safely transport other people who have been drinking.

desirable weight the weight range deemed appropriate for people, taking into consideration gender, age, and frame size.

diaphragm a soft rubber cup designed to cover the cervix.

diastolic pressure (**dye** uh stol ick) the blood pressure against blood vessel walls when the heart relaxes.

dietary supplements nutrients taken in addition to those obtained through the diet: includes powdered protein, vitamins, and mineral extracts.

dilation the gradual expansion of an opening or passageway, such as the cervix.

dilation and curettage (D & C) (kyoo re taage) a surgical procedure in which the cervical canal is dilated to allow the uterine wall to be scraped.

dissonance a feeling of uncertainty that occurs when a person believes two equally attractive but opposite ideas.

distress stress that diminishes the quality of life; commonly associated with disease, illness, and maladaptation.

double-blind study a scientific study in which both the researchers and the study participants are said to be "blind" because neither group knows the makeup of the test and control groups during the actual course of the experiment; this information is revealed only at the study's conclusion.

drug any natural or artificial substance, other than food, that by its chemical or physical nature alters structure or function in the living organism.

drug synergism (**sin** er jism) enhancement of a drug's effect as a result of the presence of additional drugs within the system.

duration the length of exercise time of each training session; for aerobic fitness, 20–60 minutes is recommended.

dynamic therapy an intensive therapy based upon the belief that effective treatment must focus on the psychological forces underlying the individual's problems.

E

ectopic pregnancy a pregnancy in which the fertilized ovum implants at a site other than the uterus, typically in the fallopian tubes.

electrical impedence a method used to measure the percentage of body fat using a harmless electrical current.

embolism a potentially fatal condition in which a circulating blood clot lodges in a smaller vessel.

emergency contraception contraceptive measures used to prevent pregnancy within 72 hours after unprotected intercourse; also called post-coital or morning after contraception.

emotional intelligence the ability to understand others and act wisely in human relations and measure how well you know your emotions, manage your emotions, motivate yourself, recognize emotions in others, and handle relationships.

empowerment the nurturing of an individual's or group's ability to be responsible for their own health and well-being.

empty calories calories obtained from foods that lack most other important nutrients.

enriched the process of returning to foods some of the nutritional elements (B vitamins and iron) removed during processing.

enucleated egg an ovum with the nucleus removed.

environment the physical conditions (temperature, humidity, light, presence of substances) and other living organisms that exist around your body.

environmental tobacco smoke tobacco smoke, regardless of source, that stays within a common source of air.

enzymes organic substances that control the rate of physiological reactions but are not altered in the process.

epinephrine (epp i **neff** rin) a powerful adrenal hormone whose presence in the bloodstream prepares the body for maximal energy production and skeletal muscle response.

epitaph an inscription on a grave marker or monument.

erection the engorgement of erectile tissue with blood; characteristic of the penis, clitoris, nipples, labia minora, and scrotum.

ergogenic aids supplements that are taken by athletes to improve performance.

erotic dreams dreams whose content elicits a sexual response.

eustress (**yoo** stress) stress that enhances the quality of life.

exercise a subcategory of physical activity; it is planned, structured, repetitive, and purposive in the sense that an improvement or maintenance of physical fitness is an objective (Casperson, et al., 1985).

excitement stage initial arousal stage of the sexual response pattern.

exhaustion stage the point at which the physical and psychological resources used to deal with stress have been consumed.

exocrine glands glands whose secretions are released through tubes or ducts, such as sweat glands.

F

fat density the percentage of a food's total calories that are derived from fat; above 30% reflects higher fat density.

FDA Schedule I a list of drugs that have a high potential for abuse but have no medical use.

fecal coliform bacteria a category of bacteria that live within the intestines of warm-blooded animals; the presence of these bacteria is used as an indicator that water has been contaminated by feces.

fellatio (feh **lay** she oh) oral stimulation of the penis.

fermentation a chemical process whereby plant products are converted into alcohol by the action of yeast cells on carbohydrate materials.

fertility the ability to reproduce.

fetal alcohol syndrome (FAS) the characteristic birth defects noted in the children of some women who consume alcohol during their pregnancies.

fiber the plant material that cannot be digested; found in cereal, fruits, and vegetables.

fight-or-flight response the physiological reaction to a stressor that prepares the body for confrontation or avoidance.

fistula a fissure, break, or hole in the wall of an organ.

flaccid (**fla** sid) nonerect; the state of erectile tissue when vasocongestion is not occurring.

flexibility the ability of joints to function through an intended range of motion.

folacin (**foe** la sin) folic acid; a vitamin of the B-complex group; used in the treatment of nutritional anemia.

food additives chemical compounds intentionally added to food to change some aspect of it, such as color or texture.

food allergy a reaction in which the immune system attacks an otherwise harmless food or ingredient; allergic reactions can range from mildly unpleasant to life-threatening.

food intolerance an adverse reaction to a specific food that does not involve the immune system; usually caused by an enzyme deficiency.

foreplay activities, often involving touching and caressing, that prepare individuals for sexual intercourse.

frequency the number of exercise sessions per week; for aerobic fitness, 3–5 days are recommended.

FSH (follicle-stimulating hormone) a gonadotrophic hormone required for initial development of ova (in the female) and sperm (in the male).

functional foods foods capable of contributing to the improvement/prevention of specific health problems.

G

gaseous phase portion of tobacco smoke containing carbon monoxide and many other physiologically active gaseous compounds.

gateway drug an easily obtainable legal or illegal drug that represents a user's first experience with a mind-altering drug; this drug can serve as the "gateway" to the use of other drugs.

gender the general term reflecting a biological basis of sexuality; the male gender or the female gender.

gender adoption the long process of learning the behavior that is traditional for one's gender.

gender identification the achievement of a personally satisfying interpretation of one's masculinity or femininity.

gender identity recognition of one's gender.

gender preference emotional and intellectual acceptance of one's own gender.

general adaptation syndrome (GAS) sequenced physiological responses to the presence of a stressor, involving the alarm, resistance, and exhaustion stages of the stress response.

generalized anxiety disorder (GAD) an anxiety disorder that involves experiencing intense and nonspecific anxiety for at least six months, in which the intensity and frequency of worry is excessive and out of proportion to the situation.

gene replacement therapy an experimental therapy in which a healthy human gene is incorporated into a harmless virus to be delivered to cells that have an abnormal version of the gene.

generic name the common or nonproprietary name of a drug.

green space areas of land that are dominated by domesticated or natural vegetation, including rural farmland, city lawns and parks, and nature preserves.

greenhouse gases a category of gases in the atmosphere that allow solar radiation to pass through the atmosphere to the Earth, but then trap the heat that is radiated from the Earth back toward space;

Greenhouse gases include water vapor, carbon dioxide, methane, nitrous oxide, and tropospheric ozone.

H

hallucinogens psychoactive drugs capable of producing hallucinations (distortions of reality).

health claims the liable statements attesting to a food's contribution to the improvement/prevention of specific health problems.

health maintenance organizations (HMOs) groups that supply prepaid comprehensive health care with an emphasis on prevention.

health promotion movement in which knowledge, practices, and values are transmitted to people for use in lengthening their lives, reducing the incidence of illness, and feeling better.

herbalism an ancient form of healing in which herbal preparations are used to treat illness and disease.

high-density lipoprotein (HDL) the type of lipoprotein that transports cholesterol from the bloodstream to the liver, where it is eventually removed from the body; high levels of HDL are related to a reduction in heart disease.

high-risk health behavior a behavioral pattern, such as smoking, associated with a high risk of developing a chronic illness.

holistic health a view of health in terms of its physical, emotional, social, intellectual, spiritual and occupational makeup.

homeopathy (hoe mee **op** ah the) the use of minute doses of herbs, minerals, or other substances to stimulate healing.

homicide the intentional killing of one person by another.

hormone replacement therapy (HRT) the use of medically administered estrogen to replace estrogen lost as the result of menopause.

host negligence a legal term that reflects the failure of a host to provide reasonable care and safety for people visiting the host's residence or business.

hot flashes temporary feelings of warmth experienced by women during and after menopause, caused by blood vessel dilation.

human cloning the replication of a human being.

human papilloma virus (HPV) sexually transmitted viruses, some of which are capable of causing precancerous

changes in the cervix; causative agent for genital warts.

humanistic therapy a treatment approach based on the belief that people, left to their own devices, will naturally grow in positive and constructive ways.

hydrostatic weighing weighing the body while it is submerged in water.

hypercellular obesity a form of obesity that results from having an abnormally large number of fat cells.

hyperglycemia the condition of having an abnormally high blood glucose level.

hypertonic saline solution a salt solution with a concentration higher than that found in human fluids.

hypertrophic obesity a form of obesity in which there are a normal number of fat cells, but the individual fat cells are enlarged.

hypervitaminosis excessive accumulation of vitamins within the body; associated with the fat-soluble vitamins.

hypoglycemia the condition of having an abnormally low blood glucose level.

hypothyroidism a condition in which the thyroid gland produces an insufficient amount of its hormone, thyroxin.

hypoxia oxygenation deprivation at the cellular level.

I

ICSH (interstitial cell stimulating hormone) a gonadotropic hormone of the male required for the production of testosterone.

identity theft a crime involving the fraudulent use of a person's name, social security number, credit line, or other personal, financial, or identifying information.

immune system the system of cellular chemical elements that protects the body from invading pathogens and foreign protein and abnormal cells.

indoor air quality characteristics of air within homes, workplaces, and public buildings, including the presence and amount of oxygen, water vapor, and a wide range of substances that can have adverse effects on your health.

infatuation an often shallow, intense attraction to another person.

inhalants psychoactive drugs that enter the body through inhalation.

inhibitions inner controls that prevent a person from engaging in certain types of behavior.

insulin a hormone produced by the islet cells of the pancreas that is necessary for the normal utilization of glucose.

intensity the level of effort put into an activity; for aerobic fitness, 50–80% of heart rate range is recommended.

intentional injuries injuries that are purposefully committed by a person.

intimacy any close, mutual, verbal, or nonverbal behavior within a relationship.

intimate partner violence violent victimizations committed by current or former spouses, boyfriends, or girlfriends.

intrauterine device (IUD) a small, plastic, medicated or unmedicated contraceptive device that prevents pregnancy when inserted in the uterus.

ionizing radiation electromagnetic radiation that is capable of breaking chemical bonds, such as x-rays and gamma rays.

isokinetic exercises (eye so kin **et** ick) muscular strength training exercises in which machines are used to provide variable resistances throughout the full range of motion.

isometric exercises (eye so **met** rick) muscular strength training exercises in which the resistance is so great that the object cannot be moved.

isotonic resistance exercises muscular strength training exercises in which traditional barbells and dumbbells are used to provide variable resistances throughout the full range of motion.

L

learned helplessness a theory of motivation explaining how individuals can learn to feel powerless, trapped, or defeated.

learned optimism an attribution style, comprised of permanence, pervasiveness, and personalization; how people explain both positive and negative events in their lives, accounting for success and failure.

low-density lipoprotein (LDL) the type of lipoprotein that transports the largest amount of cholesterol in the bloodstream; high levels of LDL are related to heart disease.

lumpectomy a surgical treatment for breast cancer in which a minimal amount of breast tissue is removed; when appropriate, this procedure is an alternative to mastectomy, in which the entire breast and underlying tissue are removed.

luteinizing hormone (LH) (**loo** ten eye zing) a gonadotropic hormone of the female required for fullest development and release of ova; ovulating hormone.

Lyme disease a bacterial infection transmitted by deer ticks.

M

macrocytic anemia (mac roe **sit** ick uh **nee** mee a) the form of anemia in which large red blood cells predominate, but in which total red blood cell count is depressed.

mainstream smoke smoke inhaled and then exhaled by a smoker.

mania an extremely excitable state characterized by excessive energy, racing thoughts, impulsive and/or reckless behavior, irritability, and being prone to distraction.

masturbation self-stimulation of the genitals.

maximum contaminant level the highest concentration of a contaminant that is allowed in drinking water, as established and regulated by the U.S. Environmental Protection Agency.

medical abortion an abortion caused by the use of prescribed drugs.

medical power of attorney for health care a legal document that designates who will make health care decisions for people unable to do so for themselves.

menopause the decline and eventual cessation of hormone production by the female reproductive system.

metaneeds secondary concerns, such as spirituality, creativity, curiosity, beauty, philosophy, and justice, that can be addressed only after the basic needs are met.

metabolic rate (met uh **bol** ick) the rate or intensity at which the body produces energy.

metastasis (muh **tas** ta sis) the spread of cancerous cells from their site of origin to other areas of the body.

minipills low-dose progesterone oral contraceptives.

misuse the inappropriate use of legal drugs intended to be medications.

monogamous (mo **nog** a mus) a paired relationship with one partner.

mononucleosis ("**mono**") a viral infection characterized by weakness, fatigue, swollen glands, sore throat, and low-grade fever.

morbidity pertaining to illness and disease.

mortality pertaining to death.

MRI scan magnetic resonance imaging scan; an imaging procedure that uses a giant magnet to generate an image of body tissue.

mucus the clear, sticky material produced by specialized cells within the mucous membranes of the body; mucus traps much of the suspended particulate matter within tobacco smoke.

multifactorial requiring the interplay of many factors; refers to the cause of a disease or condition.

multiorgasmic capacity potential to have several orgasms within a single period of sexual arousal.

murmur an atypical heart sound that suggests a backflow of blood into a chamber of the heart from which it has just left.

muscular endurance the aspect of muscular fitness that deals with the ability of a muscle or muscle group to repeatedly contract over a long period of time; supported by the respiratory and circulatory systems.

muscular strength the aspect of muscular fitness that deals with the ability to contract skeletal muscles to a maximal level; the maximal force that a muscle can exert.

mutual monogamy a pattern of dating in which a person is involved exclusively with one partner.

myocardial infarction heart attack; the death of heart muscle as a result of a blockage in one or more of the coronary arteries.

N

narcolepsy a sleep-related disorder in which a person has a recurrent, overwhelming, and uncontrollable desire to sleep, often at inappropriate times.

narcotics opiates; psychoactive drugs derived from the Oriental poppy plant; narcotics relieve pain and induce sleep.

nature the innate factors that genetically determine personality traits.

naturally acquired immunity (NAI) a type of acquired immunity resulting from the body's response to naturally occurring pathogens.

naturopathy (na chur **op** ah thee) a system of treatment that avoids drugs and surgery and emphasizes the use of natural agents to correct underlying imbalances.

neuron a nerve cell.

neurotransmitters chemical messengers that transfer electrical impulses across the synapses between nerve cells.

nicotine physiologically active, dependence-producing drug found in tobacco.

nocturnal emission ejaculation that occurs during sleep; "wet dream."

nomogram a graphic means of finding an unknown value.

non-ionizing radiation electromagnetic radiation that cannot break chemical bonds, but may excite electrons (ultraviolet radiation) or heat biological materials (infrared, radio frequency, and microwave radiation).

nontraditional-age students administrative term used by colleges and universities for students who, for whatever reason, are pursuing undergraduate work at an age other than that associated with traditional college years (18–24).

norepinephrine (nor epp in **eff** rin) an adrenalin-like chemical produced within the nervous system.

nurture the effect that the environment, people, and external factors have on personality.

nutrient density quantity of selected nutrients in 1,000 calories of food.

nutrients elements in foods that are required for the growth, repair, and regulation of body processes.

O

obesity a condition in which a person's body weight is 20% or more above desirable weight as determined by standard height/weight charts.

obsessive-compulsive disorder an anxiety disorder characterized by obsessions—intrusive thoughts, images, or impulses causing a great deal of distress—and compulsions—repetitive behaviors aimed at reducing anxiety or stress that is associated with the obsessive thoughts.

oncogenes faulty regulatory genes that are believed to activate the development of cancer.

oral contraceptive pill a pill taken orally, composed of synthetic female hormones that prevent ovulation or implantation; "the pill."

orgasmic platform expanded outer third of the vagina, which grips the penis during sexual intercourse.

orgasmic stage the third stage of the sexual response pattern; the stage during which neuromuscular tension is released.

orthodontics a dental specialty that focuses on the proper alignment of the teeth.

osteoarthritis arthritis that develops with age; largely caused by weight bearing and deterioration of the joints.

osteopathy (os tee **op** ah thee) a system of medical practice in which allopathic principles are combined with specific attention to postural mechanics of the body.

osteoporosis loss of calcium from the bone, seen primarily in postmenopausal women.

outercourse sexual activity that does not involve intercourse.

overload principle the principle whereby a person gradually increases the resistance load that must be moved or lifted; this principle also applies to other types of fitness training

overweight a condition in which a person's body weight is 1–19% above desirable weight.

ovolactovegetarian diet (oh voe **lack** toe veg a **ter** ee in) a diet that excludes all meat but does allow the consumption of eggs and dairy products.

ovulation the release of a mature egg from the ovary.

oxidation the process that removes alcohol from the bloodstream.

oxygen debt a physical state in which one's activity exceeds the body's ability to produce energy aerobically, causing the body to switch to anaerobic energy production. This produces an excess buildup of by-products, especially lactic acid, and a feeling of inability to "catch one's breath." Respiration and heart rate remain increased until the excess by-products are cleared and the body can return to aerobic energy production.

P

panic disorder an anxiety disorder characterized by panic attacks, in which individuals experience severe physical symptoms. These episodes can seemingly occur "out of the blue" or because of some trigger, and can last for a few minutes or for hours.

Pap test a cancer screening procedure in which cells are removed from the cervix and examined for precancerous changes.

particulate phase the portion of tobacco smoke composed of small suspended particles.

passively acquired immunity (PAI) a temporary immunity achieved by providing extrinsic antibodies to a person exposed to a particular pathogen.

pathogen a disease-causing agent.

pelvic inflammatory disease (PID) a generalized infection of the pelvic cavity that results from the spread of an infection through a woman's reproductive structures.

perfectionism a tendency to expect perfection in everything one does, with little tolerance for mistakes.

periodic abstinence birth control methods that rely on a couple's avoidance of intercourse during the ovulatory phase of a woman's menstrual cycle; also called fertility awareness or natural family planning.

periodontal disease destruction of soft tissue and bone that surround the teeth.

peripheral artery disease (PAD) atherosclerotic blockages that occur in arteries that supply blood to the legs and arms.

peritonitis (pare it ton **eye** tis) inflammation of the peritoneum, or lining of the abdominopelvic cavity.

permanence the first dimension of an individual's attribution style, related to whether certain events are perceived as temporary or long-lasting.

personality a specific set of consistent patterns of behavior and traits that helps to identify and characterize an individual; personality is comprised of thoughts, feelings, behaviors, motivation, instinct, and temperament.

personalization the final dimension of attribution style, related to whether an individual takes things personally or is more balanced in accepting responsibility for positive and negative events.

pervasiveness the second dimension of an individual's attribution style, related to whether they perceive events as specific or general.

pesco-vegetarian diet a vegetarian diet that includes fish, dairy products, and eggs along with plant foods.

physical activity any bodily movement produced by skeletal muscles that results in energy expenditure (Casperson, et al., 1985).

physical fitness a set of attributes that people have or achieve that relates to the ability to perform physical activity (Casperson, et al., 1985).

phenylpropanolamine (PPA) (**fen** ill **pro** pan **ol** ah meen) the active chemical compound still found in some over-the-counter diet products.

placebo pills (pla **see** bo) pills that contain no active ingredients.

placenta the structure through which nutrients, metabolic wastes, and drugs (including alcohol) pass from the bloodstream of the mother into the bloodstream of the developing fetus.

plateau stage the second stage of the sexual response pattern; a leveling off of arousal immediately before orgasm.

platelet adhesiveness tendency of platelets to clump together, thus enhancing the speed at which the blood clots.

platonic close association between two people that does not include a sexual relationship.

positive caloric balance caloric intake greater than caloric expenditure.

postpartum depression a form of depression that affects women in the weeks and months following childbirth.

post-traumatic stress disorder an anxiety disorder that sometimes develops following exposure to an extreme stressor involving threat of death or serious injury; symptoms include recurrent and distressing thoughts or nightmares about the event, emotional numbness, feelings of detachment, sleep disturbance, hypervigilance, and irritability.

potentiated effect a phenomenon whereby the use of one drug intensifies the effect of a second drug.

preventive or prospective medicine physician-centered medical care in which areas of risk for chronic illnesses are identified so that they might be lowered.

primary care health providers health care providers who generally see patients on a routine basis, particularly for preventive health care.

primary prevention measures intended to deter first-time drug use.

problem drinking an alcohol use pattern in which a drinker's behavior creates personal difficulties or difficulties for other people.

Prochaska's stages of change the six predictable stages—precontemplation, contemplation, preparation, action, maintenance, and termination—people go through in establishing new habits and patterns of behavior.

procreation reproduction.

procrastination a tendency to put off completing tasks until some later time, sometimes resulting in increased stress.

prophylactic mastectomy surgical removal of the breasts to prevent breast cancer in women who are at high risk of developing the disease.

prophylactic oophorectomy surgical removal of the ovaries to prevent ovarian cancer in women at high risk of developing the disease.

prostate-specific antigen (PSA) test a blood test used to identify prostate-specific antigen, an early indicator that the immune system has recognized and mounted a defense against prostate cancer.

prosthodontics a dental specialty that focuses on the construction and fitting of artificial appliances to replace missing teeth.

proteins compounds composed of chains of amino acids; primary components of muscle and connective tissue.

proto-oncogenes (pro toe **on** co genes) normal regulatory genes that may become oncogenes.

psychiatrist a medical doctor with specialized training in the diagnosis and treatment of psychological disorders through the use of biological and medical interventions.

psychoactive drug any substance capable of altering one's feelings, moods, or perceptions.

psychological health a broadly based concept pertaining to cognitive functioning in conjunction with the way people express their emotions, cope with stress, adversity, and success, and adapt to changes in themselves and their environment.

psychologist a doctoral level practitioner with specialized training in the diagnosis and treatment of psychological disorders through the use of psychotherapy.

psychoneuroimmunology the biomedical science field that studies the interrelationship of the mind, nervous system, and immune system and its influence on illness and disease.

psychosocial sexuality masculine and feminine aspects of sexuality.

psychosomatic disorders physical illnesses of the body generated by the effects of stress.

pulmonary emphysema an irreversible disease process in which the alveoli are destroyed.

purging using vomiting, laxatives, diuretics, enemas or other medications, or such means as excessive exercise to eliminate food.

R

radio frequency radiation electromagnetic radiation with frequency in the range of 3 kilohertz to 300 megahertz, emitted by cell phones, radios, communications transmitters, and other electronic devices.

radon a naturally occurring radioactive gas that is emitted during the decay of uranium in soil, rock, and water.

recessive inheritance pattern the inheritance of traits whose expression requires that they be carried by both biological parents.

reflexology massage applied to specific areas of the feet in order to treat illness and disease in other areas of the body.

refractory errors abnormal patterns of light wave transmission through the structures of the eye.

refractory phase that portion of the male's resolution stage during which sexual arousal cannot occur.

regulatory genes genes that control cell specialization replication, DNA repair, and tumor suppression.

resistance stage the second stage of a response to a stressor, during which the body attempts to reestablish its equilibrium or internal balance.

resolution stage the fourth stage of the sexual response pattern; the return of the body to a preexcitement state.

retinal hemorrhage uncontrolled bleeding from arteries within the eye's retina.

rheumatic heart disease chronic damage to the heart (especially the heart valves) resulting from a streptococcal infection within the heart; a complication of rheumatic fever.

rigor mortis the rigidity of the body that occurs after death.

risk factor a biomedical index such as serum cholesterol level, or a behavioral pattern such as smoking, associated with a chronic illness.

rubella German or 3-day measles.

rubeola (roo **bee** oh luh) red or common measles.

S

salt sensitive the term used to describe people whose bodies overreact to the presence of sodium by retaining fluid, thus increasing blood pressure.

satiety value (suh TIE uh tee) a food's ability to cause a feeling of fullness.

saturated fats fats that promote cholesterol formation; they are in solid form at room temperature; primarily animal fats.

sclerotic changes (skluh rot ick) thickening or hardening of tissues.

schizophrenia one of the most severe mental disorders, characterized by profound distortions in one's thought processes, emotions, perceptions, and behavior; symptoms may include hallucinations, delusions, disorganized thinking, and/or maintaining a rigid posture and not moving for hours.

seasonal affective disorder (SAD) a form of depression that develops in relation to the changes in the seasons.

secondary prevention measures aimed at early detection, intervention, and treatment of drug abuse before severe physical, psychological, emotional, or social consequences can occur.

secondary virginity the discontinuation of sexual intercourse after initial exploration.

self-actualization the highest level of psychological health—at which one reaches his or her highest potential and values truth, beauty, goodness, spirituality, love, humor, and ingenuity.

self-antigens the cells and tissues that stimulate the immune system's autoimmune response.

self-care movement the trend toward individuals taking increased responsibility for prevention or management of certain health conditions.

self-concept an individual's internal picture of him or herself; the way one sees oneself.

self-esteem an individual's sense of pride, self-respect, value, and worth.

self-fulfilling prophecy the tendency to inadvertently make something more likely to happen as a result of your own expectations and attitudes.

semen a secretion containing sperm and nutrients discharged from the urethra at ejaculation.

semivegetarianism a diet that significantly reduces but does not eliminate meat consumption and allows consumption of dairy products and eggs.

serial monogamy a pattern of dating in which a person is involved in a series of exclusive relationships, one after the other.

set point a genetically programmed range of body weight beyond which a person finds it difficult to gain or lose additional weight.

sex chromosomes the X and Y chromosomes that determine sex; chromosomes other than the autosomes.

sex flush the reddish skin response that results from increasing sexual arousal.

sexual fantasies fantasies with sexual themes; sexual daydreams or imaginary events.

sexually transmitted diseases (STDs) infectious diseases that are spread primarily through intimate sexual contact.

shingles painful fluid-filled skin erruptions along underlying sensory nerve pathways—due to reactivation of once-sequestered herpes zoster (chickenpox) virus.

shock the profound collapse of many vital body functions; evident during acute alcohol intoxication and other serious health emergencies.

sidestream smoke the smoke that comes from the burning end of a cigarette, pipe, or cigar.

skinfold measurement a measurement to determine the thickness of the fat layer that lies immediately beneath the skin; this measurement is used to calculate body composition.

sleep apnea a condition in which abnormalities in the structure of the airways lead to periods of greatly restricted air flow during sleeping, resulting in reduced levels of blood oxygen and placing greater strain on the heart to maintain adequate tissue oxygenation.

sliding scale a method of payment by which patient fees are scaled according to income.

smegma cellular discharge that can accumulate beneath the clitoral hood or the foreskin of an uncircumcized penis.

social phobia a phobia characterized by feelings of extreme dread and embarrassment in situations in which public speaking or social interaction is involved.

social worker a professional with a master's degree in social work; social workers provide both mental health and social services to the community and are the largest group of professionals to provide psychological services.

sodomy generally refers to anal or oral sex; a legal term whose definition varies from state to state.

solid waste pollutants that are in solid form, including non-hazardous household trash, industrial wastes, mining wastes, and sewage sludge from wastewater treatment plants.

solution-focused approach a goal-oriented counseling approach that helps clients change by looking for solutions rather than dwelling on problems.

specific phobia an excessive and unreasonable fear that causes anxiety and distress and interferes with a person's functioning.

spermatogenesis (sper mat oh jen uh sis) the process of sperm production.

spermicides chemicals capable of killing sperm.

stalking a crime involving an assailant's planned efforts to pursue an intended victim.

static stretching the slow lengthening of a muscle group to an extended stretch; followed by a holding of the extended position for a recommended time period.

stem cells premature cells that have the potential to turn into any kind of body cell.

sterilization generally permanent birth control techniques that surgically disrupt the normal passage of ova or sperm.

stimulants psychoactive drugs that stimulate the function of the central nervous system.

stress the physiological and psychological state of disruption caused by the presence of an unanticipated, disruptive, or stimulating event.

stress response the physiological and psychological responses to positive or negative events that are disruptive, unexpected, or stimulating.

stressors factors or events, real or imagined, that elicit a state of stress.

sudden cardiac death immediate death resulting from a sudden change in the rhythm of the heart.

synapse (sinn aps) the location at which an electrical impulse from one neuron is transmitted to an adjacent neuron; also referred to as a *synaptic junction*.

synergistic effect a heightened, exaggerated effect produced by the concurrent use of two or more drugs.

synesthesia a sensation of combining of the senses, such as perceiving color by hearing or perceiving taste by touching.

systemic (sis tem ic) distributed or occurring throughout the entire body system.

systolic pressure (sis tol ick) the blood pressure against blood vessel walls when the heart contracts.

T

tachycardia excessively rapid heartbeat, as evidenced by a resting pulse rate of greater than 100 beats per minute.

tar a chemically rich, syrupy, blackish-brown material obtained from the particulate matter within cigarette smoke when nicotine and water are removed.

target heart rate (THR) the number of times per minute the heart must contract to produce a cardiorespiratory training effect.

tertiary prevention the treatment and rehabilitation of drug-dependent people to limit physical, psychological, emotional, and social deterioration or prevent death.

test anxiety a form of performance anxiety that generates extreme feelings of distress in exam situations.

therapeutic cloning the use of certain human replication techniques to reproduce body tissues and organs.

titration (tie **tray** shun) the particular level of a drug within the body; adjusting the level of nicotine by adjusting the rate of smoking.

tolerance an acquired reaction to a drug in which the continued intake of the same dose has diminishing effects.

toxic shock syndrome (TSS) a potentially fatal condition caused by the proliferation of certain bacteria in the vagina that enter the general blood circulation.

trace elements minerals whose presence in the body occurs in very small amounts; micronutrient elements.

transcenders self-actualized people who have achieved a quality of being ordinarily associated with higher levels of spiritual growth.

transcervical balloon tuboplasty the use of inflatable balloon catheters to open blocked fallopian tubes; a procedure used for some women with fertility problems.

trans fatty acid an altered form of an unsaturated fat molecule in which the hydrogen atoms on each side of the double bond(s) are on opposite sides.

transient ischemic attack (TIA) (**tran** see ent iss **key** mick) strokelike symptoms caused by the temporary spasm of cerebral blood vessels.

transsexualism a sexual variation in which a person rejects his or her biological sexuality.

transvestism atypical behavior in which a person derives sexual pleasure from dressing in the clothes of the opposite gender.

tropospheric ozone ozone is comprised of three oxygen atoms that are bound into a single molecule. Tropospheric ozone refers to this substance as it occurs in the lower layer of the atmosphere, close to the ground.

tumor a mass of cells; may be cancerous (malignant) or noncancerous (benign).

type A personality a personality type that tends to be competitive, ambitious, and impatient; often associated with heart attacks and other stress-related conditions.

type B personality a personality type that tends to be more relaxed and patient.

U

unbalanced diet a diet lacking adequate representation from each of the food groups.

underweight a condition in which body weight is below desirable weight.

unintentional injuries injuries that have occurred without anyone's intending that harm be done.

unipolar disorder depressed state during which people experience periods of lack of motivation and other symptoms—depression.

urethra (yoo **ree** thra) the passage-way through which urine leaves the urinary bladder.

V

vasectomy a surgical procedure in which the vasa deferens are cut to prevent the passage of sperm from the testicles; the most common form of male sterilization.

vegan vegetarian diet a vegetarian diet that excludes all animal products, including eggs and dairy products.

virulent (**veer** yuh lent) capable of causing disease.

vitamins organic compounds that facilitate the action of enzymes.

volatile organic compounds a wide variety of chemicals that contain carbon and readily evaporate into the air.

W

wellness the promotion and achievement of optimal health, including physical, emotional, social, spiritual, intellectual, and occupational well-being.

withdrawal illness an uncomfortable, perhaps toxic response of the body as it attempts to maintain homeostasis in the absence of a drug; also called *abstinence syndrome*.

X

xenotransplant a transplant of tissue from an animal, such as a pig, to a human recipient.

Y

young adult years segment of the life cycle from ages 18 to 24; a transitional period between adolescence and adulthood.

Yerkes-Dodson Law a bell-shaped curve demonstrating that there is an optimal level of stress for peak performance. This law states that too little or too much stress is not helpful, while a moderate level of stress is positive and beneficial.

Z

zero tolerance laws laws that severely restrict the right to operate motor vehicles for underage drinkers who have been convicted of driving under the influence of alcohol or any other drug.

zoonosis the transmission of diseases from animals to humans.

shaping your health

Multiple Choice

_____ 1. The popular health-related term, which views a person's lifestyle not in terms of reduced morbidity or mortality but from the point of view of increased human potential is
A. wellness.
B. preventive medicine.
C. health promotion.
D. episodic health care.

_____ 2. This familiar form of health care utilizes physician-delivered risk assessment and risk reduction/management practices to reduce the likelihood of serious illness and premature death.
A. Wellness.
B. Preventive medicine.
C. Health promotion.
D. Episodic health care.

_____ 3. Which health care practitioner is least likely to engage in episodic health care delivery?
A. Physician (primary care)
B. Chiropractor
C. Clinical psychologist
D. Naturopathic physician

_____ 4. Which of the following is not one of Prochaska's Stages of Change?
A. Precontemplation
B. Preparation
C. Acceptance
D. Action

_____ 5. This term refers to the process in which individuals or groups are assisted in gaining a greater measure of control over their own health care.
A. Self-actualization
B. Empowerment
C. A wellness lifestyle
D. Entitlement

_____ 6. The developmental task most closely associated with the central question of young adulthood—"Who am I?"—is
A. forming an initial adult identity.
B. securing entry-level employment.
C. nurturing intimacy.
D. broadening skills for social interaction.

_____ 7. A young adult's ability to establish independence is measured by his or her movement toward
A. home ownership.
B. better health.
C. academic success.
D. self-sufficiency.

_____ 8. From a developmental perspective, middle-aged persons should be focused on
A. repaying society for its past and future support.
B. preparing financially and emotionally for retirement.
C. fighting the bodily changes brought on by the aging process.
D. learning how to take time for themselves.

_____ 9. This dimension of health relates most closely to the individual's relationships to nature and other people, as well as his or her most profound beliefs.
A. Spiritual
B. Intellectual
C. Emotional
D. Social

_____ 10. Most forms of organized health care focus the vast majority of their time and expertise on this dimension of health.
A. Physical
B. Emotional
C. Intellectual
D. Social

True/False

_____ 11. Preventive medicine strives to lower the individual's risk of future illness and premature death through health risk factor identification and reduction.

_____ 12. Health promotion specialists are prevented, in most states, from engaging in any form of risk-assessment or risk-reducing behavioral change intended to reduce morbidity.

_____ 13. The presence of observable self-sufficiency is a recognized marker of independence.

_____ 14. The salient questions "Did my life make sense?" and "If I could live my life again, would I live it in the same way?" are most closely related to middle-age developmental task mastery.

_____ 15. For resourcefulness to be developed within the spiritual dimension of health, people must first espouse agnosticism or atheism.

Critical Thinking

1. The leading causes of death in the United States are presented in Figure 1.1. What are the most changeable behaviors that individuals could make that would decrease the likelihood of each occurring?

2. Why do you think episodic care has been prioritized over more prevention-oriented forms of health care?

3. What life-enhancing lessons do you believe nontraditional-age students can offer to their traditional-age classmates?

4. What would be an example of a resource in each of the six dimensions of health?

5. Why do your authors contend that you will not know what constitutes a health resource until you know what you want your health to make possible?

achieving psychological health

Multiple Choice

_____ 1. The psychological model that addresses the way that biological, psychological, and social factors interact and affect health is called the
  A. biological model.
  B. biopsychological model.
  C. sociological model.
  D. Maslow's hierarchy of needs.

_____ 2. Which of the following would not typically characterize a person with a high level of psychological health?
  A. Experiences the full range of human emotions but is not overcome by them
  B. Stays on task until obligations are met
  C. Sets goals that are far above his or her ability to accomplish
  D. Feels and expresses concern over the well-being of others

_____ 3. Which of the following rests at the base of Maslow's hierarchy of needs pyramid?
  A. Physiological needs
  B. Safety and security needs
  C. Belonging and love needs
  D. Self-actualization

_____ 4. Personality traits related to temperament, such as quietness and shyness, are thought to be _____ in origin.
  A. psychosocial
  B. societal
  C. biological
  D. an equal portion of psychosocial and biological

_____ 5. A form of depression that often affects women in the months following childbirth is called
  A. post-traumatic stress disorder.
  B. seasonal affective disorder.
  C. clinical depression.
  D. postpartum depression.

_____ 6. What is the first step toward taking a proactive approach to life?
  A. Undertaking new experiences
  B. Constructing mental perceptions of self, other, and objects
  C. Accept the validity of mental perceptions
  D. Reframing mental perceptions based on newly gained insights of self

_____ 7. Anxiety (or an anxiety disorder) is characterized by
  A. envy in response to the successes of others.
  B. profound fear expressed in relation to the everyday demands of living.
  C. persistent and unfocused concerns.
  D. irreversible physical deterioration.

_____ 8. _____ are more likely to commit suicide and _____ are more likely to attempt suicide.
  A. Men, men
  B. Women, women
  C. Women, men
  D. Men, women

_____ 9. Which of the following would least likely be seen in a college student displaying consistent suicidal tendencies?
  A. An internal locus of control
  B. The giving away of possessions
  C. A sense of hopelessness
  D. Signs of depression

_____ 10. This mental health professional is professionally trained and licensed to use not only an array of psychotherapies but medications as well.
  A. Psychiatric social worker
  B. Psychologist
  C. Clergy member
  D. Psychiatrist

True/False

_____ 11. An individual's level of psychological health is determined by the way that individual expresses emotions and copes with stress, as well as by the way he or she functions cognitively.

_____ 12. In your textbook's four-step prescription for a proactive approach to living, the first step involves the undertaking of a new experience.

_____ 13. The motivational theory explaining how individuals can learn to feel powerless is called learned optimism.

_____ 14. The most common phobia is a fear of snakes.

_____ 15. Of the several types of mental health practitioners licensed to practice, only psychiatrists are medical doctors.

Critical Thinking

1. How does having a sense of humor affect psychological health?

2. What aspect of personality is thought to be most biological in its origins?

3. What, if any, are the possible problems that can arise out of having an extremely high level of self-esteem?

4. How is an experience determined to be new enough to be of use in a proactive approach to living?

5. What are some risk factors associated with suicidal behavior?

managing stress

Multiple Choice

_____ 1. Which of the following is not a stage in Selye's general adaptation syndrome?
   A. Alarm stage
   B. Relaxation stage
   C. Exhaustion stage
   D. Recovery stage

_____ 2. The theory that a certain degree of stress can be beneficial to an individual's performance is expressed by
   A. the Yerkes-Dodson Law.
   B. the three stages of stress.
   C. stress management techniques.
   D. the fight or flight response.

_____ 3. Which of the following can contribute to an individual's overall stress level?
   A. A perfectionistic personality
   B. An illness in the family
   C. A new job
   D. All of the above

_____ 4. Which of the following is not typically part of the fight or flight response?
   A. Quickening of the pulse
   B. Dilation of the pupils
   C. An increase in salivation
   D. An increase in adrenaline

_____ 5. The deterioration of this body system during prolonged periods of stress results in greater susceptibility to infections.
   A. Immune system
   B. Renal system
   C. Cardiovascular system
   D. Endocrine system

_____ 6. Irritable bowel disease (IBD) is influenced by stress in which of the following ways?
   A. In no apparent way
   B. Completely eliminated
   C. Increased to some degree
   D. Decreased to some degree

_____ 7. PMR is a coping procedure that utilizes _____ to moderate the stress response.
   A. The repetition of a mantra
   B. Self-hypnosis
   C. Focused relaxation of various muscle groups
   D. Strenuous exercise

_____ 8. Regularly scheduled aerobic exercise serves as an effective coping strategy by
   A. reducing the high energy state generated by the stress response.
   B. producing a highly unappealing body odor.
   C. decreasing the body's production of biological opiates.
   D. permitting more successful escapes from potentially stressful situations.

_____ 9. Which of the following traits are _not_ associated with type A personalities?
   A. Patient
   B. Time pressured
   C. Annoyance
   D. Competitive

_____ 10. This form of stress is likely generated in conjunction with the four-step proactive approach to emotional development described in Chapter 2.
   A. Distress
   B. Astress
   C. Eustress
   D. Convoluted stress

True/False

_____ 11. Each stressor elicits its own unique form of stress response on a given part of the body.

_____ 12. The production of epinephrine by cells in the adrenal medulla occurs in response to stimulation by sympathetic fibers of the autonomic nervous system.

_____ 13. Deep breathing exercises can be an effective way to counter the stress response.

_____ 14. Increase in cardiac output, respiratory rate, and clotting time occur during the alarm stage of the stress response.

_____ 15. Prolonged periods of stress appear to strengthen the body's immune protection, thus freeing persons from the need to deal with routine infections, such as colds, while engaging stressors.

Critical Thinking

1. From what areas of the college experience do stressors most often arise?

2. What strategies are generally recommended for structuring the most effective use of time?

3. In what ways can stress be beneficial?

4. What health problems develop during periods of stress or are exacerbated by stress?

5. Identify several coping strategies that have been found to be effective in decreasing the intensity and duration of stress.

becoming physically fit

Multiple Choice

_____ 1. Which of the following areas of physical fitness do exercise physiologists say is most important?
A. Muscular strength
B. Muscular endurance
C. Cardiorespiratory endurance
D. Flexibility

_____ 2. Anaerobic, or oxygen-deprived, energy production is the result of
A. low-intensity activity.
B. short-duration activities that quickly cause muscle fatigue.
C. activities such as walking, distance jogging, and bicycle touring.
D. none of the above.

_____ 3. Which of the following types of training exercises is based on the *overload principle*?
A. Isometric exercises
B. Progressive resistance exercises
C. Isokinetic exercises
D. All of the above

_____ 4. The American College of Sports Medicine recommends six significant areas to emphasize in improving cardiorespiratory fitness. Which of these is not one of the areas?
A. Mode of activity
B. Frequency of training
C. Intensity of training
D. Popularity of training

_____ 5. What is target heart rate (THR)?
A. An intensity level of 65% to 90% of maximum heart rate
B. An intensity level of 70% to 100% of maximum heart rate
C. The maximum number of times your heart can contract each minute
D. The rate at which you become so fatigued that you must stop exercising

_____ 6. Which of these is an abnormal warning sign during or after exercise?
A. A delay of more than one hour in your body's return to a fully relaxed, comfortable state after exercise
B. Difficulty sleeping

C. Noticeable breathing difficulties or chest pains
D. All of the above

_____ 7. Which of the following is not an activity that will improve cardiovascular fitness?
A. Rollerblading
B. Rowing
C. Bowling
D. Brisk walking

_____ 8. Which of the following is not a potential side effect of steroid use?
A. Aggressive, psychotic episodes
B. Liver complications
C. Thinning of the blood
D. Cancer

_____ 9. Androstendione and creatine are most appropriately classified as
A. steroids.
B. osteoporosis medications.
C. fluid replacements.
D. ergogenic aids.

_____ 10. The Female Athlete Triad is a syndrome comprised of disordered eating, osteoporosis, and
A. lactic acid buildup.
B. amenorrhea.
C. diarrhea.
D. muscle tissue breakdown.

True/False

_____ 11. When the oxygen demands of the muscles cannot be met, oxygen debt occurs.

_____ 12. Isometric exercises incorporate variable resistances throughout the full range of motion.

_____ 13. Experts recommend static stretching activities over ballistic stretching activities.

_____ 14. People should exercise at their maximum heart rates.

_____ 15. Creatine is an over-the-counter, steroidlike hormone.

Critical Thinking

1. What are the components of a well-designed fitness program for adults?

2. How does performance-related physical fitness differ from health-related physical fitness? Which type of fitness is more important to you?

3. Explain what steps you would take to develop a cardiorespiratory fitness program, incorporating all areas recommended by the American College of Sports Medicine.

4. Describe some of the newest trends in physical activity. Which most appeals to you, and why?

5. Why is steroid use dangerous?

Understanding nutrition and your diet

Multiple Choice

_____ 1. Which of the following nutrients fails to provide the body with needed energy?
   A. Carbohydrate
   B. Fat
   C. Dietary fiber
   D. Protein

_____ 2. Which of the following fails to accurately describe carbohydrate?
   A. Supplies 4 calories per gram
   B. Body's preferred energy source
   C. Comprised of amino acids
   D. Found in monosaccharide, disaccharide, and poly-saccharide forms

_____ 3. Which form of dietary fat is believed to contribute most strongly to the development of cardiovascular disease?
   A. Saturated
   B. Monounsaturated
   C. Supersaturated
   D. Polyunsaturated

_____ 4. The "building blocks" of protein are chemical compounds known as
   A. macronutrients.
   B. ketone bodies.
   C. heavy metals.
   D. amino acids.

_____ 5. Which of the following statements regarding minerals is not true?
   A. Minerals can be obtained through supplementation.
   B. Minerals are inorganic elements that contribute to growth, repair, and regulatory processes in the body.
   C. Minerals make up less than 5% of the body's weight.
   D. Some minerals can be synthesized within the body upon exposure to sunlight.

_____ 6. Which of the following nutrients could the body not live without for more than a week?
   A. Water
   B. Salt
   C. Dietary fiber
   D. Micronutrients

_____ 7. Which of the following is not a source of dietary fiber?
   A. Cereal grains
   B. Dairy products
   C. Fruits
   D. Raw vegetables

_____ 8. What recommendation is not in keeping with the currently adopted _USDA Food Pyramid_?
   A. Adults should consume 6 to 11 servings daily from the breads and cereals group.
   B. Adults should consume 5 to 6 servings daily from the dietary fats, sweets, and alcohol group.
   C. Adults should consume 2 to 3 servings daily from the milk, yogurt, and cheese group.
   D. Adults should consume 2 to 3 servings daily from meat, poultry, fish, eggs, and nuts.

_____ 9. An ovovegetarian would not consume which of the following foods?
   A. Fruit
   B. Dairy products
   C. Eggs
   D. Cereal grains

_____ 10. A large group of food-based physiologically active compounds that deactivate carcinogens are known as
   A. anticoagulants.
   B. soluble dietary fibers.
   C. trace elements.
   D. phytochemicals.

True/False

_____ 11. Dietary fats supply 9 calories per gram.

_____ 12. Carbohydrates should supply 25 to 30% of our daily caloric intake.

_____ 13. Relatively few American adults need protein supplementation.

_____ 14. Today the only source of vitamin D is that obtained through use of vitamin supplements.

_____ 15. In comparison to the *USDA Food Pyramid* recommendations, the *Dietary Guidelines for Americans 2000* contains no recommendations related to serving size or number of daily servings.

Critical Thinking

1. Name five familiar food items that an ovolactovegetarian would not eat.

2. What are the perceived health benefits associated with the Mediterranean diet?

3. What are the health concerns associated with the use of margarines?

4. What factors make consistent use of the food pyramid-based dietary recommendations difficult for many people?

5. What reasons, other than dietary health reasons, might stimulate a person to adopt vegan vegetarianism?

maintaining a healthy weight

Multiple Choice

_____ 1. Which of the following factors is (are) known to affect weight?
A. Genetic factors
B. Metabolic factors
C. Environmental factors
D. All of the above

_____ 2. The hunger and satiety centers that control eating behavior are located within which body system?
A. Nervous system
B. Endocrine system
C. Digestive system
D. Immune system

_____ 3. At what point is overweightness first considered to be obesity?
A. 20% above ideal or desirable weight
B. 50% above ideal or desirable weight
C. 100% above ideal or desirable weight
D. 150% above ideal or desirable weight

_____ 4. Which assessment technique fails to provide information pertaining to body composition?
A. BODPOD
B. Skin calipers
C. Hydrostatic weighing
D. Balance beam scale

_____ 5. Which assessment technique is most pertinent to the concern of the cardiologist?
A. Scale weight
B. Waist-to-hip ratio (WHR)
C. Body mass index (BMI)
D. Skin calipers

_____ 6. The process of storing or burning more energy to maintain the body optimum weight is called
A. set point.
B. adaptive thermogenesis.
C. hypercellular obesity.
D. hypothyroidism.

_____ 7. What relationship exists between basal metabolic rate (BMR) and aging?
A. As age increases, BMR decreases.
B. As age increases, BMR increases.
C. As age increases, BMR ceases.
D. There is no relationship between aging and BMR.

_____ 8. What is hypercellular obesity?
A. Obesity characterized by the virtual absence of fat cells
B. Obesity characterized by a normal number of fat cells filled to capacity
C. Obesity characterized by an excessive number of fat cells
D. Obesity characterized by a lower than normal number of fat cells filled beyond their normal capacity

_____ 9. A negative caloric balance in this amount would be necessary to reduce body weight by one pound.
A. 1000 calories
B. 2250 calories
C. 3500 calories
D. 5000 calories

_____ 10. Which of the following represents the most effective and sustainable means of weight reduction and management?
A. Caloric reduction through self-induced hypnosis
B. Caloric reduction based on sound dietary practices
C. Caloric reduction based on sound dietary practices in combination with regular planned exercise, including aerobic activity and weight training
D. Regular planned exercise, including aerobic activity and weight training

True/False

_____ 11. The overconsumption of fat-dense foods, such as fast foods, and sedentary living are now known to be critically important factors in the development of childhood obesity.

_____ 12. Today there is growing concern over childhood obesity and the development of type 1 diabetes mellitus during late adolescence and adulthood.

_____ 13. More than 75% of all American adults are now considered to be obese.

_____ 14. Excessive food consumption during infancy (12 to 18 months of age) is believed to contribute strongly to the development of hypercellular obesity.

_____ 15. The majority of persons enrolled in a nationally
advertised weight reduction program will find both
initial success and successful long-term management
of weight loss to be easily achieved.

Critical Thinking

1. What health problems would be prevented or improved upon by the long-term maintenance of desirable weight?

2. Why is family involvement an important factor in a person's quest for successful loss and maintenance of weight?

3. What steps might a person take to successfully control weight throughout a lifetime?

4. What does it mean to exercise compulsively?

5. How does anorexia nervosa differ from bulimia nervosa?

making decisions about drug use

Multiple Choice

_____ 1. Which of these is an aspect of addictive behavior?
A. Denial
B. Compulsion
C. Loss of control
D. All of the above

_____ 2. Which type of dependence creates *full* withdrawal symptoms when the drug use is stopped?
A. Psychological
B. Physical
C. Cross-tolerant
D. None of the above

_____ 3. What are neurotransmitters?
A. Chemical messengers that transmit electrical impulses
B. Proteins that carry the chemicals in drugs directly to the brain
C. Hallucinogenic drugs that are currently popular with college students
D. None of the above

_____ 4. What is "crack"?
A. Powdered cocaine that is alkalized in benzene or ether and smoked through a water pipe
B. A small, rocklike crystalline material made from cocaine hydrochloride and baking soda
C. A white powder that is snorted in "lines" through a rolled dollar bill or tube
D. A pure form of methamphetamine that looks like rock candy

_____ 5. What type of psychoactive drug *slows down* the function of the central nervous system (CNS)?
A. Stimulants
B. Hallucinogens
C. Cannabis
D. Depressants

_____ 6. What is THC?
A. A hallucinogen derived from the peyote cactus plant
B. A drug popular in the 1960s
C. The active ingredient in marijuana
D. A new "designer" drug

_____ 7. Which category of drug prevention focuses on persons who are just starting to become involved in drug use?
A. Primary prevention
B. Secondary prevention
C. Tertiary prevention
D. Comprehensive prevention

_____ 8. The combined drug effect that occurs when one drug intensifies the action of a second drug is called a(n) ——— drug effect.
A. additive
B. deadly
C. potentiated
D. antagonistic

_____ 9. The club drug GHB is classified as a central nervous system
A. depressant.
B. hallucinogen.
C. roofie.
D. stimulant.

_____ 10. "Ecstasy" continues to be a popular, but dangerous drug commonly used at all-night dance parties called
A. hip-hops.
B. square shooters.
C. promenades (or "proms").
D. raves.

True/False

_____ 11. Ritalin has been used to treat ADHD in school children.

_____ 12. The largest portion of the federal dollars spent to fight the drug war in the United States has been used for drug prevention and treatment.

_____ 13. When errors occur in the testing of persons for possible drug use, the most likely source for errors is poor technology.

_____ 14. Rohypnol has been labeled the "date rape" drug.

_____ 15. Designer drugs are drugs manufactured by Ralph Lauren, Ann Taylor, Armani, and Tommy Hilfiger.

Critical Thinking

1. What is the difference between drug *misuse* and drug *abuse?*

2. How has cocaine use affected society?

3. What are possible long-term effects of marijuana use?

4. What is a synergistic effect, and why is it dangerous?

5. What do you think about the legalization of drugs and about drug testing?

taking control of alcohol use

Multiple Choice

_____ 1. What is binge drinking?
   A. The practice of drinking and then purging
   B. A harmless activity popular among college students
   C. The practice of consuming five or more drinks in a row, at least once in the previous two-week period
   D. The practice of consuming two drinks in a row, at least once a day

_____ 2. What is the alcohol content of a bottle of 140-proof gin?
   A. 140% alcohol per fluid ounce
   B. 70% alcohol per fluid ounce
   C. 14% alcohol per fluid ounce
   D. 1.4% alcohol per fluid ounce

_____ 3. What type of drug is alcohol?
   A. Stimulant
   B. Hallucinogen
   C. Depressant
   D. Narcotic

_____ 4. What should be done with people who become unconscious as a result of alcohol consumption?
   A. They should be given a cold shower to wake them up.
   B. They should be made to drink coffee.
   C. They should be taken to bed and left undisturbed for several hours.
   D. They should be placed on their side and monitored frequently.

_____ 5. Which of the following leading causes of accidental death has connections to alcohol use?
   A. Motor vehicle collisions
   B. Falls
   C. Drownings
   D. All of the above

_____ 6. Which of the following is a good guideline to follow for responsibly hosting a party?
   A. Make alcohol the primary entertainment, especially with a keg or other popular way to serve alcohol.
   B. Ridicule those who are afraid to drink.
   C. If friends say they are just fine to drive home even though they have been drinking, let them go.
   D. None of the above is a good guideline.

_____ 7. Which support group focuses on the children of alcoholics?
   A. Al-Anon
   B. Antabuse
   C. Alateen
   D. MADD

_____ 8. Which of the following does not affect the absorption of alcohol from the stomach?
   A. Use of birth control pills
   B. Presence of food
   C. Gender
   D. Quality of the liquor

_____ 9. Which of the following is a common trait of adult children of alcoholics?
   A. Have difficulty identifying normal behavior
   B. Tend to be able to drink alcohol without being affected by it
   C. Have difficulty with intimate relationships
   D. A and C are common traits

_____ 10. The inability to remember events that occurred during a period of alcohol use is called
   A. a blackout.
   B. problem drinking.
   C. alcohol dementia.
   D. a binge.

True/False

_____ 11. Denial and enabling frequently occur simultaneously among persons trying to help alcoholics.

_____ 12. For virtually everyone, alcohol oxidation occurs at a constant level.

_____ 13. For virtually everyone, alcohol absorption occurs at a constant level.

_____ 14. BACCHUS promotes alcohol abstinence among college students.

_____ 15. Alcoholism among women tends to start later and progresses more quickly than alcoholism among men.

Critical Thinking

1. In spite of their similarities to alcoholic beverages, why do nonalcoholic beverages fail to sell as well?

2. What physiological differences in women make them more susceptible to the effects of alcohol?

3. What are the possible effects of drinking alcohol while pregnant?

4. What role does alcohol use play in violent crime, family violence, and suicide?

5 Explain *denial, enabling,* and *codependence* as they occur with alcoholism.

rejecting tobacco use

Multiple Choice

_____ 1. When comparing incidence of smoking and levels of education completed, what type of relationship has been consistently observed?
A. A direct relationship
B. An indirect relationship
C. A convoluted relationship
D. No apparent relationship

_____ 2. Which of the following is not a component of habituation or emotional dependency?
A. Reliance
B. Withdrawal
C. Compulsion
D. Self-indulgence

_____ 3. When nicotine and water are extracted from the particulate phase of tobacco smoke, this material remains.
A. Tar
B. Carbon monoxide
C. Carboxyhemoglobin
D. Steam

_____ 4. This component of the gaseous phase of tobacco smoke has a deleterious influence on red blood cell function.
A. Phenol
B. Glucosamine
C. Nicotine
D. Carbon monoxide

_____ 5. This form of tobacco smoke is defined as the smoke that lingers in a room recently used by smokers or upon the clothing recently worn by smokers.
A. Sidestream smoke
B. Environmental smoke
C. Ambient smoke
D. Mainstream smoke

_____ 6. Which observable sign first suggests the development of tissue changes within the airways of the smoker?
A. Leukoplakia
B. Difficulty breathing (shortness of breath)
C. Smoker's cough
D. Blood-tinged sputum

_____ 7. Which of the following is the end stage of the progression through chronic obstructive lung disease (COLD)?
A. Emphysema
B. Chronic bronchitis
C. Asthma
D. Smoker's cough

_____ 8. Women who choose to both smoke and use oral contraceptives are at increased risk of
A. miscarriages.
B. obesity.
C. early menopause.
D. myocardial infarction (heart attack).

_____ 9. The massive and successful class-action suit brought against the tobacco industry by the Attorney Generals of 46 states was pursued in an attempt to reclaim Medicaid money spent by the states in
A. paying funeral expenses of persons dying from the effects of tobacco smoke.
B. mandating the installation of smoke alarms in the homes of smokers.
C. paying health care costs resulting from smoking-induced illnesses.
D. purchasing life insurance for tobacco users.

_____ 10. Today it is known that spouses, children, and coworkers of smokers are
A. at no particular risk of illnesses from their association with smokers.
B. at far less risk of illnesses than was once assumed.
C. actually in better health because of their association with a smoker.
D. at greater risk of illnesses than was initially assumed.

True/False

_____ 11. Since the Surgeon General's first report on _Smoking and Health_, men have been impressively successful in reducing their incidence of cigarette use.

_____ 12. Smokeless tobacco is now considered to be a clearly safer form of tobacco use than are cigarettes.

_____ 13. Smoking during pregnancy is now considered to be a reasonably safe practice since little evidence exists that harmful components found in tobacco smoke can actually cross the placental barrier.

_____ 14. The majority of adult smokers have both stated a desire to quit smoking and have on at least one occasion actually attempted to stop cigarette smoking.

_____ 15. The smoker's cough primarily results from the over-production of mucus by the goblet cells found within the tissue lining the airways.

Critical Thinking

1. Through what mechanism or series of events was the massive class action suit brought by 46 states against the tobacco industry won?

2. Through what mechanisms has the tobacco industry targeted children and members of specific minority groups?

3. For which forms of cancer is tobacco use now considered to be the most important causative agent?

4. What aspects of tobacco use enhance the development of cardiovascular disease?

5. What outcome should be anticipated by cigarette smokers when their pathology reports indicate the existence of bronchogenic carcinoma?

enhancing your cardiovascular health

Multiple Choice

_____ 1. What is the nation's number-one "killer"?
   A. AIDS
   B. Cardiovascular disease
   C. Cancer
   D. Lung disease

_____ 2. Which of the following is a function of the blood?
   A. Regulation of the water content of body cells and fluids
   B. Transportation of nutrients, oxygen, wastes, and hormones
   C. Buffering to help maintain appropriate pH balance
   D. All of the above

_____ 3. Which of the following are three cardiovascular risk factors that cannot be changed?
   A. Increasing age, male gender, heredity
   B. Heredity, weight, glandular production
   C. Age, heredity, smoking
   D. None of the above

_____ 4. Which of the following is a risk factor that can be changed?
   A. Cigarette/tobacco use
   B. Physical inactivity
   C. High blood pressure
   D. All of the above

_____ 5. Which form of cardiovascular disease involves damage to the vessels that supply blood to the heart muscle?
   A. Hypertension
   B. Stroke
   C. Coronary heart disease
   D. Congenital heart disease

_____ 6. What is hypertension?
   A. A consistently elevated blood pressure
   B. Stress on arterial walls resulting from plaque buildup
   C. The tendency of blood to clot
   D. Abnormally low blood pressure

_____ 7. What is the name of the cardiovascular disease that begins as a streptococcal infection of the throat?
   A. Peripheral artery disease
   B. Rheumatic heart disease
   C. Phlebitis
   D. Congestive heart failure

_____ 8. Which type of fat-related substance is thought to be beneficial for a person's cardiovascular health?
   A. Low-density lipoproteins
   B. High-density lipoproteins
   C. Cholesterol
   D. Triglycerides

_____ 9. A heart attack is also called a
   A. stroke.
   B. TIA.
   C. myocardial infarction.
   D. stent.

_____ 10. An alternative approach to coronary bypass surgery that involves inserting a tiny inflatable balloon into the coronary artery is called
   A. angioplasty.
   B. angiography.
   C. heart catheterization.
   D. EKG or ECG.

True/False

_____ 11. High blood levels of homocysteine in the blood are related to a decreased risk of cardiovascular disease.

_____ 12. The systolic blood pressure represents the pressure when the heart contracts.

_____ 13. Over half of American adults have cholesterol levels that exceed 200 mg/dl.

_____ 14. In comparison to white Americans, African Americans have disproportionately lower rates of hypertension.

_____ 15. According to the American Heart Association, *physical inactivity* is as important a risk factor for cardiovascular disease as *cigarette smoking*.

Critical Thinking

1. What components make up the cardiovascular system? How does the system work?

2. Do you exhibit any risk factors for cardiovascular disease? What steps can you take to change them, if they can be changed?

3. What is the difference between HDLs and LDLs?

4. How can hypertension be prevented?

5. What are the different causes of stroke?

living with cancer

Multiple Choice

_____ 1. Today the search for the genetic basis of cancer is particularly focused on genes that
   A. attempt to suppress cancerous activity once it has begun.
   B. control specialization of cells that arise as unspecialized replacement cells.
   C. oversee divisional activity in cells that are designed to copy themselves.
   D. stimulate the body's own production of pharmacological-like agents.

_____ 2. The term "proto-oncogene" is assigned to a gene that
   A. repairs cancer-causing genes.
   B. is a cancer-causing gene.
   C. once was a cancer-causing gene.
   D. has the potential to become a cancer causing gene.

_____ 3. Cancerous cells, unlike noncancerous cells, produce this enzyme that blocks the cell's biological clock, which informs normal cells that it is time to die.
   A. Telomerase
   B. Dimutase
   C. Lipase
   D. Protease

_____ 4. This form of cancer is the most prevalent form of cancer in women.
   A. Lung cancer
   B. Ovarian cancer
   C. Breast cancer
   D. Cervical cancer

_____ 5. More women die of this form of cancer than any other form.
   A. Ovarian cancer
   B. Cervical cancer
   C. Uterine cancer
   D. Lung cancer

_____ 6. The PSA screening test is designed to provide early detection of this cancer.
   A. Lung cancer
   B. Colorectal cancer
   C. Testicular cancer
   D. Prostate cancer

_____ 7. This screening test is largely responsible for the decline in deaths from cervical cancer observed over the last 35 years.
   A. Glucose tolerance test
   B. Pap smear
   C. Mammography
   D. Needle biopsy

_____ 8. This behavior is more responsible for the development of cancer than any other alterable human behavior.
   A. Sun tanning
   B. Alcohol use
   C. Consumption of red meat
   D. Tobacco use

_____ 9. Cancer is considered cured when patients have lived symptom-free for 5 years beyond
   A. their time of diagnosis and treatment.
   B. their normal life expectancy.
   C. the average age of death for persons with that particular form of cancer.
   D. the initial prognosis given to them by their physician.

_____ 10. Many of today's most impressive cancer treatment strategies are centered in the "powering up" of this important body system.
   A. Nervous system
   B. Immune system
   C. Digestive system
   D. Reproductive system

True/False

_____ 11. The inheritance of either the BRCA1 or BRCA2 gene predisposes a woman to the development of breast and/or ovarian cancer.

_____ 12. Lung cancer has never been reported in a nonsmoker.

_____ 13. Human papillomavirus (HPV) infections are most closely associated with the eventual development of reproductive system cancers, such as cervical cancer.

_____ 14. Penetrating sunburns during childhood are strongly associated with the development of basal cell carcinoma later in life.

_____ 15. Exposure to high levels of radiation is no longer
believed to be a causative factor in the development
of cancer.

Critical Thinking

1. Explain the term *survivability* as it relates to cancer.

2. What lifestyle changes can be undertaken that would lower the risk of developing lung cancer? breast cancer? colorectal cancer? prostate
   cancer?

3. In terms of prevention and early detection of cancer, what meaning can be assigned to the statement, "Choose your parents very carefully"?

4. In what ways can employment-related decisions influence a person's risk of developing cancer?

5. How can the typical person participate in the "War Against Cancer"?

managing Chronic Conditions

Multiple Choice

_____ 1. When used in the context of health conditions, the term "chronic" implies
A. untreatable at this time.
B. infectious in nature.
C. of long duration.
D. sudden onset with rapid resolution.

_____ 2. When used in describing the first appearance of a health problem, the term "congenital" implies
A. resulting from an error during embryonic development and present at birth.
B. inherited but expressed much later in life.
C. developed during infancy and expressed during early childhood.
D. self-inflicted.

_____ 3. Klinefelter's is a genetic abnormality expressed by which of the following chromosomal configurations?
A. 44XY
B. 44XXY
C. 44X0
D. 45XY

_____ 4. This chronic condition reflects the inability of the body to regulate the chloride content of secretions from various exocrine glands, such as the tear glands.
A. diabetes mellitus type 1
B. Tay-Sachs disease
C. Multiple sclerosis
D. Cystic fibrosis

_____ 5. Persons with this chronic condition suffer from the gradual loss of skeletal muscle innervation due to loss of insulation covering the motor nerves leading to these muscles.
A. Muscular dystrophy
B. Crohn's disease
C. Multiple sclerosis
D. Parkinson's disease

_____ 6. This chronic condition reflects an autoimmune-based deterioration of connective tissues in various organs of the body.
A. Diabetes mellitus type 2
B. Asthma
C. Fibromyalgia
D. Systemic lupus erythematosus

_____ 7. Exposure to a wide array of allergens underlies this frequently seen respiratory condition.
A. Cleft lip or cleft palate
B. Chronic obstructive lung disease
C. Cystic fibrosis
D. Extrinsic asthma

_____ 8. Persons with patent foramen ovale may experience distress for the first time in conjunction with this recreational sport.
A. Scuba diving
B. Sky diving
C. Roller coaster riding
D. Jogging

_____ 9. This chronic condition of older adulthood occurs as the brain's ability to produce the neurotransmitter dopamine deteriorates.
A. Muscular dystrophy
B. Parkinson's disease
C. Depression
D. Alzheimer's disease

_____ 10. Ulceration, fissuring, and invasive deterioration of the intestinal wall are the pathological hallmarks of this chronic condition.
A. Peptic ulcers
B. Irritable bowel disease
C. Crohn's disease
D. Tay-Sachs disease

True/False

_____ 11. Underlying the development of Alzheimer's disease is the brain's gradual loss of the ability to produce the neurotransmitter dopamine.

_____ 12. Experimental procedures, such as xenotransplants involving transplanting of brain cells from fetal pigs, have been attempted in the treatment of Alzheimer's disease.

_____ 13. Diabetes mellitus (both types 1 and 2) is a condition reflecting the body's inability to utilize blood glucose in the normal manner.

_____ 14. The autoimmune condition, systemic lupus erythematosus, is primarily seen in younger adult women.

_____ 15. Males displaying the chromosomal configuration 44XYY are no longer believed to be abnormally prone to antisocial behavior.

Critical Thinking

1. What reproductively based choices are available to a person who most likely carries a genetic predisposition to have children afflicted with an inherited abnormality?

2. What might be some of the earliest behavioral symptoms related to the onset of Alzheimer's disease?

3. What lifestyle modification might prevent or delay the onset of diabetes mellitus type 2 in a person with a strong family history of developing the condition?

4. What concerns, if any, exist in the use of animal organs for human transplantation (xenotransplantation)?

5. If you were writing a lifestyle-based behavioral prescription for lowering the risk of developing or transmitting chronic conditions, what would the prescription include?

preventing infectious diseases

Multiple Choice

_____ 1. The containment of semen carrying an infectious agent by the man's use of a condom breaks the chain of infection at the
   A. agent.
   B. portal of exit.
   C. mode of transmission.
   D. new host.

_____ 2. Agents from this family of organisms are still largely untreatable by current prescription medications, such as antibiotics.
   A. Bacteria
   B. Round worms
   C. Viruses
   D. Fungi

_____ 3. These thymus-derived cells are responsible for monitoring the immune response in order that it not continue unabated for an unnecessarily long period of time.
   A. T-suppressor cells
   B. Plasma cells
   C. T-killer cells
   D. Natural killer cells

_____ 4. Artificially acquired immunity is achieved by
   A. self-imposed isolation from all potentially infectious persons.
   B. contracting an infectious disease and surviving it.
   C. immunization.
   D. dietary supplement use.

_____ 5. Immunization against this infectious disease is now being strongly recommended for entering college students, particularly if they will be living in residence halls.
   A. Hantavirus infection
   B. Bacterial meningitis
   C. Mononucleosis
   D. HIV

_____ 6. Considerable debate has arisen over the past two decades regarding whether this condition is an infectious disease or, rather, a psychogenic disorder.
   A. Hypoglycemia
   B. Chronic fatigue syndrome
   C. Mononucleosis
   D. Toxic shock syndrome

_____ 7. This infectious condition was first reported in 1999, almost entirely in states along the Eastern seaboard.
   A. West Nile virus disease
   B. Lyme disease
   C. Hantavirus pulmonary syndrome
   D. Drug-resistant tuberculosis

_____ 8. The wide array of agents responsible for this common condition almost precludes protection from subsequent episodes through naturally acquired immunity.
   A. Genital herpes
   B. Influenza
   C. Common cold
   D. Measles

_____ 9. The development and use of several protease inhibitors has significantly altered the course of this infectious disease.
   A. Oral herpes
   B. Hepatitis C
   C. Mumps
   D. HIV/AIDS

_____ 10. This infectious condition places hunters, hikers, and people who enjoy recreational activities in the out-of-doors at elevated levels of risk.
   A. Hantavirus
   B. Bacterial meningitis
   C. Lyme disease
   D. Common colds

True/False

_____ 11. Toxic shock syndrome is most commonly associated with the use of cosmetics borrowed from other people.

_____ 12. Passively acquired immunity is primarily used when a person's immune status is inadequate or unknown.

_____ 13. The incidence of HIV/AIDS is increasing at alarming and uncontrollable rates in many areas of Africa.

_____ 14. Hantavirus infections in this country have not yet been linked to any particular reservoir or mode of transmission.

_____ 15. Some particular strains of human papillomavirus have been linked to the development of cervical cancer.

Critical Thinking

1. What is the current state of childhood immunizations in this country?

2. What are the cellular responses made by the immune system to the presence of a new antigen?

3. What behavioral patterns contribute to a heightened level of risk for contracting sexually transmitted diseases?

4. What concerns seem reasonable when immunosuppressing drugs are used in the treatment of conditions that have clear autoimmune aspects, such as multiple sclerosis, systemic lupus erythematosus, and Crohn's disease?

5. What factors might account for the failure of some parents to have their infants and young children fully immunized?

exploring the origins of sexuality

Multiple Choice

_____ 1. Which basis for biological sexuality refers to the growing embryo's development of gonads?
   A. Genetic
   B. Gonadal
   C. Structural
   D. None of the above

_____ 2. What part of the testis produces sperm?
   A. Seminiferous tubules
   B. Scrotum
   C. Epididymis
   D. Interstitial cells

_____ 3. Which is the most sexually sensitive part of the female body?
   A. Mons pubis
   B. Vagina
   C. Clitoris
   D. Prepuce

_____ 4. During which phase of the menstrual cycle does the corpus luteum develop?
   A. Menstrual
   B. Preovulation
   C. Postovulation
   D. None of the above

_____ 5. Why are the testes housed in the scrotum, outside the body?
   A. To reduce the distance the sperm must travel in their attempt to fertilize the egg
   B. To increase the male's sexual responsiveness
   C. To reduce the risk of injury
   D. Because spermatogenesis requires a lower temperature than the body core temperature

_____ 6. The lower third of the uterus is called the
   A. vagina.
   B. cervix.
   C. endometrium.
   D. clitoris.

_____ 7. What term describes the blending of traditionally male and female qualities within an individual?
   A. Homosexuality
   B. Bisexuality
   C. Androgyny
   D. Asexuality

_____ 8. What is endometriosis?
   A. A condition that typically affects postmenopausal women; characterized by brittle, weak bones.
   B. A condition in which tissue that normally lines the uterus is found growing within the pelvic cavity.
   C. A condition that typically affects women who have delivered multiple babies.
   D. A condition in which a fertilized ovum implants in the fallopian tube rather than the uterus.

_____ 9. Which of the following categories of sexuality refers to the nonreproductive use of the genitals?
   A. Genital sexuality
   B. Reproductive sexuality
   C. Expressionistic sexuality
   D. Bisexuality

_____ 10. The female structures that serve as passageways for the ovum's movement from the ovary to the uterus are called the
   A. fallopian tubes.
   B. vas deferens.
   C. urethra.
   D. inguinal canals.

True/False

_____ 11. Premenstrual syndrome (PMS) occurs in the days just before ovulation.

_____ 12. Hormone replacement therapy helps to reduce hot flashes.

_____ 13. The male accessory glands that produce a clear, lubricating fluid at the tip of the penis during sexual excitement are the seminal vesicles.

_____ 14. The chromosomal structure of a male fertilized ovum is XX.

_____ 15. The onset of menstruation in a young girl is called menarche.

Critical Thinking

1. How do biological and psychosocial factors contribute to the complex expression of our sexuality?

2. How has a blending of feminine and masculine qualities benefited society?

3. Why might the "withdrawal" method of contraception not work?

4. What changes, both physiological and psychological, might menopause create in a woman's life?

5. Which female reproductive structures are "similar" in function to male reproductive structures?

Understanding sexual behavior and relationships

Multiple Choice

_____ 1. Which of the following statements about the effects of aging on sexuality is *true*?
   A. Male production of testosterone increases steadily from age 20 to 60.
   B. Vaginal lubrication increases as women age.
   C. Sexual desire typically disappears entirely by age 70.
   D. The capacity to enjoy sex is not altered.

_____ 2. What is the current view of masturbation among sex therapists and researchers?
   A. Masturbation is a sign of emotional immaturity.
   B. Masturbation should not be necessary when one is in a committed, intimate relationship.
   C. Masturbation is a harmless, normal source of self-pleasure.
   D. Masturbation is an unhealthy form of sexual expression.

_____ 3. Which type of marriage is characterized by a loss of the signs of life?
   A. The conflict-habituated marriage
   B. The passive-congenial marriage
   C. The total marriage
   D. The devitalized marriage

_____ 4. Which of the following statements is *not* true about celibacy?
   A. Celibate people may have intimate relationships without sex.
   B. It is defined as the self-imposed avoidance of sexual contact.
   C. Psychological complications often result from a celibate lifestyle.
   D. All are true.

_____ 5. Which type of oral-genital stimulation involves kissing and licking a woman's vulva?
   A. Foreplay
   B. Fellatio
   C. Cunnilingus
   D. None of the above

_____ 6. Which type of love is enduring and capable of sustaining long-term mutual growth?
   A. Infatuation
   B. Passionate love
   C. Companionate love
   D. Devotional love

_____ 7. Recent estimates place the incidence of homosexuality in America at what percentage of the population?
   A. 5%
   B. 10%
   C. 18%
   D. 22%

_____ 8. In the year 2000, which state passed the nation's first "civil union" law?
   A. California
   B. Vermont
   C. Kentucky
   D. Idaho

_____ 9. Which of the following dating practices *reduces* the likelihood of contracting infectious diseases?
   A. Mutual monogamy
   B. Serial monogamy
   C. Using oil-based lubricants
   D. Avoiding condoms

_____ 10. Which of the following is responsible for the inability of most males to experience more than one orgasm in a short time?
   A. Resolution stage
   B. Plateau stage
   C. Refractory phase
   D. Flaccid stage

True/False

_____ 11. During the sexual response pattern, both males and females show a sex flush.

_____ 12. Transsexuals are uncomfortable with their biological sexuality.

_____ 13. Women who dress like males can be accurately labeled transvestites.

_____ 14. People practicing secondary virginity have never had sexual intercourse.

_____ 15. If a couple wants to improve their sexual relationship, better communication is not particularly important.

Critical Thinking

1. If you wish to marry someday, what type of marriage do you wish to have? If you are already married, how could you improve your marriage?

2. What are your attitudes and expectations toward dating? What do you expect from a date?

3. What is your relationship history? How do you think you could improve it?

4. How do you define intimacy?

5. What is your sexual orientation? What is your attitude toward those who differ from you in their sexual orientation or gender expression?

managing your fertility

Multiple Choice

_____ 1. Which form of birth control does not prevent the spread of STDs?
   A. Withdrawal
   B. Calendar method
   C. IUD
   D. All of the above

_____ 2. Which two forms of birth control, when used together, provide a high degree of contraceptive protection and disease control?
   A. IUD and spermicides
   B. Spermicides and condoms
   C. Calendar method and spermicides
   D. Oral contraceptives and spermicides

_____ 3. Which of the following statements about oral contraceptives is false?
   A. The use of antibiotics lowers oral contraceptive effectiveness.
   B. They regulate a woman's menstrual cycle.
   C. The user may experience more frequent vaginal infections, weight gain, mild headaches, and mild depression.
   D. They are useful in the prevention of STDs.

_____ 4. What are "minipills"?
   A. Smaller versions of the regular oral contraceptives that can be swallowed more easily
   B. The placebo pills taken between cycles
   C. Oral contraceptives that contain no estrogen—only low-dose progesterone
   D. Less expensive versions of the pill

_____ 5. Which of the following birth control methods use(s) synthetic hormones to prevent ovulation and/or fertilization?
   A. Oral contraceptives
   B. Contraceptive patch
   C. Contraceptive ring
   D. All of the above

_____ 6. The most common form of emergency contraception (postcoital or "morning after" contraception) is the use of certain types of _____ following unprotected vaginal intercourse.
   A. oral contraceptives
   B. injectable contraceptives
   C. saline solutions
   D. foaming suppositories

_____ 7. The Progestasert, Mirena, and the ParaGard are examples of which type of contraceptive?
   A. Oral contraceptives
   B. Diaphragms
   C. Intrauterine devices (IUDs)
   D. Polyurethane condoms

_____ 8. Which type of abortion is performed in the earliest stages of the first trimester?
   A. Menstrual extraction
   B. Dilation and curettage
   C. Dilation and evacuation
   D. Hypertonic saline procedure

_____ 9. Periodic abstinence approaches attempt to determine when
   A. menstruation starts.
   B. a women ovulates.
   C. the cervix dilates.
   D. the uterus contracts.

_____ 10. The following are all contraindications to taking oral contraceptives except
   A. a history of regular menstrual cycles.
   B. high blood pressure.
   C. a history of blood clotting.
   D. cigarette smoking.

True/False

_____ 11. The greatest health concern for women who use the oral contraceptive is the development of cardiovascular complications.

_____ 12. Research indicates that the female condom provides greater contraceptive protection than does the male condom.

_____ 13. RU 486 is a prescription drug that produces a medical abortion.

_____ 14. Although many individual states have passed laws that prohibit the so-called "partial birth abortions," the U.S. Supreme Court has not ruled this procedure to be unconstitutional.

_____ 15. Vasectomy and tubal ligation are forms of abortion used during the second trimester.

Critical Thinking

1. What factors should you consider when choosing a method of birth control?

2. Which of the available methods of birth control would you be most likely to use, if you needed to?

3. What are the guidelines set forth under *Roe v. Wade,* the landmark 1973 Supreme Court case?

4. If an oral contraceptive were developed for males, can you envision any possible drawbacks?

5. What role do you expect your partner to play in birth control?

becoming a parent

Multiple Choice

_____ 1. Which of the following is an obstacle to pregnancy?
   A. 200 to 500 million sperm cells are deposited in each ejaculation.
   B. Sperm cells are capable of moving quickly.
   C. The acidic level of the vagina is destructive to sperm.
   D. Once inside the fallopian tubes, sperm can live for days.

_____ 2. Which of the following agents can damage a fetus?
   A. Tobacco smoke
   B. Alcohol
   C. Radiation
   D. All of the above

_____ 3. All of the following are potential complications of pregnancy except
   A. osteoporosis.
   B. gestational diabetes.
   C. preeclampsia.
   D. miscarriage.

_____ 4. A couple should seek genetic counseling if which of the following factors is present?
   A. Maternal age of 35 years or greater
   B. History of adoption in maternal or paternal families
   C. History of spontaneous abortions
   D. A and C

_____ 5. An incision made in a woman's perineum to keep it from tearing during delivery is a(n)
   A. salpingostomy.
   B. thoracotomy.
   C. episiotomy.
   D. vagotomy.

_____ 6. Which of the stages of childbirth is the longest?
   A. Effacement and dilation
   B. Delivery of the placenta
   C. Delivery of the fetus
   D. Vernix stage

_____ 7. The time period in which the mother's uterus returns to its prepregnancy size and shape is called
   A. prepartum.
   B. reduction.
   C. postpartum.
   D. cesarean time.

_____ 8. The following are all methods a man can use to increase his fertility except to
   A. take folate supplements.
   B. periodically apply cold packs to the scrotum.
   C. wear boxer shorts.
   D. have surgery to repair a structural problem.

_____ 9. Fathers-to-be can reduce their own anxiety and concern through which of the following methods?
   A. Educate themselves about pregnancy
   B. Take a course in infant care
   C. Talk with their partner about what they are feeling
   D. All of the above

_____ 10. The process of removing an ovum, fertilizing it, then replacing it in the mother's uterus is called
   A. embryo freezing.
   B. gamete intrafallopian transfer (GIFT).
   C. balloon tuboplasty.
   D. in vitro fertilization.

True/False

_____ 11. About half of all pregnancies end in a spontaneous abortion that takes place during the second trimester of pregnancy.

_____ 12. Effacement refers to an enlargement of the uterus during the first stage of labor.

_____ 13. Down syndrome can be detected as early as the first trimester of pregnancy.

_____ 14. Nearly all fertility problems are caused by sperm abnormalities.

_____ 15. One sound reason for a cesarean delivery is when a fetus is improperly positioned in the uterus.

Critical Thinking

1. Name three methods of reproductive technology. What do you think are the ethical issues of these methods?

2. Have you ever used a home-pregnancy test? If so, did you follow the directions carefully?

3. Do you think cloning of humans should be legal or illegal? Why?

4. If you had a child, would you want the baby to breast-feed? Why or why not?

5. Describe the birth process from beginning to end.

beComing an informed health Care Consumer

Multiple Choice

_____ 1. On the basis of a study conducted by AARP, this medium is the primary source of health-related information for middle-age and older adults.
   A. Television
   B. Magazines
   C. Home reference books
   D. Neighbors

_____ 2. Osteopathic medicine differs from allopathic medicine principally in terms of osteopathy's historical relationship to the use of
   A. bleeding as a means of cleansing the body.
   B. wind, sunshine, and other environmental agents.
   C. manipulation.
   D. mud baths.

_____ 3. Chiropractors that consider themselves as being aligned with the historical roots of their discipline
   A. utilize surgery in combination with spinal manipulation.
   B. prescribe over-the-counter medications.
   C. utilize food supplementation, massage, and other noninvasive techniques in combination with spinal manipulation.
   D. use only spinal manipulation.

_____ 4. This form of alternative medicine is based on balancing the active and passive forces that reside within the body.
   A. Homeopathy
   B. Chiropractic
   C. Acupuncture
   D. Herbalism

_____ 5. Medications formulated for use by this alternative form of health care are compounded on the basis of tenets derived through the _Law of Similarities._
   A. Osteopathy
   B. Homeopathy
   C. Herbalism
   D. Allopathic medicine

_____ 6. Which level of education prepares nurses to provide communities with additional primary care providers?
   A. Advance practice nursing
   B. Registered nursing
   C. Certified nursing assistance
   D. Licensed practical nursing

_____ 7. Medicaid and Medicare are both
   A. military service-based programs.
   B. prepaid fee-for-service organizations.
   C. commercial insurance programs.
   D. governmental insurance programs.

_____ 8. The estimated amount that the insured must pay before the insurer begins reimbursing for services is the
   A. fixed indemnity.
   B. deductible.
   C. premium.
   D. coinsurance portion.

_____ 9. Approximately what number of Americans have no health insurance benefits?
   A. None, as the federal government provides universal health care coverage
   B. Less than one hundred thousand
   C. About one million
   D. In excess of forty one million

_____ 10. Which set of terms reflects the FDA's focus in exercising control over the OTC drug market?
   A. Safe and effective
   B. Safe and affordable
   C. Effective and affordable
   D. Sensible and savory

True/False

_____ 11. Naturopathic medications are diluted to the point at which there are virtually no molecules of the purported active ingredient.

_____ 12. Medical quacks frequently contend that their healing technology is so revolutionary that it is not yet available to the established health care industry, thus only they can provide it to the public.

_____ 13. At this time no attempt is underway (or even being considered) by the federal government to determine in an objective and carefully controlled manner the effectiveness of the several alternative medical care fields that can be found in this country.

_____ 14. The laws of virtually every state prevent the prescribing of prescription medication by dentists, optometrists, and podiatrists.

_____ 15. While Medicare excludes coverage of virtually all persons under the age of 65 years, Medicaid covers qualified persons of all ages.

Critical Thinking

1. Considering how HMOs are operated today, what are the advantages and disadvantages to HMO membership?

2. How can continued expansion of the self-care movement be of benefit to both individuals and the established health care industry?

3. What rights do patients have upon entering the hospital, and what obligations do they have to the hospital providing their care?

4. What is meant by the term "fast-track" as it applies to the pharmaceutical industry?

5. What differentiations can be made between the terms "alternative," "complementary," and "integrative" as they apply to the array of health care philosophies that exist today?

protecting your safety

Multiple Choice

_____ 1. Which of the following would be considered a self-inflicted intentional injury?
   A. Rape
   B. Homicide
   C. Suicide
   D. Battery

_____ 2. In _____, between 25 and 50% of all homicides are drug related.
   A. homes
   B. rural settings
   C. small towns
   D. large cities

_____ 3. On the basis of current reports, who is the most likely victim of intimate partner violence?
   A. A white woman
   B. A white man
   C. An African American or Hispanic woman
   D. An African American or Hispanic man

_____ 4. To which governmental agency should suspected child abuse be reported?
   A. The Board of Health
   B. The Child Protective Services Division of the local Department of Welfare
   C. The nearest EMS service
   D. The administrative offices of the child's school district

_____ 5. On the basis of current reports, who is the most likely abuser of an elderly person?
   A. A neighbor
   B. An adult child of the elderly person
   C. A visiting home health aid
   D. The elderly person's spouse

_____ 6. Which of the following is least likely a characteristic of persons who become increasingly violent toward their dating partners?
   A. They have a history of showing jealousy and possessiveness toward partners.
   B. They are generally nonaggressive, rarely engaging in roughhousing-type behavior with others.
   C. When explaining past aggressiveness and violence they often project blame for their behavior onto others.
   D. They become confrontational when confronted by others.

_____ 7. This substance is now known to play a predominant role in cases of acquaintance or date rape as it occurs on the college campus.
   A. Tobacco
   B. Marijuana
   C. Cocaine
   D. Rohypnol

_____ 8. Which of the following would least likely increase your safety when bicycling?
   A. Use lights and reflective clothing when riding at night.
   B. Wear an approved bicycle helmet.
   C. Bicycle with at least one other person.
   D. Bicycle against the flow of oncoming traffic.

_____ 9. For all students, but particularly women, which of the following is not advised when leaving a night class?
   A. Travel alone as group noise attracts unwanted attention.
   B. Utilize campus escort services.
   C. Use only well-lighted walks and pathways.
   D. Ride university shuttle buses.

_____ 10. Which of the following is not considered prudent in terms of enhancing residential safety?
   A. Installing peep holes in all outside doors
   B. Using your full name in phone book listings
   C. When away for an extended period of time, having paper and mail delivery stopped
   D. Requiring full and valid identification from all persons doing in-home services

True/False

_____ 11. Crime statistics suggest that homicide rates are declining in this country.

_____ 12. Sexual orientation is rarely a factor associated with hate crimes.

_____ 13. Although much talked about, less than 5% of college women will experience any behavior that could be construed as acquaintance or date rape.

_____ 14. Unlike auto accidents, boating accidents rarely involve excessive alcohol use.

_____ 15. When comparing the rate of fatal accidents per 100,000 operators, motorcycles are far safer to operate than automobiles.

Critical Thinking

1. What precautions can college women take to reduce the likelihood that they will experience acquaintance or date rape?

2. When moving into a new campus apartment, the presence of what safety features should be immediately assessed?

3. How can adult children increase the safety of their elderly parents, particularly when living some distance away?

4. How can parents of young children impart important safety education to their children, when busy schedules often keep family members apart?

5. What steps can you take to protect yourself from identity theft?

the environment and your health

Multiple choice

_____ 1. Your personal health is affected by environmental factors working on several spatial scales. On which of the following spatial scales is your impact on the environment, and conversely the environment's impact on your health, the most direct?
  A. Your personal environment
  B. Your community/regional environment
  C. Your national environment
  D. Your global environment

_____ 2. Bacteria, molds, mildew, and viruses are all examples of
  A. biological air pollutants.
  B. allergens.
  C. air toxics.
  D. volatile organic compounds.

_____ 3. How can you determine if your home has unsafe levels of radon exposure?
  A. Presence of a foul odor in the basement
  B. Positive result from a radon detection kit
  C. Presence of black mold
  D. All of the above

_____ 4. Which of the following is not an example of a greenhouse gas?
  A. carbon dioxide
  B. methane
  C. tropospheric ozone
  D. oxygen

_____ 5. The chemical interaction of hydrocarbons, nitrogen oxides, and other small particulate matter in the presence of sunlight produces_____.
  A. stratospheric ozone
  B. tropospheric ozone
  C. volatile organic compounds
  D. formaldehyde

_____ 6. If you live in an older home (built before 1970) and notice cracking paint around the door trim, what should you do to minimize your family's exposure to lead?
  A. Scrape the flaking paint and repaint over it with non-lead based paint.
  B. Leave it alone.
  C. Call a certified contractor to remove it.
  D. Clean it off with soap and water.

_____ 7. What can you do to protect yourself from the damaging ultraviolet rays of the sun?
  A. Limit your exposure to direct sunlight.
  B. Always wear sunscreen when you are outside.
  C. Wear UV-blocking sunglasses when you are outside.
  D. All of the above.

_____ 8. A "yellow" air pollution alert means people who suffer from respiratory or cardiac diseases, or hypersensitivity to allergens, should
  A. avoid physical activity.
  B. wear a respirator.
  C. stay indoors.
  D. install air filters in their homes.

_____ 9. Carbon monoxide is an indoor air pollutant that is potentially lethal. Which of the following is a source of indoor carbon monoxide?
  A. Refrigerator
  B. Furnace
  C. Air conditioner
  D. Household cleaning chemicals

_____ 10. Which of the following locations is most likely to expose residents to the greatest risk of adverse health consequences?
  A. Next to a nuclear power plant
  B. Close to high voltage power lines
  C. Next to an oil refinery
  D. All of the above pose equal risk to health

True/False

_____ 11. Formaldehyde is a volatile organic compound commonly associated with decaying uranium beneath the earth's surface.

_____ 12. Asbestos-containing products must be removed from the home, even if they are intact and undisturbed.

_____ 13. The _Biophilia hypothesis_ proposes that human evolution predisposes us to desire areas with vegetation and diverse biological systems.

_____ 14. Climate and natural vegetation can increase the formation of "smog" in urban areas.

_____ 15. Noise pollution can have adverse effects not only on hearing, but also on sleep, digestion, and blood pressure.

Critical Thinking

1. In what ways can you change your daily routine to lessen the effects of environmental pollutants and other hazards on your personal health?

2. If you were to purchase a home in the coming year, what kind of health-related questions might you have as a result of reading this chapter?

3. Many believe that rapid growth of the human population, both regionally and globally, is the most important environmental problem. How is human population growth related to environmental degradation?

4. Do you consider environmental issues when you vote in local and national elections? Are the environmental issues important in local elections different from the issues important in national elections?

5. Can taking steps to protect the environment—recycling, carpooling, installing energy efficient appliances in your home—make an impact on your personal health? Explain.

Answers

Chapter 1

1.	A	6.	A	11.	T
2.	B	7.	D	12.	F
3.	D	8.	A	13.	T
4.	C	9.	A	14.	F
5.	B	10.	A	15.	F

Chapter 2

1.	B	6.	B	11.	T
2.	C	7.	C	12.	F
3.	A	8.	D	13.	F
4.	C	9.	A	14.	F
5.	D	10.	D	15.	T

Chapter 3

1.	B	6.	C	11.	F
2.	A	7.	C	12.	T
3.	D	8.	A	13.	T
4.	C	9.	A	14.	F
5.	A	10.	C	15.	F

Chapter 4

1.	C	6.	D	11.	T
2.	B	7.	C	12.	F
3.	D	8.	C	13.	T
4.	D	9.	D	14.	F
5.	A	10.	B	15.	F

Chapter 5

1.	C	6.	A	11.	T
2.	C	7.	B	12.	F
3.	A	8.	B	13.	T
4.	D	9.	B	14.	F
5.	D	10.	D	15.	T

Chapter 6

1.	D	6.	B	11.	T
2.	A	7.	A	12.	F
3.	A	8.	C	13.	F
4.	D	9.	C	14.	T
5.	B	10.	C	15.	F

Chapter 7

1.	D	6.	C	11.	T
2.	B	7.	B	12.	F
3.	A	8.	C	13.	F
4.	B	9.	A	14.	T
5.	D	10.	D	15.	F

Chapter 8

1.	C	6.	D	11.	T
2.	B	7.	C	12.	T
3.	C	8.	D	13.	F
4.	D	9.	D	14.	F
5.	D	10.	A	15.	T

Chapter 9

1.	B	6.	C	11.	T
2.	B	7.	A	12.	F
3.	A	8.	D	13.	F
4.	D	9.	C	14.	T
5.	B	10.	D	15.	T

Chapter 10

1.	B	6.	A	11.	F
2.	D	7.	B	12.	T
3.	A	8.	B	13.	T
4.	D	9.	C	14.	F
5.	C	10.	A	15.	T

Chapter 11

1.	A	6.	D	11.	T
2.	D	7.	B	12.	F
3.	A	8.	D	13.	T
4.	C	9.	A	14.	T
5.	D	10.	B	15.	F

Chapter 12

1.	C	6.	D	11.	F
2.	A	7.	D	12.	F
3.	B	8.	A	13.	T
4.	D	9.	B	14.	T
5.	C	10.	C	15.	T

Chapter 13

1.	B	6.	B	11.	F
2.	C	7.	A	12.	T
3.	A	8.	C	13.	T
4.	C	9.	D	14.	F
5.	D	10.	C	15.	T

Chapter 14

1.	B	6.	B	11.	F
2.	A	7.	C	12.	T
3.	C	8.	B	13.	F
4.	C	9.	A	14.	F
5.	D	10.	A	15.	T

Chapter 15

1.	D	6.	C	11.	T
2.	C	7.	B	12.	T
3.	D	8.	B	13.	F
4.	C	9.	A	14.	F
5.	C	10.	C	15.	F

Chapter 16

1.	D	6.	A	11.	T
2.	B	7.	C	12.	F
3.	D	8.	A	13.	T
4.	C	9.	B	14.	T
5.	D	10.	A	15.	F

Chapter 17

1.	C	6.	A	11.	F
2.	D	7.	C	12.	F
3.	A	8.	A	13.	T
4.	D	9.	D	14.	F
5.	C	10.	D	15.	T

Chapter 18

1.	A	6.	A	11.	F
2.	C	7.	D	12.	T
3.	D	8.	B	13.	F
4.	C	9.	D	14.	F
5.	B	10.	A	15.	T

Chapter 19

1.	C	6.	B	11.	T
2.	D	7.	D	12.	F
3.	C	8.	D	13.	F
4.	B	9.	A	14.	F
5.	B	10.	B	15.	F

Chapter 20

1.	A	6.	C	11.	F
2.	A	7.	D	12.	F
3.	B	8.	C	13.	T
4.	D	9.	B	14.	T
5.	B	10.	C	15.	T

Credits

Chapter One: p. 5 (Star box), Data from Yankelovich Monitor 1997, as reported in What is success? *USA Today* Jan 19:1A.
Chapter Two: p. 35 (Figure 2-1), based on "Hierarchy of Needs" from *Motivation and Personality,* 3rd ed. by Abraham H. Maslow. Revised by Robert Frager, et al., Harper & Row, Publishers 1954, 1987.; **p. 58 (Figure),** Data from Yankelovich Partners for Lutheran Brotherhood; **p. 61 (Personal Assessment),** From Study Guide and Personal Exploration for *Psychology applied to modern life; adjustment in the 80s,* by Wayne Weiten. Copyright © 1983 by Wadworth, inc. Reprinted by permission of Brooks/ Cole Publishing, Pacific Grove, CA 93950.
Chapter Three: p. 70 (Figure 3-3), Hebb, D.O. (1955). *Drive and the CNS (Conceptual Nervous System).* Psychological Review, 62 (4), 243–245; **p. 80 (Figure 3-5),** Data from the Wirthlin Report; **p. 93 (Personal Assessement),** Modified from Holmes TH, Rahe RH: The social adjustment rating scale, *Journal of Psychosomatic Research* 11:213218, 1967; **p. 95 (Personal Assessment),** Adapted with the permission of The Free Press, a Division of Simon and Schuster Adult Publishing Group, from *Never Good Enough: Freeing Yourself From The Chains of Perfectionism* by Monica Ramirez Basco, Ph.D. Copyright © 1999 by Monica Ramirez Basco. All rights reserved.
Chapter Four: p. 102 (Figure 4-1) Data from the Wirthlin Report; pp. 116–117 (Star box), Copyright 1986, USA Today, excerpted with permission, art by Donald O'Connor; **p. 122, (Table 4.1),** Prentice, WE: *Fitness for college and life.* ed 5; New York, 1997, McGraw Hill; **pp. 127–128 (Personal Assessment),** Data from the National Fitness Foundation.
Chapter Five: p. 138 (Table 5.2), Modified from Food and Nutrition Board, National Research Council: *Recommended dietary allowances,* ed 10, Washington DC, 1989, National Academy of Sciences; **p. 147 (Figure 5-4),** Reprinted with permission of Simon & Schuster Adult Publishing Group from *Eat, Drink, and Be Healthy: The Harvard Medical School Guide to Healthy Eating* by Walter C. Willet, M.D. Copyright © 2001 by President and Fellows of Harvard College; **pp. 148–149 (Table 5.5),** US Department of Agriculture; **pp. 154–155 (Figure 5-5),** Data from US Food and Drug Administration and Wardlow G, Insel P: *Perspectives in Nutrition,* ed 3, St. Louis, 1986, Mosby.; **p. 159 (Star box),** Duyff, R. *American Dietetic Association Complete Food and Nutrition Guide,* 2nd ed., © John Wiley & Sons. This material is used by permission of John Wiley and Sons, Inc.; **p. 161 (Figure 5-6),** US Department of Agriculture. **p. 173 (Personal Assessment)** From *Nutrition for a healthy life,* Courtesy of March Leeds.
Chapter Six: p. 177 (Table 6.1), From Wadlaw G, Insel P, and Seyler M: Contemporary nutrition: issues and *insights,* ed 2, St. Louis, 1994, Mosby; (Star Box), Data from C. Everett Coop Foundation, American Diabetes Association; **p. 180 (Table 6.2),** National Institutes of Health; Modified from George A. Bray; **p. 182 (Table 6.3)** Based on data from Bannister EW, Brown SR: The relative energy requirements of physical activity. In HB Falls, editor: *Exercise physiology,* New York, 1968; **(Table 6.4),** Adapted from Najjar MF, Rowland M: Anthropometric reference data and prevalence of overweight, United States 1976–1980. Vital and Health Statistics, series 11, no. 238, (PHS) 87-1688, Public Health Service, Washington, DC, 1987. US Government Printing Office; **(Table 6.5)** Reprinted with permission of Metropolitan Life Insurance Company; **p. 192 (Table 6.6),** Adapted from Guthrie H: Introductory nutrition, ed 7, St. Louis, 1989, Mosby-Year Book, pp. 226–227; **p. 184 (Figure 6-4),** Opinion Research Institue for *Simply Lite Foods;* **pp. 196–197 (Table 6.7),** Adapted from Guthrie H: Introductory nutrition, ed 7, St. Louis, 1989, Mosby.
Chapter Seven: p. 235 (Table 7.2), Modified from Muncie Star © 1987. Reprinted with permission. **p. 237 (Figure 7-2),** Source: American Management Association Survey; **p. 255 (Personal Assessment),** US Department of Education, A parent's guide to prevention.
Chapter Eight: p. 263 (Figure 8-2), Data from Core Institute: *2000 Statistics on alcohol and other drug use on American campuses,* Center for Alcohol and other Drug Studies, Student Health Programs, Southern Illinois University at Carbondale, 2000; **p. 267 (Table 8.2),** Reprinted from *Cecil Textbook of Medicine,* 18/e, Wyngardener, JB, and Smith, LH, copyright 1988, with permission from Elsevier.
p. 268 (Figure 8-3), Feldman, Understanding Psychology 5e, 2002, McGraw-Hill;
p. 270 (Figure 8-4), From Wardlaw G: Perspectives in nutrition, ed 3, St. Louis, Mosby;
p. 277 (Changing for the Better), Modified from brochure of the Indiana Alcohol Countermeasure Program; **p. 291 (Personal Assessment),** From *Are You Troubled by someone's drinking?* 1980, by Al-Anon Family Group Headquarters, Inc. Reprinted by permission of Al-Anon Family Group Headquarters, Inc.
Chapter Nine: p. 295 (Table 9.1), Data from *MMWR* 1999, 48(45): 1034–1039 and *MMWR* 2000, 49(SS-2):1-60; **p. 329 (Personal Assessment),** Reproduced with permission of the American Cancer Society.
Chapter Ten: p. 334 (Figure 10-1 and Table 10.1), Data from American Heart Association, *2001 Heart and stroke statistical update,* 2000, The Association; **p. 341 (Figure 10-3),** Reproduced with permission, © 1988, American Heart Association: Heart Facts; **p. 345 (Figure 10-4),** 1990 *Heart facts,* art by Donald O'Connor; **p. 359 (Personal Assessment),** From Howard E: *Health risks,* Tucson, 1985, Body Press.
Chapter Eleven: P. 365 (Figure 11-1), Data from National Cancer Institute: Horizons of cancer research, NIH Pub. No. 89-3011 © 1989; **pp. 369, 372, 378 (Changing for the Better),** American Cancer Society; **p. 383 (Changing for the Better),** Courtesy of the American Academy of Dermatology;

p. 393 (**Personal Assessment**), American Cancer Society.

Chapter Twelve: p. 400 (Star box) and **pp. 407, 412 (Changing for the Better)**, © Health Letter Associates, 1996, 1997 www.wellnessletter.com.

Chapter Thirteen: p. 438 (Table 13.3), Courtesy of the National Institute of Allergy and Infectious Diseases; **p. 469 (Personal Assessment)**, Centers for Disease Control and Prevention, Atlanta.

Chapter Fifteen: p. 519 (Personal Assessment), Modified from USA Today.

Chapter Sixteen: p. 525 (Table 16.1), Adapted from Hatcher et al., *Contraceptive technology.* 17th rev. ed, 1998, Ardent Media, Inc; **p. 548 (Personal Assessment)**, From Haas K, Haas A: Understanding sexuality, ed 3, St. Louis, 1993, Mosby.

Chapter Eighteen: p. 587 (Changing for the Better), Source: Pell, AR: *Making the most of Medicare,* DCI Publishing, 1990, in *insynch,* Erie PA Spring 1994, Erie Insurance; **p. 608 (Changing for the Better)**, The National Kidney Foundation Uniform Donor Card is reprinted with permission from the National Kidney Foundation, Inc. Copyright 2000, New York, NY.

Chapter Nineteen: p. 622 (Figure 19-1), Courtesy of the National Committee to Prevent Child Abuse, Chicago, IL; p. 628 (Changing for the Better), From the American college Health Association; p. 633 (Changing for the Better), Reprinted with permission of the American Academy of Ophthalmology, *Preventing eye injuries;* **p. 628 (Figure 19-2)**, National Safety Council; **p. 637 (Changing for the Better)**, Adapted from Pynoos J, Cohen E: *Creative ideas for a safe and livable home,* Washington DC, American Association of Retired Persons, 1992, and Van Tassel D: *Home safe home,* St. Louis, 1996, GenCare Health Systems.

Chapter Twenty: p. 657 (Figure 20-2), Environmental Protection Agency.

Photo Credits

Chapter 1 p. 8, Ryan McVay/PhotoDisc/Getty Images; p. 15, Digital Vision; p. 17, Geoff Manasse/PhotoDisc/Getty Images; p. 18, Joaquin Palting/PhotoDisc/Getty Images; p. 20, Keith Brofsky/Getty Images/PhotoDisc; p. 21, Don Farrall/PhotoDisc/Getty Images

Chapter 2 p. 34, Mel Curtis/PhotoDisc/Getty Images; p. 35, Buccina Studios/PhotoDisc/Getty Images; p. 44, Mel Curtis/PhotoDisc/Getty Images; p. 46, Michael Matisse/PhotoDisc/Getty Images; p. 48, PhotoDisc Collection/Getty Images

Chapter 3 p. 70, © Jean-Paul Chassenet/Photo Researchers, Inc.; p. 73, PhotoDisc Collection/Getty Images; p. 74, PhotoLink/PhotoDisc/Getty Images; p. 76, Keith Brofsky/Getty Images/PhotoDisc; p. 81, Ryan McVay/PhotoDisc/Getty Images; p. 72, © Image Source/Corbis

Chapter 4 p. 100, 103, 105, 111, Ryan McVay/Getty Images/PhotoDisc; p. 117, Courtesy Stewart Halperin; p. 125, Bruno Herdt/PhotoDisc/Getty Images

Chapter 5 p. 127, 128, Courtesy Stewart Halperin; p. 141, Ryan McVay/PhotoDisc/Getty Images; p. 143, PhotoLink/PhotoDisc/Getty Images; p. 152, © Royalty-Free/Corbis; p. 156, F. Schussler/PhotoLink/PhotoDisc/Getty Images; p. 161, Ryan McVay/PhotoDisc/Getty Images

Chapter 6 p. 178, Suza Scalora/Getty Images/PhotoDisc; p. 179T, © Davis Barber/PhotoEdit; p. 179B, © Custom Medical Stock Photo; p. 204, Ryan McVay/PhotoDisc/Getty Images; p. 205, Jack Star/PhotoLink/PhotoDisc/Getty Images

Chapter 7 p. 228, Image100; p. 238, Jack Star/PhotoLink/PhotoDisc/Getty Images; p. 242T, Doug Menuez/PhotoDisc/Getty Images; p. 242B, © The Cover Story/Corbis; p. 251, © Royalty-Free/Corbis

Chapter 8 p. 261, Jim Arbogast/Getty Images/PhotoDisc; p. 263, SW Productions/Getty Images/PhotoDisc; p. 271T, © George Steinmetz; p. 271B, Courtesy Mothers Against Drunk Driving; p. 275, Doug Menuez/PhotoDisc/Getty Images

Chapter 9 p. 295, Emma Lee/Life File/PhotoDisc/Getty Images; p. 298, Jonnie Miles/PhotoDisc/Getty Images; p. 300, Jack Star/PhotoLink/PhotoDisc/Getty Images; p. 303, © Royalty-Free/Corbis; p. 309T, Courtesy Wayne Jackson; p. 309B, © Custom Medical Stock Photo; p. 312, © Photick/Superstock

Chapter 10 p. 339, Karl Weatherley/Getty Images/PhotoDisc; p. 340, Ryan McVay/PhotoDisc/Getty Images; p. 349, Keith Brofsky/PhotoDisc/Getty Images; p. 356, Ryan McVay/Getty Images/PhotoDisc

Chapter 11 p. 362, © Kevin Laubacher/Getty Images/Taxi; p. 380, © AP/Wide World Photos; p. 382, From Thibodeau G., Patton, K. *Anatomy and Physiology*, 3/e, St. Louis, 1996. Mosby

Chapter 12 p. 399, 401, 402, 403, © Custom Medical Stock Photo; p. 415, © Rufus F. Folkks/Corbis

Chapter 13 p. 437, Janis Christie/Getty Images/PhotoDisc; p. 445, © Touhig Sion/Corbis Sygma; p. 447, © Reuters/Corbis; p. 448, © Roger Ressmeyer/Corbis; p. 457, © Phototake; p. 458, © Custom Medical Stock Photo

Chapter 14 p. 476, Digital Vision/Getty Images

Chapter 15 p. 508, Ryan McVay/Getty Images/PhotoDisc; p. 509, Buccina Studios/Getty Images/PhotoDisc; p. 510, Digital Vision/Getty Images

Chapter 16 p. 529, PhotoDisc Collection/Getty Images; p. 530, Courtesy Stewart Halperin; p. 531, © Laura J. Edwards; p. 533, Linsley Photographics; p. 534L, © Laura J. Edwards; p. 534R, Courtesy Stewart Halperin; p. 535, Courtesy of Alza Corp.; p. 538, Courtesy Organon USA

Chapter 17 p. 553, E. Dygas/Getty Images/PhotoDisc; p. 557, © Science Photo Library/Photo Researchers, Inc.; p. 559, Digital Vision/Getty Images; p. 560, © Science Photo Library/Photo Researchers, Inc.; p. 565, Keith Brofsky/Getty Images/PhotoDisc

Chapter 18 p. 586, Ryan McVay/Getty Images/PhotoDisc; p. 591, Anthony Saint James/Getty Images/PhotoDisc; p. 593, Mitch Hrdlicka/Getty Images/PhotoDisc; p. 604, Ryan McVay/Getty Images/PhotoDisc

Chapter 19 p. 621, Getty Images/PhotoDisc; p. 622, Courtesy of the Ad Council; p. 623, Jack Star/PhotoLink/Getty Images/PhotoDisc; p. 629, Ryan McVay/Getty Images/PhotoDisc; p. 632, Ryan McVay/Getty Images/PhotoDisc; p. 634, Ryan McVay/Getty Images/PhotoDisc

Chapter 20 p. 648, Digital Vision/Getty Images; p. 654, Nick Koudis/Getty Images/PhotoDisc; p. 658, Kent Knudson/Getty Images/PhotoDisc; p. 661, D. Falconer/PhotoLink/PhotoDisc/Getty Images; p. 668, Digital Vision/Getty Images; p. 670, Tomi/PhotoLink/Getty Images/PhotoDisc

index

Cohabitation, 513–514
Coinsurance, 599
Coitus, 497, 505
Coitus interruptus, 525–526
Cold, common, 437–440
COLD (chronic obstructive lung disease), 311
Cold turkey, defined, 244
College students
    alcohol use, 225, 261–263
    cigarette smoking, 295–296
    with disabilities, 13
    drug use, 225
    minority students, 12–13
    nontraditional-age, 12
    traditional-age, 11
Colonoscopy, 380
Colorectal cancer, 369, 379–380
Columbine High School shootings, 622–623
Combination drug effects, 233–234
Combined pill, as birth control method, 526, 535
Commercial weight reduction programs, 197–199
Commercials. See Advertising
Common cold, 437–440
Communication
    and birth control, 524
    with health care providers, 586
    in relationships, 512, 514
    for resolving conflict, 507
    of sexual needs, 495
    skills, 34–36, 54
    between smokers and nonsmokers, 322
    and stress, 63
    with students with disability, 65
Community environment, 646, 655–665, 671
Community health centers, 697
Community health promotion, 6–7
Companionate love, 508–509
Compatibility assessment, 503, 519
Complementary medicine, 13
    acupuncture for alcoholism, 280
    acupuncture for drug abuse, 247
    antioxidant supplementation, 163
    aphrodisiacs, 501
    biofeedback for panic disorder, 51
    Canada, 697
    Chinese herbal medicine for fertility problems, 528

DHEA, 480
    hypnotherapy for irritable bowel disease, 413
    hypnotism and smoking cessation, 321
    macrobiotic diet for cancer, 387
    meditation for hypertension, 348
    melatonin for sleep, 86
    midwifery, 563
    practitioners, 588–589, 591–594
    safety and health care decisions, 630
    therapeutic touch, 591
Compliance, 582
Compulsion, 49, 228
Compulsive overeating, 207–208
Computer waste, 662
Computerized axial tomography (CAT) scan, 350
Condoms
    as birth control method, 525–526, 530–531, 532
    female, 525–526, 531, 533
    and oral sex, 504
    use, 472–473
Conflict management, 36, 507
Conflict-habituated marriage, 510
Confrontation, for drug dependence, 246
Congenital abnormalities, 401–404
Congenital heart disease, 351
Congestive heart failure, 352
Consultations, 586–587
Consumer advocacy groups, as health information source, 583, 585
Consumer fraud, 606–607, 608, 613–614
Consumerism, 607, 609, 615
Contact inhibition, and cancer cells, 364
Contemplation stage, of change, 9
Contraception. See also Birth control
    versus birth control, 522–523
    defined, 522
    emergency, 538–539
    selecting method, 524, 537, 549
Contraceptive patch, 526, 538
Contraceptive ring, 526, 538
Contraceptive sponge, 533–534
"Contract for Life," 275
Contraindications, 536
Controlled fasting, 195, 197
Convalescence stage, of infection, 431
Convulsive seizures, first aid for, 683

Cooldown phase, 112
Cord blood (stem) cells, 435
Corona, 480
Coronary arteries, 335
Coronary arteriography, 344
Coronary artery bypass surgery, 345
Coronary heart disease, 341–347
    diagnosis, 344–345
    emergency response to heart crises, 344
    treatment, 345–347
Corpus, 483
Corpus luteum, 484
Cortisol, and stress, 66–67
Coué, Emil, 83
Counseling
    for depression, 43–44
    for emotional growth, 30
    genetic, 400, 567–568
Counselors, 51
Couples therapy, 53–54
Couric, Katie, 380
Cowper's glands, 479
CPR (cardiopulmonary resuscitation), 344, 624
Crabs, 454–455, 460
Crack cocaine, 238
Cramps, menstrual, 485
C-reactive protein, 342
Creatine, 119
Creativity, 38
Crime. See also Violence
    and alcohol use, 272–273, 286–287
    ATM crimes, 619
    bias and hate crimes, 624–625
    preventing violent crime, 619
Crises, in sickle-cell disease, 399
Crohn's disease, 412–413, 418
Cross-dressing, 503
Cross-tolerance, 230
Crosstraining, 115–117
Crosstraining shoes, 116–117
Crowning, during childbirth, 563
Cruciferous vegetables, 142
Crystal methamphetamine, 237
C-section delivery, 564–565
Cultural factors, in obesity, 187
Cunnilingus, 504
Curette, 541
CVD. See Cardiovascular disease
Cyanosis, 402
Cycle, menstrual, 483–484, 527, 528

CYP17 gene, 371
Cystic fibrosis (CF), 398–399
Cystitis, 461

D

Dancing, as aerobic exercise, 114
Date rape, 239–240, 262, 627, 628
Dating, 507–508
Death, causes of, 8, 10, 333
Death rates, cancer, 366, 367, 384
Decline stage, of infection, 431
Deductibles, health insurance, 599
Degenerative, defined, 396
Degenerative diseases, 415–418
Dehydration, 139
Delirium tremens (DTs), 277
Delivery. *See also* Childbirth
    of fetus, 563–564
    of placenta, 564
Dementia, 417
Dendrite, 227
Dengue, 466
Denial, 278
Dental dams, 504
Dentists, 594
Dependence
    defined, 230, 299
    on drugs, 230–231, 246–248
    on nicotine, 296, 302–303
Depo-Provera, 526, 537
Depressants, 235, 239–240
Depression, 42–44, 45
DES (diethylstilbestrol), 376
Desertification, 669
Designated drivers, 259, 274–275
Designer drugs, 241
Desirable weight, defined, 178
Developmental tasks
    middle adulthood, 16–17
    older adulthood, 17–18
    young adulthood, 13–16
Devitalized marriage, 510
Dexfenfluramine, 199
Dextrose, 131
DHEA, 480
Diabetes mellitus
    and cardiovascular disease, 340
    gestational, 565
    insulin-dependent, 406, 408
    non-insulin-dependent, 205,
        404–406, 407, 408
    resources for, 418
    risk of, 409

Diaphragm, for birth control,
    525, 531–532
Diastolic pressure, 347
Diet
    and cancer prevention, 385
    and diabetes prevention, 407
    and obesity, 189
    and weight management,
        193–197, 204
Dietary Guidelines for Americans,
    157–159, 180, 181–182
Dietary Supplement and Education Act
    (DSHEA), 199
Dietary supplements, 150–151, 163,
    592, 605
Dieting, and weight gain, 186–187
Digestive system, 690
Dilation, 541
Dilation and curettage (D & C), 541
Dilation and evacuation (D & E), 542
Dilation of cervix, 561–563
Dionne quintuplets, 573
Diphtheria immunization, 436
Dirty bombs, 664
Disabilities
    versus chronic conditions, 395
    developmentally disabled
        athletes, 101
    and physical activity, 193
    students with, 13, 65
    and violence, 624
Disaccharides, 131
Disaster reactions, 85
Dissonance, and tobacco use, 303
Distant cancer, 365
Distillation, 265
Distress, 65
Diuretic drugs, 349
Diversity
    Americans with Disabilities Act, 585
    college students, 34
    developmentally disabled
        athletes, 101
    heart disease prevention, 336
    kosher laws, 157
    menopause, 487
    Native Americans and the
        environment, 663
    nontraditional-age students, 12
    pregnancy and parenting after
        forty, 555
    staying sober for women, 282
    students with disabilities, 65

violence against the disabled, 624
    World No-Tobacco Day, 302
Divorce, 512–513
Dogs, watch, 631
Dole, Bob, 491
Domestic violence, 286, 617, 620–622
Dopamine
    and nicotine addiction,
        300–301, 319
    and Parkinson's disease, 415, 416
Drinking games, 263
Drinking water safety, 653–655
Drivers
    aggressive, 641–642
    designated, 259, 274–275
Driving. *See also* Drunk driving
    and cell phones, 635
Dronabinol, 244
Drownings, alcohol-related, 272
Drowsy driving, 636
Drug abuse
    defined, 231
    dynamics, 231–233
    environmental factors, 232–233
    and homicide, 620
    hot lines, 248
    individual factors, 231–232
    national groups, 248
    prevention scare tactics, 224–225
    societal factors, 233
Drug awareness assessment, 255
Drug classifications, 234–244
    cannabis, 235, 241–243
    depressants, 235, 239–240
    hallucinogens, 235, 240–241
    inhalants, 235, 244
    narcotics, 235, 243–244
    stimulants, 234, 235, 236–239
Drug Free Workplace Act, 245
Drug interactions, 630
Drug misuse, 231
Drug synergism, 274
Drug terminology, 229–231
Drug testing, 245–246
Drug use
    athletes against, 240
    college students, 225
    defined, 231
    prevention, 225–226
    society's response to, 244–248
Drugs
    brand-name, 603
    club, 234, 239–240

Heterosexuality, 500
HGE (human granulocytic ehrlichiosis), 444
Hierarchy of needs, 36–38
High-carbohydrate diet, 196
High-density lipoprotein (HDL), 133, 134, 343
High-fiber, low-calorie diets, 197
Highly active antiretroviral therapy (HAART), 452
High-protein, low-carbohydrate diets, 196
High-risk health behaviors, 5
Hindu views on environment, 649
HIV (human immunodeficiency virus). *See also* AIDS
  cross-system transmission, 431
  media coverage, 428
  prevalence, 450
  reducing risk of contracting, 456
  source, 466
  spread, 448–450
  transmission and condom use, 473
HIV infection
  diagnosis, 451–452
  prevention, 453
  signs and symptoms, 450–451
  stages, 431
  treatment, 452–453
HMOs (health maintenance organizations), 13, 599–601
Hodgkin's disease, 381
Holistic health, 18
Holmes, Thomas, 69, 93
Home care, 596
Home fitness equipment, 118
Home pregnancy tests, 559
Home safety, 619, 631–632, 633, 637, 638
Homeopathy, 592
Homeostasis, and older adults, 105, 107
Homesickness, 71
Homicide, 619–620, 634
Homocysteine, 342
Homosexuality, 501. *See also* Gays and lesbians
HONcode Principles, 614
Hooked On Nicotine Checklist, 296
Hormonal factors, in obesity, 186
Hormone replacement therapy (HRT)
  alternatives to, 486
  and breast cancer, 370
  and endometrial cancer, 376

  in menopause, 487–488
  and Parkinson's disease, 416
Hospitals, 588, 596–597
Host negligence, 274
Hot flashes, 486, 487
HRT. *See* Hormone replacement therapy
Human chorionic gonadotropin (hCG), 559
Human Genome Project, and cancer, 363, 364
Human granulocytic ehrlichiosis (HGE), 444
Human papillomavirus (HPV), 374, 375, 454–455, 457–458
Human-environment relationships, religious views on, 649
Humanistic therapy, 53
Humidifier fever, 651
Humor, sense of, 34, 82, 229
Humoral immunity, 432
Hydrostatic weighing, 184
Hydroxyurea, 399
Hymen, 482
Hypercellular obesity, 189
Hyperemesis gravidarum, 566
Hyperglycemia, 405
Hypersensitivity/autoimmune disorders, 409–415
Hypertension, 347–349
  African Americans, 337, 356–358
  and cardiovascular disease, 340
  and diabetes, 406
  and salt, 159, 348
  and stress, 356–357
Hypertonic saline abortion, 542
Hypertrophic obesity, 189
Hyperventilation, first aid for, 682
Hypervitaminosis, 137–138
Hypnosis
  for irritable bowel disease, 413
  and smoking cessation, 321
  for stress management, 84
Hypoglycemia, 408–409
Hypothyroidism, 186
Hypoxia, 312
Hysterectomy, 540, 542

I

Ice beers, 265
Identity formation, and young adults, 13–14
Identity theft, 629, 630

Idiopathic, defined, 403
Immune response, 433–435
Immune system divisions, 432–433
Immunizations, 435–437, 439
Impotence, 491, 492, 500
In situ cancer, 365
In vitro fertilization and embryo transfer (IVF-ET), 569
Incubation stage, of infection, 431
Independence, and young adults, 14
Independent practice associations (IPAs), 601
Indoor air quality, 648–652
Infatuation, 508
Infection
  body defenses against, 431–433
  chain of, 429–431
  stages, 431
Infectious diseases. *See also specific diseases*
  changing picture of, 466–467
  living with, 442
  older adults, 435
  and pathogens, 429
  transmission, 428–431
Infertility, 568–570
  causes, 568
  herbal medicine for, 528
  options for infertile couples, 569–570
  and smoking, 312
  surgical remedies, 568–569
Inflammatory bowel disease (IBD), 412–413
Influenza, 438, 440
Infomercials, 98–99, 582
Inhalants, 235, 244
Inherited genetic mutations, 398–400
Inhibitions, 260
Injectable contraceptives, 526, 537
Injuries. *See also specific injuries*
  intentional, 619–631
  unintentional, 631–638
In-line skating, 114, 125, 126
Insoluble fiber, 139–140
Institutes of Medicine, priority health concerns, 7–8
Insulin, 130, 404–406, 408
Insurance
  extended care, 601
  health, 13, 598, 599, 600
Integrative care. *See* Complementary medicine

Plateau stage, of sexual response, 496, 498
Platelet adhesiveness, and nicotine, 308
Platelet inhibitors, and heart disease, 346
Platonic cohabitation, 513–514
Pleconaril, 438
PMS (premenstrual syndrome), 484–485
Pneumococcal infection immunization, 436, 437
Pneumocystis carinii, 441
Pneumonia, 441
Podiatrists, 594
Point pollution sources, 656, 659
Poisoning, first aid for, 682
Polio immunization, 436
Pollution
    air, 653, 656–658
    land, 660–662
    noise, 655, 656
    nonpoint sources, 656, 659
    point sources, 656, 659
    water, 654, 658–660
Polyps, 379
Polysaccharides, 131, 132
Polyunsaturated fats, 133–134
Population explosion, 665–666, 667
Portal of entry, and chain of infection, 431
Portal of exit, and chain of infection, 430
Portion control, 194–195, 215–217
Positive caloric balance, 176, 179
Postovulation phase, of menstrual cycle, 484
Postpartum, defined, 564
Postpartum depression, 45
Post-traumatic stress disorder, 49–50, 627
Posture, 33, 36
Potentiated effect, 234
Power lines, health effects of, 676
PPOs (preferred provider organizations), 601
Preconceptional counseling, 400, 567–568
Precontemplation stage, of change, 9
Preeclampsia, 566
Preferred provider organizations (PPOs), 601
Pregnancy
    after forty, 555
    and alcohol use, 269–271

complications, 565–567
emotional aspects, 562
and exercise, 113–114
fathers-to-be, 557
home pregnancy tests, 559
intrauterine development, 559–560
planning for, 567
signs of, 558
and smoking, 312
and weight gain, 186
Pregnancy-induced hypertension, 566
Prehypertension, 347, 348
Premature labor, 566
Premature rupture of the membranes (PROM), 566
Premeasured food plans, 197
Premenstrual syndrome (PMS), 484–485
Preovulation phase, of menstrual cycle, 484
Preparation stage, of change, 9
Prepuce, 480
Prescription drugs, 230, 602–603
    Canada, 604
    learning about, 600
    Medicare coverage, 599, 601
President's Council on Physical Fitness and Sports, 127–128
Preventive medicine, 4–5, 587
Primary amenorrhea, 486
Primary care health providers, 587
Primary prevention, 225–226
Prion, and infectious diseases, 429
Private hospitals, 596–597
Proactive approach to life, 41–42
Probiotics, 150, 151
Problem drinking, 276. *See also* Alcohol abuse; Alcoholism
Prochaska's Stages of Change, 9
Procrastination, 77–78
Procreation, 488, 505
Prodromal stage, of infection, 431
Professional journals, as health information source, 3
Professional nurses, 595
Progestasert IUD, 534
Progesterone, 484, 485
Progressive Muscle Relaxation, 83
Proliferative breast disease, 485
Prophylactic mastectomy, 371
Prophylactic oophorectomy, 376–377
Proprietary hospitals, 596–597
Prospective medicine, 4–5, 587

Prostaglandin abortion procedure, 542
Prostaglandin hormones, 485
Prostate cancer, 369, 377–378
Prostate gland, 479
Prostate-specific antigen (PSA) test, 377–378
Prosthodontics, 594
Protease inhibitors, 452
Protein, 136, 162
Protein-sparing modified fast, 197
Proto-oncogenes, 363
Protozoa, and infectious diseases, 429
PSA (prostate-specific antigen) test, 377–378
Psychedelic drugs, 235, 240–241
Psychiatrists, 50–51
Psychoactive drugs, defined, 230
Psychological dependence, 230–231
Psychological disorders, 42–50. *See also specific disorders*
    health providers involved in treatment of, 50–52
    treatment approaches, 52–54
Psychological factors, in obesity, 188–189
Psychological health. *See also* Emotional health
    and the body, 97
    characteristics, 30
    defined, 29
    and the mind, 27
Psychologists, 51, 594
Psychoneuroimmunology, 69, 386
Psychosocial sexuality, 474–476
Psyllium, 140
Puberty, 474
Pubic lice, 454–455, 460
Public hospitals, 597
Pulmonary emphysema, 311
Pulmonary hypertension, 199
Purging, 207

Q
Quaaludes, 239
Quackery, 606–607, 608, 613–614
Quadriceps contusion, 122
Quasisynthetic narcotics, 243–244

R
Radiation, as pollutant, 664–665
Radiation sickness, 664
Radio, as health information source, 2–3

Radio frequency radiation (RFR), 676
Radon, 652
Rahe, Richard, 69, 93
Raloxifene, 371
Rape
    acquaintance rape, 627
    awareness guidelines, 627
    date rape, 239–240, 262, 627, 628
    myths about, 626
Rapid ejaculation, 500
RAS oncogene, 364
Rational Recovery, 279, 282
Reactive hypoglycemia, 408–409
Reality female condom, 533
Recessive inheritance pattern, 399
Recommended dietary allowances
        (RDAs), 137, 138, 139, 142, 190
Recovery stage, of infection, 431
Recreational safety, 632–634
Redux, 199
Reference libraries, as health
        information source, 583
Reflexology, 591–592
Refractory errors, 594
Refractory phase, of sexual
        response, 496–497
Regional cancer, 365
Regional environment, 646, 655–665
Registered nurses (RNs), 594–595
Regulatory genes, 363
Rehabilitation, for older adults, 17
Relationship problems, 71–72
Relationship Satisfaction Test, 503
Relative survivability, 362
Relaxation response, 83
Religious views on environment, 649
Remediation, for older adults, 17
Reproduction, and smoking, 312–313
Reproductive sexuality, 488
Reproductive systems, 476–484
    female, 480–484
    male, 477–480
Reservoir, and chain of
        infection, 429–430
Resistance stage, of stress, 67
Resistance training, 110–111
Resolution stage, of sexual response,
        496, 499
Respiratory system, 686
Respiratory tract cancer, 310–311
Responsibility, and young adults, 14
Restaurant eating, 150, 215, 216–217
Resting energy requirement (RER), 219

Resting metabolic rate (RMR), 191
Restricted-calorie, balanced food
        plans, 196
Restricted-practice health care
        providers, 594–595
Retinal hemorrhage, 347
Reverse-transcriptase inhibitors, 452
Reye's syndrome, 440
Rheumatic fever, 351–352
Rheumatic heart disease, 351–352
Rice, genetically modified, 170
Rice bran, 140
Rickettsia, and infectious
        diseases, 429
Risk factors, defined, 5
Risk reduction, 7, 618
Ritalin, 237, 238
RNs (registered nurses), 594–595
Road rage, 641–642
Roe v. Wade, 540–541
Rogers, Carl, 53
Rollerblading, 114, 125, 126
Romantic love, 508
Rosenman, Roy, 79–80
Rowing machines, 118
RU-486 (mifepristone), 541–542
Rubella, 351, 436
Runner's high, 82, 113, 263
Running shoes, 116, 117

S
SAD (seasonal affective
        disorder), 44–45
SADD (Students Against Destructive
        Decisions), 275
Safe Campuses Now, 630–631
Safety, 617–643
    ATM, 619
    campus, 286, 629–631
    car, 619, 633, 634–636
    cell phones, 635, 676
    complementary care, 630
    and consumer health, 579
    and fear, 625
    food, 153–157, 158
    gun, 634
    home, 619, 631–632, 633, 637, 638
    motorcycle, 637–638
    personal assessment, 643
    recreational, 632–634
    reducing risk factors, 618
Salmonella, 154
Salt, and hypertension, 159, 348

Same-sex marriage, 517–518
Sarcoma, 365
SARS (Sudden Acute Respiratory
        Syndrome), 428, 446–447
Satiety, 132
Saturated fats, 133–134, 158
Schizophrenia, 50
Sclerotic changes, 366
Scoliosis, 403–404
Screening, 586
Scrotum, 477
Scuba divers, and patent foramen
        ovale, 403
Seasonal affective disorder
        (SAD), 44–45
Secondary amenorrhea, 487
Secondary prevention, 226
Secondary virginity, 505–506
Secondhand smoke, 297, 298,
        314, 337–338
Secondhand tobacco smoke,
        337–338, 651
Secular Organizations for Sobriety
        (SOS), 279
Secular recovery programs, for
        alcoholism, 279
Sedatives, 235, 239–240
Seizures, first aid for, 683
Selenium, 150, 163
Self-actualization, 37
Self-antigens, 413
Self-care movement, 233, 595–596,
        600, 605
Self-concept, 31
    assessing, 43, 61
    and body image, 177–178
    defined, 30
    improving, 33
Self-esteem, 30–31
    defined, 30
    and drug abuse, 232
    enhancing, 33
    gays, 502
    and procrastination, 78–79
Self-fulfilling prophecy, 75,
        85–86, 87
Self-medication theory, of nicotine
        addiction, 300–301
Self-talk, 84–87
Seligman, Martin, 40
Selye, Hans, 64, 67
Semen, 479
Seminal vesicles, 479